THIRD EDITION

RADIOLOGY OF SYNDROMES, METABOLIC DISORDERS, AND SKELETAL DYSPLASIAS

RADIOLOGY OF SYNDROMES, METABOLIC DISORDERS, AND SKELETAL DYSPLASIAS

Hooshang Taybi, M.D., M.Sc.
Radiologist, Children's Hospital Medical Center
Oakland, California
Clinical Professor of Radiology
University of California School of Medicine
Attending Radiologist
University of California Medical Center
San Francisco, California

Ralph S. Lachman, M.D.
Professor of Radiology and Pediatrics
UCLA School of Medicine
Associate Chairman and Pediatric Radiologist
Department of Radiology
Harbor-UCLA Medical Center
Torrance, California
Senior Consultant
Cedars-Sinai Medical Genetics—Birth Defects Center and
    the International Skeletal Dysplasia Registry
Los Angeles, California

YEAR BOOK MEDICAL PUBLISHERS, INC.
CHICAGO • LONDON • BOCA RATON • LITTLETON, MASS.

2   3   4   5   6   7   8   9   0   YC   94   93   92   91   90

Library of Congress Cataloging-in-Publication Data
Taybi, Hooshang, 1919-
   Radiology of syndromes, metabolic disorders, and skeletal dysplasias / Hooshang Taybi, Ralph S. Lachman.—3rd ed.
      p.   cm.
   Rev. ed. of: Radiology of syndromes and metabolic disorders. 2nd ed. c1983.
   Includes bibliographical references.
   ISBN 0-8151-8742-4
   1. Diagnosis, Radioscopic.   2. Syndromes—Diagnosis.
3. Metabolism—Disorders—Diagnosis.   4. Human
skeleton—Abnormalities—Diagnosis.   I. Lachman,
Ralph S., 1935-   .   II. Taybi, Hooshang, 1919-
Radiology of syndromes and metabolic disorders.   III. Title.
   [DNLM: 1. Bone and Bones—radiography.   2. Metabolic
Diseases—radiography.   3. Radiography.   WN 200 T236r]
RC78.T25   1990   89-22437
616.07'572—dc20   CIP
DNLM/DLC
for Library of Congress

Sponsoring Editor: James D. Ryan
Associate Managing Editor, Manuscript Services: Deborah Thorp
Production Project Coordinator: Carol A. Reynolds
Proofroom Supervisor: Barbara M. Kelly

DEDICATION

To my devoted wife, Alice, with deep affection and respect.
To my sons, Paul and Claude, with best wishes for bright futures.
To my great and inspiring teacher, Dr. Frederic N. Silverman.
                                        Hooshang Taybi

To the memory of my mother.
To Rose, Nicole, and Monette, continuing sources of inspiration.
To the memory of Joe St. Geme, M.D., a wonderful friend.
                                        Ralph S. Lachman

PREFACE TO THE THIRD EDITION

The first edition of this book published in 1975 contained clinical and radiologic manifestations of about 540 "syndromes." The second edition covered 700 subjects. In this edition, nearly 1,000 entities have been described. The book is divided into three sections: Syndromes, Metabolic Disorders, and Skeletal Dysplasias. The Gamuts section (Appendix A) has been expanded, and references on some of the very rare conditions not included in the text have been added at the end of the Gamuts section. The names of the physicians associated with various disease entities are included in the index for easy reference. The Appendix C on the subject of the eponyms may be of interest to some readers.

The author of the first two chapters (H.T.) would like to extend his deep gratitude to Mrs. Alice Taybi for her excellent secretarial work and editorial contributions. The help of Mr. Leonard Shapiro at the Medical Library of Children's Hospital—Oakland, is much appreciated.

The author of the third chapter (R.S.L.) extends his appreciation to David L. Rimoin, M.D., for his friendship, encouragement, and help over the past 20 years, and extends his gratitude to the research librarians of the Parlow Library, Harbor/UCLA Medical Center, and to Savona B. Hutchings for secretarial work and general support.

Our special thanks to James D. Ryan, Deborah Thorp, and Carol A. Reynolds at Year Book Medical Publishers for their help and full cooperation in the publication of this book.

HOOSHANG TAYBI, M.D.
RALPH S. LACHMAN, M.D.

PREFACE TO THE FIRST EDITION

There has been a steady increase in the contribution radiology has made to the establishment of accurate diagnosis in syndromes of known and unknown etiologies. In most textbooks describing syndromes, brief references to the roentgenologic manifestations are usually made. For more detailed information about the radiologic aspects of the syndromes, an extensive and often time-consuming search of the literature becomes necessary. In this book, the author presents the clinical and radiologic manifestations of 541 syndromes in a short and concise form. It is hoped that this contribution will be of value to clinicians and radiologists alike.

In addition to the reference cards and several thousand reprints collected by the author over the past 20 years, the sources indicated in the Selected References have been consulted in the preparation of this book. An editorial note from the *American Journal of Roentgenology, Radium Therapy and Nuclear Medicine,* which appears in the Introduction, reflects the author's general view about the place of syndromology in medicine.

The author would like to express his appreciation to his associate, Dr. Peter E. Kane, who, during the final stage of the preparation of this book, carried the major load of our radiology practice at the Children's Hospital Medical Center. My special thanks go to my secretary, Mrs. Marilyn Merrell, for all the time and effort she contributed in the preparation of this handbook.

HOOSHANG TAYBI, M.D.

Notes on the Use of the Book

1. The most important clinical and radiologic manifestations of the syndromes appear in italics in the text.

2. A "gamut" system, arranged according to organ system, is presented in Appendix A. The headings for the contents of the "gamut" appear in the front section of Appendix A, with the page numbers directing the reader to the specific subject in the "gamut." The headings are also included in the Index section of the book.

3. Under the heading of "Frequency" in Parts I and II, the available figures in the literature are quoted. Where such figures were not available, the author's use of terms such as "rare," and "uncommon" are based on his personal experience and/or his impression from the review of literature. In the Part III, the terms used are based on the reported cases as follows: very rare, less than 10; rare, 10–40; uncommon, 40–100; common, 100–500; very common, more than 500.

CONTENTS

PART I

Syndromes

Hooshang Taybi, M.D., M.Sc.

A

AARSKOG SYNDROME

Synonyms: Aarskog-Scott syndrome; facio-digito-genital syndrome.

Mode of Inheritance: Possible heterogeneity: X-linked; autosomal dominant.

Frequency: About 100 male cases reported (Nielsen, 1988).

Clinical Manifestations: (a) *short stature;* (b) *peculiar facies* (round face, hypertelorism, antimongoloid slanting of the palpebral fissures, ptosis, maxillary hypoplasia, broad nasal bridge, short stubby nose, long philtrum), linear dimple inferior to the lip, fleshy earlobes, abnormal placement and/or malrotation of the ears; (c) *saddle abnormality of the scrotum;* (d) small hands; short fingers; small, broad, and flat feet; short thumbs with limited abduction; (e) dental malocclusion; (f) mild mental retardation; (g) joint hypermobility; (h) characteristic dermatoglyphic pattern: simian creases, distal axial triradii, etc.; (i) other reported abnormalities: blue sclerae, hypermetropia, strabismus, synophrys, short and broad neck, malocclusion, cleft palate, cleft lip, pectus excavatum, clubbing of the toes, penile hypospadias, cryptorchidism, inguinal hernia, umbilical protrusion, joint restriction, macrocytic anemia associated with hepatomegaly and hemochromatosis, Hirschsprung disease, bowel malrotation, dental anomalies, isolated growth hormone deficiency.

Radiologic Manifestations: (a) *abnormalities of the hands and feet:* short fingers, clinodactyly of the fifth fingers, mild syndactyly, camptodactyly, hypoplasia of the terminal phalanges of the fingers, fusion of the middle and distal phalanges of the fifth toes, hypoplasia of the middle phalanges of the toes; (b) cervical spine anomalies, mild laxity of the C_1–C_2 ligament, calcification of a thoracic intervertebral disk, 13 pairs of ribs; (c) maxillary hypoplasia; (d) retarded bone age (Fig SY−A−1).

Differential Diagnosis: Noonan syndrome; Robinow syndrome.

REFERENCES

Aarskog D: A familial syndrome of short stature associated with facial dysplasia and genital anomalies. *J. Pediatr.* 77:856, 1970.
Bawle E, et al.: Aarskog syndrome: Full male and female expression associated with an X-autosome translocation. *Am. J. Med. Genet.* 17:595, 1984.
Grier RE, et al.: Autosomal dominant inheritance of the Aarskog syndrome. *Am. J. Med. Genet.* 15:39, 1983.
Hassinger DD, et al.: Aarskog's syndrome with Hirschsprung's disease, midgut malrotation, and dental anomalies. *J. Med. Genet.* 17:235, 1980.
Hurst DL: Metatarsus adductus in two brothers with Aarskog syndrome. *J. Med. Genet.* 20:477, 1983.
Kodama M, et al.: Aarskog syndrome with isolated growth hormone deficiency. *Eur. J. Pediatr.* 135:273, 1981.
Nielsen KB: Aarskog syndrome in a Danish family: An illustration of the need for dysmorphology in paediatrics. *Clin. Genet.* 33:315, 1988.
Scott CI, Jr: Unusual facies, joint hypermobility, genital anomaly and short stature: A new dysmorphic syndrome. *Birth Defects* 7(6):240, 1971.
Teebi AS, et al: New autosomal recessive faciodigitogenital syndrome. *J. Med. Genet.* 25:400, 1988.
van den Bergh P, et al.: Anomalous cerebral venous drainage in Aarskog syndrome. *Clin. Genet.* 25:288, 1984.
van de Vooren MJ, et al.: The Aarskog syndrome in a large family, suggestive for autosomal dominant inheritance. *Clin. Genet.* 24:439, 1983.

AASE SYNDROME

Mode of Inheritance: X-linked recessive and autosomal recessive traits have been suggested.

Frequency: Very rare.

Clinical Manifestations: (a) *mild intrauterine growth retardation;* (b) *congenital anemia* (hypoplastic, normocytic, normochromic), increased amount of fetal hemoglobin, leukocytopenia, thrombocytopenia (rare), decreased erythropoiesis, failure of the precursors of the erythrocytic cell line (BFU-E and CFU-E) to grow in the bone marrow culture. (c) *bilateral triphalangeal thumb;* (d) other reported abnormalities: antimongoloid palpebral fissure, retinopathy, cleft lip, cleft palate, late closure of the fontanelles, web neck, narrow shoulders, congenital heart disease (ventricular septal defect, coarctation of the aorta), hepatosplenomegaly, abnormal dermatoglyphics: radial loops (thumbs and index fingers).

Radiologic Manifestations: (a) *triphalangeal thumb;* (b) other reported abnormalities: parietal foramina, scoliosis, mild radial hypoplasia, absence of navicular bones (Fig SY−A−2).

Differential Diagnosis: Fanconi anemia, thrombocytopenia−absent radius (TAR) syndrome.

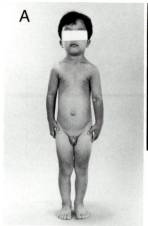

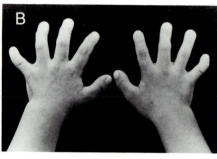

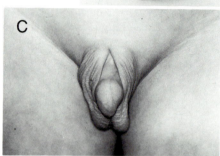

FIG SY—A—1.
Aarskog syndrome. A 5½-year-old boy with a short stature and round face with several characteristic findings **(A)**, hypoplasia and clinodactyly of the fifth finger **(B)**, and a cleft scrotum with a scrotal skin fold extending ventrally around the base of the penis **(C)**. (From Shinkawa T, Yamauchi Y, Osada Y, et al.: Aarskog syndrome. *Urology* 22:624, 1983. Used by permission.)

REFERENCES

Aase J, Smith DW: Congenital anemia and triphalangeal thumbs: A new syndrome. *J. Pediatr.* 74:471, 1969.
Muis N, et al.: The Aase syndrome. Case report and review of the literature. *Eur. J. Pediatr.* 145:153, 1986.
Murphy S, et al.: Triphalangeal thumbs and congenital erythroid hypoplasia: Report of a case with unusual features. *J. Pediatr.* 81:987, 1972.
Pfeiffer RA, et al.: Das Aase-Syndrom: Autosomal-rezessiv Vererbte, konnatal insuffiziente Erythropoese und Triphalangie der Daumen. *Monatsschr. Kinderheilkd.* 131:235, 1983.
van Weel-Sipman M, et al.: A female patient with "Aase syndrome." *J. Pediatr.* 91:753, 1977.

AASE-SMITH SYNDROME

Mode of Inheritance: Autosomal dominant.

Frequency: Very rare.

Clinical and Radiologic Manifestations: (a) hydrocephalus, Dandy-Walker malformation; (b) cleft palate; (c) joint contractures; (d) absence of dermal ridge patterning on the fingertips; (e) other reported abnormalities: feeding difficulties, thickening of the calvarium, shortened terminal phalanges, dislocated radial heads.

REFERENCES

Aase JM, Smith DW: Dysmorphogenesis of joints, brain and palate: A new dominantly inherited syndrome. *J. Pediatr.* 73:606, 1968.
Patton MA, et al.: The Aase-Smith syndrome. *Clin. Genet.* 28:521, 1985.

ABSENT TIBIAE—TRIPHALANGEAL THUMBS—POLYDACTYLY

Mode of Inheritance: Autosomal dominant has been suggested.

Clinical and Radiologic Manifestations: (a) absent tibiae; (b) triphalangeal fingerlike thumbs; (c) preaxial polydactyly of the feet; (d) severe bowing of both lower limbs.

REFERENCE

Canún S, et al: Absent tibiae, triphalangeal thumbs and polydactyly: Description of a family and prenatal diagnosis. *Clin. Genet.* 25:182, 1984.

ACANTHOCYTOSIS—NEUROLOGICAL DISEASE

Synonyms: Neuroacanthocytosis; choreoacanthocytosis; Levine-Critchley syndrome; amyotrophic chorea and acanthocytosis.

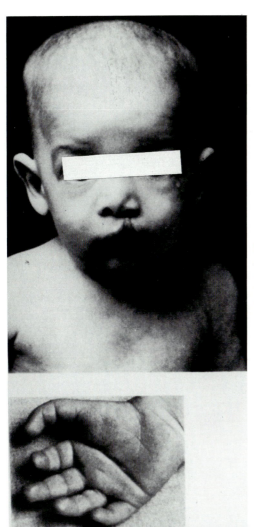

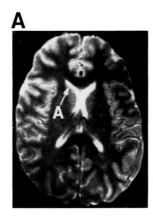

FIG SY–A–2.
Aase syndrome in a male infant with a cleft of the lip, a triphalangeal thumb, and a simian crease. (From Muis N, Beemer FA, van Dijken P, et al.: The Aase syndrome. Case report and review of the literature. *Eur. J. Pediatr.* 145:153, 1986. Used by permission.)

A

B

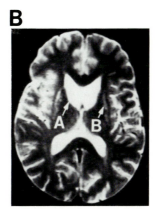

FIG SY–A–3.
Acanthocytosis—neurological disease. Magnetic resonance imaging of the caudate and putamen in control subjects **(A)** and patients with chorea-acanthocytosis **(B)**. *Arrow A* refers to the caudate. Note the atrophy in chorea-acanthocytosis **(B)** vs. the normal control **(A)**. The white linear line noted by *arrow B* is putamen atrophy not seen on the control scan **(A).** (From Vance JM, Pericak-Vance MA, Bowman MH, et al.: Chorea-acanthocytosis: A report of three new families and implications for genetic counselling. *Am. J. Med. Genet.* 28:403, 1987. Used by permission.)

Mode of Inheritance: Most likely autosomal recessive.

Clinical and Radiologic Manifestations: (a) *choreiform movements, limb-wasting, areflexia;* (b) *acanthocytosis;* (c) cardiomyopathy: (d) computed tomography, magnetic resonance imaging: bilateral caudate and putamen atrophy (Fig SY–A–3).

Differential Diagnosis: Huntington chorea.

REFERENCES

Faillace RT, et al.: Cardiomyopathy associated with the syndrome of amyotrophic chorea and acanthocytosis. *Ann. Intern. Med.* 96:616, 1982.

Levine IM, et al.: Heredity neurological disease with acanthocytosis: A new syndrome. *Arch. Neurol.* 19:403, 1968.

Vance JM, et al: Chorea-acanthocytosis: A report of three new families and implications for genetic counselling. *Am. J. Med. Genet.* 28:403, 1987.

ACHALASIA-ADRENAL-ALACRIMA SYNDROME

Synonyms: Achalasia-ACTH insensitivity-alacrima syndrome; achalasia-adrenocortical insufficiency-alacrima syndrome; Addison-achalasia-alacrimation syndrome.

Mode of Inheritance: Consistent with autosomal recessive.

Frequency: Rare.

Clinical Manifestations: (a) lethargy, chronic vomiting; (b) *decreased tear production;* (c) acquired *adrenocortical insufficiency,* adrenocorticotropic hormone (ACTH) insensitivity; (d) manometric evidence of *achalasia* of the gastroesophageal junction and dysmotility; (e) other reported abnormalities: failure to gain weight, short stature, progressive impairment of the nervous system (ataxia, optic atrophy, developmental delay, motor polyneuropathy, episodically dilated and unequal pupils, autonomic neuropathy, parkinsonian features, mild mental deterioration, etc.), abnormality of mineralocorticoid function, microcephaly, association with familial hypophosphatemic rickets, etc.

Radiologic Manifestation: *Achalasia of the esophagus.*

Differential Diagnosis: Riley-Day syndrome; Sjögren syndrome ("achalasia sicca"); adrenoleukodystrophy; familial achalasia; familial acquired glucocorticoid deficiency; etc.

REFERENCES

Allgrove J, et al.: Familial glucocorticoid deficiency with achalasia of the cardia and deficient tear production. *Lancet* 1:1284, 1978.

Ambrosino MM, et al.: The syndrome of achalasia of the esophagus, ACTH insensitivity and alacrima. *Pediatr. Radiol.* 16:328, 1986.

Ehrich E, et al.: Familial achalasia associated with adrenocortical insufficiency, alacrima, and neurological abnormalities. *Am. J. Med. Genet.* 26:637, 1987.

Kalifa G, et al.: La maladie d'Addison chez l'enfant. Anomalies associées. *Ann. Radiol. (Paris)* 29:329, 1986.

Nussinson E, et al.: Familial achalasia with absent tear production. *J. Pediatr. Gastroenterol. Nutr.* 7:284, 1988.

Roubergue A, et al.: Insuffisance isolée en glucocorticoides avec achalasie et alacrymie. Une nouvelle observation avec revue de la littérature. *Ann. Pediatr. (Paris)* 33:321, 1986.

Shah BR, et al.: Familial glucocorticoid deficiency in a girl with familial hypophosphatemic rickets. *Am. J. Dis. Child.* 142:900, 1988.

Stuckey BG, et al.: Glucocorticoid insufficiency, achalasia, alacrima with autonomic and motor neuropathy. *Ann. Intern. Med.* 106:62, 1987.

ACHALASIA, FAMILIAL ESOPHAGEAL

Mode of Inheritance: Autosomal recessive; most familial cases diagnosed in childhood; incidence in childhood: 4% to 5% of the reported cases.

Frequency: Rare.

Clinical Manifestations: (a) recurrent respiratory infection, coughing episodes, aspiration pneumonia, wheezing (compression of the trachea by the dilated esophagus); (b) recurrent emesis; (c) failure to thrive; (d) manometric studies: absence of peristalsis in the entire esophagus, increased lower esophageal sphincter pressure.

Radiologic Manifestations: (a) esophageal dilation, absent normal esophageal peristalsis, tertiary contractions, beaklike narrowing of the very distal portion of the esophagus, intermittent passage of contrast material into the stomach; (b) tracheal compression by the dilated esophagus; (c) pneumonias.

Notes: Two sporadic cases of infantile achalasia associated with other anomalies have been reported (one with narrowing of the duodenum, narrowing of the descending colon and rectosigmoid, abnormal small-bowel motility, pulmonic stenosis, and odontomatosis of the gums and the other with microgastria, a giant duodenum, and asplenia. Familial achalasia also has been reported in association with microcephaly and mental retardation.

REFERENCES

Bosher LP, et al.: Achalasia in siblings. Clinical and genetic aspects. *Am. J. Dis. Child.* 135:709, 1981.

Kaye MD, et al.: Achalasia and diffuse oesophageal spasm in siblings. *Gut* 20:811, 1979.

Khalifa MM: Familial achalasia, microcephaly, and mental

retardation. Case report and review of literature. *Clin. Pediatr. (Phila).* 27:509, 1988.

Mahboubi S, et al.: Multiple congenital anomalies associated with infantile achalasia. *Gastrointest. Radiol.* 5:225, 1980.

Vaughan WH, et al.: Familial achalasia with pulmonary complications in children. *Radiology* 107:407, 1973.

ACHARD SYNDROME

Clinical Manifestations: (a) *mandibular hypoplasia;* (b) *slender fingers, ligament laxity,* hypermobility of the joints, in particular, the hands and feet, joint subluxation.

Radiologic Manifestations: (a) brachycephaly, thick calvaria, *short mandibular rami and increased gonial angle;* (b) other reported abnormalities: absence of the ulnar styloid process, coxa valga, heel valgus, metatarsus varus, flat feet, absence of a normal thoracic kyphotic curve.

REFERENCES

Achard C: Arachnodactylie. *Bull. Mem. Soc. Med. Hop. (Paris)* 19:834, 1902.

Duncan PA: The Achard syndrome. *Birth Defects* 11:69, 1975.

Parish JG: Heritable disorders of connective tissue with arachnodactyly. *Proc. R. Soc. Med.* 53:515, 1960.

ACHEIROPODIA (BRAZIL TYPE)

Mode of Inheritance: Autosomal recessive; high incidence of consanguinity of parents.

Frequency: Extremely rare.

Clinical and Radiologic Manifestations: (a) absence of hands and feet; (b) an elongated small bone in the tip of the upper limb remnant (Bohomoletz bone) or the presence of one or more fingers in some cases.

REFERENCES

Freire-Maia A, et al.: Genetics of acheiropodia ("the handless and footless families of Brazil"): X. Roentgenologic study. *Am. J. Med. Genet.* 2:321, 1978.

Grimaldi A, et al.: Variable expressivity of the acheiropodia gene (Letter). *Am. J. Med. Genet.* 16:631, 1983.

ACQUIRED IMMUNODEFICIENCY SYNDROME

Synonym: AIDS

Definition:

(A) AIDS: (a) *the presence of a disease that is at least moderately indicative of a defect in cell-mediated immunity;* (b) *absence of known causes for diminished resistance to diseases, protozoal infections, helminthic infections, fungal infections, bacterial infections, viral infections, cancer (Kaposi sarcoma, lymphoma limited to brain).*

(B) PEDIATRIC AIDS (children under 13 years of age): (a) *primary and secondary immunodeficiencies excluded;* (b) *positive antibody test reaction for human immunodeficiency virus (HIV);* (c) *lymphoid interstitial pneumonitis.*

Etiology: Human T-cell lymphotropic retrovirus known as human immunodeficiency virus (HIV), lymphoadenopathy-associated virus (LAV), or AIDS-related virus (ARV). The high-risk groups include homosexual/bisexual males and intravenous drug abusers; maternal transmission and transfusion-related transmission form smaller groups of patients with the disease.

Clinical Manifestations:

(A) INFECTION: (a) protozoal: *Pneumocystis carinii* pneumonia, *Toxoplasma gondii* encephalitis or disseminated infection, *Cryptosporidium* enteritis; (b) helminthic: strongyloidiasis (pneumonia; central nervous system [CNS] infections, disseminated), other digestive helminths; (c) fungal: aspergillosis (CNS, disseminated), candidiasis (esophagitis, laryngitis), cryptococcosis (lung, CNS, disseminated); (d) bacterial: atypical mycobacteriosis, *Salmonella, Nocardia, Legionella,* (e) viral (noncongenital): herpes simplex (mucosa, skin, lungs, alimentary tract, disseminated), cytomegalovirus (lungs, alimentary tract, CNS, retina), progressive multifocal leukoencephalopathy (PMFL).

(B) CANCER (a) Kaposi sarcoma; (b) primary brain lymphoma; (c) oral or rectal squamous cell carcinoma in association with herpes virus infection.

(C) FETAL AIDS SYNDROME (HIV embryopathy): (a) positive serologic test results for HIV; (b) dysmorphism: growth failure, microcephaly, prominent boxlike forehead, flattened nasal bridge, short nose, increased inner and outer canthal distances, mild obliquity of the eyes (upward or downward), patulous lips, prominent triangular philtrum.

(D) AIDS-RELATED COMPLEX (ARC): Combination of any two clinical and two laboratory abnormalities: (a) clinical: fever, weight loss, fatigue, diarrhea, night sweats, lymphadenopathy; (b) helper T cell level, <400/μL; helper-suppressor ratio, <1.0; leukothrombocytopenia and anemia; elevated serum globulin levels; depressed blastogenesis; anergy to skin tests.

(E) LABORATORY TESTS: (a) hematologic abnormalities: anemia, leukopenia, thrombocytopenia, pancytopenia, a left shift in the granulocyte series, lymphopenia, atypical lymphocytes, vacuolated monocytes, increased plasma cells in bone marrow aspirates, atypical lymphocytes in the bone marrow, necrosis in the marrow specimen, etc; (b) often elevated immunoglobulin levels, occasionally normal immunoglobulin levels or panhypogammaglobulinemia; (c) antibody to HIV.

Radiologic Manifestations:

(A) CENTRAL NERVOUS SYSTEM: (a) toxoplasmosis—computed tomography (CT): low-density areas on noncontrast studies that usually enhance as an irregular nodular or ring-shaped pattern; magnetic resonance imaging (MRI): more sensitive than CT is in the early phase of the disease, ill-defined regions of low signal intensity on T_1-weighted images, isodense to high intensity signals on T_2-weighted images; (b) other nonviral infections: abscess, granuloma, meningoencephalitis with nonspecific CT and MRI manifestations as to etiologic agent; (c) viral infections: (1) subacute encephalitis—CT: normal or atrophy; MR: normal or abnormal (high intensity in the white matter on T_2-weighted images), atrophy; (2) progressive multifocal leukoencephalopathy (a papovavirus)—MR more sensitive than CT is in the detection of demyelination and edema, most common in the occipitoparietal regions; infratentorial brain and grey matter are less often affected; (3) cytomegalovirus: CT-enhancing areas in the subependymal regions; MRI: high signal intensity in the periventricular regions with irregular extension of the abnormal signal into the white matter; (4) herpes simplex encephalitis; unilateral or bilateral temporal lobe low-density lesions on CT; MRI is more sensitive in detecting the lesions; (d) lymphoma: CT and MRI imaging are nonspecific and resemble inflammatory CNS masses in AIDS—CT: low density on the precontrast study, irregular nodular or ring-shaped multicentric density on postcontrast examination; MRI: low intensity on T_1-weighted images, high intensity on T_2-weighted images; (e) leptomeningeal spread of systemic lymphoma—CT and MRI are usually negative; (f) progressive encephalopathy in children: cerebral atrophy, hydrocephalus, basal ganglia calcification, white matter calcification adjacent to the frontal horns, contrast enhancement of the basal ganglia in association with basal ganglia calcification.

(B) CHEST: (a) congestive cardiomyopathy: cardiomegaly, signs of congestive heart failure, pericardial effusion; (b) intrathoracic adenopathy; (c) opportunistic pulmonary infections, in particular, *Pneumocystis carinii* pneumonia; (d) spontaneous pneumothorax with *Pneumocystis carinii* pneumonia; (e) nonspecific interstitial pneumonitis; (f) pulmonary lymphocytic infiltration and interstitial changes with radiographic findings indistinguishable from *Pneumocystis carinii* pneumonia.

(C) DIGESTIVE TRACT: (a) esophagitis (cystomegalovirus, *Candida*); (b) cytomegalovirus gastritis (large nodular rugal folds in the fundus or as a circumferentially narrowed antrum); (c) cytomegalovirus colitis: superficial erosions, thickened folds, mucosal granularity, spasticity; (d) multifocal abnormalities, most common site in the duodenum: thickened folds, nodularity, superficial erosions, ulcerations, increased secretions, plaque formation, tumor mass; (e) abdominal CT in AIDS-related complex: mild retroperitoneal and mesenteric adenopathy, splenomegaly, perirectal inflammation; (f) abdominal CT in AIDS: adenopathy related to non-Hodgkin lymphoma, Kaposi sarcoma, or disseminated *Mycobacterium avium-intracellulare* infection.

(D) LIVER AND SPLEEN: (a) hepatosplenomegaly; (b) neoplasm; (c) cholangitis with intrahepatic and extrahepatic bile duct changes: dilatation of the common bile duct to the level of the papilla, dilated intrahepatic ducts, thickening of the duct walls and/or periductal anechoic areas in the adjacent

liver parenchyma, terminal ductal narrowing, thickened gallbladder walls, pancreatic duct dilatation.

(E) KIDNEYS: hyperechoic kidneys (focal glomerulonephritis).

REFERENCES

Amodio JB, et al.: Pediatric AIDS. *Semin. Roentgenol.* 22:66, 1987.

Barbour SD: Acquired immunodeficiency syndrome of childhood. *Pediatr. Clin. North Am.* 34:247, 1987.

Belman AL, et al.: Neurological complications in infants and children with acquired immune deficiency syndrome. *Ann. Neurol.* 18:560, 1985.

Bradford BF, et al.: Usual and unusual radiologic manifestations of acquired immunodeficiency syndrome (AIDS) and human immunodeficiency virus (HIV) infection in children. *Radiol. Clin. North Am.* 26:341, 1988.

Corboy JR, et al.: Congestive cardiomyopathy in association with AIDS. *Radiology* 165:139, 1987.

Cummings MA, et al.: Acquired immunodeficiency syndrome presenting as schizophrenia. *West. J. Med.* 146:615, 1987.

Dolmatch BL, et al.: AIDS-related cholangitis: Radiographic findings in nine patients. *Radiology* 163:313, 1987.

Epstein LG, et al.: Neurologic manifestations of human immunodeficiency virus infection in children. *Pediatrics* 78:678, 1987.

Epstein LG, et al.: Unilateral calcification and contrast enhancement of the basal ganglia in a child with AIDS encephalopathy. *A.J.N.R.* 8:163, 1987.

Federle MP: A radiologist looks at AIDS: Imaging evaluation based on symptom complexes. *Radiology* 166:553, 1988.

Goodman PC, et al.: Spontaneous pneumothorax in AIDS patients with *Pneumocystis carinii* pneumonia. *A.J.R.* 147:29, 1986.

Greene LW, et al.: Adrenal insufficiency as a complication of the acquired immunodeficiency syndrome. *Ann. Intern. Med.* 101:497, 1984.

Grody WW, et al.: Thymus involution in the acquired immunodeficiency syndrome. *Am. J. Clin. Pathol.* 84:85, 1985.

Jacobs MB: The acquired immunodeficiency syndrome and hypercalcemia. *West. J. Med.* 144:469, 1986.

Jeffrey RB, et al.: Abdominal CT in acquired immunodeficiency syndrome. *A.J.R.* 146:7, 1986.

Jeffrey RB Jr, et al.: Radiologic imaging of AIDS. *Curr. Probl. Diagn. Radiol.* 17:79, 1988.

Laine L, et al.: Protein-losing enteropathy in acquired immunodeficiency syndrome due to intestinal Kaposi's sarcoma. *Arch. Intern. Med.* 147:1174, 1987.

Levy RM, et al.: Neurological manifestations of the acquired immunodeficiency syndrome (AIDS): Experience at UCSF and review of the literature. *J. Neurosurg.* 62:475, 1985.

Maloney MJ, et al.: Pediatric acquired immune deficiency syndrome with panhypogammaglobulinemia. *J. Pediatr.* 110:266, 1987.

Marcusen DC, et al.: Otolaryngologic and head and neck manifestations of acquired immunodeficiency syndromes (AIDS). *Laryngoscope* 95:401, 1985.

Marion RW, et al.: Craniofacial dysmorphism in children

with human immunodeficiency virus infection. *J. Pediatr.* 113:784, 1988.

Marion RW, et al.: Fetal AIDS syndrome score. *Am. J. Dis. Child.* 141:429, 1987.

Megibow AJ, et al.: Radiology of nonneoplastic gastrointestinal disorders in acquired immune deficiency syndrome. *Semin. Roentgenol.* 22:31, 1987.

Naidich DP, et al.: Radiographic manifestations of pulmonary disease in the acquired immunodeficiency syndrome (AIDS). *Semin. Roentgenol.* 22:14, 1987.

Nyberg DA, et al.: Abdominal CT findings of disseminated *Mycobacterium avium-intracellulare* in AIDS. *A.J.R.* 145:297, 1985.

Nyberg DA, et al.: AIDS-related Kaposi sarcoma and lymphomas. *Semin. Roentgenol.* 22:54, 1987.

Post MJD, et al.: Cytomegalic inclusion virus encephalitis in patients with AIDS: CT, clinical, and pathologic correlation. *A.J.R.* 146:1229, 1986.

Qazi Q, et al.: Lack of evidence for craniofacial dysmorphism in perinatal human immunodeficiency virus infection. *J. Pediatr.* 112:7, 1988.

Randazzo RF, et al.: Cytomegaloviral epididymitis in a patient with the acquired immune deficiency syndrome. *J. Urol.* 136:1095, 1986.

Riechert C, et al.: Pathologic features of AIDS, in DeVita V, et al. (eds.): *AIDS.* Philadelphia, J.B. Lippincott, 1985, pp. 111–161.

Rotbart HA, et al.: Noma in children with severe combined immunodeficiency. *J. Pediatr.* 109:596, 1986.

Ruben FL, et al.: Secondary pulmonary alveolar proteinosis occurring in two patients with acquired immune deficiency syndrome. *Am. J. Med.* 80:1187, 1986.

Schaffer RM, et al.: Renal ultrasound in acquired immune deficiency syndrome. *Radiology* 153:511, 1984.

Simmons JT, et al.: Nonspecific interstitial pneumonitis in patients with AIDS: Radiologic features. *A.J.R.* 149:265, 1987.

Smith R: Liver-spleen scintigraphy in patients with acquired immunodeficiency syndrome. *A.J.R.* 145:1201, 1985.

Solinger AM, et al.: Acquired immune deficiency syndrome—an overview. *Semin. Roentgenol.* 22:9, 1987.

Spivak JL, et al.: Hematologic abnormalities in the acquired immune deficiency syndrome. *Am. J. Med.* 77:224, 1984.

Stern RG, et al.: Intrathoracic adenopathy: Differential feature of AIDS and diffuse lymphadenopathy syndrome. *A.J.R.* 142:689, 1984.

Sze G, et al.: The neuroradiology of AIDS. *Semin. Roentgenol.* 22:42, 1987.

Tapper ML, et al.: Adrenal necrosis in the acquired immunodeficiency syndrome. *Ann. Intern. Med.* 100:239, 1984.

Tong TK, et al.: Childhood acquired immune deficiency syndrome manifesting as acrodermatitis enteropathica. *J. Pediatr.* 108:426, 1986.

Wall SD, et al.: Multifocal abnormalities of the gastrointestinal tract in AIDS. *A.J.R.* 146:1, 1986.

Winchester R, et al.: The co-occurrence of Reiter's syndrome and acquired immunodeficiency. *Ann. Intern. Med.* 106:19, 1987.

Woolfenden JM, et al.: Acquired immunodeficiency syndrome: Ga-67 citrate imaging. *Radiology* 162:383, 1987.

Zimmerman BL, et al.: Children with AIDS—is pathologic diagnosis possible based on chest radiographs? *Pediatr. Radiol.* 17:303, 1987.

ACROCALLOSAL SYNDROME

Mode of Inheritance: Autosomal recessive.

Frequency: Ten published cases (Schinzel, 1988).

Clinical Manifestations: (a) *craniofacial dysmorphism: macrocephaly, prominent forehead, hypertelorism, preauricular tag, upslanting or downslanting palpebral fissures, cleft lip, cleft palate,* etc.; (b) *mental retardation;* (c) *growth retardation;* (d) *foot anomalies: duplicated halluces, postaxial polydactyly of the toes,* etc.; (e) *hand anomalies: postaxial polydactyly of the fingers, bifid terminal phalanges of the thumbs, clinodactyly and brachymesophalangia of the little fingers,* etc.; (f) *other reported abnormalities: hernias (inguinal, umbilical, epigastric), cryptorchidism, seizures,* etc.

Radiologic Manifestations: (a) *agenesis or hypoplasia of the corpus callosum, hydrocephalus,* partial absence of the tentorium, cyst between the cerebrum and cerebellum; (b)

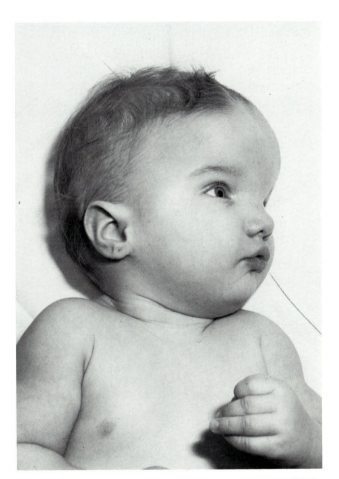

FIG SY–A–4.
Acrocallosal syndrome. A high and prominent forehead, frontal upsweep, hypertelorism, and creases in the right earlobe are seen. (From Schinzel A, Kaufman U: The acrocallosal syndrome in sisters. *Clin. Genet.* 30:399, 1986. Used by permission.)

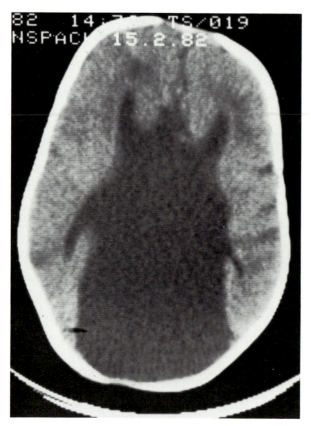

FIG SY—A—5.
Acrocallosal syndrome. Agenesis of the corpus callosum associated with lateralization of the anterior horns of the lateral ventricles is shown (From Schinzel A, Kaufmann U: The acrocallosal syndrome in sisters. *Clin. Genet.* 30:399, 1986. Used by permission.)

missing pericallosal artery on sonography (Figs SY—A—4 and SY—A—5).

    Differential Diagnosis: Greig syndrome; hydrolethalus syndrome; cranio-fronto-nasal dysplasia.

REFERENCES

Baarsma R, et al.: The missing pericallosal artery on sonography: A sign of agenesis of the corpus callosum in the neonatal brain? *Neuroradiology* 29:47, 1987.

Lassemann I, et al.: Syndrome acro-callosal. A propos de 2 observations. *J. Radiol.* 67:653, 1986.

Philip N, et al.: The acrocallosal syndrome. *Eur. J. Pediatr.* 147:206, 1988.

Schinzel A: The acrocallosal syndrome in first cousins: Widening of the spectrum of clinical features and further support for autosomal recessive inheritance. *J. Med. Genet.* 25:332, 1988.

Schinzel A, et al.: The acrocallosal syndrome in sisters. *Clin. Genet.* 30:399, 1986.

Schinzel A, Schmid W: Hallux duplication, postaxial polydactyly, absence of the corpus callosum, severe mental

retardation, and additional anomalies in two unrelated patients: A new syndrome. *Am. J. Med. Genet.* 6:241, 1980.

ACROCEPHALOPOLYSYNDACTYLY, CARPENTER TYPE

    Synonym: Carpenter syndrome.

    Mode of Inheritance: Autosomal recessive.

    Frequency: 28 published cases (Cohen et al.).

    Clinical Manifestations: (a) *acrocephaly;* (b) *peculiar facies,* broad cheeks and temples, depressed nasal bridge, lateral displacement of the medial canthi, epicanthal folds, downward thrust of the upper lids; (c) *obesity;* (d) *hypogenitalism;* (e) *brachysyndactyly of the hands;* (f) *preaxial polydactyly and syndactyly of the feet;* (g) *mental retardation* (variable); (h) *other reported abnormalities:* cardiac defects, microcornea, corneal opacities, low-set and malformed ears, postaxial polydactyly of the hands, etc.

    Radiologic Manifestations: (a) *premature closure of cranial sutures;* (b) *brachymesophalangia and soft-tissue syndactyly of the hands,* two ossification centers for the proximal phalanx of the thumb in childhood developing into duplication of the thumb in adulthood; (c) *preaxial polydactyly and syndactyly of the feet;* (d) *other reported associated abnormalities:* coxa valga, genu valgum, pes varus, flared ilia, displaced patellae, congenital heart diseases, hernias, etc.

    Differential Diagnosis: Goodman syndrome; Summitt syndrome.

    Note: It has been suggested that Goodman and Summitt syndromes are variations of Carpenter syndrome and fall within the spectrum of this disorder.

REFERENCES

Carpenter G: Two sisters showing malformations of the skull and other congenital abnormalities. *Rep. Soc. Study Dis. Child. London* 1:110, 1901.

Cohen DM, et al.: Acrocephalopolysyndactyly type II—Carpenter syndrome: Clinical spectrum and an attempt at unification with Goodman and Summitt syndromes. *Am. J. Med. Genet.* 28:311, 1987.

DerKaloustian VM, et al.: Acrocephalopolysyndactyly type II (Carpenter syndrome). *Am. J. Dis. Child.* 124:716, 1972.

Eaton AP, et al.: Carpenter syndrome—Acrocephalopolysyndactyly type II. *Birth Defects* 10(9):249, 1974.

Pfeiffer RA, et al.: Akrozephalopolysyndaktylie. *Klin. Paediatr.* 189:120, 1977.

Robinson LK, et al.: Carpenter syndrome: Natural history and clinical spectrum. *Am. J. Med. Genet.* 20:461, 1985.

Temtany S, McKusick V: Acrocephalopolysyndactyly (Carpenter syndrome). *Birth Defects* 14(3):413, 1978.

ACROCEPHALOPOLYSYNDACTYLY, GOODMAN TYPE

Synonyms: Acrocephalopolysyndactyly, type IV; Goodman syndrome.

Mode of Inheritance: Three siblings from a consanguineous family.

Clinical and Radiologic Manifestations: (a) craniofacial dysmorphism: acrocephaly, high-arched eyebrows, downward slant of the palpebral fissures, epicanthal folds, prominent nose, flared nares, high-arched palate, crowding of teeth, micrognathia, facial hirsutism, protruding deformed ears; (b) upper limbs: polydactyly, syndactyly, brachydactyly, clinodactyly, camptodactyly, ulnar deviation of the fingers, angulation of the elbow; (c) lower limbs: genu valgum, muscle hypoplasia, pes cavus, pes equinovarus, syndactyly; (d) pectus carinatum, scoliosis, thoracic asymmetry; (e) congenital heart disease.

REFERENCE

Goodman RM, et al.: Acrocephalopolysyndactyly type IV: A new genetic syndrome in 3 sibs. *Clin. Genet.* 15:209, 1979.

ACROCEPHALOPOLYSYNDACTYLY, SAKATI TYPE

Synonym: Sakati-Nyhan syndrome.

Clinical and Radiologic Manifestations: A single case report with the following anomalies: (a) cranial synostosis and acrocephaly; (b) unusual facies, dysplastic ears; (c) brachydactyly of the hands, polydactyly and syndactyly of the feet; (d) an unusual malformation of the knee region consisting of bowed femora, hypoplastic tibias, and posterior displacement of the fibulas on the femora; (e) other abnormalities: alopecia, skin atrophy, congenital heart disease, small penis, cryptorchidism, inguinal hernia.

REFERENCE

Sakati N, Nyhan WL: A new syndrome with acrocephalopolysyndactyly, cardiac disease, and distinctive defects of the ear, skin, and lower limbs. *J. Pediatr.* 79:104, 1971.

ACROCEPHALOSYNDACTYLY, APERT TYPE

Synonym: Apert syndrome.

Modes of Inheritance: Most cases are sporadic; some cases are reported as parent-to-child transmission (autosomal dominant); germinal mosaicism (two sisters born to normal unrelated parents); parental consanguinity; male transmission.

Frequency: Estimated to occur in 1 in 160,000 births (Patton).

Clinical Manifestations: (a) *deformed head with high, broad and flat forehead, brachycephaly, hypertelorism, depressed nasal bridge, antimongoloid slant of eyes, bulging eyes, open mouth, high-arched narrow palate, trapezoidal-shaped mouth with an associated high-arched palate and occasional cleft palate, relative prognathism, crowded teeth, various dental anomalies, cloverleaf skull anomaly;* (b) *"mitten hand"* and *"sock foot"*; (c) *mental retardation* (in many); (d) other reported abnormalities: conductive hearing loss, congenital fixation of stapes, otitis and its sequelae, dehiscent jugular bulb, acne vulgaris, polyhydramnios, anomalies of visceral organs (cardiovascular, respiratory, and renal

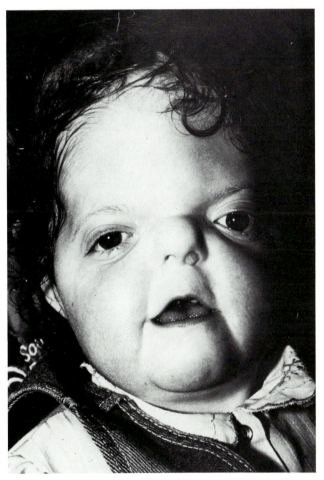

FIG SY—A—6.
Acrocephalosyndactyly, Apert type, with typical facies: high, broad, and flat forehead; hypertelorism; depressed nasal bridge; antimongoloid slant of the eyes; bulging eyes; and an open mouth. (From Allanson JE. Germinal mosaicism in Apert syndrome. *Clin. Genet.* 29:429, 1986. Used by permission.)

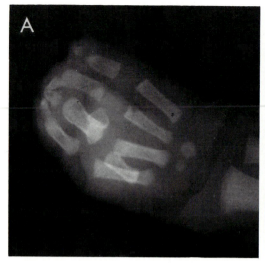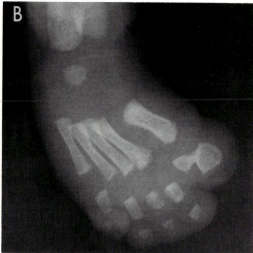

FIG SY–A–7.
Acrocephalosyndactyly, Apert type, in a 4-day-old male with turri-brachycephaly, bulging eyes, "mitten hand," and "sock foot." **A,** two ossification centers are present in carpal region. Digits are de-formed and fused. **B,** fusion of the toes, two phalanges for each toe, and fusion of deformed proximal and distal phalanges of the great toe are seen.

systems), tracheoesophageal fistula, advanced paternal age, embryonal rhabdomyosarcoma of the hand, frontonasal en-cephalocele, absence of the superior rectus muscle.

Radiologic Manifestations: (a) *turribrachycephaly, pre-mature closure of sutures* (coronals in particular), shallow or-bits, hypoplasia of the maxillae, prominent mandible, unilat-eral or bilateral canting of the temporal bone (upward tilting); (b) *complete syndactyly involving the second to fifth digits (mitten hand and sock foot)*, partial or complete duplication of the proximal phalanx of the great toes and first metatarsals, hallux varus, ankylosis of the major joints, fusion of the long bones, subluxed humeral head, flattened humeral head, fused vertebrae, irregular glenoid fossa, etc.; (c) other re-ported anomalies: hydrocephalus, convolutional atrophy, ab-sence of the corpus callosum, absence of the septum pelluci-dum, hydromyelia, arhinoencephaly, etc.; (d) prenatal ultra-sonographic diagnosis: acrocephaly, cupped hands, fusion of the digits.

Note: Two patients with manifestations resembling Apert syndrome (polydactyly of the hands and feet) who were re-ported by Maroteaux et al. may represent a distinct syndrome to be differentiated from Apert syndrome ("apparent Apert syndrome") (Figs SY–A–6 and SY–A–7).

REFERENCES

Allanson JE: Germinal mosaicism in Apert syndrome. *Clin. Genet.* 29:429, 1986.
Apert ME: De l'acrocephalosyndactylie. *Bull. Mem. Soc. Med. Hop. (Paris)* 23:1310, 1906.
Beligere N, et al.: Progressive bone dysplasia in Apert syn-drome. *Radiology* 139:593, 1981.
de León GA, et al.: Agenesis of the corpus callosum and limbic malformation in Apert syndrome. (Type I acroceph-alosyndactyly). *Arch. Neurol.* 44:979, 1987.
Gould HJ, et al.: Hearing and otopathology in Apert syn-drome. *Arch. Otolaryngol.* 108:347, 1982.
Hill LM, et al.: The ultrasonic detection of Apert syndrome. *J. Ultrasound Med.* 6:601, 1987.
Hoover GH, et al.: The hand and Apert's syndrome. *J. Bone Joint Surg. [Am.]* 52:878, 1970.
Kim H, et al.: Apert syndrome and fetal hydrocephaly. *Hum. Genet.* 73:93, 1986.
Leonard CO, et al.: Prenatal fetoscopic diagnosis of the Ap-ert syndrome. *Am. J. Med. Genet.* 11:5, 1982.
Maroteaux P, et al.: Apparent Apert syndrome with polydac-tyly: Rare pleiotropic manifestation or new syndrome? *Am. J. Med. Genet.* 28:153, 1987.
Morax S, et al.: Absence du muscle droit supérieur dans le syndrome d'Apert. *J. Fr. Ophthalmol.* 5:323, 1982.
Noetzel MJ, et al.: Hydrocephalus and mental retardation in craniosynostosis. *J. Pediatr.* 107:885, 1985.
Patton MA, et al: Intellectual development in Apert's syn-drome: A long term follow up of 29 patients. *J. Med. Genet.* 25:164, 1988.
Pflanzer K: Apert's syndrome. *Radiol. Clin. North Am.* 47:233, 1978.
Phillips SG, et al.: Congenital conductive hearing loss in Apert syndrome. *Otolaryngol. Head Neck Surg.* 95:429, 1986.
Rollnick BR: Male transmission of Apert syndrome. *Clin. Genet.* 33:87, 1988.
Schauerte EW, et al.: Progressive synostosis in Apert's syndrome (acrocephalosyndactyly). *A.J.R.* 97:67, 1966.
Sidhu SS, et al: Recessive inheritance of apparent Apert syn-drome with polysyndactyly? *Am. J. Med. Genet.* 31:179, 1988.
Temtamy S, McKusick V: Apert syndrome. *Birth Defects* 14(3):329, 1978.
Vollmer DG, et al.: Hydromyelia complicating Apert's syn-drome: A case report. *Neurosurgery* 17:70, 1985.

Waterson JR, et al.: Apert syndrome with frontonasal encephalocele. *Am. J. Med. Genet.* 21:777, 1985.

Wheaton SW: Two specimens of congenital cranial deformity in infants associated with fusion of the fingers and toes. *Trans. Pathol. Soc. London* 45:238, 1894.

ACROCEPHALOSYNDACTYLY, HERRMANN-OPITZ TYPE

Synonym: Herrmann-Opitz syndrome.

Frequency: Two published cases.

Clinical and Radiologic Manifestations: (a) *acrocephaly,* brachycephaly, peculiar facies (prominent eyes, hypoplasia of the supraorbital ridges, micrognathia, small and low-set malformed ears); (b) *brachysyndactyly of the hands;* (c) *monodactyly of the feet;* (d) short stature; (e) other abnormalities: mental retardation, cryptorchidism, rectal prolapse, absent fifth metatarsals, absent first rib, urethral atresia, webs (nuchal, antecubital, popliteal), wide occipitoparietal sutures, etc.

REFERENCES

Anyane-Yeboa K, et al.: Herrmann-Opitz syndrome: Report of an affected fetus. *Am. J. Med. Genet.* 27:467, 1987.

Herrmann J, Opitz JM: An unusual form of acrocephalosyndactyly. *Birth Defects* 5(3):39, 1969.

ACROCEPHALOSYNDACTYLY, PFEIFFER TYPE

Synonym: Pfeiffer syndrome.

Mode of Inheritance: Autosomal dominant; variability of phenotypic expression.

Clinical Manifestations: (a) *Acrocephaly, brachycephaly, hypertelorism, downward slant of the palpebral fissures, strabismus, proptosis, beaked nose, highly arched palate;* (b) *minimal soft-tissue syndactyly;* (c) *broad thumbs and great toes;* (d) normal intelligence; (e) other reported anomalies: cloverleaf skull, atresia of the external auditory canals, corectopia, scleralization of the cornea, hypoplasia of the optic nerve, hypertrophic pyloric stenosis.

Radiologic Manifestations: (a) *premature closure of the sagittal and coronal sutures,* hypertelorism, shallow anterior cranial fossa, flattened nasal bridge, hydrocephalus; Arnold-Chiari malformation; (b) *varus deformity of the great toes, broad first metatarsals, trapezoid shape of the first phalanx of the great toes;* (c) *partial membranous syndactyly of the proximal phalanx of the thumbs,* short fingers, hypoplasia or absence of the middle phalanges; (d) other reported anomalies: small iliac angle and iliac index, radial-ulnar synostosis, radiohumeral synostosis, cloverleaf skull, hydrocephalus, hearing loss (Fig SY−A−8).

Note: Noack syndrome (enlarged thumbs and great toes with duplication of the latter) and Pfeiffer types of acrocephalosyndactyly are considered the same entity (McKusick).

REFERENCES

Cremer CW: Hearing loss in Pfeiffer's syndrome. *Int. J. Pediatr. Otorhinolaryngol.* 3:343, 1981.

Kroczek RA, et al.: Cloverleaf skull associated with Pfeiffer syndrome: Pathology and management. *Eur. J. Pediatr.* 145:422, 1986.

Lanteri M, et al.: Syndrome de Pfeiffer. *Arch. Fr. Pédiatr.* 42:717, 1985.

Martsolf JT, et al.: Pfeiffer syndrome: An unusual type of acrocephalosyndactyly with broad thumbs and great toes. *Am. J. Dis. Child.* 121:257, 1971.

McKusick VA: *Mandelian Inheritance in Man,* ed. 8. Baltimore, Johns Hopkins University Press, 1988, p. 11.

Noack M: Ein Beitrag zum Krankheitsbild der Akrozephalosyndakylie (Apert). *Arch. Kinderheilkd.* 160:168, 1959.

Noetzel MJ, et al.: Hydrocephalus and mental retardation in craniosynostosis. *J. Pediatr.* 107:885, 1985.

Pfeiffer RA: Dominant erbliche Akrozephalosyndaktylie. *Z. Kinderheilkd.* 90:301, 1964.

Rasmussen SA, et al: Mild expression of the Pfeiffer syndrome. *Clin. Genet.* 33:5, 1988.

Saldino RM, et al.: Familial acrocephalosyndactyly (Pfeiffer syndrome). *A.J.R.* 116:609, 1972.

Sanchez JM, et al.: Variable expression in Pfeiffer syndrome. *J. Med. Genet.* 18:73, 1981.

Van Dyke DC, et al.: Clinical observation: Ocular abnormalities in a patient with Pfeiffer syndrome (acrocephalosyndactyly type V). *J. Clin. Dysmorphol.* 1:2, 1983.

Vaněk J, et al.: Pfeiffer's type of acrocephalosyndactyly in two families. *J. Med. Genet.* 19:289, 1982.

ACROCEPHALOSYNDACTYLY, ROBINOW-SORAUF TYPE

Synonym: Robinow-Sorauf syndrome.

Mode of Inheritance: Autosomal dominant, interfamilial variation.

Clinical and Radiologic Manifestations: (a) *craniosynostosis;* (b) *cutaneous syndactyly of the fourth and fifth toes, duplication of the great toes (distal phalanx).*

REFERENCES

Carter CO, et al.: A family study of craniosynostosis, with probable recognition of a distinct syndrome. *J. Med. Genet.* 19:280, 1982.

Robinow M, Sorauf TJ: Acrocephalopolysyndactyly, type Noack, in a large kindred. *Birth Defects* 11(5):99, 1975.

Young ID, et al.: An unusual form of familial acrocephalosyndactyly. *J. Med. Genet.* 19:286, 1982.

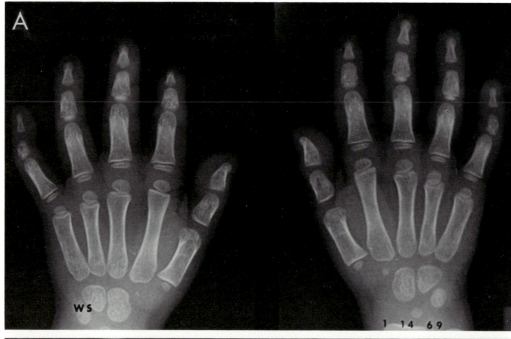

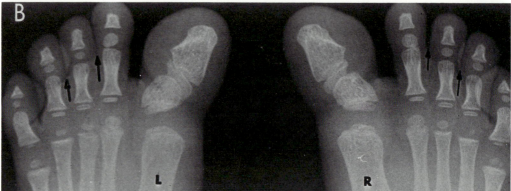

FIG SY—A—8.
Acrocephalosyndactyly, Pfeiffer type, in a 4-year-old male. **A,** shortened middle phalanges of all digits, soft-tissue hypertrophy of the thumbs, and partial membranous syndactyly between digits 2, 3, and 4 bilaterally. **B,** marked shortening of the middle phalanges, varus deformity of the great toes, trapezoid proximal phalanges of the great toes, partial membranous syndactyly of the toes *(arrows),* and soft-tissue hypertrophy of the great toes bilaterally. (From Martsolf JT, Cracco JB, Carpenter GG, et al.: Pfeiffer syndrome: An unusual type of acrocephalosyndactyly with broad thumbs and great toes. *Am. J. Dis. Child.* 121:257, 1971. Used by permission.)

ACROCEPHALOSYNDACTYLY, SAETHRE-CHOTZEN TYPE

Synonym: Saethre-Chotzen syndrome.

Mode of Inheritance: Autosomal dominant with marked penetrance and variable expressivity; occasional lack of penetrance.

Frequency: Rare.

Clinical Manifestations: (a) *brachycephaly and/or acrocephaly,* facial asymmetry, visual defects, esotropia, exotropia, ptosis of the eyelids, lacrimal duct abnormalities, mal-formed ears, impaired hearing, flattened nasofrontal angle, beaked nose, cleft palate, highly arched palate, dental malformations, malocclusion, low-set frontal hairline, labial pits at the corners of the mouth; (b) mental subnormality; (c) *syndactyly (partial, soft tissue);* (d) other reported abnormalities: renal anomalies, congenital heart disease, cryptorchidism, simian palmar creases, dermatoglyphic alterations, short arms, short and broad hands, fingerlike thumbs, clinodactyly, short feet and toes, hallux valgus, imperforate anus, recurrent infections, seizures, neoplasm, optic atrophy, etc.

Radiologic Manifestations: (a) *variable degrees of craniosynostosis* associated with plagiocephaly and facial asymmetry, microcephaly, absent or underdeveloped frontal sinuses and mastoids, abnormal cephalometric findings, dilatation of lateral ventricles, increased intracranial pressure; (b) *syndactyly;* (c) other reported abnormalities: short clavicles with distal hypoplasia, clinodactyly of the fifth fingers, hypoplastic distal phalanges of the hands, partially bifid distal phalanges of the great toes, hallux valgus, small ilia, large ischia, coxa valga, enlarged sella turcica, parietal foramina, etc.

REFERENCES

Bianchi E, et al.: A family with the Saethre-Chotzen syndrome. *Am. J. Med. Genet.* 22:649, 1985.
Chotzen F: Eine eigenartige familiäre Entwicklungsstörung (Akrocephalosyndaktylie). *Monatsschr. Kinderheilkd.* 55:97, 1933.
Evans CA, et al.: Cephalic malformations in Saethre-Chotzen syndrome: Acrocephalosyndactyly type III. *Radiology* 121:399, 1976.
Kopysc Z, et al.: The Saethre-Chotzen syndrome with partial bifid of the distal phalanges of the great toes: Observation of three cases in one family. *Hum. Genet.* 56:195, 1980.
LeMerrer M, et al.: Une observation d'acrocéphalosyndactylie. *Ann. Pediatr. (Paris)* 30:695, 1983.
McKeen EA, et al.: The concurrence of Saethre-Chotzen syndrome and malignancy in a family with in vitro immune dysfunction. *Cancer* 54:2946, 1984.
Saethre M: Ein Beitrag zum Turmschädelproblem (Pathogenese, Erblichkeit und Symptomatologie). *Dtsch. Nervenheilkd.* 119:533, 1931.
Temtamy S, McKusick VA: Saethre-Chotzen syndrome. *Birth Defects* 14:331, 1978.
Thompson EM, et al.: Parietal foramina in Saethre-Chotzen syndrome. *J. Med. Genet.* 21:369, 1984.

ACROCEPHALOSYNDACTYLY, SUMMITT TYPE

Synonym: Summitt syndrome.

Mode of Inheritance: Autosomal recessive.

Clinical and Radiologic Manifestations: (a) *acrocephaly, peculiar facies;* (b) *syndactyly of the hands and feet;* (c) *normal intelligence;* (d) *obesity, hypogenitalism.*

Note: It has been suggested that Summitt syndrome is the same as Carpenter syndrome.

REFERENCES

Sells CJ, et al.: The Summitt syndrome: Observations on a third case. *Am. J. Med. Genet.* 3:27, 1979.
Summitt RL: Recessive acrocephalosyndactyly with normal intelligence. *Birth Defects* 5:35, 1969.

ACROCEPHALOSYNDACTYLY, WAARDENBURG TYPE

Synonym: Waardenburg syndrome.

Clinical Manifestations: (a) acrocephaly; hypertelorism; hydrophthalmos; strabismus; cleft palate; thin, long, and pointed nose; (b) brachydactyly with mild soft-tissue syndactyly, contracture of elbows and knees; (c) congenital heart disease; (d) pseudohermaphroditism.

Radiologic Manifestations: (a) *plagiocephaly, acrocephaly;* (b) *bifid terminal phalanges of digits 2 and 3* and an absence of the first metatarsals; (c) contracture of the elbows and knees.

REFERENCES

Waardenburg PJ (ed.): *Genetics and Ophthalmology.* Springfield, Ill., Charles C Thomas Publishers, 1961.
Waardenburg PJ: Eine merkwürdige Kombination von angeborenen Missbildungen: Doppelseitiger Hydrophthalmos verbunden mit Akrokephalosyndaktylie, Herzfehler, Pseudohermaphroditismus und anderen Abweichungen. *Klin. Monatsbl. Augenheilkd.* 92:29, 1934.

ACRO-CRANIO-FACIAL DYSOSTOSIS

Mode of Inheritance: Autosomal recessive suggested (sisters with consanguineous parents).

Clinical Manifestations: (a) short stature; (b) acrocephaly, hypertelorism, proptosis, ptosis, downslanting palpebral fissures, high nose bridge, anteverted nares, short philtrum, cleft palate, micrognathia, abnormal external ears, preauricular pits; (c) sensorineural and conductive deafness; (d) proximally placed first toes, digitalized thumbs, bulbous digits, metatarsus adductus; (e) pectus excavatum.

Radiologic Manifestations: (a) craniosynostosis, increased mandibular angle, antegonial notching of the mandible; (b) hypoplastic first metacarpals and metatarsals, hypoplastic distal phalanges, partial duplication of the distal phalanx of the thumb; (c) malformed malleus and incus; (d) tall lumbar vertebrae, increased interpedicular distance and posterior scalloping, flared iliac wings, narrow supra-acetabular regions, acetabular "dysplasia," coxa valga.

REFERENCE

Kaplan P, et al: A new acro-cranio-facial dysostosis syndrome in sisters. *Am. J. Med. Genet.* 29:95, 1988.

ACRODERMATITIS ENTEROPATHICA

Mode of Inheritance: Autosomal recessive.

Clinical Manifestations: Onset of symptoms in infancy or early childhood: (a) *acral and orificial vesicobullous, pustular, and eczamatoid skin lesions;* recurrent infections of the skin and mucous membrane with *Candida albicans,* bacteria, or both; esophagitis; (b) *hair loss;* (c) *paronychia;* (d) *ocular lesions* (blepharitis, conjunctivitis, corneal opacities); (e) *diarrhea;* (f) failure to thrive; (g) emotional disturbances; (h) *low serum zinc and alkaline phosphatase levels,* dramatic clinical response to zinc therapy, impaired enteral absorption of linoleic acid, low urinary zinc levels; (i) small-bowel biopsy: loss of villous architecture, flattening of villi, cuboid intestinal epithelial cells with enlarged nuclei and open chromatin distribution, autopsy findings: pancreatic islet hyperplasia, absence of the thymus and germinal centers, plasmocytosis of the lymph nodes and spleen; (j) other reported abnormalities: childhood acquired immunodeficiency syndrome presenting as acrodermatitis enteropathica.

Radiologic Manifestations: (a) roentgenologic findings of malabsorption syndrome; (b) cerebral atrophy, reversible with zinc therapy.

Differential Diagnosis: Variant acrodermatitis enteropathica (normal plasma zinc values with clinical symptoms of acrodermatitis enteropathica that respond to treatment with pancreatin).

REFERENCES

Baudon J-J, et al.: Acrodermatitis enteropathica. *Arch. Fr. Pediatr.* 35:63, 1978.

Brandt T: Dermatitis in children with disturbance of the general condition and the absorption of food elements. *Acta Derm. Venereol. (Stockh.)* 17:513, 1936.

Danbolt N, Closs K: Akrodermatitis enteropathica. *Acta Derm. Venereol. (Stockh.)* 23:127, 1942.

Kelly R, et al.: Reversible intestinal mucosal abnormality in acrodermatitis enteropathica. *Arch. Dis. Child.* 51:219, 1976.

Koletzko B, et al.: Fatty acid composition of plasma lipids in acrodermititis enteropathica before and after zinc supplementation. *Eur. J. Pediatr.* 143:310, 1985.

Krieger I, et al.: Zinc dependency as a cause of chronic diarrhea in variant acrodermatitis enteropathica. *Pediatrics* 69:773, 1982.

Ohlsson A: Acrodermatitis enteropathica: Reversibility of cerebral atrophy on zinc therapy. *Acta Paediatr. Scand.* 70:269, 1981.

Rubin IL, et al.: Acrodermatitis enteropathica—A zinc deficiency state. *South Afr. Med. J.* 53:497, 1978.

Tong TK, et al.: Childhood acquired immune deficiency syndrome manifesting as acrodermatitis enteropathica. *J. Pediatr.* 108:426, 1986.

Wallis K, et al.: Acrodermatitis enteropathica associated with low density lipoprotein deficiency. *Clin. Pediatr. (Phila.)* 13:749, 1974.

ACRO-FRONTO-FACIO-NASAL DYSOSTOSIS SYNDROME

Mode of Inheritance: Most likely autosomal recessive (two siblings born to a consanguineous couple).

Frequency: Two siblings.

Clinical Manifestations: (a) *mental retardation;* (b) *short stature;* (c) *facial anomalies: hypertelorism, broad notched nasal tip, cleft lip/palate;* (d) *limb anomalies: camptopolysyndactyly, hypoplasia of the toenails,* etc.

Radiologic Manifestations: (a) hand anomalies: *postaxial polysyndactyly, hypoplasia of the distal phalanges of the digits, camptodactyly, brachymetacarpalia,* hamate-capitate fusion, disorganization of the structure of the carpal bones, etc.; (b) fibular hypoplasia; (c) *foot anomalies.*

Differential Diagnosis: Frontonasal dysplasia.

REFERENCE

Richieri-Costa A, Colletto G, Gollop TR, et al.: A previously undescribed autosomal recessive multiple congenital anomalies/mental retardation (MCA/MR) syndrome with fronto-nasal dysostosis, cleft lip/palate, limb hypoplasia, and postaxial poly-syndactyly: Acro-fronto-facio-nasal dysostosis syndrome. *Am. J. Med. Genet.* 20:631, 1985.

ACROGERIA

Mode of Inheritance: Not certain, reported in siblings and a mother and son; female preponderance.

Frequency: Very rare.

Clinical Manifestations: (a) *thin and wrinkled skin, mottled skin pigmentation, prominent veins over the dorsa of the hands and feet and the upper part of the trunk;* (b) *short stature;* (c) *midfacial duskiness, pointed chin and nose;* (d) *thickened or dystrophic nails;* (e) pathology: atrophy of the dermis and subcutaneous fat, loose and sparse collagen fibers, fragmented elastic fibers.

Radiologic Manifestations: (a) *acro-osteolysis of distal phalanges;* (b) *micrognathia, antegonial notching of the mandible;* (c) *delayed cranial suture closure, wormian bones;* (d) other reported abnormalities: broad and poorly tubulated metaphyses, gracile bones, coxa valga deformity, tubular lucencies in the long bones, aseptic necrosis of the femoral head, cortical thickening, ankylosis of the interphalangeal joints of the hands, congenital hip dislocation, mild bone demineralization, hourglass deformity of the distal phalanges of the hands and feet, short femoral neck, hypoplasis of the iliac wing, craniostenosis (adult), hypoplasia of the terminal

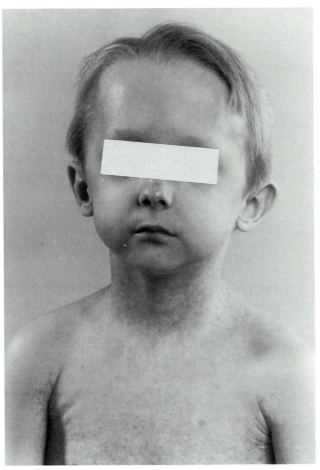

FIG SY—A—9.
Acrogeria. A pointed chin and nose and hyperpigmented skin over the neck and shoulders are present. (From Ho A, White SJ, Rasmussen JE: Skeletal abnormalities of acrogeria, a progeroid syndrome. *Skeletal Radiol.* 16:463, 1987. Used by permission.)

phalanges of the hands, absent distal phalanx of a toe, slightly short forearm, hallux valgus, etc. (Fig SY—A—9).

Differential Diagnosis: Progeria; Hajdu-Cheney syndrome; pycnodysostosis; mandibuloacral dysplasia; cleidocranial dysplasia.

REFERENCES

De Groot WP, et al.: Familial acrogeria (Gottron). *Br. J. Dermatol.* 103:213, 1970.
Gottron H: Familiare akrogerie. *Arch. Dermatol. Syph.* 181:571, 1940.
Ho A, et al.: Skeletal abnormalities of acrogeria, a progeroid syndrome. *Skeletal Radiol.* 16:463, 1987.

ACRORENAL SYNDROME

Synonym: Dieker-Opitz acrorenal syndrome.

Clinical Manifestations: (a) *acral anomalies;* (b) *urinary tract dysgenesis.*

Radiologic Manifestations: (a) *acral anomalies* (oligodactyly, ectrodactyly, brachydactyly, and polydactyly in varying combinations; syndactyly; various anomalies of the carpal and tarsal bones; split hands and feet); (b) *urinary tract dysgenesis* (unilateral renal agenesis, duplication of the collecting system, renal hypoplasia leading to renal insufficiency, vesicoureteral reflux with hydronephrosis).

Note: Under the title of acrorenal-ocular syndrome seven individuals from three generations of a family have been reported to have various combinations of acral, renal, and ocular defects (Halal): hypoplasia of the thumb, preaxial polydactyly, renal malrotation, crossed renal ectopia, vesicoureteral reflux, bladder diverticula, complete eye coloboma, coloboma of the optic nerve, ptosis, Duane anomaly, abnormal dermatoglyphics.

REFERENCES

Curran AS, et al.: Associated acral and renal malformations: A new syndrome? *Pediatrics* 49:716, 1972.
Dieker H, Opitz JM: Associated acral and renal malformations: *Birth Defects* 5(3):68, 1969.
Halal F, et al.: Acro-renal-ocular syndrome: Autosomal dominant thumb hypoplasia, renal ectopia, and eye defect. *Am. J. Med. Genet.* 17:753, 1984.
Miltényi M, et al.: A new variant of the acrorenal syndrome associated with bilateral oligomeganephronic hypoplasia. *Eur. J. Pediatr.* 142:40, 1984.
Temtamy S, McKusick VA: Acrorenal syndrome. *Birth Defects* 14(3):171, 1978.

ADAMS-STOKES SYNDROME

Clinical Manifestations: (a) *sudden change in heart rate with a transient and abrupt loss of consciousness* with or without convulsions; (b) *decrease in cardiac output;* (c) *fall in blood pressure;* (d) *paleness;* (e) *flushing of the face with resumption of heart beats.*

Radiologic Manifestations: *Depend on etiologic factors:* congenital heart anomalies, myocarditis, acquired valvular diseases, myocardial infarction, metabolic diseases, infiltrative diseases of the myocardium, toxic agents, electrolyte disturbances, metastatic and primary neoplastic diseases.

REFERENCES

Adams R: Cases of diseases of the heart, accompanied with pathological observations. *Dublin Hosp. Rep.* 4:353, 1827.
Lim CH, et al.: Stokes-Adams attacks due to acute nonspecific myocarditis. *Am. Heart J.* 90:172, 1975.

O'Rourke RA: The Stokes-Adams syndrome. *Calif. Med.*
117:96, 1972.
Stokes W: Observations on some cases of permanently slow
pulse. *Dublin Q.J. Med. Soc.* 2:73, 1846.

ADDUCTED THUMB SYNDROME

Synonym: Christian adducted thumb syndrome.

Mode of Inheritance: Probably autosomal recessive.

Frequency: Nine cases reported to 1983 (Kunz et al.).

Clinical and Radiologic Manifestations: (a) *microcephaly, asymmetrical head, prominent occiput*; (b) *arthrogryposis*; (c) *myopathic face, ophthalmoplegia, downward slanting
of the palpebral fissures, abnormal ear placement, bifid
uvula, cleft palate, highly arched palate*; (d) *adducted
thumbs*; short first metacarpal; camptodactyly; limited extension of the elbows, wrists, and knees; *talipes equinovarus;
calcaneovalgus*; (e) *muscular hypotonia*, swallowing difficulties; (f) *mental retardation*; (g) early death; (h) other reported
abnormalities: respiratory problems, microgenia, pectus excavatum, hirsutism, laryngomalacia, seizures, torticollis,
muscle abnormalities, dysmyelination, enlargement of the
occipital and basal cisterns and the lateral and third ventricles, myopathic pattern (biopsy), etc.

Differential Diagnosis: Freeman-Sheldon syndrome,
contractural arachnodactyly, congenital clasped thumb, inherited ulnar drift syndrome, X-linked hydrocephalus, MASA
syndrome, Gareis-Mason syndrome (bilateral clasped thumbs
and mental retardation).

REFERENCES

Bianchine JW, et al.: The MASA syndrome: A new heritable
mental retardation syndrome. *Clin. Genet.* 5:298, 1974.
Christian JC, Andrews PA, Conneally PM, et al.: The adducted thumbs syndrome: An autosomal recessive disease
with arthrogryposis, dysmyelination, craniostenosis, and
cleft palate. *Clin. Genet.* 2:95, 1971.
Fisk J: Congenital ulnar deviation of the fingers with clubfoot
deformities. *Clin. Orthop.* 104:200, 1974.
Gareis FJ, Mason JD: X-linked mental retardation associated
with bilateral clasp thumb anomaly. *Am. J. Med. Genet.*
17:333, 1984.
Hall JG, et al.: The distal arthrogryposes: Delineation of new
entities—review and nosologic discussion. *Am. J. Med.
Genet.* 11:185, 1982.
Kunze J, et al.: Adducted thumb syndrome. *Eur. J. Pediatr.*
141:122, 1983.

ADULT RESPIRATORY DISTRESS SYNDROME

Synonyms: ARDS; shock lung; stiff lung syndrome; blast
lung; DaNang lung; respirator lung; white lung syndrome;
capillary leak syndrome; nonhydrostatic (noncardiogenic)

pulmonary edema; traumatic wet lung; congestive atelectasis; acute alveolar failure; etc.

Etiology: (a) hypoperfusion states; (b) tissue injury,
trauma, chest radiation, burns; (c) sepsis and infections
(pneumonia, pancreatitis, etc.); (d) fat embolism, amniotic
fluid embolism; (e) intravascular coagulation; (f) aspiration;
(g) near drowning, near strangulation; (h) drugs; (i) toxic gas
inhalation, oxygen toxicity; (j) others: head stroke, pheochromocytoma, percutaneous nephrolithotripsy, adult Still disease, peritoneovenous shunt, talc inhalation, lymphangiography, venous air emboli, central nervous system disturbances,
myocardial infarction, high altitude, dead fetus syndrome,
cardiopulmonary bypass, diabetic ketoacidosis.

Clinical Manifestations and Criteria for Diagnosis: (a) *an
appropriate etiologic factor*; (b) *refractory hypoxemia (dyspnea, tachypnea, cyanosis) while breathing high oxygen concentrations*; (c) *increased pulmonary shunt fraction*; (d) *reduced lung compliance*; (e) *no evidence of cardiac failure*; (f)
previously normal lungs; (g) other reported abnormalities:
transient leukopenia, pulmonary artery hypertension, idiopathic pulmonary fibrosis.

Radiologic Manifestations: (a) clear lung at the onset of
the latent period, development of diffuse pulmonary infiltration, air bronchogram; (b) air leak, lung cysts (small and
large); (c) lung abscesses, empyema.

Note: Lung cysts (in particular, small ones) are not often
seen on plain chest radiographs but are well shown on computed tomographic examination and indicate a poor prognosis (Table SY−A−1).

REFERENCES

Addington WW, et al.: The pulmonary edema of heroin
toxicity—An example of the stiff lung syndrome. *Chest*
62:199, 1972.
Amato JJ, et al.: Post-traumatic adult respiratory distress syndrome. *Orthop. Clin. North Am.* 9:693, 1978.
Anderson HF, et al.: Adult respiratory distress syndrome in
obstetrics and gynecology. *Obstet. Gynecol.* 55:291,
1980.
Ashbaugh DG, et al.: Acute respiratory distress in adults.
Lancet 2:319, 1967.
Ashbaugh DG, et al.: Idiopathic pulmonary fibrosis in adult
respiratory distress syndrome. *Arch. Surg.* 120:530, 1985.
Bass J, et al.: Intralipid causing adult respiratory distress syn-
drome. *J. Natl. Med. Assoc.* 76:401, 1984.
Berman IR, et al.: Intravascular microaggregation and the
respiratory distress syndromes. *Pediatr. Clin. North Am.*
22:275, 1975.
Blaisdell FW, et al.: The respiratory distress syndrome: A
review. *Surgery* 74:251, 1973.
Divertie MB: The adult respiratory distress syndrome. *Mayo
Clin. Proc.* 57:371, 1982.
Dyer RA, et al.: The adult respiratory distress syndrome and

TABLE SY—A—1.

Typical Characteristics of Adult Respiratory Distress Syndrome*

Characteristic	Stage I	Stage II	Stage III
Duration	First 12–24 hr	Days 2–5	After day 5
Pathological findings	Capillary congestion, endothelial cell swelling	Fluid leakage, fibrin deposition, vascular obstruction	Alveolar cell hyperplasia, collagen deposition, microvascular destruction
Clinical findings	Acute respiratory failure, shunt due to microatelectasis, hypoxemia relieved by PEEP†	Respiratory failure, shunt due to consolidation, hypoxemia not relieved by PEEP	Respiratory failure, hypoxemia due to V̇/Q̇ imbalance
Prototypical radiographic appearance	Low lung volumes, clear lungs	Diffuse consolidation, pulmonary artery filling defects	Less dense, ground-glass opacification, cortical lucencies if ischemic infarcts
Radiographic modifiers	Opacities if pulmonary inciting process	Local lucencies or densities if complication by infection or hemorrhage	Same as stage II
Differential diagnosis	Neuromuscular hypoventilation, airway obstruction, pulmonary embolism	Cardiogenic pulmonary edema, fluid overload, massive aspiration, nosocomial infection, lung hemorrhage	Same as stage II

*Modified from Greene R: Adult respiratory distress syndrome: Acute alveolar damage. *Radiology* 163:57, 1987. Used by permission.

†PEEP = positive end-expiratory pressure.

bronchogenic pulmonary tuberculosis. *Thorax* 39:383, 1984.

Effmann EL, et al.: Adult respiratory distress syndrome in children. *Radiology* 157:69, 1985.

El-Kassimi FA, et al.: Adult respiratory distress syndrome and disseminated intravascular coagulation complicating heat stroke. *Chest* 90:571, 1986.

Fenster LF, et al.: Acute respiratory distress syndrome after peritoneovenous shunt. *Am. Rev. Respir. Dis.* 125:244, 1982.

Fulkerson WJ, et al.: Adult respiratory distress syndrome after limited thoracic radiotherapy. *Cancer* 57:1941, 1986.

Greene R: Adult respiratory distress syndrome: Acute alveolar damage. *Radiology* 163:57, 1987.

Greene R, et al.: Pulmonary vascular obstruction in severe ARDS: Angiographic alterations after IV fibrinolytic therapy. *A.J.R.* 148:501, 1987.

Hirohata S, et al.: Adult Still's disease complicated with adult respiratory distress. *Arch. Intern. Med.* 146:2409, 1986.

Joffe N: The adult respiratory distress syndrome. *A.J.R.* 122:719, 1974.

Keren A, et al.: Adult respiratory distress syndrome in the course of acute myocardial infarction. *Chest* 77:161, 1980.

Lyrene RK, et al.: Adult respiratory distress syndrome in a pediatric intensive care unit. *Pediatrics* 67:790, 1981.

O'Hickey S, et al.: Phaeochromocytoma associated with adult respiratory distress syndrome. *Thorax* 42:157, 1987.

Ostendorf P, et al.: Pulmonary radiographic abnormalities in shock. *Radiology* 115:257, 1975.

Petty TL, et al.: Adult respiratory distress syndrome. *West. J. Med.* 128:399, 1978.

Poe RH, et al.: Adult respiratory distress syndrome related to ampicillin sensitivity. *Chest* 77:449, 1980.

Rayet I, et al.: Le syndrome de détresse respiratoire de "type adulte" en pédiatrie. *Arch. Fr. Pediatr.* 43:29, 1986.

Rudy DC, et al.: Adult respiratory distress syndrome complicating percutaneous nephrolithotripsy. *Urology* 23:376, 1984.

Russell J, et al.: Adult respiratory distress syndrome complicating diabetic ketoacidosis. *West. J. Med.* 135:148, 1981.

Shale DJ: The adult respiratory distress syndrome—20 years on. *Thorax* 42:641, 1987.

Silvestri RC, et al.: Respiratory distress syndrome from lymphangiography contrast medium. *Am. Rev. Respir. Dis.* 122:543, 1980.

Stark P, et al.: CT-findings in ARDS. *Radiologe* 27:367, 1987.

Thommasen HV, et al.: Transient leucopenia associated with adult respiratory distress syndrome. *Lancet* 1:809, 1984.

Wegenius G, et al.: Determinants of early adult respiratory distress syndrome with special reference to chest radiography. A retrospective analysis of 220 patients with major skeletal injuries. *Acta. Radiol. [Diagn] (Stockh)* 26:649, 1985.

Zapol WM, et al.: Vascular components of ARDS. Clinical pulmonary hemodynamics and morphology. *Am. Rev. Respir. Dis.* 136:471, 1987.

AFFERENT LOOP SYNDROME

Clinical Manifestations: Symptoms presenting following gastrectomy and gastrojejunostomy; altered afferent loop emptying with acute or chronic symptoms; in about 50% of the cases organic causes (perivisceritis, obstruction due to internal herniation or a kink, recurrent tumor, etc.) identified: (a) epigastric distress; (b) *upper abdominal pain;* (c) abdominal distension; (d) *bilious vomiting;* (e) diarrhea; (f) weight loss; (g) anemia; (h) symptoms usually relieved by copious bilious vomiting; (i) endoscopy: bile gastritis, bile esophagitis.

Radiologic Manifestations: (a) *prominent filling of the dilated proximal jejunal segment;* (b) *marked active contractions* of the distended proximal jejunal limb; (c) dilution of barium in the afferent loop by pancreatic and biliary juices; (d) jejunogastric regurgitation; (e) *retention of contrast medium in the proximal jejunal limb;* (f) ultrasound and computed tomography: U-shaped cystic mass with location of the distal portion posterior to the superior mesenteric artery, valvulae conniventes, tracing of bile ducts into the cystic structure, gallbladder and biliary duct distension; (g) hepatobiliary scanning: altered afferent loop emptying, atonic distension of the gallbladder; (h) percutaneous transhepatic biliary catheterization and drainage.

Differential Diagnosis: Acute pancreatitis; pancreatic pseudocyst; abscess; cystic metastases.

REFERENCES

Gale ME, et al.: CT appearance of afferent loop obstruction. *A.J.R.* 138:1085, 1982.

Ho CS, et al.: Selective intubation of the afferent loop. *A.J.R.* 130:481, 1978.

Hopens T, et al.: Sonographic diagnosis of afferent loop obstruction. *A.J.R.* 138:967, 1982.

Lee LI, et al.: Refractory afferent loop problems: Percutaneous transhepatic management of two cases. *Radiology* 165:49, 1987.

Peretz G, et al.: A case of afferent loop syndrome. *Australas. Radiol.* 27:22, 1983.

Roux G, et al.: Le syndrome de l'anse afferent des gastrectomisés. *Lyon Chir.* 45:773, 1950.

Sivelli R, et al.: Technetium-99m HIDA hepatobiliary scanning in evaluation of afferent loop syndrome. *Am. J. Surg.* 148:262, 1984.

AICARDI SYNDROME

Mode of Inheritance: Female (probable X-linked dominant with male lethality); reported in a girl with a de novo balanced X/3 translocation (46,t(X;3) (p22:q12); reported in one dizygotic twin; very rarely male (47XXY,46XY).

Frequency: Approximately 100 published cases (Constad et al).

Clinical Manifestations: (a) *infantile spasm,* convulsions; (b) *subnormal intelligence;* (c) *lacunar chorioretinopathy,* microphthalmos, colobomas, iris synechia, optic atrophy, etc.; (d) electroencephalography: *hypsarrhythmia,* etc.; (e) other reported abnormalities: plagiocephaly, facial asymmetry, cleft lip and palate.

Radiologic Manifestations: (a) cerebral anomalies: *agenesis of the corpus callosum,* heterotopic gray matter, hydrocephalus, Arnold-Chiari malformation, Dandy-Walker syndrome; porencephalia, holoprosencephaly, choroid plexus papilloma, lissencephaly, polygyria, microgyria, multiple intracerebral fluid collections with higher signal density than cerebrospinal fluid (magnetic resonance imaging), mi-

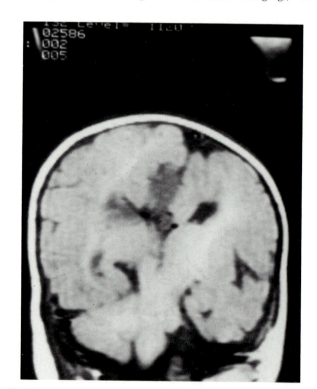

FIG SY—A—10.
Aicardi syndrome. A coronal T_2-weighted image (TR, 2,000 ms; TE, 30 ms) shows widely separated, parallel lateral ventricles consistent with agenesis of the corpus callosum. The interhemispheric fissure extends upward, between the lateral ventricles. The interhemispheric cyst on the right displays higher signal intensity than cerebrospinal fluid does. (From Igidbashian V, Mahboubi S, Zimmerman RA: CT and MR findings in Aicardi syndrome. *J. Comput. Assist. Tomogr.* 11:357, 1987. Used by permission.)

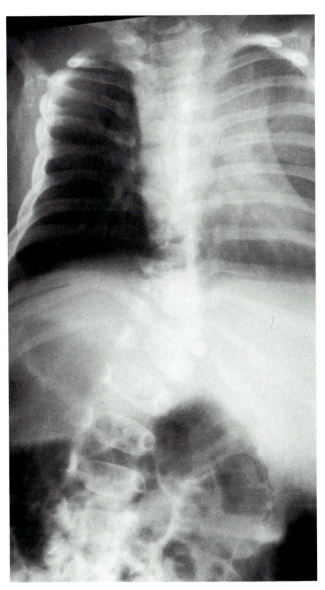

FIG SY—A—11.
Aicardi syndrome. Scoliosis of the thoracic spine with multiple rib and vertebral anomalies is shown. (From Igidbashian V, Mahboubi S, Zimmerman RA: CT and MR findings in Aicardi syndrome. *J. Comput. Assist. Tomogr.* 11:357, 1987. Used by permission.)

crophthalmos, cystic intraorbital lesions; (b) costovertebral malformations: block vertebrae, hemivertebrae, butterfly vertebrae, spina bifida, abnormal costovertebral articulations, scoliosis (Figs SY—A—10 and SY—A—11).

REFERENCES

Aicardi J, et al.: Le syndrome spasme en fléxion, agénesie calleuse, anomalies chorio-retiniennes. *Arch. Fr. Pediatr.* 26:1103, 1969.
Aicardi J, et al.: Spasms in flexion, callosal agenesis, ocular abnormalities: A new syndrome. *Electroencephalogr. Clin. Neurophysiol.* 19:609, 1965.

Baiert P, et al.: MR imaging in Aicardi syndrome. *A.J.N.R.* 9:805, 1988.
Bešenski N, et al.: Cortical heterotopia in Aicardi's syndrome—CT findings. *Pediatr. Radiol.* 18:391, 1988.
Canstad WH, et al.: Aicardi syndrome in one dizygotic twin. *Pediatrics* 76:450, 1985.
Curatolo P, et al.: Aicardi syndrome in a male infant. *J. Pediatr.* 96:286, 1980.
Igidbashian V, et al.: CT and MR findings in Aicardi syndrome. *J. Comput. Assist. Tomogr.* 11:357, 1987.
Phillips HE, et al.: Aicardi's syndrome; radiologic manifestations. *Radiology* 127:453, 1978.
Rao KC, et al.: The Aicardi syndrome: Demonstration of brain anomalies by ultrasound. *J. Clin. Ultrasound* 10:457, 1982.
Robinow M, et al.: Aicardi syndrome, papilloma of the choroid plexus, cleft lip, and cleft of the posterior palate. *J. Pediatr.* 104:404, 1984.
Ropers HH, et al.: Agenesis of corpus callosum, ocular, and skeletal anomalies (X-linked dominant Aicardi's syndrome) in a girl with balanced X/3 translocation. *Hum. Genet.* 61:364, 1982.
Sato N, et al.: Aicardi syndrome with holoprosencephaly and cleft lip and palate. *Pediatr. Neurol.* 3:114, 1987.

AINHUM

Synonyms: Dactylolysis spontanea; dactylolysis essentialis; ainhoum; ombanja (Bantu).

Mode of Inheritance: Familial cases have been reported.

Clinical Manifestations: Toes and fingers involved—*deep soft-tissue groove* corresponding to a hyperkeratotic band *partially or totally encircling the digit*.

Radiologic Manifestations: (a) *sharply demarcated thinning and narrowing of bone, then fracture and resorption;* (b) autoamputation of the digit in some cases.

Differential Diagnosis: Pseudoainhum occurring in association with several hereditary and acquired dermatoses (palmoplantar keratoderma, pachyonychia congenita, Vohwinkel disease, mal de Meleda syndrome, pityriasis rubra pilaris, fungal infection, leprosy, psoriasis, after trauma, erythropoietic protoporphyria) (Fig SY—A—12).

REFERENCES

Bertoli CL, et al.: Ainhum—An unusual presentation involving the second toe in a white male. *Skeletal Radiol.* 11:133, 1984.
Christopher AP, et al.: Pseudoainhum and erythropoietic protoporphyria. *Br. J. Dermatol.* 118:113, 1988.
Cole GJ: Ainhum: An account of fifty-four patients with special reference to etiology and treatment. *J. Bone Joint Surg. [Br.]* 47:43, 1965.
da Silva Lima JF: Estudo sobre o "Ainhum." *Gaz. Med. da Bahia* 1:146, 1867 (cited by Cole, 1965).

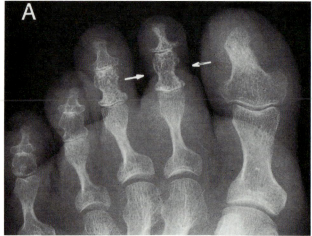

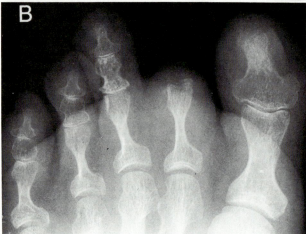

FIG SY—A—12.
Ainhum. **A,** constricting soft-tissue band *(arrows)* at the middle phalanx of the second toe and acro-osteolysis of the distal phalanx of the same toe. **B,** a radiograph of the toes 2 years later shows amputation of the distal and most of the middle phalanx of the second toe. (From Bertoli CL, Stassi J, Rifkin MD: Ainhum—an unusual presentation involving second toe in a white male. *Skeletal Radiol.* 11:133, 1984. Used by permission.)

Fetterman LE, et al.: The clinico-roentgenologic features of Ainhum. *A.J.R.* 100:512, 1967.
Maass E: Beobachtungen über Ainhum. *Arch. Schiffs-U. Tropenhygiene* 30:32, 1926.
Simon KMB: Ainhum, a family disease. *J.A.M.A.* 76:560, 1921.

ALAGILLE SYNDROME

Synonyms: Arteriohepatic syndrome; Watson-Alagille syndrome; syndromic hepatic ductular hypoplasia.

Mode of Inheritance: Consistent with an autosomal dominant gene with reduced penetrance and variable expressivity; partial syndrome in some cases.

Frequency: Uncommon.

Clinical Manifestations: Major features are presented in *b, c, d,* and *e.* (a) *retarded growth,* low birth weight; (b) *dysmorphic facies:* (95%), small triangular face, broad forehead, pointed mandible, flattened cheeks, mild ocular hypertelorism, deep-set eyes, prominent or malformed ears; (c) ocular abnormalities: *posterior embryotoxon* (88%), Axenfeld anomaly (attachment of iris processes to the Descemet membrane), ectopic and/or eccentrically shaped pupils, *chorioretinal atrophy, pigment clumping,* myopia, strabismus, cataract; (d) cardiovascular anomalies (85%): *peripheral pulmonary stenosis or hypoplasia,* pulmonary valvular stenosis, patent ductus arteriosus, atrial septal defect, ventricular septal defect, etc.; (e) *neonatal cholestasis* (91%), neonatal hypercholesterolemia, hypoplasia of the intrahepatic bile ducts, attenuated extrahepatic bile duct, hepatomegaly, abnormal liver function test results; (f) other reported abnormalities: renal function defects (decreased creatinine clearance, increased blood urea nitrogen, increased uric acid), endocrine disorders (decreased thyroxine, increased testosterone, hypogonadism, spermatogenic hypoplasia), absent reflexes, normal or mild to moderate mental retardation (16%); behavioral problems, high-pitched voice, signs of progressive portal hypertension, cirrhosis, liver failure, severely reduced thromboxane B_2 synthesis by platelets, chromosome abnormality [46,XX,del (20) (p11.2)], hepatoma, hepatocarcinoma, renal structural and parenchymal abnormalities in 10% of the cases (tubulointerstitial nephropathy, membranous glomerular lipid

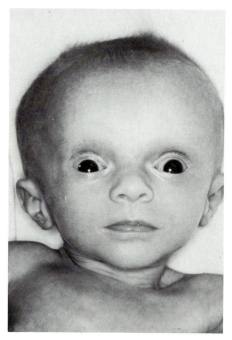

FIG SY—A—13.
Alagille syndrome with dysmorphic facies: triangular face, broad forehead, pointed chin, flattened cheeks, hypertelorism, deep-set eyes. (From Alagille D, Estrada A, Hadchouel M, et al.: Syndromic paucity of interlobular bile ducts (Alagille syndrome or arteriohepatic dysplasia): Review of 80 cases. *J. Pediatr.* 110:195, 1987. Used by permission.)

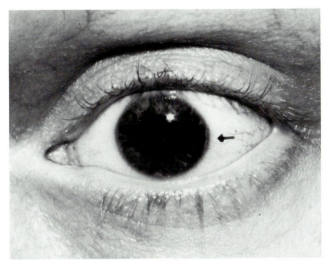

FIG SY—A—14.
Alagille syndrome: the posterior embryotoxon *(arrow)*. (From Mueller RF: The Alagille syndrome (arteriohepatic dysplasia). *J. Med. Genet.* 24:621, 1987. Used by permission.)

deposits with renal failure, proliferative glomerulonephritis with transient renal tubular acidosis, cystic disease, etc.)

Radiologic Manifestations: (a) *cardiovascular anomalies;* (b) *vertebral defects: butterfly vertebrae,* small vertebral bodies, narrow interpedicular distances, irregular end plates, pointed anterior process of the first cervical spine, fused vertebral bodies, spina bifida occulta, etc.; (c) limb deformities; short ulna, short distal phalanges, long and thin fingers, proximally placed thumbs, radioulnar synostosis, multiple lacunae possibly representing intraosseous xanthomas, etc.; (d) diffuse hepatic increase in echogenicity and loss of normal texture due to parenchymal disease, regenerative liver nodules, etc.; (e) renal structural abnormalities (hypoplastic kidneys, renal artery stenosis, unilateral absence of a kidney, medullary cystic disease with prominent renal echoes, duplicated ureters), renal stones; (f) other reported abnormalities: osteopenia, hypertelorism, craniostenosis, rib anomalies (11 ribs, 13 ribs, rib synostosis, bifid rib), narrow-waisted ilium, retarded bone age, hepatobiliary scintigraphic findings similar to those usually associated with biliary atresia (Figs SY—A—13 to SY—A—15).

REFERENCES

Alagille D, et al.: L' atrésie des voies biliaires intrahépatiques avec voies biliaires extrahépatiques perméables chez l'enfant. *Rev. Med. Chir. Mal. Foie.* 45:93, 1970.

Alagille D, et al.: Syndromic paucity of interlobular bile ducts (Alagille syndrome or arteriohepatic dysplasia): Review of 80 cases. *J. Pediatr.* 110:195, 1987.

Brunelle F, et al.: Skeletal anomalies in Alagille's syndrome. Radiographic study in eighty cases. *Ann. Radiol. (Paris)* 29:687, 1986.

Byrne JLB, et al.: del(20p) with manifestations of arteriohepatic dysplasia. *Am. J. Med. Genet.* 24:673, 1986.

Deprettere A, et al.: Syndromic paucity of the intrahepatic bile ducts: Diagnostic difficulty; severe morbidity throughout early childhood. *J. Pediatr. Gastroenterol. Nutr.* 6:865, 1987.

Dupont J, et al.: Eicosanoid synthesis in Alagille syndrome. *N. Engl. J. Med.* 314:718, 1986.

Kaufman SS, et al.: Hepatocarcinoma in a child with the Alagille syndrome. *Am. J. Dis. Child.* 141:698, 1987.

Mueller RF: The Alagille syndrome (arteriohepatic dysplasia). *J. Med. Genet.* 24:621, 1987.

Oestreich AE, et al.: Renal abnormalities in arteriohepatic

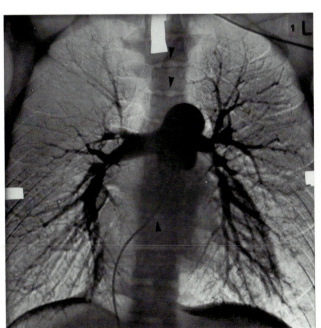

FIG SY—A—15.
Alagille syndrome. Peripheral pulmonary stenosis and "butterfly" thoracic vertebrae *(arrowheads)* are shown. (From Singcharoen T, Patridge J, Jeans WD, et al.: Arteriohepatic dysplasia. *Br. J. Radiol.* 59:509, 1986. Used by permission.)

dysplasia and nonsyndromic intrahepatic biliary hypoplasia. *Ann. Radiol. (Paris)* 26:203, 1983.

Ong E, et al.: MR imaging of a hepatoma associated with Alagille syndrome. *J. Comput. Assist. Tomogr.* 10:1047, 1986.

Riely CA, et al.: A father and son with cholestasis and peripheral pulmonic stenosis: A distinct form of intrahepatic cholestasis. *J. Pediatr.* 92:406, 1978.

Singcharoen T, et al.: Arteriohepatic dysplasia. *Br. J. Radiol.* 59:509, 1986.

Shulman SA, et al.: Arteriohepatic dysplasia (Alagille syndrome): Extreme variability among affected family members. *Am. J. Med. Genet.* 19:325, 1984.

Summerville DA, et al.: Hepatobiliary scintigraphy in arteriohepatic dysplasia (Alagille's syndrome). *Pediatr. Radiol.* 18:32, 1988.

Tolia V, et al.: Renal abnormalities in paucity of interlobular bile ducts. *J. Pediatr. Gastroenterol. Nutr.* 6:971, 1987.

Watson GH, et al.: Arteriohepatic dysplasia: Familial pulmonary arterial stenosis with neonatal liver disease. *Arch. Dis. Child.* 48:459, 1973.

ALEXANDER DISEASE

Mode of Inheritance: Possibly autosomal recessive. A child with the disease had four siblings with macrocephaly who died without proven diagnoses.

Pathology: A leukodystrophy of unknown etiology; *widespread dymyelination; progressive fibrinoid degeneration of fibrillary astrocytes.*

Frequency: Uncommon.

Clinical Manifestations: A progressive neurodegenerative disease with an onset of symptoms usually in early infancy and death in early childhood; less common is an onset in later childhood or adult life: (a) *megalencephaly;* (b) *psychomotor retardation, seizures, spasticity.*

Radiologic Manifestations: (a) computed tomographic findings variable at different progressive stages of the disease; typical findings in the advanced stage of the disease are *white matter lucency in the frontal lobe with extension into the peripheral zone, involvement of the external capsules, relatively lesser involvement of the internal capsules, increased density of the optic chiasm, optic radiations, columns of fornices, basal ganglia, subependymal rim and medial portions of the forceps minor; marked enhancement of the dense areas after contrast medium injection;* mild to moderate dilatation of the lateral and third ventricles; (b) ultrasonography: mild ventricular dilation in the early stage of disease associated with some loss of definition of sulci, abnormal increase in brain size, loss of definition of sulci, and uniform appearance of cerebral tissues.

REFERENCES

Alexander WS: Progressive fibrinoid degeneration of fibrillary astrocytes associated with mental retardation in a hydrocephalic infant. *Brain* 72:373, 1949.

Farrell K, et al.: Computed tomography in Alexander's disease. *Ann. Neurol. (Paris)* 15:605, 1984.

Harbord MG, et al.: Alexander's disease: Cranial ultrasound findings. *Pediatr. Radiol.* 18:227, 1988.

Riggs JE, et al.: Asymptomatic adult Alexander's disease: Entity or nosological misconception? *Neurology* 38:152, 1988.

Trommer BL, et al.: Noninvasive CT diagnosis of infantile Alexander disease: Pathologic correlation. *J. Comput. Assist. Tomogr.* 3:509, 1983.

Walls J, et al.: Alexander's disease with Rosenthal fibre formation in an adult. *J. Neurol. Neurosurg. Psychiatry* 47:399, 1984.

ALPORT SYNDROME

Mode of Inheritance: Genetic heterogeneity; autosomal dominant; X-linked recessive; possibly also autosomal recessive.

Frequency: Over 200 families reported (Crawfurd).

Clinical Manifestations: (a) *nephropathy* (hematuria, proteinuria, progressive renal failure); (b) *sensorineural deafness,* loss of high-frequency auditory perception (in 30% to 40% of cases); (c) ocular abnormalities (in about 20% of cases): posterior polymorphous dystrophy of the cornea, anterior lenticonus, perimacular and retinal flecks, arcus juvenalis, spherophakia, cataract, pigment dispersion syndrome, optic disc drusen, anisocoria, iris atrophy, iris heterochromia; (d) urinary excretion of glomerular basement antigen (immunoelectrophoresis), glomerular basement changes (thinning, irregularity, focal thickening, etc.); (e) other reported abnormalities: inguinal hernia, anomalies of fingers, cryptorchidism, central nervous system tumors, myasthenia, decreased sensibility for vibration and position, decreased memory of recent events, megathrombocytopenia.

Radiologic Manifestations: (a) roentgenologic findings of renal failure; (b) congestive cardiac failure secondary to hypertension; (c) renal arteriography: poor cortical opacification, severe tortuosity and crowded appearance at corticomedullary junction, pruning of interlobar arteries, indistinctness of corticomedullary junction; (d) other reported abnormalities: anomalies of urinary system, diffuse renal enlargement, minimal blunting of the calices, small and contracted kidney, pectus excavatum, spina bifida, renal cortical calcification.

Note: Fechtner syndrome represents a variant of Alport syndrome (nephritis, hearing loss, eye abnormalities, macrothrombocytopenia, and leukocyte inclusions).

REFERENCES

Alport AC: Hereditary familial congenital haemorrhagic nephritis. *Br. Med. J.* 1:504, 1927.

Atkin CL, et al.: Mapping of Alport syndrome to the long arm of the X chromosome. *Am. J. Hum. Genet.* 42:249, 1988.

Chuang VP, et al.: Angiographic features of Alport's syndrome: Hereditary nephritis. *A.J.R.* 121:539, 1974.

Crawfurd M d'A: Alport's syndrome. *J. Med. Genet.* 25:623, 1988.

Flinter FA, et al.: Genetics of classic Alport's syndrome. *Lancet* 2:1005, 1988.

Gershoni-Baruch R, et al.: Fechtner Syndrome: Clinical and genetic aspects. *Am. J. Med. Genet.* 31:357, 1988.

Grünfeld JP, et al.: The clinical spectrum of hereditary nephritis. *Kidney Int.* 27:83, 1985.

Gubler M: Alport's syndrome: A report of 58 cases and a review of the literature. *Am. J. Med.* 70:493, 1981.

Hasstedt SJ, et al.: Genetic heterogeneity among kindreds with Alport syndrome. *Am. J. Hum. Genet.* 38:940, 1986.

Hasstedt SJ, et al.: X-linked inheritance of Alport syndrome: Family P revisited. *Am. J. Hum. Genet.* 35:1241, 1983.

Lalli AF: Renal parenchyma calcifications. *Semin. Roentgenol.* 17:101, 1982.

Lubec G, et al.: Urinary excretion of glomerular basement antigen in Alport's syndrome. *Arch. Dis. Child.* 53:401, 1978.

Roussel B, et al.: Léiomyomatose oesophagienne familiale associée a un syndrome d'Alport chez un garçon de 9 ans. *Helv. Paediat. Acta* 41:359, 1986.

Thompson SM, et al.: Ocular signs in Alport's syndrome. *Eye* 1:146, 1987.

AMELOGENESIS IMPERFECTA– NEPHROCALCINOSIS SYNDROME

Synonym: Enamel-renal syndrome.

Mode of Inheritance: Autosomal recessive.

Frequency: Two sibships (Lubinsky et al.).

Clinical and Radiologic Manifestations: (a) amelogenesis imperfecta; (b) lifelong nocturnal enuresis; (c) decreased calcium and phosphate excretion over 24 hours and after an acute load, increased serum osteocalcin and decreased urine δ-carboxyglutamic acid; (d) renal function deterioration after early teens (renal failure); (e) progressive punctate nephrocalcinosis.

REFERENCES

Lubinsky M, et al.: Syndrome of amelogenesis imperfecta, nephrocalcinosis, impaired renal concentration, and possible abnormality of calcium metabolism. *Am. J. Med. Genet.* 20:233, 1985.

MacGibbon D: Generalized enamel hypoplasia and renal dysfunction. *Aust. Dent. J.* 17:61, 1972.

AMINOPTERIN FETOPATHY

Synonym: Fetal aminopterin syndrome.

Etiology: Due to teratogenic effects of aminopterin and amethopterin used in the first trimester of pregnancy.

Clinical Manifestations: (a) *low birth weight;* (b) *cranial dysplasia;* (c) *abnormal facies:* low-set ears, prominent eyes, hypertelorism, flat nasal bridge, micrognathia, cleft palate, upswept frontal hair pattern, shallow supraorbital ridges; (d) miscellaneous limb anomalies; (e) mental retardation in some survivors; (f) physical retardation, progressive improvement of clinical picture with growth; (g) other reported abnormalities: myopia, hydrocephalus, anencephaly, meningoencephalocele, cardiac anomalies, renal anomalies.

Radiologic Manifestations: (a) *cranial dysplasia:* lack of normal ossification of the cranial vault at birth, poor ossification of the cranium and development of multiple wormian bones in follow-up studies, cranium bifidum, aberrant longitudinal suture in the parietal bones, partial craniosynostosis; (b) other reported anomalies: shortness of limbs, in particular the forearms; congenital stenosis of the medullary space of the long bones; subluxation of the radial heads; clubfoot deformity; synostosis of the bones of the hands and feet; hip dislocation; slender ribs; low iliac indices; retarded ossification of the pubis and ischium; skeletal maturation retardation.

Differential Diagnosis: Aminopterin-like syndrome without aminopterin (Fig SY–A–16).

REFERENCES

Brandner M, et al.: Foetopathie due à l'aminopterine avec sténose congénitale de l'espace médullaire des os tubulaires longs. *Ann. Radiol. (Paris)* 12:703, 1969.

Char F: Picture of the month: Aminopterin embryopathy syndrome. *Am. J. Dis. Child.* 133:1189, 1979.

Reich EW, et al.: Recognition in adult patients of malformations induced by folic acid antagonists. *Birth Defects* 4:139, 1978.

Shaw EB: Fetal damage due to aminopterin ingestion: Follow-up at 17½ years of age. *Am. J. Dis. Child.* 134:1172, 1980.

Shaw EB, et al.: Aminopterin-induced fetal malformation: Survival of infant after attempted abortion. *Am. J. Dis. Child.* 115:477, 1968.

Thiersch JB: Therapeutic abortions with folic acid antagonist, 4-aminopteroylglutamic acid (4-amino P.G.A.) administered by oral route. *Am. J. Obstet. Gynecol.* 63:1298, 1952.

AMINOPTERIN-LIKE SYNDROME WITHOUT AMINOPTERIN

Mode of Inheritance: Possibly autosomal recessive.

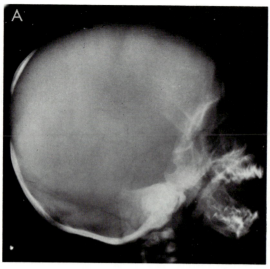

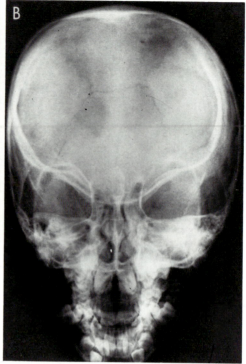

FIG SY–A–16.
Aminopterin fetopathy. **A,** delayed ossification of the frontal and parietal bones produces large coronal and sagittal sutures at 3½ months of age. A dense bone is seen within the posterior part of the sagittal suture. The metopic suture is wide, and the mandible is short. **B,** at 53 months of age in the same patient bone in the sagittal suture has enlarged and produced two anomalous sutures on either side of the midline. (From Shaw EB, Steinbach HL: Aminopterin-induced fetal malformation: Survival of infant after attempted abortion. *Am. J. Dis. Child.* 115:477, 1968. Used by permission.)

FIG SY–A–17.
Aminopterin-like syndrome without aminopterin. Ocular hypertelorism, a prominent nasal root, and low-set posteriorly rotated ears are present. (From Fraser FC, Anderson RA, Mulvihill JI, et al.: An aminopterin-like syndrome without aminopterin (ASSAS). *Clin. Genet.* 32:28, 1987. Used by permission.)

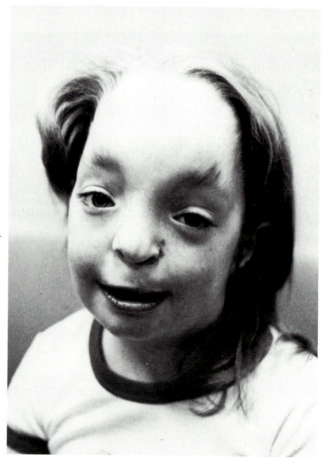

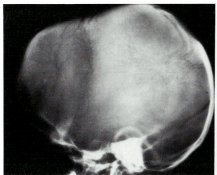 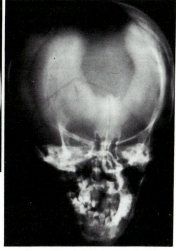

FIG SY–A–18.
Aminopterin-like syndrome without aminopterin. Ossification defects of the cranium are shown. (From Fraser FC, Anderson RA, Mulvihill JJ, et al.: An aminopterin-like syndrome without aminopterin (ASSAS). *Clin. Genet.* 32:28, 1987. Used by permission.)

Clinical Manifestations: Very similar to aminopterin syndrome with no evidence of maternal exposure to the drug: (a) *craniofacial dysmorphism: temporal recession of the hairline with an upswept frontal hair pattern, ocular hypertelorism, prominent nasal root, low-set posteriorly rotated ear lobes, highly arched cleft palate;* (b) *dermatoglyphic anomalies;* (c) limited elbow movement; (d) *short stature;* (e) *psychomotor retardation* (mild to moderate); (f) other reported abnormalities: seizures, hearing defect, distal shortening of the limbs, cryptorchidism.

Radiologic Manifestations: (a) *parietal cranial bone defects,* small orbits, ossification defect of the orbital roof, facial asymmetry, micrognathia, hydrocephalus; (b) other reported abnormalities: mild scoliosis, spina bifida, small iliac wings, a tapering mildly hypoplastic thumb (Figs SY–A–17 and SY–A–18).

REFERENCE

Fraser FC, et al.: An aminopterin-like syndrome without aminopterin (ASSAS). *Clin. Genet.* 32:28, 1987.

AMNIOTIC BAND SEQUENCE

Synonym: Streeter dysplasia; amniotic band disruption complex; amniotic band syndrome; ring constriction; etc.

Mode of Inheritance: Sporadic; familial amniotic bands and amniotic band disruption in twins have rarely been reported.

Pathogenesis: Compression-related deformities due to amnion rupture with retained chorion integrity are most likely the cause of the anomalies; a possibility of chorionic villus biopsy as a cause of the amniotic band syndrome has been suggested.

Pathology: *Triad of amniotic-denuded placenta, fetal attachment to or entanglement by amniotic remnants and fetal malformations.*

Clinical and Radiologic Manifestations: (a) head: facial clefts, calvarial defects, hydrocephalus, anencephaly, encephalocele, microphthalmos, microcephaly, sutural synostosis, hypertelorism, etc.; (b) limbs: *single or multiple ring constrictions, most common distally,* varying in severity from minor grooves to total amputation, digital fusion, clubfoot deformity, pseudoarthrosis, etc.; (c) trunk: gastroschisis, omphalocele, malformed genitalia, imperforate anus, hypoplastic lungs, chest deformity, scoliosis, meningomyelocele, ectopia cordis, strangulation of the umbilical cord, etc.; (d) other reported abnormalities: association with Ehlers-Danlos syndrome, type IV, and osteogenesis imperfecta; transient oligohydramnios (ultrasound imaging); etc. (Fig SY–A19 and SY–A–20).

Differential Diagnosis: The "Michelin tire baby" syndrome; accidental or purposeful band formation around the extremities.

REFERENCES

Askins G, et al.: Congenital constriction band syndrome. *J. Pediatr. Orthop.* 8:461, 1988.
Bieber FR, et al.: Amniotic band sequence associated with ectopia cordis in one twin. *J. Pediatr.* 105:817, 1984.
Chen H, et al.: Amniotic band sequence and its neurocutaneous manifestations. *Am. J. Med. Genet.* 28:661, 1987.

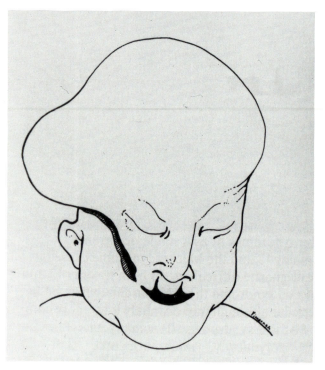

FIG SY—A—19.
Diagrammatic representation of the facial appearance of an infant with the amniotic band disruption complex. Note the right-sided parietal soft-tissue mass, the oblique deep facial furrow, and the cleft lip. (From McCarthy S, Sarwar M, Virapongse C, et al.: Craniofacial anomalies in amniotic band disruption complex. *Pediatr. Radiol.* 14:44, 1984. Used by permission.)

Donnenfeld AE, et al.: Discordant amniotic band sequence in monozygotic twins. *Am. J. Med. Genet.* 20:685, 1985.

Fisher RM, et al.: Limb defects in the amniotic band syndrome. *Pediatr. Radiol.* 5:24, 1976.

Fried AM, et al.: Omphalocele in limb/body wall deficiency syndrome: Atypical sonographic appearance. *J. Clin. Ultrasound* 10:400, 1982.

Heifetz SA: Strangulation of the umbilical cord by amniotic bands: Report of 6 cases and literature review. *Pediatr. Pathol.* 2:285, 1984.

Herva R, et al.: Cluster of severe amniotic adhesion malformations in Finland. *Lancet* 1:818, 1980.

Hill LM, et al.: Prenatal ultrasound diagnosis of a forearm constriction band. *J. Ultrasound Med.* 7:293, 1988.

Hudgins RJ, et al.: Pediatric neurosurgical implications of the amniotic band disruption complex. Case reports and review of the literature. *Pediatr. Neurosci.* 12:232, 1985.

Hunter AGW, et al.: Implications of malformations not due to amniotic bands in the amniotic band sequence. *Am. J. Med. Genet.* 24:691, 1986.

Johnson CF: Constricting bands. Manifestations of possible child abuse. Case reports and a review. *Clin. Pediatr. (Phila.)* 27:439, 1988.

Kunze J, et al.: A new genetic disorder: Autosomal-dominant multiple benign ring-shaped skin creases. *Eur. J. Pediatr.* 138:301, 1982.

Lubinsky M, et al.: Familial amniotic bands. *Am. J. Med. Genet.* 14:81, 1983.

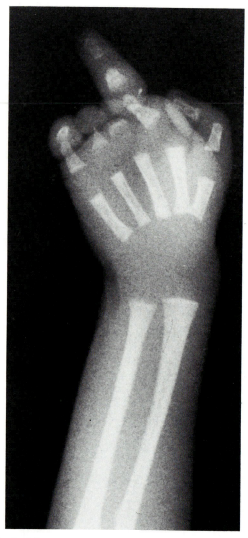

FIG SY—A—20.
Amniotic band syndrome in a newborn male: partial and near total amputation of the digits.

McCarthy S, et al.: Craniofacial anomalies in the amniotic band disruption complex. *Pediatr. Radiol.* 14:44, 1984.

Planteydt HT, et al.: Amniotic bands and malformations in child born after pregnancy screened by chorionic villus biopsy. *Lancet* 2:756, 1986.

Streeter GL: Focal deficiencies in fetal tissues and their relationship to intra-uterine amputations. *Contrib. Embryol. Carnegie Inst.* 22:1, 1930.

Wiedemann, H-R: Multiple benign circumferential skin creases on limbs—a congenital anomaly existing from the beginning of mankind (Letter). *Am. J. Med. Genet.* 28:225, 1987.

Young ID, et al.: Amniotic bands in connective tissue disorders. *Arch. Dis. Child.* 60:1061, 1985.

Zionts LE, et al.: Congenital annular bands in identical twins. *J. Bone Joint Surg. [Am.]* 66:450, 1984.

Zych GA, et al.: Congenital band causing pseudarthrosis and impending gangrene of the leg. *J. Bone Joint Surg. [Am.]* 65:410, 1983.

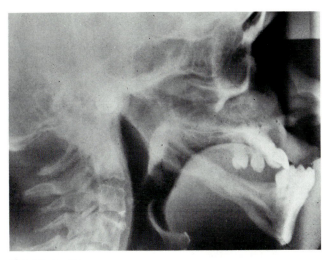

FIG SY—A—21.
Anderson syndrome in a 23-year-old female. A lateral view of the facial structure shows the mandible to be thick in the mental region. The ramus is thin and wavy in contour, and the gonial angle is markedly obtuse. (From Buchignani JS, Cook AJ, Anderson LG: Roentgenographic findings in familial osteodysplasia. *A.J.R.* 116:602, 1972. Used by permission.)

ANDERSON SYNDROME

Synonym: Familial osteodysplasia.

Mode of Inheritance: Probably autosomal recessive.

Clinical Manifestations: (a) *unusual facies:* recessed, flattened midface with diminished malar prominence, prominent brows, narrow and prognathic jaw, flat nasal bridge, large ear lobes; (b) elevated serum uric acid level; (c) other reported abnormalities: repeated mandibular fracture, elevated diastolic blood pressure, dental malocclusion.

Radiologic Manifestations: (a) *marked diminution in size of the maxilla and zygomatic bones, calvarial thinning, brachycephaly,* pointed configuration of the mastoids, hypoplasia of petrous bone; (b) prominently pointed small spinous process of the cervical vertebrae, *thoracic scoliosis;* (c) thick cortex of clavicles; (d) *thinning of ribs;* (e) thinning of superior pubic rami; (f) *cortical thickening of the long bones and tubular bones of the hands and feet* (Fig SY—A—21).

REFERENCES

Anderson LG, et al.: Familial osteodysplasia. *J.A.M.A.* 220:1687, 1972.
Buchighani JS, et al.: Roentgenographic findings in familial osteodysplasia. *A.J.R.* 116:602, 1972.

ANEURYSM, INTRACRANIAL FAMILIAL

Synonym: Familial intracranial aneurysm.

Mode of Inheritance: Autosomal dominant or multifactorial trait.

Clinical Manifestations: (a) intracranial hemorrhage; (b) other reported abnormalities: coarctation of the aorta, polycystic kidneys, Ehlers-Danlos syndrome.

Radiologic Manifestations: Intracranial aneurysm(s) with a tendency to rupture at a younger age (peak incidence, 30 to 39 years) than in the general population (nonfamilial aneurysms).

REFERENCES

Halal F, et al.: Intracranial aneurysms: a report of a large pedigree. *Am. J. Med. Genet.* 15:89, 1983.
Jankowicz E, et al.: Intracranial familial aneurysms associated with polycystic kidneys. *Neurol. Neurochir. Pol.* 5:263, 1971.
Pope FM, et al.: Some patients with cerebral aneurysms are deficient in type III collagen. *Lancet* 1:973, 1981.
ter Berg JWM, et al.: Detection of unruptured familial intracranial aneurysms by intravenous digital subtraction angiography. *Neuroradiology* 29:272, 1987.
Ulrich DP, et al.: Familial cerebral aneurysms including one extracranial carotid aneurysm. *Neurology* 10:288, 1960.

ANGELMAN SYNDROME

Synonym: "Happy puppet" syndrome.

Mode of Inheritance: Sporadic; familial cases in siblings; autosomal recessive inheritance has been considered; low recurrence risk (about 5%).

Frequency: Approximately 60 published cases (Willems et al., Fisher et al., and others).

Clinical Manifestations: (a) *mental retardation;* (b) *microbrachycephaly;* (c) *ataxia;* (d) *stiff, jerky puppetlike movements and gait;* (e) paroxysmal laughter, salaam seizures; (f) protruding tongue; (g) inability to speak; (h) ocular anomalies: faulty pigmentation, optic atrophy, strabismus, abnormal eye movements, congenital cataract; (i) abnormal electroencephalographic findings: 2 to 3 counts per second spike and wave activity.

Radiologic Manifestations: (a) *microbrachycephaly,* vertical inclination of the base of the skull, horizontal occipital depression, prognathism; (b) brain atrophy.

REFERENCES

Angelman H: "Puppet" children: A report of three cases. *Dev. Med. Child Neurol.* 7:681, 1965.
Baraitser M, et al.: The Angelman (happy puppet) syndrome: Is it autosomal recessive? *Clin. Genet.* 31:323, 1987.

Boyd SG, et al.: The EEG in early diagnosis of the Angelman (happy puppet) syndrome. *Eur. J. Pediatr.* 147:508, 1988.

Fisher JA, et al.: Angelman (happy puppet) syndrome in a girl and her brother. *J. Med. Genet.* 24:294, 1987.

Pelc S, et al.: "Happy puppet" syndrome ou syndrome du "pantin hilare." *Helv. Paediatr. Acta* 31:183, 1976.

Willems PJ, et al.: Recurrence risk in the Angelman ("happy puppet") syndrome. *Am. J. Med. Genet.* 27:773, 1987.

Williams CA, et al.: The Angelman ("happy puppet") syndrome. *Am. J. Med. Genet.* 11:453, 1982.

ANIRIDIA–WILMS TUMOR ASSOCIATION

Frequency: Incidence of 1 in 43 to 91 cases of Wilms tumor (Narahara et al.).

Clinical and Radiologic Manifestations: (a) *Wilms tumor* high incidence of bilateral tumor (in about one third); (b) *congenital aniridia* (sporadic type); (c) other reported associated abnormalities: mental retardation, skull or craniofacial dysmorphism, various skeletal defects, deformities of the pinna, genitourinary anomalies, hamartomatous lesions, umbilical and inguinal hernias, hyperkinesis, genitourinary anomalies (hypospadias, undescended testes, etc.), cataracts, glaucoma, etc.; (d) chromosome abnormality (deletion 11p 13–14.1), the mother of a child with the association with an 11p deletion involving the p13 band (Nakagome), high incidence in males, advanced maternal age, familial isolated aniridia reported in association with a translocation involving chromosomes 11 and 22.

Recommended Management of Children with Sporadic Aniridia: (a) initial evaluation: a complete history and physical examination, urinalysis, chromosome analysis, excretory urography, abdominal ultrasonography; (b) follow-up: physical examination, urinalysis, and ultrasonography every 4 to 6 months until 8 years of age, following which the physical, laboratory, and imaging evaluation is performed at 6- to 12-month intervals; if ultrasonography is unsatisfactory or questionable or shows an abnormality, computed tomography is recommended.

Note: (a) the presence of an 11p13 deletion increases the likelihood of the development of Wilms tumor; (b) 80% of all Wilms tumors occur before 5 years of age.

REFERENCES

Friedman AL: Wilms' tumor detection in patients with sporadic aniridia. Successful use of ultrasound. *Am. J. Dis. Child.* 140:173, 1986.

Miller R, et al.: Association of Wilms' tumor with aniridia, hemihypertrophy and other congenital malformations. *N. Engl. J. Med.* 270:922, 1964.

Moore JW, et al.: Familial isolated aniridia associated with a translocation involving chromosomes 11 and 22 [t(11;22)(p13;q12.2)]. *Hum. Genet.* 72:297, 1986.

Nakagome Y, et al.: High-resolution studies in patients with aniridia–Wilms tumor association, Wilms tumor or related congenital abnormalities. *Hum. Genet.* 67:245, 1984.

Narahara K, et al.: Regional mapping of catalase and Wilms tumor–aniridia, genitourinary abnormalities, and mental retardation triad loci to the chromosome segment 11p1305→p1306. *Hum. Genet.* 66:181, 1984.

Palmer N, et al.: The association of aniridia and Wilms' tumor: Methods of surveillance and diagnosis. *Med. Pediatr. Oncol.* 11:73, 1983.

Pendergrass TW: Congenital anomalies in children with Wilms' tumor. A new survey. *Cancer* 37:403, 1976.

Riccardi VM, et al.: Chromosomal imbalance in the aniridia–Wilms' tumor association: 11 p interstitial deletion. *Pediatrics* 61:604, 1978.

Riccardi VM, et al.: Wilms tumor with aniridia/iris dysplasia and apparently normal chromosomes. *J. Pediatr.* 100:574, 1982.

Shannon RS, et al.: Wilms's tumour and aniridia: Clinical and cytogenetic features. *Arch. Dis. Child.* 57:685, 1982.

Tank ES, et al.: Neoplasms associated with hemihypertrophy, Beckwith-Wiedemann syndrome and aniridia. *J. Urol.* 124:266, 1980.

Turleau C, et al.: Del 11p/aniridia complex. Report of three patients and review of 37 observations from the literature. *Clin. Genet.* 26:356, 1984.

Yunis JJ, et al.: Familial occurrence of the aniridia–Wilms tumor syndrome with deletion 11 p 13–14.1. *J. Pediatr.* 96:1027, 1980.

ANKYLOSED TEETH–CLINODACTYLY

Mode of Inheritance: Autosomal dominant.

Frequency: 12 persons in four generations (Pelias et al. 1985).

Clinical and Radiologic Manifestations: (a) ankylosed teeth; (b) cephalometric abnormalities: mild mandibular prognathism, decreased lower facial height, bone deficiencies caused by abnormal tooth eruption and migration; (c) bilateral clinodactyly of the fifth fingers.

REFERENCE

Pelias MZ, et al.: Autosomal dominant transmission of ankylosed teeth, abnormalities of the jaws and clinodactyly. A four-generation study. *Clin. Genet.* 27:496, 1985.

ANKYLOSING SPONDYLITIS

Synonym: Bechterew syndrome.

Mode of Inheritance: Aggregation in families; high percentage have been reported to be HLA-B27–positive (in 85% to 90% of patients).

Clinical Manifestations: (a) onset typically in young adults, onset in childhood in about 10% to 15%, males predominate; (b) onset in adult male often with central joints and with peripheral joints in children and female patients; (c) pain and tenderness at the site of tendinous and ligamentous insertion to bone (enthesopathy) in association with soft-tissue swelling and local temperature increase; (d) juxta-articular masses; (e) cardiovascular system: aortic incompetence (in 3% to 10% of cases), cardiac conduction defects, mitral regurgitation, arteritis of large vessels (aortic arch branches), cardiomyopathy, pericardial effusion; (f) iritis; (g) ulcerative colitis; (h) pleuropulmonary diseases; (i) cauda equina syndrome.

Radiologic Manifestations: (a) sacroiliitis the most common early radiologic finding, present in all cases in the advanced stage: indistinct joint borders in early phase, followed by a wide joint space with reactive sclerotic margins, then progressive narrowing of the joint, and finally bony ankylosis of the joint; (b) bone erosions, periostitis at the tendon attachment sites resulting in irregular bony borders of pelvis; (c) spine: squaring of the vertebral bodies, syndesmophytes and ossification of the outer layers of the annulus fibrosus (bamboo spine), ossification of the ligaments, ankylosis of the apophyseal joints, osteoporosis, spontaneous or traumatic spinal fracture, pseudoarthrosis, spinal canal stenosis, atlantoaxial subluxation, basilar invagination, atrophy of the posterior spinal and psoas muscles, laminar erosions of the posterior elements of the vertebrae in association with cauda equina syndrome, etc; (d) peripheral joints (large proximal joints, in particular, hips): soft-tissue swelling, erosions, periostitis, osteophyte formation (such as an "apron osteophyte" around the femoral neck), spurs (calcaneous); (e) increased skeletal uptake on scintigraphic examinations, in particular, in the early phase of sacroiliac joint involvement; (f) pleuropulmonary disease (in particular, in the upper lobes): nodular and linear infiltrates, progressive parenchymal fibrosis, pleural fibrosis, cyst formation, cavitation, underventilation of the upper lobes of the lungs in the presence of fibrosis, secondary pulmonary infection, bronchocenteric granulomatosis.

REFERENCES

Abelló R, et al.: MRI and CT of ankylosing spondylitis with vertebral scalloping. *Neuroradiology* 30:272, 1988.

Braunstein EM, et al.: Ankylosing spondylitis in men and women: A clinical and radiographic comparison. *Radiology* 144:91, 1982.

Brewerton DA, et al.: The myocardium in ankylosing spondylitis. A clinical, echocardiographic, and histopathological study. *Lancet* 1:995, 1987.

Chan FL, et al.: Spinal pseudarthrosis complicating ankylosing spondylitis: Comparison of CT and conventional tomography. *A.J.R.* 150:611, 1988.

Ginsburg WW, et al.: Peripheral arthritis in ankylosing spondylitis. A review of 209 patients followed up for more than 20 years. *Mayo Clin. Proc.* 58:593, 1983.

Grosman H, et al.: CT of long-standing ankylosing spondylitis with cauda equina syndrome. *A.J.N.R.* 4:1077, 1983.

Hull RG, et al.: Ankylosing spondylitis and an aortic arch syndrome. *Br. Heart J.* 51:663, 1984.

Lindsley HB, et al.: Ankylosing spondylitis presenting as juxta-articular masses in females. *Skeletal Radiol.* 16:142, 1987.

Menkes CJ, et al.: Les spondylarthrites ankylosantes à début juvénile. *Ann. Pediat. (Paris)* 30:593, 1983.

Møller P, et al.: Family studies in Bechterew's syndrome (ankylosing spondylitis) III. Genetics. *Clin. Genet.* 24:73, 1983.

Møller P, et al.: Ankylosing spondylitis is part of a multifactorial syndrome: Hereditary multifocal relapsing inflammation (HEMRI). *Clin. Genet.* 26:187, 1984.

Nance EP, et al.: The rheumatoid variants. *Semin. Roentgenol.* 17:16, 1982.

Paolaggi JB, et al.: Les enthésopathies dans la spondylarthrite ankylosante et les rhumatismes inflammatoires séronégatifs. 28 observations. *Presse Med.* 12:2229, 1983.

Parkin A, et al.: Regional lung ventilation in ankylosing spondylitis. *Br. J. Radiol.* 55:833, 1982.

Rohatgi P, et al.: Bronchocentric granulomatosis and ankylosing spondylitis. *Thorax* 39:317, 1984.

Rumancik WM, et al.: Fibrobullous disease of the upper lobes: An extraskeletal manifestation of ankylosing spondylitis. *J. Comput. Tomogr.* 8:225, 1984.

Sage MR, et al.: Muscle atrophy in ankylosing spondylitis: CT demonstration. *Radiology* 149:780, 1983.

Schörner W, et al.: Die Spondylitis ankylosans beim weiblichen Geschlecht: Ein Vergleich szintigraphischer Ergebnisse mit klinischen und röntgenologischen Befunden. *Radiologe* 22:524, 1982.

Shah A: Echocardiographic features of mitral regurgitation due to ankylosing spondylitis. *Am. J. Med.* 82:353, 1987.

Shah A, et al.: Pericardial changes and left ventricular function in ankylosing spondylitis. *Am. Heart J.* 113:529, 1987.

Tucker CR, et al.: Aortitis in ankylosing spondylitis: Early detection of aortic root abnormalities with two dimensional echocardiography. *Am. J. Cardiol.* 49:680, 1982.

Vandermarcq P, et al.: Érosions lamaires: Aspect tomodensitométrique dans le syndrome de la queue de cheval au cours de la spondylarthrite ankylosante. *Ann. Radiol. (Paris)* 29:486, 1986.

Weinstein RP, et al.: Spinal cord injury, spinal fracture, and spinal stenosis in ankylosing spondylitis. *J. Neurosurg.* 57:609, 1982.

ANONYCHIA-ECTRODACTYLY SYNDROME

Mode of Inheritance: Probable autosomal dominant transmission.

Clinical Manifestations: (a) *partial or complete absence of nails*; (b) *variable absence of phalanges and carpal and tarsal bones.*

Radiologic Manifestations: (a) asymmetrical digital anomalies presented in the form of failure or absence of normal segmentation; (b) crooked fingers and toes; (c) partial absence of metacarpals, metatarsals, and phalanges; (d) syndactyly; (e) polydactyly.

REFERENCES

Charteris F: Case of partial hereditary anonychia. *Glasg. Med. J.* 89:207, 1918.

Hobbs ME: Hereditary onychial dysplasia. *Am. J. Med. Sci.* 190:200, 1935.

Lees DH, et al.: Anonychia with ectrodactyly: Clinical and linkage data. *Ann. Hum. Genet.* 22:69, 1957.

ANORECTAL MALFORMATION, HEREDITARY

Mode of Inheritance: Autosomal dominant.

Clinical and Radiologic Manifestations: (a) anorectal anomalies: stenosis, imperforate anus, rectovaginal fistula; (b) other reported abnormalities: relatives with nephritis and nerve deafness (?Alport syndrome), preauricular skin tag, renal anomalies, etc.

REFERENCES

Cozzi F, et al.: Familial incidence of congenital anorectal anomalies. *Surgery* 64:669, 1968.

Lowe J, et al.: Dominant ano-rectal malformation, nephritis and nerve-deafness: A possible new entity? *Clin. Genet.* 24:191, 1983.

ANOREXIA NERVOSA

Clinical Manifestations: Onset often prior to 25 years of age: (a) anorexia with weight loss; (b) a "distorted, implacable attitude toward eating, food, or weight that overrides hunger, admonitions, reassurance, and threats"; apparent enjoyment in losing weight and being thin; (c) no known medical or overt psychiatric illnesses; (d) hormonal abnormalities: thyroid dysfunction; low basal plasma levels of follicular stimulating hormone (FSH), luteinizing hormone (LH), and estradiol; elevated resting levels of growth hormone (GH); elevated basal plasma cortisol levels; defective urinary concentrating function (partial diabetes insipidus); (e) hematologic abnormalities: anemia, acanthocytosis, leukopenia, mild thrombocytopenia, low erythrocyte sedimentation rate (ESR), decreased fibrinogen levels, bone marrow changes (hypoplasia, increased ground substance, abnormal histiocytes); (f) immunologic abnormalities: granulocyte bacterial defect, chemotactic defect, hypocomplementemia, decreased cellular immunity (?); (g) decreased voltage on electrocardiogram, pericardial effusion; (h) other reported abnormalities: hyperactivity despite severe weight loss, bulimia and self-induced vomiting, bradycardia, hypotension, lanugo, abnormalities in thermoregulation, negative growth (shrinkage) assessed by knemometry.

Radiologic Manifestations: (a) superior mesenteric artery syndrome; (b) small cardiac image on the chest roentgenogram, pericardial effusion; (c) cerebral dystrophic changes: reversible enlargement of cerebrospinal fluid spaces (subarachnoid, ventricular), the cerebellum less involved in the dystrophic changes; (d) spontaneous pneumomediastinum, pneumoretroperitoneum.

REFERENCES

Altmeyer RB, et al.: Spontaneous pneumomediastinum as a complication of anorexia nervosa. *W. Va. Med. J.* 77:189, 1981.

Artmann H, et al.: Reversible and non-reversible enlargement of cerebrospinal fluid spaces in anorexia nervosa. *Neuroradiology* 27:304, 1985.

Bryant-Waugh R, et al.: Long term follow up of patients with early onset anorexia nervosa. *Arch. Dis. Child.* 63:5, 1988.

Datlof S, et al.: Ventricular dilation on CAT scans of patients with anorexia nervosa. *Am. J. Psychiatry* 143:96, 1986.

Feighner JP, et al.: Diagnostic criteria for use in psychiatric research. *Arch. Gen. Psychiatry* 26:57, 1972.

Golden N, et al.: An overview of the etiology, diagnosis, and management of anorexia nervosa. *Clin. Pediatr. (Phila.)* 23:209, 1984.

Hermanussen M, et al.: "Negative growth" in anorexia nervosa assessed by knemometry. *Eur. J. Pediatr.* 146:561, 1987.

Kay J, et al.: Hematologic and immunologic abnormalities in anorexia nervosa. *South Med. J.* 76:1008, 1983.

Overby KJ, et al.: Mediastinal emphysema in an adolescent with anorexia nervosa and self-induced emesis. *Pediatrics* 31:134, 1988.

Silverman JA, et al.: Anorexia nervosa: A cause of pericardial effusion? *Pediatr. Cardiol.* 4:125, 1983.

ANTERIOR TIBIAL COMPARTMENT SYNDROME

Etiology: Due to strenuous muscle activity, ergotamine ingestion, androgen therapy, surgery, hemorrhage, gunshot wound, compressive dressing, crush injury.

Clinical Manifestations: (a) *pain;* (b) *sensory changes;* (c) *swelling;* (d) tenderness; (e) increased tension and circulatory deficiency in the anterior tibial compartment; (f) ischemic necrosis.

Radiologic Manifestations: (a) *fracture site (if it is the cause);* (b) *soft-tissue swelling,* ectopic calcification; (c) *arteriography: vascular obstruction;* (d) ultrasonographic demonstration of hemorrhage.

REFERENCES

Elliott MJ, et al.: Anterior tibial compartment syndrome associated with ergotamine ingestion. *Clin. Orthop.* 118:44, 1976.

Greenbaum EI, et al.: Value of delayed filming in the anterior tibial compartment syndrome secondary to trauma. *Radiology* 93:373, 1969.

Halpern AA, et al.: Bilateral compartment syndrome associated with androgen therapy. *Clin. Orthop.* 128:243, 1977.

Matsen FA III, Clauson DK (eds.): Compartmental

syndromes: Symposium. *Clin. Orthop.* 113:2–110, 1975.
Palmer BV, et al.: Anterior tibial compartment syndrome following femoral artery perfusion. *Thorax* 28:492, 1973.
Rosengart R, et al.: Anterior tibial compartment syndrome in a child: An unusual complication of cardiac catheterization. *Pediatrics* 58:456, 1976.
Viau MR, et al.: Ectopic calcification as a late sequela of compartment syndrome. *Clin. Orthop.* 176:178, 1983.

APLASIA CUTIS CONGENITA

Synonym: Adams-Oliver syndrome (aplasia cutis and transverse terminal limb defect).

Classification and Mode of Inheritance: Heterogeneous group of disorders with various clinical manifestations. Sybert classification: type I—aplasia cutis congenita (ACC) *limited to the scalp:* sporadic and familial (autosomal dominant gene with incomplete penetrance, variable intrafamilial expression); type II—*ACC involving the body with or without the scalp:* sporadic and familial (autosomal dominant gene with reduced penetrance or autosomal recessive, sporadic, environmental origin); type IIA represents *ACC involving the body with or without limb defects;* type III—*ACC limited to the scalp with or without limb defects:* sporadic and familial (autosomal dominant gene); type IV—*ACC with epidermolysis bullosa* (EB letalis, dystrophic EB, EB simplex); type IVA (Bart syndrome), which has variable skin defects and nail abnormalities, may be an autosomal dominant condition.

Frequency: More than 40 published cases of Adams-Oliver syndrome.

Clinical Manifestations: (a) *usually occurs in the midline of the scalp,* less often on the trunk and limbs; often round or oval, sharply marginated; *ulcerated or covered by thin membrane at birth;* gradual closure over a few months with scar formation; (b) may be multiple sites; (c) *limb anomalies:* absent nails, nail deformities, simian creases, absent interphalangeal creases, skin tags on the deformed toes, polydactyly,

restricted finger motion, clubbing of hands and feet; (d) superior sagittal sinus hemorrhage; (e) other reported abnormalities: trisomy 13–15, cutis marmorata, spastic paralysis, cerebral atrophy, monozygotic twin with "fetus papyraceus," joint contracture, pyloric obstruction, cleft lip, cleft palate, colobomas, ambiguous genitalia, absent or deformed ear lobes, microphthalmos, meningocele, congenital heart disease, omphalocele, imperforate anus, epidermolysis bullosa–like lesions, focal dermal hypoplasia, Johanson-Blizzard syndrome, hemangioma, urogenital anomalies, association with therapy for maternal thyroid disease, association with fetus papyraceus in a triplet pregnancy; (f) complications: venous thrombosis, local infection, hemorrhage, meningitis, cosmetic management problems.

Radiologic Manifestations: (a) skull defect underlying the skin lesion (in some), multiple wormian bones, anomalous scalp veins, drainage of scalp veins into intracranial venous sinuses, anomalous vessels of the face and eyes, hydrocephalus, cerebral atrophy, meningocele, dural defects, etc.; (b) *limb anomalies:* acral reduction defects (partial or total absence of the digits, absent metacarpals, rudimentary terminal phalanges, short feet), absent lower limb below the midcalf, polydactyly, syndactyly, cavus foot deformity; (c) other reported abnormalities: intestinal lymphangiectasia, clubbing of the hands and feet, hemangiomas, anomalous scalp veins draining into intracranial venous sinuses, vascular lesions of the face and eyes, hydrocephalus, cerebral malformations, dural defects, polycystic kidneys, meningocele, tracheoesophageal fistula, patent ductus arteriosus, occult spinal dysrhaphia underlying the cutaneous anomaly, etc. (Figs SY–A–22 and SY–A–23).

REFERENCES

Adams FH, Oliver P: Hereditary deformities in man due to arrested development. *J. Hered.* 36:3, 1945.
Buttiëns M, et al.: Scalp defect associated with postaxial

FIG SY–A–22.
Aplasia cutis congenita. The vertex of a 3½-year-old boy shows an oval area of thin, cicatricial skin. The area was mostly hairless, with occasional fine scales or rare, thin, short hairs. (From Bronspiegel N, Zelnick N, Robinowitz H, et al.: Aplasia cutis congenita and intestinal lymphangiectasia. An unusual association. *Am. J. Dis. Child.* 139:509, 1985. Used by permission.)

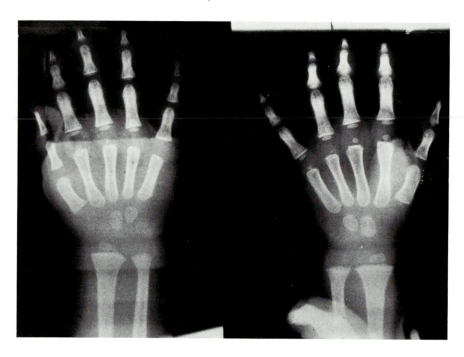

FIG SY—A—23.
Aplasia cutis and distal limb reduction anomalies: hypoplasia of the distal phalanges of the hands. (From Fryns JP: Congenital

polydactyly: Confirmation of a distinct entity with autosomal dominant inheritance. *Hum. Genet.* 71:86, 1985.

Bronspiege N, et al.: Aplasia cutis congenita and intestinal lymphangiectasia. An unusual association. *Am. J. Dis. Child.* 139:509, 1985.

Campbell W: Case of congenital ulcer on the cranium of a fetus. *Edinb. J. Med. Sci.* 2:82, 1826.

Fowler GW, et al.: Cutis aplasia and cerebral malformation. *Pediatrics* 52:861, 1973.

Fryns JP: Congenital scalp defects with distal limb reduction anomalies. *J. Med. Genet.* 24:493, 1987.

Higginbottom MC, et al.: Aplasia cutis congenita: A cutaneous marker of occult spinal dysrhaphism. *J. Pediatr.* 96:687, 1980.

Kalb RE, et al.: The association of aplasia cutis congenita with therapy of maternal thyroid disease. *Pediatr. Dermatol.* 3:327, 1986.

Koiffmann CP, et al.: Congenital scalp skull defects with distal limb anomalies (Adams-Oliver syndrome—McKusick 10030): Further suggestion of autosomal recessive inheritance. *Am. J. Med. Genet.* 29:263, 1988.

Küster W, et al.: Congenital scalp defects with distal limb anomalies (Adams-Oliver syndrome): Report of ten cases and review of the literature. *Am. J. Med. Genet.* 31:99, 1988.

Markman L, et al.: Association of aplasia cutis congenita and fetus papyraceus in a triplet pregnancy. *Aust. Paediatr. J.* 18:294, 1982.

Schneider BM, et al.: Aplasia cutis congenita complicated by sagittal sinus hemorrhage. *Pediatrics* 66:948, 1980.

Sybert VP: Aplasia cutis congenita: A report of 12 new families and review of the literature. *Pediatr. Dermatol.* 3:1, 1985.

Toriello HV, et al.: Scalp and limb defects with cutis mar-

scalp defects with distal limb reduction anomalies. *J. Med. Genet.* 24:493, 1987. Used by permission.)

morata telangiectatica congenita: Adams-Oliver syndrome? *Am. J. Med. Genet.* 29:269, 1988.

Yagupsky P, et al.: Aplasia cutis congenita in one of monozygotic twins. *Pediatr. Dermatol.* 3:403, 1986.

APPLE PEEL SYNDROME

Synonyms: Familial apple peel jejunal atresia; "Christmas tree" deformity of the small intestine.

Mode of Inheritance: Not definitely known; familial aggregation of cases; an autosomal recessive gene has been suggested.

Pathology: (a) *proximal intestinal atresia, multiple atresias;* (b) *bowel malrotation;* (c) *absence of the distal superior mesenteric artery and the dorsal mesentery, retrograde blood supply from the right colic vessels to the distal portion of the small bowel;* (d) other reported anomalies: imperforate anus, biliary atresia, intestinal duplication, spina bifida, hydrocephalus, microcephaly, microphthalmos, atrial septal defect, ureteropelvic junction obstruction.

Clinical Manifestations: (a) high incidence of prematurity; (b) *signs and symptoms of bowel obstruction;* (c) *polyhydramnios;* (d) *short-bowel syndrome;* (e) high mortality rate.

Radiologic Manifestations: (a) *high intestinal obstruction;* (b) *short bowel, microcolon;* (c) *malrotation;* (d) coiled or spiral-like distal segment of the ileum; (e) prenatal ultrasonographic diagnosis of intestinal obstruction (Fig SY—A—24).

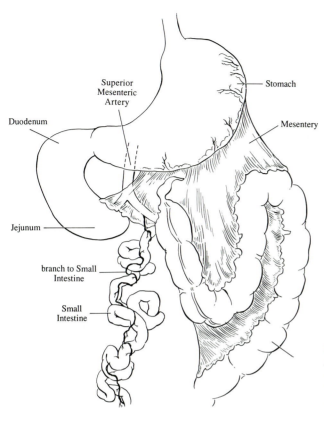

FIG SY–A–24.
Apple peel jejunal atresia (familial): schematic drawing of typical apple peel atresia. (From Seashore JH, Collins FS, Markowitz RI, et al.: Familial apple peel jejunal atresia: Surgical, genetic, and radiographic aspects. *Pediatrics* 80:540, 1987. Used by permission.)

REFERENCES

Leonidas JC, et al.: Duodenojejunal atresia with "apple peel" small bowel. *Radiology* 118:661, 1976.
Schiavetti E, et al.: "Apple peel" syndrome: A radiological study. *Pediatr. Radiol.* 14:380, 1984.
Seashore JH, et al.: Familial apple peel jejunal atresia: Surgical, genetic, and radiographic aspects. *Pediatrics* 80:540, 1987.
Weitzman JJ, et al.: Jejunal atresia with agenesis of the dorsal mesentery: With "Christmas tree" deformity of the small intestine. *Am. J. Surg.* 111:443, 1966.

ARTERIAL CALCIFICATION OF INFANCY

Synonyms: Idiopathic infantile arterial calcification; idiopathic arterial calcification of infancy; occlusive infantile arteriopathy.

Mode of Inheritance: Occurrence in siblings; the pattern of inheritance not definitely known.

Frequency: More than 80 cases have been reported.

Pathology: Patchy destruction and disruption of the internal elastic membrane and deposition of calcium hydroxyapatite (systemic and pulmonary arteries of all sizes), periarticular ligamentous calcification, stippled calcification of the epiphyseal cartilage, renal calcification (tubules, glomeruli, interstitial), enlarged heart due to hypertrophy of both ventricles or only the left ventricle, myocardial infarction, coronary artery abnormalities (calcification, thickened wall, tortuosity, thrombosis).

Clinical Manifestations: (a) *congestive heart failure* (cyanosis, tachypnea, etc.), hypertension, myocardial ischemia; (b) periarticular hard swelling; (c) other reported abnormalities: gangrene of the extremities, abdominal crisis and ileus, visceral infarction, premature aging, motor and mental retardation, convulsions, association with endocardial fibroelastosis; (d) death in about 85% of cases within the first 6 months of life, spontaneous regression of calcification extremely rare (2 out of 80 cases).

Radiologic Manifestations: (a) *arterial wall calcification* shown by radiographic examination and sonography (very prominent echogenicity of the arterial wall and acoustic shadowing from the vessel walls); (b) diffuse hyperechogenicity of the kidney; (c) *cardiomegaly, congestive heart failure;* (d) periarticular calcification, epiphyseal calcification, cerebral infarction.

Differential Diagnosis: Metastatic calcification (renal disease, hyperparathyroidism, hypervitaminosis D), aortic and pulmonary calcification with congenital heart disease, etc. (Fig SY–A–25).

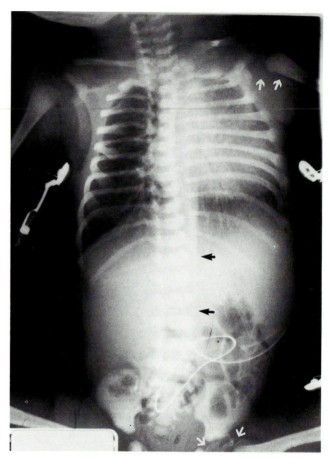

FIG SY−A−25.
Arterial calcification of infancy in a newborn male. Cardiomegaly and calcification in the left axillary region and abdominal aorta are present. Note the calcification in the left hip joint area. A subsequent female sibling also was affected.

REFERENCES

Maayan C, et al.: Idiopathic infantile arterial calcification: A case report and review of the literature. *Eur. J. Pediatr.* 142:211, 1984.
Rosenbaum DM, et al.: Sonographic recognition of idiopathic arterial calcification of infancy. *A.J.R.* 146:249, 1986.
Sholler GF, et al.: Generalized arterial calcification of infancy: Three case reports, including spontaneous regression with long-term survival. *J. Pediatr.* 105:257, 1984.
Van Dyck M, et al.: Idiopathic infantile arterial calcification with cardiac, renal and central nervous system involvement. *Eur. J. Pediatr.* 148:374, 1989.

ARTHROGRYPOSIS

Synonym: Congenital contractures.

Definition: A descriptive term, not a specific disease entity that refers to a hetergenous group of conditions associated with multiple congenital joint contractures (syndromic and nonsyndromic) (Table SY−A−2).

Mode of Inheritance: Table SY−A−3 shows the genetic breakdown of 350 cases with congenital contracture.

Laboratory Tests: Electromyography and muscle biopsy showing myopathic diseases, variation in muscle fiber size associated with an abnormal fiber type distribution suggesting abnormal innervation, etc.

Radiologic Manifestations: (a) brachycephaly; (b) hypoplasia of the mandible; temporomandibular fusion; (c) *small muscle masses, excess subcutaneous fat, increased fat between muscle bundles;* (d) *slender bones;* (e) osteoporosis; (f) propensity to fractures; (g) dislocated joints; (h) carpal and tarsal fusion (occurring after 10 years of age); (i) polydactyly, syndactyly; (j) coxa vara or valga; (k) short tibia and femur; (l) *vertical talus, rocker-bottom foot;* (m) other reported abnormalities: absent corpus callosum, microcephaly, agenesis of the vermis, porencephaly, hydrocephaly, lissencephaly, micropolygyria, brain atrophy, heterotopic gray matter, moya moya, congenital spinal epidural hemorrhage, caudal duplication, multiple intestinal atresia associated with amyoplasia congenita; (n) prenatal diagnosis of distal arthrogryposis by ultrasound.

REFERENCES

Baty BJ, et al.: Prenatal diagnosis of distal arthrogryposis. *Am. J. Med. Genet.* 29:501, 1988.

TABLE SY—A—2.

Specific Known Causes of Multiple Congenital Contractures*

	Areas of Involvement	
Primarily Limbs	Limbs Plus Other Body Areas	Limbs Plus CNS
Absence of dermal ridges	Antley-Bixler syndrome	Adducted thumbs
Absence of distal interpha-langeal (DIP) creases	Camptomelic dysplasia	"C" syndrome
Amniotic bands (Streeter)	Conradi-Hunermann (chondrodys-plasia punctata)	Cerebro-oculofacioskeletal (COFS)
Amyoplasia	Contractural arachnodactyly	Cloudy corneas, diaphrag-matic defects, distal limb deformities
Antecubital webbing	Craniocarpotarsal dystrophy (whis-tling face, Freeman-Sheldon)	Craniofacial/brain anomalies/IUGR
Camptodactyly	Diastrophic dysplasia	
Clasped thumbs, congenital	Focal femoral dysplasia	Cryptorchidism, chest defor-mity, contractures
Coalition	G syndrome	Faciocardiomelic syndrome
Contractures, continuous muscle discharge, and titu-bation	Gordon syndrome	Fetal alcohol syndrome
	Hand muscle wasting and senso-rineural deafness	FG syndrome
Distal arthrogryposis	Holt-Oram syndrome	Lenz microphthalmos syndrome
Humeroradial synostosis (HRS)	Kneist syndrome	Marden-Walker syndrome
Impaired pronation, supina-tion of the forearm (familial)	Kuskokwim	Meckel syndrome
	Larsen dysplasia	Meningomyelocele
Liebenberg syndrome	Leprechaunism	Mietens
Nievergelt-Pearlman	Megalocornea with multiple skeletal anomalies	Miller-Dieker (lissencephaly)
Poland anomaly	Metaphyseal dysostosis (Jansen)	Multiple pterygium—lethal
Radioulnar synostosis	Metatropic dysplasia	Myotonic dystrophy—severe congenital (SCMD)
Symphalangia	Möbius syndrome	
Symphalangia/brachydactyly	Moore-Federman syndrome	Neu-Laxova
Tel Hashomir camptodactyly	Multiple pterygium syndrome	Neuromuscular disease of the larynx
Trismus pseudocamptodactyly	Multiple synostosis syndrome	
X-linked resolving	Nail-patella syndrome (hereditary onycho-osteodysplasia)	Nezelof syndrome
	Nemaline myopathy	Pena-Shokeir (ankylosis, facial anomalies, and pulmonary hypoplasia)
	Neurofibromatosis	
	Oculo-dento-digital syndrome	Popliteal pterygium with facial clefts
	Ophthalmo-mandibulo-melic dyspla-sia	Potter syndrome
	Oral-cranial-digital syndrome	Pseudotrisomy 18
	Osteogenesis imperfecta: congenital, lethal, "crumpled-bone" type (type II)	X-linked, lethal
		Zellweger syndrome (cerebro-hepatorenal)
	Otopalatodigital	46XXY/48XXXY
	Pfeiffer syndrome	49XXXXX and 49XXXXY
	Popliteal pterygium	Trisomy 4 p
	Prader-Willi habitus, osteoporosis, hand contractures	Trisomy 8/trisomy 8 mosaicism
	Pseudothalidomide syndrome (Robert syndrome)	Trisomy 9
	Puretic syndrome	Trisomy 9q
	Sacral agenesis	Trisomy 10q
	Schwartz-Jampel	Trisomy 10p
	SED congenita	Trisomy 11q
	Sturge-Weber	Trisomy 13
	Tuberous sclerosis	Partial trisomy 14 (proximal)
	VATER association	Trisomy 15 (proximal)
	Weaver syndrome	Trisomy 18
	Winchester syndrome	Many other chromosomal anomalies
	X-linked involving facies and dimple over skin	

*From Hall JG: Genetic aspects of arthrogryposis. *Clin. Orthop.* 194:47, 1985. Used by permission.

TABLE SY–A–3.

Genetic Breakdown of Cases*

	Areas of Involvement				
	Primarily Limbs	Limbs Plus Other Body Areas	Limbs Plus CNS	Total	
Autosomal dominant	24	24	—	48 (14%)	
Autosomal recessive	3	16	7	26 (7%)	
X-linked recessive	3	2	1	6 (2%)	28%
Chromosomal	—	3	6	9 (3%)	
Multifactorial	—	5	—	5 (2%)	
Environmental	4	4	14	22 (6%)	
Known syndrome with no recurrence risk	139	24	1	164 (46%)	
Unknown condition—not a recognized syndrome	13	51	6	70 (20%)	
Total	186	129	35	350	

*From: Hall JG: Genetic aspects of arthrogryposis. *Clin. Orthop.* 194:47, 1985. Used by permission.

Collins DL, et al.: Multiple intestinal atresia and amyoplasia congenita in four unrelated infants: A new association. *J. Pediatr. Surg.* 21:331, 1986.

Gericke GS, et al.: Diagnostic considerations in arthrogryposis syndromes in South Africa. *Clin. Genet.* 25:155, 1984.

Hageman G, et al.: Arthrogryposis multiplex congenita. Review with comment. *Neuropediatrics* 14:6, 1983.

Hall JG: Arthrogryposis, in Spranger J, Tolksdorf M (eds.): *Klinische Genetik in der Paediatrie.* 2. Symposion in Mainz. New York, Georg Thieme Verlag, 1980, pp. 105–121.

Hall JG, et al.: Three distinct types of X-linked arthrogryposis seen in 6 families. *Clin. Genet.* 21:81, 1982.

Hall JG, et al.: The distal arthrogryposes: Delineation of new entities—Review and nosologic discussion. *Am. J. Med. Genet.* 11:185, 1982.

Hall JG, et al.: Part I. Amyoplasia: A common, sporadic condition with congenital contractures. *Am. J. Med. Genet.* 15:571, 1983.

Hall JG, et al.: Part II. Amyoplasia: Twinning in amyoplasia—a specific type of arthrogryposis with an apparent excess of discordantly affected identical twins. *Am. J. Med. Genet.* 15:591, 1983.

Hall JG, et al.: Genetic aspects of arthrogryposis. *Clin. Orthop.* 194:47, 1985.

Jacobson HG, et al.: Arthrogryposis multiplex congenita. *Radiology* 65:8, 1955.

Livingstone IR, et al.: Arthrogryposis multiplex congenita occurring with maternal multiple sclerosis. *Arch. Neurol.* 41:1216, 1984.

Matthews JG, et al.: Arthrogryposis in caudal duplication. An anatomical and histological study or arthrogrypotic limbs. *J. Bone Joint Surg. [Br.]* 64:88, 1982.

Pagnan NAB, et al.: Distal arthrogryposis type II D in three generations of a Brazilian family. *Am. J. Med. Genet.* 26:613, 1987.

Poznanski AK, et al.: Radiographic manifestations of the arthrogryposis syndrome. *Radiology* 95:353, 1970.

Reed SD, et al.: Chromosomal abnormalities associated with congenital contractures (arthrogryposis). *Clin. Genet.* 27:353, 1985.

Reiss JA, et al.: Distal arthrogryposis type II: A family with varying congenital abnormalities. *Am. J. Med. Genet.* 24:255, 1986.

Strehl E, et al.: EMG and needle muscle biopsy studies in arthrogryposis multiplex congenita. *Neuropediatrics* 16:225, 1985.

Sul YC, et al.: Neurogenic arthrogryposis in one identical twin. *Arch. Neurol.* 39:717, 1982.

Thompson GH (ed): Arthrogryposis multiplex congenita. *Clin. Orthop.* 194:2, 1985.

Uchida T, et al.: Arthrogryposis multiplex congenita: Histochemical study in biopsied muscles. *Pediatr. Neurol.* 1:169, 1985.

Yonenobu K, et al.: Arthrogryposis of the hand. *J. Pediatr. Orthop.* 4:599, 1984.

ARTHROGRYPOSIS-ADVANCED SKELETAL MATURATION-UNUSUAL FACIES

Clinical Manifestations: (a) facial features: round face, low-set hairline, small nose, prominent nostrils, abnormal ears, puffy eyelids, coloboma; (b) short neck; (c) contracture of all the large joints.

Radiologic Manifestations: (a) shortening and broadening of the long bones, multiple bone excrescences ("spurs"), wide ribs; (b) nonuniformly advanced bone age (femoral head).

REFERENCE

Jequier S, et al.: Unusual facies, arthrogryposis, advanced skeletal maturation and unique bone changes. *Pediatr. Radiol.* 17:405, 1987.

ASPLENIA SYNDROME

Synonyms: Ivemark syndrome; absent spleen syndrome.

Mode of Inheritance: Sporadic, male excess, recessive and dominant, X-linked recessive; occurrence of asplenia and polysplenia in the same family; exposure to warfarin.

Pathology: (a) *absent spleen*, rarely hypoplastic spleen; (b) chest: *thoracic isomerism, right-sided appearance of left-sided organs* in the form of bilateral trilobed lungs, bilateral epiarterial bronchi (90% of cases), extralobulation of the lungs, isomerism of the atria; (c) *complex cyanotic heart diseases*: bilateral superior venae cavae, a common hepatic vein, *anomalous pulmonary venous drainage* (in about 70%, 10% infradiaphragmatic), *transposition of the great arteries* (about 70%), *pulmonary stenosis or atresia* (about 90%), *abdominal aorta and inferior vena cava on the same side,* some form of endocardial cushion defect, often only one functioning ventricle; (d) *alimentary system anomalies*: right-sided or midline location of stomach, hiatal hernia, *incomplete rotation of intestine,* annular pancreas, pancreatic malformation, volvulus of the stomach, volvulus of the colon, imperforate anus, diaphragmatic hernia, right and left lobes of the liver of almost equal size (symmetrical liver), midline gallbladder, agenesis of the gallbladder; (e) genitourinary anomalies: renal dysplasia, cystic kidneys, fused kidneys, bicornuate uterus, etc.; (f) endocrine anomalies: fused or horseshoe adrenals, unilateral absence of the adrenal gland; (g) other reported abnormalities: hydrocephalus, meningocele, cerebellar hypoplasia, arhinencephalia, etc.

Clinical Manifestations: (a) weight and length below normal; (b) feeding difficulties, respiratory distress, cyanosis, congestive heart failure; (c) polycythemia, *Howell-Jolly bodies and Heinz bodies in the peripheral blood*; (d) high incidence of sepsis (about 25%), isolated deficiency of IgM, isolated deficiency of IgE; echocardiographic manifestations of various anomalies, purulent pericarditis, etc.

Radiologic Manifestations: (a) abdomen: horizontal liver, absent spleen (computed tomography, dual radiopharmaceutical imaging with the use of ^{99m}Tc–sulfur colloid and with the ^{99m}Tc-PIPIDA: similarity of the images suggesting asplenia and a discrepancy in organ morphology between the two scans indicates the presence of a spleen); radiological diagnosis of various alimentary tract anomalies enumerated under "Pathology"; vena cava and aorta on the same side of the spine in a "piggyback" fashion shown by computed tomography, ultrasonography, and angiography; absent splenic vein; midline portal vein; (b) chest: bilateral pulmonary three lobes, bilateral epiarterial bronchi, congenital heart anomalies demonstrated by various imaging modalities; (c) other reported abnormalities: increased incidence of radiographic visibility of ossification of the hyoid bone (100% vs. 71% in the control group) and humeral capital epiphysis (71.4% vs. 16.1% in the control group) (Fig SY–A–26).

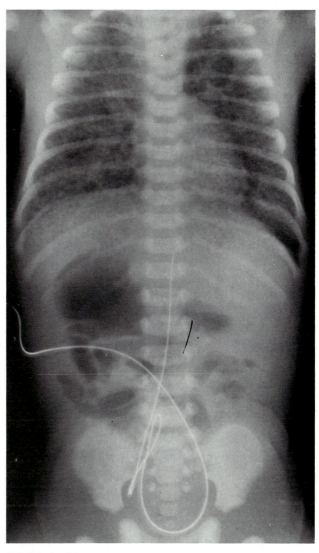

FIG SY–A–26.
Asplenia syndrome in a cyanotic newborn male in respiratory distress. Extensive bilateral venous engorgement, a normal-sized heart with an abnormal contour, a wide upper mediastinum, a horizontal liver, and a right-sided stomach are present. A common atrium, single ventricle, pulmonary artery atresia, pulmonary venous atresia, pulmonary lymphangiectasia, bilateral superior vena cavae, trilobed lungs with bilateral epiarterial bronchi, malrotation of the bowel, and a midline gallbladder were the major findings at the postmortem study.

Note: The occurrence of asplenia and polysplenia in the members of the same family suggests that the two syndromes are pathogenetically related and most likely the same and should be categorized as a developmental field complex.

REFERENCES

Aoyama K, et al.: Gastric volvulus in three children with asplenic syndrome. *J. Pediatr. Surg.* 21:307, 1986.

Berman W, et al.: Asplenia syndrome with atypical cardiac anomalies. *Pediatr. Cardiol.* 3:35, 1982.

Cox DR, et al.: Asplenia syndrome after fetal exposure to warfarin. *Lancet* 2:1134, 1977.

Crawford Md'A: Renal dysplasia and asplenia in two sibs. *Clin. Genet.* 14:338, 1978.

Di Donato R, et al.: Palliation of cardiac malformations associated with right isomerism (asplenia syndrome) in infancy. *Ann. Thorac. Surg.* 44:35, 1987.

Hausdorf G: Das sonographische Bild des Asplenia-Syndroms. *Fortschr. Rontgenstr.* 138:548, 1983.

Hurwitz RC, et al.: Ivemark syndrome in siblings. *Clin. Genet.* 22:7, 1982.

Ivemark BI: Implications of agenesis of the spleen on the pathogenesis of cono-truncus anomalies in childhood: An analysis of the heart malformations in the splenic agenesis syndrome, with 14 new cases. *Acta Paediatr. Scand.* 44(suppl. 104):1, 1955.

Kim K-M, et al.: Asplenia syndrome complicated by purulent pericarditis. *Pediatr. Cardiol.* 6:114, 1985.

Lochte: Beitrag zur Kenntniss des Situs transversus partialis und der angeborenen Dextrocardie. *Beitr. Pathol. Anat.* 16:189, 1894. Cited by Van Mierop LHS, et al.: Asplenia and polysplenia syndromes, in Bergsma D, et al. (eds.): *The Clinical Delineation of Birth Defects. The Cardiovascular System.* New York: Alan R Liss, Inc. 1972, vol. 8, pp. 36–44.

Markowitz RI, et al.: Volvulus·of the colon in a child with congenital asplenia (Ivemark syndrome). *Radiology* 122:442, 1977.

Mathias RS, et al.: X-linked laterality sequence: Situs inversus, complex cardiac defects, splenic defects. *Am. J. Med. Genet.* 28:111, 1987.

Mishalany H, et al.: Congenital asplenia and anomalies of the gastrointestinal tract. *Surgery* 91:38, 1982.

Niikawa N, et al.: Familial clustering of situs inversus totalis, and asplenia and polysplenia syndromes. *Am. J. Med. Genet.* 16:43, 1983.

Rao BK, et al.: Dual radiopharmaceutical imaging in congenital asplenia syndrome. *Radiology* 145:805, 1982.

Robinson RG, et al.: Congenital hypoplastic anemia (CHA) associated with congenital absence of the spleen. *Am. J. Pediatr. Hematol. Oncol.* 4:341, 1982.

Soto B, et al.: Identification of thoracic isomerism from the plain chest radiograph. *A.J.R.* 131:995, 1978.

Tonkin ILD, et al.: Visceroatrial situs abnormalities: Sonographic and computed tomographic appearance. *A.J.R.* 138:509, 1982.

Waldman JD, et al.: Sepsis and congenital asplenia. *J. Pediatr.* 90:555, 1977.

Wells TR, et al.: Ossification centre of the hyoid bone in complete transposition of great vessels, Ivemark asplenia syndrome, and Down's syndrome with congenital heart disease: Correlation with the humeral capital epiphysis. *Br. J. Radiol.* 59:1069, 1986.

ATAXIA-TELANGIECTASIA SYNDROME

Synonyms: Louis-Bar syndrome; Border-Sedgwick syndrome; cephalo-oculocutaneous telangiectasis.

Mode of Inheritance: Autosomal recessive; genetic heterogeneity.

Frequency: Uncommon.

Pathology: Cerebellar cortical atrophy with marked reduction in the number of Purkinje and granule cells and some loss of stellate and basket cells; increase in the number of Golgi epithelial cells; degenerative changes in the dentate and olivary nuclei and in the spinal cord; neurochemical abnormalities in the cerebellum; embryonic-like thymus.

Clinical Manifestations: Onset of symptoms in childhood: (a) *oculocutaneous telangiectasia;* (b) *progressive cerebellar ataxia,* nystagmus, strabismus, failure of purposive eye movement, choreoathetosis, dysarthria, progressive mental deterioration, generalized muscle weakness, etc. (c) recurrent sinopulmonary infections; (d) premature graying, atrophic and sclerodermatous skin changes, follicular and solar keratoses, basal cell epithelioma, eczema, generalized skin pigmentation; (e) endocrinopathies: gonadal agenesis or hypoplasia, decreased 17-ketosteroid excretion, abnormal glucose metabolism, elevated plasma insulin levels, pituitary dysfunction (growth retardation); (f) *high susceptibility to irradiation,* enhanced in vitro radiosensitivity of cultured skin cells, defect in DNA repair; (g) *predisposition to malignancies,* in particular, lymphoreticular neoplasms and leukemia (more than 120 times greater than that of age-matched controls); heterozygous carriers of the gene for ataxia-telangiectasia have been reported to have an excess risk of cancer, particularly breast cancer in women; (h) *abnormal humoral and cellular immunity,* decreased or absent serum or secretory IgA, decreased or absent IgE, deficiency of IgG2 and IgG4, increased IgG1 levels, aplastic or rudimentary thymus at autopsy; (i) chromosomal instability; (j) elevated α-fetoprotein levels.

Radiologic Manifestations: (a) *sinusitis;* (b) *recurrent pulmonary infections, bronchiectasis, pulmonary fibrosis,* tracheomegaly; (c) *lack of a thymic shadow in infancy, diminished or absent nasopharyngeal lymphoid tissues, absent nodal enlargement in pulmonary hili;* (d) diffuse cerebellar atrophy, vermian atrophy, cerebellar hemispheric atrophy; (e) radiological findings associated with neoplastic lesions.

REFERENCES

Assencio-Ferreira VJ, et al.: Computed tomography in ataxia-telangiectasia. *J. Comput. Assist. Tomogr.* 5:660, 1981.

Brown LR, et al.: Ataxia-telangiectasia (Louis-Bar syndrome). *Semin. Roentgenol.* 11:67, 1976.

Cox R, et al.: Ataxia telangiectasia: Evaluation of radiosensitivity in cultured skin fibroblasts as a diagnostic test. *Arch. Dis. Child.* 53:386, 1979.

Gatti RA, Swift M: *Ataxia-Telangiectasia Genetics, Neuropathology, and Immunology of a Degenerative Disease of Childhood.* New York: Alan R Liss Inc, 1985.

Hecht F, et al.: Chromosome changes connect immunodeficiency and cancer in ataxia-telangiectasia. *Am. J. Pediatr. Hematol. Oncol.* 9:185, 1987.

Huang PC, et al.: Genetic and biochemical studies with ataxia telangiectasia. A review. *Hum. Genet.* 59:1, 1981.

Lallemand D, et al.: Tracheomegalie et déficit immunitaire chez l'enfant. *Ann. Radiol. (Paris)* 24:67, 1981.

Louis-Bar D: Sur syndrome progressif comprenant des télangiectasies capillaires cutanées et conjonctivales symétriques, a disposition naevoïde et des troubles cérébelleux. *Confin. Neurol.* 4:32, 1941.

McKinnon PJ: Ataxia-telangiectasia: An inherited disorder of ionizing-radiation sensitivity in man. Progress in the elucidation of the underlying biochemical defect. *Hum. Genet.* 75:197, 1987.

Ohta S, et al.: Ataxia-telangiectasia with papillary carcinoma of the thyroid. *Am. J. Pediatr. Hematol. Oncol.* 8:255, 1986.

Oxelius VA, et al.: IgG2 deficiency in ataxia-telangiectasia. *N. Engl. J. Med.* 306:515, 1982.

Paula-Barbosa MM, et al.: Cerebellar cortex ultrastructure in ataxia-telangiectasia. *Ann. Neurol* 13:297, 1983.

Perry TL, et al.: Neurochemical abnormalities in a patient with ataxia-telangiectasia. *Neurology* 34:187, 1984.

Richkind KE, et al.: Fetal proteins in ataxia-telangiectasia. *J.A.M.A.* 248:1346, 1982.

Scheres JMJC, et al.: Chromosome 7 in ataxia-telangiectasia. *J. Pediatr.* 97:440, 1980.

Swift M, et al.: Breast and other cancers in families with ataxia-telangiectasia. *N. Engl. J. Med.* 316:1289, 1987.

Syllaba L, et al.: Contribution a' l'indépendance de l'athétose double idiopathique et congénitale. *Rev. Neurol. (Paris)* 1:541, 1926.

Taylor AMR, et al.: Variant forms of ataxia telangiectasia. *J. Med. Genet.* 24:669, 1987.

Tsukahara M, et al.: Ataxia telangiectasia with generalized skin pigmentation and early death. *Eur. J. Pediatr.* 145:121, 1986.

Waldmann TA, et al.: Ataxia-telangiectasia: A multisystem heredity disease with immunodeficiency, impaired organ maturation, x-ray hypersensitivity, and a high incidence of neoplasia. *Ann. Intern. Med.* 99:367, 1983.

Yount WJ: IgG2 deficiency and ataxia-telangiectasia. *N. Engl. J. Med.* 306:541, 1982.

AURICULO-OSTEODYSPLASIA

Mode of Inheritance: Autosomal dominant.

Clinical Manifestations: (a) *short stature;* (b) *auricular dysplasia* (elongated and attached external ear lobe, accompanied by a small, slightly posterior lobule); (c) *limited motion of elbows.*

Radiologic Manifestations: (a) *dysplasia of radiocapitellar joint* with radial-head dislocation; (b) *enlargement of the base of the acromion;* (c) *ulnarward sloping and absence of normal volar tilt of the distal part of the radius;* (d) shortness of the metacarpals in some; (e) *concave and often scalloped axillary border of the scapula;* (f) hip dysplasia and dislocation, precocious arthritic changes.

REFERENCE

Beals RK: Auriculo-osteodysplasia: A syndrome of multiple osseous dysplasia, ear anomaly and short stature. *J. Bone Joint Surg. [Am.]* 49:1541, 1967.

AXIAL OSTEOMALACIA

Mode of Inheritance: Reported in a mother and her son in association with polycystic liver and kidney disease.

Clinical Manifestations: (a) axial skeletal pain; (b) normal circulating calcium, inorganic phosphate, and vitamin D metabolite levels; elevated alkaline phosphate activity; (c) bone biopsy: osteomalacia, intense alkaline phosphatase activity in the osteoblasts along most trabecular bone surfaces; (d) muscle weakness and myopathy in one individual.

Radiologic Manifestations: Increase in bone density and coarse trabecular pattern of the axial skeleton (spine, pelvis, ribs).

REFERENCE

Frame B, et al.: Atypical osteomalacia involving the axial skeleton. *Ann. Intern. Med.* 55:632, 1961.

Whyte MP, et al.: Axial osteomalacia. Clinical, laboratory and genetic investigation of an affected mother and son. *Am. J. Med.* 71:1041, 1981.

AZOREAN NEUROLOGICAL DISEASE

Synonyms: Machado-Joseph-Azorean disease; Joseph disease; Machado-Joseph disease; nigrospinodentate degeneration.

Mode of Inheritance: Autosomal dominant; Portuguese or people of Portuguese ancestry.

Pathology: Degeneration with severe neuronal loss in caudate, putamen, substantia nigra, red nucleus, dentate, and anterior horn cells of the spinal cord; the cerebral cortex and interior olives are intact.

Clinical Manifestations: (a) three types: (1) *extrapyramidal and pyramidal signs:* dystonia, athetosis, rigidity, spasticity, etc.; (2) *cerebellar, pyramidal, and extrapyramidal signs;* (3) *cerebellar signs and peripheral amyotrophy;* (b) other manifestations: decreased peripheral sensation, distal weakness, etc.

Radiologic Manifestations: *Atrophy of the pons and cerebellum* (Fig SY−A−27).

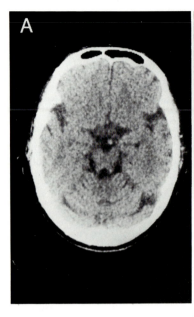
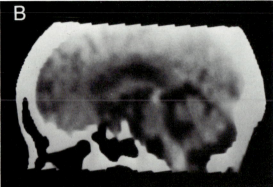

FIG SY—A—27.
Azorean neurological disease. Computed tomographic scans of the head shows cerebellar atrophy and moderate enlargement of the cisterns around the brain stem. (From Yuasa T, Ohama E, Harayama H, et al.: Joseph's disease: Clinical and pathological studies in a Japanese family. *Ann. Neurol.* 19:152, 1986. Used by permission.)

REFERENCES

Bharucha NE, et al.: Machado-Joseph-Azorean disease in India. *Arch. Neurol.* 43:142, 1986.

Nakano K, et al.: Machado disease: A hereditary ataxia in Portuguese emigrants to Massachusetts. *Neurology* 22:49, 1972.

Sakai T, et al.: Joseph disease in a non-Portuguese family. *Neurology* 33:74, 1983.

Yuasa T, et al.: Joseph's disease: Clinical and pathological studies in a Japanese family. *Ann. Neurol.* 19:152, 1986.

BALLER-GEROLD SYNDROME

Synonym: Craniosynostosis–radial aplasia syndrome.

Mode of Inheritance: Probably autosomal recessive.

Clinical Manifestations: (a) *acrocephaly*, prominent nasal bridge, low-set dysplastic ears, prominent mandible, ocular hypotelorism, epicanthal folds, unusual hair pattern; (b) *bilateral forearm deformity;* (c) *oligodactyly;* (d) other reported abnormalities: small for gestational age, postnatal growth retardation, polymicrogyria, midline capillary hemangioma, dry scaly skin, imperforate anus, congenital heart disease (ventricular septal defect, subaortic valvular hypertrophy), etc.

Radiologic Manifestations: (a) *craniosynostosis* (coronal, metopic, lambdoidal); (b) *radial hypoplasia or aplasia;* shortening and curvature of the ulna; radial deviation of the hand; *hypoplastic or absent thumbs;* missing phalanges, metacarpals, and/or carpal bones; fused carpal bones; (c) other reported anomalies: vertebral anomalies, rib anomalies, crossed renal ectopia.

Differential Diagnosis: Craniosynostosis–ulnar aplasia.

REFERENCES

Anyane-Yeboa K, et al.: Baller-Gerold syndrome: Craniosynostosis–radial aplasia syndrome. *Clin. Genet.* 17:161, 1980.
Baller F: Radiusaplasie und Inzucht. *Z. Menschl. Vereb. Konstit. Lehre* 29:782, 1950.
Calabro A, et al.: Craniosynostosis and unilateral ulnar aplasia. *Am. J. Med. Genet.* 20:203, 1985.
Feingold M, et al.: Craniosynostosis–radial aplasia: Baller-Gerold syndrome. *Am. J. Dis. Child.* 133:1279, 1979.
Gerold M: Frakturheilung bei einem seltenen Fall kongenitaler Anomalie der oberen Gliedmassen. *Zentralbl. Chir.* 84:831, 1959.
Ladda RL, et al.: Craniosynostosis associated with limb reduction malformations and cleft lip/palate: A distinct syndrome. *Pediatrics* 61:12, 1978.
Pelias MZ, et al.: Brief clinical report: A sixth report (eighth case) of craniosynostosis–radial aplasia (Baller-Gerold) syndrome. *Am. J. Med. Genet.* 10:133, 1981.

BANNAYAN SYNDROME

Synonym: Bannayan-Zonana syndrome.

Mode of Inheritance: Autosomal dominant; male predominance.

Frequency: 11 published cases (Okumura et al.).

Clinical Manifestations: (a) *macrocephaly;* (b) increased birth size, *postnatal growth deceleration;* (c) *tumors:* lipoma, hemangioma, lymphangioma, thyroid follicular cell, meningothelial meningioma, angioleiomyoma, mixed; (d) localized overgrowth; (e) mild neurological dysfunction, mild mental retardation, seizures; (f) other reported abnormalities: downslanting of the palpebral fissures, high palate, joint hyperextensibility, pectus excavatum, strabismus, amblyopia, prolonged drooling, hyperplasia of the small intestinal mucosa, colonic polyp.

Radiologic Manifestations: (a) *macrocephaly without ventricular enlargement;* (b) *tumors (mesodermal hamartomas:* subcutaneous, intracranial, visceral, intestinal, thoracic, skeletal).

Differential Diagnosis: Riley-Smith syndrome; Klippel-Trenaunay syndrome; neurofibromatosis; cutis marmorata–telangiectasia congenita; Ruvalcaba-Myhre-Smith syndrome.

REFERENCES

Bannayan GA: Lipomatosis, angiomatosis, and macrencephalia. *Arch. Pathol.* 92:1, 1971.
Miles JH, et al.: Macrocephaly with hamartomas: Bannayan-Zonana syndrome. *Am. J. Med. Genet.* 19:225, 1984.
Okumura K, et al.: Bannayan syndrome—generalized lipomatosis associated with megalencephaly and macrodactyly. *Acta Pathol. Jpn.* 36:269, 1986.
Zonana J, et al.: Macrocephaly with multiple lipomas and hemangiomas. *J. Pediatr.* 89:600, 1976.

BANTI SYNDROME

Clinical Manifestations: (a) *splenomegaly;* (b) *leukopenia;* (c) *anemia;* (d) *moderate thrombocytopenia* (frequent); (e) upper alimentary tract hemorrhage; (f) various manifestations of hepatic failure.

Radiologic Manifestations: (a) *esophageal and/or gastric varices;* (b) splenoportographic or arteriographic demonstration of *portal system obstruction: intrahepatic* (cirrhosis of the liver) or *extrahepatic* (splenic vein thrombosis, cavernous transformation of the portal venous system, pancreatic fibrosis, tumor) aneurysms of branches of the splenic artery, etc.

REFERENCES

Banti G: Splenomegalie mit Lebercirrhose. *Beitr. Pathol. Anat. Allg. Pathol.* 24:21, 1898.

Baron M, et al.: Splenoportography. *J.A.M.A.* 206:629, 1968.

Girardet J-P, et al.: Syndrome de Banti au cours d'une maladie angiomateuse. *Arch. Fr. Pediatr.* 35:308, 1978.

Ruzicka FF, et al.: Arterial portography: Pattern of venous flow. *Radiology* 92:777, 1969.

BARDET-BIEDL SYNDROME

Mode of Inheritance: Autosomal recessive.

Frequency: Less than 1:160,000; 500 published cases of Bardet-Biedl syndrome and approximately 20 cases of Laurence-Moon syndrome to 1982 (Schachat et al.).

Clinical Manifestations: (a) *pigmentary retinal degeneration*; (b) *polydactyly*; (c) *obesity*; (d) *genital hypoplasia*; (e) *mental retardation*; (f) other reported abnormalities: syndactyly, dwarfism, congenital heart disease, microphthalmos, cataract, strabismus, deafness, dental anomalies, nephropathy (glomerular sclerosis, interstitial sclerosis, uremia), hypertension, anal atresia, diabetes insipidus, genu valgum, ataxia, cystic dilatation of intrahepatic and common bile ducts, microstomia, cleft lip and palate, hypertrichosis, webbed neck, hepatic fibrosis.

Radiologic Manifestations: (a) *polydactyly*, syndactyly, clinodactyly of the fifth finger; (b) *urinary tract anomalies*: cysts, calyceal diverticula, lobulated renal outlines of the fetal type, diffuse renal cortical loss, hypoplasia of the kidney, hydronephrosis, persistent urogenital sinus, vesicovaginal fistula; (c) other reported abnormalities: congenital cardiovascular defects, left ventricular hypertrophy, skull defects, hip dysplasia, dilatation of intrahepatic bile ducts and common bile duct, enlargement of the lateral ventricles.

Differential Diagnosis: (a) Laurence-Moon syndrome: the cases reported by Laurence and Moon had mental retardation, hypogenitalism, pigmentary retinopathy, and spastic paraplegia. Bardet-Biedl and Laurence-Moon syndromes are considered different but interrelated autosomal recessive disorders; (b) Biemond syndrome (Fig SY−B−1).

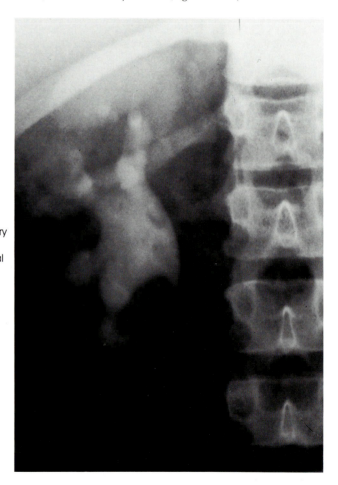

FIG SY−B−1.
Bardet-Biedl syndrome in a boy aged 9 years 10 months. Excretory urography shows mild calyceal dilation and paracalyceal diverticula. (Courtesy of Ronald A. Cohen, M.D., Children's Hospital Medical Center, Oakland, Calif.)

REFERENCES

Ammann F: Investigations cliniques et génétiques sur le syndrome de Bardet-Biedl en Suisse. *J. Genet. Hum.* 18(suppl.):1, 1970.

Bardet G: *Sur un Syndrome d'Obesité Congénitale Avec Polydactylie et Rétinite Pigmentaire* (thesis). Paris, 1920.

Biedl A: Ein Geschwisterpaar mit adiposogenitaler Dystrophie. *Dtsch. Med. Wochenschr.* 48:1630, 1922.

Brault B: *Les Signes Radiologiques du Syndrome de Laurence-Moon-Bardet-Biedl* (thesis). Paris, 1972.

Farag TI, et al.: Bardet-Biedl and Laurence-Moon syndromes in a mixed Arab population. *Clin. Genet.* 33:78, 1988.

Harnett JD, et al.: The spectrum of renal disease in Laurence-Moon-Biedl syndrome. *N. Engl. J. Med.* 319:615, 1988.

Klein D, et al.: Syndrome of Laurence-Moon-Bardet-Biedl and allied diseases in Switzerland: Clinical, genetic and epidemiologic studies. *J. Neurol. Sci.* 9:497, 1969.

Labrune M, et al.: Urographic findings in the Laurence-Moon-Bardet-Biedl syndrome. *Ann. Radiol. (Paris)* 17:385, 1974.

Laurence JZ, Moon RC: Four cases of "retinitis pigmentosa" occurring in the same family and accompanied by general imperfections of development. *Ophthalmol. Rev.* 2:32, 1866.

Linne T, et al.: Renal involvement in the Laurence-Moon-Biedl syndrome. Functional and radiological studies. *Acta Paediatr. Scand.* 75:240, 1986.

Michel JR, et al.: Une nouvelle entité radio-clinique: La dysplasie rénale multidiverticulaire. Rapport avec le syndrome de Laurence-Moon-Bardet-Biedl. *Ann. Radiol. (Paris)* 18:533, 1975.

Pagon RA, et al.: Hepatic involvement in the Bardet-Biedl syndrome. *Am. J. Med. Genet.* 13:373, 1982.

Truchiya R, et al.: Congenital cystic dilatation of the bile duct associated with Laurence-Moon-Biedl-Bardet syndrome. *Arch. Surg.* 112:82, 1977.

BARNES SYNDROME

Synonym: Thoracolaryngopelvic dysplasia.

Mode of Inheritance: Autosomal dominant.

Clinical Manifestations: (a) small, rigid, "bell-shaped" thorax; (b) laryngeal stenosis; (c) asthenic build.

Radiologic Manifestations: (a) narrow thorax; (b) small iliac wing and pelvis, shallow sacroiliac notch, etc.

Differential Diagnosis: Asphyxiating thoracic dysplasia; thoracic-pelvic dysostosis.

REFERENCES

Bankier A, et al.: Thoracic-pelvic dysostosis: A "new" autosomal dominant form. *J. Med. Genet.* 20:276, 1983.

Barnes ND, Hull D, Symons JS: Thoracic dystrophy. *Arch. Dis. Child.* 44:11, 1969.

Burn J, et al.: Autosomal dominant thoracolaryngopelvic dysplasia: Barnes syndrome. *J. Med. Genet.* 23:345, 1986.

BARTTER SYNDROME

Mode of Inheritance: Autosomal recessive most likely; obligatory carriers reported to have the same pattern of platelet aggregation inhibition as their affected children.

Frequency: More than 100 published cases to 1984 (Ohlsson et al.).

Clinical Manifestations: (a) growth retardation, mental retardation; (b) craniofacial features: large head, prominent forehead, triangular face, large eyes, drooping mouth, large pinnae; (c) muscle weakness, tetany, vomiting, polydipsia, polyuria, *normal blood pressure;* (d) *hypokalemic alkalosis, hyperaldosteronism,* renal sodium wasting, plasma volume contraction, hypomagnesemia, defect in platelet aggregation, inability to concentrate urine, elevated plasma renin and angiotensin levels, diminished pressor response to infused angiotensin, rise in aldosterone levels following the infusion of renin, hypophosphatemia due to hyperparathyroidism; (e) renal biopsy: *hyperplasia of the juxtaglomerular apparatus;* (f) excessive prostaglandin activity; (g) other reported abnormalities: fetal polyuria leading to polyhydramnios, amniotic fluid having a high chloride concentration, premature birth, low urinary calcium excretion, hypercalciuria and nephrocalcino-

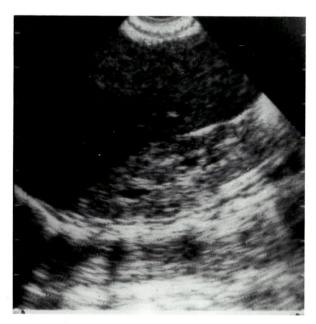

FIG SY−B−2.
Bartter syndrome. A longitudinal sonogram of the right kidney shows markedly increased echogenicity of the parenchyma in a normal-sized kidney. (From Strauss S, Robinson G, Lotan D, et al.: Renal sonography in Bartter syndrome. *J. Ultrasound Med.* 6:265, 1987. Used by permission.)

sis, cystinosis presenting with features suggesting Bartter syndrome, trisomy 3 mosaicism.

Radiologic Manifestations: (a) *nephromegaly,* marked renal medullary and minimal cortical hypertrophy, splayed minor calices, pyelectasis, hydroureters without obstruction, loss of cortical substance in the absence of vesicoureteral reflux; (b) arteriography: splaying of interlobar and arcuate arteries; (c) *increased renal parenchymal echogenecity with a loss of corticomedullary differentiation,* small cortical cysts, nephrocalcinosis; (d) rickets/osteomalacia (hypophosphatemia due to hyperparathyroidism) (Fig SY–B–2).

REFERENCES

Bartter FC, et al.: Hyperplasia of the juxtaglomerular complex with hyperaldosteronism and hypokalemic alkalosis. *Am. J. Med.* 33:811, 1962.

Bold AM, et al.: Hypokalaemia presenting with leg pain in Bartter's syndrome. *Lancet* 2:989, 1984.

Cha EM, et al.: Bartter's syndrome: With angiographic evaluation. *Radiology* 113:703, 1974.

Cumming WA, et al.: Nephrocalcinosis in Bartter's syndrome. *Pediatr. Radiol.* 14:125, 1984.

De Keyser F, et al.: Trisomy 3 mosaicism in a patient with Bartter syndrome. *J. Med. Genet.* 25:358, 1988.

Girardin E, et al.: Familial Bartter's syndrome: Report of a case with early manifestations and persistent hypercalciuria. *Helv. Paediatr. Acta* 41:221, 1986.

James T, et al.: Bartter syndrome: Typical facies and normal plasma volume. *Am. J. Dis. Child.* 129:1205, 1975.

Jones BF, et al.: Unusual radiological changes associated with probable Bartter's syndrome. *J. Urol.* 127:306, 1982.

Ohlsson A, et al.: A variant of Bartter's syndrome. Bartter's syndrome associated with hydramnios, prematurity, hypercalciuria and nephrocalcinosis. *Acta Paediatr. Scand.* 73:868, 1984.

Pereira RR, et al.: Inheritance of Bartter syndrome. *Am. J. Med. Genet.* 15:79, 1983.

Proesmans W, et al.: Prenatal diagnosis of Bartter syndrome. *Lancet* 1:394, 1987.

Rudin A, et al.: Low urinary calcium excretion in Bartter's syndrome. *N. Engl. J. Med.* 310:1190, 1984.

Sann L, et al.: Hypophosphatemia and hyperparathyroidism in a case of Bartter's syndrome. *Helv. Paediatr. Acta* 33:299, 1978.

Stoff JS, et al.: A defect in platelet aggregation in Bartter's syndrome. *Am. J. Med.* 68:171, 1980.

Strauss S, et al.: Renal sonography in Bartter syndrome. *J. Ultrasound Med.* 6:265, 1987.

Watson MI, et al.: Systemic prostaglandin I₂ synthesis is normal in patients with Bartter's syndrome. *Lancet* 2:368, 1983.

Whyte MP, et al.: Cystinosis presenting with features suggesting Bartter syndrome. *Clin. Pediatr. (Phila.)* 24:447, · 1985.

BECKWITH-WIEDEMANN SYNDROME

Synonyms: Wiedemann-Beckwith syndrome; EMG syndrome (exomphalos, macroglossia, gigantism).

Mode of Inheritance: Most consistent with autosomal dominant, multifactorial inheritance; variability of expression; occurrence in one of a pair of monozygotic twins.

Frequency: Not very uncommon; 388 published cases to 1986 (Koh et al.).

Clinical Manifestations: (a) *craniofacial dysmorphism:* normal head size with prominent occiput or microcephaly, midfacial hypoplasia, hypertelorism, mandibular prognathism, ear anomalies (pits and/or creases), nevus flammeus, macroglossia; (b) *omphalocele, umbilical hernia or diastasis recti;* (c) *gigantism;* (d) *visceromegaly;* (e) increased incidence of neoplasms (7.5%), especially if associated with asymmetry: nephroblastoma, adrenal cortical carcinoma, hepatoblastoma, hepatocellular carcinoma, nesidioblastosis of the pancreas, pancreatoblastoma, neuroblastoma, gonadoblastoma, glioma, lymphoma; (f) other reported abnormalities: hemihypertrophy, congenital hypothyroidism, conductive hearing loss, chronic alveolar hypoventilation secondary to macroglossia, bowel malrotation, undescended testes, hydrocephalus, renal failure, systemic hypertension, association with prune-belly syndrome.

Pathologic Findings: *visceromegaly* (liver, kidneys, pancreas, heart, etc), *cellular hyperplasia* (interstitial gonadal cells, pancreatic islet cells, parganglia, adrenal fetal cortex, etc), adrenal cortical cyst, fetal lobulation of the kidneys, renal medullary dysplasia with sparse and immature collecting tubules, corticomedullary renal cysts, pyelocalyceal diverticula, clitoromegaly, hyperplasic uterus, bicornuate uterus, thymic hyperplasia, neoplasms including nephroblastomatosis, congenital pancreatoblastoma.

Laboratory Findings: Trisomy 11p15, *hypoglycemia* (hyperinsulinism), neonatal polycythemia, increased serum α-fetoprotein level, thyroxine-binding globulin deficiency, abnormal urinary excretion of polyamines, high or low levels of circulating somatomedin activity; hyperlipemia, hypercholesterolemia, hypocalcemia, combined immune deficiency.

Radiologic Manifestations: (a) *large tongue;* (b) *omphalocele or umbilical hernia;* (c) *nephromegaly,* diffuse increased echogenicity of the cortex, normal or proportionately enlarged nondilated calices, lobulated renal margin, corticomedullary cysts, nodules of mixed echogenecity, pelvocalyceal distension, pelvocalyceal diverticula, duplex collecting system, etc.; (d) *hepatomegaly;* (e) *advanced skeletal maturation (in some);* (f) other, less common manifestations: widening of the metaphyses and cortical thickening of the long bones, hemihypertrophy, neonatal cardiomegaly, posterior eventration of the diaphragm, microcephaly, malignant growths, rapid growth, adrenal calcification.

Note: The incidence of the occurrence of tumor (mainly malignant) in the patients with Beckwith-Wiedemann syndrome has been estimated to be 7.5%. In 12.5% of children with this syndrome hemihypertrophy was present, in 40% of

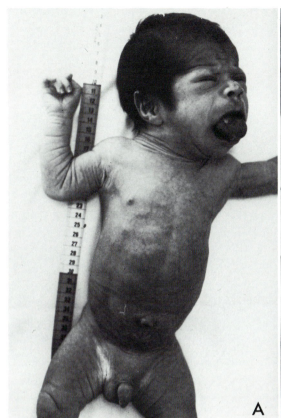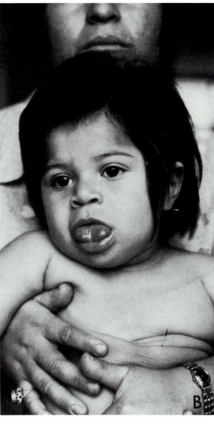

FIG SY−B−3.
Beckwith-Wiedemann syndrome in association with hypothyroidism in a 35-day-old infant **(A).** Note the midfacial hypoplasia and the remarkable macroglossia (in contrast, the macroglossia in congenital hypothyroidism is never so accentuated). The swollen skin suggests incipient myxedema. Cutis marmorata and lanugo in the forehead are signs of hypothyroidism. The patient at 21 months of age **(B)** still shows macroglossia in spite of the thyroid therapy. (From Martínez RM, Ocampo-Campos R, Pérez-Arroyo R, et al.: The Wiedemann-Beckwith syndrome in four sibs including one with associated congenital hypothyroidism. *Eur. J. Pediatr.* 143:233, 1985. Used by permission.)

children with the Beckwith-Wiedemann syndrome and tumor, hemihypertrophy was present. The following recommendation has been made (Wiedemann): every child with Beckwith-Wiedemann syndrome needs to be examined with renal sonography, first at 3-month intervals and after the third year of life at 6-month intervals (Figs SY−B−3 to SY−B−5).

REFERENCES

Barlow GB: Excretion of polyamines by children with Beckwith's syndrome. *Arch. Dis. Child.* 55:40, 1980.

Beckwith JB, et al.: Hyperplastic fetal visceromegaly with macroglossia, omphalocele, cytomegaly of adrenal fetal cortex, postnatal somatic gigantism, and other abnormalities: Newly recognized syndrome (abstracted, no. 41). Presented at the American Pediatric Society, Seattle, 1964.

Bose B, et al.: Wiedemann-Beckwith syndrome in one of monozygotic twins. *Arch. Dis. Child.* 60:1191, 1985.

Bronk JB, et al.: Pyelocalyceal diverticula in the Beckwith-Wiedemann syndrome. *Pediatr. Radiol.* 17:80, 1987.

Daugbjerg P, et al.: A case of Beckwith-Wiedemann syndrome with conductive hearing loss. *Acta Paediatr. Scand.* 73:408, 1984.

Drut R, et al.: Congenital pancreatoblastoma in Beckwith-Wiedemann syndrome: An emerging association. *Pediatr. Pathol.* 8:331, 1988.

Emergy LG, et al.: Neuroblastoma associated with Beckwith-Wiedemann syndrome. *Cancer* 52:176, 1983.

Engstrom W, et al.: Wiedemann-Beckwith syndrome. *Eur. J. Pediatr.* 147:450, 1988.

Greenwood RD, et al.: Cardiovascular abnormalities in the Beckwith-Wiedemann syndrome. *Am. J. Dis. Child.* 131:293, 1977.

Grundy H, et al.: Beckwith-Wiedemann syndrome: Prenatal ultrasound diagnosis using standard kidney to abdominal circumference ratio. *Am. J. Perinatol.* 2:236, 1985.

Ichiba Y, et al.: Adrenal calcification in Beckwith-Wiedemann syndrome. *Am. J. Dis. Child.* 131:1296, 1977.

Journel H, et al.: Trisomy llp15 and Beckwith-Wiedemann syndrome. Report of two new cases. *Ann. Genet. (Paris)* 28:97, 1985.

Knight JA, et al.: Association of the Beckwith-Wiedemann and prune belly syndromes. *Clin. Pediatr. (Phila.)* 19:485, 1980.

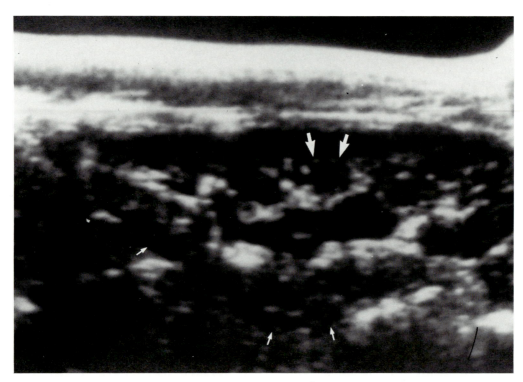

FIG SY–B–4.
Beckwith-Wiedemann syndrome. A prone longitudinal ultrasound scan reveals nephromegaly (*thin arrows* outline the lobulated anterior margin), medullary nodules of mixed echogenecity (*thick arrows* point to a nodule), and a distended renal pelvis. (From Shah KJ: Beckwith-Wiedemann syndrome: Role of ultrasound in its management. *Clin. Radiol.* 34:313, 1983. Used by permission.)

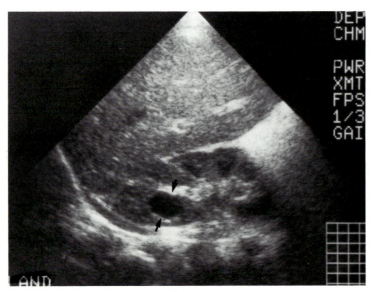

FIG SY–B–5.
Beckwith-Wiedemann syndrome in a 2-year-old male. A cyst of the right kidney measured 2 cm in diameter. (Courtesy of Peter E. Kane, M.D., Children's Hospital Medical Center, Oakland, Calif.)

Koh THHG, et al.: Pancreatoblastoma in a neonate with Wiedemann-Beckwith syndrome. *Eur. J. Pediatr.* 145:435, 1986.

Labbe A, et al.: Le syndrome de Wiedemann-Beckwith. A propos de six observations dont trois cas familiaux. *Ann. Pediatr. (Paris)* 28:665, 1981.

Lee FA: Radiology of the Beckwith-Wiedemann syndrome. *Radiol. Clin. North Am.* 10:261, 1972.

Martínez RM, et al.: The Wiedemann-Beckwith syndrome in four sibs including one with associated congenital hypothyroidism. *Eur. J. Pediatr.* 143:233, 1985.

Olney AH, et al.: Wiedemann-Beckwith syndrome in apparently discordant monozygotic twins. *Am. J. Med. Genet.* 29:491, 1988.

Pettenati MJ, et al.: Wiedemann-Beckwith syndrome: Presentation of clinical and cytogenetic data on 22 new cases and review of the literature. *Hum. Genet.* 74:143, 1986.

Potts SR, et al.: Pancreoblastoma in a neonate associated with Beckwith-Wiedemann syndrome. *Z. Kinderchir.* 41:56, 1986.

Shah KJ: Beckwith-Wiedemann syndrome: Role of ultrasound in its management. *Clin. Radiol.* 34:313, 1983.

Smith DF, et al.: Chronic alveolar hypoventilation secondary to macroglossia in the Beckwith-Wiedemann syndrome. *Pediatrics* 70:695, 1982.

Turleau C, et al.: Trisomy 11p15 and Beckwith-Wiedemann syndrome. A report of two cases. *Hum. Genet.* 67:219, 1984.

Waziri M, et al.: Abnormality of chromosome 11 in patients with features of Beckwith-Wiedemann syndrome. *J. Pediatr.* 102:873, 1983.

Weinstein JM, et al.: Optic glioma associated with Beckwith-Wiedemann syndrome. *Pediatr. Neurol.* 2:308, 1986.

Wiedemann HR: Complexe malformatif familial avec hernie ombilicale et macroglossie: "Un syndrome nouveau"? *J. Genet. Hum.* 13:223, 1964.

Wiedemann HR: Tumours and hemihypertrophy associated with Wiedemann-Beckwith syndrome. *Eur. J. Pediatr.* 141:129, 1983.

BEHÇET SYNDROME

Synonyms: Behçet disease; Adamentiades-Behçet syndrome; Gilbert-Behçet syndrome; Halushi-Behçet syndrome; l'aphthose de Touraine.

Etiology: Unknown, some familial cases have been reported; proposed etiological factors: immunologic, genetic, viral, bacterial, fibrinolytic, ecological; highest incidence reported from the Mediterranean region, Middle East, and Japan.

Clinical Manifestations: Occurrence most commonly in young male adults, rare in children (usually incomplete form); exacerbations and remission of various duration and frequency; (a) mucocutaneous lesions: *aphthous stomatitis,* absent or scanty lingual fungiform papillae, cutaneous and mucosal ulcerations, erythema nodosum, subungual infarction; (b) *genital ulcer,* ureteral obstruction with bladder involvement, epididymitis, urethritis, orchitis, nephrotic syndrome, glomerulonephritis; (c) alimentary system involvement: esophageal lesions, ulceration and perforation of the small bowel, colitis, diarrhea, pancreatitis, hepatomegaly; (d) ocular manifestations present in 70% to 85% of cases, *iridocyclitis with hypopyon,* localized retinal edema, macular edema, disc edema, retinal pigmentary changes, accumula-

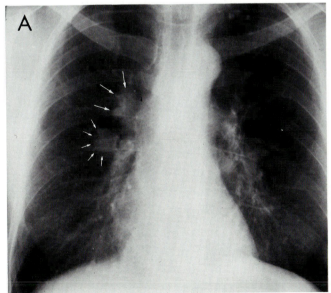
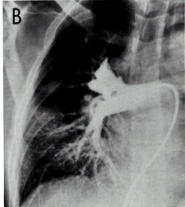

FIG SY–B–6.
Behçet syndrome. **A,** plain film, and **B,** right pulmonary angiogram: right suprahilar lobulated opacities *(arrows)* on the plain film correspond to two pulmonary aneurysms with a lack of perfusion of the right upper lobe. The rounded parahilar opacity was subpleural on the lateral film. (From Grenier P, Bletry O, Cornud F, et al.: Pulmonary involvement in Behçet disease. *A.J.R.* 137:565, 1981. Used by permission.)

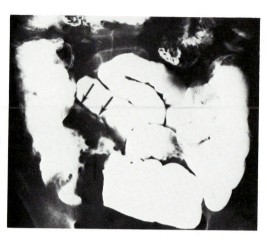

FIG SY–B–7.
Behçet syndrome in an 11-year-old girl. An irregularly narrowed, ulcerated terminal ileum *(lower arrow)*, and fistulous tract to the ascending colon *(upper arrows)* are shown. (From Vlymen WJ, Moskowitz PS: Roentgenographic manifestations of esophageal and intestinal involvement in Behçet's disease in children. *Pediatr. Radiol.* 10:193, 1981. Used by permission.)

tion of exudative material in the deep part of the retina, occlusion of retinal vessels, cranial nerve palsies, homonymous hemianopic field aspect, papillitis, subretinal neovascular membrane and disciform scars; (e) neurological manifestations, meningoencephalitis, cranial nerve palsies, peripheral neuropathy, polyneuropathy, palatal myoclonus, hemiplegia due to vascular obstruction, intracranial hypertension (headaches, papilledema, etc.); (f) respiratory system manifesta-

tions: hemoptysis, recurrent pneumonia; (g) oligoarthritis, polyarthritis, soft-tissue swelling, Baker cyst (ruptured simulating thrombophlebitis); (h) pericarditis, myocarditis, myocardial infarction, cardiac dilation, gallop rhythm, conduction defects, pulseless disease due to subclavian artery occlusion, hypertension (renal artery stenosis); (i) other reported abnormalities: lymphadenopathy, fever, syndrome of Hughes-Stovin, development of lymphoma, inner-ear involvement

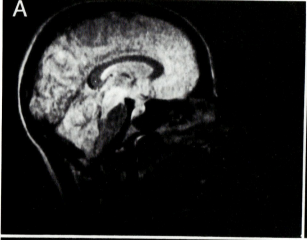

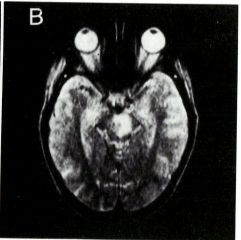

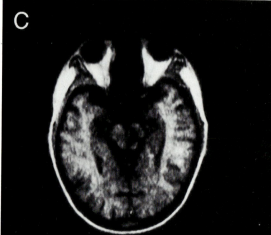

FIG SY–B–8.
Behçet syndrome. **A** and **B,** in the T$_2$-weighted images (TR, 2,320 ms; TE, 40 ms) an area of high signal intensity is recognized in the upper portion of the brain stem, mostly on the left. **C,** a focus of low signal intensity in the left upper portion of the brain stem is clearly shown with an inversion recovery sequence (TR, 1,900 ms; TI, 500 ms). (From Willeit J, Schmutzhard E, Aichner F, et al.: CT and MR imaging in neuro-Behçet disease. *J. Comput. Assist. Tomogr.* 10:313, 1986. Used by permission.)

(hearing disturbances, vertigo, cochlear and vestibular abnormalities on audiological examination), blood coagulation problems, Budd-Chiari syndrome as a complication of the disease, coexistence with manifestations of relapsing polychondritis reported as "mouth and genital ulcers with inflamed cartilage (MAGIC) syndrome."

Pathology: *Necrotizing arteritis,* aneurysmal dilatation of minor and major arteries, thrombotic occlusions of arteries, *thrombophlebitis.*

Radiologic Manifestations: (a) pulmonary parenchymal infiltrate, recurrent pneumonia, hilar adenopathy; (b) arterial aneurysm, venous thrombosis, pulmonary embolism, pseudoaneurysm, rupture of the coronary artery with false aneurysm formation, arterial thrombosis, Budd-Chiari syndrome; (c) esophageal ulceration, stenosis, perforation and functional disorder (poor peristalsis), enterocolitis, inflammatory polyposis of colon; (d) central nervous system abnormalities: vascular occlusion, infarct, edema, "mass lesions" (pseudotumor), intracranial hypertension due to cerebral venous thrombosis, etc.; (e) osteoporosis, joint space narrowing, osseous erosions, spontaneous atlantoaxial subluxation, sacroiliitis, avascular necrosis of the femoral head, enthesopathy (calcaneal spurs, etc.) (Figs SY−B−6 to SY−B−8).

REFERENCES

Adamantiades B: Sur un cas d'iritis à hypopyon recidivant. *Ann. Ocul. (Paris)* 168:271, 1931.

Adler OB, et al.: Vascular aspects of Behçet disease. Case presentations and review of literature. *Ann. Radiol. (Paris)* 27:371, 1984.

Ammann AJ, et al.: Behçet syndrome. *J. Pediatr.* 107:41, 1985.

Behçet H: Uber rezidivierende aphthöse, durch ein Virus verursachte Geschwüre am Mund, am Auge und an den Genitalen. *Dermatol. Wochenschr. (Leipzig)* 105:1152, 1937.

Ben-Itzhak J, et al.: Intracranial venous thrombosis in Behçet's syndrome. *Neuroradiology* 27:450, 1985.

Brama I, et al.: Inner ear involvement in Behçet's disease. *Arch. Otolaryngol.* 106:215, 1980.

Caporn N, et al.: Arthritis in Behçet's syndrome. *Br. J. Radiol.* 56:87, 1983.

Carswell GF: A case of Behçet's disease involving the bladder. *Br. J. Urol.* 48:199, 1976.

Chong SKF, et al.: Infantile colitis: A manifestation of intestinal Behçet's syndrome. *J. Pediatr. Gastroenterol. Nutr.* 7:622, 1988.

Colvard DM, et al.: The ocular manifestations of Behçet's disease. *Arch. Ophthalmol.* 95:1813, 1977.

Firestein GS, et al.: Mouth and genital ulcers with inflamed cartilage: MAGIC syndrome. Five patients with features of relapsing polychondritis and Behçet's disease. *Am. J. Med.* 79:65, 1985.

Gilbert W: Über chronische Verlaufsform der metastatischen Ophthalmie ("Ophthalmia lenta"). *Arch. Augenh.* 96:119, 1925.

Grenier P, et al.: Pulmonary involvement in Behçet disease. *A.J.R.* 137:565, 1981.

Grenier P, et al.: Syndrome de Hughes-Stovin: A propos d'une cas revélant une maladie de Behçet. *Ann. Radiol. (Paris)* 23:509, 1980.

Hamza M, et al.: Pseudo thrombophlébite par rupture de kyste poplité au cours de la maladie de Behçet. *Ann. Radiol. (Paris)* 28:53, 1985.

Harper CM, et al.: Intracranial hypertension in Behçet's disease: Demonstration of sinus occlusion with use of digital subtraction angiography. *Mayo Clin. Proc.* 60:419, 1985.

Herreman G, et al.: Behçet's syndrome and renal involvement: A histological and immunofluorescent study of eleven renal biopsies. *Am. J. Med. Sci.* 284:10, 1982.

Hutchison SJ, et al.: Behçet's syndrome presenting as myocardial infarction with impaired blood fibrinolysis. *Br. Heart J.* 52:686, 1984.

James DJ: Silk route disease (Behçet's disease). *West J. Med.* 148:433, 1988.

James DG, et al.: Recognition of the diverse cardiovascular manifestations in Behçet's disease. *Am. Heart J.* 103:457, 1982.

Kaseda, S, et al.: Huge false aneurysm due to rupture of the right coronary artery in Behçet's syndrome. *Am. Heart J.* 103:569, 1982.

Koss JC, et al.: Atlantoaxial subluxation in Behçet's syndrome. *A.J.R.* 134:392, 1980.

Larrue V, et al.: Polyneuropathie inflammatoire chronique et syndrome de Behçet. *Presse Med.* 16:732, 1987.

Litvan I, et al.: Behçet's syndrome masquerading as tumor. *Neuroradiology* 29:103, 1987.

Lewis MA, et al.: Transient neonatal Behçet's disease. *Arch. Dis. Child.* 61:805, 1986.

McLean AM, et al.: Ileal ring ulcers in Behçet syndrome. *A.J.R.* 140:947, 1983.

Nojiri C, et al.: Conduction disturbance in Behçet's disease. Association with ruptured aneurysm of the sinus of valsalva into the left ventricular cavity. *Chest* 86:636, 1984.

Park JH, et al.: Arterial manifestations of Behçet disease. *A.J.R.* 143:821, 1984.

Pedinielli FJ, et al.: Maladie de Behçet avec anticoagulant circulant. *Presse Med.* 13:1157, 1984.

Rosenberger A, et al.: Radiological aspects of Behçet disease. *Radiology* 144:261, 1982.

Shuttleworth EC, et al.: Palatal myoclonus in Behçet's disease. *Arch Intern. Med.* 145:949, 1985.

Stringer DA, et al.: Behçet's syndrome involving the gastrointestinal tract—a diagnostic dilemma in childhood. *Pediatr. Radiol.* 16:131, 1986.

Vlyman WJ, et al.: Roentgenographic manifestation of esophageal and intestinal involvement in Behçet's disease in children. *Pediatr. Radiol.* 10:193, 1981.

Wilkey D, et al.: Budd-Chiari syndrome and renal failure in Behçet disease. *Am. J. Med.* 75:541, 1983.

Willeit J, et al.: CT and MR imaging in neuro-Behçet disease. *J. Comput. Assist. Tomogr.* 10:313, 1986.

Williams AL, et al.: Computed tomography in Behçet disease. *Radiology* 131:403, 1979.

Yim CW, et al.: Behçet's syndrome in a family with inflammatory bowel disease. *Arch. Intern. Med.* 145:1047, 1985.

BENCZE SYNDROME

Mode of Inheritance: Autosomal dominant.

Clinical Manifestations: Mild facial asymmetry, esotropia, amblyopia, submucous cleft palate, growth deficiency, mental deficiency, primary telecanthus, hyperextensible knees.

Radiologic Manifestations: Mild pectus carinatum, mild scoliosis, asymmetrical frontal sinus development, coxa valga, narrow iliac wings.

REFERENCES

Bencze JA, et al.: Dominant inheritance of hemifacial hyperplasia associated with strabismus. *Oral Surg.* 35:489, 1973.
Kurnit D, et al.: An autosomal dominantly inherited syndrome of facial asymmetry, esotropia, amblyopia, and submucous cleft palate (Bencze syndrome). *Clin. Genet.* 16:301, 1979.

BERK-TABATZNIK SYNDROME

Clinical and Radiologic Manifestations: (a) linear growth deficiency; (b) congenital optic atrophy; (c) cervical kyphosis (hemivertebrae, vertebral wedging); (d) small distal phalanges; (e) spastic quadriparesis.

REFERENCES

Berk ME, Tabatznik B: Cervical kyphosis from posterior hemivertebrae with brachyphalangy and congenital optic atrophy. *J. Bone Joint Surg. [Br.]* 43:77, 1961.
Hartwell EA, et al.: Congenital optic atrophy and brachytelephalangy: The Berk-Tabatznik syndrome. *Am. J. Med. Genet.* 29:383, 1988.

BERNHEIM SYNDROME

Pathology: *Left ventricular hypertrophy and dilatation, encroachment of the interventricular septum into the right ventricle* resulting in stenosis or a barrier to blood flow and finally systemic venous engorgement (right-heart failure).

Clinical Manifestations: Catheterization: lower pulmonary pressure when compared with the right ventricle.

Radiologic Manifestations: (a) cardiomegaly with a left ventricular contour; (b) *encroachment of the left ventricle on the right ventricle,* relatively small right ventricular chamber; (c) *demonstration of primary disease:* left ventricular hypertrophy due to supravalvular aortic stenosis, aortic valvular stenosis, aortic hypoplasia, coarctation of the aorta, etc.

REFERENCES

Bernheim: De l'asytolie veineuse dans l'hypertrophie du coeur gauche. *Rev. Med. (Paris)* 30:785, 1910.
Drago EE, et al.: Bernheim's syndrome. *Am. J. Cardiol.* 14:568, 1964.
Herbst M, et al.: Klinische und angiocardiographische Bestätigung des Bernheim-Syndroms. *Fortschr. Roentgenstr.* 91:679, 1959.

BIEMOND SYNDROME, I

Mode of Inheritance: Reported in one family in four generations.

Clinical Manifestations: (a) *brachydactyly;* (b) *nystagmus;* (c) *cerebellar ataxia;* (d) mental deficiency; (e) strabismus.

Radiologic Manifestations: *Brachydactyly due to one short metacarpal and metatarsal.*

REFERENCES

Biemond A: Brachydactylie, nystagmus en cerebellaire ataxie als familiair syndroom. *Ned. Tijdschr. Geneeskl.* 78:1423, 1934.
Temtamy S, McKusick VA: Synopsis of hand malformations with particular emphasis on genetic factors. *Birth Defects* 5:125, 1969.

BIEMOND SYNDROME, II

Mode of Inheritance: Irregular autosomal dominant inheritance.

Clinical Manifestations: (a) *obesity;* (b) *hypogenitalism;* (c) *coloboma of the iris;* (d) *polydactyly;* (e) mental retardation; (f) other reported anomalies: hypospadias, hydrocephalus.

Radiologic Manifestations: (a) *postaxial polydactyly;* (b) hydrocephalus (in some).

REFERENCES

Biemond A: Het syndroom van Laurence-Biedl en een aanverwant nieuw syndroom. *Ned. Tijdschr. Geneeskl.* 78:1801, 1934.
Temtamy S, McKusick VA: Synopsis of hand malformations with particular emphasis on genetic factors. *Birth Defects* 5:125, 1969.
Van Bogaert L, Delhaye A: Observation d'un syndrome familial nouveau (Biemond) proche de la maladie de Laurence-Moon-Bardet. *Bull. Soc. Med. Hop. Paris* 52:683, 1936.

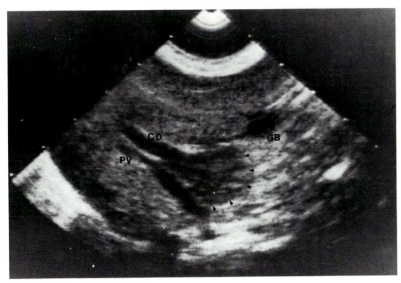

FIG SY–B–9.
Bile plug syndrome. An oblique sonographic scan through the upper portion of the abdomen shows a common duct *(CD)* anterior to the portal vein *(PV)* with distal focal dilatation *(arrowheads)*. GB = gallbladder. (From Pfeiffer WR, Robinson LH, Balsara VJ: Sonographic features of bile plug syndrome. *J. Ultrasound Med.* 5:161, 1986. Used by permission.)

BILE PLUG SYNDROME

Synonym: Inspissated bile syndrome.

Pathology: Impacted, thickened secretions and bile in the extrahepatic ducts; bile duct dilatation.

Clinical Manifestations: (a) association with total parenteral nutrition, dehydration, massive hemolysis due to Rh or ABO incompatibility, cystic fibrosis, etc; (b) obstructive jaundice in infancy.

Radiologic Manifestations: (a) ultrasonographic demonstration of dilated bile ducts and inspissated bile (low-level echoes); (b) nuclear medicine hepatobiliary imaging: lack of excretion of the radionuclide into the bowel indicates bile duct obstruction; (c) dilation of the ducts and the intraluminal "mass" causing obstruction are demonstrated by an intraoperative cholangiogram (Figs SY–B–9 and SY–B–10).

Differential Diagnosis: hepatitis; choledochal cyst; stenosis of the common bile duct.

REFERENCES

Bernstein J, et al.: Bile-plug syndrome: A correctable cause of obstructive jaundice in infants. *Pediatrics* 43:273, 1969.
Pfeiffer WR, et al.: Sonographic features of bile plug syndrome. *J. Ultrasound Med.* 5:161, 1986.
Rickham PP, et al.: Neonatal jaundice. Surgical aspects. *Clin. Pediatr. (Phila.)* 3:197, 1964.

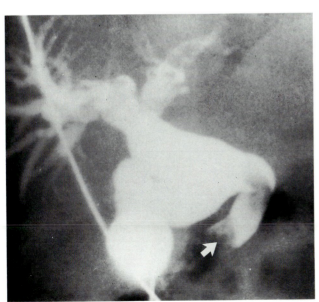

FIG SY–B–10.
Bile plug syndrome. An intraoperative cholangiogram demonstrates obstruction of the common bile duct by an intraluminal mass (bile plug). (From Pfeiffer WR, Robinson LH, Balsara VJ: Sonographic features of bile plug syndrome. *J. Ultrasound Med.* 5:161, 1986. Used by permission.)

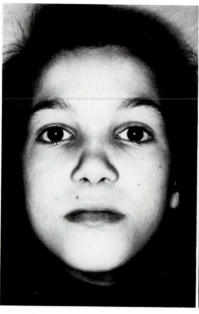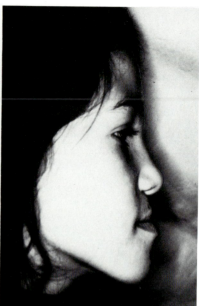

FIG SY–B–11.
Binder syndrome. Nasal anomalies (absent
frontonasal angle, nasal kyphosis, rounded
appearance of the nares) and projection of the
chin are noted. (From Delaire J, Tessier P, Tulasne
JF: Clinical and radiologic aspects of maxillonasal
dysostosis (Binder syndrome). *Head Neck Surg.*
3:105, 1980. Used by permission.)

Sty JR, et al.: Comparative imaging bile-plug syndrome.
  Clin. Nucl. Med. 12:489, 1987.

BINDER SYNDROME

Synonyms: Maxillonasal dysplasia; nasomaxillovertebral
syndrome.

Clinical Manifestations: (a) *craniofacial dysmorphism:
nasal anomalies* (obtuse or almost totally absent frontonasal
angle, downward angling of the nasal pyramid, nasal kyphosis, hypoplasia of the alar cartilage, rounded appearance of
the nares, hypoplastic and ptotic columella, "half-moon" appearance of the external nares, atrophy of the nasal mucosa),
outward projection of the upper lip, projection of the chin,
flatness of the mental area, aplasia of the maxilla and premaxilla around and under the nares and the columella, atrophy of
the frenulum of the upper lip, dental occlusion problems
(obliquity of the upper incisors toward the tongue or mouth,
etc.); (b) cervical kyphosis and scoliosis; (c) other reported
abnormalities: small stature, short legs, thick-set and "square"
feet, strabismus, cleft lip, cleft maxilla, cleft palate, dental
agenesis (incisors, molars), amelogenesis imperfecta, association with Down syndrome, esophageal achalasia (megae-
sophagus).

Radiologic Manifestations: (a) *craniofacial anomalies:*
small glabella, flat nasofrontal angle, vertical position of the
nasal bones, hypoplasia of the frontal process of the maxilla,
thinness of the alveolar bone on the labial side of the upper

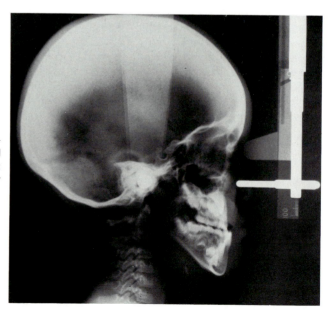

FIG SY–B–12.
Binder syndrome. Maxillonasal hypoplasia, absent nasal spine, severe mandibular prognathism, and hypoplasia of the odontoid
process are demonstrated. (From Delaire J, Tessier P, Tulasne JF:
Clinical and radiologic aspects of maxillonasal dysostosis (Binder
syndrome). *Head Neck Surg.* 3:105, 1980. Used by permission.)

incisors, vestibular version of the incisors, inversion of the incisors, pseudoprognathism or true mandibular prognathism, wide gonial angle; (b) cervical spine anomalies (in about one half of the cases): abnormality of the arch of C_1, ossiculum terminale, separate odontoid process, spina bifida, block vertebrae, persistent chorda dorsalis (central canal of defective mineralization) (Figs SY–B–11 and SY–B–12).

REFERENCES

Binder KH: Dysostosis maxillo-nasalis, ein arhinencephaler Missbildungskomplex. *Dtsch. Zahnärztl. Z.* 17:438, 1962.

Delaire J, et al.: Clinical and radiologic aspects of maxillo-nasal dysostosis (Binder syndrome). *Head Neck Surg.* 3:105, 1980.

Narcy C, et al.: Association méga-oesophage, syndrome de Binder et dysautonomie: une nouvelle neurocristopathie? *Arch. Fr. Pediatr.* 44:119, 1987.

Noyes FB: Case report. *Angle Orthod.* 9:160, 1939.

Olow-Nordenram MAK, et al.: Maxillo-nasal dysplasia (Binder syndrome) and associated malformations of the cervical spine. *Acta. Radiol. [Diagn.] (Stockh.)* 25:353, 1984.

BLIND LOOP SYNDROME

Synonym: Blind pouch syndrome.

Pathology: Formation of a pouch after side-to-side intestinal anastomosis.

Clinical Manifestations: (a) *weight loss;* (b) *growth retardation;* (c) *abdominal cramps;* (d) *malnutrition;* (e) abdominal distension; (f) melena; (g) malabsorption; (h) *macrocytic anemia;* (i) multiple vitamin deficiencies; (j) bacterial overgrowth in the intestine, bile salt inactivation; (k) breath hydrogen test: high basal excretion of breath hydrogen after overnight fasting, an earlier and greater breath hydrogen value after oral lactose administration than is formed in lactose malabsorption alone, sustained hydrogen concentration rise over a period of several hours.

Radiologic Manifestations: (a) spherical, tubular, or club-shaped gas-containing structure on a plain film of the abdomen; (b) pseudotumor if filled with fluid or food debris; (c) *demonstration of a pouch by contrast study of the bowel.*

REFERENCES

Bayes BJ, et al.: Blind loop syndrome in children. *Arch. Dis. Child.* 44:76, 1969.

Brin MF, et al.: Blind loop syndrome, vitamin E malabsorption, and spinocerebellar degeneration. *Neurology (N.Y.)* 35:338, 1985.

Cannon WB, et al.: The movements of the stomach and intestines in some surgical conditions. *Ann. Surg.* 43:512, 1907.

Fromm D: Ileal resection, or disease, and the blind loop syndrome: Current concepts of pathophysiology. *Surgery* 73:639, 1973.

LeVine M, et al.: Blind pouch formation secondary to side to side intestinal anastomosis. *A.J.R.* 89:706, 1963.

Nose O, et al.: Breath hydrogen test in infants and children with blind loop syndrome. *J. Pediatr. Gastroenterol. Nutr.* 3:364, 1984.

Whitaker WG Jr, et al.: Late sequela of blind intestinal pouch. *Am. J. Surg.* 120:752, 1970.

BLOOM SYNDROME

Synonym: Bloom-German syndrome.

Mode of Inheritance: Autosomal recessive; predominance in males.

Frequency: Uncommon.

Clinical Manifestations: (a) *telangiectatic erythema of the face;* (b) *dolichocephaly with malar hypoplasia;* (c) *low birth weight and dwarfism* (well-proportioned minuteness); (d) sensitivity to sunlight; (e) unspecific and variable immunodeficiency (IgA, IgG, IgM); (f) high risk of malignancy: leukemia, lymphoma, carcinoma, Wilms tumor, etc.; (g) *chromosomal breakages and rearrangement,* high frequency of sister chromatid exchanges, cultured fibroblasts of homozygotes and heterozygotes for the syndrome exhibiting an enhanced formation of micronuclei; (h) other reported abnormalities: hypogonadism, porokeratosis of Mibelli, mental retardation, body asymmetry, clinodactyly, microdactyly, etc.

Radiologic Manifestations: Nonspecific: (a) recurrent infections; (b) limb anomalies (syndactyly, supernumerary digits, clinodactyly, absence of toes, short lower limbs, pes equinus).

Differential Diagnosis: Silver-Russell syndrome; Rothmund-Thomson syndrome (Fig SY–B–13).

REFERENCES

Bloom D: Congenital telangiectatic erythema resembling lupus erythematosus in dwarfs. *Am. J. Dis. Child.* 88:754, 1954.

Bloom D: The syndrome of congenital telangiectatic erythema and stunted growth. *J. Pediatr.* 68:103, 1966.

Cairney AEL, et al.: Wilms tumor in three patients with Bloom syndrome. *J. Pediatr.* 111:414, 1987.

Emerit I, et al.: Chromosome breakage factor in the plasma of two Bloom's syndrome patients. *Hum. Genet.* 61:65, 1982.

Frorath B, et al.: Heterozygous carriers for Bloom syndrome exhibit a spontaneously increased micronucleus formation in cultured fibroblasts. *Hum. Genet.* 67:52, 1984.

German J: Bloom's syndrome: I. Genetical and clinical observations in the first twenty-seven patients. *Am. J. Hum. Genet.* 21:196, 1969.

German J, et al.: The Bloom's syndrome registry: Current

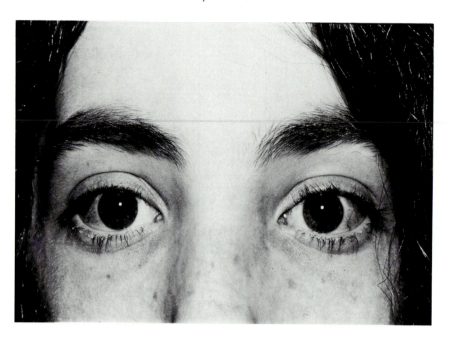

FIG SY−B−13.
Bloom syndrome. Note the telangiectatic lesions on both temporal sides of the conjunctivae. (From Vanderschueren-Lodeweyckx M, Fryns J-P: Bloom's syndrome. Possible pitfalls in clinical diagnosis. *Am. J. Dis. Child.* 138:812, 1984. Used by permission.)

status and incidence of cancer. *Clin. Genet.* 27:310, 1985.

Mulcahy M, et al.: Pregnancy in Bloom's syndrome. *Clin. Genet.* 19:156, 1981.

Rosin MP, et al.: Evidence for chromosome instability in vivo in Bloom syndrome: increased numbers of micronuclei in exfoliated cells. *Hum. Genet.* 71:187, 1985.

Takemiya M, et al.: Bloom's syndrome with porokeratosis of Mibelli and multiple cancers of the skin, lung and colon. *Clin. Genet.* 31:35, 1987.

Vanderschueren-Lodeweyckx M, et al.: Bloom's syndrome. Possible pitfalls in clinical diagnosis. *Am. J. Dis. Child.* 138:812, 1984.

Van Kerckhove CW, et al: Bloom's syndrome. Clinical features and immunologic abnormalities of four patients. *Am. J. Dis. Child.* 142:1089, 1988.

Werner-Favre C, et al.: Cytogenetic study in a mentally retarded child with Bloom syndrome and acute lymphoblastic leukemia. *Am. J. Med. Genet.* 18:215, 1984.

BLUE DIGIT SYNDROME

Synonym: Blue toe syndrome.

Etiology: Embolization of cholesterol-containing material.

Clinical Manifestations: Abrupt appearance of symptoms in the distal parts of extremities (lower portion of the leg, toes, hands, fingers): (a) focal, painful, cyanotic areas with sharp demarcation from the adjacent normally perfused skin; (b) preservation of distal pulses; (c) peripheral gangrene.

Radiologic Manifestations: Angiography: (a) atheroma(s) in a major artery; (b) small distal emboli.

REFERENCES

Brewer ML, et al.: Blue toe syndrome: Treatment with anticoagulants and delayed percutaneous transluminal angioplasty. *Radiology* 166:31, 1988.

Hoye SJ, et al.: Atheromatous embolization: A factor in peripheral gangrene. *N. Engl. J. Med.* 261:128, 1959.

Kermody AM, et al.: "Blue toe" syndrome: An indication for limb salvage surgery. *Arch. Surg.* 111:1263, 1976.

Kumpe DA, et al.: Blue digit syndrome: Treatment with percutaneous transluminal angioplasty. *Radiology* 166:37, 1988.

BLUE RUBBER BLEB NEVUS SYNDROME

Synonym: Bean syndrome.

Mode of Inheritance: Most cases sporadic; autosomal dominant in some families.

Clinical Manifestations: (a) rubbery, raised bluish to black cutaneous *nevi* (cavernous hemangioma, 0.1 to 5 cm in diameter); (b) gastrointestinal bleeding due to *mucosal hemangiomas;* (c) other rare sites of hemangioma: lungs, liver, spleen, joint capsule, deep subcutaneous tissues, thyroid, heart, kidney, brain, spinal cord, meninges, cranial bones, muscles; (d) other reported abnormalities: anemia, chronic consumption coagulopathy, association with Maffucci syn-

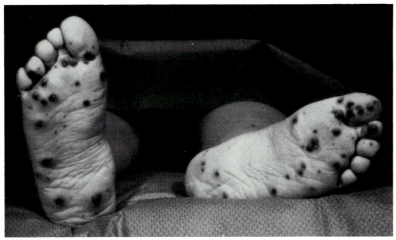

FIG SY–B–14.
Blue rubber bleb nevus syndrome in a 13-year-old girl with blue-black nevi of the feet. Similar lesions were present all over the body, particularly on her trunk and perineum. (From McCauley RGK, Leonadias JC, Bartoshesky LE: Blue rubber bleb nevus syndrome. *Radiology* 133:375, 1979. Used by permission.)

drome (Bean-Maffucci syndrome), association with neoplasms (leukemia, medulloblastoma, hypernephroma, squamous cell carcinoma), intussusception, hypercalcemia, fractures, thrombophlebitis, convulsions, limb asymmetry.

Radiologic Manifestations: (a) *single or multiple polypoid filling defects of the bowel of varying sizes;* (b) phlebolith; (c) *angiographic demonstration of visceral hemangiomas* (early opacification that then increases in the venous phase); (d) magnetic resonance imaging: bright signal on T_2-weighted images that is probably due to slow flow or thrombosis; (e) central nervous system involvement: hemangioma, intracranial calcification, venous thrombosis, brain atrophy, frontal sinus pericranii, venous angioma.

Differential Diagnosis: Glomangiomatosis; multiple cavernous hemangiomatosis involving only the skin; gastrointestinal lesions in Peutz-Jeghers syndrome; Gardner syndrome; Cronkhite-Canada syndrome; Cowden syndrome; Osler-Weber-Rendu syndrome (Figs SY–B–14 and SY–B–15).

REFERENCES

Bean WB: *Vascular Spiders and Related Lesions of the Skin.* Springfield, Ill., Charles C Thomas, Publishers, 1958, pp. 178–185.

Browne AF, et al.: Blue rubber bleb nevi as a cause of intussusception. *J. Pediatr. Surg.* 18:7, 1983.

Jorizzo JR, et al.: MR imaging of blue rubber bleb nevus syndrome. *J. Comput. Assist. Tomogr.* 10:686, 1986.

McCarthy JC, et al.: Orthopaedic dysfunction in the blue rubber–bleb nevus syndrome. *J. Bone Joint Surg. [Am.]* 64:280, 1982.

McCauley RGK, et al.: Blue rubber bleb nevus syndrome. *Radiology* 133:375, 1979.

Oranje AP: Blue rubber bleb nevus syndrome. *Pediatr. Dermatol.* 3:304, 1986.

Satya-Murti S, et al.: Central nervous system involvement in blue-rubber–bleb-nevus syndrome. *Arch. Neurol.* 43:1184, 1986.

Sherry RG, et al.: Sinus pericranii and venous angioma in the blue-rubber bleb nevus syndrome. *A.J.N.R.* 5:832, 1984.

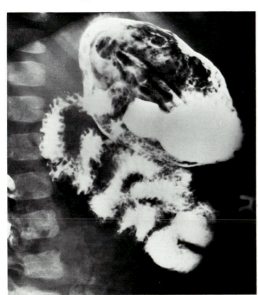

FIG SY–B–15.
Blue rubber bleb nevus syndrome in a 5-year-old boy with multiple cutaneous hemangiomas and chronic gastrointestinal bleeding. Several polypoid filling defects of various sizes are present in the fundus and body of the stomach. (From McCauley RGK, Leonadias JC, Bartoshesky LE: Blue rubber bleb nevus syndrome. *Radiology* 133:375, 1979. Used by permission.)

Travis RC: An unusual cause of gastrointestinal haemorrhage. *Br. J. Radiol.* 60:933, 1987.

BOBBLE-HEAD DOLL SYNDROME

Synonym: Head-bobbling "tic."

Pathology: (a) *suprasellar arachnoid cyst, third ventricle cyst;* (b) *dilated lateral ventricles;* (c) other reported abnormalities: aqueductal stenosis, large cavum vellum interpositum, slow-growing mass in the anterior part of the third ventricle.

Clinical Manifestations: (a) *to-and-fro bobbing or nodding of head and trunk;* (b) other reported abnormalities: precocious puberty, memory loss, delayed developmental milestones, macrocephaly, hyperreflexia, truncal ataxia, mild to moderate mental retardation, optic palor, optic atrophy.

Radiologic Manifestations: *cystic mass; aqueductal stenosis; hydrocephalus.*

REFERENCES

Benton JW, et al.: The bobble-head doll syndrome: Report of a unique truncal tremor associated with third ventricular cyst and hydrocephalus in children. *Neurology (NY)* 16:725, 1966.

Dell S: Further observations on the "Bobble-headed doll syndrome." *J. Neurol. Neurosurg. Psychiatry* 44:1046, 1981.
Jensen HP et al.: Head bobbing in a patient with a cyst of the third ventricle. *Childs Brain* 4:235, 1978.
Kirkham TH: Optic atrophy in the bobble-head doll syndrome. *J. Pediatr. Ophthalmology* 14:299, 1977.
Oubergue A, et al.: Syndrome de la poupée a tête ballotante. Bobble-head doll syndrome. *Arch. Fr. Pediatr.* 42:377, 1985.

BOERHAAVE SYNDROME

Clinical Manifestations: Rupture of all layers of wall of esophagus (posterolateral wall of the distal segment on the left side); triad of (a) *vomiting;* (b) *epigastric and chest pain;* (c) *subcutaneous emphysema;* (d) dyspnea, cyanosis, painful swallowing, abdominal rigidity, etc.

Radiologic Manifestations: (a) *early phase: "V sign"* of Naclerio (localized mediastinal emphysema in the left retrocardiac region corresponding to the fascial planes of the mediastinal and diaphragmatic pleurae); (b) *late phase: pleural effusion or hydropneumothorax, mediastinitis,* spontaneous formation of an esophageal-bronchial fistula; (c) demonstration of the site of tear by contrast study of the esophagus.

Differential Diagnosis: Myocardial infarction; dissecting aneurysm; perforated ulcer (pain as a presenting manifestation) (Fig SY–B–16).

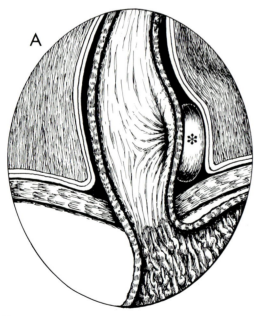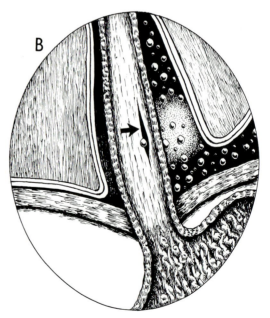

FIG SY–B–16.
Boerhaave syndrome. **A,** a mucosal bubble *(asterisk)* protrudes through the muscular wall and dissects the surrounding mediastinal tissues. **B,** a vertical linear tear in the left posterolateral wall of the esophagus is created. Air is present in the mediastinum. A "pocket" is adjacent to the tear *(arrow)*. (From Rogers LF, Paig AW,

Dooley BN, et al.: Diagnostic consideration in mediastinal emphysema: A pathophysiologic-roentgenologic approach to Boerhaave's syndrome and spontaneous pneumomediastinum. *A.J.R.* 115:495, 1972. Used by permission.)

REFERENCES

Boerhaave H: Atrocis, nec descripti prius, morbi historia: Secundum medicae artis leges conscripta. *Boutesteniana* 1724.

Cadranel JF, et al.: Perforation oesophagienne spontanée. Diagnostic radiologique. *J. Radiol.* 69:45, 1988.

Graeber GM, et al.: A comparison of patients with endoscopic esophageal perforations and patients with Boerhaave's syndrome. *Chest* 92:995, 1987.

Han SY, et al.: Perforation of the esophagus: Correlation of site and cause with plain film findings. *A.J.R.* 145:537, 1985.

Jaworski A, et al: Boerhaave's syndrome. Computed tomographic findings and diagnostic considerations. *Ann. Intern. Med.* 148:223, 1988.

Naclerio EA: The "V sign" in the diagnosis of spontaneous rupture of the esophagus (an early roentgen clue). *Am. J. Surg.* 93:291, 1957.

Patton AS, et al.: Re-evaluation of the Boerhaave syndrome. A review of fourteen cases. *Am. J. Surg.* 137:560, 1979.

Rogers LF, et al.: Diagnostic consideration in mediastinal emphysema: A pathophysiologic-roentgenologic approach to Boerhaave's syndrome and spontaneous pneumomediastinum. *A.J.R.* 115:495, 1972.

Zenone EA, et al.: Boerhaave's syndrome: Spontaneous formation of an esophageal-bronchial fistula. *J.A.M.A.* 238:2048, 1977.

BÖÖK SYNDROME

Synonym: "PHC" syndrome.

Mode of Inheritance: Autosomal dominant with strong penetrance.

Clinical and Radiologic Manifestations: (a) *hypodontia* of the premolar region (P); (b) *hyperhidrosis* of the palms and soles (H); (c) *canities prematura* (premature whitening of the hair) (C).

REFERENCE

Böök JA: Clinical and genetical studies of hypodontia: I. Premolar aplasia, hyperhidrosis, and canities prematura: A new hereditary syndrome in man. *Am. J. Hum. Genet.* 2:240, 1950.

BÖRJESON-FORSSMAN-LEHMANN SYNDROME

Mode of Inheritance: Probably X-linked.

Frequency: Ten published cases (Ardinger et al.).

Clinical Manifestations: (a) *craniofacial features*: microcephaly, prominent supraorbital ridge, deep-set eyes, ptosis, nystagmus, large ears, "coarse" facial appearance; (b) *mental retardation, seizures, hypotonia*; (c) *obesity*; (d) *short stature*; (e) *hypogonadism*; (f) *small hands with tapering hyperextensible fingers*.

Radiologic Manifestations: (a) brain atrophy; (b) *skeletal abnormalities*: steep radiocarpal angle, small femoral and/or humeral heads, narrow cervical spinal canal, scoliosis, Scheurmann-like vertebral changes.

Differential Diagnosis: Prader-Willi syndrome; Coffin-Lowry syndrome; Bardet-Biel syndrome; etc.

REFERENCES

Ardinger HH, et al.: Börjeson-Forssman-Lehmann syndrome: Further delineation in five cases. *Am. J. Med. Genet.* 19:653, 1984.

Börjeson M, Forssman H, Lehmann O: An X-linked recessively inherited syndrome characterized by grave mental deficiency, epilepsy and endocrine disorder. *Acta Med. Scand.* 173:12, 1962.

Robinson LK, et al.: The Börjeson-Forssman-Lehmann syndrome. *Am. J. Med. Genet.* 15:457, 1983.

BOUVERET SYNDROME

Clinical and Radiologic Manifestations: (a) impacted gallstone in duodenal bulb; (b) gastric outlet obstruction.

REFERENCES

Maglinte DDT, et al.: Sonography of Bouvereht's syndrome. *J. Ultrasound Med.* 6:675, 1987.

Patel NM, et al.: Gastric outlet obstruction secondary to a gallstone (Bouveret's syndrome). *J. Clin. Gastroenterol.* 7:277, 1985.

BOWED LONG BONES (FAMILIAL)

Clinical and Radiologic Manifestations: (a) bilateral symmetrical bowing of femora, mild bowing of humeri; (b) self-corrective course.

Differential Diagnosis: Hypophosphatasia; camptomelic dysplasia.

REFERENCES

Conway TJ: Prenatal bowing and angulation of long bones: A description of its occurrence in a brother and sister. *Am. J. Dis. Child.* 95:305, 1958.

Hall BD, et al.: Congenital bowing of the long bones: A review and phenotype analysis of 13 undiagnosed cases. *Eur. J. Pediatr.* 133:131, 1980.

Kapur S, et al.: Isolated congenital bowed long bones. *Clin. Genet.* 29:165, 1986.

Kozlowski K, et al.: Syndromes of congenital bowing of the long bones. *Pediatr. Radiol.* 7:40, 1978.

Mahloudji M, et al.: Prenatal bowing of long bones in two sibs. *Birth Defects* 10:121, 1974.

BRACHYDACTYLY SYNDROME, TYPE E

Mode of Inheritance: Autosomal dominant.

Clinical Manifestations: (a) mild to moderate dwarfism; (b) short hands and feet.

Radiologic Manifestations: Shortness of the metacarpals and metatarsals, in particular, the fourth and fifth; cone-shaped epiphyses; shortness of the phalanges of variable degrees.

REFERENCE

Riccardi VM, et al.: Brachydactyly, type E. *J. Pediatr.* 84:251, 1974.

BRACHYMESOPHALANGIA—NAIL DYSPLASIA

Synonym: Brachydactyly, type A4.

Mode of Inheritance: Autosomal dominant.

Clinical Manifestations: Brachymesodactyly, nail dysplasia.

Radiologic Manifestations: Absence of the middle phalanges in the fingers and lateral four toes; duplicated distal phalanges of the thumbs.

REFERENCE

Bass HN: Familial absence of middle phalanges with nail dysplasia: A new syndrome. *Pediatrics* 42:318, 1968.

BRANCHIO-GENITO-SKELETAL SYNDROME

Synonyms: Branchio-skeleto-genital syndrome; Unger-Trott syndrome; Elsahy-Waters syndrome; craniofacial, genital, dental syndrome (CFGD).

Mode of Inheritance: Probably autosomal recessive or X-linked.

Frequency: Rare.

Clinical Manifestations: (a) mental retardation, seizures; (b) craniofacial features: brachycephaly, ocular hypertelorism, midfacial hypoplasia, wide nasal tip, flared alae, nystagmus, strabismus, mild ptosis, submucous cleft palate, dysplastic dentin, unerupted teeth in adolescents; (c) hypospadias.

Radiologic Manifestations: (a) dentigerous cyst, dysplastic dentine, partial obliteration of pulp chambers; (b) fusion of the second and third cervical vertebrae.

Note: Since there is no evidence of a failure of development of the first branchial arch and its derivatives, the suggestion has been to use the name of craniofacial, genital, dental syndrome (Wedgwood et al.).

REFERENCES

Elsahy NI, Waters WR: The branchio-skeleto-genital syndrome. *Plast. Reconstr. Surg.* 48:542, 1971.
Shafai J, et al.: The branchio-skeleto-genital syndrome: Report of a further case and confirmation of the syndrome. Presented at a Birth Defect Conference, San Diego, 1981.
Wedgwood DL, et al.: Cranio-facial and dental anomalies in the branchio-skeleto-genital (BSG) syndrome with suggestions for more appropriate nomenclature. *Br. J. Oral Surg.* 21:94, 1983.
Witkop CJ: Hereditary defects of dentin. *Dent. Clin. North Am.* 19:25, 1975.

BRANCHIO-OTO-RENAL SYNDROME

Synonyms: BOR syndrome; Melnick-Fraser syndrome.

Mode of Inheritance: Autosomal dominant, variable expressivity and penetrance.

Frequency: Estimated to be approximately 1:40,000; 2% of profoundly deaf children (Heimler et al.).

Clinical Manifestations: (a) asthenic appearance; (b) long and narrow facies, cup-shaped anteverted pinnae, bilateral prehelical pits, deep overbite, constricted palate, bilateral branchial fistulas; (c) mixed hearing deficit, stapes fixation; (d) myopia, aplasia of the lacrimal ducts; (e) other reported abnormalities: association with hemifacial microsomia, Potter syndrome (absent kidneys), gustatory lacrimation, diminished glomerular filtration rate, oligomeganephronic renal hypoplasia and multicystic renal dysplasia (biopsy).

Radiologic Manifestations: (a) renal anomalies (dysplasia, aplasia, polycystic kidney, etc.); (b) middle-ear and inner-ear malformations (Mondini type of cochlear malformation) (Fig SY—B—17).

REFERENCES

Carmi R, et al.: The branchio-oto-renal (BOR) syndrome: Report of bilateral agenesis in three sibs. *Am. J. Med. Genet.* 14:625, 1983.
Heimler A, et al.: Branchio-oto-renal syndrome: Reduced penetrance and variable expressivity in four generations of a large kindred. *Am. J. Med. Genet.* 25:15, 1986.
Melnick M, et al.: Autosomal dominant brancho-oto-renal dysplasia. *Birth Defects* 11:121, 1975.
Preisch JW, et al.: Gustatory lacrimation in association with the branchio-oto-renal syndrome. *Clin. Genet.* 27:506, 1985.

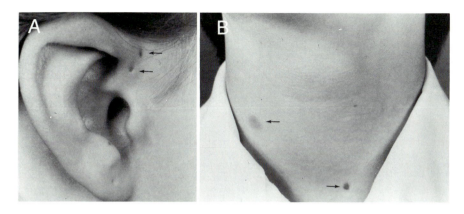

FIG SY–B–17.
Branchio-oto-renal syndrome. **A,** preauricular sinuses *(arrows)*. **B,** note the opening of the branchial arch sinus on either side *(arrows)*. (From Widdershoven J, Monnes L, Assmann K, et al.: Renal disorder in the branchio-oto-renal syndrome. *Helv. Paediatr. Acta* 38:513, 1983. Used by permission.)

Rollnick BR, et al.: Branchio-oto-renal syndrome: Reduced penetrance and variable expressivity in four generations of a large kindred (Letter). *Am. J. Med. Genet.* 27:233, 1987.

Stoll C, et al.: La dysplasie branchio-oto-renale. Un syndrome héréditaire autosomique dominant à expression variable. *Arch. Fr. Pediatr.* 40:763, 1983.

Widdershoven J, et al.: Renal disorders in the branchio-oto-renal syndrome. *Helv. Paediatr. Acta* 38:513, 1983.

BRANCHIO-OTO-URETERAL SYNDROME

Synonym: BOU syndrome.

Mode of Inheritance: Autosomal dominant inheritance has been suggested.

Clinical and Radiologic Manifestations: (a) bilateral sensorineural hearing loss; (b) preauricular pit or tag; (c) duplication of the ureters or bifid renal pelvices.

REFERENCE

Fraser FC, et al.: Autosomal dominant duplication of the renal collecting system, hearing loss, and external ear anomalies: A new syndrome? *Am. J. Med. Genet.* 14:473, 1983.

BROWN SYNDROME

Synonym: Superior oblique tendon sheath syndrome (congenital, acquired).

Definition: Impaired ability to vertically elevate the eye in an adducted position.

Clinical Manifestations: (a) diplopia during upward gaze, especially with the eye in adducted position; (b) pseudopalsy (apparent inferior oblique "palsy"); (c) "clicking" in the area of the trochlea.

Etiology: Congenital or acquired ("simulated Brown syndrome") caused by a mechanical obstacle to the passage of the superior oblique tendon through the trochlea: (a) congenitally short or taut superior oblique tendon sheath complex; (b) swelling of the tendon (trauma, sinusitis, rheumatoid arthritis, etc.).

Radiologic Manifestations: Computed tomography: thickening of the superior oblique tendon; edema of the tendon in acute inflammation and trauma (Fig SY–B–18).

REFERENCES

Brown HW: Congenital structural muscle anomalies, in Allen JH (ed.): *Strabismus Ophthalmic Symposium.* St. Louis, Mosby Co, 1950, pp. 205–236.

Brown HW: True and simulated superior oblique tendon sheath syndromes. *Doc. Ophthalmol.* 34:123, 1973.

Mafee MF, et al.: Computed tomography in the evaluation of Brown syndrome of the superior oblique tendon sheath. *Radiology* 154:691, 1985.

Roifman CM, et al.: Tenosynovitis of the superior oblique muscle (Brown syndrome) associated with juvenile rheumatoid arthritis. *J. Pediatr.* 106:617, 1985.

BROWN-SÉQUARD SYNDROME

Pathology: Unilateral lesion of the spinal cord due to different etiologic factors: trauma, neoplasm, inflammation, degenerative disorders, delayed radiation myelopathy, acute herniated cervical disk, cervical spondylosis, ischemia (embolization, systemic lupus erythematosus, Behçet syndrome, etc.), hemorrhage, cyst, congenital dysraphia, contrast agents, etc.).

Clinical Manifestations: (a) ipsilateral paresis or paralysis below the lesion, associated atrophy, loss of vibratory joint and tendon sensations; (b) contralateral loss of pain and temperature sensibilities.

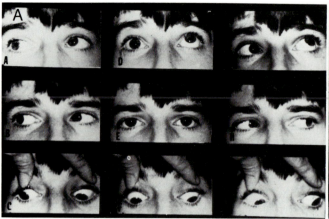

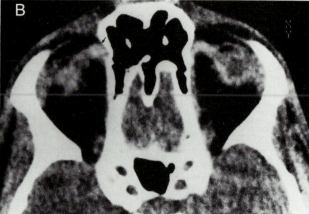

FIG SY−B−18.

A, acquired Brown syndrome with the eyes in various gazing positions. The eyes are normal in the primary (phoria) *(E)*, right lateral *(B)*, left lateral *(H)*, down and right *(C)*, downward midline *(F)*, and down and left positions *(I)*. However, in the upward midline *(D)* and up and left positions (adduction of the right eye) *(G)*, elevation of the right eye is lacking. As the eye is adducted, the level of elevation remains the same until the midline is reached *(D, G)*, at which point full elevation is usually possible *(A)*. When the eye is adducted nasally *(G)* from the primary position *(E)*, the primary action of the inferior oblique muscle is elevation; thus a lack of elevation of the right eye during adduction *(G)*, as in this patient, sim-ulates paralysis of the right inferior oblique tendon, which is the hallmark of Brown syndrome. This actually represents "pseudoparalysis" since the cause is not dysfunction of the right inferior oblique muscle but rather inadequate relaxation of its antagonist, the right superior oblique muscle. **B,** an axial computed tomographic scan demonstrates marked thickening of the reflected tendon *(arrow).* (From Mafee MF, Folk ER, Langer BG, et al.: Computed tomography in the evaluation of Brown syndrome of the superior oblique tendon sheath. *Radiology* 154:691, 1985. Used by permission.)

Radiologic Manifestations: Etiologic factor demonstrated by various imaging modalities.

Note: The term *Brown-Séquard-plus* syndromes has been used for the cases with spinal damage differing widely in extension (e.g., asymmetrical paraplegia).

REFERENCES

Brown-Séquard CE: De la transmission croisée des impressions sensitives par la moelle épinière. *Compt. Rend. Soc. Biol.* 2:33, 1850.

Dundas R: Case of concussion of the spine, tending to confirm the opinion that the nerves of sensation and of motion are distinct. *Edinburgh Med. Surg. J.* 23:304, 1825.

Khardori N et al: Brown-Séquard syndrome secondary to soft tissue infection in a patient with acute lymphocyte leukemia. *Neuroradiology* 30:348, 1988.

Koehler PJ, et al.: Brown-Séquard syndrome due to spinal cord infarction after subclavian vein catheterisation. *Lancet* 2:914, 1985.

Koehler PJ, et al.: The Brown-Séquard syndrome. True or false? *Arch. Neurol.* 43:921, 1986.

BUDD-CHIARI SYNDROME

Synonym: Chiari syndrome.

Pathology: Obstruction of major hepatic veins or obstruction in the intrahepatic portion of the inferior vena cava or ostium of a hepatic vein; concomitant portal vein thrombosis in about 20% of cases.

Etiology: In almost two thirds the etiology not determined; primary (congenital obstruction due to a web or diaphragm) or secondary: thrombus (oral contraceptives, dehydration, septicemia, polycythemia rubra, paroxysmal nocturnal hemoglobinuria), tumor, hydatid cyst of the liver, amebiasis, sickle cell anemia, sarcoidosis, trauma, association with nephrotic syndrome and renal vein thrombosis, leukemia, hepatic torsion, etc.

Clinical Manifestations: (a) abdominal pain; (b) jaundice; (c) hematemesis; (d) edema of the legs; (e) *ascites;* (f) *hepatomegaly;* (g) laboratory manifestations of *hepatocellular dysfunction;* (h) other reported abnormalities: liver failure and shock, association with Behçet syndrome, association with pregnancy.

Radiologic Manifestations: (a) *ascites;* (b) *esophageal varices;* (c) *ultrasonography:* thickened wall of hepatic veins, stenosis, irregularity of the venous wall, proximal dilatation, thrombosis, intrahepatic collateral circulation, slow flow and site of obstruction shown by Doppler technique, compression of the inferior vena cava by the enlarged liver, tumor and/or clot in the inferior vena cava, cirrhosis, etc; (d) *computed tomography:* hepatomegaly, cirrhosis, hypodensity on a plain scan, absence of opacification of the hepatic veins on a postcontrast injection scan that is associated with a central "fan-shaped" patchy zone of increased attenuation followed by a

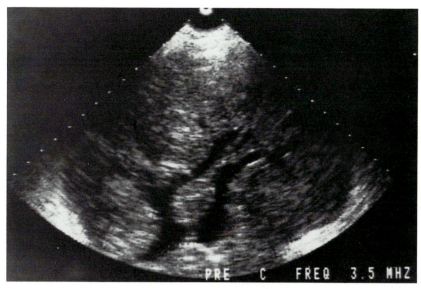

FIG SY–B–19.
Budd-Chiari syndrome. A longitudinal sonogram shows irregular hepatic veins with focal areas of dilatation. (From Murphy FB, Steinberg HV, Shire GT, et al.: The Budd-Chiari syndrome: A review. *A.J.R.* 147:9, 1986. Used by permission.)

decrease in attenuation, inhomogeneous liver density (slow blood flow and collateral venous opacification), etc; (e) *magnetic resonance imaging:* reduction in the caliber or complete absence of the hepatic veins, "comma-shaped" intrahepatic collateral vessels, slow flow, thrombosis, laminar clot, tumor, hepatomegaly, inhomogeneity of the liver parenchyma, constriction of the vena cava, cirrhosis, varices, splenomegaly, etc; (f) *venography:* inferior vena constriction due to hepatomegaly, irregular filling defects in the inferior vena cava or the hepatic veins, web, clot, occlusion of the inferior vena cava with or without collateral vessels, "spider-web"-type collateral intrahepatic veins shown by hepatic wedge venography, pressure measurement demonstrating a gradient at the site of obstruction; (g) *arteriography:* stretching, narrowing, and pruning of the hepatic arteries; decreased hepatopedal flow or hepatofugal flow; varices; etc.; (h) *nuclear medicine* (⁹⁹ᵐTc sulfur colloid): normal or abnormal (decreased activity in the right and left lobes; caudate lobe appearing as a "hot spot," possibly due to a separate venous drainage into the inferior vena cava, etc.) (Figs SY–B–19 to SY–B–21).

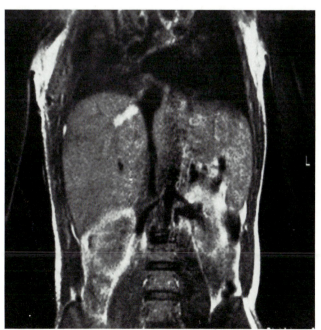

FIG SY–B–20.
Budd-Chiari syndrome. A coronal magnetic resonance image shows a high-intensity signal in an obstructed middle hepatic vein. The inferior vena cava is minimally narrowed secondary to hepatomegaly. (From Murphy FB, Steinberg HV, Shire GT, et al.: The Budd-Chiari syndrome: A review. *A.J.R.* 147:9, 1986. Used by permission.)

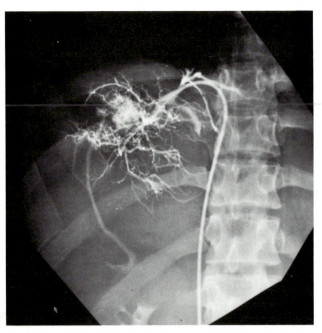

FIG SY—B—21.
Budd-Chiari syndrome. A selective hepatic wedge venogram shows the characteristic "spider-web" pattern of collateral intrahepatic veins. (From Murphy FB, Steinberg HV, Shire GT, et al.: The Budd-Chiari syndrome: A review. *A.J.R.* 147:9, 1986. Used by permission.)

REFERENCES

Brunelle F, et al.: Familial Budd Chiari disease: Angiographic study in two sisters. *Pediatr. Radiol.* 11:91, 1981.

Budd G: *On Diseases of the Liver,* ed. 7. London, J. & A. Churchill Ltd, 1845, p. 146.

Chiari H: Ueber die selbständige Phlebitis obliterans der Haupstamme der Venae hepaticae als Todesursache. *Beitr. Pathol. Anat.* 26:1, 1899.

Gentil-Kocher S, et al.: Budd-Chiari syndrome in children: Report of 22 cases. *J. Pediatr.* 113:30, 1988.

Kobayashi A, et al.: Calcification in caval membrane causing primary Budd-Chiari syndrome: CT demonstration. *J. Comput. Assist. Tomogr.* 12:401, 1988.

Makuuchi M, et al.: Primary Budd-Chiari syndrome: Ultrasonic demonstration. *Radiology* 152:775, 1984.

Mathieu D, et al.: Budd-Chiari syndrome: Dynamic CT. *Radiology* 165:409, 1987.

Montagnac R, et al.: Le syndrome de Budd-Chiari, complication inhabituelle de la maladie de Behçet. *Presse Med.* 15:1427, 1986.

Murphy FB, et al.: The Budd-Chiari syndrome: A review. *A.J.R.* 147:9, 1986.

Natalino MR, et al.: The Budd-Chiari syndrome in sarcoidosis. *J.A.M.A.* 239:2657, 1978.

Schraut WH, et al.: Metastatic Wilms' tumor causing acute hepatic vein occlusion (Budd-Chiari syndrome). *Gastroenterology* 88:576, 1985.

Sequeira FW, et al.: Budd-Chiari syndrome caused by hepatic torsion. *A.J.R.* 137:393, 1981.

Stark DD, et al.: MRI of the Budd-Chiari syndrome. *A.J.R.* 146:1141, 1986.

Van Beers B, et al.: Hepatic heterogeneity on CT in Budd-Chiari syndrome: Correlation with regional disturbances in portal flow. *Gastrointest. Radiol.* 13:61, 1988.

Vogelzang RL, et al.: Budd-Chiari syndrome: CT observations. *Radiology* 163:329, 1987.

BURNING HANDS SYNDROME

Etiology: Probably due to a concussion of the spinal cord resulting in spinothalamic tract dysfunction.

Clinical Manifestations: (a) *burning dysesthesias and paresthesia in the hands;* (b) *somatosensory evoked potentials (SSEPs): decrease in amplitude of positive waves.*

Radiologic Manifestations: (a) cervical spine trauma; (b) magnetic resonance imaging: *widening of the spinal cord, increase in the signal intensity from the cord parenchyma.*

REFERENCES

Maroon JC: Burning hands in football spinal cord injuries. *J.A.M.A.* 238:2051, 1977.

Wilberger JE, et al.: Burning hands syndrome revisited. *Neurosurgery* 19:1038, 1986.

C SYNDROME

Synonym: Opitz trigonocephaly syndrome.

Mode of Inheritance: Autosomal recessive has been suggested.

Frequency: Rare.

Clinical Manifestations: (a) *short stature at birth;* (b) *craniofacial dysmorphism:* trigonocephaly, microcephaly, broad nasal bridge, epicanthus, short nose, upward-slanting palpebral fissures, micrognathia, thick anterior alveolar ridges, multiple oral frenula, low simple philtrum, macrostomia, abnormal ear (abnormal shape, reduced cartilage, low-set and/or posteriorly rotated), anterior "cowlick," strabismus; (c) *limb anomalies:* short limbs, polysyndactyly, cutaneous syndactyly of the toes, varus or equinovarus deformities, ulnar deviation of the fingers, contracture, hyperextensibility; (d) other reported abnormalities: pectus deformities, congenital heart disease, cryptorchidism, prominent clitoris, neonatal loose skin, hemangiomas, mental retardation in surviving children, multiple gingival frenula, joint contractures, renal cortical cysts, terminal transverse limb reduction defects, severe hypotonia, seizures, psychomotor retardation, etc.

Radiologic Manifestations: (a) *trigonocephaly,* "heaped-up" sagittal and metopic cranial sutures, incomplete bony fusion, bone defect between the orbits, microcephaly; (b) trunk: anomalous ribs, fused sternal ossification centers, scoliosis; (c) limbs: hypoplasia of the metacarpals and phalanges, polydactyly, syndactyly, radial head dislocation, hip dislocation, cupping of the metaphyses of the metacarpal bones, skeletal maturation retardation, terminal transverse limb reduction (absence of the distal phalanges of the hand and foot), etc. (Fig SY−C−1).

REFERENCES

Flatz SD, et al.: Opitz trigonocephaly syndrome: Report of two cases. *Eur. J. Pediatr.* 141:183, 1984.
Fryns JP, et al.: Opitz trigonocephaly syndrome and terminal transverse limb reduction defects. *Helv. Paediatr. Acta* 40:485, 1985.
Opitz JM, et al.: The C syndrome of multiple congenital anomalies. *Birth Defects* 5:161, 1969.

CAFFEY DISEASE

Synonyms: Infantile cortical hyperostosis; de Toni-Caffey disease; Caffey-Silverman disease; Caffey-Smyth disease; Röske-de Toni-Caffey-Smyth disease.

Mode of Inheritance: An autosomal dominant transmission has been suggested in some cases.

Clinical Manifestations: Onset of symptoms in early infancy, prenatal onset rare; (a) irritability, fever, pallor; (b) soft-tissue swelling adjacent to involved bones; (c) pseudoparalysis, Erb palsy, diaphragmatic paralysis and eventration, radial nerve palsy, absence of biceps and triceps reflexes; (d) increase in the erythrocyte sedimentation rate (ESR), thrombocythemia, elevated serum alkaline phosphatase level, raised immunoglobulin concentration, in particular IgA and IgM, elevated white blood cell level, increased C-reactive protein levels; (e) other reported abnormalities: nasal obstruction, vitamin E deficiency, orbital swelling and ocular proptosis, maternal herpes zoster, dysphagia, association with the Wiskott-Aldrich syndrome, good response to high-dose immunoglobulin, etc.

Radiologic Manifestations: (a) *subperiosteal cortical hyperostosis* (slight periosteal thickening, dense laminated subperiosteal new bone formation or a marked increase in the width and density of the cortex); (b) *epiphyses of the long bones spared;* (c) *mandible, clavicle, and ribs* most often involved; (d) lytic skull lesions uncommon (frontal, parietal, nasal, and zygomatic bones); carpal, tarsal, and vertebral bodies very rarely involved; (e) prominent uptake of bone-seeking radionuclide agent before lesions become detectable by radiographic technique; (f) sequelae: mandibular asymmetry, undergrowth of the mandible, synostosis of the ribs and bones of the forearms and legs, bowing of long bones, leg-length discrepancy, recurrence of disease in childhood; (g) other reported abnormalities: disappearing intramedullary lytic bone lesions, monostotic disease, disease limited to the ribs, association with osteomyelitis, etc.

Differential Diagnosis: Osteomyelitis; congenital syphilis; skeletal dysplasias with osteosclerosis (Fig SY−C−2).

REFERENCES

Abinuun M, et al.: Infantile cortical hyperostosis associated with the Wiskott-Aldrich syndrome. *Eur. J. Pediatr.* 147:518, 1988.
Berthier M, et al.: Caffey disease responding to high-dose immunoglobulin. *Eur. J. Pediatr.* 147:443, 1988.
Blank E: Recurrent Caffey's cortical hyperostosis and persistent deformity. *Pediatrics* 55:856, 1975.
Blasier RB, et al.: Infantile cortical hyperostosis with osteomyelitis of the humerus. *J. Pediatr. Orthop.* 5:222, 1985.
Caffey J, Silverman WA: Infantile cortical hyperostosis: Preliminary report on a new syndrome. *A.J.R.* 54:1, 1945.

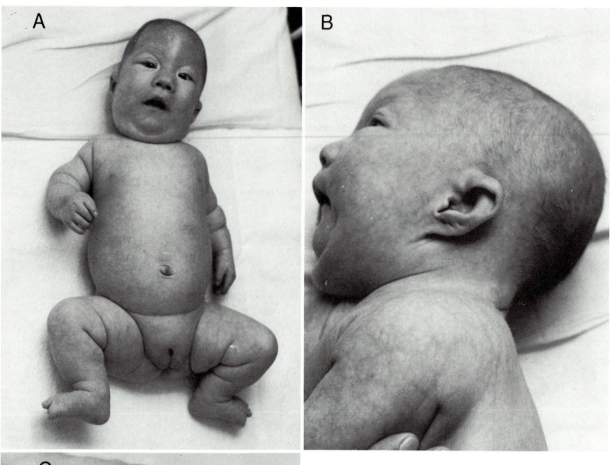

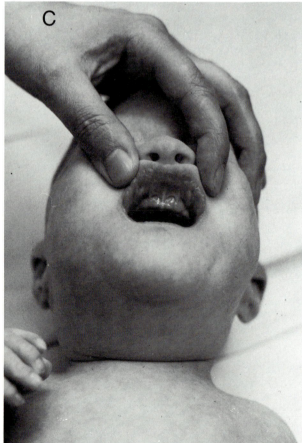

FIG SY–C–1.
A–C, C syndrome (Opitz trigonocephaly syndrome) in an 8-week-old infant with trigonocephaly, upslanted palpebral fissures, inner epicanthic folds, abnormally located and shaped ears, broad alveolar ridges, numerous labiogingival frenula, and a small chin. (From Flatz SD, Schinzel A, Doehring E, et al.: Opitz trigonocephaly syndrome. *Eur. J. Pediatr.* 141:183, 1984. Used by permission.)

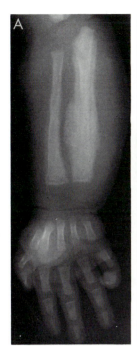
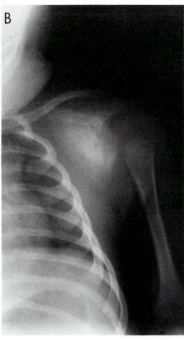

FIG SY—C—2.
Caffey disease. A 5-week-old female had intermittent fever, hyperirritability, and swelling of her right forearm. This was followed by development of swelling over the left scapulum, mandible, and bridge of the nose. She had an elevated ESR, leukocytosis, and thrombocythemia. **A,** subperiosteal cortical hyperostosis of the shaft of the radius and ulna. **B,** hyperostosis of the scapulum and subperiosteal cortical reaction of the mandible.

Claëssan I: Infantile cortical hyperostosis: Report of a case with late manifestations. *Acta Radiol. [Diag.] (Stockh.)* 17:594, 1976.

Fauré C, et al.: Predominant or exclusive orbital and facial involvement in infantile cortical hyperostosis (de Toni-Caffey's disease). *Pediatr. Radiol.* 6:103, 1977.

Gentry RR, et al.: Infantile cortical hyperostosis of the ribs (Caffey's disease) without mandibular involvement. *Pediatr. Radiol.* 13:236, 1983.

Harris V, et al.: Caffey's disease: A case originating in the first metatarsal and review of a 12 year experience. *A.J.R.* 130:335, 1978.

Kaufmann HJ, et al.: Monosteal infantile cortical hyperostosis. *Skeletal Radiol.* 2:109, 1977.

Keeton BR: Vitamin E deficiency and thrombocytosis in Caffey's disease. *Arch. Dis. Child.* 51:393, 1976.

Leung VC, et al.: Infantile cortical hyperostosis with intramedullary lesions. *J. Pediatr. Orthop.* 5:354, 1985.

Marshall GS, et al.: Sporadic congenital Caffey's disease. *Clin. Pediatr. (Phila.)* 26:177, 1987.

Ramchander V, et al.: Infantile cortical hyperostosis with raised immunoglobulins. *Arch. Dis. Child.* 53:426, 1978.

Röske G: Eine eigenartige Knochenerkrankung im Saüglingsalter. *Monatsschr. Kinderheilkd.* 47:385, 1930.

Sheppard JJ, et al.: Dysphagia in infantile cortical hyperostosis (Caffey's disease): A case study. *Dev. Med. Child Neurol.* 30:108, 1988.

Smyth FS, et al.: Periosteal reaction, fever, and irritability in young infants: A new syndrome? *Am. J. Dis. Child.* 71:333, 1946.

Tabardel Y, et al.: Maladie de Caffey-Silverman néonatale avec thrombocytose, augmentation de la C-réactive protéine et des immunoglobulines. *Arch. Fr. Pediatr.* 45:263, 1988.

Taillefer R, et al.: Aspect scintigraphique de l'hyperostose corticale infantile (maladie de Caffey). *J. Can. Assoc. Radiol.* 34:12, 1983.

Tien R, et al.: Caffey's disease: Nuclear medicine and radiologic correlation: A case of mistaken identity. *Clin. Nucl. Med.* 13:583, 1988.

Yousefzadeh DK, et al.: Infantile cortical hyperostosis, Caffey's disease, involving two cousins. *Skeletal Radiol.* 4:141, 1979.

CALCINOSIS UNIVERSALIS

Clinical Manifestations: Onset usually before the age of 20 years, more common in females: (a) fatigue; (b) difficulty in locomotion; (c) muscular pain; (d) low-grade fever; (e) *palpable calcific plaques in subcutaneous or deeper tissues;* (f) high levels of γ-carboxyglutamic acid in involved tissues and in the urine.

Radiologic Manifestations: (a) *long bands of symmetrical subcutaneous calcification with progressive spread to deeper connective tissues* (tendons, ligaments, nerve sheaths); (b) leak of calcium deposits through the skin; (c) extraskeletal uptake of technetium 99m—high-density polyethylene oxidronate.

Note: Calcinosis universalis in about one third of cases is secondary to scleroderma or dermatomyositis.

REFERENCES

Berger RG, et al.: Treatment of calcinosis universalis with low-dose warfarin. *Am. J. Med.* 83:72, 1987.

Hilbish TF, et al.: Roentgen findings in abnormal deposition of calcium in tissues. *A.J.R.* 87:1128, 1962.

Simons M, et al.: La calcinose idiopathique. *Ann. Pediatr. (Paris)* 32:501, 1985.

Teissier LJ: *Du Diabéte Phosphatique* (thesis). Paris, 1876.

CALVARIAL DOUGHNUT LESIONS-OSTEOPOROSIS-DENTINOGENESIS IMPERFECTA

Mode of Inheritance: Probably autosomal dominant.

Frequency: Very rare.

Clinical Manifestations: (a) multiple fractures; (b) lumps on the head; (c) dental caries, underdeveloped teeth; (d) elevated serum alkaline phosphatase level.

Radiologic Manifestations: (a) osteoporosis; (b) calvarial doughnut lesions (round radiolucency surrounded by a dense

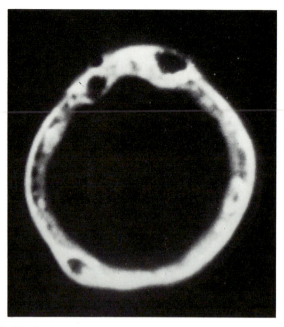

FIG SY—C—3
Calvarial doughnut syndrome. CT scan of the skull in a 21-year-old man shows radiolucent lesions in the diploë with sclerotic rims. There is localized expansion of the outer and inner tables at the level of the lesions. (From Colavita N, Kozlowski K, LaVecchia G, et al.: Calvarial doughnut lesions with osteoporosis, multiple fractures, dentinogenesis imperfecta and tumorous changes in the jaws: Report of a case. *Australas. Radiol.* 28:226, 1984. Used by permission.)

ring of sclerotic bone); (c) dentinogenesis imperfecta; (d) other reported abnormalities: "bone-in-bone" appearance of the vertebral bodies, lateral bowing of the femora, deformities related to the old fractures (long bones, vertebrae), tubulation defects of the diaphyses of the long bones, squaring of metacarpal bones, high uptake of calvarial lesions on bone scintigraphy, etc. (Fig SY—C—3).

REFERENCES

Aubé L, et al.: Lésions en beignet de la voûte crânienne: Une dysplasie osseuse héréditaire. *J. Can. Assoc. Radiol.* 39:204, 1988.
Bartlett JE, et al.: Familial "doughnut" lesions of the skull. *Radiology* 119:385, 1976.
Colavita N, et al: Calvarial doughnut lesions with osteoporosis, multiple fractures, dentinogenesis imperfecta and tumorous changes in the jaws: Report of a case. *Australas. Radiol.* 28:226, 1984.

CALVARIAL HYPEROSTOSIS, FAMILIAL

Mode of Inheritance: X-linked recessive: three males in two generations.

Clinical and Radiologic Manifestations: (a) bony prominence in the frontoparietal regions (lateral frontal horn); (b) calvarial hyperostosis (frontal, parietal, occipital) with thickened diploic spaces, prominent bony trabeculae; (c) normal skeletal survey (excluding the skull).

Pathology: Dense trabecular bone separated by stroma packed with large, morphologically unusual histiocytes, etc.

Differential Diagnosis: Frontometaphyseal dysplasia; thickened calvarium associated with a hematologic disorder (thalassemia, etc).

REFERENCES

Pagon RA, et al.: Calvarial hyperostosis: A benign X-linked recessive disorder. *Clin. Genet.* 29:73, 1986.

CAMPTODACTYLY-ICHTHYOSIS SYNDROME

Mode of Inheritance: Autosomal recessive.

Clinical and Radiologic Manifestations: (a) distal arthrogryposis: windmill vane camptodactyly affecting all limbs, ulnar deviation of the fingers, vertical talus, calcaneovalgus deformity; (b) motor delay, generalized muscular hypoplasia; (c) generalized ichthyosis involving flexures; (d) reduced facial mobility.

REFERENCES

Baraitser M, et al.: A recessively inherited windmill-vane camptodactyly/ichthyosis syndrome. *J. Med. Genet.* 20:125, 1983.

CAMPTODACTYLY—SENSORINEURAL HEARING LOSS SYNDROME

Mode of Inheritance: Autosomal dominant with complete penetrance and variable expressivity.

Clinical and Radiologic Manifestations: (a) *camptodactyly;* congenital flexion contracture of the digits; wasting of thenar, hypothenar, and interosseous muscles; (b) *sensorineural hearing loss;* (c) limitation of motion of the toes.

REFERENCE

Stewart JM, et al.: Familial hand abnormality and sensorineural deafness. A new syndrome. *J. Pediatr.* 78:102, 1971.

CANAVAN DISEASE

Synonyms: Spongy degeneration of the van Bogaert-Bertrand type; Canavan-van Bogaert-Bertrand disease.

Mode of Inheritance: Autosomal recessive.

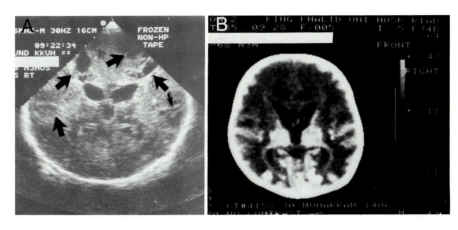

FIG SY−C−4.
Canavan disease in a 3-month-old female. **A,** a coronal cranial sonogram shows diffuse leukomalacia and multiple anechoic areas. **B,** an axial computed tomography scan shows diffuse, low-attenuation white matter in both hemispheres. (From Patel PJ, Ko-lawole TM, Mahdi AH, et al.: Sonographic and computed tomographic findings in Canavan's disease. *Br. J. Radiol.* 59:1226, 1986. Used by permission.)

Pathology: *Spongy change predominantly affecting the white matter (lipid-filled glial cells).*

Clinical Manifestations: Onset of symptoms in early infancy: (a) *megaloencephaly;* (b) *initial hypotonia followed by spasticity;* (c) *progressive psychomotor degeneration;* (d) *blindness;* (e) *increased amount of N-acetylaspartic acid in the urine and plasma.*

Radiologic Manifestations: (a) ultrasonography: *increased sonolucency of the white matter, multiple anechoic cavitary lesions* (lack of myelin, increased water content); (b) computed tomography (CT) and magnetic resonance imaging: diffuse *low CT attenuation due to demyelinating white matter disease, increase in signal intensity on T_2-weighted spin-echo sequences* (demyelination effect), brain atrophy (Fig SY−C−4).

REFERENCES

Andriola MR: Computed tomography in the diagnosis of Canavan's disease. *Ann. Neurol.* 11:323, 1982.
Brown LW, et al.: Psychomotor retardation and macrocephaly in an infant. *Pediatr. Neurosci.* 12:266, 1985.
Matalon R, et al.: Aspartoacylase deficiency and N-acetylaspartic aciduria in patients with Canavan disease. *Am. J. Med. Genet.* 29:463, 1988.
Patel PJ, et al.: Sonographic and computed tomographic findings in Canavan's disease. *Br. J. Radiol.* 59:1226, 1986.

CANTRELL SYNDROME

Synonyms: Septum transversum syndrome; thoracoabdominal wall defect; pentalogy of Cantrell.

Frequency: Uncommon.

Pathology: (a) *Combined anterior abdominal wall, diaphragmatic, sternal, pericardial, and intracardiac defects;* (b) other reported abnormalities: anencephaly, hydrocephalus, cleft palate, absent lung, asphyxiating thoracic dysplasia, Turner syndrome.

Clinical Manifestations: (a) *diastasis, omphalocele or umbilical hernia;* (b) *chest wall defect,* ectopia cordis through the defect in the distal portion of the sternum; (c) congenital heart disease.

Radiologic Manifestations: (a) *sternal defect;* (b) *dextroposition of the heart;* (c) *intrapericardial herniation of abdominal organs;* (d) *cardiac anomalies* (ventricular septal defect, atrial septal defect, pulmonary stenosis, tetralogy of Fallot, anomalous pulmonary venous drainage, ventricular diverticulum, etc. (Fig SY−C−5).

REFERENCES

Abu-Yousef MM, et al.: Antenatal ultrasound diagnosis of variant of pentalogy of Cantrell. *J. Ultrasound Med.* 6:531, 1987.
Cantrell JR, et al.: A syndrome of congenital defects involving the abdominal wall, sternum, diaphragm, pericardium and heart. *Surg. Gynecol. Obstet.* 107:602, 1958.
Casey BM, et al.: Syndrome of mesodermal defects involving the abdominal wall, diaphragm, sternum, heart and pericardium. *Br. J. Radiol.* 48:52, 1975.
Fox JE, et al.: Trisomy 18 with Cantrell pentalogy in a stillborn infant. *Am. J. Med. Genet.* 31:391, 1988.
Garson A Jr, et al.: Thoracoabdominal ectopia cordis with mosaic Turner's syndrome: Report of a case. *Pediatrics* 62:218, 1978.
Ghidini A, et al.: Prenatal diagnosis of pentalogy of Cantrell. *J. Ultrasound Med.* 7:567, 1988.
Wesselhoeft CW, et al.: Neonatal septum transversum diaphragmatic defects. *Am. J. Surg.* 147:481, 1984.

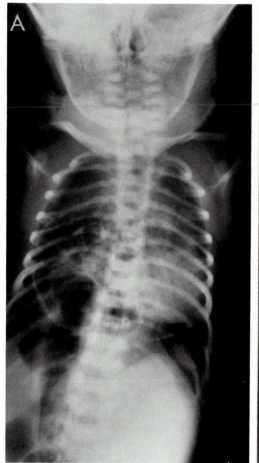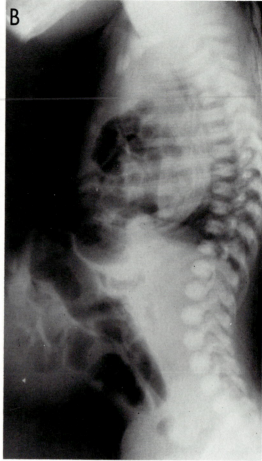

FIG SY–C–5.
Cantrell syndrome. Roentgenograms of the chest and abdomen in the anteroposterior, **(A)** and lateral, **(B)** projections demonstrate a midline defect of the abdominal wall and intrapericardial her-niation of the bowel in a newborn. (Courtesy of Dr. James J. Du Bois, Letterman General Hospital, San Francisco.)

Zachariou Z, et al.: Das Cantrellsche Syndrom. *Z. Kinder-chir.* 42:255, 1987.

CAPLAN SYNDROME

Clinical Manifestations: (a) signs and symptoms of rheumatoid arthritis; (b) cough, dyspnea; (c) biopsy of lung nodules: dust particles, necrosis; (d) energy-dispersive x-ray microanalysis of the dust particles that demonstrates silicon and other materials.

Radiologic Manifestations: (a) disseminated lung nodules, some with cavitation, pleural thickening and calcification, calcification within some nodules, pulmonary fibrotic changes; (b) roentgenologic findings of rheumatoid arthritis.

REFERENCES

Anttila S, et al.: Rheumatoid pneumoconiosis in a dolomite worker: A light and electron microscopic, and x-ray microanalytical study. *Br. J. Dis. Chest* 78:195, 1984.

Caplan JA: Certain unusual radiological appearances in the chest of coal-miners suffering from rheumatoid arthritis. *Thorax* 8:29, 1953.
Greaves IA: Rheumatoid "pneumoconiosis" (Caplan syndrome) in an asbestos worker: A 17 years' followup. *Thorax* 34:404, 1979.
Mattson S-B: Caplan's syndrome in association with asbestosis. *Scand. J. Respir. Dis.* 52:153, 1971.

CARCINOID SYNDROME

Etiology: The syndrome occurs when the humoral output of tumors (primary and metastases) exceeds the capacity of monoamine oxidase present in the liver and lung for metabolism of serotonin; rare occurrence of "carcinoid syndrome" reported in noncarcinoid malignant tumors and dermatomyositis; the syndrome is usually associated with *liver metastasis*.

Pathology: Deposition of fibrous tissue on cardiac valves and endocardium resulting in tricuspid stenosis and insufficiency, pulmonary stenosis, and rarely, left-sided valvular in-

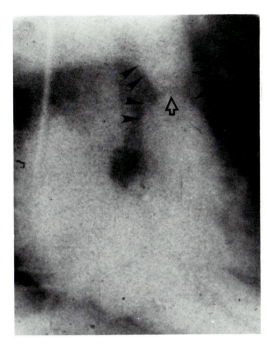

FIG SY−C−6.
Carcinoid syndrome with cardiac involvement in a 56-year-old man with clinical manifestations of carcinoid syndrome, tricuspid valvar stenosis, and insufficiency. Cardioangiography in right anterior oblique view with injection of contrast material into the right atrium shows that the pulmonic valve annulus is narrowed *(arrow);* the proximal pulmonary artery and subvalvar right ventricular infundibulum taper toward the valve (hourglass appearance) *(arrowheads).* (From Holt RG, Gross R, Carlsson E: Angiographic features of carcinoid heart disease. *Radiology* 127:601, 1978. Used by permission.)

volvement, loss of trabeculation of the ventricle due to endocardial fibrosis.

Mode of Inheritance: Familial cases reported in a father and daughter and in a brother and sister.

Clinical Manifestations: (a) *flushing of the skin,* telangiectasia of the face and neck; (b) *episodes of diarrhea and abdominal cramps,* digestive tract bleeding, bowel obstruction; (c) deficiency syndromes; (d) attacks of *wheezing;* (e) intractable right-sided congestive heart failure, valvular heart disease (usually right sided), pericarditis; (f) *hypertension;* (g) *secretion of pharmacologically active substances:* serotonin, kallikrein, substance P, prostaglandins; (h) other reported abnormalities: arthropathy, psychiatric symptoms, pellagra.

Radiologic Manifestations: (a) small bowel most common site of tumor; *atypical intramural defect in earlier stage and intraluminal lobulated growth in later stage;* direct extension of tumor into the mesentery with a resultant fanlike appearance of the mucosa; bowel obstruction; intussusception; bowel perforation; rapid transit time of barium; angiographic demonstration of a stellate arterial pattern, narrowing of deep mesenteric branches, poor to moderate tumor stain, and lack of visualization of draining veins; *computed tomography demonstration of a mesenteric soft-tissue mass with radiating linear strands, primary tumor (often in the distal portion of the ileum), retroperitoneal lymph node enlargement, liver metastasis;* (b) bronchial tree tumor; (c) *carcinoid heart disease:* (1) cardiomegaly, right-sided heart failure; (2) two-dimensional echography: *thickening, shortening, and immobility of the tricuspid valve leaflets in association with valvular regurgitation; thickening and doming of the tricuspid valve in association with stenosis,* no evidence of commissural fusion, *pulmonary valvular abnormalities similar to the*

tricuspid valve disease; (3) cardioangiography: *tricuspid stenosis and insufficiency, pulmonary stenosis (hourglass tapering toward the valve:* proximal pulmonary artery and subvalvular right ventricular outflow tract); (d) *scintiscanning with the use of* ^{131}I *meta*-iodobenzylguanidine (MIBG): intense tracer uptake in the tumor and metastasis (Figs SY−C−6 and SY−C−7).

REFERENCES

Adolph JMG, et al.: Carcinoid tumors: CT and I-131 meta-iodo-benzylguanidine scintigraphy. *Radiology* 164:199, 1987.

Bancks NH, et al.: The roentgenologic spectrum of small intestinal carcinoid tumor. *A.J.R.* 123:274, 1975.

Carrasco CH, et al.: The carcinoid syndrome: Palliation by hepatic artery embolization. *A.J.R.* 147:149, 1986.

Forman MB, et al.: Two-dimensional echocardiography in the diagnosis of carcinoid heart disease. *Am. Heart J.* 107:492, 1984.

Holt RG, et al.: Angiographic features of carcinoid heart disease. *Radiology* 127:601, 1978.

Oates JA: The carcinoid syndrome. *N. Engl. J. Med.* 315:702, 1986.

Picus D, et al.: Computed tomography of abdominal carcinoid tumors. *A.J.R.* 143:581, 1984.

Ricci C, et al.: Carcinoid syndrome in bronchial adenoma. *Am. J. Surg.* 126:671, 1973.

Rich LL, et al.: Carcinoid pericarditis. *Am. J. Med.* 54:522, 1973.

Stephan E, et al.: Carcinoid heart disease from primary carcinoid tumour of the ovary. Haemodynamic and cine coronary angiocardiographic study after operation. *Br. Heart J.* 36:613, 1974.

Yang D, et al.: Dermatomyositis, myocardial involvement and carcinoid syndrome. *J.A.M.A.* 239:1067, 1978.

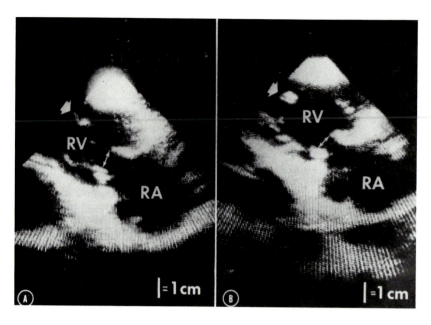

FIG SY–C–7.
Carcinoid heart disease: **A,** parasternal long-axis view of the right atrium *(RA)* and right ventricle *(RV)*. Both chambers are enlarged, and the tricuspid valve is thick, shortened, and immobile; the *small arrow* indicates the reduced valve orifice measured at the time of maximal opening. The *large arrow* indicates the papillary muscle, which has increased echo density compatible with endocardial thickening. **B,** the same view 2 months later shows progression of the tricuspid valve lesions with a further reduction in the tricuspid valve opening *(small arrow)* and more papillary muscle endocardial thickening *(large arrow)*. (From Forman MB, Byrd BF, Oates JA, et al.: Two-dimensional echo-cardiography in the diagnosis of carcinoid heart disease. *Am. Heart J.* 107:492, 1984. Used by permission.)

CARDIOAUDITORY SYNDROMES (DEAFNESS AND HEART DISEASES)

Clinical and Radiologic Manifestations: (a) extraordinarily long Q–T interval and deaf mutism (Jervell and Lange-Nielsen syndrome); (b) pulmonary stenosis (valvular, infundibular, or both) and deaf mutism; (c) left ventricular hypertrophy, right ventricular hypertrophy (in some), and deaf mutism (cardioauditory syndrome of Sanchez-Cascos); (d) mitral insufficiency, conductive deafness, dwarfism, and pigmentary changes of the iris.

REFERENCES

Forney WR, et al.: Congenital heart disease, deafness, and skeletal malformations: A new syndrome? *J. Pediatr.* 68:14, 1966.
Sanchez-Cascos A, et al.: Cardio-auditory syndromes: Cardiac and genetic study of 511 deaf-mute children. *Br. Heart J.* 31:26, 1969.

CARDIOFACIAL SYNDROME

Synonym: Cayler syndrome.

Clinical and Radiologic Manifestations: (a) mild to marked *unilateral partial lower facial weakness in the neonate;* (b) *congenital heart disease* (ventricular septal defect, patent ductus arteriosus, tetralogy of Fallot, right aortic arch, pulmonary stenosis, coarctation of the aorta, atrial septal defect, atrioventricular canal, etc.); (c) other reported abnormalities: genitourinary, musculoskeletal, respiratory.

REFERENCES

Alexiou D, et al.: Frequency of other malformations in congenital hypoplasia of depressor anguli oris muscle syndrome. *Arch. Dis. Child.* 51:891, 1976.
Bodard M, et al.: Les paralysies faciales néonatales. Étude clinique, étiologique et thérapeutique. *Ann. Pediatr. (Paris)* 31:329, 1984.
Cayler GG: An "epidemic" of congenital facial paresis and heart disease. *Pediatrics* 40:666, 1967.
Levin SE, et al.: Hypoplasia or absence of the depressor anguli oris muscle and congenital abnormalities, with special reference to the cardiofacial syndrome. *S. Afr. Med. J.* 61:227, 1982.

CARDIOMYOPATHIES

Synonym: Myocardiopathies.

Classification:

(A) HEART MUSCLE DISEASES OF UNKNOWN CAUSE: (a) dilated cardiomyopathy: dilatation of one or both ventricles, impaired systolic function, congestive heart failure may develop, small percentage familial; (b) hypertrophic cardiomyopathy (idiopathic hypertrophic subaortic stenosis, muscular subaortic stenosis, obstructive cardiomyopathy, asymmetrical hypertrophy, asymmetrical septal hypertrophy, etc.): disproportionate hypertrophy of the left ventricle and occasionally also of the right ventricle, septum more prominently involved, ventricular chamber normal or small, systolic gradients often present; autosomal dominant mode of inheritance with incomplete penetrance; (c) restrictive cardiomyopathy: endomyocardial fibrosis, eosinophilic endomyocardial disease (Löffler cardiomyopathy, endocarditis parietalis fibroplastica); (d) unclassified cardiomyopathy.

(B) HEART MUSCLE DISEASES WITH KNOWN CAUSE OR ASSOCIATED WITH DISORDERS OF OTHER SYSTEMS: (a) infections; (b) metabolic disorders: endocrinopathies (hypothyroidism, thyrotoxicosis, acromegaly, adrenal cortical insufficiency, pheochromocytoma), storage diseases and infiltrations (glycogen storage disease, mucopolysaccharidosis, hemochromatosis, Refsum syndrome, Niemann-Pick disease, Fabry-Anderson disease, mucopolysaccharidoses, Hand-Schüller-Christian disease, etc.), deficiencies (potassium metabolic disorders, magnesium deficiency, anemia, beriberi, kwashiorkor, etc.), amyloidosis, etc.

(C) GENERAL SYSTEM DISEASES: connective tissue disorders (systemic lupus erythematosus, polyarthritis nodosa, rheumatoid arthritis, dermatomyositis, scleroderma, etc.), infiltrations and granulomas (leukemia, sarcoidosis, etc.), heredofamilial diseases (muscular dystrophies, Friedreich ataxia, etc.), sensitivity and toxic reactions (sulfonamides, alcohol, antimony, irradiation, etc.).

Note: The definition of cardiomyopathies as reflected in the report of the World Health Organization and International Society and Federation of Cardiology Task Force is as follows: "Cardiomyopathies are heart muscle diseases of unknown cause."

REFERENCES

Berko BA, et al.: X-linked dilated cardiomyopathy. *N. Engl. J. Med.* 316:1186, 1987.

Brigden W: Hypertrophic cardiomyopathy. *Br. Heart J.* 58:299, 1987.

Calderon A, et al: Subsarcolemmal vermiform deposits in skeletal muscle, associated with familial cardiomyopathy: Report of two cases of a new entity. *Pediatr. Neurosci.* 13:108, 1987.

Davies MJ: The cardiomyopathies: A review of terminology, pathology and pathogenesis. *Histopathology* 8:363, 1984.

Edwards WD: Cardiomyopathies: *Hum. Pathol.* 18:625, 1987.

Fitzpatrick AP, et al.: Familial neurofibromatosis and hypertrophic cardiomyopathy. *Br. Heart J.* 60:247, 1988.

Gini A, et al.: Focusing on peripartum cardiomyopathy using radionuclide cardiac imaging. *Clin. Nucl. Med.* 12:941, 1987.

Keller BB, et al.: Oncocytic cardiomyopathy of infancy with Wolff-Parkinson-White syndrome and ectopic foci causing tachydysrhythmias in children. *Am. Heart J.* 114:782, 1987.

Lombes A, et al.: Myocardiopathies primitives, d'apparence idiopathique, chez l'enfant. Place des étiologies métaboliques. *Arch. Fr. Pediatr.* 44:569, 1987.

Moene RJ, et al.: Unclassified familial cardiomyopathy with ventricular dysrhythmia. *Pediatr. Cardiol.* 8:177, 1987.

Netter JC, et al.: Cardiomyopathie hypertrophique et encéphalopathie néonatale associées à une acidurie 3-méthylglutaconique. *Ann. Pediatr. (Paris)* 34:741, 1987.

Oakley CM: Report of the WHO/ISFC task force on the definition and classification of cardiomyopathies. *Br. Heart J.* 44:672, 1980.

Pochmalicki G, et al.: Cardiomyopathie hypertrophique familiale à révélation précoce. *Ann. Pediatr. (Paris)* 34:307, 1987.

Schmidt MA, et al.: Familial dilated cardiomyopathy. *Am. J. Med. Genet.* 31:135, 1988.

Servidei S, et al.: Fatal infantile cardiopathy caused by phosphorylase b kinase deficiency. *J. Pediatr.* 113:82, 1988.

Servidei S, et al.: Severe cardiopathy in branching enzyme deficiency. *J. Pediatr.* 111:51, 1987.

Zeviani M, et al.: Myopathy and fatal cardiopathy due to cytochrome c oxidase deficiency. *Arch. Neurol.* 43:1198, 1986.

CARDIOVOCAL SYNDROME

Synonym: Ortner syndrome.

Frequency: Uncommon.

Clinical and Radiologic Manifestations: (a) hoarseness, unilateral (most common) or bilateral cord paralysis; (b) cardiovascular disease, cardiomegaly (high output failure, mitral stenosis); (c) return to normal (laryngeal cords) reported after surgery for congenital cardiovascular defects.

REFERENCES

Condon LM, et al.: Cardiovocal syndrome in infancy. *Pediatrics* 76:22, 1985.

Newman B, et al.: Vocal cord paralysis and cardiovascular disease in children. *Ann. Radiol. [Diagn.] (Stockh.)* 29:697, 1986.

Ortner N: Recurrenslähmung bei Mitralstenose. *Wien. Klin. Wochenschr.* 10:753, 1897.

Polaner DM, et al.: Cardiovocal syndrome. *Pediatrics* 78:380, 1986.

Robida A, et al.: Cardiovocal syndrome in an infant with a double outlet of the right ventricle. *Eur. J. Pediatr.* 148:15, 1988.

CARNEY SYNDROME

Synonym: Carney triad.

Frequency: Over 30 published cases (Danoff et al., Carney).

Clinical and Radiologic Manifestations: Predilection for young women. (a) *pulmonary chondroma* (smoothly lobulated nodules, computed tomographic demonstration of calcification in the periphery of the nodules); (b) *extra-adrenal paraganglioma*; (c) *gastric epithelioid leiomyosarcoma*.

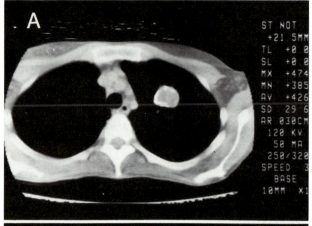

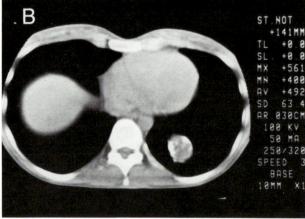

FIG SY–C–8.
Carney syndrome. **A** and **B,** computed tomography demonstrates lobulated pulmonary chondromas with peripheral calcification and normal-appearing mediastinum. (From McGahan JP: Carney syndrome: Usefulness of computed tomography in demonstrating pulmonary chondromas. *J. Comput. Assist. Tomogr.* 7:137, 1983. Used by permission.)

Note: (a) only two of the three tumors may be present in some patients; (b) another entity under the title of Carney syndrome is myxomas, spotty pigmentation and endocrine over-activity (Fig SY–C–8).

REFERENCES

Carney JA: The triad of gastric epithelioid leiomyosarcoma, functioning extra-adrenal paraganglioma, and pulmonary chondroma. *Cancer* 43:374, 1979.
Carney JA: The triad of gastric epithelioid leiomyosarcoma, pulmonary chondroma, and functioning extra-adrenal paraganglioma: A five-year review. *Medicine (Baltimore)* 62:159, 1983.
Carney JA, et al.: Dominant inheritance of the complex of myxomas, spotty pigmentation, and endocrine overactivity. *Mayo Clin. Proc.* 61:165, 1986.
Carney JA, et al.: The triad of gastric leiomyosarcoma, functioning extra-adrenal paraganglioma and pulmonary chondroma. *N. Engl. J. Med.* 296:1517, 1977.

Dajee A, et al.: Pulmonary chondroma, extra-adrenal paraganglioma, and gastric leiomyosarcoma. Carney's triad. *J. Thorac. Cardiovasc. Surg.* 84:377, 1982.
Danoff A, et al.: Adrenocortical micronodular dysplasia, cardiac myxomas, lentigines, and spindle cell tumors. *Arch. Intern. Med.* 147:443, 1987.
Messina MS, et al.: Carney's triad: Role of transthoracic needle biopsy. *Am. Rev. Respir. Dis.* 128:311, 1983.

CAROLI SYNDROME

Synonym: Caroli disease.

Pathology: *Segmental saccular dilatation of intrahepatic bile ducts with extension to the hepatic periphery; absence of liver cirrhosis or portal hypertension in the pure form of the disease; cholangitis, liver abscess, hepatic fibrosis, renal tubular ectasia, or other renal cystic lesions; intrahepatic calculi.*

Clinical Manifestations: (a) recurrent crampy upper *abdominal pain;* (b) *intermittent obstructive jaundice;* (c) fever.

Radiologic Manifestations: (a) intraductal biliary calculi; (b) *saccular dilatation* of bile ducts demonstrable by various methods: ultrasonography, computed tomography (CT) *(CT before and after the infusion of cholangiographic contrast material demonstrating a significant rise in CT number of the cystic lesions),* endoscopic retrograde cholangiopancreatography, transhepatic or operative cholangiography, radionuclide hepatocholangiography; (c) other reported abnormalities: cholangiocarcinoma.

Note: The syndrome has been classified into two types: with and without fibrosis; the fibrotic type is more common (Fig SY–C–9).

REFERENCES

Caroli J, et al.: La dilatation polykystique congénitale des voies biliaires intra-hépatiques: Essai de classification. *Sem. Hop. Paris* 34:128, 1958.
Dayton MT, et al.: Caroli's disease: A premalignant condition? *Am. J. Surg.* 145:41, 1983.
Grumbach R, et al.: La maladie fibrokystique due foie avec hypertension portale chez l'enfant. *Arch. Anat. Pathol.* 74:30, 1954.
Kaiser JA, et al.: Diagnosis of Caroli disease by computed tomography: Report of two cases. *Radiology* 132:661, 1979.
Marchal GJ, et al.: Caroli disease: High-frequency US and pathologic findings. *Radiology* 158:507, 1986.
Musante F, et al.: CT cholangiography in suspected Caroli's disease. *J. Comput. Assist. Tomogr.* 6:482, 1982.
Perisic V: Role of PTC and ERCP in diagnostic imaging of the hepatobiliary tree: Caroli's disease in two siblings. *J. Pediatr. Gastroenterol. Nutr.* 6:647, 1987.
Puech JL, et al.: Diagnostic de maladie de Caroli par les ex-

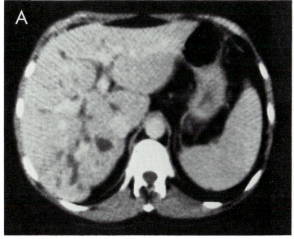
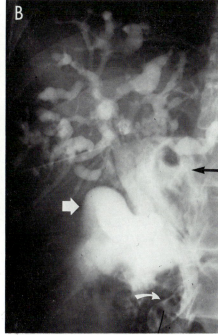
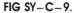

FIG SY–C–9.

Caroli syndrome in a 40-year-old man with a 2-year history of recurrent right upper quadrant abdominal pain and low-grade fever. **A,** a computed tomographic scan through the liver after the intravenous administration of contrast material demonstrates multiple branching, low density, and tubular structures that extend to the periphery and communicate with localized ectatic areas. **B,** a percutaneous transhepatic cholangiogram demonstrates dilated intrahepatic biliary radicles as well as a large cystic area in the right lobe *(black arrow)* with filling defects. Radiolucent stones are present in the distal common bile duct *(curved arrow)*. The gallbladder is also filled *(arrowhead)*. An excretory urogram demonstrated deformed calices and "brushlike" collections of contrast material in the renal pyramids that were consistent with renal tubular ectasia. (From Kaiser JA, Mall JC, Salmen BJ, et al.: Diagnosis of Caroli disease by computed tomography: Report of two cases. *Radiology* 132:661, 1979. Used by permission.)

plorations radiologiques non invasives: Intérêt du cholangio-scanner. *Ann. Radiol. (Paris)* 30:387, 1987.

Sorensen KW, et al.: Diagnosis of cystic ectasia of intrahepatic bile ducts by computed tomography. *J. Comput. Assist. Tomogr.* 6:486, 1982.

Sty JR, et al.: 99m Tc-PIPIDA biliary imaging in children. *Clin. Nucl. Med.* 4:315, 1979.

CARPAL BONE DEFORMITY, HEREDITARY

Mode of Inheritance: Reported in a mother and her son.

Clinical and Radiologic Manifestations: (a) limitation of movement of the hand, ulnar deviation of the hand; (b) unilateral carpal deformity: absence of most of the proximal carpal bones, dysplasia of the distal row of carpal bones; (c) other reported abnormalities: retrognathic mandible; protruding maxillary incisors; open lip at rest; highly arched palate; malocclusion; problems with speech, reading, and motor skills.

REFERENCE

Krauss CM, et al.: Unilateral carpal bone deformity in mother and son. *Am. J. Med. Genet.* 26:557, 1987.

CARPAL TUNNEL SYNDROME

Etiology: Various causes: trauma; tumor; endocrine disorders (diabetes mellitus, acromegaly, myxedema); pregnancy; rheumatoid arthritis; amyloidosis; sarcoidosis; systemic lupus erythematosus; gout; pseudogout; anomalous muscles, tendons, and blood vessels; infections (tuberculosis, fungi, pyogenic, etc.); mucopolysaccharidoses; Paget disease; Raynaud disease; vascular (thrombosis, vascular shunt for hemodialysis, arterial puncture in the newborn); association with tennis elbow; familial, athetoid-dystonic cerebral palsy; work-related (grocery checker); anomalous distal end of the radius; toxic shock syndrome; rubella, etc.

Clinical Manifestations: (a) numbness, paresthesia, weakness, burning pain on the anterior aspect of the wrist with extension to the fingers; (b) *abnormal clinical signs (wrist flexion, nerve percussion, and tourniquet tests) and abnormal electrophysiological test results.*

Radiologic Manifestations: (a) *computed tomography: abnormal cross-sectional area of the carpal canal;* (b) *magnetic resonance imaging: segmental and diffuse swelling of the median nerve, distortion of the nerve, thickening of the tendon sheaths;* (c) thermography helpful in comparing pretreatment and post-treatment findings (Fig SY–C–10).

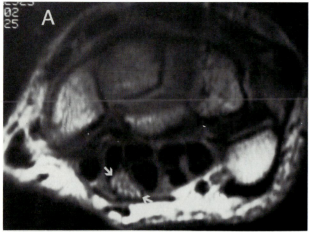

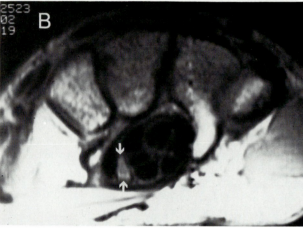

FIG SY–C–10.
Carpal tunnel syndrome with segmental swelling of the median nerve *(arrows)*. Axial magnetic resonance images (TR 2,000, TE 20) were taken at levels of the pisiform **(A)** and hook of the hamate **(B)**. The left wrist is viewed toward the elbow with the palm down. Note the enlargement of the nerve proximally **(A)** as compared with a normal caliber of the nerve distally **(B)**. (From Middleton WD, Kneeland JB, Kellman GM, et al.: MR imaging of the carpal tunnel: Normal anatomy and preliminary findings in the carpal tunnel syndrome. *A.J.R.* 148:307, 1987. Used by permission.)

REFERENCES

Alvarez N, et al.: Carpal tunnel syndrome in athetoid-dystonic cerebral palsy. *Arch. Neurol.* 39:311, 1982.
Barnhart S, et al.: Carpal tunnel syndrome in grocery checkers. A cluster of a work-related illness. *West J. Med.* 147:37, 1987.
Bleecker ML, et al.: Carpal tunnel syndrome: Role of carpal canal size. *Neurology* 35:1599, 1985.
Blennow G, et al.: Transient carpal tunnel syndrome accompanying rubella infection. *Acta Paediatr. Scand.* 71:1025, 1982.
Cuhadar M, et al.: Carpal tunnel syndrome in childhood. *Z. Kinderchir.* 38:330, 1983.
Editorial: Diagnosis of the carpal tunnel syndrome. *Lancet* 1:854, 1985.

Gellman H, et al.: Carpal tunnel syndrome. An evaluation of the provocative diagnostic tests. *J. Bone Joint Surg. [Am.]* 68:735, 1986.
Gilbert MS, et al.: Carpal tunnel syndrome in patients who are receiving long-term renal hemodialysis. *J. Bone Joint Surg. [Am.]* 70:1145, 1988.
Hodgkins ML, et al.: Carpal tunnel syndrome. *West J. Med.* 148:217, 1988.
Izhar-Ul-Haque: Carpal tunnel syndrome due to an anomalous distal end of the radius. *J. Bone Joint Surg. [Am.]* 64:943, 1982.
Jain VK, et al.: Carpal tunnel syndrome in patients undergoing maintenance hemodialysis. *J.A.M.A.* 242:2868, 1979.
Klofkorn RW, et al.: Carpal tunnel syndrome as the initial manifestation of tuberculosis. *Am. J. Med.* 60:583, 1976.
Marie P, et al.: Atrophie isolée de l'éminence thenar d'origine névritique, role du ligament anulaire antérior du carpe dans la pathogénie de la lesion. *Rev. Neurol. (Paris)* 26:647, 1913.
McDonnell JM, et al.: Familial carpal-tunnel syndrome presenting in childhood. *J. Bone Joint Surg. [Am.]* 69:928, 1987.
Merhar GL, et al.: High-resolution computed tomography of the wrist in patients with carpal tunnel syndrome. *Skeletal Radiol.* 15:549, 1986.
Middleton WD, et al.: MR imaging of the carpal tunnel: Normal anatomy and preliminary findings in the carpal tunnel syndrome. *A.J.R.* 148:307, 1987.
Roger B, et al.: Apport de la thermographie en plaque dans l'évaluation du canal carpien idiopathique. *J. Radiol.* 66:361, 1985.
Sahs AL, et al.: Carpal tunnel syndrome. Complication of toxic shock syndrome. *Arch. Neurol.* 40:414, 1983.
Spiegel PG, et al.: Acute carpal tunnel syndrome secondary to pseudogout. *Clin. Orthop.* 120:185, 1976.

CARRARO SYNDROME

Mode of Inheritance: Four of six siblings in the original report.

Clinical and Radiologic Manifestations: (a) *congenital deafness;* (b) *absence or hypoplasia of the tibias.*

REFERENCES

Carraro A: Assenza congenita della tibia e sordomutismo nel quattro fratelli. *Chir. Organi. Mov.* 16:429, 1931.
Wendler H, Schwartz R: Carraro-Syndrom. *Fortschr. Roentgenstr.* 133:43, 1980.

CAST SYNDROME

Etiology: Obstruction of the third segment of the duodenum, probably caused by compression by the superior mesenteric artery in patients who are undergoing treatment for scoliosis with or without the use of a body cast; factors contributing to the development of obstruction: diminished compliance of the abdominal wall, lumbar hyperextension, primary lumbar hyperlordosis, traction on or distraction of the spine, asthenic body build, prolonged bed rest in the supine position, rapid weight loss, etc.

Clinical Manifestations: *Nausea; vomiting; abdominal distension.*

Radiologic Manifestations: *Gastroduodenal dilatation* extending to the third portion of duodenum.

REFERENCES

Ehrlich HG, et al.: Das Spinal-Traction-Syndrom (Cast-Syndrom) - Ätiologie, Diagnose, Therapie und Prophylase. *Beitr. Orthop. Traumatol.* 32:234, 1985.

Evarts CM, et al.: Vascular compression of the duodenum associated with the treatment of scoliosis: Review of the literature and report of eighteen cases. *J. Bone Joint Surg. [Am.]* 53:431, 1971.

Griffiths GJ, et al.: Radiological features of vascular compression of the duodenum occurring as a complication of the treatment of scoliosis (the cast syndrome). *Clin. Radiol.* 29:77, 1978.

Munns SW, et al.: Hyperalimentation for superior mesenteric-artery (cast) syndrome following correction of spinal deformity. *J. Bone Joint Surg. [Am.]* 66:1175, 1984.

CATARACT-CEREBELLAR ATROPHY-MENTAL RETARDATION-MYOPATHY

Mode of Inheritance: Probably autosomal recessive.

Clinical and Radiologic Manifestations: (a) infantile hypotonia; (b) ataxia; (c) cataract; (d) mental retardation; (e) cerebellar atrophy; (f) muscle biopsy: vacuolar degeneration, adipose tissue proliferation, autophagic vacuoles, and myelin bodies on electron microscopy.

Differential Diagnosis: Marinesco-Sjögren syndrome.

REFERENCE

Herva R, et al.: A syndrome with juvenile cataract, cerebellar atrophy, mental retardation and myopathy. *Neuropediatrics* 18:164, 1987.

CATEL-MANZKE SYNDROME

Mode of Inheritance: Probably X-linked.

Clinical and Radiologic Manifestations: (a) *Robin anomaly* (mandibular hypoplasia, glossoptosis, U-shaped cleft pal-

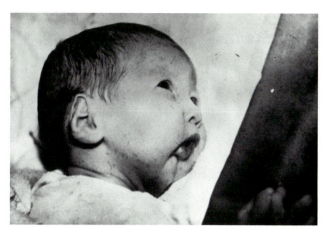

FIG SY–C–11.
Catel-Manzke syndrome in an 11-day-old boy with severe micrognathia, full cheeks, epicanthus, a low frontal hair line, a malformed ear with a prominent anthelix, and a short neck. (From Sundaram V, Taysi K, Hartmann AF Jr, et al.: Hyperphalangy and clinodactyly of the index finger with Pierre Robin anomaly: Catel-Manzke syndrome. A case report and review of the literature. *Clin. Genet.* 21:407, 1982. Used by permission.)

ate; (b) *congenital heart disease;* (c) *malformation of the index finger:* (accessory ossicle at the base, ulnar deviation); (d) other reported abnormalities: dislocatable knees, ossicle between the base of the proximal phalanges of the third and fourth digits (Figs SY–C–11 and SY–C–12).

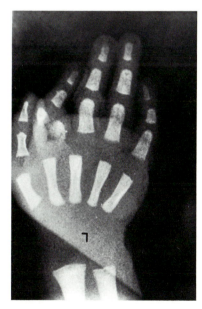

FIG SY–C–12.
Catel-Manzke syndrome in an 11-day-old male. Radiograph of the hand shows an accessory ossicle in the base of the index finger with ulnar angulation of the involved digit. (From Sundaram V, Taysi K, Hartmann AF Jr, et al.: Hyperphalangy and clinodactyly of the index finger with Pierre Robin anomaly: Catel-Manzke syndrome. A case report and review of the literature. *Clin. Genet.* 21:407, 1982. Used by permission.)

REFERENCES

Brude E: Pierre Robin sequence and hyperphalangy—a genetic entity (Catel-Manzke syndrome). *Eur. J. Pediatr.* 142:222, 1984.

Catel W: *Differentialdiagnose von Krankheitssymptomen bei Kindern und Jugendlichen,* ed 3. Stuttgart, West Germany, Georg Thieme Verlag, 1961, vol. 1, pp. 218–220.

Manzke VH: Symmetrische Hyperphalangie des zweiten Fingers durch ein akzessorisches Metacarpale. *Fortschr. Rontgenstr.* 105:425, 1966.

Sundaram V, et al.: Hyperphalangy and clinodactyly of the index finger with Pierre Robin anomaly: Catel-Manzke syndrome. A case report and review of the literature. *Clin. Genet.* 21:407, 1982.

Thompson WM, et al.: A male infant with the Catel-Manzke syndrome and dislocatable knees. *J. Med. Genet.* 23:271, 1986.

CAT-EYE SYNDROME

Synonym: Coloboma of the iris and anal atresia syndrome.

Clinical Manifestations: (a) *anorectal anomalies* (anal atresia, rectovestibular fistula); (b) *lower, vertical iridal and choroidal coloboma (cat eyes);* (c) *auricular abnormalities* (preauricular tag/fistula, low-set ears); (d) *ocular hypertelorism with antimongoloid slant;* (e) *genitourinary anomalies;* (f) *chromosome evaluation:* presence of a supernumerary marker, the origin of which has been controversial; partial tetrasomy for 22q11 in most cases; (g) *other reported abnormalities:* cardiovascular anomalies, skeletal anomalies (ribs, vertebrae, hip dislocation, etc.), psychomotor retardation, physical retardation, oral-palatal anomalies, unusual dermatoglyphics, Hirschsprung disease, phenotypic and cytogenic variability.

Radiologic Manifestations: (a) *anorectal anomalies;* (b) *skeletal anomalies;* (c) *genitourinary anomalies.*

REFERENCES

Duncan AMV, et al.: Re-evaluation of the supernumerary chromosome in an individual with cat eye syndrome (Letter). *Am. J. Med. Genet.* 27:225, 1987.

Franklin RC, et al.: The cat-eye syndrome. *Acta Paediatr. Scand.* 61:581, 1972.

Freedom RM, et al.: Congenital cardiac disease and the "cat eye" syndrome. *Am. J. Dis. Child.* 126:16, 1973.

Haab O: Beitrage zu den angeborenen Fehlern des Auges: *Graefes Arch. Klin. Ophthalmol.* 24:257, 1878.

Magenis RE, et al: Parental origin of the extra chromosome in the cat eye syndrome: Evidence from heteromorphism and in situ hybridization analysis. *Am. J. Med. Genet.* 29:9, 1988.

Mahboubi S, et al.: Association of Hirschsprung's disease and imperforate anus in a patient with "cat-eye" syndrome. *Pediatr. Radiol.* 14:441, 1984.

Pierson M, et al.: Syndrome dit de l'oeil de chat avec nanisme hypophysaire et développement mental normal. *Arch. Fr. Pediatr.* 32:835, 1975.

CAUDA EQUINA SYNDROME

Synonym: Pseudoclaudication syndrome.

Pathogenesis: *Narrowing of the sagittal diameter of the distal spinal canal* secondary to various factors: enlarged apophyseal joints, shortened pedicles, thickened ligamenta flava, disk protrusion, marginal osteophytes, capillary hemangioma of the filum terminale, rheumatoid spondylitis, ankylosing spondylitis, familial lumbar stenosis, following chemonucleolysis, lumbar diskectomy, chiropraxis, acromegaly, etc.

Clinical Manifestations: (a) *intermittent "claudication" induced either by activity or by posture,* lasting a few seconds to several minutes, manifested by numbness, coldness, or burning in areas of distribution of the lower lumbar and sacral dermatomes; (b) muscle atrophy, minor degree of muscle weakness, reflex asymmetry, sensory abnormalities.

Radiologic Manifestations: (a) *abnormalities of the vertebrae and spinal canal:* ankylosing spondylitis, spondylolisthesis, herniated disk, narrow lumbar spinal canal, etc.; (b) *magnetic resonance imaging:* demonstration of the neural elements' compression; (c) epidural venous stasis in spinal stenosis.

REFERENCES

Dorwart RH, et al.: Spinal stenosis. *Radiol. Clin. North Am.* 21:301, 1983.

Floman Y, et al.: Cauda equina syndrome presenting as a herniated lumbar disk. *Clin. Orthop.* 147:234, 1980.

Freeman RE, et al.: An unusual compressive syndrome of the cauda equina. *Mayo Clin. Proc.* 50:139, 1975.

Grosman H, et al.: CT of long-standing ankylosing spondylitis with cauda equina syndrome. *A.J.N.R.* 4:1077, 1983.

Kaiser MC, et al.: Epidural venous stasis in spinal stenosis. CT appearance. *Neuroradiology* 26:435, 1984.

Malmievaara A, et al.: Cauda equina syndrome caused by chiropraxis on a patient previously free of lumbar spine symptoms. *Lancet* 2:986, 1982.

McLaren AC, et al.: Cauda equina syndrome: A complication of lumbar discectomy. *Clin. Orthop.* 204:143, 1986.

Postacchini F, et al.: Familial lumbar stenosis. Case report of three siblings. *J. Bone Joint Surg. [Am.]* 67:321, 1985.

Smith S, et al.: Acute herniated nucleus pulposus with cauda equina compression syndrome following chemonucleolysis. *J. Neurosurg.* 66:614, 1987.

Prusick VR, et al.: Cauda equina syndrome as a complication of free epidural fat-grafting. A report of two cases and a review of the literature. *J. Bone Joint Surg. [Am.]* 70:1256, 1988.

Rubenstein DJ, et al: Case report 477: Cauda equina syndrome (CES) complicating long-standing ankylosing spondylitis (AS). *Skeletal Radiol.* 17:212, 1988.

CAUDAL DYSPLASIA SEQUENCE

Synonym: Caudal regression syndrome.

Frequency: Uncommon.

Etiology: Small number of familial cases have been reported; association with maternal diabetes or maternal prediabetic condition; association with a small marker chromosome of unknown origin, full trisomy 22, or partial trisomy for the upper part of chromosome 22; association with monozygotic twinning, 7q terminal deletion; infant born to a pancreatectomized mother.

Clinical Manifestations: (a) *flat buttocks;* (b) *short intergluteal cleft;* (c) *dimpling of the buttocks;* (d) *"siren" or "mermaid" configuration in most severe cases;* (e) *froglike deformity of the lower limbs in moderately severe cases;* (f) other reported abnormalities: association with Goldenhar syndrome (axial mesodermal dysplasia spectrum), congenital heart disease, myelomeningocele, sacral lipoma, anorectal anomalies, genitourinary anomalies, bladder and bowel dysfunction, upper limb anomalies, Dandy-Walker defect, absence of the pituitary gland, hydrocephalus, etc.

Radiologic Manifestations: (a) *vertebral agenesis that may vary from partial sacral agenesis to total agenesis below* the first lumbar vertebra; (b) limb anomalies of various types and severities such as hip dislocation, equinovarus deformities of the feet; (c) fused iliac bones in severe forms; (d) bowel dysfunction; (e) neurogenic bladder; (f) intraspinal anomalies; (g) intrauterine diagnosis by ultrasonography (Fig SY−C−13).

REFERENCES

Abraham E: Sacral agenesis with associated anomalies (caudal regression syndrome): Autopsy case report. *Clin. Orthop.* 145:168, 1979.

Anderton JM, et al.: Absence of the pituitary gland in a case of congenital sacral agenesis. *J. Bone Joint Surg. [Br]* 65:182, 1983.

Bléry M, et al.: Agénésie dorso-lombo-sacrée. A propos de 2 cas. Revue de la littérature. *J. Radiol.* 64:171, 1983.

Bruyere HJ, et al.: A fetus with upper limb amelia, "caudal regression" and Dandy-Walker defect with an insulin-dependent diabetic mother. *Eur. J. Pediatr.* 134:139, 1980.

Duhamel B: From the mermaid to anal imperforation: The syndrome of caudal regression. *Arch. Dis. Child.* 36:152, 1961.

Finer NN, et al.: Caudal regression anomalad (sacral agenesis) in siblings. *Clin. Genet.* 13:353, 1978.

Gonzalez CH, et al.: Caudal "regression" anomaly in a boy

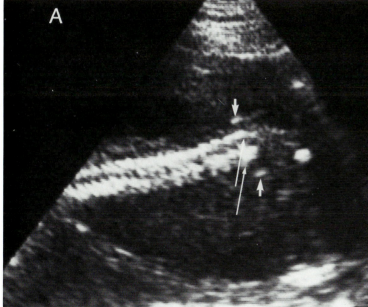

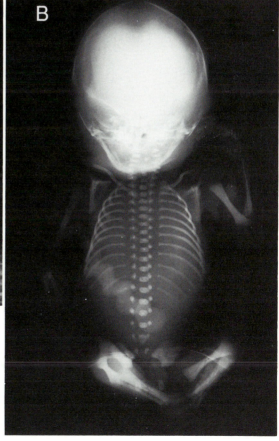

FIG SY−C−13.
Caudal regression syndrome. **A,** fetal ultrasonogram at 19 week's gestation. Note the absence of the sacral ossification centers. The *lower arrows* indicate the lower-most vertebra, probably L$_4$, and *short arrows* indicate the iliac crests. **B,** postmortem radiograph showing an abnormal L$_5$ vertebra and an absent sacrum. (From Loewy JA, Richards DG, Toi A: In-utero diagnosis of the caudal regression syndrome. Report of three cases. *J. Clin. Ultrasound* 15:469, 1987. Used by permission.)

born to a pancreatectomized mother. *Am. J. Med. Genet.* 21:205, 1985.

Jensen PKA, et al.: A bisatellited marker chromosome in an infant with the caudal regression anomalad. *Clin. Genet.* 19:126, 1981.

Loewy JA, et al.: In-utero diagnosis of the caudal regression syndrome: Report of three cases. *J. Clin. Ultrasound* 15:469, 1987.

Riedel F, et al.: Caudal dysplasia and femoral hypoplasia—unusual facies syndrome: Different manifestations of the same disorder? *Eur. J. Pediatr.* 144:80, 1985.

Scanlan KA: Sacral agenesis with crossed fused renal ectopia (caudal regression syndrome). *A.J.R.* 146:1074, 1986.

Schrander-Stumpel C, et al.: Caudal deficiency sequence in 7q terminal deletion. *Am. J. Med. Genet.* 30:757, 1988.

Sparnon AL, et al.: Urological anomalies in the caudal regression syndrome. *Aust. N.Z. J. Surg.* 54:365, 1984.

Tihansky DP, et al.: CT findings in lumbosacral agenesis. *J. Comput. Tomogr.* 8:325, 1984.

Welch JP, et al.: The syndrome of caudal dysplasia: A review, including etiologic considerations and evidence of heterogeneity. *Pediatr. Pathol.* 2:313, 1984.

CELIAC AXIS COMPRESSION SYNDROME

Synonyms: Arcuate ligament syndrome; celiac artery entrapment syndrome; celiac artery compression syndrome; median arcuate ligament syndrome.

Pathology: *Compression of the celiac artery against the aorta by the median arcuate ligament of the diaphragm.* This may cause a "stealing" of blood from the mesenteric artery via collaterals.

Clinical Manifestations: (a) *periumbilical pain, epigastric discomfort,* nausea, vomiting; (b) malabsorption (occasionally); (c) weight loss; (d) *systolic epigastric bruit.*

Radiologic Manifestations: (a) lateral abdominal aortogram: *narrowing of the celiac trunk with smooth eccentric compression of the anterior wall; dorsocaudal displacement of the celiac artery;* (b) selective superior mesenteric arteriography: opacification of the celiac artery bed through collaterals, delayed washout of contrast medium from the celiac artery territory; (c) other reported abnormalities: complete occlusion of the celiac axis combined with narrowing of the superior mesenteric artery.

Note: Compression of celiac axis and resulting ischemia as a cause of abdominal pain has been questioned (Brandt).

REFERENCES

Brandt LJ, et al.: Celiac axis compression syndrome: A critical review. *Am. J. Dig. Dis.* 23:633, 1978.

Harjola PT: A rare obstruction of the celiac artery. *Ann. Chir. Gynaecol. Fenn.* 52:547, 1963.

Lawson JD, et al.: Median arcuate ligament syndrome with severe two-vessel involvement. *Arch. Surg.* 119:226, 1984.

Warter J, et al.: La maladie phréno-coelique. *Ann. Radiol. (Paris)* 19:361, 1976.

Williams S, et al.: Celiac axis compression syndrome: Factors predicting a favorable outcome. *Surgery* 98:879, 1985.

CENTRAL CORD SYNDROME

Etiology: Cervical spondylosis; hyperextension injuries; fracture; fracture-dislocation; congenital abnormality.

Clinical and Radiologic Manifestations: (a) motor impairment, most pronounced in the upper limbs, variable degree of sensory loss below the level of the cord lesion, Lhermitte sign (sudden shooting paresthesia-like electric shocks spreading down the body or into the limbs on flexion of the neck); (b) radiological manifestations of traumatic injuries and other etiologic factors.

REFERENCES

Brodkey JS, et al.: The syndrome of acute central cervical spine cord injury revisited. *Surg. Neurol.* 14:251, 1980.

Merriam WF, et al.: A reappraisal of acute traumatic central cord syndrome. *J. Bone Joint Surg. [Br.]* 68:708, 1986.

Schneider RC, et al.: Syndrome of acute central cervical spinal cord injury with special reference to mechanisms involved in hyper-extension injuries of cervical spine. *J. Neurosurg.* 11:546, 1954.

CENTRAL HYPOVENTILATION SYNDROME (CONGENITAL)

Synonym: Ondine's curse.

Etiology: Diminished sensitivity of the respiratory center to reduced oxygen or increased carbon dioxide.

Clinical Manifestations: (a) persistent hypoventilation; (b) recurrent apnea and cyanosis; (c) difficulty in feeding and swallowing; (d) seizures related to hypoventilation; (e) abnormal brainstem auditory evoked responses during sleep: delays in peak latencies pIII and interpeak latencies pI–III that imply a functional disturbance of brainstem control of ventilation during sleep; (f) arterial blood gas analysis in sleep: respiratory acidosis and hypercapnia; (g) other reported abnormalities: association with Hirschsprung disease and neural crest tumors (neurocristopathy), occurrence in monozygotic twins.

Radiologic Manifestations: (a) normal brain computed tomography; (b) associated lesions (neurocristopathy).

REFERENCES

Beckerman R, et al.: Brain-stem auditory response in Ondine's syndrome. *Arch. Neurol.* 43:698, 1986.

Bower RJ, et al.: Ondine's curse and neurocristopathy. *Clin. Pediatr. (Phila.)* 19:665, 1980.

Khalifa MM, et al.: Congenital central hypoventilation syndrome in monozygotic twins. *J. Pediatr.* 113:853, 1988.

Mellins RB, et al.: Failure of automatic control of ventilation (Ondine's curse). *Medicine (Baltimore)* 49:487, 1970.

Poceta JS, et al.: Ondine curse and neurocristopathy. *Pediatr. Neurol.* 3:370, 1987.

Yasuma F, et al.: Congenital central alveolar hypoventilation (Ondine's curse): A case report and review of the literature. *Eur. J. Pediatr.* 146:81, 1987.

CEPHALOSKELETAL DYSPLASIA

Synonym: Taybi-Linder syndrome.

Mode of Inheritance: Probably autosomal recessive.

Frequency: Very rare.

Pathology: Brain dysgenesis; severe enchondral growth disorders.

Clinical Manifestations: (a) *low birth weight;* (b) *microcephaly;* (c) unusual facies with bulging eyes, flat bridge of the nose, high-arched palate; (d) *spadelike hands and feet;* (e) *mental and physical retardation;* (f) other reported abnormalities: clubfoot deformity, cleft palate, absent hair.

Radiologic Manifestations: (a) *severe microcephaly,* small fontanelles; (b) *deep intervertebral spaces* with a relative decrease in vertical diameter of the vertebral bodies; (c) *shortness of all long bones, splayed and irregular margins of the metaphyses of long bones and cup-shaped ends of the short tubular bones of the hands and feet;* (d) delayed ossification of tali, calcanei, and epiphyses at the knees; (e) short iliac wings, near-zero acetabular angles, irregular ossification of acetabular roofs, narrow sciatic notches; (f) computed tomography: microcephaly, ventricular dilatation, large sub-

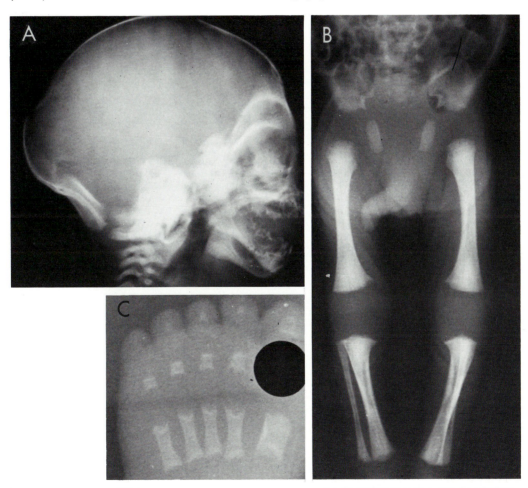

FIG SY–C–14.
Cephaloskeletal dysplasia in newborn siblings: male **(A and B)** and female **(C). A,** microcephaly, small anterior fontanelle, and open sutures. **B,** the interpedicular distances are not narrow, the iliac wings are short, the acetabular angles are near zero, the acetabular roofs are irregular, the sciatic notches are narrow, and the metaphyseal margins are irregular, particularly in the knee re-gion. **C,** concave ossified ends of the metatarsals and the metaphysis of the phalanges, with nonossification of several phalanges. (From Taybi H, Linder D: Congenital familial dwarfism with cephalo-skeletal dysplasia. *Radiology* 89:275, 1967. Used by permission.)

arachnoid space; (g) other reported abnormalities: long clavicles, hydronephrosis (Fig SY–C–14).

REFERENCES

Lavollay B, et al.: Nanisme familial congenital avec dysplasie céphalo-squelettique (syndrome de Taybi-Linder). *Arch. Fr. Pediatr.* 41:57, 1984.
Majewski F, et al.: Studies of microcephalic primordial dwarfism III: An intrauterine dwarf with platyspondyly and anomalies of pelvis and clavicles—Osteodysplastic primordial dwarfism type III. *Am. J. Med. Genet.* 12:37, 1982.
Taybi H, Linder D: Congenital familial dwarfism with cephalo-skeletal dysplasia. *Radiology* 89:275, 1967.
Thomas PS, et al.: Congenital familial dwarfism with cephalo-skeletal dysplasia (Taybi-Linder syndrome). *Ann. Radiol. (Paris)* 19:187, 1976.

CEREBRO-COSTO-MANDIBULAR SYNDROME

Synonym: Rib gap defect–micrognathia syndrome.

Modes of Inheritance: Majority of cases are sporadic; genetic heterogeneity; autosomal dominant and autosomal recessive transmissions have been suggested; consanguinity (father-daughter union); father and daughter with rib gap.

Frequency: 33 published cases (Merlob et al.).

Pathology: Rib gaps consisting of fibrous or cartilaginous tissues.

Clinical Manifestations: (a) *micrognathia;* (b) *respiratory distress due to flail chest;* (c) mental handicaps; (d) *palatal defect;* (e) other reported abnormalities: microcrania, pterygium colli, clubfoot deformity, congenital heart disease, conductive deafness, feeding difficulties, speech disorders, prenatal and postnatal growth deficiency, malformed auricles, low-set ears, prominent eyes, pectus carinatum, pectus excavatum, dental anomalies, hypotonia, forked tongue tip, undescended testes, microstomia, long philtrum, short internipple distance, depressed sacral region, etc.

Radiologic Manifestations: (a) *micrognathia;* (b) *gaps in the dorsal portion of the ribs,* fragmented ossification of the ribs, absence of normal costovertebral articulations; (c) other reported anomalies: *brain defects,* vertebral anomalies, subluxation of the elbows, dental defects, laryngeal and tracheal abnormalities, internal rotation of the iliac bones, hip dislocation, gastroesophageal reflux, renal anomalies (medullary cysts, renal ectopia), vesicoureteral reflux, persistent urinary tract infection, abnormal phalanges of the toes, polyhydramnios, ultrasonographic demonstration of brain dysgenesis and rib anomalies, association with cystic fibrosis, hydrocephalus, and multiple ossification centers of the calcaneus (a case report) (Figs SY–C–15 and SY–C–16).

REFERENCES

Burton EM, et al.: Cerebro-costo-mandibular syndrome with stippled epiphysis and cystic fibrosis. *Pediatr. Radiol.* 18:365, 1988.
Clark EA, et al.: Cerebro-costo-mandibular syndrome with consanguinity. *Pediatr. Radiol.* 15:264, 1985.

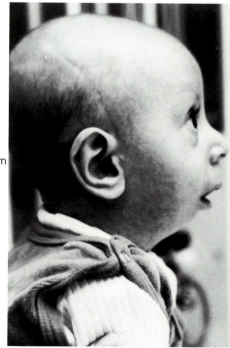

FIG SY–C–15.
Cerebro-costo-mandibular syndrome. Micrognathia and large ears are evident. (From Hennekam RCM, Beemer FA, Huijbers WAR, et al.: The cerebro-costo-mandibular syndrome: Third report of familial occurrence. *Clin. Genet.* 28:118, 1985. Used by permission.)

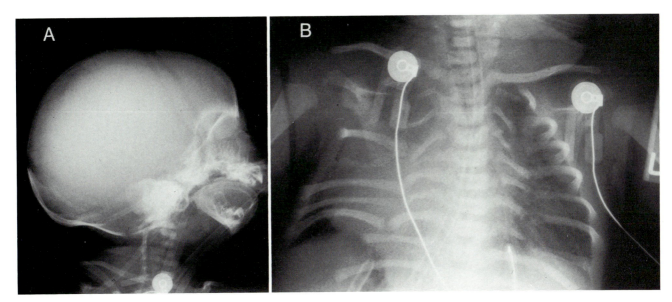

FIG SY–C–16.
Cerebro-costo-mandibular syndrome. Micrognathia **(A)** and extensive rib defects **(B)** are present. (Courtesy of Peter E. Kane, M.D., Children's Hospital Medical Center, Oakland, Calif.)

Hennekam RCM, et al.: The cerebro-costo-mandibular syndrome: Third report of familial occurrence. *Clin. Genet.* 28:118, 1985.

Merlob P, et al.: Autosomal dominant cerebro-costo-mandibular syndrome: Ultrasonographic and clinical findings. *Am. J. Med. Genet.* 26:195, 1987.

Miller KE, et al.: Rib gap defects with micrognathia: The syndrome with rib dysplasia. *A.J.R.* 114:253, 1972.

Silverman FN, et al.: Cerebro-costo-mandibular syndrome. *J. Pediatr.* 97:406, 1980.

Smith DW, et al.: Rib-gap defect with micrognathia, malformed tracheal cartilages, and redundant skin: A new pattern of defective development. *J. Pediatr.* 69:799, 1966.

Smith KG, et al.: Cerebrocostomandibular syndrome. *Clin. Pediatr. (Phila.)* 24:223, 1985.

Trautman MS, et al.: Cerebro-costo-mandibular syndrome: A familial case consistent with autosomal recessive inheritance. *J. Pediatr.* 107:990, 1985.

Walizadeh Gh-R: Pierre-Robin-Syndrom mit Rippenanomalien. *Fortsch. Rontgenstr.* 129:275, 1978.

CEREBRO-OCULO-FACIO-SKELETAL SYNDROME

Synonyms: COFS syndrome; Pena-Shokeir syndrome, type II.

Frequency: Rare.

Clinical Manifestations: (a) *prenatal growth retardation;* (b) *craniofacial dysmorphism:* microcephaly, sloping forehead, prominent bony ridge of the nose, high nose bridge, upper lip overhanging the lower lip, micrognathia or retrognathia, narrow palpebral fissures; (c) *microphthalmos, cataract,* blepharophimosis, cloudy corneas; (d) kyphosis, scoliosis; (e) *contracture, mainly at the elbows and knees, perma-nently clenched fists,* camptodactyly, simian crease, longitudinal foot groove folding, *foot deformities;* (f) *hypotonia;* (g) other reported abnormalities: failure to thrive, oligohydramnios, widely set nipples, extensive cell necrosis (iliac crest biopsy), etc.

Radiologic Manifestations: (a) acetabular dysplasia, hip dislocation, narrow pelvis, coxa valga; (b) *foot deformities: vertical talus, rocker-bottom feet, calcaneovalgus,* hypoplasia of the second cuneiform and proximal displacement of the second metatarsal; (c) osteoporosis; (d) renal anomalies; (e) cerebral calcification (lenticular nucleus and hemispheric white matter).

Differential Diagnosis: Neu-Laxova syndrome.

REFERENCES

Hwang WS, et al.: Chondro-osseous changes in cerebro-oculo-facial-skeletal (COFS) syndrome. *J. Pathol.* 138:33, 1982.

Insler MS: Cerebro-oculo-facio-skeletal syndrome. *Ann. Ophthalmol.* 19:54, 1987.

Linna, SL, et al.: Intracranial calcification in cerebro-oculo-facio-skeletal (COFS) syndrome. *Pediatr. Radiol.* 12:28, 1982.

Pena DJ, Shokeir MHK: Autosomal recessive cerebro-oculo-facio-skeletal (COFS) syndrome. *Clin. Genet.* 5:285, 1974.

Piussan Ch, et al.: Le syndrome cérébro-oculo-facio-squelettique. *Arch. Fr. Pediatr.* 36:379, 1979.

Preus M, et al.: Renal anomalies and oligohydramnios in the cerebro-oculo-facio-skeletal syndrome. *Am. J. Dis. Child.* 131:62, 1977.

Silengo MC, et al.: The NEU-COFS (cerebro-oculo-facio-skeletal) syndrome: Report of a case. *Clin. Genet.* 25:201, 1984.

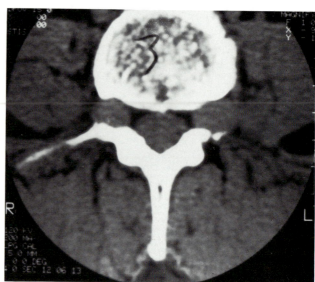

FIG SY–C–17.
Neuropathy of Charcot-Marie-Tooth disease. Note the bilateral nerve root enlargement at the L₃ level. These symmetrical changes have enlarged and eroded the intervertebral neural foramina and extend into the spinal canal in a manner similar to "dumbbell"-shaped lesions. (From Morano JU, Russell WF: Nerve root enlargement in Charcot-Marie-Tooth disease: CT appearance. *Radiology* 161:784, 1986. Used by permission.)

CHARCOT-MARIE-TOOTH DISEASE

Synonyms: Peroneal muscular atrophy; hereditary motor and sensory neuropathy (HNSN).

Modes of Inheritance: Sporadic; autosomal dominant (most cases of type I), autosomal recessive, and X-linked recessive forms have also been reported; genetic linkage evidence of heterogeneity; type I linked to the Duffy blood group locus and chromosome 1.

Clinical Manifestations: (a) *chronic, slowly progressive demyelinating motor and sensory neuropathy* (peripheral nerves and roots) resulting in distal muscular atrophy (feet and legs at first, hands later); (b) *slow nerve conduction in type I, normal conduction in type II;* (c) other reported abnormalities: association with sensorineural deafness, scoliosis, pes cavus, hammertoes, diaphragmatic dysfunction, respiratory failure.

Radiologic Manifestations: (a) *nerve root enlargement;* (b) muscle atrophy; (c) other reported abnormalities: posterior scalloping of the lumbar vertebrae, scoliosis, enlargement and erosion of intervertebral neural foramina, hip dysplasia in older children and adolescents (steep acetabular roof, irregular ossification of the acetabular roof, flat hypoplastic femoral head, subluxation of the femoral head), coxa valga, etc. (Fig SY–C–17).

REFERENCES

Bird TD, et al.: Genetic linkage evidence for heterogeneity in Charcot-Marie-Tooth neuropathy (HMSN type I). *Ann. Neurol.* 14:679, 1983.

Chan CK, et al.: Diaphragmatic dysfunction in siblings with hereditary motor and sensory neuropathy (Charcot-Marie-Tooth disease) *Chest* 91:567, 1987.

Chance PF, et al.: Genetic linkage relationships of Charcot-Marie-Tooth disease (HMSN-Ib) to chromosome 1 markers. *Neurology* 37:325, 1987.

Charcot JM, Marie P: Sur une forme particulière d'atrophie musculaire progressive souvent familiale debutante par les pieds et les jambes et atteignant plus tard les mains. *Rev. Med.* 6:97, 1886.

Cornell J, et al.: Autosomal recessive inheritance of Charcot-Marie-Tooth disease associated with sensorineural deafness. *Clin. Genet.* 25:163, 1984.

Daher YH, et al.: Spinal deformities in patients with Charcot-Marie-Tooth disease. A review of 12 patients. *Clin. Orthop.* 202:219, 1986.

Griffiths LR, et al.: Chromosome 1 linkage studies in Charcot-Marie-Tooth neuropathy type I. *Am. J. Hum. Genet.* 42:756, 1988.

Kumar SJ, et al.: Hip dysplasia associated with Charcot-Marie-Tooth disease in the older child and adolescent. *J. Pediatr. Orthop.* 5:511, 1985.

Mann RA, et al.: Pathophysiology of Charcot-Marie-Tooth disease. *Clin. Orthop.* 234:221, 1988.

Miura T, et al.: Radiological findings in a case of Charcot-Marie-Tooth disease. *Br. J. Radiol.* 58:1017, 1985.

Morano JU, et al.: Nerve root enlargement in Charcot-Marie-Tooth disease: CT appearance. *Radiology* 161:784, 1986.

Ouvrier RA, et al: The hypertrophic forms of hereditary motor and sensory neuropathy. A study of hypertrophic Charcot-Marie-Tooth disease (HMSN Type I) and Dejerine-Sottas disease (HMSN Type III) in childhood. *Brain* 110:121, 1987.

Ruiz C, et al.: A distinct congenital motor and sensory neuropathy (neuronal type) with dysmorphic features in a father and two sons. A variant of Charcot-Marie-Tooth disease. *Clin. Genet.* 31:109, 1987.

Sabir M, et al.: Pathogenesis of Charcot-Marie-Tooth disease. Gait analysis and electrophysiologic, genetic, histopathologic, and enzyme studies in a kinship. *Clin. Orthop.* 184:223, 1984.

Tooth HH: *The Peroneal Type of Progressive Muscular Atrophy.* London, H.K. Lewis, 1886.

CHARGE ASSOCIATION

Synonym: CHARGE syndrome.

Mode of Inheritance: sporadic; dominant transmission in some families.

Frequency: Approximately 150 published cases (Oley et al.).

Clinical and Radiologic Manifestations: (a) congenital anomalies: *coloboma of the eye* (C); *heart disease* (H); *atresia of the choana* (A); *retarded growth, development, and/or central nervous system anomalies* (R); *genital hypoplasia* (G); *ear anomalies and/or deafness* (E); (b) other reported abnormalities: retrogenia, orofacial clefts, antimongoloid slanting of the palpebral fissures, anteverted nares, facial paralysis, feeding problems, malar flattening, long philtrum or prominent nasal columella, "wedge"-shaped audiogram, hypopituitarism, tracheoesophageal fistula, esophageal atresia, anal atresia/stenosis, renal anomalies, the VATER association.

Differential Diagnosis: Velocardiofacial syndrome.

REFERENCES

August GP, et al.: Hypopituitarism and the CHARGE association. *J. Pediatr.* 103:424, 1983.
Cyran SE, et al.: Spectrum of congenital heart disease in CHARGE association. *J. Pediatr.* 110:576, 1987.
Davenport SJH, et al.: The spectrum of clinical features in CHARGE syndrome. *Clin. Genet.* 29:298, 1986.
Koletzko B, et al.: Congenital anomalies in patients with choanal atresia: CHARGE-association. *Eur. J. Pediatr.* 142:271, 1984.
Lin AE: Charge association vs. velo-cardio-facial syndrome. *Am. J. Med. Genet.* 29:951, 1988.
Metlay LA, et al.: Familial CHARGE syndrome: Clinical report with autopsy findings. *Am. J. Med. Genet.* 26:577, 1987.
Oley CA, et al.: A reappraisal of the CHARGE association. *J. Med. Genet.* 25:147, 1988.
Pagon RA, et al.: Coloboma, congenital heart disease, and choanal atresia with multiple anomalies: CHARGE association. *J. Pediatr.* 99:223, 1981.
Stewart G, et al.: CHARGE association in neonates presenting with choanal atresia. *Z. Kinderchir.* 42:12, 1987.
Valente A, et al.: Oesophageal atresia and the CHARGE association. *Pediatr. Surg.* 2:93, 1987.
Weaver DD, et al.: The VATER association. Analysis of 46 patients. *Am. J. Dis. Child.* 140:225, 1986.

CHEDIAK-HIGASHI SYNDROME

Mode of Inheritance: Autosomal recessive.

Clinical Manifestations: (a) *partial albinism*; sparse melanine granules in hair shafts; (b) fragile appearance; (c) predisposition to infections; (d) development of lymphoma-like illness in the accelerated phase of the disease; (e) *massive lysosomal inclusions in the white blood cells* (formation related to a combined process of fusion, cytoplasmic injury, and phagocytosis), the inclusions exhibit both azurophilic and specific granular markers; (f) neutropenia; anemia; thrombocytopenia; high zinc concentration in plasma, erythrocytes, lymphocytes, and granulocytes; defective neutrophil, monocyte, and lymphocyte locomotion; (g) *hepatosplenomegaly*; (h) other reported abnormalities: presentation with neurological disorder that resembled a spinocerebellar degeneration and parkinsonism, hypertriglyceridemia, etc.

Radiologic Manifestations: Nonspecific: (a) hilar and mediastinal lymphadenopathy; (b) hepatosplenomegaly; (c) lymphangiography: reticular pattern of enlarged inguinal and para-aortic lymph nodes.

REFERENCES

Barak Y, et al.: Chédiak-Higashi syndrome. *Am. J. Pediatr. Hematol. Oncol.* 9:42, 1987.
Chédiak M: Nouvelle anomalie leucocytaire de caractère constitutionnel et familial. *Rev. Hematol. (Paris)* 7:362, 1952.
Higashi O: Congenital gigantism of peroxidase granules. *Tohoku J. Exp. Med.* 59:315, 1954.
McLelland R, et al.: The Chédiak-Higashi syndrome. *J. Can. Assoc. Radiol.* 19:78, 1968.
Pettit RE, et al.: Chédiak-Higashi syndrome. *Arch. Neurol.* 41:1001, 1984.
Rubin CM, et al.: The accelerated phase of Chédiak-Higashi syndrome. An expression of the virus-associated hemophagocytic syndrome? *Cancer* 56:524, 1985.
Yegin O, et al.: Defective lymphocyte locomotion in Chédiak-Higashi syndrome. *Am. J. Dis. Child.* 137:771, 1983.
Yip WCL, et al.: Chédiak-Higashi syndrome in a Chinese infant. *Aust. Paediatr. J.* 19:51, 1983.

CHEIRO-ORAL SYNDROME

Pathology: Lesion in the inferior medial portion of the posterolateral ventral nucleus and lateral part of posteromedial ventral nucleus of the thalamus, brain stem, etc.

Clinical Manifestations: Sensory disturbance around the corner of the mouth and the palm of the hand on the same side.

Radiologic Manifestations: Infarct; hematoma.

REFERENCES

Iwasaki Y, et al.: The cranial computed tomographic findings in patients with cheiro-oral syndrome. *Comput. Med. Imag. Graph.* 12:237, 1988.
Sittig O: Klinische Beiträge zur Lehre von den Lokalisation der sensiblen Rindenzentren. *Prager. Med. Wochenschr.* 45:548, 1914.

CHILAIDITI SYNDROME

Clinical Manifestations: (a) *abdominal pain,* vomiting, anorexia, constipation, frequent passage of flatus; (b) *marked diurnal abdominal distension;* (c) absence of liver dullness, displaced liver edge; (d) posterior hepatodiaphragmatic interposition of the colon has been reported in association with incarceration of the colon, obesity, lung cancer, paralytic ileus, volvulus of the sigmoid colon, etc.

Radiologic Manifestations: (a) *complete or incomplete interposition of the bowel between the liver and diaphragm;* (b) mimicking a posterior hepatic lesion, posterior retroperitoneal masses, or a disrupted diaphragm on sonography.

REFERENCES

Auh YH, et al.: Posterior hepatodiaphragmatic interposition of the colon: Ultrasonographic and computed tomographic appearance. *J. Ultrasound Med.* 4:113, 1985.

Chilaiditi D: Zur Frage der Hepatoptose im allgemeinen Anschluss an drei Fälle von temporärer partieller Leberverlagerung. *Fortschr. Rontgenstr.* 16:173, 1910.

Lekkas CN, et al.: Symptom-producing interposition of the colon: Clinical syndrome in mentally deficient adults. *J.A.M.A.* 240:747, 1978.

Melester T, et al.: Chilaiditi's syndrome. Report of three cases. *J.A.M.A.* 254:944, 1985.

Vessal K, et al.: Hepatodiaphragmatic interposition of the intestine (Chilaiditi's syndrome). *Clin. Radiol.* 27:113, 1976.

CHILD SYNDROME

Synonyms: Unilateral ichthyosiform erythroderma; syndrome of unilateral ectromelia, psoriasis, and central system anomalies; ichthyosis–limb reduction syndrome; etc.

Mode of Inheritance: Majority female; possibly X-linked dominant gene.

Frequency: Rare.

Clinical Manifestations: Onset at birth or early childhood. (a) *ichthyosiform erythroderma* (present at birth or soon after birth, erythema, scaling with distinct demarcation at the midline of the trunk, face always spared), impaired hair growth and linear areas of alopecia on the affected side, destruction of nails and replacement by keratotic clawlike material, onychorrhexis; (b) *limb deformity (ipsilateral):* varies from digital hypoplasia to complete absence of an extremity; (c) *ipsilateral hypoplasia of other parts* of the skeleton, brain, spinal cord, viscera; (d) other reported abnormalities: minor skin and visceral anomalies on the contralateral side, cleft lip, umbilical hernia, minimal hearing loss.

Radiologic Manifestations: (a) *unilateral hypoplasia or aplasia of a limb;* (b) *unilateral hypoplasia of the calvaria, mandible, scapula, clavicle, and ribs;* (c) vertebral defects, scoliosis; (d) visceral anomalies: cardiovascular (single ventricle, single coronary ostium, Shone syndrome, etc.), renal (ipsilateral absent kidney, hydronephrosis), hypoplasia of the lung; (e) endocrine defects (unilateral hypoplasia of the thyroid, adrenal, ovary, and fallopian tube); (f) punctate epiphyseal calcification.

Differential Diagnosis: Chondrodysplasia punctata.

Note: The term *CHILD* originates from Congenital *h*emidysplasia with *i*chthyosiform erythroderma and *l*imb *d*efects (Fig SY–C–18).

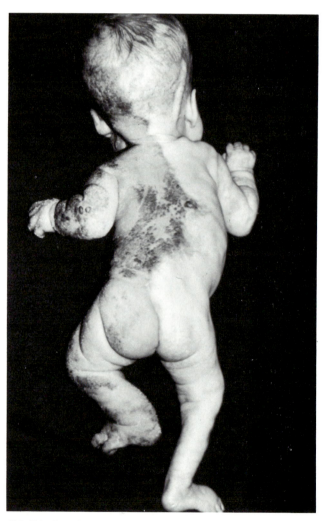

FIG SY–C–18.
The CHILD syndrome. Marked unilateral hyperkeratosis and erythema involving the left side of the trunk, scalp, and left arm are present. (From Hebert AA, Esterly NB, Holbrook KA, et al.: The CHILD syndrome. Histologic and ultrastructural studies. *Arch. Dermatol.* 123:503, 1987. Used by permission.)

REFERENCES

Happle R, et al.: The CHILD syndrome: Congenital hemidysplasia with ichthyosiform erythroderma and limb defects. *Eur. J. Pediatr.* 134:27, 1980.

Hebert AA, et al.: The CHILD syndrome. Histologic and ultrastructural studies. *Arch. Dermatol.* 123:503, 1987.

CHILD ABUSE SYNDROME

Synonyms: Battered child syndrome; the shaken baby syndrome; le syndrome de Silverman; the syndrome of Ambroise Tardieu; Caffey-Kempe syndrome.

Clinical Manifestations: (a) *mucocutaneous lesions:* tears of the floor of the mouth, bruises, burns, lacerations, bite marks, scars, traumatic alopecia, etc.; (b) *head trauma:* subgaleal hemorrhage, seizures, coma, increased intracranial pressure, retinal hemorrhage, retinal detachment, residual permanent brain damage, mental retardation, unilateral ear bruising ("tin ear syndrome") associated with ipsilateral cerebral edema, obliteration of the basilar cisterns, hemorrhagic retinopathy; (c) *internal organ lesions,* elevated amylase concentration, etc.; (d) other reported manifestations; hypernatremia, dehydration, failure to thrive, jittery baby, repeated poisoning, genital injuries, hypopituitarism, performing below normal on the Wechsler Intelligence Scale and delay in language development and reading ability on the follow-up evaluation several years after the abuse period, rhabdomyolysis and myoglobulinuria associated with renal failure, simulated "acquired" imperforate hymen following the genital trauma of sexual abuse, muscular trauma simulating myositis, residual neurological deficits, polymicrobial bacteremia due to "Polle syndrome" (the child abuse variant of Munchausen by proxy).

Radiologic Manifestations: (a) *skeletal system:* epiphyseal, metaphyseal, and diaphyseal fractures (microtraumatic, macrotraumatic fractures); traumatized multiple bones often in different stages of healing; bone sclerosis (healing fracture); intramedullary necrosis and periosteal new bone formation secondary to traumatic pancreatitis; costal and vertebral fractures; anterior dislocation of a vertebral body; scoliosis; sternal fracture; sequelae of skeletal trauma (growth disturbance, defective joint alignment, etc.); skull fracture (multiple fractures, bilateral fractures, and fractures crossing sutures occurring significantly more often in child abuse cases than in accidental injury); (b) *central nervous system abnormalities:* infarction, intracranial hemorrhage (epidural, subdural, cerebral, interhemispheric), brain edema, brain tear, hydrocephalus, porencephaly, brain atrophy, subdural hygroma, spinal cord injury, etc.; (c) *visceral trauma:* pulmonary trauma, mesenteric tears, intraperitoneal hematoma, duodenal and proximal jejunal hematomas, bowel rupture, liver lacerations, bile peritonitis, pancreatic laceration, pseudocyst formation, chylous ascites, ruptured bladder, renal trauma, retroperitoneal hematoma, etc.; (d) other reported abnormalities: acute gastric dilatation following feeding of nutritionally abused children, acute renal failure secondary to rhabdomyolysis with myoglobulinuria (bilateral dense prolonged nephrogram after the injection of contrast medium, increased renal echogenecity).

Differential Diagnosis: Menkes syndrome; congenital syphilis; hemophilia; mongolian spots; "Cao-Gio" (Vietnamese traditional medicine), cupping lesions, moxibustion (Chinese and Southeast Asian traditional medicine); near-miss sudden infant death syndrome (retinal hemorrhages due to thoracic compression associated with resuscitation); subdural hematoma due to Mexican folk remedy for caida de mollera ("fallen fontanelle").

REFERENCES

Alexander RC, et al.: Magnetic resonance imaging of intracranial injuries from child abuse. *J. Pediatr.* 109:975, 1986.

Ben-Youssef L, et al.: Battered child syndrome simulating myositis. *J. Pediatr. Orthop.* 3:392, 1983.

Berkowitz CD, et al.: A simulated "acquired" imperforate hymen following the genital trauma of sexual abuse. *Clin. Pediatr. (Phila.)* 26:307, 1987.

Bird RC, et al.: Strangulation in child abuse: CT diagnosis. *Radiology* 163:373, 1987.

Caffey J: Multiple fractures in the long bones of infants suffering from chronic subdural hematoma. *A.J.R.* 56:163, 1946.

Caffey J: The parent-infant traumatic stress syndrome: (Caffey-Kempe syndrome), (battered baby syndrome). *A.J.R.* 114:217, 1972.

Caffey J: The whiplash shaken infant syndrome: Manual shaking by the extremities with a whiplash-induced intracranial and intraocular bleedings, linked with residual permanent brain damage and mental retardation. *Pediatrics* 54:396, 1974.

Cohen H, et al.: Pancreatitis, child abuse, and skeletal lesions. *Pediatr. Radiol.* 10:175, 1981.

Cohen RA, et al.: Cranial computed tomography in the abused child with head injury. *A.J.R.* 146:97, 1986.

David A, et al.: Une observation de "Cao-Gio," confusion possible avec des sevices. *Arch. Fr. Pediatr.* 43:147, 1986.

Fauré C, et al.: La vertèbre vagabonde. *Ann. Radiol. (Paris)* 22:96, 1979.

Green HG: Child abuse presenting as chylothorax. *Pediatrics* 66:620, 1980.

Guillois B, et al.: Insuffisance rénale par rhabdomyolyse secondaire à des morsures et des griffures de chien chez un nourrisson victime de négligence. *Ann. Pediatr. (Paris)* 34:337, 1987.

Halstead CC, et al.: Child abuse: Acute renal failure from ruptured bladder. *Am. J. Dis. Child.* 133:861, 1979.

Hanigan WC, et al.: Tin ear syndrome: Rotational acceleration in pediatric head injuries. *Pediatrics* 80:618, 1987.

Jaudes PK: Comparison of radiography and radionuclide bone scanning in the detection of child abuse. *Pediatrics* 73:166, 1984.

Kempe CH, et al.: The battered-child syndrome. *J.A.M.A.* 181:17, 1962.

Kirschner RH, et al.: The mistaken diagnosis of child abuse. A form of medical abuse? *Am. J. Dis. Child.* 139:873, 1985.

Kleinman PK, et al.: Avulsion of the spinous processes caused by infant abuse. *Radiology* 151:389, 1984.

Kleinman PK, et al.: Resolving duodenal-jejunal hematoma in abused children. *Radiology* 160:747, 1986.

Kleinman PK, et al.: The metaphyseal lesion in abused infants: A radiologic-histopathologic study. *A.J.R.* 146:895, 1986.

Liston TE, et al.: Polymicrobial bacteremia due to Polle syndrome: The child abuse variant of Munchausen by proxy. *Pediatrics* 72:211, 1983.

Mallet JF, et al.: Le syndrome de Silverman ou syndrome des enfants battus. *Ann. Pediatr. (Paris)* 31:117, 1984.

Merten DF, et al.: The abused child: A radiological reappraisal. *Radiology* 146:377, 1983.

Meservy CJ, et al.: Radiographic characteristics of skull fractures resulting from child abuse. *A.J.R.* 149:173, 1987.

Miller WL, et al.: Child abuse as a cause of posttraumatic hypopituitarism. *N. Engl. J. Med.* 302:724, 1980.

Mukherji SK, et al.: Rhabdomyolysis and renal failure in child abuse. *A.J.R.* 148:1203, 1987.

Oates RK, et al.: The development of abused children. *Dev. Med. Child Neurol.* 26:649, 1984.

Shulman BH, et al.: Acute gastric dilatation following feeding of nutritionally abused children. *Clin. Pediatr. (Phila.)* 23:108, 1984.

Silverman FN: Child abuse: The conflict of underdetection and overreporting. *Pediatrics* 80:441, 1987.

Silverman FN: The roentgen manifestations of unrecognized skeletal trauma in infants. *A.J.R.* 69:413, 1953.

Silverman FN: Unrecognized trauma in infants: The battered child syndrome and the syndrome of Ambroise Tardieu. Rigler lecture. *Radiology* 104:337, 1972.

Strassburg HM, et al.: Not "Polle syndrome", please. *Lancet* 1:166, 1984.

Sty JR, et al.: The role of bone scintigraphy in the evaluation of the suspected abused child. *Radiology* 146:369, 1983.

CHROMOSOME 1 LONG ARM DELETION

Chromosomal Abnormality: Interstitial deletion of chromosome 1 (1q24–25→1q32).

Clinical and Radiologic Manifestations: (a) *low birth weight, growth, and psychomotor retardation;* (b) *craniofacial dysmorphism:* microcephaly, epicanthus, broad/flat nasal bridge, cleft lip/palate, low-set ears, malformed auricles, anteverted nostrils, micrognathia; (c) short neck; (d) brachydactyly, short toes, clinodactyly; (e) other reported abnormalities: renal agenesis, cryptorchidism, hypospadias, congenital heart disease, partially fused cervical vertebrae.

REFERENCE

Hamano S, et al.: A case of interstitial 1q deletion [46,XY, del(q25q32.1)] *Ann. Genet. (Paris)* 30:105, 1987.

CHROMOSOME 1, PARTIAL DELETION SYNDROME

Clinical and Radiologic Manifestations: (a) *craniofacial dysmorphism:* microbrachycephaly, frontal bossing, exophthalmos, epicanthus, abnormal ears, micrognathia, cleft lip and palate, highly arched palate; (b) *skeletal anomalies:* short broad hands and feet, hypoplastic fingers, clinodactyly of the fifth digit, coxa vara, pes valgus, knee dislocation, 11 pairs of ribs; (c) transverse palmar crease; (d) delayed growth, mental retardation, hypotonia; (e) retarded bone age.

REFERENCES

Callahan DJ, et al.: Congenital dislocation of the knees associated with a partial chromosome I deletion. *J. Pediatr. Orthop.* 5:593, 1985.

Estévez de Pablo C, et al.: Interstitial deletion in the long arms of chromosome I: 46,XY, del(1) (pter q22::q25 qter). *J. Med. Genet.* 17:483, 1980.

Sekhon GS, et al.: Deletion in the long arm of chromosome I from a subject with multiple congenital anomalies. *Cytogenet. Cell Genet.* 21:176, 1978.

CHROMOSOME 3 TRISOMY SYNDROME

Chromosome Abnormality: Trisomy of the distal end of the short arm of chromosome 3 (either segment 3p23→27 or 3p21→27).

Clinical and Radiologic Manifestations: (a) craniofacial dysmorphism: microcephaly, frontal bossing, temporal indentation, square facies, prominent cheeks, micrognathia and/or retrognathia, hypertelorism, horizontal palpebral fissures, epicanthus, depressed nasal bridge, long and prominent philtrum, prominent middle upper lip; (b) short neck; (c) increased number of whorls on the digits, deep creases on the soles; (d) congenital heart defects; (e) renal malformation, hypoplastic penis, undescended testes; (f) gastrointestinal malformations; (g) cutaneous syndactyly, clinodactyly, camptodactyly.

REFERENCE

Yunis JJ: Trisomy for the distal end of the short arm of chromosome 3: A syndrome. *Am. J. Dis. Child.* 132:30, 1978.

CHROMOSOME 3 TRISOMY (3q+) SYNDROME

Clinical and Radiologic Manifestations: (a) craniofacial dysmorphism: microcephaly, trigonocephaly, square-shaped face, prominent maxilla, synophrys, bushy eyebrows, mongoloid slant of the eyes, epicanthus, cloudy cornea, strabismus, ocular hypertelorism, malformed ear lobes, depressed nasal bridge, short nose with anteverted nostrils, long philtrum, cleft palate; (b) skeletal anomalies: proximally placed thumbs, clinodactyly of the fifth digit, syndactyly, hemivertebrae; (c) hypertrichosis; (d) transverse palmar creases; (e) congenital heart disease; (f) urogenital anomalies: renal anomalies, renal cyst, bicornuate uterus, vaginal duplication, cryptorchidism; (g) other reported abnormalities: hearing loss, edema of the hands and feet, hypotonia, abnormal cry, deformed chest wall, widely spaced nipples, omphalocele, umbilical hernia, mental and physical retardation, etc.

Differential Diagnosis: de Lange syndrome.

REFERENCES

Steinbach P, et al.: The dup(3q) syndrome: Report of eight cases and review of the literature. *Am. J. Med. Genet.* 10:159, 1981.

Tranebjaerg L, et al.: Partial trisomy 3q syndrome inherited from familial t(3;9)(q26.1;p23). *Clin. Genet.* 32:137, 1987.

Wilson GN, et al.: Further delineation of the dup(3q) syndrome. *Am. J. Med. Genet.* 22:117, 1985.

CHROMOSOME 4p TRISOMY (4p+) SYNDROME

Clinical Manifestations: (a) severe mental and growth retardation, hypotonia, seizures; (b) craniofacial dysmorphism: microcephaly, prominent glabella, horizontal eyebrows and palpebral fissures, broad nose with a bulbous tip, ocular hypertelorism, pointed chin, large mouth, large tongue, low-set, slanted, and malformed ears; (c) widely spaced nipples; (d) flexion deformities of the hands and feet; (e) abnormal dermatoglyphics; (f) micropenis, hypospadias, small scrotum, cryptorchidism.

Radiologic Manifestations: (a) microcephaly, small sella turcica, hypertelorism, blunt mandibular angle, malocclusion; (b) scoliosis, "square" vertebral bodies, hypoplasia of the 1st or 12th rib; (c) narrow iliac wings, narrow acetabular angle, hip dislocation; (d) limb deformities: flexion deformities of the fingers, clinodactyly of the fifth fingers, pseudoepiphysis of the metacarpals, plantar flexion of the toes, hallux valgus, camptodactyly, prominent heel; (e) retarded bone age.

REFERENCES

Dallapiccola B, et al.: The radiological pattern associated with the trisomy of the short arm of chromosome No. 4. *Pediatr. Radiol.* 3:34, 1975.

Mastroiacova P, et al.: Picture of the month. *Am. J. Dis. Child.* 130:1119, 1976.

CHROMOSOME 4p− SYNDROME

Synonyms: Wolf syndrome; Wolf-Hirschhorn syndrome; del (4p) syndrome.

Clinical Manifestations: (a) *mental and growth retardation;* (b) *craniofacial anomalies: microcephaly, prominent glabella, ocular hypertelorism,* broad-beaked nose, micrognathia, short philtrum with a down-turned mouth, *cleft lip and/or cleft palate;* (c) other reported anomalies: congenital heart disease, midline scalp defects, genital anomalies, clubfoot deformity, low birth weight, hypotonia, seizures, congenital hip dysplasia, extra toes, sacral dimple or a pilonidal sinus, iris coloboma, hemangioma, antimongoloid slant of the eyes, epicanthal folds, preauricular sinus or tags, hypoplastic dermal ridges, simian crease, various renal anomalies, renal cystic dysplasia, ptosis of the eyelids; (d) dermatographic abnormalities; (e) *partial deletion of the short arm of chromosome 4.*

Radiologic Manifestations: (a) *microcephaly, hypertelorism, micrognathia;* (b) retarded skeletal maturation; (c) clubfoot; (d) other reported anomalies: scaphocephaly, prognathism, kyphoscoliosis, small pelvis with underdeveloped pubic rami, separation of pubic bones, increased iliac angles, flexion deformity of the fingers, clinodactyly, malformed great toes, proximal radio-ulnar synostosis, fused vertebrae, bifid vertebrae, 13 rib−bearing vertebrae, rib anomalies, anomalous sternal ossification, thin fibula, underossification of the middle and distal phalanges of the hands and feet, thin diaphyses of the long bones, diaphragmatic hernia, intestinal malrotation, central nervous system anomalies (dilated ventricles, cavum septum pellucidum, absent septum pellucidum, intraventricular cysts, microgyria, flattening of gyri), abnormal lung lobulation, accessory spleen, absence of the gallbladder, abnormal shape of the pancreas, urogenital anomalies, enlarged adrenals.

REFERENCES

Battini J, et al.: Monosomie 4p− (syndrome de Wolf-Hirschhorn). *Arch. Fr. Pediatr.* 34:876, 1977.

Dunbar RD, et al.: Radiologic signs of the 4p− (Wolf) syndrome. *Radiology* 117:395, 1975.

Hirschhorn K, et al.: Apparent deletion of short arms of one chromosome (4 or 5) in a child with defects of midline fusion. *Hum. Chrom. Newslett.* 4:14, 1961.

Kitsious S, et al.: Unusual pathologic findings in a girl with Wolf-Hirschhorn syndrome, del (4p). *Pediatr. Pathol.* 6:161, 1986.

Lazjuk GI, et al.: The Wolf-Hirschhorn syndrome. II. Pathologic anatomy. *Clin. Genet.* 18:6, 1980.

Léonard C, et al: A photometer used for diagnosing a small-sized 4p deletion in Wolf syndrome. *Clin. Genet.* 34:276, 1988.

Magill HL, et al.: 4p− (Wolf-Hirschhorn) syndrome. *A.J.R.* 35:283, 1980.

Martsolf JT, et al.: Familial transmission of Wolf syndrome resulting from specific deletion 4p16 from t(4;8)(p16;p21) mat. *Clin. Genet.* 31:366, 1987.

Wolf U, et al.: Defizienz an den kurzen Armen eines Chromosoms 4. *Hum. Genet.* 1:397, 1965.

CHROMOSOME 4q— SYNDROME

Clinical and Radiologic Manifestations: (a) preterm delivery, small for date, growth retardation, developmental delay; (b) craniofacial dysmorphism: microcephaly, earlobe anomalies, hypertelorism, epicanthic folds, upward slanting of the palpebral fissures, short nose, flat nasal bridge, cleft lip/palate, micrognathia, anteverted nostrils; (c) skeletal anomalies: various digital anomalies, malposition of the toes, hip dislocation, clubfoot deformity; (d) other reported abnormalities: oropharyngeal incoordination, congenital heart defects, altered palmar creases, skeletal maturation retardation, hypospadias, cryptorchidism.

REFERENCE

Jefferson RD, et al.: A terminal deletion of the long arm of chromosome 4 [46,XX,del(4)(q33)] in an infant with phenotypic features of Williams syndrome. *J. Med. Genet.* 23:474, 1986.

CHROMOSOME 5p— SYNDROME

Synonyms: Cri-du-chat syndrome; cat-cry syndrome.

Clinical Manifestations: (a) *severe growth and mental retardation;* (b) *catlike cry* (not present in all cases, not pathognomonic), (c) round-moon facies, micrognathia, retrognathia, *microcephaly,* low-set ears, *antimongoloid slant of the eyes,* hypertelorism, strabismus; (d) *muscular hypotonia;* (e) other reported abnormalities: congenital heart disease, simian crease, distal axial triradius, facial asymmetry.

Radiologic Manifestations: (a) *microcephaly, micrognathia;* (b) abnormal development of the long bones related to muscular hypotonia; (c) hands smaller than normal; disproportionate shortness of the third, fourth, and fifth metacarpals; elongation of the second, third, fourth, and fifth proximal phalanges; (d) other reported abnormalities: scoliosis, small iliac wings, etc.

REFERENCES

Fenger K, et al.: Measurement on hand radiographs from 32 cri-du-chat probands. *Radiology* 129:137, 1978.
Gebauer HJ, et al.: Cri-du-chat syndrome in a child with a 5/15 translocation and interstitial centromeric heterochromatin. *Clin. Genet.* 14:345, 1978.
James AE Jr, et al.: Radiological features of most common autosomal disorders. *Clin. Radiol.* 22:417, 1971.
James AE Jr, et al.: The cri du chat syndrome. *Radiology* 92:50, 1969.
Labrune M, et al.: Etude de signes radiologiques de la maladie du cri du chat. *Ann. Radiol. (Paris)* 10:303, 1967.
Lejeune J, et al.: Trois cas de deletion partielle du bras court d' un chromosome 5. *C. R. Acad. Sci. (Paris)* 257:3098, 1963.
Niebuhr E: Anthropometry in the cri du chat syndrome. *Clin. Genet.* 16:82, 1979.

Suerinck E, et al.: Ring chromosome 5 in two malformed boys with cri du chat syndrome. *Clin. Genet.* 14:125, 1978.
Tolksdorf M, et al.: Male infant with cat cry syndrome and apparent absence of the Y chromosome. *Eur. J. Pediatr.* 133:293, 1980.
Wilkins LE, et al.: Psychomotor development in 65 home-reared children with cri-du-chat syndrome. *J. Pediatr.* 97:401, 1980.

CHROMOSOME 7q+ SYNDROME

Chromosomal Variants: 7q32→qter; 7q31→qter; 7q22→q31.

Clinical and Radiologic Manifestations: (a) low birth weight, retardation of development; (b) *craniofacial dysmorphism:* asymmetrical skull, frontal bossing and occipital prominence, wide open fontanelle, low-set ears, external ear anomalies, hypertelorism, epicanthus, small palpebral fissures, strabismus, small nose, cleft palate, large tongue, microretrognathia; (c) skeletal abnormalities: syndactyly, rib aplasia, kyphoscoliosis, hip dislocation; (d) other reported abnormalities: hypotonia, hypertonia, death in early infancy, hyperconvex nails.

REFERENCE

Couzin DA, et al.: Partial trisomy 7 (q32→qter) syndrome in two children. *J. Med. Genet.* 23:461, 1986.

CHROMOSOME 8 TRISOMY SYNDROME

Clinical Manifestations: (a) *mild to moderate psychomotor retardation;* (b) *craniofacial dysmorphism:* scaphocephaly, cranial asymmetry, broad-based pug nose, low-set ears, dysplastic ears, strabismus, everted lower lip, high-arched palate, cleft palate, micrognathia; (c) *slender appearance* with narrow shoulders and pelvic girdle; (d) *contracture of large and small joints,* in particular, fingers and toes; (e) congenital cardiovascular anomalies (septal defects, large vessel anomalies); (f) characteristic dermatoglyphics; (g) other reported abnormalities: thickened and bulging skin with deep furrows, renal anomalies, cryptorchidism, etc.; (h) chromosome 8 trisomy, chromosomal mosaicism often present; (i) may live to adult life.

Radiologic Manifestations: (a) macrocephaly, frontal bossing, micrognathia, absent corpus callosum; (b) osteoporosis; (c) vertebral anomalies (number, shape), kyphosis, scoliosis, narrow interpediculate distances in the lower lumbar region; (d) underdeveloped glenoid fossae, flaring of the metaphyses of the long bones, narrow diaphyses of the long bones, radial head dislocation, clinodactyly, radial deviation of the fingers with or without contractures, cone-shaped epiphyses of the first metacarpals, hypoplasia of iliac bones, vertical iliac wings, wide interpubic distance, absent or hypoplastic patellas, toe anomalies; (e) advanced bone age.

REFERENCES

Anneren G, et al.: Trisomy 8 syndrome. *Helv. Paediatr. Acta* 36:465, 1981.

Cassidy SB, et al.: Trisomy 8 syndrome. *Pediatrics* 56:826, 1975.

Fineman RM, et al.: Trisomy 8 mosaicism syndrome. *Pediatrics* 56:762, 1975.

Grünebaum M, et al.: Etude radiologique de la trisomie 8 en mosaique. *Ann Radiol. (Paris)* 19:593, 1976.

Lai CC, et al.: Trisomy 8 syndrome. *Clin. Orthop.* 110:239, 1975.

Lewandowski RC Jr, et al.: New chromosomal syndromes. *Am. J. Dis. Child.* 129:515, 1975.

Silengo M, et al.: Radiological features in trisomy 8. *Pediatr. Radiol.* 8:116, 1979.

CHROMOSOME 9 TRISOMY SYNDROME

Clinical Manifestations: (a) low birth weight; (b) psychomotor retardation, muscular hypotonia, feeding problems; (c) craniofacial dysmorphism: microcephaly, micrognathia, wide cranial sutures, occipital bossing, narrow temples, prominent nose with a bulbous tip, pouched cheeks, enophthalmos, small palpebral fissures, mongolian slant of the eyes, low-set ears, malformed ears, high-arched or cleft palate, gingival hyperplasia, webbing of the neck, brain malformation (cystic); (d) cardiovascular anomalies, single umbilical artery; (e) urogenital malformations: cryptorchidism, abnormal scrotum and penis, renal anomalies, microcysts of the kidneys; (f) clenched hands, overlapping fingers; (g) other reported abnormalities: widely spaced nipples, hyperconvex nails, simian creases, deep palmar and/or plantar creases; (h) single cell line or trisomy 9 mosaicism; (i) death often in infancy.

Radiologic Manifestations: (a) skeletal anomalies: malformed hands, phalangeal aplasia, pelvic malformations, hip dislocation, knee dislocation, talipes calcaneovalgus, malformed toes, vertebral anomalies, rib anomalies.

REFERENCES

Annerén G, et al.: Trisomy 9 syndrome. *Acta Paediatr. Scand.* 70:125, 1981.

Bowen P, et al.: Trisomy 9 mosaicism in a newborn infant with multiple malformations. *J. Pediatr.* 85:95, 1974.

Lewandowski RC Jr: New chromosomal syndromes. *Am. J. Dis. Child.* 129:515, 1975.

Mace SE, et al.: The trisomy 9 syndrome: Multiple congenital anomalies and unusual pathological findings. *J. Pediatr.* 92:446, 1978.

CHROMOSOME 9(p+) TRISOMY SYNDROME

Clinical Manifestations: (a) low birth weight, short stature, growth and mental retardation, delayed puberty; (b) craniofacial dysmorphism: microcephaly and/or brachycephaly, parietal or frontal bossing, antimongoloid slant of the eyes, deep-set eyes, hypertelorism (real or pseudo), epican-thal folds, Brushfield spots in the iris, coloboma, pupil eccentricity, strabismus, vision abnormalities, prominent and globular nose with anteverted nostrils, down-turned mouth, micrognathia, highly arched palate, simple low-set ears, preauricular dimple, short, thick, and/or webbed neck; (c) unusual cry (flutter-purr); (d) limb anomalies: small hands and feet, shortness of digits, contracture of the fingers, clinodactyly, dysplasia or hypoplasia of the nails, syndactyly of the toes; (e) abnormal dermatoglyphics; (f) other reported abnormalities: café-au-lait spots, hemangiomas, hypertrichosis, cryptorchidism, sacral dimple, narrow pelvis, scoliosis and/or kyphosis, congenital heart disease, etc.; (g) trisomy for the short arm of chromosome 9(p+).

Radiologic Manifestations: (a) osteoporosis; (b) clinodactyly, brachymesophalangia of the little fingers, thick epiphyses of the terminal phalanges, hypoplastic distal phalanges, pseudoepiphysis of the metacarpals, slender metacarpals and phalanges, short and broad first metacarpals, etc.; (c) slender metatarsals, triangular distal phalanges of the toes, absent or hypoplastic middle phalanges of the toes, etc.; (d) delayed ossification of the pubic bones, broad ischial tuberosities, wide interpubic distance, etc.; (e) bone age retardation.

REFERENCES

Mattina T, et al.: Duplication 9p due to unequal sister chromatid exchange. *J. Med. Genet.* 24:303, 1987.

Pilling DW, et al.: Radiological abnormalities associated with anomalies of the ninth chromosome. *Pediatr. Radiol.* 6:215, 1978.

Preus M, et al.: Trisomy 9 (pter→q1 to q3): The phenotype as an objective aid to karyotypic interpretation. *Clin. Genet.* 26:52, 1984.

Rethoré M-O, et al.: Sur quatre cas de trisomie pour le bras court du chromosome 9. Individualisation d'une nouvelle entité morbide. *Ann. Genet. (Paris)* 13:217, 1970.

Schinzel A: Trisomy 9p, a chromosome aberration with distinct radiographic findings. *Radiology* 130:125, 1979.

CHROMOSOME 13 TRISOMY SYNDROME

Synonym: Patau syndrome.

Clinical Manifestations: (a) *low birth weight,* (b) *typical facies:* microcephaly, large broad nose, cleft lip and palate, hypertelorism or hypotelorism, malformed and low-set ears, micrognathia, anophthalmia, or microphthalmos, etc.; (c) *digital anomalies:* long hyperconvex fingernails, camptodactyly, fifth finger overlapping the fourth, polydactyly, syndactyly; (d) *rocker-bottom feet;* (e) soft-tissue defects of the head and neck; (f) *severe mental defect;* (g) capillary hemangiomas; (h) *trisomy 13–15;* (i) other reported abnormalities: undescended testes, capillary hemangiomas, jitteriness and apneic spells, congenital heart disease, extra skin of the nape of the neck, short neck, retroflexible thumbs, single palmar crease, hypotonia, hypertonia, seizures, web neck, cervical cystic hygroma, hydrops fetalis, nuclear projections of the polymorphonuclear neutrophils, sparse/absent eyebrows, etc.

Radiologic Manifestations: (a) *microcephaly with a sloping forehead,* hypotelorism or hypertelorism, holoprosencephaly, poor ossification of the calvaria, small orbits; (b) *hand and foot deformities;* (c) hypoplasia of the ribs; (d) various cardiovascular and renal anomalies; (e) hypoplasia of the pelvis, low acetabular angles; (f) double vagina, bicornuate uterus.

REFERENCES

Agbata IA, et al.: Holoprosencephaly and trisomy 13 in a cyclops. *J.A.M.A.* 241:1109, 1979.
Cabin HS, et al.: Congenital heart disease with trisomy 13. *Am. Heart J.* 100:563, 1980.
Franceschini P, et al.: First rib hypoplasia in Patau's disease. *Pediatr. Radiol.* 2:65, 1974.
Greenberg F, et al.: Cystic hygroma and hydrops fetalis in a fetus with trisomy 13. *Clin. Genet.* 24:389, 1983.
James AE Jr, et al.: Radiological features of most common autosomal disorders. *Clin. Radiol.* 22:417, 1971.
Ming P-ML, et al.: Cytogenetic variants in holoprosencephaly. Report of a case and review of the literature. *Am. J. Dis. Child.* 130:864, 1976.
Nakazato Y, et al.: Fetal cystic hygroma, web neck and trisomy 13 syndrome. *Br. J. Radiol.* 58:1011, 1985.
Patau K, et al.: Multiple congenital anomaly caused by an extra chromosome. *Lancet* 1:790, 1960.
Singleton EB, et al.: The radiographic manifestations of chromosomal abnormalities. *Radiol. Clin. North Am.* 2:281, 1964.

CHROMOSOME 18q− SYNDROME

Clinical and Radiologic Manifestations: (a) low birth weight, short stature, mental retardation, generalized hypotonia, generalized ligament laxity, incoordination; (b) craniofacial dysmorphism: microcephaly, midface hypoplasia, deep-set eyes, prominent antihelix and antitragus of the ears, carp-shaped mouth (angles below the midpoint of the upper margin of the lower lip), narrow or atretic ear canals, conductive hearing loss, horizontal nystagmus, anomalies of the fundi (posterior staphylomas, temporal tilting of the optic discs), subcutaneous nodules at the site of a cheek dimple; (c) skeletal anomalies: clubfoot, abnormal toe implantation, proximally implanted or short thumb, atlantoaxial rotatory fixation, long-tapered fingers; (d) genital anomalies: cryptorchidism, small penis, hypoplasia or absence of the labia minora and clitoris; (e) congenital heart disease; (f) partial deletion of the long arm (18q− or partial 18q monosomy); (g) other reported abnormalities: widely spaced nipples, cleft lip/palate, increased transverse palmar creases, diminished IgA levels, decrease in activity of the enzyme peptidase A, seizures, extraskeletal Ewing sarcoma, etc.

REFERENCES

de Grouchy J, et al.: Deletion partielle des bras longs du chromosome 18. *Pathol. Biol.* 12:579, 1964.
Felding I, et al.: Contribution to the 18q− syndrome. A patient with del (18) (q22.3qter). *Clin. Genet.* 31:206, 1987.
Valtuena MM, et al.: 18q− syndrome and extraskeletal Ewing's sarcoma. *J. Med. Genet.* 23:426, 1986.
Wertelecki W, et al.: Clinical and chromosomal studies of the 18q− syndrome. *J. Pediatr.* 78:44, 1971.
Wolf JW Jr, et al.: Atlanto-axial rotatory fixation associated with the 18q− syndrome. Case report. *J. Bone Joint Surg. [Am.]* 62:295, 1980.

CHROMOSOME 18p− SYNDROME

Clinical and Radiologic Manifestations: (a) short stature, mental deficiency, muscular hypotonia; (b) craniofacial dysmorphism: flat occiput, flat face, hypertelorism, ptosis, epicanthal folds, strabismus, short broad-based nose, wide mouth, irregular dentition, dental caries, small chin, big protruding ears, deep hair line, short and broad neck; (c) skeletal system: broad chest, pectus excavatum, kyphoscoliosis, incurved fifth fingers, etc.; (d) deletion of the short arm of chromosome 18.

REFERENCES

Christensen MF, et al.: Deletion short arm 18 and Silver-Russell syndrome. *Acta Paediatr. Scand.* 67:101, 1978.
Schinzel A, et al.: Structural aberrations of chromosome 18. The 18-p− syndrome. *Arch. Genet.* 47:1, 1974.

CHROMOSOME 18 TRISOMY SYNDROME

Synonym: Edwards syndrome.

Clinical Manifestations: (a) *low birth weight;* (b) *physical and mental retardation;* (c) muscular hypotonia followed by hypertonia; (d) *characteristic facies:* (elongated skull with prominent occiput, micrognathia, small triangular mouth with short upper lip, low-set malformed ears, high-arched palate); short neck; (e) shield deformity of the chest; (f) *flexion deformity of the fingers* (first digit adducted and second digit overlapping the third); (g) *foot deformities* (rocker-bottom, short first digit, dorsiposed hallux); (h) low-arched dermal ridge patterning on fingertips; (i) other reported anomalies: cardiovascular, genitourinary, gastrointestinal, hernias, feeding difficulty, single umbilical artery, limited hip abduction, inguinal or umbilical hernia, retroflexible thumb, distally implanted thumb, Meckel diverticulum, biliary atresia, absent gallbladder, hypertrophy of the clitoris, central nervous system neoplasia, Wilms tumor, liver neoplasia, polyhydramnios, ectopia cordis, limb reduction malformations, discontinuous eyebrows, distichiasis, blue sclerae.

Radiologic Manifestations: (a) thin calvaria with frontal bossing, *prominent occiput,* J-shaped sella turcica, *hypopla-*

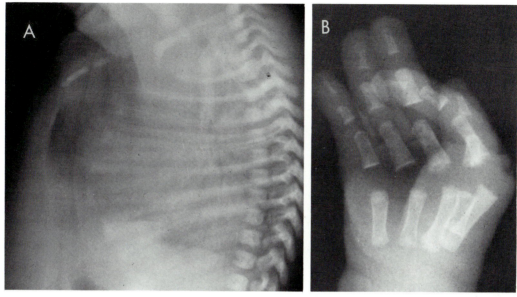

FIG SY–C–19.

Chromosome 18 trisomy syndrome in a 2-day-old female with an abnormal craniofacial appearance (prominent occiput, low-set ears, hypertelorism, high-arched palate, and micrognathia), congenital heart disease, deformed fingers, and rocker-bottom feet.

A, the sternum is short and the anteroposterior diameter of the chest abnormally wide. **B,** ulnar deviation of the digits and the second digit overlapping the third.

sia of the mandible and maxilla; (b) *thin hypoplastic ribs, 11 pairs of ribs, short sternum;* (c) *hand deformities* (ulnar deviation of the digits, V-shaped deformity between the second and third digits, hypoplastic first metacarpal, flexion deformities); (d) *foot deformities* (rocker-bottom, short first digit, hammertoes, hypoplastic distal phalanges); (e) *small pelvis,* steep iliac angles; (f) antenatal sonographic findings: micromelia, intrauterine growth retardation, foot deformity, polyhydramnios or oligohydramnios, agenesis of the corpus callosum, hydrops fetalis, choroid plexus cyst, nuchal skin thickening, etc.; (g) other reported abnormalities: chondrodysplasia punctata, protrusio acetabuli, kyphoscoliosis, etc. (Fig SY–C–19).

Note: A scoring system for the diagnosis of trisomy 18 in the immediate neonatal period has been presented (Marion et al.). Points are assigned for the presence of features known to occur in this disease: (a) 5 points for the presence of features reported to occur in 50% or more of the affected infants; 3 points for features reported to occur in 10% to 50% of affected infants, and 1 point for features known to occur in fewer than 10% of newborns with trisomy 18; (1) the 5-point features are intrauterine growth retardation, prematurity or postmaturity, a single umbilical artery, a prominent occiput, a narrow bifrontal region, short palpebral fissures, low-set malformed auricles, small oral opening, micrognathia, narrow palatal arch, characteristic hand posture, absent distal interphalangeal (DIP) crease, low-arch pattern on five fingers, nail hypoplasia, short hallux, short sternum, small nipples, systolic heart murmur, cardiomegaly, hernia (inguinal, umbilical, or omphalocele) or diastasis recti, female sex; (2) the 3-point features are microcephaly, hypoplastic supraorbital ridges, epicanthal folds, corneal opacification, simian crease(s), hypoplastic or absent thumb(s), ulnar or radial deviation of hand(s), syndactyly of the toes or fingers, equinovarus, rocker-bottom feet, malposed or funnel-shaped anus, eventration or hernia of the diaphragm, hypoplasia of the labia majora, cryptorchidism, hypotonia or hypertonia, small pelvis, limited hip abduction; (3) the 1-point features are upward or downward obliquity of the eyes, coloboma of the iris, choanal atresia, cleft lip and/or palate, radial aplasia, short fifth metacarpals, ectodactyly, pectus excavatum, dextrocardia, imperforate anus, dislocated hip(s), vertebral anomaly, meningomyelocele, scoliosis, rib anomaly, thrombocytopenia; (b) in the infants without trisomy 18 the score was 60 or less (average, 41.4); in the patients with trisomy 18 the score range was 70 to 113 (average, 94.3).

REFERENCES

Alpert LI, et al.: Neonatal hepatitis and biliary atresia associated with trisomy 17–18 syndrome. *N. Engl. J. Med.* 280:16, 1979.

Benacerraf BR, et al.: Abnormal facial features and extremities in human trisomy syndromes: Prenatal US appearance. *Radiology* 159:243, 1986.

Bundy AL, et al.: Antenatal sonographic findings in trisomy 18. *J. Ultrasound Med.* 5:361, 1986.

Cabin HS, et al.: Congenital heart disease in trisomy 13. *Am. Heart J.* 100:563, 1980.

Christianson AL, et al.: Four cases of trisomy 18 syndrome

with limb reduction malformations. *J. Med. Genet.* 21:293, 1984.

Dasouki M, et al.: Trisomy 18 and hepatic neoplasia. *Am. J. Med. Genet.* 27:203, 1987.

Edwards JH, et al.: A new trisomic syndrome. *Lancet* 1:787, 1960.

Franceschini P, et al.: Skeletal alterations in Edward's disease (trisomy 18 syndrome). *Ann. Radiol. (Paris)* 17:361, 1974.

James AE Jr, et al.: Radiological features of most-common autosomal disorders. *Clin. Radiol.* 22:417, 1971.

Karayalcin G, et al.: Wilms' tumor in a 13-year-old girl with trisomy 18. *Am. J. Dis. Child.* 135:665, 1981.

Le Marec B, et al.: A propos de 20 cas de trisomie 18. Considération sur le sex-ratio en fonction de l'âge maternel. *Ann. Pediatr. (Paris)* 24:125, 1977.

Le Marec B, et al.: Epiphyses ponctuées et aberrations chromosomiques. *Ann. Radiol. (Paris)* 19:599, 1976.

Le Marec B, et al.: La phénocopie de la trisomie 18: Une maladie autosomique récessive? *Arch. Fr. Pediatr.* 38:253, 1981.

Marion RW, et al.: Trisomy 18 score: A rapid, reliable diagnostic test for trisomy 18. *J. Pediatr.* 113:45, 1988.

Mehta L, et al.: Trisomy 18 in a 13 year old girl. *J. Med. Genet.* 23:256, 1986.

Poon CCS, et al.: Eleven pairs of ribs in E-trisomy. *Arch. Dis. Child.* 50:84, 1975.

Ray S, et al.: Arthrokatadysis in trisomy 18. *J. Pediatr. Orthop.* 6:100, 1986.

Robinson MG, et al.: Trisomy 18 and neurogenic neoplasia. *J. Pediatr.* 99:428, 1981.

Soper SP, et al.: Trisomy 18 with ectopia cordis, omphalocele, and ventricular septal defect. *Pediatr. Pathol.* 5:481, 1986.

CHROMOSOME 20p TRISOMY SYNDROME

Clinical Manifestations: (a) prenatal and postnatal growth failure; (b) mental retardation, poor coordination, speech impediment; (c) microcephaly, unusual facial appearance, occipital flattening, coarse hair, strabismus, dental abnormalities.

Radiologic Manifestations: (a) various nonspecific bone anomalies: reduced intervertebral disk spaces, partial fusion of the vertebrae, small pelvis, flaring of the proximal femoral metaphysis; (b) chronic lung disease.

REFERENCES

Centerwall W, et al.: Familial trisomy 20p: Five cases and two carriers in three generations. *Ann. Genet. (Paris)* 20:77, 1977.

Rudd N, et al.: Partial trisomy 20 confirmed by gene dosage studies. *Am. J. Med. Genet.* 4:357, 1979.

CHROMOSOME 21 TRISOMY SYNDROME

Synonyms: Down syndrome; "mongolism"; mongoloidism.

Etiology: (a) chromosomal abnormality: nondisjunction in about 92% (maternal age dependent, i.e., higher risk with older mothers), translocation in about 5%, mosaicism in about 3%; (b) chance of recurrence in general is about 1%.

Clinical Manifestations and Pathology: (a) *craniofacial dysmorphism:* brachycephaly, flat occiput, short neck with a skin fold, straight hair, upward slanting of the palpebral fissures, epicanthal folds, small mouth, protruding tongue, narrow palate, fissured tongue, ear deformity (small low-set ears, small earlobes, angular overlapping helix, prominent anthelix); (b) *dental manifestations:* delayed tooth eruption, small teeth, irregular tooth placement, abnormal sequence of tooth eruption, partial anodontia, low susceptibility to dental caries; (c) *ocular manifestations:* Brushfield spots of the iris, strabismus, abnormalities of refraction, cataract, keratoconus, blepharoconjunctivitis, ectropion, iris hypoplasia, fundus changes; (d) *mental and motor retardation,* Alzheimer disease in patients beyond the age of 30 or 40 years, association with Tourette syndrome, predisposition to moyamoya disease, compression of the spinal cord resulting in cervical myelopathy (quadriparesis, incontinence, etc.); (e) *short stature, hypotonia, obesity, dry skin, alopecia, excess or loose skin of the hands, acromicria, brachydactyly, clinodactyly, small middle phalanx,* second and fifth digits partial adactyly, wide space between the first and second toes, syndactyly of the second and third toes, simian creases; (f) *endocrine disorders:* thyroid dysfunction (hypothyroidism, hyperthyroidism), diabetes mellitus, precocious or delayed puberty, sterility in males, decreased fertility in females, primary gonadal dysfunction in females, elevated serum levels of follicle-stimulating hormone and luteinizing hormone in institutionalized male patients; (g) *immune disorders:* thymic hormone deficiency, immunodeficiency; (h) *blood disorders/neoplasm:* blood test abnormalities in newborns with benign natural history (increased hematocrit, decreased hematocrit, decreased platelet count, increased white cell count), platelets smaller than normal with reduced numbers and volumes of electron-dense bodies, transient neonatal leukemoid reactions, leukemia (18-fold increased risk), testicular cancer, retinoblastoma, etc. (i) *cardiovascular abnormalities:* congenital heart disease (cushion defects, ventricular septal defect, etc.), high frequency (57%) of mitral valve prolapse in asymptomatic adults, tricuspid valve prolapse and aortic regurgitation less common, high incidence of aberrant right subclavian artery (10% to 20% as compared with 0.5% to 1.5% of the normal population), abnormal radial artery pattern (16% of patients with Down syndrome), intimal arterial fibrodysplasia; (j) *respiratory system:* pulmonary hypoplasia (diminished volume, diminished number of alveoli in relation to acini, enlarged alveoli and alveolar ducts, small alveolar surface area), cystic lung disease, congenital pleural effusion, sleep apnea, upper airway obstruction associated with midfacial hypoplasia (cor pulmonale and congestive heart failure), epiglottic enlargement (nonbacterial), bacterial tracheitis; (k) *alimentary system:* duodenal atresia, duodenal stenosis, annular pancreas, intraluminal duodenal diverticulum, Hirschsprung disease, anorectal anomalies, esophageal dysfunction (reduced number of neurons in esophageal plexus ganglia), celiac disease, biliary atresia; (l) *genitourinary system:* mean stretched penile length and the mean testicular volume below the mean value of normal men, dorsal urethral duplication and/or glandular hypospadias, cryptorchidism; (m) low maternal serum α-fetoprotein levels; (n) other reported abnormalities: premature aging, lordosis, kyphosis, diastasis recti, umbilical hernia, hearing loss, Turner-Down polysyndrome, nonimmune fetal hydrops, short umbilical cord, in association with prune-belly anomaly, etc.

Radiologic Manifestations: (a) *craniofacial anomalies:* brachycephalic microcephaly, hypoplasia of the facial bones and sinuses, short hard palate, high cribriform plate, thin calvaria with wide sutures and delay in closure, orbital hypotelorism, high orbital roofs, soft-tissue thickening of the neck and back of the fetal occiput (ultrasonography) in the second trimester (not a specific sign, not present in all cases of Down syndrome); (b) *central nervous system:* high incidence (about 11%) of bilateral calcification of the basal ganglia, small posterior fossa, small cerebellum, small brain stem, large sylvian fissure in those under 1 year of age, high incidence of midline cava (cavum septi pellucidi, cavum vergae, cavum veli interpositi), posterior fossa ependymal cyst, spinal cord compression due to atlantoaxial dislocation (narrow canal); (c) *spine:* atlanto-occipital instability and dislocation, atlantoaxial instability and dislocation (10% to 20% of individuals with Down syndrome have atlantoaxial instability), subluxation at cervical interspaces other than C_1-C_2, congenital vertebral fusion, flattening of the cervical vertebrae, degenerative arthritis of the cervical vertebrae and intervertebral disks (patients usually over 20 years of age), upper cervical ossicles, increased height and decreased anteroposterior diameter of the lumbar vertebrae in newborns, scoliosis, extreme hyperextension of the fetal head with dorsoflexions of the cervicodorsal segment in the last trimester; (d) *thorax:* 11 pairs of ribs, 2 ossification centers of the manubrium, bell-shaped chest (logistic regression analysis has indicated that if all three findings are present the probability of trisomy 21 is 58.4% [Edwards et al.]), gracile ribs, congenital pleural effusion; (e) *pelvis:* flared iliac wings with small acetabular angles and iliac index, distal tapering of the ischium in the first year of life; (f) *limbs:* short hands with stubby digits, clinodactyly with dysplasia of the middle phalanges of the fifth fingers (shortened, disproportionately wide, and frequently wedge shaped), brachymesophalangia, severe joint laxity, hip dislocation, patellofemoral instability, pes planus, metatarsus varus, genu valgum, acetabular dysplasia with or without hip dislocation, slipped capital femoral epiphysis, tibiotalar slant, pseudoepiphyses of the hands, variable skeletal maturation, stippled epiphyses, etc.

Notes:

(A) CARDINAL SIGNS IN THE NEWBORN: hypotonia, poor Moro reflex, hyperflexibility of the joints, excess skin on the back of the neck, flat facial profile, slanted palpebral fissures, anomalous auricles, dysplastic pelvis, dysplastic middle phalanx of the fifth finger, simian creases; six or more of the above present in 89% of cases (Hall).

(B) DIAGNOSTIC INDEX: eight features used in the index (Rex et al.) included three dermatoglyphic traits (hallucal and forefinger pattern, palmar triradius), two measurements of physical traits (ear length, internipple distance), and three other clinical findings (Brushfield spots, wide-spaced first toe, excess back neck skin; it has been estimated that about 95% of the patients suspected of having this syndrome can be categorized as having or not having it with 99.9% confidence.

(C) RECOMMENDATION OF THE COMMITTEE ON SPORTS MEDICINE, AMERICAN ACADEMY OF PEDIATRICS (*Pediatrics* 74:152, 1984): (a) all children with Down syndrome who wish to participate in sports that involve possible trauma to the head and neck should have lateral view roentgenograms of the cervical region in neutral, flexion, and extension positions within the patient's tolerance before beginning training or competition; this recommendation applies to all participants in the high-risk sports who have not previously had normal findings on cervical roentgenograms; some physicians may prefer to screen all patients with Down syndrome routinely at 5 to 6 years of age to rule out atlantoaxial instability; (b) when the distance between the odontoid process of the axis and the anterior arch of the atlas exceeds 4.5 mm or the odontoid is abnormal, there should be restrictions on sports that involve

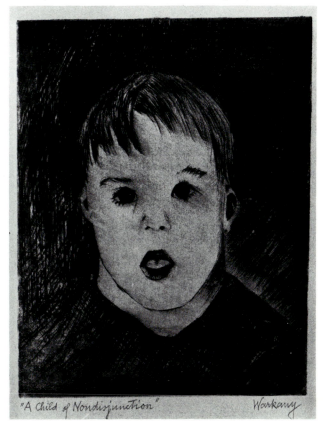

"A Child of Nondisjunction"   Warkany

FIG SY–C–20.
Down syndrome. (From Warkany J: *Congenital Malformations. Notes and Comments.* Chicago, Year Book Medical Publishers Inc, 1971. Used by permission.)

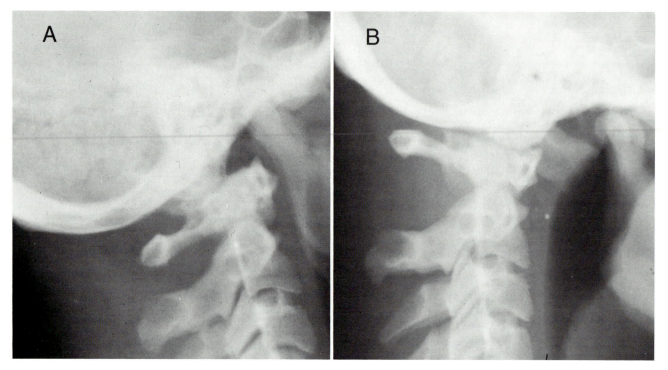

FIG SY-C-21.
Down syndrome with atlanto-occipital instability in a 17-year-old male patient. **A,** a lateral radiograph in extension shows a normal position of the occiput on C_1, with the basion directly over the odontoid. **B,** flexion results in 1.2-cm forward movement on the occiput along the relatively flat articular surface of C_1 (an audible "clunk" was noted clinically). There is no abnormal separation of the odontoid from the anterior ring of C_1. (From Rosenbaum DM, Blumhagen JD, King HA, Atlantooccipital instability in Down syndrome. *A.J.R.* 146:1269, 1986. Used by permission.)

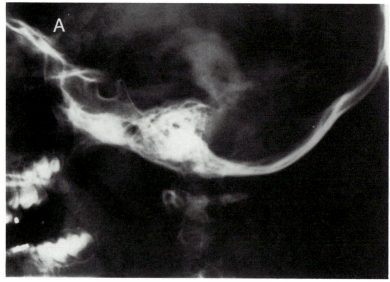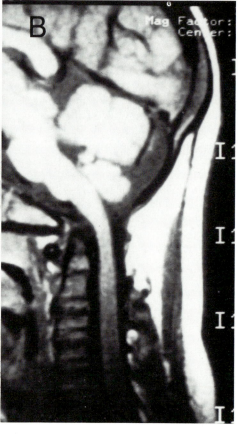

FIG SY-C-22.
Down syndrome in a 7⅓-year-old male. A distance of 4 mm is present between the odontoid process of C_2 and the anterior arch of C_1 **(A).** Magnetic resonance imaging **(B)** shows a moderate impression on the upper cervical cord and medulla by the odontoid process. Note the narrowing of the cord at this level as compared with the segment below. (Courtesy of Robert Binder, M.D., and Bent Kjos, M.D., Magnetic Imaging Affiliates, Oakland, Calif.)

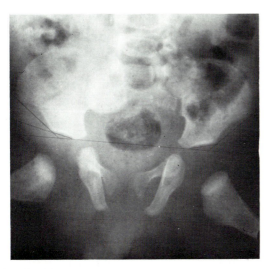

FIG SY—C—23.
Chromosome 21 trisomy syndrome with a flared iliac wing and a small acetabular angle and iliac index. (From Taybi H, Kane P: Small acetabular and iliac angles and associated diseases. *Radiol. Clin. North Am.* 6:215, 1968. Used by permission.)

trauma to the head and neck, and the patient should be followed at regular intervals; (c) at the present time, repeated roentgenograms are not indicated for those who have previously had normal findings; indications for repeated roentgenograms will be defined by research; (d) persons with atlantoaxial subluxation or dislocation and neurological signs or symptoms should be restricted in all strenuous activities, and operative stabilization of the cervical spine should be considered; (e) persons with Down syndrome who have no evidence of atlantoaxial instability may participate in all sports; follow-up is not required unless musculoskeletal or neurologic signs or symptoms develop.

Please refer to the following papers on this subject: Davidson; Pueschel, 1988 (Figs SY—C—20 to SY—C—23).

REFERENCES

Ahmad A, et al.: The fundus in mongolism. *Arch. Ophthalmol.* 94:772, 1976.

Austin JHM, et al.: Short hard palate in newborn: Roentgen sign of mongolism. *Radiology* 92:775, 1969.

Baird PA, et al.: Prune belly anomaly in Down syndrome (letter). *Am. J. Med. Genet.* 26:747, 1987.

Balkany TJ, et al.: Hearing loss in Down's syndrome. *Clin. Pediatr. (Phila.)* 18:116, 1979.

Barabas G, et al.: Coincident Down's and Tourette syndromes: Three case reports. *J. Child Neurol.* 1:358, 1986.

Benacerraf BR, et al.: Down syndrome: Sonographic sign for diagnosis in the second-trimester fetus. *Radiology* 163:811, 1987.

Bentley D: A case of Down's syndrome complicated by retinoblastoma and celiac disease. *Pediatrics* 56:131, 1975.

Braun DL, et al.: Down's syndrome and testicular cancer: A possible association. *Am. J. Pediatr. Hematol Oncol.* 7:208, 1985.

Brooke DC, et al.: Asymptomatic occipito-atlantal instability in Down syndrome (trisomy 21). *J. Bone Joint Surg. [Am.]* 69:293, 1987.

Burwood RJ, et al.: The skull in mongolism. *Clin. Radiol.* 24:475, 1973.

Caffey J, et al.: Pelvic bones in infantile mongolism. *A.J.R.* 80:458, 1958.

Campbell WA, et al.: Serum gonadotrophins in Down's syndrome. *J. Med. Genet.* 19:98, 1982.

Cant AJ, et al.: Bacterial tracheitis in Down's syndrome. *Arch. Dis. Child.* 62:962, 1987.

Chaudhry V, et al.: Symptomatic atlantoaxial dislocation in Down's syndrome. *Ann. Neurol.* 21:606, 1987.

Clark JFJ, et al.: Duodenal atresia in utero in association with Down's syndrome and annular pancreas. *J. Natl. Med. Assoc.* 76:190, 1984.

Cooney TP, et al.: Pulmonary hypoplasia in Down's syndrome. *N. Engl. J. Med.* 307:1170, 1982.

Currarino G, et al.: A developmental variant of ossification of the manubrium sterni in mongolism. *Radiology* 82:916, 1964.

Davidson RG: Atlantoaxial instability in individuals with Down syndrome: A fresh look at the evidence. *Pediatrics* 81:857, 1988.

Diamond LS, et al.: Orthopedic disorders in patients with Down's syndrome. *Orthop. Clin. North Am.* 12:57, 1981.

Down JL: Observations on an ethnic classification of idiots. *London Hosp. Clin. Lect. Rep.* 3:259, 1866.

Dugdale TW, et al.: Instability of the patellofemoral joint in Down syndrome. *J. Bone Joint Surg. [Am.]* 68:405, 1986.

Edwards DK III, et al.: Chest radiographic diagnosis of trisomy-21 in newborn infants. *Radiology* 167:317, 1988.

El-Khoury GY et al.: Posterior atlantooccipital subluxation in Down syndrome. *Radiology* 159:507, 1986.

Fabris N, et al.: Thymic hormone deficiency in normal ageing and Down's syndrome: Is there a primary failure of the thymus? *Lancet* 1:983, 1984.

Fidone GS: Degenerative cervical arthritis and Down's syndrome. *N. Engl. J. Med.* 314:320, 1986.

Fleisher GR, et al.: Primary intimal fibroplasia in a child with Down's syndrome. *Am. J. Dis. Child.* 132:700, 1978.

Foote KD, et al.: Congenital pleural effusion in Down's syndrome. *Br. J. Radiol.* 59:609, 1986.

French HG, et al.: Upper cervical ossicles in Down syndrome. *J. Pediatr. Orthop.* 7:69, 1987.

Fujimoto A, et al.: Nonimmune fetal hydrops and Down syndrome. *Am. J. Med. Genet.* 14:533, 1983.

Fukushima Y, et al.: Are Down syndrome patients predisposed to moyamoya disease? *Eur. J. Pediatr.* 144:516, 1986.

Gatrad AR: Congenital dislocation of the knees in a child with Down-mosaic Turner syndrome. *J. Med. Genet.* 18:148, 1981.

Gerald BE, et al.: Normal and abnormal interorbital distance with special reference to mongolism. *A.J.R.* 95:154, 1965.

Goldhaber SZ, et al.: High frequency of mitral valve prolapse and aortic regurgitation among asymptomatic adults with Down's syndrome. *J.A.M.A.* 258:1793, 1987.

Graham JM Jr, et al.: Choanal atresia with Down syndrome. *J. Pediatr.* 98:664, 1981.

Hall B: Mongolism in newborn infants. *Clin. Pediatr. (Phila.)* 5:4, 1966.

Hanukoglu A, et al.: Fatal aplastic anemia in a child with Down's syndrome. *Acta Paediatr. Scand.* 76:539, 1987.

Heydarian M, et al.: Cardiac tamponade heralding hypothyroidism in Down's syndrome. *Am. J. Dis. Child.* 141:642, 1987.

Hsiang YH, et al.: Gonadal function in patients with Down syndrome. *Am. J. Med. Genet.* 27:449, 1987.

Hungerford GD, et al.: Atlanto-occipital and atlanto-axial dislocations with spinal cord compression in Down's syndrome: A case report and review of the literature. *Br. J. Radiol.* 54:758, 1981.

Ieshima A, et al.: A morphometric CT study of Down's syndrome showing small posterior fossa and calcification of basal ganglia. *Neuroradiology* 26:493, 1984.

Joshi VV, et al.: Cystic lung disease in Down's syndrome. *Pediatr. Pathol.* 5:79, 1986.

Journel H, et al.: Manifestations oculaires de la trisomie 21. *Ann. Pediatr. (Paris)* 33:387, 1986.

Lang DJ, et al.: Hypospadias and urethral abnormalities in Down syndrome. *Clin. Pediatr. (Phila.)* 26:40, 1987.

Laurin S, et al.: Aberrant subclavian artery in Down's syndrome and in A-V canal defects (abstract). *Pediatr. Radiol.* 12:314, 1982.

LeClech G, et al.: La première dentition du trisomique 21. *Ann. Pediatr. (Paris)* 33:795, 1986.

Le Marec B, et al.: Epiphyses ponctuées et aberrations chromosomiques. *Ann. Radiol. (Paris)* 19:599, 1976.

Levack B, et al.: Dislocation in Down's syndrome. *Dev. Med. Neurol.* 26:122, 1984.

Levine OR: Down's syndrome, fetal alcohol syndrome, and upper airway obstruction. *Am. J. Dis. Child.* 141:478, 1987.

Lo RNS, et al.: Abnormal radial artery in Down's syndrome. *Arch. Dis. Child.* 61:885, 1986.

Loudon MM, et al.: Thyroid dysfunction in Down's syndrome. *Arch. Dis. Child.* 60:1149, 1985.

Loughlin GM, et al.: Sleep apnea as a possible cause of pulmonary hypertension in Down syndrome. *J. Pediatr.* 98:435, 1981.

McCook TA, et al.: Epiglottic enlargement in Down's syndrome: New finding? Non-bacterial enlargement of epiglottis. *Pediatr. Radiol.* 12:227, 1982.

Miller JDR, et al.: Changes at the base of skull and cervical spine in Down syndrome. *J. Can. Assoc. Radiol.* 37:85, 1986.

Miller JDR, et al.: Computed tomography of the upper cervical spine in Down syndrome. *J. Comput. Assist. Tomogr.* 10:589, 1986.

Miller M, et al.: Hematological abnormalities in newborn infants with Down syndrome. *Am. J. Med. Genet.* 16:173, 1983.

Modi N, et al: Congenital non-chylous pleural effusion with Down's syndrome. *J. Med. Genet.* 24:567, 1987.

Moessinger AC, et al.: Umbilical cord length in Down's syndrome. *Am. J. Dis. Child.* 140:1276, 1986.

More R, et al.: Platelet abnormalities in Down's syndrome. *Clin. Genet.* 22:128, 1982.

Nakazato Y, et al.: Reduced number of neurons in esophageal plexus ganglia in Down syndrome: Additional evidence for reduced cell number as a basic feature of the disorder. *Pediatr. Pathol.* 5:55, 1986.

Pueschel SM: Atlantoaxial instability and Down syndrome. *Pediatrics* 81:879, 1988.

Pueschel SM: Maternal alpha-fetoprotein screening for Down's syndrome. *N. Engl. J. Med.* 317:376, 1987.

Pueschel SM, et al.: Adolescent development in males with Down syndrome. *Am. J. Dis. Child.* 139:236, 1985.

Pueschel SM, et al.: Atlantoaxial instability in individuals with Down syndrome: Epidemiologic, radiographic, and clinical studies. *Pediatrics* 80:555, 1987.

Pueschel SM, et al: Atlantoaxial instability in persons with Down syndrome: Roentgenographic, neurologic, and somatosensory evoked potential studies. *J. Pediatr.* 110:515, 1988.

Pueschel SM, et al.: Thyroid dysfunction in Down syndrome. *Am. J. Dis. Child.* 139:636, 1985.

Pueschel SM, et al.: Unilateral partial adactyly in Down's syndrome. *Pediatrics* 54:466, 1974.

Puri P, et al.: Intrahepatic biliary atresia in Down's syndrome. *J. Pediatr. Surg.* 10:423, 1975.

Rabinowitz JG, et al.: The lateral lumbar spine in Down's syndrome: A new roentgen feature. *Radiology* 83:74, 1964.

Radetti G, et al.: Down's syndrome, hypothyroidism and insulin-dependent diabetes mellitus. *Helv. Paediat. Acta* 41:377, 1986.

Rex AP, et al.: A diagnostic index for Down syndrome. *J. Pediatr.* 100:903, 1982.

Roberts GM, et al.: Radiology of the pelvis and hips in adults with Down's syndrome. *Clin. Radiol.* 31:475, 1980.

Robison LL, et al.: Down syndrome and acute leukemia in children: A 10-year retrospective survey from children's cancer study group. *J. Pediatr.* 105:235, 1984.

Rogers PCJ, et al.: Neonate with Down's syndrome and transient congenital leukemia. In vitro studies. *Am. J. Pediatr. Hematol. Oncol.* 5:59, 1983.

Rosenbaum DM, et al.: Atlantooccipital instability in Down syndrome. *A.J.R.* 146:1269, 1986.

Ruch W et al.: Coexistent coeliac disease, Graves' disease and diabetes mellitus type 1 in a patient with Down syndrome. *Eur. J. Pediatr.* 144:89, 1985.

Rush PJ, et al.: Tibiotalar slant in Down syndrome. *J. Can. Assoc. Radiol.* 36:257, 1985.

Russell JGB, et al.: Fetal cervical hyperextension in breech presentation. *Br. J. Radiol.* 49:580, 1976.

Sampliner J, et al.: Intraluminal duodenal diverticulum associated with trisomy 21. *A.J.R.* 127:677, 1976.

Saule H, et al.: Pseudohypoaldosteronism in a child with Down syndrome. Long-term management of salt loss by ion exchange resin administration. *Eur. J. Pediatr.* 142:286, 1984.

Simon JH, et al.: Acute megakaryoblastic leukemia associated with mosaic Down's syndrome. *Cancer* 60:2515, 1987.

Spina CA, et al.: Altered cellular immune functions in patients with Down's syndrome. *Am. J. Dis. Child.* 135:251, 1981.

Taybi H, Kane P: Small acetabular and iliac angles and associated diseases. *Radiol. Clin. North Am.* 6:215, 1968.

Ugazio AG, et al.: Immunodeficiency in Down's syndrome. *Acta Paediatr. Scand.* 67:705, 1978.

Villaverde MM, et al.: Turner-mongolism polysyndrome: Review of the first eight known cases. *J.A.M.A.* 234:844, 1975.

Wang AM, et al.: Posterior fossa ependymal cyst and atlantoaxial subluxation in a patient with Down syndrome: CT findings. *J. Comput. Assist. Tomogr.* 8:783, 1984.

Weingast GR, et al: Congenital lymphangiectasia with fetal cystic hygroma: Report of two cases with coexistent Down's syndrome. *J. Clin. Ultrasound* 16:663, 1988.

Wisniewski KE, et al.: Alzheimer's disease in Down's syndrome. Clinicopathologic studies. *Neurology* 35:957, 1985.

CHROMOSOME 22 TRISOMY SYNDROME

Clinical and Radiologic Manifestations: (a) *characteristic facies*: microcephaly, micrognathia, preauricular skin tags, appendages and sinuses, low-set and/or malformed ears, cleft palate; (b) *mental and growth retardation*: (c) deformed lower extremities, fingerlike malposed thumbs, cubitus valgus; (d) abnormal and/or low-set nipples; (e) congenital heart disease.

REFERENCES

Bass HN, et al.: Probable trisomy 22 identified by fluorescent and trypsin-Giemsa banding. *Ann. Genet. (Paris)* 16:189, 1973.

Hsu LYF, et al.: Trisomy 22: Clinical entity. *J. Pediatr.* 79:12, 1971.

Uchida IA, et al.: Familial occurrence of trisomy 22. *Am. J. Hum. Genet.* 20:107, 1968.

CHROMOSOME X, FRAGILE

Synonyms: Fragile X syndrome; fra(x) syndrome; Martin-Bell syndrome.

Chromosomal Abnormality: The fragile site at Xq27.3.

Clinical Manifestations: (a) craniofacial: head circumference over the 50th percentile, long narrow face, large pro-

truding ears, prognathism, etc.; (b) language difficulties, learning disability, mild to marked mental retardation; (c) behavior disorders of various types and severity; (c) mild increase in birth weight, reduced adult height in males; (d) macro-orchidism (70% to 90% in adults); (e) other reported abnormalities: hyperextensible joints, mitral valve prolapse, mitral regurgitation, aortic and tricuspid abnormalities, mild aortic coarctation associated with hypoplasia of the descending aorta, myopia, strabismus, clubfoot deformity, high-arched palate, cleft palate, Robin sequence, seizures, abnormal dermatoglyphics (increased number of arches, decreased total ridge count on the fingertips, etc.), obesity, stubby hands and feet, diffuse hyperpigmentation, cerebral gigantism, pectus excavatum, Down syndrome, neurofibromatosis, etc.

Radiologic Manifestations: (a) mild cerebral ventricular dilatation; (b) mitral valve prolapse, aortic root dilatation; (c) metaphyseal dysostosis (irregularity of the metaphyses of the long bones) with a normal spine and skull.

Notes: (a) fragile X in males may be present without the usual clinical features (large head, macro-orchidism, mental retardation, etc.); (b) adult heterozygotes may have the typical physical features of the syndrome (long face, mandibular prognathism, prominent forehead, macrocephaly, and less frequently, large protruding ears) (Fig SY–C–24).

REFERENCES

Beemer FA, et al.: Cerebral gigantism (Sotos syndrome) in two patients with FRA(X) chromosomes. *Am. J. Med. Genet.* 23:221, 1986.

Fryns J-P, et al.: A peculiar subphenotype in the fra(X) syndrome: Extreme obesity-short stature-stubby hands and feet-diffuse hyperpigmentation. Further evidence of dis-

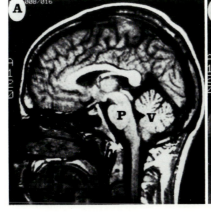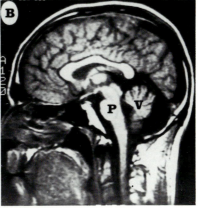

FIG SY–C–24.
Fragile X (Martin-Bell) syndrome shown on Midsagittal magnetic resonance imaging scans in a normal subject **(A)** and a fragile X subject **(B)**. Note the smallness of the cerebellar vermis *(V)* and the pons *(P)* in **B**. (From Reiss AL, Patel S, Kumar AJ, et al.: Neuroan- atomical variations of the posterior fossa in men with the fragile X (Martin-Bell) syndrome. *Am. J. Med. Genet.* 31:407, 1988. Used by permission.)

turbed hypothalamic function in the fra(X) syndrome? *Clin. Genet.* 32:388, 1987.

Fryns J-P et al.: The concurrence of Klinefelter syndrome and fragile X syndrome. *Am. J. Med. Genet.* 30:109, 1988.

Hagerman RJ: Fragile X syndrome. *Curr. Probl. Pediatr.* 17:627, 1987.

Hockey A, et al.: Early manifestations of the Martin-Bell syndrome based on a series of both sexes from infancy. *Am. J. Med. Genet.* 30:61, 1988.

Loehr JP, et al.: Aortic root dilatation and mitral valve prolapse in the fragile X syndrome. *Am. J. Med. Genet.* 23:189, 1986.

McKinley MJ, et al.: Prenatal diagnosis of fragile X syndrome by placental (chorionic villi) biopsy culture. *Am. J. Med. Genet.* 30:355, 1988.

Phelan MC, et al.: Fragile X syndrome and neoplasia. *Am. J. Med. Genet.* 30:77, 1988.

Prouty LA, et al.: Fragile X syndrome: Growth, development, and intellectual function. *Am. J. Med. Genet.* 30:123, 1988.

Thake A, et al.: Is it possible to make a clinical diagnosis of the fragile X syndrome in a boy? *Arch. Dis. Child.* 60:1001, 1985.

Waldstein G, et al.: Aortic hypoplasia and cardiac valvular abnormalities in a boy with fragile X syndrome. *Am. J. Med. Genet.* 30:83, 1988.

Williams CA, et al.: Metaphyseal dysostosis and congenital nystagmus in a male infant with the fragile X syndrome. *Am. J. Med. Genet.* 23:207, 1986.

CHROMOSOME X MONOSOMY (PARTIAL, TOTAL) SYNDROME

Synonyms: Turner syndrome; Ulrich-Turner syndrome.

Chromosome Abnormalities: Majority, 45,X (about 55%); less common: mosaicism (X/XX, X/XY, X/XX/XY), isochromosome X, ring X, partial deletion of the X chromosome.

Clinical Manifestations: (a) *short stature;* (b) relatively small mandible, narrow palate, inner canthal folds, anomalous auricles; (c) blue sclerae, strabismus, ptosis, cataract; (d) webbed neck, low posterior hairline, appearance of a short neck; (e) *transient lymphedema of the hands and feet in infancy;* (f) *shield chest;* (g) *widely spaced hypoplastic nipples;* (h) wide arm span and *cubitus valgus;* (i) hypoplastic nails, cutis laxa, keloid formation; (j) congenital cardiovascular anomalies, in particular, coarctation of the aorta (15% of all cases, 50% in patients with a 45,X karyotype); less common anomalies are septal defects, dissecting aneurysm of the aorta, hypoplastic left-heart syndrome, pulmonary stenosis (45,X), intestinal telangiectasia, hemangiomas, lymphangiectasis (cyclic), increased number of renal arteries, systemic hypertension; (k) *ovarian dysgenesis* with primary amenorrhea; infantile uterus, vagina, and breast; 5% have spontaneous menstruation; fertility rare and often associated with spontaneous abortion (structural and chromosomal defects of the fetus); (l) autoimmune disorders: hypothyroidism (20% of

adult women), diabetes mellitus, inflammatory bowel disease, Addison disease, acute Hashimito thyroiditis; (m) characteristic electroencephalographic (EEG) background activity: (1) more rapid frequency, larger amplitude, and lower amount of alpha waves; (2) higher amount of theta waves; (3) larger amplitude and higher amount of delta waves; (4) larger amplitude and higher amount of beta waves than in controls (Tsuboi et al.); (n) other reported abnormalities: mental retar-

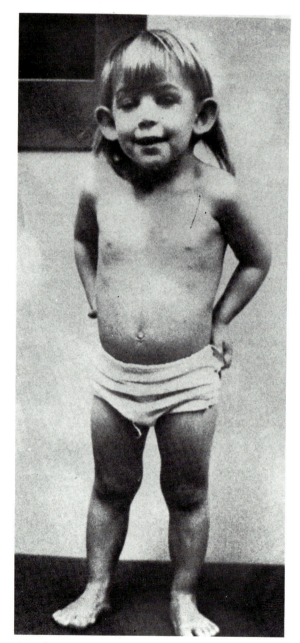

FIG SY–C–25.
Turner syndrome in a 4-year-old girl. Note the somewhat broad chest, prominent ears, and ptosis, but otherwise normal proportions. There is no pronounced neck webbing or edema. (From Hall JG, Sybert VP, Williamson RA, et al.: Turner's syndrome. *West J. Med.* 137:32, 1982. Used by permission.)

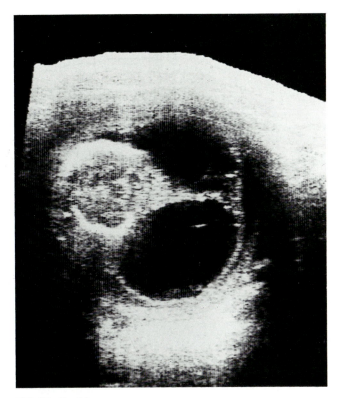

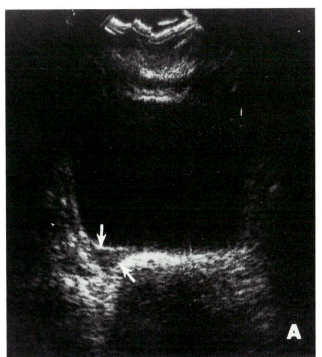

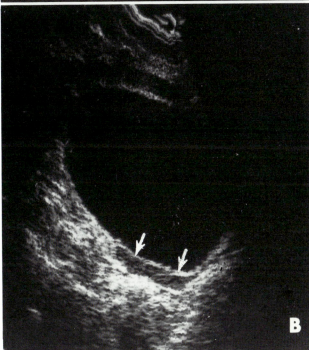

FIG SY–C–26.
Turner syndrome. An abdominal sonogram at 16 weeks' gestation shows a bilobed cystic hygroma related to the fetal neck. (From Newman DE, Cooperberg PL: Genetics of sonographically detected intrauterine fetal cystic hygromas. *J. Can. Assoc. Radiol.* 25:77, 1984. Used by permission.)

dation (Turner syndrome is almost always associated with other chromosomal abnormalities), asynchronous growth of the scalp hair, hearing defect, tendency to become obese, elevated α-fetoprotein levels in amniotic fluid, etc.

Radiologic Manifestations: (a) parietal thinning, brachycephaly, normal sellar volume or increase in size of the pituitary fossa with thinning of the posterior clinoids and dorsum sellae, double floor, abnormal bony contour of the sella turcica, decreased dimensions of the mastoid processes, small facial bones, enlargement and increased thickness of the mandible, extensive calcification of petroclinoid ligaments, excessive pneumatization of sphenoid sinuses, increased angle of the base of the skull, thin cranial vault, craniosynostosis; (b) scoliosis, Scheuermann disease, vertebral fusion, premature sternal fusion, cervical rib; (c) osteoporosis; (d) thinness of the lateral aspect of the clavicle and posterior ends of the ribs; (e) *shortening of the fourth metacarpals*, fusion of the carpal bones, radiocarpal angulation, drumstick phalanges, disproportionately long phalanges in the fourth finger, coarse reticular patterns of the carpal bones, small carpal bone surface area, Madelung deformity; (f) male configuration of the pelvic inlet, protrusio acetabuli; (g) *depression of the medial tibial condyle*, exostosis of the tibia, lateral dislocation of patellae, hypoplastic patellae, irregularity of

FIG SY–C–27.
Turner syndrome. Transverse **(A)** and longitudinal **(B)** scans of the pelvis show a prepubertal-shaped uterus *(arrows)* in this 16-year-old patient with a 45,X0 karyotype. The ovaries were not visible. (From Shawker TH, Garra BS, Loriau DL, et al.: Ultrasonography of Turner's syndrome. *J. Ultrasound Med.* 5:125, 1986. Used by permission.)

the tibial metaphysis and epiphysis, tibiotalar slant; (h) pes cavus, fusion of the tarsal bones, short fourth metatarsals; (i) skeletal maturation retardation; (j) *coarctation of the aorta,* aortic dissection, aortic dilatation, tunnel subaortic stenosis, high incidence of bicuspid aortic valves, pulmonary valvular stenosis (X/XX type), septal defects, dextrocardia, ectopia cordis, myxomatous degeneration of the mitral valve, anomalous pulmonary venous return, systemic venous anomalies, phlebectasia, multiple renal arteries, right aortic arch, intestinal telangiectasia, hemangiomas, etc.; (k) lymphangiogram: hypoplastic lymphatics; (l) pleural-pericardial effusion and ascites in the neonatal period, chylous ascites; (m) *various urinary tract anomalies (horseshoe kidneys,* bifid pelvis, malrotation, reduplication), retrocaval ureter; (n) ultrasonography: absence of ovaries in 45,X, from absent to infantile to normal adult-sized ovaries in the chromosomal mosaics, small uterus (sexual infantilism); (o) prenatal ultrasonographic findings: nuchal blebs or cystic hygroma (lymphocele), ascites, fetal hydrops, small for gestational age; (p) other reported abnormalities: esophageal duplication and hiatal hernia, synovial chondromatosis of the hip joint, etc. (Figs SY−C−25 to SY−C−27).

REFERENCES

Ayuso MC, et al.: Two fertile Turner women in a family. *Clin. Genet.* 26:591, 1984.

Barreto A, et al.: The value of abdominal angiography in Turner's syndrome: A case report. *Cardiovasc. Intervent. Radiol.* 4:97, 1981.

Bercu BB, et al.: A useful radiologic sign for the diagnosis of Turner's syndrome. *Pediatrics* 58:737, 1976.

Bozzola M, et al.: Craniosténose et syndrome de Turner: Association inhabituelle. *Ann. Pediatr. (Paris)* 33:64, 1986.

Brown BSJ, et al.: Ultrasonographic features of the fetal Turner syndrome. *J. Can. Assoc. Radiol.* 35:40, 1984.

Burge DM, et al.: Intestinal haemorrhage in Turner's syndrome. *Arch. Dis. Child.* 56:557, 1981.

Carr RF, et al.: Fetal cystic hygroma and Turner's syndrome. *Am. J. Dis. Child.* 140:580, 1986.

Cleeve DM, et al.: Retrocaval ureter in Turner syndrome. *Urology* 13:544, 1979.

Cleveland RH, et al.: Small carpal bone surface area, a characteristic of Turner's syndrome. *Pediatr. Radiol.* 15:168, 1985.

Courtecuisse V, et al.: Lymphoedème tardif dans le syndrome de Turner. *Arch. Fr. Pediatr.* 35:988, 1978.

de Papendieck LG, et al.: High incidence of thyroid disturbances in 49 children with Turner syndrome. *J. Pediatr.* 111:258, 1987.

Garson A, et al.: Thoracoabdominal ectopia cordis with mosaic Turner's syndrome: Report of a case. *Pediatrics* 62:218, 1978.

Gelfand RA: Cushing's disease associated with ovarian dysgenesis. *Am. J. Med.* 77:1108, 1984.

Hall JG, et al.: Turner's syndrome. *West J. Med.* 137:32, 1982.

Herman TE, et al.: Premature sternal fusion in gonadal dysgenesis with coarctation. *Pediatric. Radiol.* 15:350, 1985.

Huseman CA: Mosaic Turner syndrome with precocious puberty. *J. Pediatr.* 102:892, 1983.

Iinuma K, et al.: "Knuckle sign" in Turner's syndrome. *Lancet* 2:322, 1980.

Keats TE, et al.: The radiographic manifestations of gonadal dysgenesis. *Radiol. Clin. North Am.* 2:297, 1964.

Lacro RV, et al.: Coarctation of the aorta in Turner syndrome: A pathologic study of fetuses with nuchal cystic hygromas, hydrops fetalis, and female genitalia. *Pediatrics* 81:445, 1988.

Lebecque P, et al.: Myxomatous degeneration of the mitral valve in a child with Turner syndrome and partial anomalous pulmonary venous return. *Eur. J. Pediatr.* 141:228, 1984.

Lie JT: Aortic dissection in Turner's syndrome. *Am. Heart J.* 103:1077, 1982.

Lin AE, et al.: Aortic dilation, dissection, and rupture in patients with Turner syndrome. *J. Pediatr.* 109:820, 1986.

Litvak AS, et al.: The association of significant renal anomalies with Turner's syndrome. *J. Urol.* 120:671, 1978.

Lyon AJ, et al.: Growth curve for girls with Turner syndrome. *Arch. Dis. Child.* 60:932, 1985.

Mazzanti L, et al: Heart disease in Turner's syndrome. *Helv. Paediatr. Acta* 43:25, 1988.

Miller MJ, et al.: Echocardiography reveals a high incidence of biscuspid aortic valve in Turner syndrome. *J. Pediatr.* 102:47, 1983.

Natowicz M, et al.: Association of Turner syndrome with hypoplastic left-heart syndrome. *Am. J. Dis. Child.* 141:218, 1987.

Necič S, et al.: Diagnostic value of hand x-rays in Turner's syndrome. *Acta Paediatr. Scand.* 67:309, 1978.

Newman DE, et al.: Genetics of sonographically detected intrauterine fetal cystic hygromas. *J. Can. Assoc. Radiol.* 35:77, 1984.

Pai GS, et al.: Thyroid abnormalities in 20 children with Turner syndrome. *J. Pediatr.* 91:267, 1977.

Paller AS, et al.: Pedal hemangiomas in Turner syndrome. *J. Pediatr.* 103:87, 1983.

Pidcock FS: Intellectual functioning in Turner syndrome. *Dev. Med. Child. Neurol.* 26:539, 1984.

Platt LD, et al.: Altered fetal growth and development in a patient with Turner's syndrome. *Am. J. Perinatol.* 3:175, 1986.

Polychronakos C, et al.: Carbohydrate intolerance in children and adolescents with Turner syndrome. *J. Pediatr.* 96:1009, 1980.

Richart RC, et al.: Turner syndrome, a further cause of tibiotalar slant. *Radiologia* 24:467, 1982.

Robinow M, et al.: Turner syndrome: Sonography showing fetal hydrops simulating hydramnios. *A.J.R.* 135:846, 1980.

Rzymski K, et al.: The skull in gonadal dysgenesis: A roentgenometric study. *Clin. Radiol.* 26:379, 1975.

Salomonowitz E, et al.: Angiographic demonstration of phlebectasia in a case of Turner's syndrome. *Gastrointest. Radiol.* 8:279, 1983.

Savino AW, et al.: Synovial chondromatosis in association with Turner's syndrome. *Clin. Orthop.* 144:183, 1979.

Shawker TH, et al.: Ultrasonography of Turner's syndrome. *J. Ultrasound Med.* 5:125, 1986.

Smith DW, et al.: Asynchronous growth of scalp hair in XO Turner syndrome. *J. Pediatr.* 87:659, 1975.

Smith MA, et al.: Bone demineralisation in patients with Turner's syndrome. *J. Med. Genet.* 19:100, 1982.

Tamburrini O, et al.: Epicardial oesophageal duplication

with hiatal hernia in a case of Turner's syndrome. *Pediatr. Radiol.* 13:342, 1983.

Tommaso CL, et al.: Tunnel subaortic stenosis in XO Turner's syndrome. *Am. J. Cardiol.* 53:1731, 1984.

Treisman J, et al.: Adult Turner syndrome associated with chylous ascites and vascular anomalies. *Clin. Genet.* 31:218, 1987.

Tsuboi T, et al: Turner's syndrome: A qualitative and quantitative analysis of EEG background activity. *Hum. Genet.* 78:206, 1988.

Turner HH: Syndrome of infantilism, congenital webbed neck and cubitus valgus. *Endocrinology* 23:566, 1938.

CHROMOSOME 49, XXXXX SYNDROME

Synonym: Penta-X syndrome.

Clinical Manifestations: (a) *psychomotor retardation, growth failure;* (b) *peculiar facies with coarse features, hypertelorism, mongoloid slant of the palpebral fissures, short neck;* (c) *small hands and feet, clinodactyly of the fifth finger,* talipes equinovarus, etc.; (d) other reported abnormalities: congenital heart defect.

Radiologic Manifestations: (a) *radio-ulnar synostosis,* subluxation of the elbow joint, pseudoepiphysis in the hand, brachymesophalangia of the fifth finger, coxa valga, talipes equinovarus, etc.; (b) retarded bone age.

REFERENCES

Fragoso R, et al: 49,XXXXX syndrome. *Ann. Genet. (Paris)* 25:145, 1982.

Gouyon JB, et al: Pentasomie X. A propos d'une novelle observation. *Ann. Pediatr. (Paris)* 29:584, 1982.

Kesaree N, et al.: A phenotype female with 49 chromosomes presumably XXXXX. *J. Pediatr.* 63:1099, 1963.

Sergovich F, et al.: The 49,XXXXX chromosome constitution: Similarities to the 49,XXXXY condition. *J. Pediatr.* 78:285, 1971.

Silengo MC, et al.: The 49 XXXXX syndrome. Report of a case with 48 XXXX/49 XXXXX mosaicism. *Acta Paediatr. Scand.* 68:769, 1979.

CHROMOSOME XXXXY SYNDROME

Clinical Manifestations: (a) *mental retardation;* (b) *short stature,* short neck; (c) a Down syndrome–like facial appearance; (d) hypotonia; (e) joint laxity, *limited motion at the elbows;* (f) hypogenitalism, hypogonadism; (g) clinodactyly of the fifth finger, gap between the first and second toes, short and wide distal phalanx of the great toes.

Radiologic Manifestations: Nonspecific and not constant: (a) thick cranial vault, hypertelorism, prognathism, sclerotic cranial sutures; (b) *thick sternum* with abnormal segmentation; (c) scoliosis, kyphosis, square vertebral bodies; (d) *radio-ulnar synostosis, dislocation of the radial head,* elongated upper radius, wide proximal end of the ulna, distal ulnar elongation; (e) pseudoepiphyses of the tubular bones of the hands, *brachymesophalangia of the fifth finger,* retarded ossification of the middle and distal phalanges of the fifth fingers; (f) retarded skeletal maturation; (g) narrow iliac wings, coxa valga, shallow intercondylar fossa of the distal part of the femur, pes planus.

REFERENCES

Fraccaro M, et al.: A child with 49 chromosomes. *Lancet* 2:899, 1960.

Houston CS: Roentgen findings in the XXXXY chromosome anomaly. *J. Can. Assoc. Radiol.* 18:258, 1967.

Jancu J: Radioulnar synostosis: A common occurrence in sex chromosomal abnormalities. *Am. J. Dis. Child.* 122:10, 1971.

Rehder H, et al.: The fetal pathology of the XXXXY syndrome. *Clin. Genet.* 30:213, 1986.

Shapiro LR, et al.: XXXXY boy: A 15-month-old child with normal intellectual development. *Am. J. Dis. Child.* 119:79, 1970.

Toudic L, et al.: Le syndrome 49 XXXXY. *Arch. Fr. Pediatr.* 39:247, 1982.

CHROMOSOME XXY SYNDROME

Synonym: Klinefelter syndrome.

Clinical Manifestations: (a) tall, thin-built male; (b) *eunuchoid appearance;* (c) normal or slightly underdeveloped penis, *testicular atrophy, azoospermia,* seminiferous tubule dysgenesis; (d) *gynecomastia;* (e) *elevated gonadotropin excretion in the urine, low normal or decreased 17-ketosteroid excretion in the urine;* (f) mild mental retardation common; (g) chromosome abnormality: 47,XXY in about 80% to 85%, variants and mosaics in about 15% to 20%: 46,XY/47,XXY; XX/XXY; XY/XXY; XXY/XXXY; XXXY/XXXXY; 46,XX/46,XY/47, XXY/48,XXXY/48,XXYY; XY/XXY and fragile X syndrome; (h) association with neoplastic lesions: breast cancer, embryonal carcinoma, teratoma, primary mediastinal germ cell tumor, thyroid cancer, leukemia, primary myelodysplastic syndrome, paraneoplastic syndrome, etc.; (i) other reported abnormalities: incontinentia pigmenti, subarachnoid hemorrhage (aneurysm), diabetes mellitus, pulmonary disease (bronchitis, bronchiectasis, emphysema), mitral valve prolapse, varicose veins, hypostatic leg ulcers, subacute ischemia of the lower limbs, Takayasu arteritis, venous thromboemboli, situs inversus, occurrence in identical twins, etc.

Radiologic Manifestations: Nonspecific and nonconstant: (a) radio-ulnar synostosis; (b) positive metacarpal sign; (c) phalangeal preponderance (normally the length of the fourth metacarpal is equal to length of distal plus proximal phalanges); (d) pointed appearance or squared ends of fingers; (e) brachymesophalangia with or without clinodactyly of fifth finger; (f) high metacarpal index (length/width); (g) miscellaneous anomalies (ribs, spina bifida occulta); (h) *skull* *dysmorphism;* temporal flattening, decreased width of vault, short anteroposterior diameter of skull, shortening of anterior fossa, decrease in length of base, thinning of vault at major fontanelle, premature and excessive calcification of coronal suture, deepening of posterior fossa, shortening of mandibular rami, increase in size of pituitary fossa associated with thinning of posterior clinoid and dorsum sella, and a double floor; (i) dental anomalies: short roots, elongated body, enlarged pulp chamber.

REFERENCES

Al-Awadi SA, et al.: Klinefelter's syndrome, mosaic 46,XX/ 46,XY/47,XXY/48,XXXY/48,XXYY: A case report. *Ann. Genet. (Paris)* 29:119, 1986.

Campbell WA, et al.: Venous thromboembolic disease in Klinefelter's syndrome. *Clin. Genet.* 19:275, 1981.

Chaussain J-L, et al.: Klinefelter syndrome, tumor, and sexual precocity. *J. Pediatr.* 97:607, 1980.

Danziger J, et al.: The sella turcica in primary end organ failure. *Radiology* 131:111, 1979.

Fryns JP, et al.: Klinefelter syndrome and two fragile X chromosomes. *Clin. Genet.* 26:445, 1984.

Garcin JM, et al.: Syndrome de Klinefelter associé a un situs inversus. *Presse Med.* 16:1099, 1987.

Hatch TR, et al.: Klinefelter syndrome in identical twins. *Urology* 26:396, 1985.

Jacobs PA, et al.: Klinefelter's syndrome: An analysis of the origin of the additional sex chromosome using molecular probes. *Ann. Hum. Genet.* 52:93, 1988.

Jancu J: Radioulnar synostosis: A common occurrence in sex chromosomal abnormalities. *Am. J. Dis. Child.* 122:10, 1971.

Kalifa G, et al.: Syndrome de Klinefelter et tératome médiastinal. *Ann. Radiol. (Paris)* 26:138, 1983.

Keats TE, et al.: The radiographic manifestations of gonadal dysgenesis. *Radiol. Clin. North Am.* 2:297, 1964.

Klinefelter HF Jr, et al.: Syndrome characterized by gynecomastia, aspermatogenesis without aleydigism, and increased excretion of follicle stimulating hormone. *J. Clin. Endocrinol. Metab.* 2:615, 1942.

Komatz Y, et al.: Taurodontism and Klinefelter's syndrome. *J. Med. Genet.* 15:452, 1978.

Kosowicz J, et al.: Radiological features of the skull in Klinefelter's syndrome and male hypogonadism. *Clin. Radiol.* 26:371, 1975.

Lee MW, et al.: Klinefelter's syndrome and extragonadal germ cell tumors. *Cancer* 60:1053, 1987.

Mulliez Ph, et al.: Troubles respiratoires au cours du syndrome de Klinefelter. *Presse Med.* 15:667, 1986.

Ohsawa T, et al.: Roentgenographic manifestations of Klinefelter's syndrome. *A.J.R.* 112:178, 1971.

Ormerod AD, et al.: Incontinentia pigmenti in a boy with Klinefelter's syndrome. *J. Med. Genet.* 24:439, 1987.

Phebus CK, et al.: Acute megakaryoblastic leukemia and Klinefelter's syndrome. *Am. J. Pediatr. Hematol. Oncol.* 8:260, 1986.

Sanchez AG, et al.: Lobular carcinoma of the breast in a patient with Klinefelter's syndrome. *Cancer* 57:1181, 1986.

Saupin V, et al.: Ischémie subaiguë des membres inférieurs

chez un malade atteint d'un syndrome de Klinefelter. *Presse Med.* 16:1056, 1987.

Talarmin FM, et al.: Association syndrome de Klinefelter et cancer de la thyroïde. *Presse Med.* 14:1972, 1985.

Verp MS, et al.: Hypostatic ulcers in 47,XXY Klinefelter's syndrome. *J. Med. Genet.* 20:100, 1983.

CHROMOSOME XY (46) GONADAL DYSGENESIS

Mode of Inheritance: X-linked recessive or sex-limited autosomal dominant transmission in most cases.

Clinical and Radiologic Manifestations: (a) short stature, mild developmental delay, skeletal maturation retardation, ectodermal scalp defect, peculiar facies; (b) broad hands and feet; (c) urogenital anomalies, streak gonads; (d) congenital heart disease.

REFERENCE

Brosnan DG: A new familial syndrome of 46,XY gonadal dysgenesis with anomalies of ectodermal and mesodermal structures. *J. Pediatr.* 97:586, 1980.

CHURG-STRAUSS SYNDROME

Histology: The three histological components often are not simultaneously present temporally or spatially: (a) *necrotizing vasculitis;* (b) *tissue infiltration by eosinophils;* (c) *extravascular granulomas.*

Clinical and Radiologic Manifestations: (a) *asthma;* (b) *systemic vasculitis* (c) *eosinophilia;* (d) *allergic rhinitis,* nasal polyposis, sinusitis; (e) *pulmonary infiltrates,* pleural effusion, respiratory failure; (f) hypertension, cardiac failure, pericarditis; (g) abdominal pain, diarrhea, gastrointestinal bleeding and perforation; (h) renal failure; (i) purpura, nodules, erythema, urticaria; (j) arthralgia, myalgia, arthritis; (k) cerebral hemorrhage, brain infarct, cranial nerve palsies, ischemic optic neuritis, mononeuritis multiplex, etc.

REFERENCES

Churg J, Strauss L: Allergic granulomatosis, allergic angiitis and periarteritis nodosa. *Am. J. Pathol.* 27:277, 1951.

Davison AG, et al.: Prominent pericardial and myocardial lesions in the Churg-Strauss syndrome (allergic granulomatosis and angiitis). *Thorax* 38:793, 1983.

Degesys GE, et al.: Allergic granulomatosis: Churg-Strauss syndrome. *A.J.R.* 135:1281, 1980.

Lanham JG, et al.: Systemic vasculitis with asthma and eosinophilia: A clinical approach to the Churg-Strauss syndrome. *Medicine (Baltimore)* 63:65, 1984.

Le Thi Huong Du, et al.: Facteurs pronostiques de la péri-artérite noueuse et de l'angéite de Churg et Strauss. Etude multifactorielle de la survie de 165 malades. *Presse Med.* 14:1341, 1985.

MacFadyen R, et al.: Allergic angiitis of Churg and Strauss syndrome. Response to pulse methylprednisolone. *Chest* 91:629, 1987.

CLAUDE SYNDROME

Etiology: Trauma; neoplasms; vascular disease; mesencephalic paramedian infarct.

Clinical Manifestations: *Ipsilateral fascicular third nerve palsy; contralateral ataxia.*

Radiologic Manifestations: Demonstration of the etiologic factor by computed tomography or magnetic resonance imaging.

Note: A fascicular nerve palsy in association with contralateral hemiplegia is called Weber syndrome.

REFERENCES

Claude H, Loyez: Ramollissement du noyau rouge. *Rev. Neurol. (Paris)* 23:49, 1912 (cited by Woo et al.).

Woo E, et al.: Claude's syndrome: Clinical and computed tomography correlations. *J. Comput. Tomogr.* 11:208, 1987.

CLOUSTON SYNDROME

Mode of Inheritance: Autosomal dominant.

Clinical Manifestations: Recognizable at birth; *ectodermal dysplasia*: rough, thick, easily cracked dyskeratotic skin on the palms and soles; hyperpigmentation of the skin over the knuckles, elbows, knees, axillae, areolae, and pubic areas; thickening deformity; hypoplasia and occasionally absent nails; thin and sparse hair on the head, eyebrows, and body.

Radiologic Manifestations: (a) thickening of the skull; (b) tufting of the terminal phalanges.

REFERENCES

Clouston HR: Hereditary ectodermal dystrophy. *Can. Med. Assoc. J.* 21:18, 1929.

Clouston HR: The major forms of hereditary ectodermal dysplasia (with an autopsy and biopsies on the anhydrotic type). *Can. Med. Assoc. J.* 40:1, 1939.

Escobar V, et al.: Clouston syndrome: An ultrastructural study. *Clin. Genet.* 24:140, 1983.

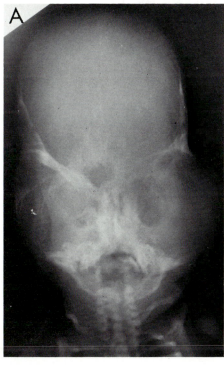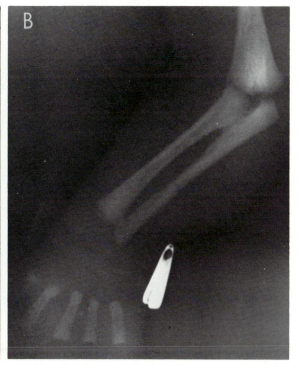

FIG SY–C–28.
Cloverleaf skull–limb anomalies in a 2-day-old male with a grotesque craniofacial appearance (trilobed skull, very low set ears, atretic external ear canals, bilateral gross exophthalmos with microcornea, ocular hypertelorism, and a beaked nose), fixed elbows in flexion, very large thumbs and great toes, syndactyly of the second and third toes. **A,** trilobed skull, orbital hypertelorism, and premature closure of sutures. **B,** marked deformity of the humerus, radius, and ulna at the elbow and flexion deformity.

CLOVERLEAF SKULL DEFORMITY

Synonym: Kleeblattschädel anomaly.

Classification: (a) Holtermuller-Wiedemann type: isolated anomaly; (b) associated with ankylosis in the large joints and bony syndactyly; (c) associated with thanatophoric dysplasia; (d) associated with generalized skeletal dysplasia; (e) associated with other conditions: craniosynostosis syndromes (Apert, Pfiefer, Carpenter, Crouzon), chromosome 13 partial trisomy, 15q partial trisomy, hypopituitarism, a form of camptomelic syndrome, severe form of achondroplasia, amniotic bands, unusual skeletal anomalies (short wide clavicles, winged scapulae, rib anomalies with prominent costovertebral junctions, widely separated ischia, angulated ulnae, polydactyly of the hands and feet, abnormal metacarpal and metatarsal bones), iatrogenic (bilateral subtemporal decompression), osteoglophonic dysplasia, etc.

Clinical Manifestations: (a) *trilobed skull;* (b) *low-set ears, beaked nose, prognathism, recessed nasal root, severe exophthalmos;* (c) limb anomalies; (d) mental retardation.

Radiologic Manifestations: (a) *premature closure of cranial sutures (coronal, lambdoid, squamous)* resulting in grotesque appearance, computed tomographic findings (near complete absence of the lateral orbital wall, thin covering over the temporal lobe, enormous protrusion of the temporal fossa, hydrocephalus), shallow orbits, ocular hypertelorism, relative prognathism; (b) *limb anomalies* (subluxation of the radial heads, bony ankylosis of the elbows, shortness and bowing of the long bones, hip dislocation, webbed toes, webbed fingers); (c) prenatal ultrasonography: polyhydramnios, trilobed skull, increased biparietal diameter, hydrocephalus, intact temporal bone, absent corpus callosum, limb deformities.

Differential Diagnosis (Intrauterine): encephalocele, meningoencephalocele (Figs SY–C–28 and SY–C–29).

REFERENCES

Benallègue A, et al.: Crâne en trèfle associé à une atteinte généralisée du squelette proche de la dysplasie thoracique asphyxiante. *Ann. Genet.* 30:113, 1987.

Cohen MM: Cloverleaf syndrome update. *Proc. Greenwood Center* 5:186, 1986.

Hall BD, et al.: Kleeblattschädel (cloverleaf) syndrome: Severe form of Crouzon's disease? *J. Pediatr.* 80:526, 1972.

Holtermuller K, Wiedemann HR: Kleeblattschädel-Syndrome. *Med. Monatschr.* 14:439, 1960.

Kozlowski K, et al.: Cloverleaf skull and bone dysplasias (report of four cases). *Australas. Radiol.* 31:309, 1987.

McCorquodale M, et al.: Kleeblattschädel anomaly and partial trisomy for chromosome 13(47,XY, +der (13), t(3,13) (q24;q14). *Clin. Genet.* 17:409, 1980.

Noetzel M, et al.: Hydrocephalus and mental retardation in craniosynostosis. *J. Pediatr.* 107:885, 1985.

Say B, et al.: Cloverleaf skull associated with unusual skeletal anomalies. *Pediatr. Radiol.* 17:93, 1987.

Stamm ER, et al.: Kleeblattschadel anomaly. In utero sonographic appearance. *J. Ultrasound Med.* 6:319, 1987.

Wodarz R, et al.: CT—Findings in a case of clover-leaf skull. *Eur. J. Pediatr.* 131:75, 1979.

Zuleta A, et al.: Cloverleaf skull syndrome. *Child Brain* 11:418, 1984.

COCKAYNE SYNDROME

Mode of Inheritance: Autosomal recessive; reported in twins.

Frequency: Over 40 cases (Moyer et al.).

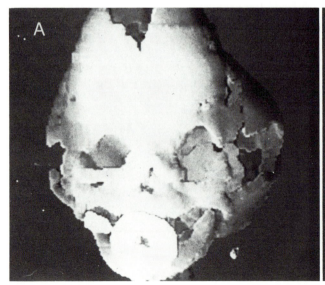
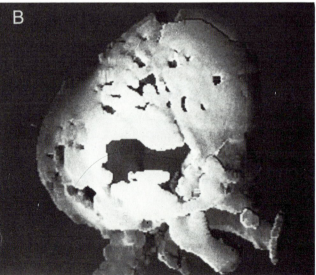

FIG SY–C–29.
Cloverleaf skull deformity in a newborn female with premature fusion of metopic, coronal, and saggital sutures. (Courtesy of Ronald A. Cohen, M.D., Children's Hospital Medical Center, Oakland, Calif.)

Description: A progressive disease that typically becomes manifested in the second year of life; prenatal onset and early postnatal onset of symptoms rare.

Clinical Manifestations: (a) *dwarfism, growth failure;* (b) progressive *mental retardation;* (c) *characteristic cachectic facies* with a loss of adipose tissues, sunken eyes, slender nose, prominent superior maxillae, *microcephaly, senilelike appearance;* (d) *short trunk and relatively large hands and feet;* (e) cool extremities; (f) retinal atrophy, retinitis pigmentosa, cataract; (g) moderate deafness; (h) thin skin, scaly eczematous dermatitis, *dermal photosensitivity;* (i) severe dental caries; (j) renal disease and hypertension; (k) peripheral neuropathy, gait disturbance, incontinence, joint contracture, ankylosis; (l) pathological changes: reduced number of spinal motor neurons and nerve cells in the myenteric plexus of the colon; siderocalcific pericapillary deposits in the cerebellum, basal ganglia, and some parts of the cerebrum; increased sensitivity of cultured skin fibroblasts to ultraviolet light; hydrocephalus; segmental demyelination and granular lysosomal inclusion on ultrastructural examination; (m) prenatal diagnosis with the use of cultured skin fibroblasts: demonstration of sensitivity to ultraviolet light in association with an anomalous response of nucleic acid synthesis in cultured fibroblasts after ultraviolet irradiation (lack of recovery); (n) other reported abnormalities: airway obstruction causing emphysema, hypogonadism, thymic hormone deficiency, low gamma globulin levels, etc.

Radiologic Manifestations: Abnormalities becoming noticeable after the first year of life: (a) *microcephaly, thick cranial vault, abnormal intracranial calcification,* hydrocephalus, demyelination of the white matter, hypoplastic brain stem and cerebellum, small sella turcica; (b) spine abnormalities: ovoid vertebral bodies with anterior notching, biconcave vertebral bodies, increase in the anteroposterior diameter of vertebral bodies, scalloping and posterior wedging, thoracic kyphosis, intervertebral calcification; (c) various nonspecific limb bone abnormalities: slender long bones with narrow medullary canal; slightly bowed fibulas; bulky metaphyses and epiphyses; large tarsal and carpal bones; large second

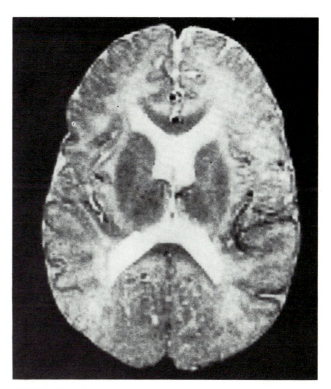

FIG SY–C–30.
Cockayne syndrome in a 39-month-old male. Note the cachetic appearance, deep-set eyes, and sparse hair. (From Dabbagh O, Swaiman KF: Cockayne syndrome: MRI correlates of hypomyelination. *Pediatr. Neurol.* 4:113, 1988. Used by permission.)

FIG SY–C–31.
Cockayne syndrome in a 39-month-old male: T$_2$-weighted axial image of brain. Note the increase in ventricular size. Myelination is limited to the basal ganglia, thalamus, internal capsule, splenium, and genu of the corpus callosum. The pattern is the equivalent of the myelination usually observed at 8 months of age. The rest of the white matter is poorly myelinated as reflected by the fact that the white matter is less intense than the gray matter is; this finding is the opposite of what is normally observed. (From Dabbagh O, Swaiman KF: Cockayne syndrome: MRI correlates of hypomyelination. *Pediatr. Neurol.* 4:113, 1988. Used by permission.)

metacarpal pseudoepiphyses; short and broad metacarpals, metatarsals, and phalanges; ivory epiphyses; cone-shaped epiphyses; asymmetrical fingers; coxa valga; flexion deformities in the elbows and knees; short second toes; (d) osteoporosis; (e) thin elongated ribs; (f) other reported abnormalities: underdevelopment and sclerosis of the mastoids, poor aeration of the paranasal sinuses, small mandible (Figs SY-C-30 and SY-C-31).

REFERENCES

Bensman A et al.: The spectrum of x-ray manifestations in Cockayne's syndrome. *Skeletal Radiol.* 7:173, 1981.

Brumbach RA, et al.: Normal pressure hydrocephalus: Recognition and relationship to neurological abnormalities in Cockayne's syndrome. *Arch. Neurol.* 35:337, 1978.

Cockayne EA: Dwarfism with retinal atrophy and deafness. *Arch. Dis. Child.* 11:1, 1936.

Cunningham M, et al.: Cockayne's syndrome and emphysema. *Arch. Dis. Child.* 53:722, 1978.

Dabbagh O, et al: Cockayne syndrome: MRI correlates of hypomyelination. *Pediatr. Neurol.* 4:113, 1988.

Gandolfi A, et al.: Deafness in Cockayne's syndrome: Morphological, morphometric, and quantitative study of the auditory pathway. *Ann. Neurol.* 15:135, 1984.

Grunnet ML, et al.: Ultrastructure and electrodiagnosis of peripheral neuropathy in Cockayne's syndrome. *Neurology (N.Y.)* 33:1606, 1983.

Higginbottom MC, et al.: The Cockayne syndrome: An evaluation of hypertension and studies of renal pathology. *Pediatrics* 64:929, 1979.

Houston CS, et al.: Identical male twins and brother with Cockayne syndrome. *Am. J. Med. Genet.* 13:211, 1982.

Julien T, et al.: Syndrome de Cockayne: Un cas avec déficity en hormone thymique. *Ann. Pediatr. (Paris)* 33:345, 1983.

Lehmann AR, et al.: Prenatal diagnosis of Cockayne's syndrome. *Lancet* 1:486, 1985.

Levinson ED, et al.: Cockayne syndrome. *J. Comput. Assist. Tomogr.* 6:1172, 1982.

Lewis JM: Cockayne's syndrome. *Clin. Pediatr. (Phila.)* 26:156, 1987.

Moyer DB, et al.: Cockayne syndrome with early onset of manifestations. *Am. J. Med. Genet.* 13:225, 1982.

Proops R, et al.: A clinical study of a family with Cockayne's syndrome. *J. Med. Genet.* 18:288, 1981.

Schmickel RD, et al.: Cockayne syndrome: A cellular sensitivity to ultraviolet light. *Pediatrics* 60:135, 1977.

Silengo MC, et al.: Distinctive skeletal dysplasia in Cockayne syndrome. *Pediatr. Radiol.* 16:264, 1986.

COFFIN-LOWRY SYNDROME

Mode of Inheritance: X-linked semidominant inheritance has been suggested; males are more severely affected than are females.

Frequency: Over 50 published cases (Gilgenkrantz et al., Young).

Clinical Manifestations: (a) *severe mental retardation* in males, less mental retardation in females; (b) *craniofacial dysmorphism:* square forehead with prominent outer lateral aspects, bitemporal narrowing, thickened supraorbital ridge and outer margins, thickened sagittal suture, thickened zygomatic arch, antimongoloid slant of the eyes, hypertelorism, broad nasal bridge, thick nasal septum, anteverted nostrils, thickened prominent lips with pouting lower lip, open-mouth facies, thick and prominent chin, prominent ears; (c) *large flabby hands and tapering fingers;* (d) other reported abnormalities: short stature, forearm fullness due to increased subcutaneous fat, transverse hypothenar crease, general hypotonia with extensible joints, persistent large anterior fontanelle beyond the age of 2 years, cardiomyopathy, pectus carinatum or excavatum, kyphosis, scoliosis.

Radiologic Manifestations: (a) thickened facial bones, hyperostosis frontalis; (b) pectus carinatum or excavatum,

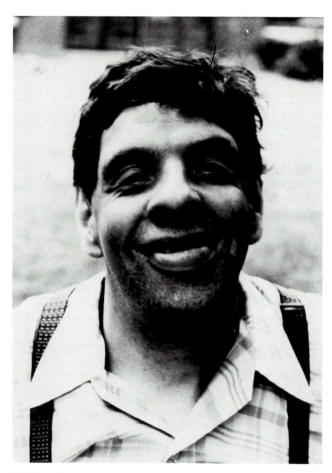

FIG SY-C-32.
Coffin-Lowry syndrome in a 35-year-old patient with coarse facial features, heavy bowed eyebrows, hypertelorism, downslanting of the somewhat narrowed palpebral fissures, big nose with a broad and flattened nasal tip and a large open mouth with full everted lips. (From Haspeslagh M, Fryns JP, Bensen L, et al.: The Coffin-Lowry syndrome. A study of two new index patients and their families. *Eur. J. Pediatr.* 143:82, 1984. Used by permission.)

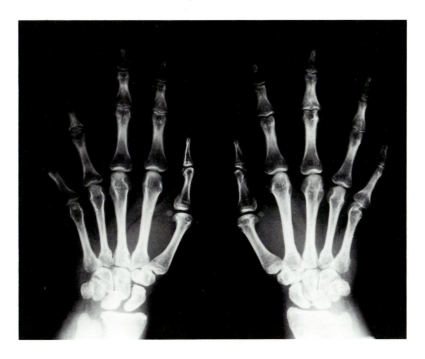

FIG SY−C−33.
Coffin-Lowry syndrome. A radiograph of the hands shows hypoplastic tufted terminal phalanges (From Haspeslagh M, et al.: The Coffin-Lowry syndrome. A study of two new index patients and their families. *Eur. J. Pediatr.* 143:82, 1984. Used by permission.)

spine deformities: kyphosis of the thoracic spine, lumbar gibbous deformity, narrowed intervertebral disk spaces; (c) drumstick-shaped terminal phalanx of the fingers and constriction of the adjacent shaft, coxa valga, lower-limb discrepancy, narrow iliac wings, short great toe; (d) skeletal maturation retardation (Figs SY−C−32 and SY−C−33).

REFERENCES

Charles S, et al: Complication cardiaque mortelle chez un enfant opéré d'une scoliose grave et atteint d'un syndrome de Coffin-Lowry. *Chir. Pediatr.* 29:36, 1988.

Coffin GS, et al.: Mental retardation with osteocartilaginous anomalies. *Am. J. Dis. Child.* 112:205, 1966.

Collacott RA, et al.: Coffin-Lowry syndrome and schizophrenia: A family report. *J. Ment. Defic. Res.* 31:199, 1987.

Gilgenkrantz S, et al.: Coffin-Lowry syndrome: A multicenter study. *Clin. Genet.* 34:230, 1988.

Hanauer A, et al.: Probable localisation of the Coffin-Lowry locus in Xp22.2-p22.1 by multipoint linkage analysis. *Am. J. Med. Genet.* 30:523, 1988.

Haspeslagh M, et al.: The Coffin-Lowry syndrome. A study of two new index patients and their families. *Eur. J. Pediatr.* 143:82, 1984.

Hersh JH, et al.: Forearm fullness in Coffin-Lowry syndrome: A misleading yet possible early diagnostic clue. *Am. J. Med. Genet.* 18:195, 1984.

Hunter AG, et al.: The Coffin-Lowry syndrome. Experience from four centres. *Clin. Genet.* 21:321, 1982.

Krajewska-Walesek M, et al.: Cardiac involvement in Coffin-Lowry syndrome. *Eur. J. Pediatr.* 147:448, 1988.

Lowry B, et al.: A new dominant gene mental retardation syndrome. *Am. J. Dis. Child.* 121:496, 1971.

Temtamy SA, et al.: The Coffin-Lowry syndrome: An inherited faciodigital mental retardation syndrome. *J. Pediatr.* 86:724, 1975.

Vles JSH, et al.: Early clinical signs in Coffin-Lowry syndrome. *Clin. Genet.* 26:448, 1984.

Young ID: The Coffin-Lowry syndrome. *J. Med. Genet.* 25:344, 1988.

COFFIN-SIRIS SYNDROME

Mode of Inheritance: Possibly autosomal recessive.

Frequency: 22 published cases (Rogers et al.).

Clinical Manifestations: (a) *prenatal and postnatal growth deficiency, mental retardation;* (b) *craniofacial dysmorphism: microcephaly, prominent lips, wide mouth, low nasal bridge, wide nose, sparse scalp hair, bushy eyebrows, synophrys;* (c) *nail hypoplasia or absence, with predominantly fifth finger and toe involvement;* (d) *body hypertrichosis;* (e) *lax joints;* (f) *feeding difficulties in infancy;* (g) *other reported abnormalities:* congenital heart disease, cleft palate, scoliosis, perforated ulcer in infancy, frequent respiratory infections, absent uterus, redundant antral/pyloric mucosa with thickened folds causing gastric outlet obstruction, hindbrain dysgenesis (inferior and medial accessory olives, large arcuate nuclei, heterotopic olivary nuclei, heterotopic nuclei in the white matter of the cerebellum), medulloblastoma, etc.

Radiologic Manifestations: (a) *absent or hypoplastic terminal phalanges of the fifth fingers and toes;* (b) *absent or hypoplastic terminal phalanges of other fingers and toes;* (c)

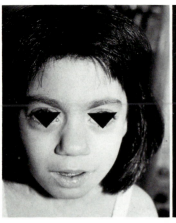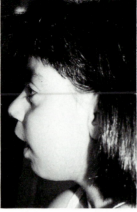

FIG SY–C–34.
Coffin-Siris syndrome in a 4-year-old female having a coarse facies with heavy eyebrows, synophrys, a bulbous nose, a prominent philtrum, and full lips (From Franceschini P, Silengo MC, Bianco R, et al.: The Coffin-Siris syndrome in two siblings. *Pediatr. Radiol.* 16:330, 1986. Used by permission.)

other limb anomalies: clinodactyly, radial head dislocation, cone-shaped epiphyses, coxa valga, foot deformities (varus, valgus), absence of middle phalangeal ossification of the toes, small or absent patellae; (d) other reported abnormalities: *retarded bone age*, absent corpus callosum, pectus excavatum, hypoplastic clavicle, scoliosis, narrow intervertebral disks, eventration of the diaphragm, ureteropelvic junction obstruction, bladder diverticula, intestinal malrotation, Dandy-Walker malformation, vertebral fusion, supernumerary vertebrae and ribs, intussusception, gastric outlet obstruction, etc. (Figs SY–C–34 and SY–C–35).

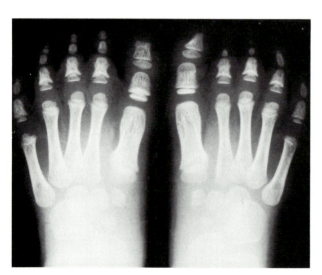

FIG SY–C–35.
Coffin-Siris syndrome in a 4-year-old female with hypoplasia/aplasia of the distal phalanges (From Franceschini P, Silengo MC, Bianco R, et al.: The Coffin-Siris syndrome in two siblings. *Pediatr. Radiol.* 16:330, 1986. Used by permission.)

REFERENCES

Bodurtha J, et al.: Distinctive gastrointestinal anomaly associated with Coffin-Siris syndrome. *J. Pediatr.* 109:1015, 1986.
Coffin GS, et al.: The Coffin-Siris syndrome. *Am. J. Dis. Child.* 139:12, 1985.
Coffin GS, Siris E: Mental retardation with absent fifth fingernail and terminal phalanx. *Am. J. Dis. Child.* 119:433, 1970.
DeBassio WA, et al.: Coffin-Siris syndrome. Neuropathologic findings. *Arch. Neurol.* 42:350, 1985.
Franceschini P, et al.: The Coffin-Siris syndrome in two siblings. *Pediatr. Radiol.* 16:330, 1986.
Haspeslagh M, et al.: The Coffin-Siris syndrome: Report of a family and further delineation. *Clin. Genet.* 26:374, 1984.
Lucaya J, et al.: The Coffin-Siris syndrome: A report of four cases and review of the literature. *Pediatr. Radiol.* 11:35, 1981.
Rogers L, et al: Medulloblastoma in association with the Coffin-Siris syndrome. *Child Nerv. Syst.* 4:41, 1988.

COGAN SYNDROME

Etiology: Vasculitis.

Frequency: Rare.

Clinical Manifestations: (a) general symptoms: headaches, myalgia, arthralgia, abdominal pain, pleuritis, fever; (b) ophthalmologic findings: *redness, photophobia,* eye discomfort, disturbance of visual acuity, *interstitial keratitis,* conjunctivitis, excess lacrimation, ciliary flush, uveitis, episcleritis, scleritis, inflamed optic papilla, muscular involvement, papilledema, thinned sclera, cells in the anterior chamber, corneal ulceration, blindness; (c) *vestibuloauditory dysfunction,* mainly cochlear; sensorineural hearing defect; vertigo; tinnitus; nausea; intralabyrinthine osteogenesis; (d) congestive heart failure, hypertension, vascular occlusion; (e) eosinophilia, nonreactive serology for syphilis; (f) other reported abnormalities: gastrointestinal hemorrhage, adenopathy, splenomegaly.

Radiologic Manifestations: (a) cardiovascular: congestive heart failure, aortic insufficiency (aortitis, inflammatory or myxoid degeneration of valves), vascular occlusion (partial or complete); (b) pleural effusion (Fig SY–C–36).

Differential Diagnosis: syphilis; tuberculosis; connective tissue disorders; sarcoidosis; etc.

REFERENCES

Cogan DG: Syndrome of nonsyphilitic interstitial keratitis and vestibuloauditory symptoms. *Arch. Ophthalmol.* 33:144, 1945.

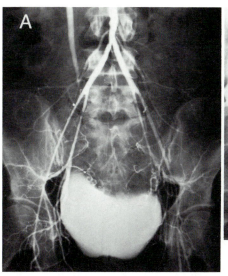
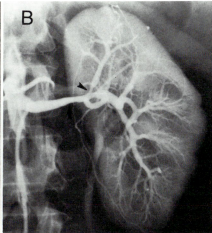

FIG SY–C–36.
Cogan syndrome. **A,** diffuse narrowing of the right external iliac artery and both internal iliac arteries. Also, the aorta is stenotic, and the left common femoral artery is occluded. **B,** segmental narrowing of the main left renal artery *(arrow)* and focal stenosis of the upper primary branch *(arrowhead).* (From Vollertsen RS, McDonald TJ, Younge BR, et al.: Cogan's syndrome: 18 cases and a review of the literature. *Mayo Clin. Proc.* 61:344, 1986. Used by permission.)

Kundell SP, et al.: Cogan syndrome in childhood. *J. Pediatr.* 97:96, 1980.

Laffin MA, et al.: Vestibuloauditory impairment in Cogan's syndrome: A case report. *J. Otolaryngol.* 16:137, 1987.

LaRaja RD: Cogan syndrome associated with mesenteric vascular insufficiency. *Arch. Surg.* 111:1028, 1976.

Rarey KE, et al.: Intralabyrinthine osteogenesis in Cogan's syndrome. *Am. J. Otolaryngol.* 7:87, 1986.

Vollertsen RS, et al.: Cogan's syndrome: 18 cases and a review of the literature. *Mayo Clin. Proc.* 61:344, 1986.

COHEN SYNDROME

Mode of Inheritance: Probably autosomal recessive.

Frequency: Uncommon.

Clinical Manifestations: (a) low birth weight for gestation, *short stature, obesity;* (b) *mental retardation;* (c) *hypotonia;* (d) *craniofacial dysmorphism:* microcephaly, high nasal bridge, hypotelorism, prominent ears, maxillary hypoplasia, malar hypoplasia, short philtrum, open mouth, micrognathia, antimongoloid slanted eyes, mottled pigment on the retina, prominent upper incisors, narrow palate, gingival hyperplasia; (e) *hyperextensibility of the joints,* cubitus valgus, genu valgum, *narrow hands and feet,* finger syndactyly (second and third), hip dislocation; (f) delayed puberty; (g) *ophthalmologic abnormalities:* decreased visual acuity, hemeralopia, constricted visual fields, chorioretinal dystrophy with bull's-eye–like maculae and pigmentary deposits, optic atrophy, isoelectric electroretinogram, strabismus, myopia, coloboma, microphthalmos.

Radiologic Manifestations: (a) mild shortening of the metacarpals and metatarsals, cubitus valgus, genu valgus; (b) mild lumbar lordosis, mild thoracic scoliosis (Fig SY–C–37).

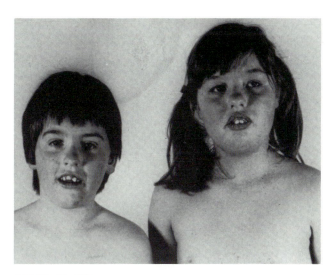

FIG SY–C–37.
Cohen syndrome. Downward-slanting palpebral fissures, a prominent nasal bridge, an open mouth due to a short philtrum, and prominent maxillary incisors are present. (From Goecke T, Majewski F, Kauter KD, et al.: Mental retardation, hypotonia, obesity, ocular, facial, dental, and limb abnormalities (Cohen syndrome). *Eur. J. Pediatr.* 138:338, 1982. Used by permission.)

REFERENCES

Carey JC, et al.: Confirmation of the Cohen syndrome. *J. Pediatr.* 93:239, 1978.

Cohen MM, et al.: A new syndrome with hypotonia, obesity, mental deficiency, and facial, ocular, and limb abnormalities. *J. Pediatr.* 83:280, 1973.

Ferré P, et al.: Le syndrome de Cohen, une affection autosomique récessive? *Arch. Fr. Pediatr.* 39:159, 1982.

Goecke T, et al.: Mental retardation, hypotonia, obesity, ocular, facial, dental, and limb abnormalities (Cohen syndrome) *Eur. J. Pediatr.* 138:338, 1982.

Koussef BG: Cohen syndrome: Futher delineation and inheritance. *Am. J. Med. Genet.* 9:25, 1981.

Méhes K, et al: Cohen syndrome: A connective tissue disorder? *Am. J. Med. Genet.* 31:131, 1988.

Norio R, et al: Are the Mirhosseini-Holmes-Walton syndrome and the Cohen syndrome identical (letter)? *Am. J. Med. Genet.* 25:397, 1986.

Norio R, et al.: Further delineation of the Cohen syndrome; report on chorioretinal dystrophy, leukopenia and consanguinity. *Clin. Genet.* 25:1, 1984.

Young ID, et al.: Intrafamilial variation in Cohen syndrome. *J. Med. Genet.* 24:488, 1987.

COMPARTMENTAL SYNDROMES

Definition: A compromise of circulation and various functions of tissue within a closed space as a result of increased intracompartmental pressure.

Locations: Forearm (dorsal, volar); hand (interosseous); leg (anterior, lateral, superficial posterior, deep posterior).

Etiology: (a) decreased compartmental size (postsurgical, external pressure); (b) increased compartmental content: hemorrhage (fracture, vascular injury, blood disorders), swelling (ischemia, exercise, trauma, burns, postsurgical, venous obstruction, nephrotic syndrome, infiltrated infusion, prolonged abnormal recumbent posture, snake bite, eclampsia, lumbar sympathectomy, disk surgery, muscular hypertrophy, pneumatic tourniquet, sepsis in the newborn, weight lifting, intraosseous infusion, etc.

Clinical Manifestations: (a) pain, sensory changes, painful passive movements; (b) swelling, increased tissue tension; (c) circulatory deficiency, ischemic necrosis.

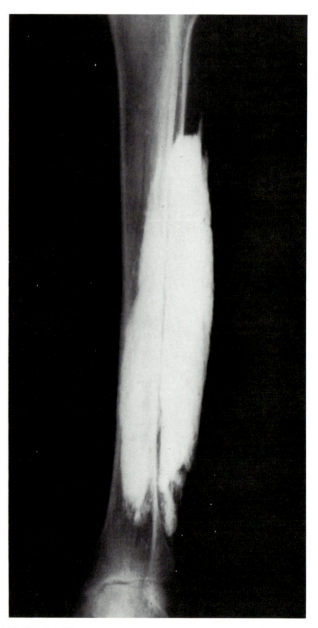

FIG SY—C—39.
Compartment syndrome. Extensive ectopic calcification in all compartments of the leg is apparent. (From Viau MR, Pedersen HE, Salciccioli GG, et al.: Ectopic calcification as a late sequela of compartment syndrome. *Clin. Orthop.* 176:178, 1983. Used by permission.)

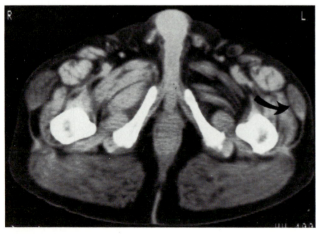

FIG SY—C—38.
Chronic compartment syndrome. A computed tomographic scan demonstrates the somewhat inhomogeneous swelling of the right tensor fascia lata compared with the normal appearance of the left tensor muscle *(arrow)*. (From Rydholm U, Brun A, Ekebunds L, et al.: Chronic compartmental syndrome in the tensor fasciae latae muscle. *Clin. Orthop.* 177:169, 1983. Used by permission.)

Radiologic Manifestations: (a) soft-tissue swelling; (b) hematoma and deep soft-tissue swelling demonstrated by computed tomography or ultrasonography; (c) arteriography: vascular obstruction; (d) ectopic calcification as a late sequela (Figs SY−C−38 and SY−C−39).

REFERENCES

Allen MJ, et al.: Exercise pain in the lower leg. Chronic compartment syndrome and medial tibial syndrome. *J. Bone Joint Surg. [Br.]* 68:818, 1986.

Christiansen SD, et al.: Ischemic extremities due to compartment syndromes in a septic neonate. *J. Pediatr. Surg.* 18:641, 1983.

Greene TL, et al.: Compartment syndrome of the arm—a complication of the pneumatic tourniquet. *J. Bone Joint Surg. [Am.]* 65:270, 1983.

Lee BY, et al.: Management of compartmental syndrome. Diagnostic and surgical considerations. *Am. J. Surg.* 148:383, 1984.

Matsen FA, et al.: Compartmental syndromes in children. *J. Pediatr. Orthop.* 1:33, 1981.

Matsen FA, et al.: Diagnosis and management of compartmental syndromes. *J. Bone Joint Surg. [Am.]* 62:286, 1980.

Rimar S, et al: Compartment syndrome in an infant following emergency intraosseous infusion. *Clin. Pediatr. (Phila.)* 27:259, 1988.

Rydholm U, et al.: Chronic compartmental syndrome in the tensor fasciae latae muscle. *Clin. Orthop.* 177:169, 1983.

Verta MJ, et al.: Adductor canal compression syndrome. *Arch. Surg.* 119:345, 1984.

Viau MR, et al.: Ectopic calcification as a late sequela of compartment syndrome. *Clin. Orthop.* 176:178, 1983.

CONTRACTURAL ARACHNODACTYLY

Synonyms: Congenital contractural arachnodactyly; Beals-Hecht syndrome.

Mode of Inheritance: Autosomal dominant with variable expressivity; many cases sporadic.

Frequency: Uncommon.

Clinical Manifestations: (a) craniofacial appearance: oval-shaped head, somewhat deep set eyes, small mouth, mild limitation in excursion of the jaw, *external ear deformity* (crumbled appearance of the anthelix, flattening of the helix and partial obliteration of the concha); (b) *progressive scoliosis in childhood;* (c) *arachnodactyly;* (d) *flexion contracture of the proximal interphalangeal joints of the fingers, flexion deformity of the elbows and knees,* adducted thumbs, ulnar deviation of the fingers, spontaneous improvement of the contracture with time; (e) *dolichostenomelia;* (f) other reported abnormalities: keratoconus, micrognathia, heart disease (mitral regurgitation, aortic aneurysmal dilatation), single umbilical artery, ankyloblepharon, hypoplastic muscles.

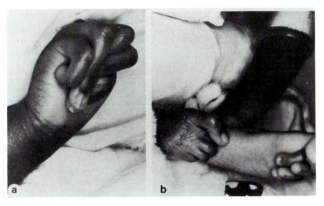

FIG SY−C−40.
Contractural arachnodactyly. Long and thin fingers **(a)** and toes **(b)** and contracture are present. (From Currarino G, Friedman JM: A severe form of congenital contractural arachnodactyly in two newborn infants. *Am. J. Med. Genet.* 25:763, 1986. Used by permission.)

Radiologic Manifestations: (a) slight osteopenia; (b) *gracile bones;* (c) mild bowing of the long bones; (d) *elongation of the proximal phalanges of the fingers and toes;* (e) other reported abnormalities: advanced bone age, vertebral malformations, restrictive lung disease resulting from kyphoscoliosis and thoracic constriction, esophageal atresia, duodenal atresia with an annular pancreas, mitral valve prolapse.

Differential Diagnosis: Marfan syndrome; arthrogryposis (amyoplasia congenita).

Notes: (a) cases reported under the title of contractural arachnodactyly may represent clinically and etiologically heterogeneous conditions; (b) a suggestion has been that the patient reported by Marfan had contractural arachnodactyly (Figs SY−C−40 and SY−C−41).

REFERENCES

Anderson RA, et al.: Cardiovascular findings in congenital contractural arachnodactyly: Report of an affected kindred. *Am. J. Med. Genet.* 18:265, 1984.

Bass HN, et al.: Congenital contractural arachnodactyly, keratoconus, and probable Marfan syndrome in the same pedigree. *J. Pediatr.* 98:591, 1981.

Beals RK, et al.: Congenital contractural arachnodactyly: A heritable disorder of connective tissue. *J. Bone Joint Surg. [Am.]* 53:987, 1971.

Currarino G, et al.: A severe form of congenital contractural arachnodactyly in two newborn infants. *Am. J. Med. Genet.* 25:763, 1986.

Hecht F, et al.: "New" syndrome of congenital contractural arachnodactyly originally described by Marfan in 1896. *Pediatrics* 49:574, 1972.

Ho NK, et al.: Congenital contractural arachnodactyly. Report of a neonate with advanced bone age. *Am. J. Dis. Child.* 133:639, 1979.

Marfan AB: Un cas de déformation congénitale des quatre

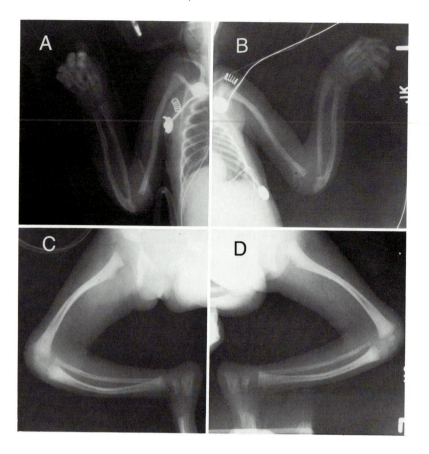

FIG SY–C–41.
Contractural arachnodactyly. Radiographs of the upper and lower limbs show severe flexion contracture at the elbows and knees. The long bones are bowed, elongated, and thin, with narrow medullary cavities. (From Currarino G, Friedman JM: A severe form of congenital contractural arachnodactyly in two newborn infants. _Am. J. Med. Genet._ 25:763, 1986. Used by permission.)

membres, plus prononcée aux extremités caracterisée par l'allongement des os avec un certain degré d'amincissement. _Bull. Mem. Soc. Med. Hop. (Paris)_ 13:220, 1896.

Ramos MA, et al.: Congenital contractural arachnodactyly. Report of four additional families and review of literature. _Clin. Genet._ 27:570, 1985.

Note: Another condition with patients' symptoms reported to be of costal origin is the "floating-rib syndrome": chronic, incapacitating loin pain mimicking renal colic in childhood, reproducible by palpation of involved (11th or 12th) rib, "cure" with subperiosteal resection of the painful rib.

COSTO-ILIAC IMPINGEMENT SYNDROME

Etiology: Impingement of the lowest rib against the iliac crest in association with loss of height.

Clinical Manifestations: (a) back pain in the region of the 12th thoracic vertebra that radiates to the loin or loin pain alone; (b) grating sensation in some cases; (c) loss of height over the years; (d) reproduction of pain by palpation under the lowest rib and by lateral flexion to the affected side, when the rib could be felt impinging on the iliac crest; (e) relief of symptoms following rib resection.

Radiologic Manifestations: (a) osteoporosis of the vertebrae; (b) long 12th ribs.

REFERENCES

Boddy S-AM, et al.: Floating rib syndrome mimicking renal colic in childhood. _J. Pediatr. Surg._ 21:199, 1986.

Wynne AT, et al.: Costo-iliac impingement syndrome. _J. Bone Joint Surg. [Br.]_ 67:124, 1985.

CÔTÉ-KATSANTONI SYNDROME

Clinical Manifestations: Retarded somatic growth; mental retardation; ectodermal dysplasia; transient neutropenia; malabsorption; etc.

Radiologic Manifestations: Osteosclerosis.

REFERENCES

Blau EB: Ectodermal dysplasia, osteosclerosis, atrial septal defect, malabsorption, neutropenia, growth, and mental retardation: The Côté-Katsantoni syndrome? *Am. J. Med. Genet.* 26:729, 1987.

Côté GB, Katsantoni A: Osteosclerosis and ectodermal dysplasia, in Papadatos CJ, Bartosocas CS (eds.): *Skeletal Dysplasia.* New York, Alan R Liss Inc, 1982, pp. 161–162.

COWDEN SYNDROME

Synonym: Multiple hamartoma syndrome.

Mode of Inheritance: Autosomal dominant with a high penetrance in males and females and interfamilial and intrafamilial differences in the expressivity of symptoms.

Frequency: 85 cases published in the English literature (1963 to 1986) (Chen et al.).

Clinical Manifestations: (a) *large head size, birdlike facies,* hypoplastic mandible and maxilla, microstomia, high-arched palate; (b) *breast lesions:* virginal hyperplasia, fibrocystic disease, neoplasm, benign gynecomastia in males; (c) *multiple facial papules, acral keratoses, palmoplantar keratoses,* acral verrucoid lesions, dermal fibromas, multiple skin tags, lipomas, cutaneous malignancies; (d) *multiple oral papillomas,* (Fig SY–C–42) oral fibromas, scrotal tongue, oral malignancies; (e) *thyroid diseases:* goiter, adenoma, hyperthyroidism, hypothyroidism, thyroiditis, thyroglossal duct cyst, follicular adenocarcinoma; (f) *genitourinary system:* menstrual irregularities, miscarriages, stillbirths, ovarian abnormalities (cysts, etc.), leiomyomas in females, vaginal and vulvar cysts, adenocarcinoma of the uterus, carcinoma of the uterine cervix, carcinoma of the ovary, hydrocele, varicocele, transitional cell carcinoma of the renal pelvis, transitional cell carcinoma of the bladder; (g) *alimentary system:* polyps (hamartomatous, juvenile, simple hyperplastic), diverticula of the colon, ganglioneuromas, neuromas, epithelioid leiomyoma of the rectosigmoid, adenocarcinoma of the colon, hepatic hamartoma; (h) *nervous system:* dullness, seizures, intention tremors, neuroma of cutaneous nerves, neurofibroma, meningioma, hearing loss; (i) *eye:* cataracts, angioid streaks, myopia, congenital blood vessel anomaly; (j) *other reported abnormalities:* vocal cord polyp, soft-tissue tumors (lipomas, fibroangiomas, angiolipoma), cavernous hemangiomas, cyst of the scalp, supernumerary digits, pectus excavatum, scoliosis, kyphosis, bone cyst, etc.

Radiologic Manifestations: (a) alimentary tract polyps; (b) thyroid tumor; (c) breast lesions.

Note: "Cowden" is the family name of the propositus.

Differential Diagnosis: Gardner syndrome; Peutz-Jeghers syndrome; Cronkhite-Canada syndrome; multiple adenomatous polyps.

REFERENCES

Brownstein MH, et al.: Trichilemmomas in Cowden's disease. *J.A.M.A.* 238:26, 1977.

Carlson HE, et al.: Cowden disease: Gene marker studies and measurements of epidermal growth factor. *Am. J. Hum. Genet.* 38:908, 1986.

Chen YM, et al.: Cowden's disease: A case report and literature review. *Gastrointest. Radiol.* 12:325, 1987.

Flageat J, et al.: La maladie de Cowden. Syndrome des hamartomes multiples. *J. Radiol.* 65:701, 1984.

Gold BM, et al.: Radiologic manifestations of Cowden disease. *A.J.R.* 135:385, 1980.

Hauser H, et al.: Radiological findings in multiple hamartoma syndrome (Cowden disease): Report of three cases. *Radiology* 137:317, 1980.

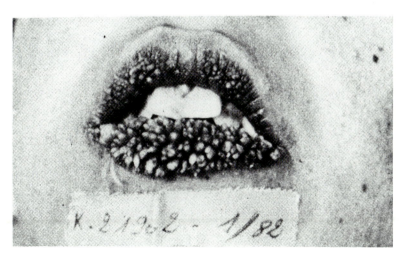

FIG SY–C–42.
Cowden syndrome. Labial papillomatosis is present (From Flageat J, Vircens JL, Binameur M, et al.: La maladie de Cowden. Syndrome des hamartomes multiples. *J. Radiol.* 65:701, 1984. Used by permission.)

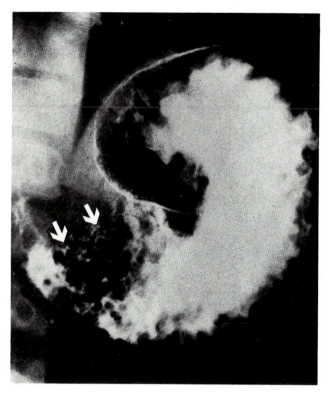

FIG SY–C–43.
Cowden syndrome. Gastric polyps are shown *(arrows)*. (From Flageat J, Vircens JL, Binameur M, et al.: La maladie de Cowden. Syndrome des hamartomes multiples. *J. Radiol.* 65:701, 1984. Used by permission.)

Lloyd KM, et al.: Cowden's disease: A possible new symptom complex with multiple system involvement. *Ann. Intern. Med.* 58:136, 1963.
Starink TM, et al.: The Cowden syndrome: A clinical and genetic study in 21 patients. *Clin. Genet.* 29:222, 1986.
Walton BJ, et al.: Cowden's disease: A further indication for prophylactic mastectomy. *Surgery* 99:82, 1986.

CRANIOECTODERMAL DYSPLASIA

Mode of Inheritance: Possibly autosomal recessive (siblings in one family).

Clinical Manifestations: (a) small stature; (b) *craniofacial dysmorphism:* large dolichocephalic head, frontal bossing, anteverted nares, full cheeks, epicanthal folds, antimongoloid slant of the eyes, posteriorly rotated ears, small helices, everted lower lips, high-arched palate, multiple oral frenula, capillary nevus on the forehead; (c) myopia, hyperopia, nystagmus; (d) *dental anomalies:* microdontia, hypodontia, fusion, widely spaced teeth, enamel dysplasia; (e) fine, sparse, and slow-growing hair; (f) short and narrow thorax, pectus excavatum, congenital heart disease; (g) limb anomalies: short limbs, hyperextensible joints, small hands, clinodactyly of the fifth fingers, cutaneous syndactyly, aberrant palmar creases, broad and short nails of the fingers, short

toes, increased space between the first and second toes, cutaneous syndactyly of the second and third toes, hallux valgus, etc.

Radiologic Manifestations: (a) osteoporosis; (b) limb anomalies: short tubular bones, especially in the hands and feet, thinness of the cortex of the tubular bones, slight widening of the metaphyses, flatness of the epiphyseal ossification center, delayed appearance of ossification of the femoral head, relative shortness of fibulas; (c) infantile type of vertebrae with biconvex upper and lower borders, narrow interpediculate distance in the lower lumbar region.

REFERENCES

Dunber D: Picture of the month (cranioectodermal dysplasia). *Am. J. Dis. Child.* 133:1276, 1979.
Levin LS, et al.: A heritable syndrome of craniosynostosis, short thin hair, dental abnormalities and short limbs: Cranioectodermal dysplasia. *J. Pediatr.* 90:55, 1977.
Sensenbrenner JA, et al.: New syndromes of skeletal, dental and hair abnormalities. *Birth Defects* 11:372, 1975.

CRANIO-FRONTO-NASAL DYSPLASIA

Mode of Inheritance: The majority of reported cases have been familial and females; the mode of inheritance has not been definitely determined, male-to-male transmissions have been reported, and the females in the familial cases are more severely affected than males are.

Frequency: Approximately 50 published cases (Young et al.).

Clinical Manifestations: (a) *craniofacial dysmorphism:* brachycephaly, plagiocephaly, acrocephaly, dolichocephaly, frontal bossing, broad forehead, facial asymmetry, midface hypoplasia, occular hypertelorism, broad nasal tip, bifid nose, esotropia or exotropia, primary telecanthus, high-arched palate, cleft lip and/or palate, bifid uvula; (b) *limb anomalies:* pseudoarthrosis of the clavicle, Sprengel shoulder deformity, short fifth finger, grooved nails, broad digits, long fingers, digital hypoplasia, syndactyly, clinodactyly, hallux valgus, polydactyly, duplicated hallux, duplicated phalanx, camptodactyly; (c) *other reported abnormalities:* short stature, developmental delay, webbed neck, pectum excavatum, scoliosis, shawl scrotum, hypospadias, hyperextensible digital joints, dental abnormalities, chromosomal abnormality (fragile site at 12q13), rounded shoulders, asymmetrical breast development, etc.

Radiologic Manifestations: (a) *coronal suture synostosis, hypertelorism, midfacial hypoplasia;* (b) other reported abnormalities: syndactyly, camptodactyly, clinodactyly, duplicated hallux, duplicated phalanx, etc.

Differential Diagnosis: Acrocallosal syndrome; frontonasal dysplasia; median cleft face syndrome; Greig syndrome.

REFERENCES

Cohen MM: Craniofrontonasal dysplasia. *Birth Defects* 15:85, 1979.

Kumar D, et al.: A family with craniofrontonasal dysplasia, and fragile site 12q13 segregating independently. *Clin. Genet.* 29:530, 1986.

Kwee ML, et al: Inheritance of cranio-fronto-nasal syndrome. *Am. J. Med. Genet.* 30:841, 1988.

Morris CA, et al.: Delineation of the male phenotype in craniofrontonasal syndrome. *Am. J. Med. Genet.* 27:623, 1987.

Sax CM, et al.: Craniofrontonasal dysplasia: Clinical and genetic analysis. *Clin. Genet.* 29:508, 1986.

Young ID: Craniofrontonasal dysplasia. *J. Med. Genet.* 24:193, 1987.

CRANIO-FRONTO-NASAL DYSPLASIA— LIKE SYNDROME

Mode of Inheritance: Report in a large Arab kindred in four generations (autosomal dominant).

Clinical and Radiologic Manifestations: (a) craniofacial: round face, prominent forehead, pronounced ocular hypertelorism, mild antimongoloid slant of the palpebral fissures, heavy and broad eyebrows, ptosis of the eyelids, broad and/ or depressed nasal bridge, widow's peak, short nose with or without anteverted nostrils, hypoplastic maxilla, long deep philtrum, dental malocclusion and/or overcrowded teeth, horizontal thin upper lip and/or pouty lower lip, prominent lower jaw, fleshy ear lobule and/or prominent anthelix; (b) acral manifestations: slightly small broad hands, clinodactyly of the fifth finger, broad flat feet with bulbous toes, mild interdigital webbing; (c) shawl scrotum.

Differential Diagnosis: Cranio-fronto-nasal dysplasia; Aarskog syndrome.

REFERENCE

Teebi AS: New autosomal dominant syndrome resembling craniofrontonasal dysplasia. *Am. J. Med. Genet.* 28:581, 1987.

CRANIOSYNOSTOSIS-RADIAL/FIBULAR APLASIA-CLEFT LIP/PALATE SYNDROME

Synonym: Craniosynostosis-limb reduction malformation-cleft lip/palate syndrome.

Clinical Manifestations: (a) craniofacial abnormalities: dysplastic ears, hypertelorism, epicanthal folds, strabismus, refractory errors, malocclusion, *cleft lip/cleft palate*, midfacial capillary hemangioma; (b) *forearm and leg deformities*; (c) other reported abnormalities: short stature, hypogonadism, pterygia, simian crease(s), mild to moderate mental retardation.

Radiologic Manifestations: (a) *craniosynostosis;* (b) *radial aplasia, fibular aplasia;* (c) other reported anomalies: hand deformities, foot deformities, vertebral anomalies.

REFERENCE

Ladda RL, et al.: Craniosynostosis associated with limb reduction malformation and cleft lip/palate: A distinct syndrome. *Pediatrics* 61:12, 1978.

CRANIOTELENCEPHALIC DYSPLASIA

Mode of Inheritance: Occurrence reported in two sisters, probably autosomal recessive transmission.

Frequency: Four published cases (Hughes et al.).

Pathology: (a) *premature closure of cranial sutures;* (b) *brain dysgenesis:* (agyria, microgyria, heterotopic gray matter, partially fused frontal lobes, hydrocephalus, absent corpus callosum, etc.); (c) optic nerve hypoplasia, etc.

Clinical Manifestations: (a) *frontal bone protusion;* (b) *neurological abnormalities,* diminished brain growth, development delay, seizures; (c) other reported abnormalities: midforehead nevus flammeus, microphthalmos.

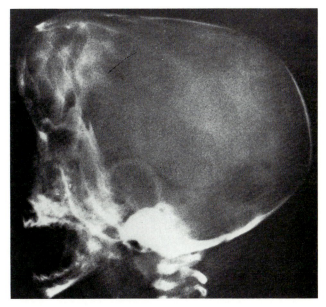

FIG SY–C–44.
Craniotelencephalic dysplasia. Six-week-old infant with large flat ears, a small nose, frontal bone protrusion, hypotelorism, and a midline hemangioma. Lateral radiograph of the skull shows frontal bone protuberance and closure of the coronal sutures, a short anterior fossa, and vertical slope of middle fossa. (From Jabbour JT, Taybi H: Unusual example of dysplasia of frontal bone. *Am. J. Dis. Child.* 108:627, 1964. Used by permission.)

Radiologic Manifestations: (a) *premature closure of cranial sutures* (metopic, sagittal, coronal) with *prominent protrusion of the frontal bone,* short anterior fossa, vertical slope of the middle fossa, orbital hypotelorism, etc; (b) *brain dysgenesis* (Fig SY—C—44).

REFERENCES

Daum S, et al.: Dysplasie telencephalique avec excroissance d'l'os frontal. *Semin. Hop. Paris* 34:1893, 1958.
Hughes HE, et al.: Craniotelencephalic dysplasia in sisters: Further delineation of a possible syndrome. *Am. J. Med. Genet.* 14:557, 1983.
Jabbour JT, Taybi H: Craniotelencephalic dysplasia. An unusual example of dysplasia of frontal bone. *Am. J. Dis. Child.* 108:627, 1964.

CREST SYNDROME

Synonyms: Calcinosis-Raynaud phenomenon-sclerodactyly-telangiectasia; CRST syndrome; Thibierge-Weissenbach syndrome.

Clinical Manifestations: Onset of symptoms at the average age of 45 years: (a) sclerodactyly with ulcerations of the skin, scleroderma, limited to the fingers and face; (b) Raynaud phenomenon; (c) telangiectasia; (d) dysphagia; (e) other reported abnormalities: pericardial effusion, minor myocardial dysfunction, association with Sjögren syndrome, pulmonary hypertension.

Radiologic Manifestations: (a) soft-tissue calcification at various sites (fingers, shoulders, thoracic wall, cervical spine,

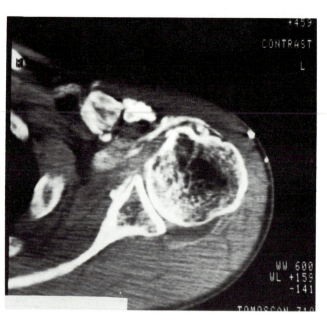

FIG SY—C—46.
CREST syndrome. Computed tomography of the shoulder shows capsuloligamentous and synovial calcification. Calcific joint effusion is also present (From Claudon M, Jacquier A, Rubini B, et al.: CRST syndrome avec calcification peri et intra-articulaires diffuses. Intérêt de la scanographie. *J. Radiol.* 66:793, 1985. Used by permission.)

etc.); (b) osteopenia; (c) bone erosions, intra-articular calcification, atlantoaxial joint destruction, subluxation of the upper cervical spine; (d) abnormal motor function of the esophagus (Figs SY—C—45 and SY—C—46).

REFERENCES

Albert J, et al.: Association d'un syndrome de Gougerot-Sjögren et d'un syndrome C.R.S.T. avec calcifications intraarticulaires et lésions ostéolytiques inhabituelles. *J. Radiol.* 63:757, 1982.
Audebert M, et al.: Complications des localisations digestives du syndrome de Thibierge-Weissenbach (syndrome CRST). *Nouv. Presse Med.* 8:1839, 1979.
Claudon M, et al.: CRST syndrome avec calcifications péri et intra-articulaires diffuses. Intérêt de la scanographie. *J. Radiol.* 66:793, 1985.
Follansbee WP, et al.: Myocardial function and perfusion in the CREST syndrome variant of progressive systemic sclerosis. Exercise radionuclide evaluation and comparison with diffuse scleroderma. *Am. J. Med.* 77:489, 1984.
Fritzler MJ, et al.: The CREST syndrome: A distinct serologic entity with anticentromere antibodies. *Am. J. Med.* 69:520, 1980.
Koch B, et al: Das Crest-Syndrom. *Radiologe* 28:228, 1988.
Leopold H, et al.: Thibierge-Weissenbach Syndrom. *Radiologe* 19:63, 1979.
Meyer E, et al.: Ungewöhnliche, tumorartige Verkalkung bei Sklerodermie. Thibièrge-Weissenbach-Syndrom. *Radiologe* 27:572, 1987.
Moilanen A, et al.: Craniovertebral lesions in patient with

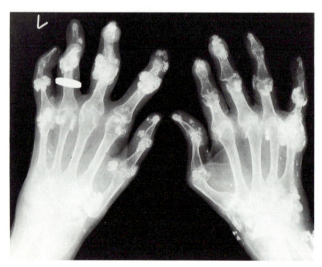

FIG SY—C—45.
CREST syndrome. The hand radiograph demonstrates extensive intraarticular and subcutaneous calcification as well as distal atrophy and flexion contracture of multiple fingers. (From Moilanen A, Vilppula A: Craniovertebral lesions in patient with CREST syndrome. *Fortschr. Rontgenstr.* 140:618, 1984. Used by permission.)

CREST syndrome. *Fortschr. Rontgenstr.* 140:618, 1984.

Page E, et al.: Crest syndrome. A propos d'une observation avec épanchement péricardique et hypertension pulmonaire sévère rapidement mortelle. *Presse Med.* 12:2400, 1983.

Thibierge G, Weissenbach RJ: Concrétions calcaires souscutanée et sclerodermie. *Ann. Dermatol. Syphiligr. (Paris)* 2:129, 1911.

Winterbauer RH: Multiple telangiectasia, Raynaud's phenomenon, sclerodactyly and subcutaneous calcinosis: A syndrome mimicking hereditary hemorrhagic telangiectasia. *Bull. Johns Hopkins Hosp.* 114:361, 1964.

CRONKHITE-CANADA SYNDROME

Mode of Inheritance: No known hereditary factors.

Frequency: 55 published cases (Daniel et al.).

Clinical Manifestations: Onset in middle or old age (a) *gastrointestinal hamartomatous polyps of the juvenile* (retention) *type*; (b) *alopecia*; (c) *onychodystrophy*; (d) *skin hyperpigmentation*; (e) abdominal pain, diarrhea with dehydration, electrolyte depletion, protein-losing enteropathy, malabsorption, edema, anemia, weight loss, anorexia, weakness, hematochezia, vomiting, hypogeusia, paresthesia, xerostomia, tetany, glossitis, cataracts, transient ischemic attacks, hypocalcemia, hypomagnesemia, hypokalemia, swallowing difficulties, fatty degeneration of the liver, thromboembolic episodes, association with systemic lupus, complete remission (rare); (f) infantile form associated with clubbing of the fingers, macrocephaly, hypotonia, hepatosplenomegaly, anemia, protein-losing enteropathy.

Radiologic Manifestations: (a) *polyps of stomach, small bowel, and colon*; esophageal polyp very rare; (b) coarsening of the mucosal folds of the small intestine with or without polypoid filling defects; (c) segmentation of barium in the

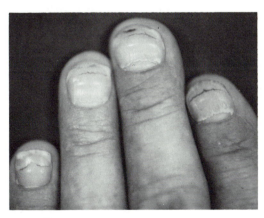

FIG SY−C−47.
Cronkhite-Canada syndrome. Onychodystrophy is manifested by new nail forming under the superficial portion of the abnormal old nail. (From Koehler PR, et al.: Diffuse gastrointestinal polyposis with ectodermal changes: Cronkhite-Canada syndrome. *Radiology* 103:589, 1972. Used by permission.)

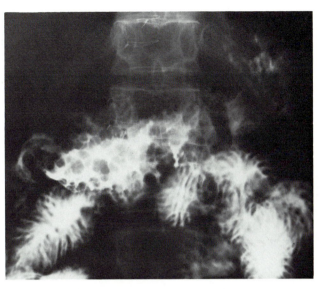

FIG SY−C−48.
Cronkhite-Canada syndrome. Polyps ranging from 0.5 to 1.5 cm are seen in the stomach of a 56-year-old male patient with Cronkhite-Canada syndrome. (From Koehler PR, et al.: Diffuse gastrointestinal polyposis with ectodermal changes: Cronkhite-Canada syndrome. *Radiology* 103:589, 1972. Used by permission.)

small bowel; (d) intussusception (rare); (e) carcinoma of the colon (rare); (f) erosive arthritis (Figs SY−C−47 and SY−C−48).

REFERENCES

Canada Diner W: The Cronkhite-Canada syndrome. *Radiology* 105:715, 1971.

Cronkhite LW Jr, Canada WJ: Generalized gastrointestinal polyposis: Unusual syndrome of polyposis, pigmentation, alopecia and onychotrophia. *N. Engl. J. Med.* 252:1011, 1955.

Daniel ES, et al.: The Cronkhite-Canada syndrome. An analysis of clinical and pathologic features and therapy in 55 patients. *Medicine (Baltimore)* 61:293, 1982.

Doyle T, et al.: Reversal of changes in Cronkhite-Canada syndrome. *Australas. Radiol.* 28:19, 1984.

Kilcheski T, et al.: The radiographic appearance of the stomach in Cronkhite-Canada syndrome. *Radiology* 141:57, 1981.

Koehler PR, et al.: Diffuse gastrointestinal polyposis with ectodermal changes: Cronkhite-Canada syndrome. *Radiology* 103:589, 1972.

Kubo T, et al.: Canada-Cronkhite syndrome associated with systemic lupus erythematosus. *Arch. Intern. Med.* 146:995, 1986.

Maurer H-J: Cronkhite-Canada Syndrom, Roentgendiagnostik. *Fortschr. Rontgenstr.* 122:399, 1975.

Sanders KM, et al.: Erosive arthritis in Cronkhite-Canada syndrome. *Radiology* 156:309, 1985.

Scharf GM, et al.: Juvenile gastrointestinal polyposis or the infantile Cronkhite-Canada syndrome. *J. Pediatr. Surg.* 21:953, 1986.

CROUZON SYNDROME

Synonym: Craniofacial dysostosis.

Mode of Inheritance: Autosomal dominant; also sporadic (about one fourth of cases).

Frequency: Uncommon.

Clinical Manifestations: (a) brachycephaly or oxycephaly, scaphocephaly and trigonocephaly less common; (b) *par-* *rot-beaked nose;* (c) *bilateral exophthalmos, bilateral divergent pseudostrabismus;* (d) *mandibular prognathism;* (e) mild to moderate mental retardation; (f) airway obstruction with cor pulmonale, sleep apnea; (g) other reported abnormalities: bifid uvula or cleft palate, atresia of the auditory meatus, spontaneous luxation of the eyes, subluxation of the radial heads, cloverleaf skull anomaly, diffuse hemangiomatous architecture identified by microscopic examination of bone specimens obtained at cranial synostectomy (Crouzon syndrome and cloverleaf skull deformity combination).

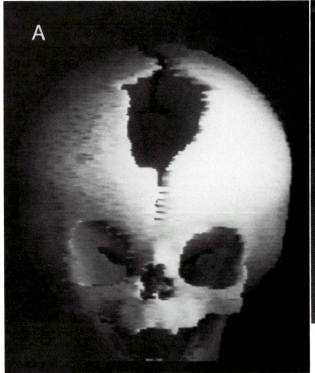

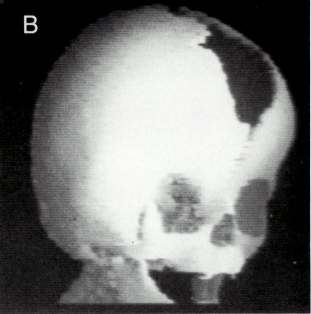

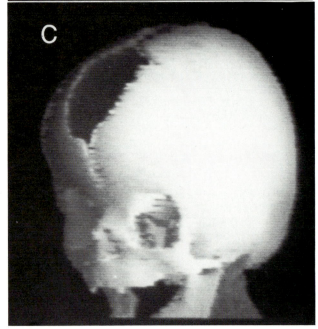

FIG SY–C–49.
Crouzon syndrome in a 5-month-old female with a high calvarial vertex, orbital hypertelorism, premature synostosis of the coronal sutures, and a flattened midface. (Three-dimensional reconstruction images courtesy of Ronald A. Cohen, M.D., Children's Hospital Medical Center, Oakland, Calif.)

Radiologic Manifestations: (a) *craniofacial deformities:* high vertex in the region of the anterior fontanelle, premature closure of any or all cranial sutures, increased digital markings, basilar kyphosis with the plane of the clivus being more near vertical than normal, sphenoidal plane inclined downward and foreward, downward displacement of the cribriform plate, medial and upward tilt of the petrous portion of the temporal bone, poor development or absence of development of the frontal sinus, shallow orbits, upward tilt of the roof of the orbit (frontal bone and lesser wing of the sphenoid), hypoplasia of the infraorbital rim, orbital hypertelorism resulting from enlarged ethmoidal air cells and lateral expansion and ballooning of the ethmoids, small and deformed optic foramina, exotropia, upward and medial tilt of the external auditory canal, poor pneumatization of the mastoids, deformity of the middle-ear ossicles in some cases, cloudy middle ears due to the presence of secretions (eustachian tube obstruction), stubby lateral and superior semicircular canals in some cases, elongated vertical portion of the carotid canal, more vertical direction of the groove of the sigmoid sinus, shallow sigmoid notch, hypoplasia of the maxillomalar facial mass, recession of the malar bone, short and distorted zygomatic arches, narrow pterygomaxillary fossa, marked thickening of the alveolar process of the maxilla, narrow V-shaped or semicircular deformity of the upper alveolar dental arch, crowding of the maxillary teeth, very short and high palate, lateral accumulation of soft tissue on the palatine processes (histological studies shown to be due to an accumulation of mucopolysaccharide acid), thick and long soft palate, relative mandibular prognathism; (b) hydrocephalus, deformed ventricular system due to skull deformity; (c) *nasopharyngeal airway constriction, narrow oropharynx;* (d) other reported abnormalities: anomalies of the craniocervical junction, basal impression, narrow trachea (completely cartilaginous trachea, cloverleaf skull deformity, calcaneocuboid coalition, etc. (Fig SY–C–49).

REFERENCES

Alpers CE, et al.: Hemangiomatous anomaly of bone in Crouzon's syndrome: Case report. *Neurosurgery* 16:391, 1985.

Blatt N, et al.: Les altérations du canal optique dans la maladie de Crouzon. *J. Radiol.* 41:645, 1960.

Craig CL, et al.: Calcaneocuboid coalition in Crouzon's syndrome (craniofacial dysostosis). *J. Bone Joint Surg. [Am.]* 59:826, 1977.

Crouzon O: Dysostose cranio-faciale héréditaire. *Bull. Soc. Med. Hop. (Paris)* 33:545, 1912.

Devine P, et al.: Completely cartilaginous trachea in a child with Crouzon syndrome. *Am. J. Dis. Child.* 138:40, 1984.

Don N, et al.: Cor pulmonale in Crouzon's disease. *Arch. Dis. Child.* 46:394, 1971.

Kaler SG, et al.: Radiographic hand abnormalities in fifteen cases of Crouzon syndrome. *J. Craniofac. Genet. Dev. Biol.* 2:205, 1982.

Lauritzen C, et al.: Airway obstruction and sleep apnea in children with craniofacial anomalies. *Plast. Reconstr. Surg.* 77:1, 1986.

Mafee MF, et al.: Radiology of the craniofacial anomalies. *Otolaryngol. Clin. North Am.* 14:947, 1981.

Noetzel MJ, et al.: Hydrocephalus and mental retardation in craniosynostosis. *J. Pediatr.* 107:885, 1985.

Powazek M, et al.: Assessment of intellectual development after surgery for craniofacial dysostosis. *Am. J. Dis. Child.* 133:151, 1979.

Rollnick BR: Germinal mosaicism in Crouzon syndrome. *Clin. Genet.* 33:145, 1988.

CRUVEILHIER-BAUMGARTEN SYNDROME

Synonym: Pegot-Cruveilhier-Baumgarten syndrome.

Clinical Manifestations: (a) *prominent umbilical or paraumbilical veins;* (b) *venous hum;* (c) *splenomegaly;* (d) *portal hypertension with esophageal varices;* (e) *liver disease (fibrosis, atrophy).*

Radiologic Manifestations: (a) esophageal varices; (b) splenomegaly; (c) intrahepatic portal venous obstruction; (d) patency of the umbilical vein in association with portal hypertension and abdominal collateral circulation demonstrable by various methods (splenoportography, percutaneous transhepatic portography, injection of superficial abdominal veins, superior mesenteric angiography, ultrasonography, and computed tomography).

REFERENCES

Aagaard J, et al.: Recanalized umbilical vein in portal hypertension. *A.J.R.* 139:1107, 1982.

Cruveilhier J: *Anatomie Pathologique du Corps Humain.* Paris, J.B. Baillière, 1829–1835, vol. 1, p. 16.

Goto A, et al.: Cruveilhier-Baumgarten disease: A case report emphasizing the diagnostic value of CT scanning and angiography. *J. Clin. Gastroenterol.* 4:59, 1982.

Park SC, et al.: Computed tomography and angiography in the Cruveilhier-Baumgarten syndrome. *J. Comput. Assist. Tomogr.* 5:19, 1981.

Pegot: Tumeur variqueuse avec anomalie du system veineux et persistence de la veine ombilicale et développement des veines souscutanées abdominales. *Bull. Soc. Anat.* 8:57, 1833.

Vigne J, et al.: Le syndrome de Pegot-Cruveilhier-Baumgarten. *J. Radiol. Electrol. Med. Nucl.* 46:763, 1965.

von Baumgarten P: Uber vollständiges; Offenbleiben der Vena umbilicalis; zugleich ein Beitrag zur Frage des Morbus. *Banti.-Baumgartens Arbeiten Leipzig* 6:93, 1907.

CURRARINO TRIAD

Mode of Inheritance: Autosomal dominant in about half of the cases.

Frequency: Uncommon.

Clinical and Radiologic Manifestations: (a) anorectal malformations (stenosis, anal ectopia, imperforate anus); (b) sacral bony abnormality (scimitar sacrum, sacral hypoplasia, etc.); (c) presacral mass (anterior meningocele, teratoma, enteric cyst; isolated or in combination); (d) other reported abnormalities: constipation, progressive neurological dysfunction, abnormalities on spinal cord imaging (computed tomography, magnetic resonance imaging, ultrasonography) such as lipomeningocele, tethered cord, low conus, dural ectasia, dysplastic conus, and dural sac stenosis.

REFERENCES

Currarino G, et al.: Triad of anorectal, sacral, and presacral anomalies. *A.J.R.* 137:395, 1981.

Janneck C, et al: Die Currarino-Trias-Beobachtung von 4 Fällen. *Z. Kinderchir.* 43:112, 1988.

Kennedy RLJ: An unusual rectal polyp: Anterior sacral meningocele. *Surg. Gynecol. Obstet.* 43:803, 1926.

Kirks DR, et al.: The Currarino triad: Complex of anorectal malformation, sacral bony abnormality, and presacral mass. *Pediatr. Radiol.* 14:220, 1984.

Tunell WP, et al.: Neuroradiologic evaluation of sacral abnormalities in imperforate anus complex. *J. Pediatr. Surg.* 22:58, 1987.

Werner JL, Taybi H: Presacral masses in childhood. *A.J.R.* 109:403, 1970.

Yates VD, et al: Anterior sacral defects: An autosomal dominantly inherited condition. *J. Pediatr.* 102:239, 1983.

CUTIS LAXA

Synonyms: Cutis pendula; chalazoderma; dermatomegaly; dermatochalasia; systemic elastosis (with internal manifestations); generalized elastosis; etc.

Mode of Inheritance: Autosomal dominant with variable penetrance (benign form); autosomal recessive present at birth or shortly after birth (malignant form, early death); X-linked recessive; acquired primary elastolysis (after dermatitis, vesicular eruptions, or systemic illness).

Frequency: Rare.

Pathology: Reduction in the amount and size of elastic fibers.

Clinical Manifestations: (a) *loose and pendulous skin,* in particular, facial skin (bloodhound appearance); (b) *growth retardation;* (c) deep voice, (d) hernias; (e) rectal and vaginal prolapse; (f) respiratory symptoms; (g) cor pulmonale, arrythmia; (h) degenerative changes in the cornea; (i) mental retardation; (j) other reported abnormalities: simian creases, high-arched palate, colobomas, oculus laxa, ruptured patellar tendon, airway obstruction due to lax and elongated vocal cords, hooked nose, generalized edema in the newborn, intrauterine growth retardation, congenital hip dislocation, short digits with absent phalanges, ambiguous genitalia, low serum copper levels, joint hyperextensibility, hypotonia, large ears, dental caries.

Radiologic Manifestations: (a) *pulmonary emphysema;* (b) *cor pulmonale;* (c) dilatation and tortuosity of blood vessels; (d) pulmonary artery stenosis; (e) coarctation of the aorta; (f) diverticula of the gastrointestinal and urogenital tracts; (g) gastric ulcer; (h) esophageal dilatation; (i) dilatation and tortuosity of the ureters; (j) hernias, diaphragmatic eventration; (k) other reported abnormalities: radial head dislocation, pectus excavatum, osteoporosis with multiple fractures and flat vertebrae (compression fractures), punctate hip calcification, vesicoureteral reflux.

Note: Subgroups: (a) DeBarsy syndrome or DeBarsy-Moens-Dierckx syndrome: dwarfism, oligophrenia, cloudy cornea, degeneration of the elastic and collagenous tissue in skin, etc.; (b) cutis laxa with ligament laxity and delayed development, congenital hip dislocation, wide patency and delayed closure of the anterior fontanelle, delayed intrauterine

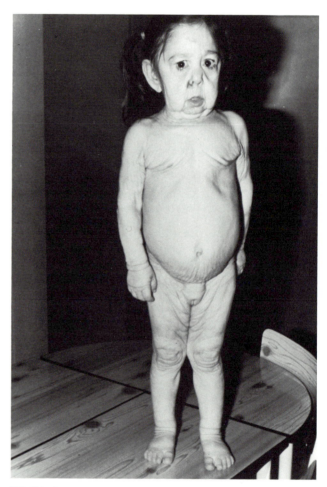

FIG SY–C–50.
Cutis laxa. Note the strikingly elderly looking features, droopy appearance of the face, huge ears, ptosis of the eyelids and cheeks, anteverted nostrils, and redundant skin folds, particularly marked in the axillary areas and on the abdomen. (From Van Maldergem L, Vamos E, Liebaers I, et al.: Severe congenital cutis laxa with pulmonary emphysema: A family with three affected sibs. *Am. J. Med. Genet.* 31:455, 1988. Used by permission.)

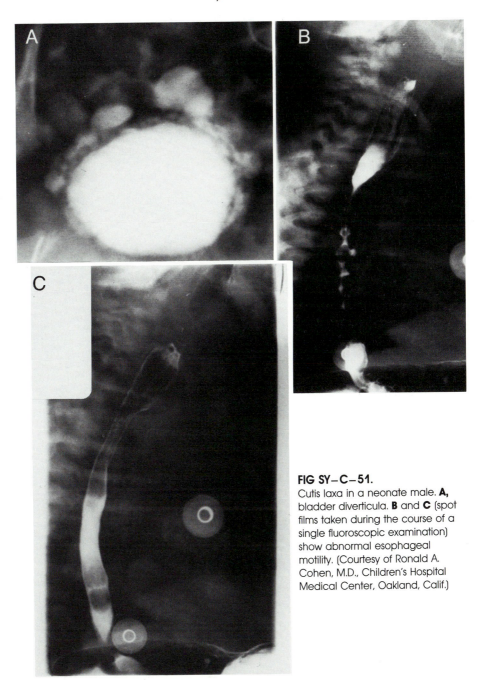

FIG SY–C–51.
Cutis laxa in a neonate male. **A,** bladder diverticula. **B** and **C** (spot films taken during the course of a single fluoroscopic examination) show abnormal esophageal motility. (Courtesy of Ronald A. Cohen, M.D., Children's Hospital Medical Center, Oakland, Calif.)

and extrauterine growth and development, females may be autosomal recessive, X-linked dominant lethal in the male (Sakati) (Figs SY–C–50 to SY–C–52).

REFERENCES

Agha A, et al.: Two forms of cutis laxa presenting in the newborn period. *Acta Paediatr. Scand.* 67:775, 1978.

Allanson J, et al.: Congenital cutis laxa with retardation of growth and motor development: A recessive disorder of connective tissue with male lethality. *Clin. Genet.* 29:133, 1986.

Fitzsimmons JS, et al.: Variable clinical presentation of cutis laxa. *Clin. Genet.* 28:284, 1985.

Kaye CI, et al.: Cutis laxa, skeletal anomalies and ambiguous genitalia. *Am. J. Dis. Child.* 127:115, 1974.

Khaldi F, et al.: Cutis laxa. A propos de deux cas a révélation néonatale. *Ann. Pediatr. (Paris)* 34:165, 1987.

Koch SE, et al.: Acquired cutis laxa: Case report and review of disorders of elastolysis. *Pediatr. Dermatol.* 2:282, 1985.

Lally JF, et al.: The roentgenographic manifestations of cutis laxa (generalized elastolysis). *Radiology* 113:605, 1974.

Meine F, Grossman H, Forman W, et al.: The radiographic findings in congenital cutis laxa. *Radiology* 113:687, 1974.

Patton MA, et al.: Congenital cutis laxa with retardation of

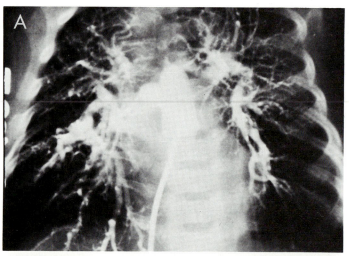

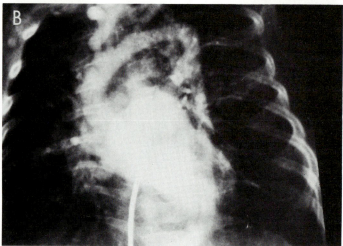

FIG SY–C–52.
Cutis laxa: pulmonary arteriogram in an infant. Marked stenosis and tortuosity of the right and left pulmonary arteries and tortuosity of the peripheral branches are present, **A,** the levo phase shows marked unfolding and tortuosity of the aortic arch and tortuosity of all brachiocephalic vessels, **B,** note the course of the lower descending thoracic aorta. (From Meine F, Grossman H, Forman W, et al.: The radiographic findings in congenital cutis laxa. *Radiology* 113:687, 1974. Used by permission.)

growth and development. *J. Med. Genet.* 24:556, 1987.
Pontz BF, et al.: Biochemical, morphological and immunological findings in a patient with a cutis laxa–associated inborn disorder (DeBarsy syndrome). *Eur. J. Pediatr.* 145:428, 1986.
Sakati NO, et al.: Congenital cutis laxa and osteoporosis. *Am. J. Dis. Child.* 137:452, 1983.
Sakati NO, et al.: Syndrome of cutis laxa, ligamentous laxity and delayed development. *Pediatrics* 72:850, 1983.

CUTIS VERTICIS GYRATA

Synonyms: Cutis sulcata; bulldog scalp; corrugated skin.

Mode of Inheritance: Majority sporadic, autosomal recessive and dominant inheritance with varying expressivity in some.

Frequency: Rare.

Clinical Manifestations: (a) corrugated or gyrate appearance of the scalp, sparse hair in the areas of the folds; (b) mental retardation frequent; (c) other reported abnormalities: seizures, microcephaly, eye abnormalities (strabismus, cata-

ract, blindness), cerebral palsy, hypotonia, development delay, etc.

Radiologic Manifestations: (a) *thick scalp folds;* (b) microcephaly and skull asymmetry; (c) small cerebellum, macroventriculy or microventriculy.

Notes: Gyrated scalp has also been reported in association with hydranencephaly and ocular abnormalities (cataracts, leukomas, optic atrophy). The secondary form of cutis verticis gyrata occurs in association with endocrine disorders, acromegaly, chronic inflammatory diseases, tumors, nevi, pachydermoperiostosis, rotational traction (long matted hair) (Fig SY–C–53).

REFERENCES

Akesson HO: Cutis verticis gyrata and mental retardation in Sweden. *Acta Med. Scand.* 175:115, 1964; 177:459, 1965.
Bauer CR, et al.: Gyrated scalp associated with hydranencephaly in a newborn infant. *J. Pediatr.* 90:492, 1977.
Bruwer A, et al.: Roentgenologic recognition of cutis verticis gyrata. *Proc. Staff Meet. Mayo Clin.* 28:635, 1953.

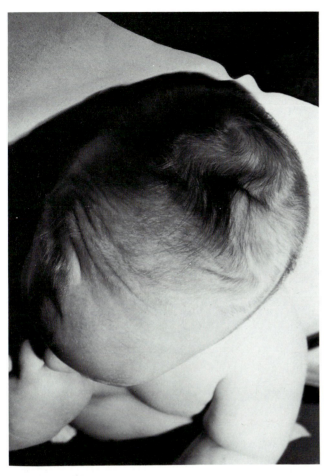

FIG SY—C—53.
Cutis verticis gyrata with a sharply demarcated, hypertrophic, folded area on the asymmetrical scalp. The head circumference and the cranial computed tomography results were normal. (Courtesy of Dr. I. Felding, Helsingborg, Sweden.)

Felding I, et al.: Picture of the month (cutis verticis gyrata) *Am. J. Dis. Child.* 142:305, 1988.

Garden JM, et al: Essential primary cutis verticis gyrata. Treatment with the scalp reduction procedure. *Arch. Dermatol.* 120:1480, 1984.

Hsieh HL, et al: Cutis verticis gyrata in a neonate. *Pediatr. Dermatol.* 1:153, 1983.

Khare AK, et al.: Acquired cutis verticis gyrata due to rotational traction. *Br. J. Dermatol.* 110:125, 1984.

Leibowitz MR, et al: Cutis verticis gyrata with metabolic abnormalities. *Dermatologica* 166:146, 1983.

McDowall TW: Case of abnormal development of the scalp. *J. Ment. Sci.* 39:62, 1893.

Palo J, et al.: Aetiological aspects of the cutis verticis gyrata and mental retardation syndrome. *J. Ment. Defic. Res.* 14:33, 1970.

CYCLIC EDEMA

Clinical Manifestations: (a) *periodic edema in women;* (b) *headaches;* (c) *cyclic oliguria;* (d) *exertional dyspnea;* (e) *constipation;* (f) *marked thirst;* (g) *asthenia;* (h) *arterial hypotension;* (i) *a defect in the regulation of antidiuretic hor-* mone has been suggested (delay in excretion of the water load and inability to decrease urinary osmolarity below 137 mOsm/L).

Radiologic Manifestations: Lymphographic demonstration of (a) *fragility and reduced number of lymph channels;* (b) *mild to marked extravasation of contrast medium* at a site where edema is clinically most pronounced (pelvis and lower limbs).

REFERENCES

Laval-Jeantet M, et al.: La lymphographie dans le syndrome d'oedèmes cycliques idiopathiques. *Ann. Radiol. (Paris)* 14:89, 1971.

Mach RS, et al.: Oedème idiopathique par rétention sodique avec hyperaldostéronurie. *Bull. Mem. Soc. Med. Hop. (Paris)* 71:726, 1955.

Zech P, et al.: Oedème cyclique idiopathique: Trouble de l'élimination hydrique à majoration orthostatique. *Nouv. Presse Med.* 6:1121, 1977.

CYSTIC FIBROSIS

Synonym: Mucoviscidosis.

Mode of Inheritance: Autosomal recessive, the gene located in the middle of the long arm of chromosome 7 (7cen-q22).

Frequency: 1 in 2000 live births.

Clinical Manifestations:

(A) MAJOR MANIFESTATIONS: (a) *meconium ileus;* (b) *pancreatic insufficiency;* (c) *chronic pulmonary disease;* (d) *sweat chloride levels >60mEq/L (>80 mEq/L in adults),* heat prostration.

(B) SUGGESTIVE CLINICAL MANIFESTATIONS: (a) positive family history; (b) rectal prolapse; (c) nasal prolapse; (d) mucoid *Pseudomonas aeruginosa* in the sputum; (e) aspermia; (f) focal biliary cirrhosis.

(C) OTHER ABNORMALITIES: (a) *respiratory system:* hemoptysis, bronchopulmonary aspergillosis; (b) *alimentary system:* meconium plug syndrome, steatorrhea, intussusception, appendicitis, chronic intestinal obstruction, meconium ileus equivalent (lower-quadrant abdominal mass), recurrent pancreatitis, malabsorption, gallstones, obstructive jaundice, hepatic dysfunction, hepatosplenomegaly, portal hypertension, (c) *cardiovascular system:* cardiomyopathy (multifocal myocardial fibrosis, lymphedema of the heart, acute cardiac failure in infants, arrhythmias); (d) *blood manifestations:* anemia, bleeding diathesis, abnormal glucose tolerance, inadequate erythroid response to hypoxia; (e) *nutritional deficit:* hypoproteinemia; various vitamin deficiencies (A, B_{12}, D, E, K) resulting in symptoms such as night blindness, xerophthalmia, increased intracranial pressure due to vitamin A deficiency, rickets, neurological deficits associated with vitamin E deficiency (abnormal eye movements, diminished reflexes, decreased vibratory and position sense, ataxia, muscle weakness); hypomagnesemia; low plasma levels of zinc and selenium; (f) *skeletal system:* kyphosis, scoliosis, clubbing, pulmonary osteoarthropathy (pain, tenderness); (g) *prenatal screening:* enzyme deficiency in the amniotic fluid: intestinal hydrolases, maltase, sucrase, palatinase, alkaline phosphatase, trehalase, and γ-glutamyltransferase; (h) *neonatal screening:* increased sweat osmolarity, elevated serum immunoreactive trypsin; (i) *other reported abnormalities (laboratory):* increased mean glomerular filtration rate and filtration fraction, serum pancreatic amylase isoenzyme activity below normal, subclinical hypothyroidism shown by thyroid function tests, elevated serum vitamin B_{12} levels, hypergammaglobulinemia, etc.; (j) *other reported abnormalities (clinical):* failure to thrive, short stature, pubertal delay, diabetes mellitus, secondary amyloidosis, polyarthritis ("reactive arthritis"), neoplasms (acute leukemia, neuroblastoma, retinoblastoma, ileal carcinoma), intradural spinal hematoma, inguinal hernia, hydrocele, brain abscess, pneumoparotid (due to attempts at cough suppression).

Radiologic Manifestations: (a) *antenatal sonographic findings:* pseudocyst, calcified mass due to a contained bowel perforation, meconium peritonitis, calcification in the peritoneal cavity, echogenic mass representing inspissated meconium, dilated fetal bowel caused by thickened meconium, ascites, hydramnios; (b) *respiratory system:* air trapping in the lungs (anterior bowing of the sternum, spinal kyphosis, diaphragm depression), prominent linear interstitial shadows, peribronchial cuffing, mottled shadows with either radiopaque or radiolucent center, segmental or lobar atelectasis or consolidation, mucoid impaction of bronchi, bronchiectasis, pneumothorax, pneumonias, abnormal perfusion and ventilation scans, cystic air spaces, distinctly visible right upper lobe bronchus on the lateral chest radiograph in adolescents, tracheomegaly, etc.; (c) *gastrointestinal system:* meconium ileus, meconium plug, meconium peritonitis, meconium ileus equivalent, thickened folds, nodular filling defects, mucosal smudging, dilatation and redundancy of the duodenum, widening of small intestinal plicae, increased intestinal diameter, decreased peristalsis, segmentation and flocculation of barium in the small bowel, filling defects and cobblestone appearance of the colonic wall, pneumatosis coli, fecalith, appendiceal nonfilling (barium enema examination), esophageal varices, scrotal calcification associated with meconium peritonitis, gastroesophageal reflux, peptic ulcer (distal smallbowel obstruction), small left-colon syndrome in the newborn, pneumatosis intestinalis, barium impaction causing small-bowel obstruction, Crohn disease; (d) *pancreas:* lithiasis, decrease in size, fatty replacement of the pancreas (computed tomographic scan), increased pancreatic echogenicity, pancreatic cyst, pancreatitis, nonvisualization of the pancreatic duct by ultrasonography, inhomogeneous attenuation on computed tomography (fibrosis, fatty replacement, calcification, and cyst(s); (e) *hepatobiliary system: liver:* hepatomegaly, textural changes of liver on computed tomography and ultrasonographic examinations; fatty liver; portal hypertension; gallstones; contracted gallbladder; irregular filling de-

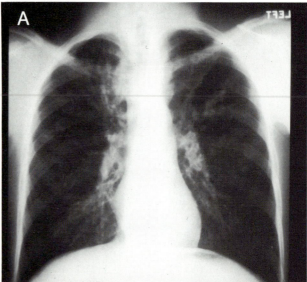

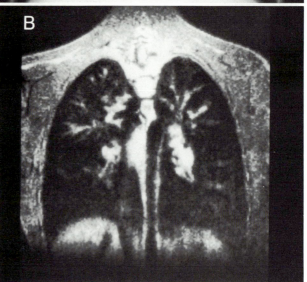

FIG SY–C–54.
Cystic fibrosis of moderate severity. **A,** a chest roentgenogram demonstrates peribronchial cuffing, bronchial plugging, and atelectasis. Pathological changes in the lungs are difficult to separate from normal pulmonary vessels. **B,** a magnetic resonance coronal image demonstrates the branching pattern of mucoid impacted bronchi, most severe in the upper lobes. (From Gooding CA, Lallemand DP, Brasch RC, et al.: Magnetic resonance imaging in cystic fibrosis. *J. Pediatr.* 105:384, 1984. Used by permission.)

fects in the biliary tree representing thickened bile, mucus, and stone; dilatation of the intrahepatic bile ducts; irregularity of the ductules due to recurrent cholangitis and/or focal biliary cirrhosis; common bile duct obstruction due to thick viscid secretions in the neonates; sludge and stones in older patients; intrapancreatic compression of the common bile duct; ultrasonographic demonstration of an irregular inferior margin of the liver; (f) *cardiovascular system:* cor pulmonale, portal hypertension, systemic-to-pulmonary anastomosis, se-

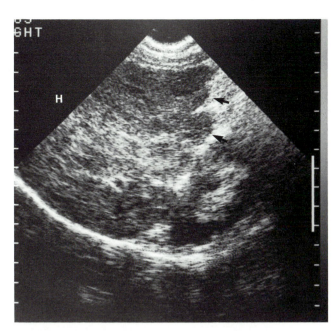

FIG SY−C−55.
The ultrasonograph in a patient with cystic fibrosis shows a markedly irregular inferior margin of the liver *(arrows)*. (From McHugo JM, McKeown C, Brown MT, et al.: Ultrasound findings in children with cystic fibrosis. *Br. J. Radiol.* 60:137, 1987. Used by permission.)

lective bronchial arteriographic demonstration of the origin of hemoptysis, vascular and extravascular calcifications; (g) *head and neck:* cloudy paranasal sinuses, nasal polyp, mucocele, pyomucocele of the ethmoid sinus, proptosis, sialolithiasis, brain abscess; (h) *skeletal system:* digital clubbing, hy-

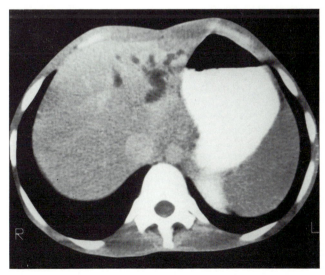

FIG SY−C−56.
Cystic fibrosis in a 23-year-old female. Computed tomography shows marked dilatation of the bile ducts peripherally that is associated with viscid material within the ducts. The patient also had fatty replacement of the pancreas, a stricture in the left hepatic duct, and a porcelain gallbladder. (Courtesy of Peter E. Kane, M.D., Children's Hospital Medical Center, Oakland, Calif.)

pertrophic osteoarthropathy, skeletal maturation retardation, demineralization, spontaneous fracture of the sternum, scoliosis, thoracic kyphosis; (i) *genital abnormalities:* absence or atresia of the vas deferens, incomplete development of epididymis and seminal vesicle, cyst formation and calcification within the prostate, cystic ovaries (Fig SY−C−54 to SY−C−56).

REFERENCES

Abramson SJ, et al.: Gastrointestinal manifestations of cystic fibrosis. *Semin. Roentgenol.* 22:97, 1987.

Amodio JB, et al.: Cystic fibrosis in childhood: Pulmonary, paranasal sinus and skeletal manifestations. *Semin. Roentgenol.* 22:125, 1987.

Ater JL, et al.: Relative anemia and iron deficiency in cystic fibrosis. *Pediatrics* 71:810, 1983.

Bass S, et al.: Biliary tree in cystic fibrosis. Biliary tract abnormalities in cystic fibrosis demonstrated by endoscopic retrograde cholangiography. *Gastroenterology* 84:1592, 1983.

Berg U, et al.: Renal function in cystic fibrosis with special reference to the renal sodium handling. *Acta Paediatr. Scand.* 71:833, 1982.

Biggs BG, et al.: Cystic fibrosis complicated by acute leukemia. *Cancer* 57:2441, 1986.

Brasfield D, et al.: Evaluation of scoring system of the chest radiograph in cystic fibrosis: A collaborative study. *A.J.R.* 134:1195, 1980.

Bruns WT, et al.: Submandibular sialolithiasis in a cystic fibrosis patient. *Am. J. Dis. Child.* 126:685, 1973.

Cassio A, et al.: Neonatal screening for cystic fibrosis by dried blood spot trypsin assay. *Acta Paediatr. Scand.* 73:554, 1984.

Castile R, et al.: Amyloidosis as a complication of cystic fibrosis. *Am. J. Dis. Child.* 139:728, 1985.

Chéron G, et al.: Cardiac involvement in cystic fibrosis revealed by a ventricular arrhythmia. *Acta Paediatr. Scand.* 73:697, 1984.

Cleghorn GJ, et al.: Treatment of distal intestinal obstruction syndrome in cystic fibrosis with a balanced intestinal lavage solution. *Lancet* 1:8, 1986.

Cohen AM, et al.: Evaluation of pulmonary hypertrophic osteoarthropathy in cystic fibrosis. A comprehensive study. *Am. J. Dis. Child.* 140:74, 1986.

Cunningham DG, et al.: Computed tomography in the evaluation of liver disease in cystic fibrosis patients. *J. Comput. Assist. Tomogr.* 4:151, 1980.

Daneman A, et al.: Pancreatic changes in cystic fibrosis: CT and sonographic appearances. *A.J.R.* 141:653, 1983.

David ML, et al: Pneumoparotid in cystic fibrosis. *Clin. Pediatr. (Phila.)* 27:506, 1988.

Davies C, et al.: Inspissated bile in a neonate with cystic fibrosis. *J. Ultrasound Med.* 5:335, 1986.

DeLuca F, et al.: Thyroid function in children with cystic fibrosis. *Eur. J. Pediatr.* 138:327, 1982.

De Lumley L, et al.: Polyarthrite chronique au cours d'une mucoviscidose. *Arch. Fr. Pediatr.* 40:723, 1983.

Dennis JL, et al.: Growth and bone-age retardation in cystic fibrosis. *J.A.M.A.* 194:113, 1965.

Ehrhardt P, et al.: Iron deficiency in cystic fibrosis. *Arch. Dis. Child.* 62:185, 1987.

Ellerbroek C, et al.: Neonatal small left colon in an infant with cystic fibrosis. *Pediatr. Radiol.* 16:162, 1986.

Erkkila JC, et al.: Spine deformities and cystic fibrosis. *Clin. Orthop.* 131:146, 1978.

Feigelson J, et al.: Anomalies du sperme, des déférents et de l'épididyme dans la mucoviscidose. *Presse Med.* 15:523, 1986.

Fernald GW, et al.: Cystic fibrosis: Overview. *Semin. Roentgenol.* 22:87, 1987.

Fiel SB, et al.: Magnetic resonance imaging in young adults with cystic fibrosis. *Chest* 91:181, 1987.

Finkel LI, et al.: Meconium peritonitis, intraperitoneal calcifications and cystic fibrosis. *Pediatr. Radiol.* 12:92, 1982.

Fischer WW, et al.: Barium impaction as a cause of small bowel obstruction in an infant with cystic fibrosis. *Pediatr. Radiol.* 14:230, 1984.

Fletcher BD, et al.: Contrast enema in cystic fibrosis: Implication of appendiceal nonfilling. *A.J.R.* 137:323, 1981.

Franckx J, et al.: The use of sweat osmolality in the diagnosis of cystic fibrosis. *Helv. Paediatr. Acta* 39:347, 1984.

Friedman PJ: Chest radiographic findings in the adult with cystic fibrosis. *Semin. Roentgenol.* 22:114, 1987.

Gibbens DT, et al: Osteoporosis in cystic fibrosis. *J. Pediatr.* 113:295, 1988.

Gillard BK, et al.: Cystic fibrosis serum pancreatic amylase. Useful discriminator of exocrine function. *Am. J. Dis. Child.* 138:577, 1984.

Gooding CA, et al.: Magnetic resonance imaging in cystic fibrosis. *J. Pediatr.* 105:384, 1984.

Green CG, et al.: Symptomatic hypomagnesemia in cystic fibrosis. *J. Pediatr.* 107:425, 1985.

Griscom NT, et al.: Radiologic and pathologic abnormalities of the trachea in older patients with cystic fibrosis. *A.J.R.* 148:691, 1987.

Gunn T, et al.: Edema as the presenting symptom of cystic fibrosis: Difficulties in diagnosis. *Am. J. Dis. Child.* 132:317, 1978.

Hen J, et al.: Meconium plug syndrome associated with cystic fibrosis and Hirschsprung's disease. *Pediatrics* 66:466, 1980.

Hernanz-Schulman M, et al.: Pneumatosis intestinalis in cystic fibrosis. *Radiology* 160:497, 1986.

Hernanz-Schulman M, et al.: Pancreatic cystosis in cystic fibrosis. *Radiology* 158:629, 1986.

Holsclaw DS, et al.: Intussusception in patients with cystic fibrosis. *Pediatrics* 48:51, 1971.

Holsclaw DS, et al.: Occult appendiceal abscess complicating cystic fibrosis. *J. Pediatr. Surg.* 11:217, 1976.

Howman-Giles R, et al.: Partial common bile duct obstruction in cystic fibrosis (CF): Detection by biliary scintigraphy and percutaneous cholangiogram (PTC). Presented at International Pediatric Radiology, Toronto, 1987.

Iannaccone G, et al.: Calcification of the pancreas in cystic fibrosis. *Pediatr. Radiol.* 9:85, 1980.

Jacobsen LE, et al.: Cystic fibrosis: A comparison of computed tomography and plain chest radiographs. *J. Can. Assoc. Radiol.* 37:17, 1986.

Katz SM, et al: Microscopic nephrocalcinosis in cystic fibrosis. *N. Engl. J. Med.* 319:263, 1988.

Kaufman DG, et al.: Cystic fibrosis presenting in a 45-year-old man with infertility. *J. Urol.* 136:1081, 1986.

Kuhn JP, et al.: Metastatic calcification in cystic fibrosis. *Radiology* 97:59, 1970.

Kumari-Subaiya S, et al.: Portal vein measurement by ultrasonography in patients with long-standing cystic fibrosis: Preliminary observations. *J. Pediatr. Gastroenterol. Nutr.* 6:71, 1987.

Landon C, et al.: Short stature and pubertal delay in male adolescents with cystic fibrosis. *Am. J. Dis. Child.* 138:388, 1984.

Ledesma-Medina J, et al.: Abnormal paranasal sinuses in patients with cystic fibrosis of the pancreas: Radiological findings. *Pediatr. Radiol.* 9:61, 1980.

Lifschitz MI, et al.: Pneumothorax as a complication of cystic fibrosis. *Am. J. Dis. Child.* 116:633, 1968.

Lindemans J, et al.: Elevated serum vitamin B_{12} in cystic fibrosis. *Acta Paediatr. Scand.* 73:768, 1984.

Logvinoff MM, et al.: Kyphosis and pulmonary function in cystic fibrosis. *Clin. Pediatr. (Phila.)* 23:389, 1984.

Loeuille GA, et al.: Étude critique de la scintigraphie pulmonaire au technetium 99m et au xenon 133 chez les malades atteints de mucoviscidose. *Ann. Pediatr. (Paris)* 30:75, 1983.

MacLusky I, et al.: Cystic fibrosis: Part 1. *Curr. Probl. Pediatr.* 15:1, 1985.

McCarthy VP, et al.: Appendiceal abscess in cystic fibrosis. A diagnostic challenge. *Gastroenterology* 86:564, 1984.

McHugo JM, et al.: Ultrasound findings in children with cystic fibrosis. *Br. J. Radiol.* 60:137, 1987.

Mischler EH, et al.: Demineralization in cystic fibrosis detected by direct photon absorptiometry. *Am. J. Dis. Child.* 133:632, 1979.

Mitchell EA, et al.: Spontaneous fracture of the sternum in a youth with cystic fibrosis. *J. Pediatr.* 97:789, 1980.

Morin PR, et al.: Prenatal detection of intestinal obstructions, aneuploidy syndromes, and cystic fibrosis by microvillar enzyme assays (disaccharidases, alkaline phosphatase, and glutamyltransferase) in amniotic fluid. *Am. J. Med. Genet.* 26:405, 1987.

Moss RB, et al.: Cystic fibrosis and neuroblastoma. *Pediatrics* 76:814, 1985.

Neve J, et al.: Plasma and erythrocyte zinc, copper and selenium in cystic fibrosis. *Acta Paediatr. Scand.* 72:437, 1983.

Nyberg DA, et al.: Dilated fetal bowel. A sonographic sign of cystic fibrosis. *J. Ultrasound Med.* 6:257, 1987.

Oestreich AE, et al.: Appendicitis as the presenting complaint in cystic fibrosis. *J. Pediatr. Surg.* 17:191, 1982.

Paling MR, et al.: Scoliosis in cystic fibrosis—an appraisal. *Skeletal Radiol.* 8:63, 1982.

Park RW, et al.: Gastrointestinal manifestations of cystic fibrosis: A review. *Gastroenterology* 81:1143, 1981.

Patrick MK, et al.: Common bile duct obstruction causing right upper abdominal pain in cystic fibrosis. *J. Pediatr.* 108:101, 1987.

Phelan MS, et al.: Radiographic abnormalities of the duodenum in cystic fibrosis. *Clin. Radiol.* 34:573, 1983.

Pitts-Tucker TJ, et al.: Finger clubbing in cystic fibrosis. *Arch. Dis. Child.* 61:576, 1986.

Porter DK, et al.: Massive hemoptysis in cystic fibrosis. *Arch. Intern. Med.* 143:287, 1983.

Rabkin CS, et al.: Brain abscess: A complication of cystic fibrosis in adults. *Ann. Neurol.* 15:608, 1984.

Reinig JW, et al.: The distinctly visible right upper lobe bronchus on the lateral chest: A clue to adolescent cystic fibrosis. *Pediatr. Radiol.* 15:222, 1985.

Reiter EO, et al.: The reproductive endocrine system in cystic fibrosis. *Am. J. Dis. Child.* 135:422, 1981.

Roach ES, et al.: Increased intracranial pressure following treatment of cystic fibrosis. *Pediatrics* 66:622, 1980.

Rosenstein BJ: Cystic fibrosis presenting with meconium plug syndrome. *Am. J. Dis. Child.* 132:167, 1978.

Rosenstein BJ, et al.: Peptic ulcer disease in cystic fibrosis: An unusual occurrence in black adolescents. *Am. J. Dis. Child.* 140:966, 1986.

Schidlow DV, et al.: Arthritis in cystic fibrosis. *Arch. Dis. Child.* 59:377, 1984.

Scott J, et al.: Rickets in adult cystic fibrosis with myopathy, pancreatic insufficiency and proximal tubular dysfunction. *Am. J. Med.* 63:488, 1977.

Scott RB, et al.: Gastroesophageal reflux in patients with cystic fibrosis. *J. Pediatr.* 106:223, 1985.

Shawker TH, et al.: Cystic ovaries in cystic fibrosis: An ultrasound and autopsy study. *J. Ultrasound Med.* 2:439, 1983.

Simpson RM, et al.: Vitamin B_{12} deficiency in cystic fibrosis. *Acta Paediatr. Scand.* 74:794, 1985.

Siraganian PA, et al.: Cystic fibrosis and ileal carcinoma. *Lancet* 2:1158, 1987.

Sitrin MD, et al.: Vitamin E deficiency and neurologic disease in adults with cystic fibrosis. *Ann. Intern. Med.* 107:51, 1987.

Steinkamp G, et al.: Renal function in cystic fibrosis: Proteinuria and enzymuria before and after tobramycin therapy. *Eur. J. Pediatr.* 145:526, 1986.

Stern RC, et al.: Rectal prolapse in cystic fibrosis. *Gastroenterology* 82:707, 1982.

Stern RC, et al.: Treatment and prognosis of nasal polyps in cystic fibrosis. *Am. J. Dis. Child.* 136:1067, 1982.

Strauss RG, et al.: Unilateral proptosis in cystic fibrosis. *Pediatrics* 43:297, 1969.

Stringer DA, et al: The association of cystic fibrosis, gastroesophageal reflux, and reduced pulmonary function. *J. Can. Assoc. Radiol.* 39:100, 1988.

Sullivan MM, et al.: Supraventricular tachycardia in patients with cystic fibrosis. *Chest* 90:239, 1986.

Swobodnik W, et al.: Ultrasound characteristics of the pancreas in children with cystic fibrosis. *J. Clin. Ultrasound* 13:469, 1985.

Vichinsky EP, et al.: Inadequate erythroid response to hypoxia in cystic fibrosis. *J. Pediatr.* 105:15, 1984.

Wainwright BJ, et al.: Localization of cystic fibrosis locus to human chromosome 7cen-q22. *Nature* 318:384, 1985.

Wang CI, et al.: Inguinal hernia, hydrocele, and other genitourinary abnormalities in boys with cystic fibrosis and their siblings. *Am. J. Dis. Child.* 119:236, 1970.

White H, et al.: Cystic fibrosis of the pancreas: Clinical and roentgenographic manifestations. *Radiol. Clin. North Am.* 1:539, 1963.

Zimmermann A, et al.: Cardiomyopathy in cystic fibrosis: Lymphoedema of the heart with focal myocardial fibrosis. *Helv. Paediatr. Acta* 37:183, 1982.

Zochodne D, et al.: Intradural spinal hematoma in an infant with cystic fibrosis. *Pediatr. Neurol.* 2:311, 1986.

CYSTIC HAMARTOMA OF THE LUNG AND KIDNEY

Clinical and Radiologic Manifestations: (a) abdominal mass detected during infancy; (b) hypertension due to bilateral multilocular renal cysts; (c) hamartomatous pulmonary cysts.

Differential Diagnosis: Weinberg-Zumwalt syndrome (multifocal cystic hamartoma of the lung with associated marked parenchymal overgrowth of the kidney).

Note: These two groups of lesions are considered to represent a spectrum of abnormal morphogenesis involving both the lung and kidney.

REFERENCES

Graham JM Jr, et al.: Cystic hamartomata of lung and kidney: A spectrum of developmental abnormalities. *Am. J. Med. Genet.* 27:45, 1987.

Weinberg AF, Zumwalt RE: Bilateral nephromegaly and multiple pulmonary cysts. *Am. J. Clin. Pathol.* 67:284, 1977.

D

DANDY-WALKER SYNDROME

Synonym: Dandy-Walker malformation.

Etiology: Occurrence as an isolated malformation or in association with various chromosomal aberrations, single gene disorders, environmentally induced malformation syndromes, or other multifactorial abnormalities.

Pathology: (a) *hydrocephalus associated with congenital anomaly of the fourth ventricle and cerebellum* with atresia of the foramen of Magendie and atresia of one or both foramina of Luschka; absence of the cerebellar vermis (partial or complete); (b) other reported abnormalities: agenesis of the corpus callosum and fornix; subdural hygroma; cranium bifidum; cerebellar heterotopias; infundibular hamartoma; malformed olives; microcephaly; aqueductal stenosis; polymicrogyria; anomalies of cerebellar folia; syringomyelia; malrotation of the bowel; association with the de Lange syndrome; Aase-Smith syndrome (hand abnormalities, joint contracture, cleft palate, and Dandy-Walker malformation); orofacial anomalies; genitourinary anomalies; omphalocele; cardiac defect; complex malformation of the cerebrum, cerebellum, and brain stem; hydromyelia with or without syringomyelia, myelomeningocele, and other cord lesions; arhinoencephalia and microphthalmos; cerebellar and brain stem malformations; aqueductal forking; etc.

Clinical Manifestations: (a) *enlargement of the skull in the occipital region* with prominent external convexity posterior to the foramen magnum; (b) other reported abnormalities: prominent posterior fontanelle, microphthalmos, macroglossia, polydactyly, syndactyly, hemangioma of the face, impaired motor function, cerebellar deficits, cleft palate, craniofacial dysostosis, abnormal electroencephalogram (EEG), abnormal gait, etc.

Radiologic Manifestations: (a) skull: *enlarged dolichocephalic skull with a deep posterior fossa, thin occiput, high position of the tentorium cerebelli, torcular Herophili, and grooves for the lateral sinuses*; (b) *dilated fourth ventricle that extends to the inner table of the skull with a finger-like extension into the upper cervical region*, torcular-lambdoid inversion, absent inferior vermis, dysplastic cerebellar hemispheres bounded posteromedially by the cyst, compression of basilar cisterns, bowing of the pericallosal artery, elevated branches of the middle cerebral artery, anterosuperior displacement of the proximal segment of the superior cerebellar artery, small or absent cerebellar blush, elongated great vein of Galen, elevated torcular Herophili, steep descent of the transverse sinuses.

Differential Diagnosis: Dandy-Walker variant; posterior fossa arachnoidal cysts; a fourth ventricle "encysted" due to hemorrhage or infection; megacisterna magna (Fig SY−D−1; Table SY−D−1).

REFERENCES

Dandy WE, et al.: Internal hydrocephalus: An experimental, clinical and pathological study. *Am. J. Dis. Child.* 8:406, 1914.

Fileni A, et al.: Dandy-Walker syndrome: Diagnosis in utero by means of ultrasound and CT correlations. *Neuroradiology* 24:233, 1983.

Golden JA, et al.: Dandy-Walker syndrome and associated anomalies. *Pediatr. Neurosci.* 13:38, 1987.

Groenhout CM, et al.: Value of sagittal sonography and direct sagittal CT of the Dandy-Walker syndrome. *A.J.N.R.* 5:476, 1984.

Hanigan WC, et al.: Magnetic resonance imaging of the Dandy-Walker malformation. *Pediatr. Neurosci.* 12:151, 1985.

Hirsch J-F, et al.: The Dandy-Walker malformation. A review of 40 cases. *J. Neurosurg.* 61:515, 1984.

Jenkyn LR, et al.: Dandy-Walker malformation in identical twins. *Neurology* 31:337, 1981.

Kaplan LC: Congenital hydrocephalus and the Dandy-Walker malformation associated with maternal warfarin use during pregnancy. Presented at a *Birth Defects Conference*, San Diego, 1981.

La Torre E, et al.: Angiographic differentiation between Dandy-Walker cyst and arachnoid cyst of the posterior fossa in newborn infants and children. *J. Neurosurg.* 38:298, 1973.

Lehman RM: Dandy-Walker syndrome in consecutive siblings: Familial hindbrain malformation. *Neurosurgery* 8:717, 1981.

Maria BL, et al.: Dandy-Walker syndrome revisited. *Pediatr. Neurosci.* 13:45, 1987.

Murray JC, et al.: Dandy-Walker malformation: etiologic heterogeneity and empiric recurrence risks. *Clin. Genet.* 28:272, 1985.

Nyberg DA, et al.: The Dandy-Walker malformation prenatal sonographic diagnosis and its clinical significance. *J. Ultrasound Med.* 7:65, 1988.

Patton MA, et al.: The Aase-Smith syndrome. *Clin. Genet.* 28:521, 1985.

Ritscher D, et al.: Dandy-Walker (like) malformation, atrioventricular septal defect and a similar pattern of minor anomalies in 2 sisters: A new syndrome? *Am. J. Med. Genet.* 26:481, 1987.

Sautreaux JL, et al.: Dandy-Walker malformation associated with occipital meningocele and cardiac anomalies: A rare complex embryologic defect. *J. Child Neurol.* 1:64, 1986.

Walker AE: A case of congenital atresia of the foramina of

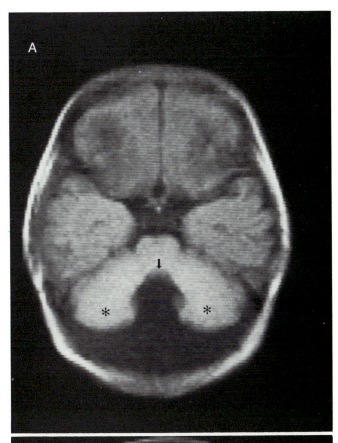

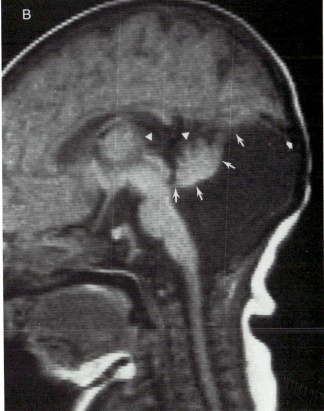

FIG SY–D–1.
Dandy-Walker malformation: magnetic resonance imaging. **A,** hypoplasia and anteriolateral displacement of the cerebellar hemispheres are seen. The fourth ventricle is directly continuous with the retrocerebellar position of the cyst through the defect created by absence of the inferior vermis. **B,** the enlargement of the posterior fossa, the cyst extending inferiorly into the upper cervical canal, and the anterior medullary velum extending into the anterior cyst wall are shown. (From Hanigan WC, Wright R, Wright S: Magnetic resonance imaging of the Dandy-Walker malformation. *Pediatr. Neurosci.* 12:151, 1985. Used by permission.)

TABLE SY–D–1.

Dandy-Walker Malformation Association With Other Abnormalities*

Mendelian	Chromosomal	Environmental	Multifactorial	Sporadic
Warburg† (AR)‡	45,X	Rubella†	Congenital heart disease†	Holoprosencephaly
Aase-Smith (Arthrogryposis) (AD)‡	6p–	Coumadin	Neural tube defects†	Cornelia de Lange
Ruvalcaba S. (AD/XL)‡	9qh+†	Alcohol	Cleft lip/palate†	Goldenhar
Coffin-Siris S.† (AR)	dup 5p†	Cytomegalo		Kidney abnormalities†
Oral-Facial Digital S.	dup 8p†	virus		Facial
Type II† (AR)	dup 8q†	Diabetes		hemangiomas†
Meckel-Gruber S.† (AR)	trisomy 9†	Isotretinoin†		Klippel-Feil†
Aicardi S.† (XL)	triploidy†			Polysyndactyly†
Joubert-Boltshauser S.† (AR)	dup 17q			
X-linked cerebellar hypoplasia† (XL)				
Ellis van Creveld (AR)				
Fraser Cryptophthalmos (AR)				

*From Murray JC, et al.: Dandy-Walker malformation: Etiologic heterogeneity and empiric recurrence risks. *Clin. Genet.* 28:272, 1985. Used by permission.
†Reported in more than one unrelated child.
‡AD = autosomal dominant; AR = autosomal recessive; XL = X-linked.

Luschka and Magendie: Surgical cure. *J. Neuropathol. Exp. Neurol.* 3:368, 1944.

DARIER DISEASE

Synonyms: Darier-White disease; keratosis follicularis.

Mode of Inheritance: Autosomal dominant.

Pathology: *Epidermal acantholysis and keratosis.*

Clinical Manifestations: (a) *multiple, firm, brown or flesh-colored greasy papules*; face, upper portion of the trunk, and flanks most common sites; (b) brittle and dry nails with longitudinal red and white stripes; (c) mucous membrane and corneal lesions; (d) other reported abnormalities: autoimmune thyroiditis, goiter, hypothyroidism, gonadal hypoplasia, testicular agenesis, diffuse pulmonary fibrosis.

Radiologic Manifestations: (a) pulmonary nodular infiltrates; (b) polycystic kidney, renal agenesis; (c) cystic bony changes.

REFERENCES

Claudy A, et al.: Maladie de Darier et polykystose renale. *Ann. Dermatol. Venereol.* 108:675, 1981.
Darier J: Psorospermose folliculaire végétante. Étude anatomo-pathologique d'une affection cutanée non décrite ou comprise dans le groupe des acnés sébacées, cornées, hypertrophiantes, des kératoses (ichthyoses) folliculaires, etc. *Ann. Dermatol. Syph. Paris* 10:597, 1889.
Larregue M, et al.: La maladie de Darier chez l' enfant. A propos de huit cas. *Ann. Pediat. (Paris)* 29:35, 1982.
Matsuoka LY, et al.: Renal and testicular agenesis in a patient with Darier's disease. *Am. J. Med.* 78:873, 1985.

Thambiah AS, et al.: Darier's disease with cystic changes in the bones. *Br. J. Dermatol.* 78:87, 1966.
White JC: A case of keratosis (ichthyosis) follicularis. *J. Cutan. Genitourin. Dis.* 7:13, 1889.

DEAF MUTISM-GOITER-EUTHYROIDISM SYNDROME

Mode of Inheritance: Three of six siblings product of consanguineous marriage.

Clinical Manifestations: (a) *deaf mutism*; (b) *goiter*; (c) *euthyroidism*; (d) *abnormally high protein-bound iodine levels.*

Radiologic Manifestations: (a) *stippled epiphyses*; (b) skeletal maturation retardation (Fig SY–D–2).

REFERENCES

Refetoff S, et al.: Familial syndrome combining deaf-mutism, stippled epiphyses, goiter and abnormally high PBI: Possible target organ refractoriness to thyroid hormone. *J. Clin. Endocrinol. Metab.* 27:279, 1967.
Refetoff S, et al.: Studies of a sibship with apparent hereditary resistance to the intracellular action of thyroid hormone. *Metabolism* 21:723, 1972.

DEAFNESS AND METAPHYSEAL DYSOSTOSIS

Mode of Inheritance: Autosomal recessive (three siblings in one family).

Clinical Manifestations: (a) *conductive hearing deficit*; (b) mild mental retardation; (c) short and broad hands and feet, loose-jointed fingers.

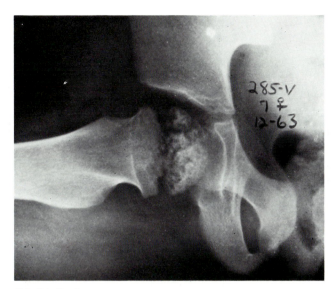

FIG SY–D–2.
Deaf mutism-goiter-euthyroidism syndrome showing a markedly stippled epiphysis of the femur and irregularity of the borders of the physis. (Courtesy of Dr. Richard R. Schreiber, Los Angeles.)

Radiologic Manifestations: (a) *fragmentation and widening of the metaphyses of tubular bones, short metacarpals and phalanges;* (b) low position of the middle ear ossicles, upward angulation of the internal auditory canals.

REFERENCE

Rimoin DL, et al.: Metaphyseal dysostosis, conductive hearing loss, and mental retardation: A recessivity inherited syndrome. *Birth Defects* 7:116, 1971.

DEGOS SYNDROME

Synonyms: Köhlmeier-Degos disease; Degos-Köhlmeier disease; malignant atrophic papulosis.

Pathology: Progressive cutaneovisceral (buccal mucosa, gastrointestinal tract, eyes, central nervous system, heart, kidneys, urinary tract, pleura, lungs, liver, pancreas) *occlusive arteriopathy*: subendothelial fibromuscular proliferation, intimal deposits of lipid-laden cells (middle-sized and small arteries), often thrombus formation.

Clinical Manifestations: Often a male patient in the third decade, rare in children: (a) *papular skin eruption progressing to ulceration*; (b) involvement of the mucous membrane; (c) *shallow ulcers of the mucosa of the stomach and bowel, bowel perforation, peritonitis;* (d) myocardial infarction, pericardial effusion, fibrous and fibrinous pericarditis, constrictive pericarditis, myocardial fibrosis, pulmonary infarct, renovascular hypertension, central nervous system manifestations (intellectual, social, and motor functions); (e) often rapidly fatal; (f) other reported abnormalities: lung abscess, subarachnoid hemorrhage.

Radiologic Manifestations: (a) bowel perforation, peritonitis, bowel infarction; (b) pleural effusion, pericardial effusion, pleural and pericardial calcification; (c) arteriographic findings: *occlusion of interlobar renal arteries,* intrarenal collateral circulation at the site of occlusion, delayed nephrographic phase at the area of intrarenal collaterals; multiple *intracerebral arterial narrowing and ectasia ("beading"), visceral arterial occlusions.*

REFERENCES

Bilbao JI, et al.: Maladie de Degos. Atteinte intestinale mise en evidence par angiographie numérique. Un cas. *J. Radiol.* 67:711, 1986.
Civatte J: Robert Degos (1904–1987). *Presse Med.* 16:1214, 1987.
Degos R, Delort J, Tricot R: Dermatite papulosquameuse atrophiante. *Ann. Dermatol. Syph.* 2:148, 281, 1942.
Köhlmeier W: Multiple Hautnekrosen bei Thromboaniitis obliterans. *Arch. Dermatol. Syph.* 181:783, 1941.
Petit WA, et al.: Degos disease: Neurologic complications and cerebral angiography. *Neurology* 32:1305, 1982.
Pierce RN, et al.: Intrathoracic manifestations of Degos disease (malignant atrophic papulosis). *Chest* 73:79, 1978.
Schade FB, et al.: Renovascular hypertension in a child with Degos-Köhlmeier disease. *Pediatr. Radiol.* 17:260, 1987.
Schneider A, et al.: Maligne atrophisierende Papulose (Degos-Syndrom) bei einem Säugling. *Helv. Paediatr. Acta* 41:447, 1986.
Sotrel A, et al.: Childhood Köhlmeier-Degos disease with atypical skin lesions. *Neurology* 33:1146, 1983.

DEJERINE-SOTTAS SYNDROME

Synonyms: Hypertrophic neuropathy of Dejerine-Sottas; HMSN, type III.

Mode of Inheritance: Autosomal dominant.

Pathology: *Thickening of affected nerves due to hyperplasia of the nerve sheath* (cranial nerves, spinal nerves, cauda equina, peripheral nerves).

Clinical Manifestations: Onset of disease usually in childhood, but often the disease is diagnosed in adult life: (a) symmetrical diffuse or localized manifestations with a picture of *progressive motor and sensory neural involvement* (muscle weakness, pain, nystagmus, etc.) and periodic phases of apparent remission, ataxia, areflexia, intention tremor, cranial nerve deficits, pupillary abnormalities, etc.); (b) enlarged and frequently palpable peripheral nerves.

Radiologic Manifestations: (a) *vertebral abnormalities:* scalloping of the dorsal aspect of vertebral bodies, enlarged interpediculate distances, triangulation of the pedicle with flattening of the superior aspect of the pedicle, erosion of the pedicle; (b) *myelography:* thickening of nerve roots, blocked

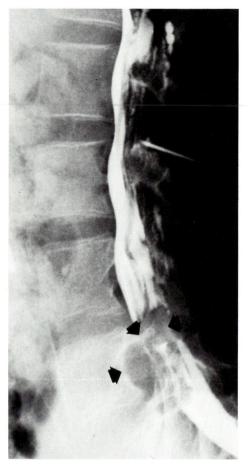

FIG SY–D–3.
Dejerine-Sottas syndrome in a 17-year-old boy with a 1-month history of pain in the right leg and lower part of the back. Marked atrophy of all extremities and decreased position sense were present. Myelographic examination demonstrates marked thickening of the nerves *(upper arrows)*. Vertical lucencies throughout the column of contrast also represent nerve root thickening. Scalloping of the dorsal portion of the fifth lumbar vertebra is also evident *(lower arrow)*. (From Patel DV, Ferguson RJL, Shey WL: Enlargement of the intervertebral foramina: An unusual cause, *A.J.R.* 131:911, 1978. Used by permission.)

flow of contrast material, distortion of contrast within the spinal canal and pooling due to large hypertrophied nerve roots (Fig SY–D–3).

Differential Diagnosis (Hypertrophic Neuropathy): Charcot-Marie-Tooth disease; Refsum disease; neurofibromatosis; leprosy; chronic Guillain-Barré syndrome; isolated peripheral nerve lesions.

REFERENCES

Appenzeller O, et al.: Macrodactyly and localized hypertrophic neuropathy. *Neurology* 24:767, 1974.
Carlin L, et al.: Hypertrophic neuropathy with spinal cord compression. *Surg. Neurol.* 18:237, 1982.
Dejerine J, Sottas J: Sur la nérvite interstitielle hypertrophique et progressive de l'enfance. *Mem. Soc. Biol.* 5:63, 1893.
Ouvrier RA, et al.: The hypertrophic forms of hereditary motor and sensory neuropathy. A study of hypertrophic Charcot-Marie-Tooth disease (HMSN type I) and Dejerine-Sottas disease (HMSN type III) in childhood. *Brain* 110:121, 1987.
Patel DV, et al.: Enlargement of the intervertebral foramina: An unusual cause. *A.J.R.* 131:911, 1978.
Rao CVGK, et al.: Dejerine-Sottas syndrome in children (hypertrophic interstitial polyneuritis). *A.J.R.* 122:70, 1974.

de LANGE SYNDROME

Synonyms: Cornelia de Lange syndrome; Brachmann—de Lange syndrome; typus degenerativus Amstelodamensis.

Mode of Inheritance: Sporadic in most cases; familial occurrence suggests a genetic disorder; recurrence rate of 2% to 5%.

Frequency: Estimated birth prevalance of 1:10,000 (Opitz, 1985).

Clinical Manifestations: (a) *low birth weight, growth failure;* (b) *characteristic facies:* low hairline; heavy confluent eyebrows; curly eyelashes; small upturned nose; micrognathia; wide, thin, and downturned upper lip; (c) *microbrachycephaly;* (d) *hirsutism;* (e) *cryptorchidism;* (f) *marked mental, motor, and social retardation;* (g) *limb anomalies,* absence or deformities of the ulnar rays, contractures and webbing of the fingers, micromelia, microdactyly, flexion contractures of the elbow and restriction of supination and pronation, prominent and palpable radial head, toe deformities, webbing, tight Achilles tendon, pes planus, valgus heel, flexion contracture of the knees, congenital hip dislocation, coxa valga; (h) *initial hypertonicity;* (i) *low-pitched weak cry;* (j) other reported abnormalities: high-arched palate, eye anomalies (optic atrophy, myopia, astigmatism, optic nerve coloboma, proptosis), cleft palate, low-set ears, congenital heart defect, cutis marmorata, hypoplastic nipples and umbilicus, nonspecific chromosomal abnormalities, microcephaly, recurrent respiratory infections, delayed eruption and wide spacing of the teeth, hypospadias, recurrent convulsions, hernias, hearing loss, feeding problems, behavioral problems, low levels of 5-OH-indole-3-acetic acid (5HIAA) in amniotic fluid, abscence of pregnancy-associated plasma protein A (PAPP-A) in the serum of the mother carrying a de Lange fetus.

Radiologic Manifestations: (a) *microbrachycephaly;* (b) *anomalies of limbs,* e.g., micromelia, phocomelia, and hemimelia; (c) *anomalies of digits,* e.g., oligodactyly, syndactyly, clinodactyly, proximally placed thumb, *hypoplasia of the first metacarpal,* pattern profiles of the hand (method of Poznanski): short first metacarpal bone, relatively long third and fourth metacarpals; (d) *dysplasia and dislocation of the radial head* with flexion and contracture of the elbow; (e)

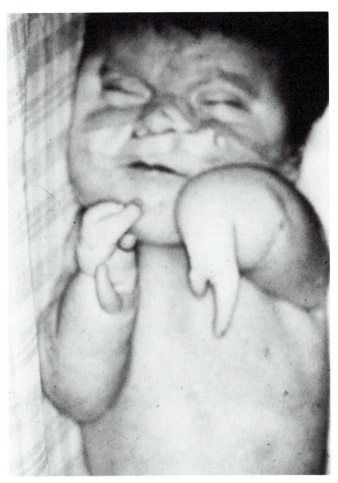

FIG SY–D–4.
de Lange syndrome in a newborn with the characteristic facies (small forehead with proximal hair implantation, synophrys, long eyelashes, small nose, thin lips and micrognathia, and upper limb deformities). (From Fryns JP, Deremaeker AM, Hoefnagels M, et al.: The Brachman-deLange syndrome in two siblings of normal parents. *Clin. Genet.* 31:413, 1987. Used by permission.)

skeletal maturation retardation; (f) flat acetabular angle; (g) abnormal thoracic configuration (rounded thoracic inlet, wide upper portion of the rib cage, short sternum, advanced development of sternal ossification centers); (h) other reported abnormalities: choanal atresia, short esophagus, hiatal hernia, intestinal duplication, bowel malrotation, pyloric stenosis, inguinal hernia, overconstruction of long bones, Kirner deformity, spurs of the mandible, cerebral ventricular dilatation, horseshoe kidneys, aseptic necrosis of the femoral head, epichondylar process of the humerus (Figs SY–D–4 and SY–D–5).

REFERENCES

Bankier A, et al: Familial occurrence of Brachmann-de Lange syndrome (letter). *Am. J. Med. Genet.* 25:163, 1986.

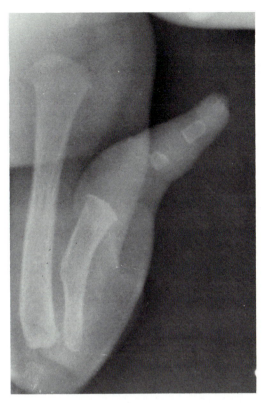

FIG SY–D–5.
de Lange syndrome in a 2-month-old male with absence of the ulna and all digits except the thumb. (From Taybi H: Cornelia de Lange syndrome. *Semin. Roentgenol.* 8:198, 1973. Used by permission.)

Beck B, et al.: Chromosomes in the Cornelia deLange syndrome. *Hum. Genet.* 59:271, 1981.

Brachmann W: Ein Fall von symmetrischer Monodaktylie durch Ulnadefekt, mit symmetrischer Flughautbildung in den Ellenbogen sowie andren Abnormalitäten (Zwerghaftigkeit, Halsrippen, Behaarung). *J. Kinderheilkd. Phys. Erzieh.* 84:225, 1916.

Curtis JA, et al.: Spurs of the mandible and supraclavicular process of the humerus in Cornelia de Lange syndrome. *A.J.R.* 129:156, 1977.

de Lange C: Sur un type nouveau de dégéneration (typus Amstelodamensis). *Arch. Med. Enf.* 36:713, 1933.

Fryns JP, et al.: The Brachmann-deLange syndrome in two siblings of normal parents. *Clin. Genet.* 31:413, 1987.

Gerald B, et al.: The Cornelia de Lange syndrome: Radiographic findings. *Radiology* 88:96, 1967.

Hawley PP, et al.: Sixty-four patients with Brachmann-deLange syndrome: A survey. *Am. J. Med. Genet.* 20:453, 1985.

Joubin J, et al.: Cornelia deLange's syndrome. *Clin. Orthop.* 171:180, 1982.

Kurlander GJ, et al.: Roentgenology of the Brachmann–de Lange syndrome. *Radiology* 88:101, 1967.

Lacourt GC, et al.: Microcephalic dwarfism with associated low amniotic fluid 5-hydroxyindole-3-acetic acid (5 HIAA): Report of a case of Cornelia de Lange syndrome. *Helv. Paediatr. Acta* 32:149, 1977.

Lee FA: Generalized overconstriction of long bones and unilateral Kirner's deformity in a de Lange dwarf. *Am. J. Dis. Child.* 116:599, 1968.

Naguib KK, et al.: Brachmann-deLange syndrome in sibs. *J. Med. Genet.* 24:627, 1987.

Opitz JM: The Brachmann-deLange syndrome. *Am. J. Med. Genet.* 22:89, 1985.

Peeters FLM: Radiological manifestations of the Cornelia de Lange syndrome. *Pediatr. Radiol.* 3:41, 1975.

Preus M, et al.: Definition and diagnosis of the Brachmann-DeLange syndrome. *Am. J. Med. Genet.* 16:301, 1983.

Taybi H: Cornelia de Lange syndrome. *Semin. Roentgenol.* 8:198, 1973.

Westergaard JG, et al.: Pregnancy-associated plasma protein A: A possible marker in the classification and prenatal diagnosis of Cornelia deLange syndrome. *Prenatal Diagn.* 3:225, 1983.

Willems PJ, et al: Activation of fatty acid oxidation in the Silver-Russell syndrome and the Brachmann–de Lange syndrome. *Am. J. Med. Genet.* 30:865, 1988.

Wilson WG, et al.: Reciprocal translocation 14q;21q in a patient with the Brachmann-deLange syndrome. *J. Med. Genet.* 20:469, 1983.

Wilson GN, et al.: The association of chromosome 3 duplication and the Cornelia de Lange syndrome. *J. Pediatr.* 93:783, 1978.

de MORSIER SYNDROME

Synonyms: Septo-optic dysplasia and pituitary dwarfism; Kaplan-Grumbach-Hoyt syndrome.

Pathology: (a) *agenesis of the septum pellucidum* (in the majority of the cases); (b) *presence of a primitive optic ventricle;* (c) *hypoplasia of the chiasm.*

Clinical Manifestations: (a) apnea, hypotonia, seizures, hypoglycemia, and prolonged jaundice in newborns; (b) *ocular disease:* amblyopia, nystagmus, hemianopia, hypoplastic optic disks, irregular field defects; (c) normal or subnormal intelligence; (d) hypothalmic and neurohypophyseal insufficiency, hypothalamic hypothyroidism, elevated prolactin levels, diabetes insipidus, etc.; (e) short stature; (f) other reported abnormalities: occurrence of panhypopituitarism in two first cousins, one of whom had septo-optic dysplasia, cerebral palsy, phalangeal anomalies (absence or hypoplasia of the distal and middle phalanges of fingers 2, 3, and 4 and the great toes; snydactyly and areas of constriction on the digits), hemiparesis, impairment of topographical orientation, route learning and kinesthetic memory in a blind patient, diabetic mother, infantile spasms, etc.

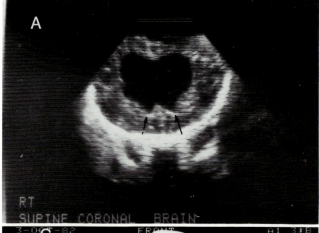
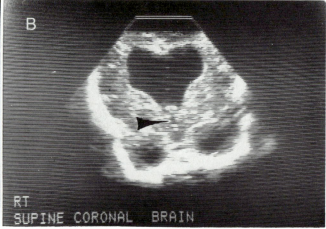
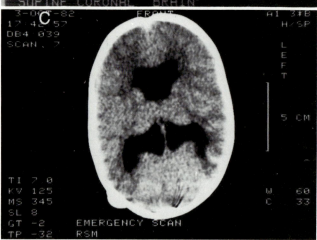

FIG SY–D–6.
de Morsier syndrome. **A,** a coronal ultrasound scan shows the inferior pointing in the anterior horns of both lateral ventricles *(arrows)*. Notice the absence of the midline septum; **B,** a coronal ultrasound scan shows a small dysmorphic third ventricle *(arrowhead)*. A corpus callosum is not present. **C,** axial CT scan illustrates flattening of the anterior portion of the dilated frontal horns; the anterior portion of the septum pellucidum is absent. (From Williams JL, Faerber EN: Septooptic dysplasia (deMorsier syndrome). *J. Ultrasound Med.* 4:265, 1985. Used by permission.)

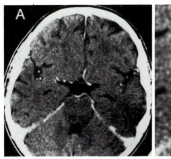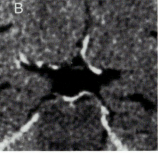

FIG SY–D–7.
de Morsier syndrome in a 12-year-old male with bilateral optic atrophy, blindness, and growth hormone deficiency. A computed tomographic scan shows a small optic chiasm. (From Wilson DM, Enzmann DR, Hintz RL, et al.: Computed tomographic findings in septo-optic dysplasia: A discordance between clinical and radiological findings. *Neuroradiology* 26:279, 1984. Used by permission.)

Radiologic Manifestations: (a) *absence of the septum pellucidum, flattening of the roof and inferior pointing of the floor of the frontal horns of lateral ventricles, hypoplasia of the anterior optic pathways, prominent optic recess of the third ventricle,* dilatation of the suprasellar and chiasmatic cisterns, small optic nerves, normal brain computed tomographic scan in the presence of typical endocrinologic and ophthalmologic manifestations of septo-optic dysplasia; (b) other reported abnormalities: agenesis of the corpus callosum, enlargement of the pituitary stalk and infundibulum when septo-optic dysplasia is associated with diabetes insipidus, cortical atrophy with dilated sulci, sphenoidal encephalocele; (c) retarded bone age (Figs SY–D–6 and SY–D–7).

REFERENCES

Blethen SL, et al.: Hypopituitarism and septooptic "dysplasia" in first cousins. *Am. J. Med. Genet.* 21:123, 1985.
de Morsier G: Etudes sur les dysraphies crânio-encéphaliques: III. Agénésie du septum lucidum avec malformations du tractus optique: La dysplasie septo-optique. *Schweiz. Arch. Neurochir. Psychiatr.* 77:267, 1956.
Donat JF: Septo-optic dysplasia in an infant of a diabetic mother. *Arch. Neurol.* 38:590, 1981.
Griffiths P, et al.: Specific spatial defect in a child with septo-optic dysplasia. *Dev. Med. Child Neurol.* 26:391, 1984.
Hoyt WF, et al.: Septo-optic dysplasia and pituitary dwarfism. *Lancet* 1:893, 1970.
Kaplan SL, et al.: A syndrome of hypopituitary dwarfism, hypoplasia of optic nerves and malformation of prosencephalon: Report of 6 patients. *Pediatr. Res.* 4:480, 1970.
Kewitz G, et al.: Septo-optic pituitary dysplasia. *Helv. Paediatr. Acta* 39:355, 1984.
Kuriyama M, et al.: Septo-optic dysplasia with infantile spasms. *Pediatr. Neurol.* 4:62, 1988.
Margalith D, et al.: Congenital optic nerve hypoplasia with hypothalamic-pituitary dysplasia. A review of 16 cases. *Am. J. Dis. Child.* 139:361, 1985.
O'Dwyer JA et al.: Radiologic features of septooptic dysplasia. *A.J.N.R.* 1:443, 1980.
Osborn RE, et al.: Schizencephaly with optic nerve hypoplasia simulating septo-optic dysplasia and other syndromes. *J. Med. Imag.* 2:240, 1988.
Pagon RA, et al.: Septo-optic dysplasia with digital anomalies. *J. Pediatr.* 105:966, 1984.
Petrus M, et al.: Le syndrome de Kaplan, Grumbach et Hoyt. *Ann. Pediatr. (Paris)* 28:409, 1981.
Reeves DL: Congenital absence of septum pellucidum. *Johns Hopkins Med. J.* 69:61, 1941.
Williams JL, et al.: Septooptic dysplasia (deMorsier syndrome). *J. Ultrasound Med.* 4:265, 1985.
Wilson DM, et al.: Computed tomographic findings in septo-optic dysplasia: Discordance between clinical and radiological findings. *Neuroradiology* 26:279, 1984.

DENTINE DYSPLASIA–SCLEROTIC BONES

Mode of Inheritance: Autosomal dominant.

Clinical and Radiological Manifestations: (a) radicular dentine dysplasia; (b) dense sclerotic bones (long bones, mandible, maxilla) with narrow or occluded marrow spaces.

REFERENCE

Morris ME, et al.: Dentine dysplasia with sclerotic bone and skeletal anomalies inherited as an autosomal dominant trait. *Oral Surg. Oral Med. Oral Pathol.* 43:267, 1977.

DERMATOMYOSITIS

This is a nonsuppurative systemic inflammatory disease (necrotizing vasculitis) that primarily involves the skin, subcutaneous tissues, and skeletal muscles; female predominance; the disease more crippling and soft-tissue calcification more extensive in the childhood form; associated neoplasms more common in adults (five- to sevenfold increase); presumed autoimmune disease triggered by exogenous factors.

Clinical Manifestations: Acute or insidious onset: (a) muscle weakness involving the proximal muscles more than the distal extremities, girdle muscles, etc.; (b) pain, atrophy, and/or contracture; (c) skin rash: periorbital heliotrope hue, erythematous rash over the extensor surfaces, V-shaped erythema of the upper part of the torso; (d) electromyelography: short, low-amplitude polyphasic motor unit action potentials and fibrillations; (e) elevated levels of muscle enzymes: aldolase, creatine kinase, pyruvate kinase, etc.; (f) muscle biopsy: perifascicular inflammatory infiltrate, fiber atrophy, capillary necrosis, necrosis of muscle endothelial cells; (g) dysphagia, abdominal pain, perforation of the digestive tract; (h) other reported manifestations: abnormal phona-

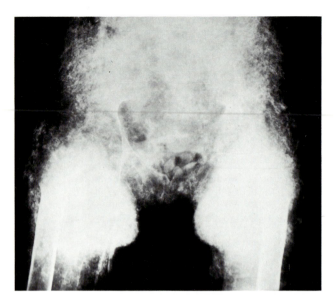

FIG SY—D—8.
Dermatomyositis. A lacy, reticular, subcutaneous pattern of calcification encases the patient. (From Blane CE, White SJ, Braunstein EM, et al.: Pattern of calcification in childhood dermatomyositis. *A.J.R.* 142:397, 1984. Used by permission.)

tion, photophobia, intermittent paresthesia, skin necrosis, interstitial lung disease, pulmonary fibrosis, involvement of respiratory muscles, decrease in ventilatory capacity, myocardial involvement (abnormal electrocardiographic findings), transient retinal exudates and "cotton-wool" spots (small-vessel occlusion), optic atrophy, nail bed telangiectasia, digital ulceration, infarction of the oral epithelium, exacerbation

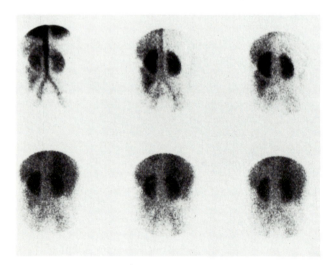

FIG SY—D—9.
Dermatomyositis and calcinosis universalis. The angiogram phase of a ⁹⁹ᵐTc glucoheptonate study demonstrates vascularity in a wedge-shaped lesion inferior to the left kidney. (From Czarnecki DJ, Schroeder BA, Sty JR: Calcinosis of child dermatomyositis with glucoheptonate angiogram. *Clin. Nucl. Med.* 12:675, 1987. Used by permission.)

of skin inflammation on exposure to sunlight, nasal speech due to soft-palate dysfunction, masseter atrophy, renal involvement (glomerular lesions), occurrence in monozygotic twins.

Radiologic Manifestations: (a) calcification: deep calcareal masses, superficial calcareal masses, deep linear deposits, and a lacy, reticular, subcutaneous calcium deposition encasing the trunk; onset of calcification often at pressure point sites (elbows, knees, buttocks); calcified necrosis of the ureters; (b) alimentary tract: difficulty in swallowing solids, pooling of secretions, pooling of barium in the hypopharynx, atonic pyriform fossae, mucosal ulceration due to vasculitis, perforation, benign pneumatosis intestinalis; (c) pulmonary disease, pulmonary fibrosis; (d) abnormal vascular pattern on a ⁹⁹ᵐTc glucoheptonate angiogram (kidney) (Figs SY—D—8 and SY—D—9).

REFERENCES

Basset N, et al.: Dermatomyosite, nécroses cutanées et fibrose pulmonaire. Nouvelle entité ou association fortuite? *Presse Med.* 16:1243, 1987.

Blane CE, et al.: Patterns of calcification in childhood dermatomyositis. *A.J.R.* 142:397, 1984.

Bohan A, et al.: A computer-assisted analysis of 153 patients with polymyositis and dermatomyositis. *Medicine (Baltimore)* 56:255, 1977.

Borrelli M, et al.: Ureteral necrosis in dermatomyositis. *J. Urol.* 139:1275, 1988.

Czarnecki DJ, et al.: Calcinosis of childhood determatomyositis with glucoheptonate angiogram. *Clin. Nucl. Med.* 12:675, 1987.

Dowsett RJ, et al.: Dermatomyositis and Hodgkin's disease. Case report and review of the literature. *Am. J. Med.* 80:719, 1986.

Fudman EJ, et al.: Dermatomyositis without creatine kinase elevation. A poor prognostic sign. *Am. J. Med.* 80:329, 1986.

Harati Y, et al.: Childhood dermatomyositis in monozygotic twins. *Neurology (N.Y.)* 36:721, 1986.

Kalmanti M, et al.: Neuroblastoma occurring in a child with dermatomyositis. *Am. J. Pediatr. Hematol. Oncol.* 7:387, 1985.

Magill HL, et al.: Duodenal perforation in childhood dermatomyositis. *Pediatr. Radiol.* 14:28, 1984.

Martini A, et al.: Calcinosis as the presenting sign of juvenile dermatomyositis in a 14-month-old boy. *Helv. Paediatr. Acta* 42:181, 1987.

Miller LC, et al.: Childhood dermatomyositis. *Clin. Pediatr. (Phila.)* 26:561, 1987.

Pachman LM: Juvenile dermatomyositis. *Pediatr. Clin. North Am.* 33:1097, 1986.

Pasquali JL, et al.: Les manifestations rénales au cours des dermatomyosites et des polymyosites. *Ann. Med. Interne (Paris)* 138:109, 1987.

Schröter HM, et al.: Juvenile dermatomyositis induced by toxoplasmosis. *J. Child Neurol.* 2:101, 1987.

Steiner RM, et al.: The radiological findings in dermatomyositis of childhood. *Radiology* 111:385, 1974.

DERMO-CHONDRO-CORNEAL DYSTROPHY OF FRANÇOIS

Synonyms: François syndrome no. 2; familial dermo-chondrocorneal dystrophy; arthropathic nodular fibromatosis.

Mode of Inheritance: Autosomal recessive.

Clinical Manifestations: (a) *cutaneous xanthomatous nodules;* (b) *corneal dystrophy;* (c) skeletal deformities with *contractures,* subluxations, and limitation of motion.

Radiologic Manifestations: Osteochondral deformities detectable in the first decade of life: (a) *defective endochondral ossification, defective and irregular ossification of some tarsal bones;* (b) rarely extensive osteoarticular destruction involving the entire skeleton except the spine and skull (Fig SY–D–10).

REFERENCES

François J: Dystrophie dermo-chondro-cornéenne familiale. *Ann. Ocul.* 182:409, 1949.

Jansen VJ: Dermo-chondro-corneal dystrophy: Report of a case. *Acta Ophthalmol.* 36:71, 1958.

Remky H, et al.: Dystrophia dermo-chondro-cornealis (François). *Klin. Monatsbl. Augenheilkd.* 151:319, 1967.

Ruiz-Maldonado R, et al.: Dystrophie dermo-chondro-cornéenne familiale (syndrome de François). *Ann. Dermatol. Vénéréol.* 104:475, 1977.

Wiedemann H-R: Zur François' schen Krankheit: Dystrophia dermo-chondro-cornealis familiaris. *Aerztl. Wochenschr.* 13:905, 1958.

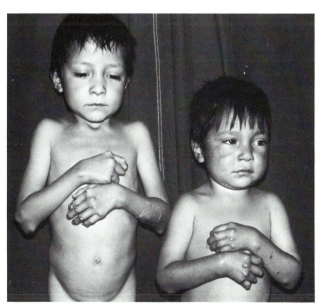

FIG SY–D–10.
Dermochondrocorneal dystrophy of François. Note the nodules of the hands and ear lobes. (From Ruiz-Maldonado R, Tamayo L, Velazques E: Dystrophie dermo-chondro-cornéenne familiale (syndrome de François). *Ann. Dermatol. Venereol.* 104:475, 1977. Used by permission.)

DE SANCTIS–CACCHIONE SYNDROME

Synonym: Xerodermic idiocy.

Mode of Inheritance: Autosomal recessive.

Clinical Manifestations: Onset in infancy or early childhood: (a) *dwarfism;* (b) *xeroderma pigmentosum;* (c) *microcephaly,* mental retardation, speech disorders, convulsions, spasticity, choreoathetosis, cerebellar ataxia; (d) *gonadal hypoplasia;* (e) other reported abnormalities: propensity for skin neoplasm, leukemia; (f) dermatoglyphic pattern: very few palmar creases and arch patterns in all the fingers except the thumbs, increased level of serum copper, low excretion of 17-ketosteroids in the urine, elevated serum cholesterol level, hepatomegaly, pneumonia.

Radiologic Manifestations: (a) microcephaly, cerebral cortical atrophy and ventricular dilatation, premature closure of cranial sutures; (b) skeletal growth retardation.

REFERENCES

de Sanctis C, Cacchione A: L'idiozia zerodermica. *Riv. Sper. Freniat.* 56:269, 1932.

Hananian J, et al.: Xeroderma pigmentosum exhibiting neurological disorders and systemic lupus erythematosus. *Clin. Genet.* 17:39, 1980.

Handa J, et al.: Cranial computed tomography findings in xeroderma pigmentosum with neurologic manifestations (de Sanctis–Cacchione syndrome). *J. Comput. Assist. Tomogr.* 2:456, 1978.

Lynch HT, et al.: Xeroderma pigmentosum, malignant melanoma, and congenital ichthyosis: A family study. *Arch. Dermatol.* 96:625, 1967.

Mimaki T, et al.: Xeroderma pigmentosum with versive seizures. *Pediatr. Neurol.* 4:58, 1988.

Mishra PC, et al.: De Sanctis–Cacchione syndrome. *Indian J. Pediatr.* 49:891, 1982.

Reed WB, et al.: Xeroderma pigmentosum with neurological complications: The de Sanctis–Cacchione syndrome. *Arch. Dermatol.* 91:224, 1965.

Tachi N, et al.: Peripheral neuropathy in four cases of group A xeroderma pigmentosum. *J. Child Neurol.* 3:114, 1988.

DESMOID SYNDROME

Clinical and Radiologic Manifestations: (a) *desmoid tumor;* (b) *bone abnormalities:* cortical thickening, cystic areas of translucency, compact bone islands, sacralization of the fifth lumbar vertebra; (c) higher frequency of bony abnormalities in the relatives of the patients than in control population.

REFERENCES

Häyry P, et al.: The desmoid tumor. III. A biochemical and genetic analysis. *Am. J. Clin. Pathol.* 77:681, 1982.

Reitamo JJ, et al.: The desmoid syndrome. New aspects in the cause, pathogenesis and treatment of the desmoid tumor. *Am. J. Surg.* 151:230, 1986.

DIAMOND-BLACKFAN SYNDROME

Synonyms: Blackfan-Diamond syndrome; congenital pure red cell aplasia; congenital (erythroid) hypoplastic anemia.

Mode of Inheritance: Autosomal recessive.

Clinical Manifestations: Insidious onset in infancy or childhood: (a) unusual facies in some (two-colored hair, wide-set eyes, snub nose, thick upper lip); (b) *normocytic, normochromic refractory anemia* with normal value of other formed elements; (c) no hepatosplenomegaly or lymph node enlargement; (d) *complete or near complete absence of cells of the erythroid series in bone marrow;* (e) musculoskeletal abnormalities (in 30% of patients): abnormalities of the thumb (particularly triphalangeal thumb and thenar muscle atrophy), Sprengel deformity, Klippel-Feil syndrome, etc.; (f) other reported abnormalities: short stature, webbed neck, Turner syndrome–like appearance, hemolysis, active erythropoiesis, tracheoesophageal fistula, chylothorax, idiopathic distal renal tubular acidosis, increased erythrocyte adenosine deaminase activities, hydrops fetalis, abnormality of chromosome 1, hypogonadotropic hypogonadism (pituitary dysfunction probably secondary to frequent transfusion therapy), acute lymphocytic leukemia.

Radiologic Manifestations: (a) skeletal, cardiac, and renal anomalies; (b) growth retardation; (c) cardiac enlargement, refractory heart failure.

REFERENCES

Balaban EP, et al.: Diamond-Blackfan syndrome in adult patients. *Am. J. Med.* 78:533, 1985.

Beck W, et al.: Endocrine studies in Blackfan-Diamond anemia: Evidence for hypothalamic-pituitary dysfunction under frequent transfusion therapy. *Eur. J. Pediatr.* 135:103, 1980.

Diamond LK, Blackfan KD: Hypoplastic anemia. *Am. J. Dis. Child.* 56:464, 1938.

Freedman MH: Diamond-Blackfan anemia. Neonatal presentation as Rh incompatibility, hemolysis, and active erythropoiesis. *Am. J. Pediatr. Hematol. Oncol.* 7:327, 1985.

Heyn R, et al.: The association of Blackfan-Diamond syndrome, physical abnormalities, and an abnormality of chromosome 1. *J. Pediatr.* 85:531, 1974.

Josephs HW: Anaemia of infancy and early childhood. *Medicine (Baltimore)* 15:307, 1936.

Lazarus KH, et al.: Multiple congenital anomalies in a patient with Diamond-Blackfan syndrome. *Clin. Pediatr. (Phila.)* 23:520, 1984.

Scimeca PG, et al.: Diamond-Blackfan syndrome: An unusual cause of hydrops fetalis. *Am. J. Pediatr. Hematol. Oncol.* 10:241, 1988.

Steinberg PG, et al.: Hepatocellular carcinoma, transfusion-induced hemochromatosis and congenital hypoplastic anemia (Blackfan-Diamond syndrome). *Am. J. Med.* 60:1032, 1976.

Whitehouse DB, et al.: Adenosine deaminase activity in Diamond-Blackfan syndrome. *Lancet* 2:1398, 1984.

DIENCEPHALIC SYNDROME

Synonym: Russell syndrome.

Pathology: Tumors in the region of the anterior hypothalamus (glioma most often); nondiencephalic tumors a less common cause of the syndrome.

Clinical Manifestations: (a) *emaciation;* (b) hyperkinesia; (c) normal or *increased appetite;* (d) *euphoria;* (e) *overalertness;* (f) *initial growth acceleration;* (g) other reported abnormalities: hypotension, hypoglycemia, skin pallor, increased urinary catecholamine excretion, pituitary insufficiency, optic nerve atrophy, strabismus, spasmus nutans as a presenting sign, cherry-red macular spot.

Radiologic Manifestations: (a) *complete absence of subcutaneous fat;* (b) sutural widening and other roentgenographic findings of *increased intracranial pressure;* (c) hydrocephalus; (d) *mass in the hypothalamic region* with indenta-

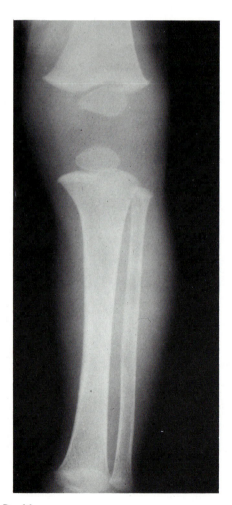

FIG SY–D–11.
Diencephalic syndrome. Note the complete absence of fat lines in this 9-month-old boy. (From Poznanski AK, Manson G: Radiographic appearance of the soft tissues in the diencephalic syndrome of infancy. *Radiology* 81:101, 1963. Used by permission.)

tion on the third ventricle; (e) increased uptake of radionuclide (^{99m}Tc) in the vicinity of the sella turcica (Fig SY−D−11).

REFERENCES

Blanc JF, et al.: Diagnostic échographique d'une tumeur diencéphalique cachectisante. *Arch. Fr. Pediatr.* 40:575, 1983.

Chynn KY, et al.: Diencephalic syndrome of emaciation. *A.J.R.* 95:917, 1965.

Eliash A, et al.: Diencephalic syndrome due to a suprasellar epidermoid cyst. *Child Brain* 10:414, 1983.

Garty BZ, et al.: Spasmus nutans as a presenting sign of diencephalic syndrome. *J. Pediatr.* 107:484, 1985.

Nagashima K, et al.: Infantile neuroaxonal dystrophy: Perinatal onset with symptoms of diencephalic syndrome. *Neurology* 35:735, 1985.

Poznanski AK, Manson G: Radiographic appearance of the soft tissues in the diencephalic syndrome of infancy. *Radiology* 81:101, 1963.

Russell A: A diencephalic syndrome of emaciation in infancy and childhood. *Arch. Dis. Child.* 26:274, 1951.

Sakura N, et al.: Cherry red macular degeneration. A clinical manifestation of the diencephalic syndrome? *Acta Paediatr. Scand.* 71:857, 1982.

Scott EW, et al.: Pediatric diencephalic gliomas—A review of 18 cases. *Pediatr. Neurosci.* 13:225, 1987.

DIETL SYNDROME

Synonyms: Dietl crisis; intermittent hydronephrosis.

Etiology: Intermittent ureteropelvic junction obstruction, often related to an aberrant vessel.

Clinical Manifestations: Recurrent symptoms: crampy upper abdominal pain, nausea, vomiting.

Radiologic Manifestations: Demonstration of the obstruction by diuretic excretory urography, ultrasonography, and renal scan (delayed double-peak pattern shown on ^{99m}Tc-diethylenetriaminepentaacetic acid diuretic renography).

REFERENCES

Dietl J: Wandernde Nieren and deren Einklemmung. *Wien. Med. Wochenschr.* 14:153−166, 579−581, 593−595, 1864.

Flotte TR: Dietl syndrome: Intermittent ureteropelvic junction obstruction as a cause of episodic abdominal pain. *Pediatrics* 82:792, 1988.

Homsy YL, et al.: Intermittent hydronephrosis: A diagnostic challenge. *J. Urol.* 140:1222, 1988.

Malek RS: Intermittent hydronephrosis: The occult ureteropelvic obstruction. *J. Urol.* 130:863, 1983.

DiGEORGE SYNDROME

Synonyms: Third and fourth pharyngeal pouch syndrome; DiGeorge sequence.

Mode of Inheritance: A few familial cases and occurrence in monozygotic twins have been reported; autosomal dominant.

Frequency: Uncommon.

Pathological Classification: (a) complete DiGeorge syndrome: absent parathyroid, no T-cell function; (b) partial DiGeorge syndrome: some T-cell function; (c) abnormalities of the third and fourth pharyngeal pouches: malformation and hypoplasia or maldescent of the thymus and parathyroid glands; (d) other reported abnormalities: hypoplasia, delayed

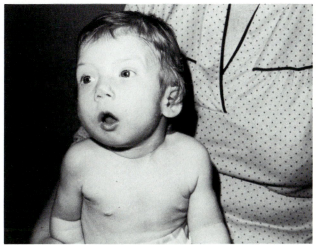

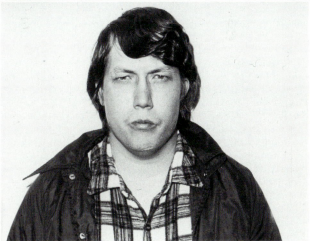

FIG SY−D−12.
DiGeorge syndrome in a father and son. Note the low-set ears, micrognathia, and hypertelorism in the child and more subtle dysmorphism in the father. (From Rohn RD, Leffell MS, Leadem P, et al.: Familial third-fourth pharyngeal pouch syndrome with apparent autosomal dominant transmission. *J. Pediatr.* 105:47, 1984. Used by permission.)

maximum growth rate, persistent fetal shape of the thyroid cartilage, shortened trachea with a reduced number of cartilage rings, abnormalities of the stapes, anomalies of the brain, alimentary tract and genitourinary tract anomalies.

Clinical Manifestations: (a) *unusual facial features:* broad nose, shortened philtrum, hypoplastic mandible, low-set ears, fused helix and anthelix, hypertelorism; (b) *hypocalcemic tetany in the newborn;* (c) *frequent infections,* particularly those of the respiratory system (especially acid-fast bacteria, virus, fungi, and *Pneumocystis carinii); (d) normal levels of all immunoglobulins,* impaired cell-mediated immunity (T- and B-cell immunodeficiency, low levels of facteur thymic serique [FTS]); (e) *cardiovascular anomalies;* (f) other reported abnormalities: failure to thrive and developmental delay, arhinencephalia, cleft lip/palate, dysfunction of the glossopharyngeal nerve, glioma, Graves disease, chromosome abnormalities (monosomy of chromosome 22), maternal alcoholism, webbed neck.

Radiologic Manifestations: (a) *absence of a thymic shadow in the first week of life* on a chest roentgenogram; (b) *cardiovascular anomalies,* especially *aortic arch anomalies,* interrupted aortic arch, truncus arteriosus, tetralogy of Fallot, high incidence of DiGeorge syndrome when aortic arch interruption is associated with a right-sided descending aorta, etc.; (c) other reported abnormalities: diaphragmatic abnormalities, hydronephrosis, malrotation of the bowel, imperforate anus, stapedial hypoplasia, esophageal atresia, tracheoesophageal fistula, significantly low incidence of visible hyoid bone ossification centers on the radiographic examination, vertebral anomalies, digital anomalies (Fig SY–D–12).

REFERENCES

Ammann AJ, et al.: The DiGeorge syndrome and fetal alcohol syndrome. *Am. J. Dis. Child.* 136:906, 1982.

Augusseau S, et al.: DiGeorge syndrome and 22q11 rearrangements. *Hum. Genet.* 74:206, 1986.

Burgio GR, et al.: Errors of morphogenesis and inborn errors of immunity 20 years after the discovery of DiGeorge anomaly. *Eur. J. Pediatr.* 144:9, 1985.

Conley ME, et al.: The spectrum of the DiGeorge syndrome. *J. Pediatr.* 94:883, 1979.

DiGeorge AM: Discussion on new concept of cellular basis of immunity. *J. Pediatr.* 67:907, 1965.

Faed MJW, et al.: Features of diGeorge syndrome in a child with 45,XX,−3,−22,+der(3),t(3;22)(p25;q11). *J. Med. Genet.* 24:225, 1987.

Goldsobel AB, et al.: Bone marrow transplantation in DiGeorge syndrome. *J. Pediatr.* 111:40, 1987.

Gosseye S, et al.: Association of bilateral renal agenesis and DiGeorge syndrome in an infant of a diabetic mother. *Helv. Paediatr. Acta* 37:471, 1982.

Greenberg F, et al: Prenatal diagnosis of deletion 17p13 associated with DiGeorge anomaly. *Am. J. Med. Genet.* 31:1, 1988.

Keppen LD, et al: Confirmation of autosomal dominant transmission of the DiGeorge malformation complex. *J. Pediatr.* 113:506, 1988.

Miller JD, et al.: DiGeorge's syndrome in monozygotic twins. *Am. J. Dis. Child.* 137:438, 1983.

Moerman P, et al.: Interrupted right aortic arch in DiGeorge syndrome. *Br. Heart J.* 58:274, 1987.

Pong AJH, et al.: DiGeorge syndrome: Long-term survival complicated by Graves disease. *J. Pediatr.* 106:619, 1985.

Müller W, et al: The DiGeorge syndrome. I. Clinical evaluation and course of partial and complete forms of the syndrome. *Eur. J. Pediatr.* 147:496, 1988.

Raatikka M, et al.: Familial third and fourth pharyngeal pouch syndrome with truncus arteriosus: DiGeorge syndrome. *Pediatrics* 67:173, 1981.

Radford DJ, et al.: Spectrum of DiGeorge syndrome in patients with truncus arteriosus: Expanded DiGeorge syndrome. *Pediatr. Cardiol.* 9:95, 1988.

Rohn RD, et al.: Familial third-fourth pharyngeal pouch syndrome with apparent autosomal dominant transmission. *J. Pediatr.* 105:47, 1984.

Rose JS, et al.: Congenital absence of the pulmonary valve associated with congenital aplasia of the thymus (DiGeorge's syndrome). *A.J.R.* 122:97, 1974.

Sein K, et al.: Short trachea, with reduced number of cartilage rings—a hitherto unrecognized feature of DiGeorge syndrome. *Pediatr. Pathol.* 4:81, 1985.

Tuvia J, et al.: Aplastic anaemia complicating adenovirus infection in DiGeorge syndrome. *Eur. J. Pediatr.* 147:643, 1988.

Van Mierop LHS, et al.: Cardiovascular anomalies in DiGeorge syndrome and importance of neural crest as a possible pathogenetic factor. *Am. J. Cardiol.* 58:133, 1986.

Wells TR, et al.: Abnormal growth of the thyroid cartilage in the DiGeorge syndrome. *Pediatr. Pathol.* 6:209, 1986.

Wells TR, et al.: Ossification centre of the hyoid bone in DiGeorge syndrome and tetralogy of Fallot. *Br. J. Radiol.* 59:1065, 1986.

Winter WE, et al.: Familial DiGeorge syndrome with tetralogy of Fallot and prolonged survival. *Eur. J. Pediatr.* 141:171, 1984.

DIGITOTALAR DYSMORPHISM

Synonym: Ulnar drift.

Mode of Inheritance: Autosomal dominant transmission has been suggested.

Frequency: Very rare.

Clinical and Radiologic Manifestations: (a) flexion deformities, ulnar deviation and narrowing of the fingers, soft-tissue web causing abnormal position of the thumbs; (b) vertical talus (Fig SY–D–13).

REFERENCES

Dhaliwal AS, et al.: Digitotalar dysmorphism. *Orthop. Rev.* 14:90, 1985.

Sallis JG, et al.: Dominantly inherited digito-talar dysmorphism. *J. Bone Joint Surg. [Br.]* 54:509, 1972.

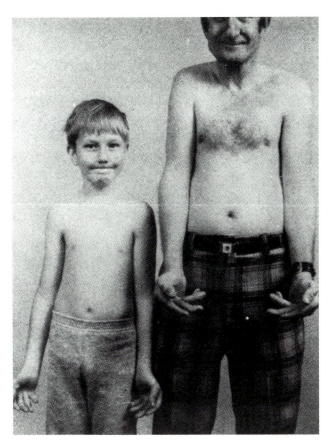

FIG SY–D–13.
Digitotalar dysmorphism in a father and son. Ulnar deviation of phalanges and adduction and flexion deformity of the thumbs are present. (From Dhaliwal AS, Myers TL: Digitotalar dysmorphism. *Orthop. Rev.* 14:90, 1985. Used by permission.)

Temtamy S, McKusick VA: Digitotalar dysmorphism. *Birth Defects* 14:466, 1978.

DISTAL OSTEOSCLEROSIS

Mode of Inheritance: Autosomal dominant.

Clinical Manifestations: (a) asymptomatic; (b) widened distal segment of the forearms.

Radiologic Manifestations: (a) mild calvarial hyperostosis, sclerosis of the base of the skull; (b) hyperostosis of the bones of the forearms and lower portions of the legs, mild sclerosis of the pelvis with striae in the ilia and femoral necks, mild expansion of the lower one third of the femora, expanded clavicles; (c) localized sclerosis of the vertebral pedicles.

REFERENCE

Beighton P, et al.: Distal osteosclerosis. *Clin. Genet.* 18:298, 1980.

DISTICHIASIS-LYMPHEDEMA SYNDROME

Mode of Inheritance: Autosomal dominant.

Clinical Manifestations: (a) *extra rows of eyelashes;* (b) partial ectropion of the lower lids (in some); (c) *lymphedema of the lower limbs;* (d) other reported abnormalities: facial dysmorphism, epicanthal folds, pterygium colli, secondary neurological complication of epidural cyst, congenital ptosis, submucous palatoschisis.

Radiologic Manifestations: (a) lymphangiography: *hypoplastic lymph channels;* (b) other reported abnormalities: kyphoscoliosis, spina bifida, spinal extradural cysts.

REFERENCES

Dale RF: Primary lymphoedema when found with distichiasis is of the type defined as bilateral hyperplasia by lymphography. *J. Med. Genet.* 24:170, 1987.
Kuhnt H: Ueber distichiasis (congenital) vera. *Z. Augenhk.* 2:46, 1899.
Pap Z, et al.: Syndrome of lymphoedema and distichiasis. *Hum. Genet.* 53:309, 1980.
Schwartz JF, et al.: Hereditary spinal arachnoid cysts, distichiasis, and lymphedema. *Ann. Neurol.* 7:340, 1980.
Shammas HJF, et al: Distichiasis of the lids and lymphedema of the lower extremities: A report of ten cases. *J. Pediatr. Ophthalmol. Strabismus* 16:129, 1979.

DIVERTICULOSIS OF JEJUNUM-MACROCYTIC ANEMIA-STEATORRHEA SYNDROME

Clinical Manifestations: *Steatorrhea; megaloblastic anemia.*

Radiologic Manifestations: (a) scattered pockets containing air-fluid levels in the upright position; (b) contrast study of the small bowel revealing many *small-bowel diverticula,* often limited to the jejunum, ranging in size from a few millimeters to several centimeters in diameter; (c) delayed motor function of the small bowel.

REFERENCES

Badenoch J, et al.: Massive diverticulosis of small intestine with steatorrhea and megaloblastic anaemia. *Q. J. Med.* 24:321, 1955.
Irwin GAL: Syndrome of jejunal diverticulosis and megaloblastic anemia. *A.J.R.* 94:366, 1965.
Polacheck AA, et al.: Diverticulosis of jejunum with macrocytic anemia and steatorrhea. *Ann. Intern. Med.* 54:636, 1961.

DOOR SYNDROME

Mode of Inheritance: Considerable heterogeneity; both autosomal recessive and autosomal dominant inheritance have been reported.

Frequency: 18 published cases to 1987 (Patton et al.)

Clinical Manifestations: (a) *neurosensory deafness* (D); (b) *onychodystrophy* (O): absent or small nails; (c) *osteodystrophy* (O) *of the terminal phalanges*; (d) *mental retardation* (R); (e) other reported abnormalities: dental anomalies, seizures, elevated plasma and urinary 2-oxoglutarate levels.

Radiologic Manifestations: (a) *phalangeal anomalies:* hypoplasia, clinodactyly, cutaneous syndactyly, cone-shaped epiphyses, proximally placed thumbs, triphalangeal thumbs, etc.; (b) other reported abnormalities: spinal anomalies, short femoral neck, metaphysial spur on the distal end of the femur, etc.

Note: It has been suggested that the acronym DOO be used for the autosomal dominant deafness and onycho-osteodystrophy and the acronym DOOR to be used for the autosomal recessive deafness, onycho-osteodystrophy, and retardation (Fig SY–D–14).

REFERENCES

Cantwell RJ: Congenital sensorineural deafness associated with onycho-osteodystrophy and mental retardation. (DOOR syndrome). *Humangenetik* 26:261, 1975.
Feinmess M, Zelig S: Congenital deafness associated with onychodystrophy. *Arch. Otolaryngol.* 74:507, 1961.
Hess RO, et al.: Additional case report of the DOOR syndrome (letter). *Am. J. Med. Genet.* 19:401, 1984.
Nevin NC, et al.: Deafness, onycho-osteodystrophy, mental retardation (DOOR) syndrome. *Am. J. Med. Genet.* 13:325, 1982.
Patton MA, et al.: DOOR syndrome (deafness, onycho-osteodystrophy, and mental retardation): Elevated plasma and urinary 2-oxoglutarate in three unrelated patients. *Am. J. Med. Genet.* 26:207, 1987.
Qazi Q, et al.: Abnormal distal phalanges and nails, deafness, mental retardation, and seizure disorder: A new familial syndrome. *J. Pediatr.* 104:391, 1984.
Thomas PS, et al.: Radiological findings in the DOOR syndrome. *Ann. Radiol. (Paris)* 25:54, 1982.

DR SYNDROME

Synonyms: Duane/radial dysplasia syndrome; Okihiro syndrome; radial ray defect; Duane anomaly.

Mode of Inheritance: An autosomal dominant transmission of radial defects has been suggested.

Clinical and Radiologic Manifestations: (a) *Duane syndrome:* congenital strabismus with a deficiency of abduction and adduction, retraction of the globe, oblique movement of the globe and narrowing of the palpebral fissure during adduction; deficiency of convergence; (b) *various limb anomalies* (radial dysplasia, etc.); (c) other reported anomalies: Klippel-Feil syndrome, Goldenhar syndrome, Wildervanck syndrome, abnormal ears, cleft palate, facial palsy, spinal meningocele, spastic diplegia, syringomyelia, genitourinary anomalies, deafness, etc.

REFERENCES

Duane A: Congenital deficiency of abduction associated with impairment of adduction retraction movements, contraction of the palpebral fissure and oblique movements of the eye. *Arch. Ophthalmol.* 34:133, 1905.
Hayes A, et al.: The Okihiro syndrome of Duane anomaly, radial ray abnormalities, and deafness. *Am. J. Med. Genet.* 22:273, 1985.
MacDermot KD, et al.: Radial ray defect and Duane anomaly: Report of a family with autosomal dominant transmission. *Am. J. Med. Genet.* 27:313, 1987.
Okihiro MM, et al.: Duane syndrome and congenital upper-limb anomalies. *Arch. Neurol.* 34:174, 1977.

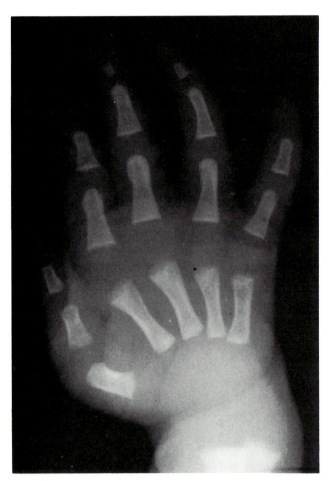

FIG SY–D–14.
DOOR syndrome. An absence of the bony terminal phalanges of the second and fifth digits and shortness of the distal phalanges of the third and fifth digits are shown. The fingernails of the hands and feet were completely absent, as were the terminal phalangeal joints of the fingers. (From Thomas PS, Nevin NC: Radiological findings in the DOOR syndrome. *Ann. Radiol. (Paris)* 25:54, 1982. Used by permission.)

Temtamy S, McKusick VA: Duane syndrome with radial malformations. *Birth Defects* 14:133, 1978.
Temtamy SA: The DR syndrome or the Okihiro syndrome (letter)? *Am. J. Med. Genet.* 25:173, 1986.
Temtamy SA, et al.: The Duane radial dysplasia syndrome: An autosomal dominant disorder. New chromosomal and malformation syndromes. *Birth Defects* 11:344, 1975.

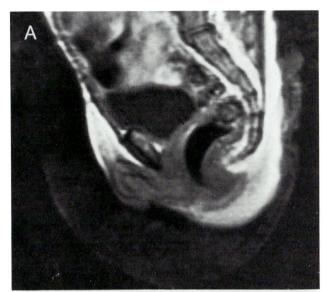

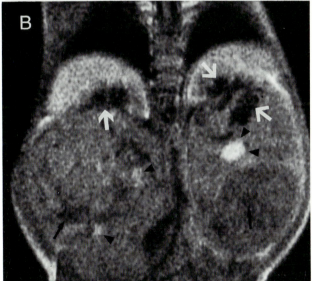

FIG SY–D–15.
Drash syndrome in an 8-month-old patient with ambiguous genitalia and bilateral Wilms tumor. **A,** magnetic resonance image of the pelvis (SE TR 500; TE 28) in the sagittal plane. This midline scan shows a small vagina but no uterus. **B,** magnetic resonance image of the abdomen (SE TR 500; TE 28) in the coronal plane shows massive enlargement of the kidneys due to Wilms tumor, areas of high-signal intensity secondary to hemorrhage *(arrowheads),* and areas of low-signal intensity due to tumor necrosis *(arrows).* The remaining normal renal parenchyma is compressed, and hydronephrosis *(white arrows)* is present in both sides. (From Boechat MI, Kangarloo H: MR imaging in Drash syndrome. *J. Comput. Assist. Tomogr.* 12:405, 1988. Used by permission.)

DRASH SYNDROME

Clinical and Pathological Manifestations: (a) male pseudohermaphroditism, dysgenetic gonads; (b) progressive glomerular disease: diffuse mesangial sclerosis, renal failure; (c) nephroblastoma; (d) other reported abnormalities: gonadoblastoma, granulosa cell tumor, metanephric hamartoma, etc.

Radiologic Manifestations: (a) increased echogenicity of the renal cortex; (b) Wilms tumor (unilateral or bilateral).

Note: The syndrome may present in partial or complete forms, and the other elements of the triad may become manifested later (Fig SY–D–15).

REFERENCES

Boechat MI, et al.: MR imaging in Drash syndrome. *J. Comput. Assist. Tomogr.* 12:405, 1988.
Denys P, et al.: Association d'un syndrome anatomo-pathologique de pseudohermaphrodisme masculin, d'une tumeur de Wilms, d'une néphropathie parenchymateuse et d'une mosaïcisme XX/XY. *Arch. Fr. Pediatr.* 24:729, 1967.
Drash A, et al.: A syndrome of pseudohermaphroditism, Wilms' tumor, hypertension, and degenerative renal disease. *J. Pediatr.* 76:585, 1970.
Gallo GE, et al.: The association of Wilms' tumor, male pseudohermaphroditism and diffuse glomerular disease (DRASH syndrome): Report of eight cases with clinical and morphologic findings and review of the literature. *Pediatr. Pathol.* 7:175, 1987.
Garel L et al.: Intérêt de l'échographie dans le syndrome de Drash. A propos de trois cas. *Ann. Radiol.* (Paris) 27:223, 1984.
Goldman SM, et al.: The Drash syndrome: Male pseudohermaphroditism, nephritis, and Wilms tumor. *Radiology* 141:87, 1981.
Manivel JC, et al.: Complete and incomplete Drash syndrome. *Hum. Pathol.* 18:80, 1987.
Stump TA, et al.: Bilateral Wilms' tumor in a male pseudohermaphrodite. *J. Urol.* 72:1146, 1954.

DUBOWITZ SYNDROME

Mode of Inheritance: Probably autosomal recessive.

Frequency: Approximately 30 cases reported from Europe and the United States (Shuper et al.).

Clinical Manifestations: (a) prenatal and postnatal *growth failure, mental retardation* (in most cases); (b) *craniofacial dysmorphism*: microcephaly, high and sloping forehead, flat supraorbital ridges, broad nasal bridge, dystopia canthorum or true ocular hypertelorism, blepharophimosis, high-arched palate, cleft palate, dysplastic ears, micrognathia, delayed dental eruption, severe dental caries; (c) *skin eruption* (eczema) on the face and limbs, sparse hair, café au lait patches; (d) other reported abnormalities: hoarse voice, high-

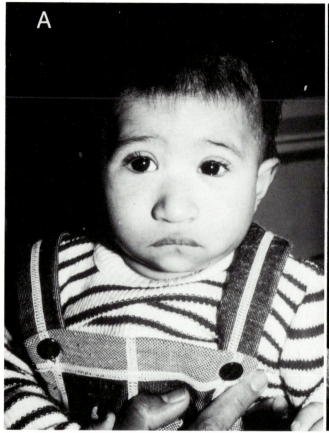 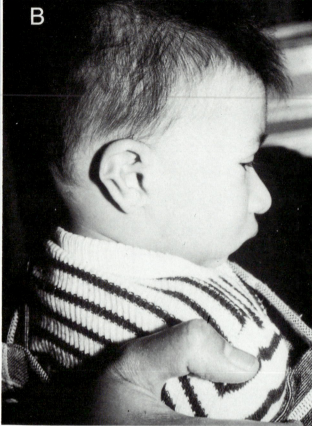

FIG SY—D—16.
A and **B,** Dubowitz syndrome. Sloping forehead, epicanthic folds, broad nose, ear dysplasia, and micrognathia are present. (From

Winter RM: Dubowitz syndrome. *J. Med. Genet.* 23:11, 1986. Used by permission.)

pitched voice, chronic diarrhea, vomiting in infancy, rectal prolapse, cryptorchidism, hypospadias, abnormal fundi, hyperactivity and behavioral problems, sacral dimple, syndactyly of the second and third toes, clinodactyly of the fifth fingers, pilonidal dimple, malignancy (lymphoma, neuroblastoma, lymphocytic leukemia), aplastic anemia—bone marrow failure, hypogammaglobulinemia.

Radiologic Manifestations: (a) skeletal anomalies: clinodactyly of the fifth fingers, preaxial polydactyly, cutaneous syndactyly of the second and third toes, pes planus, pes planovalgus, periosteal hyperostosis of the long bones; (b) retarded bone age.

Differential Diagnosis: Fetal alcohol syndrome; Bloom syndrome (Fig SY—D—16).

REFERENCES

Berthold F, et al.: Fatal aplastic anaemia in a child with features of Dubowitz syndrome. *Eur. J. Pediatr.* 146:605, 1987.
Dubowitz V: Familial low birth weight dwarfism with an unusual facies and a skin eruption. *J. Med. Genet.* 2:12, 1965.
Küster W, et al.: The Dubowitz syndrome. *Eur. J. Pediatr.* 144:574, 1986.
Shuper A, et al.: The diagnosis of Dubowitz syndrome in the neonatal period—a case report. *Eur. J. Pediatr.* 145:151, 1986.
Winter RM: Dubowitz syndrome. *J. Med. Genet.* 23:11, 1986.

DUCHENNE MUSCULAR DYSTROPHY

Synonym: Pseudohypertrophic muscular dystrophy.

Mode of Inheritance: X-linked recessive trait (males); sporadic cases in females; genetic heterogeneity.

Clinical Manifestations: Onset in early childhood: (a) *progressive muscular weakness, pseudohypertrophy,* in particular, in calf muscles; (b) progressive cardiomyopathy: electrocardiographic abnormalities (increased R/S ratio in V_1, deep but narrow Q waves, tachycardia, cardiac conduction abnormalities, etc.); (c) pulmonary complications; (d) scoliosis, kyphosis, or hyperextended spine; (e) enlarged head cir-

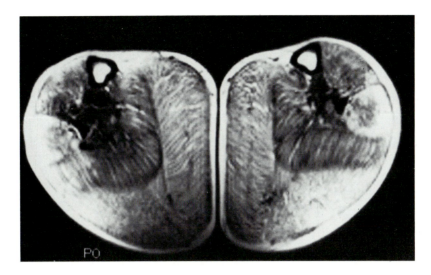

FIG SY–D–17.
Duchenne muscular dystrophy. Magnetic resonance imaging through the midcalf of a 10½-year-old boy shows massive "pseudohypertrophy" of both the soleus and gastrocnemius mus-cles. (From Schreiber A, Smith WL, Ionasescu V, et al.: Magnetic resonance imaging of children with Duchenne muscular dystrophy. *Pediatr. Radiol.* 17:495, 1987. Used by permission.)

cumference; (f) high levels of creatine kinase, pyruvate kinase, and aldolase in heterozygotes; fluctuation in serum levels of creatine kinase and myoglobin; increased long-chain acyl coenzyme A in muscle; prenatal diagnosis by DNA analysis; (g) nuclear magnetic resonance spectroscopy (phosphorus spectrum): reduced ratio of phosphocreatine to adenosine triphosphate and to inorganic phosphate; (h) other reported abnormalities: translocation involving Xp21 (an X; autosome translocation), failure to thrive, malignant hyperthermia, neuroblastoma, short stature, etc.

Radiologic Manifestations: (a) *gradual replacement of muscle by fat in form of striation* that appears between 3 and 6 years of age, increase in size of muscle mass under 6 years of age, coxa valga, osteoporosis, increased thickness in the anteroposterior diameter of the fibula with a narrow transverse diameter (fibula-tibia ratio in lateral projection, above 0.70; normal is less than 0.66), skeletal changes mimicking juvenile rheumatoid arthritis (apparent overgrowth of the epiphyses, periarticular osteoporosis, joint space narrowing, premature epiphyseal closure, etc.); (b) Ultrasonography: increased echogenicity of the muscles with a corresponding decrease in the bone echogenicity; (c) computed tomography: *total or partial replacement of normal muscle by fat density*, helpful in the detection of carriers of the disease (decreased density in various nonparetic muscles); (d) magnetic resonance imaging: *nonhomogeneous increased-intensity signal in affected muscles (fat replacement)*; (e) *scoliosis and contractures* in the late stage; (f) cardiomegaly and pulmonary edema (Fig SY–D–17).

REFERENCES

Call G, et al.: Failure to thrive in Duchenne muscular dystrophy. *J. Pediatr.* 106:939, 1985.

Cambridge W, et al.: Scoliosis associated with Duchenne muscular dystrophy. *J. Pediatr. Orthop.* 7:436, 1987.

Carroll JE, et al.: Increased long chain acyl CoA in Duchenne muscular dystrophy. *Neurology* 33:1507, 1983.

Cladera R, et al.: Les signes cardiaques de la maladie de Duchenne à évolution rapide. *Ann. Pediatr. (Paris)* 33:299, 1986.

De Visser M, et al.: Computed tomographic findings in manifesting carriers of Duchenne muscular dystrophy. *Clin. Genet.* 27:269, 1985.

Duchenne GBA: Recherches sur la paralysie musculaire pseudohypertrophique ou paralysie myo-sclérosique. *Arch. Gen. Med. (Paris)* 11:5, 179, 305, 421, 552, 1868.

Eiholzer U, et al: Short stature: A common feature in Duchenne muscular dystrophy. *Eur. J. Pediatr.* 147:602, 1988.

Emery A: Genetic heterogeneity in Duchenne muscular dystrophy (letter), *Am. J. Med. Genet.* 26:235, 1987.

Florence JM, et al.: Activity, creatine kinase, and myoglobin in Duchenne muscular dystrophy: A clue to etiology? *Neurology* 35:758, 1985.

Greenberg CR, et al.: Gene studies in newborn males with Duchenne muscular dystrophy detected by neonatal screening. *Lancet* 2:425, 1988.

Harris VJ, et al.: Increased thickness of the fibula in Duchenne muscular dystrophy. *A.J.R.* 98:744, 1966.

Hawley RJ Jr, et al: Computed tomographic patterns of muscles in neuromuscular diseases. *Arch. Neurol.* 41:383, 1984.

Heckmatt JZ, et al.: Ultrasound imaging in the diagnosis of muscle disease. *J. Pediatr.* 101:656, 1982.

Hunsaker RH, et al.: Cardiac function in Duchenne's muscular dystrophy. Results of 10-year follow-up study and noninvasive tests. *Am. J. Med.* 73:235, 1982.

Jacobs PA, et al.: Duchenne muscular dystrophy (DMD) in a female with an X/autosomal translocation: Further evidence that the DMD locus is at Xp21. *Am. J. Hum. Genet.* 33:513, 1981.

Johnston KM, et al.: Neuroblastoma in Duchenne muscular dystrophy. *Pediatrics* 78:1170, 1986.

Kelfer HM, et al.: Malignant hyperthermia in a child with Duchenne muscular dystrophy. *Pediatrics* 71:118, 1983.

Miller F, et al.: Pulmonary function and scoliosis in Duchenne dystrophy. *J. Pediatr. Orthop.* 8:133, 1988.

Muir WA, et al.: Improved detection of Duchenne muscular dystrophy heterozygotes using discriminant analysis of creatine kinase levels. *Am. J. Med. Genet.* 14:125, 1983.

Nevin NC, et al.: Duchenne muscular dystrophy in a female with a translocation involving Xp21. *J. Med. Genet.* 23:171, 1986.

Newman RJ, et al.: Nuclear magnetic resonance studies of forearm muscle in Duchenne dystrophy. *Br. Med. J.* 284:1072, 1982.

Nowak TV, et al: Gastrointestinal manifestations of the muscular dystrophies. *Gastroenterology* 82:800, 1982.

Old JM, et al.: Prenatal diagnosis of Duchenne muscular dystrophy by DNA analysis. *J. Med. Genet.* 23:556, 1986.

Richardson ML, et al.: Skeletal changes in neuromuscular disorders mimicking juvenile rheumatoid arthritis and hemophilia. *A.J.R.* 143:893, 1984.

Sanyal SK, et al.: Cardiac conduction abnormalities in children with Duchenne's progressive muscular dystrophy: Electrocardiographic features and morphologic correlates. *Circulation* 66:853, 1982.

Sanyal SK, et al.: Mitral valve prolapse syndrome in children with Duchenne's progressive muscular dystrophy. *Pediatrics* 63:116, 1979.

Schmidt B, et al.: Increased head circumference in patients with Duchenne muscular dystrophy. *Ann. Neurol.* 17:620, 1985.

Schreiber A, et al.: Magnetic resonance imaging of children with Duchenne muscular dystrophy. *Pediatr. Radiol.* 17:495, 1987.

Stern LM, et al.: Carrier detection in Duchenne muscular dystrophy using computed tomography. *Clin. Genet.* 27:392, 1985.

Xiuyuan HU, et al: Partial gene duplication in Duchenne and Becker muscular dystrophies. *J. Med. Genet.* 25:369, 1988.

DUMPING SYNDROME

Etiology: (a) rapid transit of food into the small bowel: subtotal gastrectomy, pyloroplasty, Nissen fundoplication, malplacement of a feeding gastrostomy tube, generalized autonomic dysfunction; (b) osmotic effects of foodstuffs.

Clinical Manifestations: *Postprandial symptoms:* (a) *sense of fullness;* (b) *cramps;* (c) *diarrhea;* (d) *nausea;* (e) *vasomotor symptoms* (weakness, palpitation, sweating, flushing, dizziness); (f) *fluctuation in blood glucose levels* (fainting, hypoglycemic seizures).

Radiologic Manifestations: (a) symptoms may be produced by a mixture of food and barium or 50% glucose mixed with barium; (b) *rapid gastric emptying;* (c) *dilution of a mixture within the small bowel due to a shift of fluid into the bowel.*

REFERENCES

Caulfield ME, et al.: Dumping syndrome in children. *J. Pediatr.* 110:212, 1987.

Jay BS, et al.: Iatrogenic problems following gastric surgery. *Gastrointest. Radiol.* 2:239, 1977.

Kneepkens CMF, et al: Dumping syndrome in children. Diagnosis and effect of glucomannan on glucose tolerance and absorption. *Acta Paediatr. Scand.* 77:279, 1988.

Lavine JE, et al: Dumping in infancy diagnosed by radionuclide gastric emptying technique. *J. Pediatr. Gastroenterol. Nutr.* 7:614, 1988.

Rivkees SC, et al.: Hypoglycemia pathogenesis in children with dumping syndrome. *Pediatrics* 80:937, 1987.

Whitehouse GH, et al.: The evaluation of dumping and diarrhoea after gastric surgery using physiological test meal. *Clin. Radiol.* 28:143, 1977.

DU PAN SYNDROME

Mode of Inheritance: Autosomal recessivity has been suggested.

Clinical and Radiologic Manifestations: (a) complex type of brachydactyly; (b) fibular aplasia.

REFERENCES

DuPan M: Absence congénitale due péroné sans déformation du tibia. Curieuses déformations congénitales des mains. *Rev. Orthop.* 11:227, 1924.

Temtamy S, McKusick VA: Fibular aplasia and complex brachydactyly. *Birth Defects* 14:173, 1978.

DYKE-DAVIDOFF-MASSON SYNDROME

Synonym: Davidoff-Dyke syndrome.

Clinical Manifestations: (a) *mental retardation,* seizures; (b) *facial asymmetry;* (c) *contralateral hemiplegia.*

Radiologic Manifestations: (a) *cerebral hemiatrophy with homolateral thickening and increased density of the calvaria, hypertrophy of the frontal sinuses and elevation of the sphenoid wing and petrous ridge;* (b) *computed tomography: asymmetry of the ventricles with a unilateral loss of brain substance; apparent shift of the ventricles, falx, and pineal to the atrophic side.*

REFERENCES

Brennan RE, et al.: Computed tomographic findings in cerebral hemiatrophy. *Neuroradiology* 17:17, 1979.

Dyke CG, Davidoff LM, Masson CB: Cerebral hemiatrophy with homolateral hypertrophy of the skull and sinuses. *Surg. Gynecol. Obstet.* 57:588, 1933.

Lerner MA, et al.: Radiological case of the month (Dyke-

Davidoff-Masson Syndrome). *Am. J. Dis. Child.* 142:303, 1988.

Parker CE, et al.: Dyke-Davidoff-Masson syndrome: Five case studies and deductions from dermatoglyphics. *Clin. Pediatr. (Phila.)* 11:288, 1972.

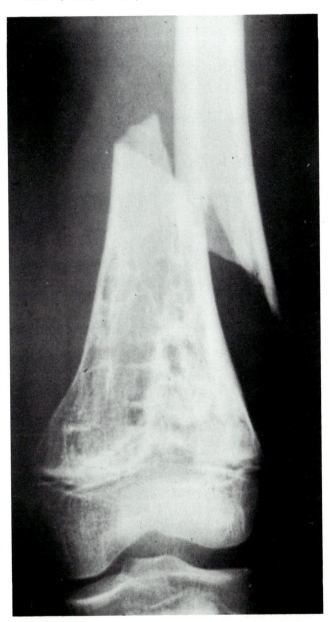

FIG SY–D–18.
Dyskeratosis congenita: femoral fracture in a 13-year-old patient. Note the lucencies proximal to the metaphysis and the coarse trabecular pattern of the metaphysis. (From Wormer R, Clark JE, Wood P, et al.: Dyskeratosis congenita: Two examples of this multisystem disorder. *Pediatrics* 71:603, 1983. Used by permission.)

DYSKERATOSIS CONGENITA

Synonym: Zinsser-Engman-Cole syndrome.

Mode of Inheritance: X-linked.

Clinical Manifestations: (a) *hyperpigmentation of the skin,* hyperkeratosis and hyperhidrosis of the palms and soles; (b) *leukoplakia of the mucous membrane;* (c) *nail dystrophy;* (d) pancytopenia; (e) other reported abnormalities: blepharitis, ectropion, nasolacrimal duct obstruction, poor dentition, sparse fine hair, testicular hypoplasia, cirrhosis, mental retardation, dysphagia, diarrhea, abnormalities of both cell-mediated and humoral immunity (diffuse hypogammaglobulinemia, decreased IgG and IgM with normal IgA, normal IgG and IgA with slightly decreased IgM, increased IgG), eye abnormalities (retinal atrophy, optic pallor, atherosclerotic changes of the retinal vessels, corneal cloudiness, cataract, angioma of the retina), postnatal growth retardation, etc.

Radiologic Manifestations: (a) osteoporosis, bone fragility, aseptic necrosis of the femoral head, radiolucent areas in the shafts of the long bones, coarse trabeculation in the metaphyses of the long bones; (b) intracranial calcification (Fig SY–D–18).

REFERENCES

Cole HN, et al.: Dyskeratosis congenita with pigmentation, dystrophia unguis and leukokeratosis. *Arch. Dermatol. Syph.* 21:71, 1930.

Engman M: A unique case of reticular pigmentation of the skin with atrophy. *Arch. Dermatol. Syph.* 13:685, 1926.

Friedland M, et al.: Dyskeratosis congenita with hypoplastic anemia: A stem cell defect. *Am. J. Hematol.* 20:85, 1985.

Kalb RE, et al.: Avascular necrosis of bone in dyskeratosis congenita. *Am. J. Med.* 80:511, 1986.

Kelly TE, et al.: Dyskeratosis congenita: Radiologic features. *Pediatr. Radiol.* 12:31, 1982.

Lieblich LM, et al.: Dyskeratosis congenita and intracranial calcifications (letter). *Arch. Dermatol.* 117:523, 1981.

Menon V, et al.: Zinsser-Cole-Engman syndrome (dyskeratosis congenita) with cataract—a rare association. *Jpn. J. Ophthalmol.* 30:192, 1986.

Olsen TG, et al.: Acute urinary tract obstruction in dyskeratosis congenita. *J. Am. Acad. Dermatol.* 4:556, 1981.

Womer R, et al.: Dyskeratosis congenita: Two examples of this multisystem disorder. *Pediatrics* 71:603, 1983.

Zinsser F: Atrophia cutis reticularis cum pigmentatione, dystrophia unguium et leukoplakia oris. *Iconogr. Dermatol.* 219, 1906.

EAGLE SYNDROME

Etiology: (a) the classic syndrome in tonsillectomized patients, dense scar tissue in the tonsillar fossa; (b) carotodynia: external compression of the carotid arteries by the ossified stylohyoid process.

Clinical Manifestations: (a) the classic syndrome: *spastic and nagging pain in the pharynx with radiation into the mastoid region, dysphagia,* a feeling of a foreign body in the throat, *a palpable hard mass* in the tonsillar fossa (ossified stylohyoid ligament), a complete relief of the symptoms following surgical removal of the ossified stylohyoid ligament; (b) *carotodynia:* pain along the distribution of the carotid artery, subsidence of the symptoms following surgical resection of the stylohyoid process.

Radiologic Manifestations: (a) a smooth or bulky *ossified stylohyoid process of varying length and degree of segmentation extending to the area of the lesser cornu of the hyoid bone;* (b) external impression of the ossified ligament on the carotid artery (Fig SY−E−1).

REFERENCES

Eagle WW: Elongated styloid process. *Arch. Otolaryngol.* 25:584, 1937.

Eagle WW: Symptomatic elongated styloid process. *Arch. Otolaryngol.* 49:490, 1949.

Frommer J: Anatomic variations in the stylohyoid chain and their possible clinical significance. *Oral Surg.* 38:659, 1974.

Lorman JG, et al.: The Eagle syndrome. *A.J.R.* 140:881, 1983.

ECTODERMAL DYSPLASIA (HYPOHIDROTIC)

Synonym: Hypohidrotic ectodermal dysplasia.

Mode of Inheritance: X-linked recessive; the gene locus is on the proximal part of the long arm of the X chromosome.

Frequency: Uncommon.

Clinical Manifestations: (a) *hypohidrosis;* (b) *hypotrichosis;* (c) *oligodontia or anodontia;* (d) *unusual facies:* dish face, frontal bossing, saddle-shaped nose, prominent supraorbital ridges, protuberant lips, protruding ears; (e) *fever of unknown origin,* seizures associated with hyperpyrexia; (f) mucus gland deficiencies: recurrent respiratory infections, upper airway obstruction, tenacious nasal secretions, crusts of nasal secre-

tions causing obstruction of nasal passages, nasal infections, sinusitis, vestibulitis, epistaxis, feeding problems in infancy; (g) hearing problems, accumulation of wax in the auditory canals; (h) dry and peeling skin at birth, eczema; (i) deficiency of saliva, dental decay related to salivary gland dysfunction; (j) lacrimation deficiency; (k) female carriers recognizable by dental abnormalities and examination of sweat pores, patchiness of body or scalp hair, dental defects and sweating abnormalities in female heterozygotes, heat intolerance, respiratory infections in some of the females; (1) other reported abnormalities: absence of nipples and mammary glands, gonadal abnormalities, finger abnormalities, microphthalmos, corneal dysplasia, hypothyroidism, cleft lip/palate (Rapp-Hodgkin ectodermal dysplasia).

Radiologic Manifestations: (a) *deficient dentition;* (b) upper and lower respiratory tract infections (sinusitis, pneumonia, etc.).

Differential Diagnosis: More than 100 varieties of ectodermal dysplasia have been recognized, some with the autosomal dominant or autosomal recessive modes of inheritance; the genetic features and clinical manifestations are considered in the classification of the various forms of ectodermal dysplasia (Figs SY−E−2 and SY−E−3).

REFERENCES

Burck U, et al.: Athelia in a female infant—heterozygous for anhidrotic ectodermal dysplasia. *Clin. Genet.* 19:117, 1981.

Capitanio MA, et al.: Congenital anhidrotic ectodermal dysplasia. *A.J.R.* 103:168, 1968.

Chautard-Freire-Maia EA, et al.: Further evidence against linkage between Christ-Siemens-Touraine (CST) and XG loci. *Hum. Genet.* 57:205, 1981.

Christ J: Ueber die Korrelationen der kongenitalen Defekte des Ektoderms untereinander mit besonderer Berücksichtigung ihrer Beziehungen zum Auge. *Z. Haut. Geschlechtskr.* 40:1, 1932.

Clarke A: Hypohidrotic ectodermal dysplasia. *J. Med. Genet.* 24:659, 1987.

Clarke A, et al.: Clinical aspects of X-linked hypohidrotic ectodermal dysplasia. *Arch. Dis. Child.* 62:989, 1987.

Familusi JB, et al.: Hereditary anhidrotic ectodermal dysplasia: Studies in a Nigerian family. *Arch. Dis. Child.* 50:642, 1975.

Freire-Maia N, Pinheiro M: *Ectodermal Dysplasias: A Clinical and Genetic Study.* New York, Alan R Liss Inc, 1984.

Hanauer A, et al.: Genetic mapping of anhidrotic ectodermal dysplasia: DXS159, a closely linked proximal marker. *Hum. Genet.* 80:177, 1988.

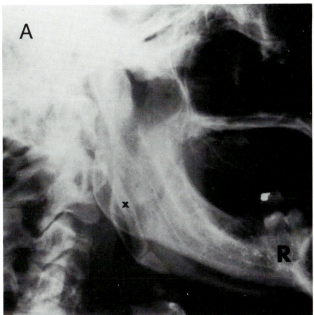

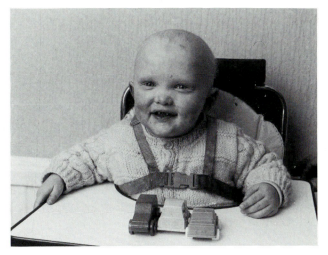

FIG SY−E−2.
Hypohidrotic ectodermal dysplasia. (From Clarke A: Hypohidrotic ectodermal dysplasia. *J. Med. Genet.* 24:659, 1987. Used by permission.)

ations: An apparently new genetic ectodermal dysplasia of the tricho-odonto-onychial subgroup. *Clin. Genet.* 29:332, 1986.

Schroeder HW, et al.: Rapp-Hodgkin ectodermal dysplasia. *J. Pediatr.* 110:72, 1987.

Siemens HW: Studien ueber Vererbung von Hautkrankheiten: XII. Anhidrosis hypotrichotica. *Arch. Dermatol. Syph.* 175:565, 1937.

Smith DW, et al.: Aberrant scalp hair patterning in hypohidrotic ectodermal dysplasia. *J. Pediatr.* 90:248, 1977.

Söderholm AL, et al.: Expression of X-linked hypohidrotic

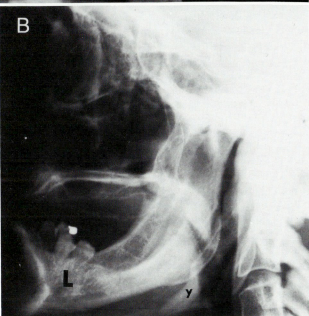

FIG SY−E−1.
Eagle syndrome. **A,** styloid process *(x)* is as long as in **B,** but thinner. Pseudoarticulations and segmentation are not unusual. **B,** thick, elongated ossified process *(y)* was easily palpated in the tonsillar fossa. (From Lorman JG, Biggs JR: The Eagle syndrome. *A.J.R.* 140:881, 1983. Used by permission.)

Myer CM: The role of an otolaryngologist in the care of ectodermal dysplasia. *Pediatr. Dermatol.* 4:34, 1987.

Pabst HF, et al.: Hypohidrotic ectodermal dysplasia with hypothyroidism. *J. Pediatr.* 98:223, 1981.

Pike MG, et al.: A distinctive type of hypohidrotic ectodermal dysplasia featuring hypothyroidism. *J. Pediatr.* 108:109, 1986.

Pinheiro M, et al.: Trichodermodysplasia with dental alter-

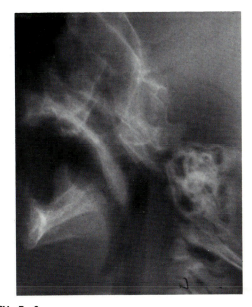

FIG SY−E−3.
Ectodermal dysplasia (hypohidrotic) in a 5-month-old boy with clinical manifestations of pneumonia and a history of recurrent respiratory infections. Sparse hair and absent eyebrows were noted. The teeth buds are absent.

ectodermal dysplasia in six males and in their mothers. *Clin. Genet.* 28:136, 1985.

Thurnam J: Two cases in which the skin, hair and teeth were very imperfectly developed. *Proc. R. Med. Chir. Soc. (Lond.)* 31:71, 1848.

Touraine A: L'anidrose avec hypotrichose et anodontie. *Presse Med.* 44:145, 1936.

Viljoen DL, et al.: A new form of hypohidrotic ectodermal dysplasia. *Am. J. Med. Genet.* 31:25, 1988.

Weech AA: Hereditary ectodermal dysplasia. *Am. J. Dis. Child.* 37:766, 1929.

EEC SYNDROME

Synonyms: Ectrodactyly-ectodermal dysplasia-clefting syndrome; Rudiger syndrome; EECUT syndrome.

Mode of Inheritance: Sporadic; autosomal dominant.

Frequency: Uncommon.

Clinical Manifestations: (a) *ectodermal dysplasia*: hypopigmentation, absence or reduction of the sebaceous glands, hypoplastic nails, sparse scalp hair and eyebrows, sparse eyelashes, pigmented nevi, albinoid changes in the skin and hair, abnormal dermatoglyphics (dysplastic ridges with multiple irregular furrows, disorganized sweat pore arrangement), etc; (b) *ectrodactyly*: clawhand and clawfoot, syndactyly, polydactyly; (c) facial dysmorphism: midfacial hypoplasia, *bilateral cleft lip, cleft palate,* prominent supraorbital ridges and nasal bridge, telecanthus, flat nasal tip, prominent ears, low position of the ears, hypoplasia of the earlobes; (d) xerostomia, absence of Stensen ducts, oral moniliasis, anodontia, oligodontia, enamel hypoplasia, dental caries; (e) absent lacrimal puncta, photophobia, chronic blepharitis, decreased tear formation, narrowing of the palpebral fissures, corneal vascularization, strabismus, astigmatism, ectropion; (f) other reported abnormalities: microcephaly, mental retardation, conduction deafness, inguinal hernia, cryptorchidism, incomplete forms (combination of two of the three major manifestations), prune-belly syndrome, transverse vaginal septum, etc.

Radiologic Manifestations: (a) *clawhand, clawfoot;* various abnormalities of the carpals, tarsals, metacarpals, and metatarsals; (b) genitourinary anomalies: renal agenesis, hydronephrosis, hydroureter, bladder diverticulum, etc.; (c) other reported abnormalities: scoliosis, coxa vara, spina bifida, cervical vertebrae, growth hormone deficiency, etc.

Differential Diagnosis:

(A) Ectrodactyly and Cleft Lip/Palate: (a) ECP syndrome: ectrodactyly, cleft palate, autosomic dominant transmission; (b) Fontaine syndrome: cleft palate, ectrodactyly and syndactyly of the feet, micrognathia, ear dysplasia, mental retardation, autosomal dominant transmission; (c) Weyer oligodactyly syndrome: cleft lip, ectrodactyly, sternal and renal malformations, etc.; (d) Roberts syndrome; (e) orofaciodigital syndromes.

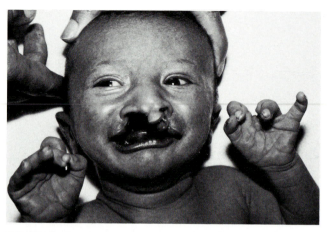

FIG SY–E–4.
EEC syndrome. A cleft lip/palate and ectrodactyly are seen. (From Parent P, Castel Y, Guillet G, et al.: Le syndrome EEC. *Ann. Pediatr. (Paris)* 34:293, 1987. Used by permission.)

(B) Ectrodactyly and Ectodermal Dysplasia: (a) odontotrichomelic syndrome: hypotrichosis, hypodontia, limb anomalies, mental retardation, autosomal recessive; (b) ectrodactyly-ectodermal dysplasia-muscular dystrophy (EEM syndrome): autosomal recessive, macular dystrophy; (c) Robinson type of ectodermal dysplasia: partial anodontia, nail dystrophy, neurosensory deafness, syndactyly and polydactyly in some, autosomal dominant; (d) LARD syndrome (lacrymo-auriculo-radio-dental syndrome): lacrymal system atresia, ear deformities, dental anomalies, radial ray digital anomalies; (e) tricho-odonto-onycho-dermal syndrome: facial dysmorphism, distal extremity abnormalities, etc;

(C) Ectodermal Dysplasia and Cleft Lip/Palate: (a) Rapp-Hodgkin syndrome: ectodermal dysplasia, cleft lip/palate, ocular anomalies (cataract, ectropion, absent lacrimal puncta), hypospadias, syndactyly, autosomal dominant mode of inheritance; (b) popliteal pterygium syndrome.

Notes: (a) the acronym EEC derives from ectrodactyly, ectodermal dysplasia, and cleft lip/palate; (b) due to the high occurrence of urinary tract abnormalities, EECUT has been suggested and included under "Synonyms" (Fig SY–E–4).

REFERENCES

Gemme G, et al.: La sindrome EEC. *Minerva Pediatr.* 28:36, 1976.

Hecht F: Updating a diagnosis. The EEC/EECUT syndrome. *Am. J. Dis. Child.* 139:1185, 1985.

Ivarsson S, et al.: Coexisting ectrodactyly-ectodermal dysplasia-clefting (EEC) and prune belly syndromes. *Acta Radiol.* 23:287, 1982.

Knudtzon J, et al.: Growth hormone deficiency associated with the ectrodactyly-ectodermal dysplasia-clefting syndrome and isolated absent septum pellucidum. *Pediatrics* 79:410, 1987.

Küster W et al.: EEC syndrome without ectrodactyly? Report of 8 cases. *Clin. Genet.* 28:130, 1985.

Leibowitz MR, et al.: A newly recognized feature of ectrodactyly, ectodermal dysplasia, clefting (EEC) syndrome: Comedone naevus. *Dermatologica* 169:80, 1984.

Majewski F, et al.: EEC syndrome sine sine? Report of a family with oligosymptomatic EEC syndrome. *Clin. Genet.* 33:69, 1988.

Parent P, et al.: Le syndrome EEC (ectrodactyly, ectodermal dysplasia, cleft lip and palate. *Ann. Pediatr. (Paris)* 34:293, 1987.

Parkash H, et al.: Ectrodactyly, ectodermal dysplasia, cleft lip and palate (E.E.C.) a rare syndrome. *Indian J. Pediatr.* 50:337, 1983.

Pashayan HM: The EEC syndrome. *Am. J. Dis. Child.* 130:653, 1976.

Pinheiro M, et al.: EEC and odontotrichomelic syndromes. *Clin. Genet.* 17:363, 1980.

Predine-Hug F, et al.: Dysplasie ectodermique et ectrodactylie familiale. *Arch. Fr. Pediatr.* 41:49, 1984.

Rollnick BR, et al.: Genitourinary anomalies are a component manifestation in the ectodermal dysplasia, ectrodactyly, cleft lip/palate (EEC) syndrome. *Am. J. Med. Genet.* 29:131, 1988.

Rudiger RA, et al.: Association of ectrodactyly, ectodermal dysplasia, cleft lip-palate: The EEC syndrome. *Am. J. Dis. Child.* 120:160, 1970.

Schnitzler L, et al.: Le syndrome de Rüdiger (Syndrome EEC): A propos d'un cas associe a un eczema atopique. *Ann. Dermatol. Venereol.* 105:201, 1978.

Wallis CE: Ectrodactyly (split-hand/split-foot) and ectodermal dysplasia with normal lip and palate in a four-generation kindred. *Clin. Genet.* 34:252, 1988.

EFFERENT LOOP (GASTROJEJUNOSTOMY) SYNDROME

Etiology: Functional disturbance of the efferent loop of the jejunum after gastrojejunostomy that causes a temporary delay in emptying; this may last a few days to several weeks.

Clinical Manifestations: *Bile-stained vomiting* after a postsurgical lag period of 8 to 10 days.

Radiologic Manifestations: (a) *poor filling of the flaccid efferent segment* about 2 to 10 cm below the site of gastroenterostomy; (b) *marked delay in emptying;* (c) normal mucosal pattern; (d) absence of generalized paralytic ileus.

REFERENCES

Bodon GR, et al.: The gastrojejunostomy efferent loop syndrome. *Surg. Obstet. Gynecol.* 134:777, 1972.

Bortolotti M, et al.: Effect of Billroth II operation on the intestinal interdigestive motor activity. *Digestion* 31:194, 1985.

Glenn F, et al.: The surgical treatment of peptic ulcers. *Ann. Surg.* 132:36, 1950.

Golden R: Functional obstruction of the efferent loop of jejunum following partial gastrectomy. *J.A.M.A.* 148:721, 1952.

Koehler R, et al.: Radiographic abnormalities after gastric bypass. *A.J.R.* 138:267, 1982.

EHLERS-DANLOS SYNDROME(S)

Synonym: Arthrochalasis multiplex congenita.

Frequency: Uncommon.

Clinical Manifestations: (a) connective tissue disorders with common clinical manifestations of joint hyperextensibility, abnormal stretchability of the skin, excessive bruisability, fragility of blood vessels (Table SY–E–1); (b) other reported abnormalities: α_2-macroglobulin deficiency, defective platelet function.

Radiologic Manifestations: (a) *calcified subcutaneous spheroids* (2- to 15-mm ringlike shells); (b) *subluxation or dislocation of joints;* (c) osteoarthritic changes in adults; (d) other reported abnormalities: (1) *skull:* delayed ossification of the vault, flattened orbits, micrognathia, hypertelorism; (2) *spine:* scoliosis, kyphosis, thoracic lordosis, platyspondyly; (3) *chest wall:* thoracic asymmetry, subluxation of the sternoclavicular joints, pectus recurvatum, pectus carinatum, elongated chest, costovertebral subluxations; (4) *limbs:* elongated ulnar styloid process, radio-ulnar synostosis, acro-osteolysis, flexion deformity of small hand joints, congenital hip dislocation, claw and hammertoes, distraction of the pubic symphysis during delivery, ectopic bone formation around hip joints, clubfoot, flatfoot, pes cavus, navicular-cuneiform synostosis, clinodactyly of the fifth finger, arachnodactyly, syndactyly, carpal fusion, recurrent subluxation and dislocation; (5) *alimentary system:* dilatation of the alimentary tract, spontaneous rupture, hemorrhage, mural hematoma, diverticula, malabsorption due to diverticula, constipation, rectal prolapse, diaphragmatic hernia, malabsorption; (6) *cardiovascular:* spontaneous rupture of the main arteries, aortic dissection, aneurysms, arteriovenous fistulas, elongated aortic arch, tortuous systemic or pulmonary arteries, arterial stenosis, cystic medial necrosis, pseudoaneurysm, varicose veins, perforation of the superior vena cava (angiography complication), renovascular hypertension, congenital heart defects (septal defects, tetralogy of Fallot, dextrocardia, arch anomalies, bicuspid aortic valve, pulmonary artery anomalies, bicuspid tricuspid valve), mitral prolapse, mitral insufficiency, aortic valve stenosis, aortic valve insufficiency, spontaneous left ventricular rupture, aneurysm of the sinus of Valsalva, aortic or coronary tortuosity, tricuspid insufficiency, pulmonary valve stenosis, pulmonary valve insufficiency, pulmonary artery dilatation, papillary muscle dysfunction, etc; (7) *respiratory system:* mediastinal emphysema, spontaneous pneumothorax, subpleural blebs, transient multiple fluid-filled pulmonary cysts, hyperinflation, tracheomegaly, bronchiectasis, severe irreversible obstructive pulmonary disease, pulmonary hypertension; (8) *genitourinary system:* hydronephrosis, infantile polycystic disease of the kidneys, bladder diverticulum, bladder neck obstruction, medullary sponge kidney, adult polycystic kidney disease, pregnancy complications in type IV (rupture of the uterus, bowel, aorta, or vena cava; vaginal laceration; postpartum uterine hemorrhage); (9) *teeth:* malformed stunted roots, pulp stones; (10) *central nervous system:* vascular malformations, dilatation of the fourth ventri-

TABLE SY–E–1.

Clinical Features, Modes of Inheritance, Biochemical Abnormalities, and Ultrastructural Characteristics of Different Types of Ehlers-Danlos Syndrome*

Type	Clinical Features	Inheritance	Biochemical Disorder	Ultrastructural Findings
I Gravis	Soft, velvety skin; marked skin hyperextensibility, fragility, and easy bruisability; "cigarette paper" scars; large- and small-joint hypermobility; frequent venous varicosities; hernia; prematurity due to ruptured fetal membranes common	AD†	Not known	Large collagen fibrils, many irregular in shape
II Mitis	Soft skin, moderate skin hyperextensibility, and easy bruisability; moderate joint hypermobility; varicose veins and hernia occur, but less commonly than in type I; prematurity rare	AD	Not known	Large collagen fibrils, many irregular in shape
III Benign familial hypermobility	Skin soft but otherwise minimally affected; joint mobility markedly increased and affecting large and small joints; dislocation common	AD	Not known	Large collagen fibrils, many irregular in shape
IV Ecchymotic or arterial	Skin thin, translucent, or both; veins readily visible over the trunk, arms, legs, and abdomen; repeated ecchymosis with minimal trauma; skin not hyperextensible; joints (except the small joints in the hands) usually of normal mobility; frequent bowel (usually affecting the colon) and arterial rupture, often leading to death; uterine rupture during pregnancy	AD AR†	Decreased or absent secretion of type III collagen; structurally abnormal type III collagen	Thin dermis, small fibers; often engorged cells in the dermis; fibrils of variable size
V X-linked	Similar to EDS† II, with bruising possibly more extensive	XR†	Not known	Not known
VI Ocular	Soft, velvety, hyperextensible skin; hypermobile joints; scoliosis, scarring less severe than in EDS I; ocular fragility and keratoconus in some patients	AR	Lysyl hydroxylase deficiency	Small collagen bundles; fibrils normal or similar to those in EDS I
VII Arthrochalasis multiplex congenita	Soft skin, scars near normal; marked joint hyperextensibility, congenital hip dislocation	AD AR	Amino acid substitution near the NH_2-terminal cleavage site of pro-$\alpha2$(I) NH_2-terminal protease deficiency	Not known
VIII Periodontal form	Marked skin fragility with abnormal, atrophic, pigmented scars; minimal skin extensibility and moderate joint laxity; asthenic habitus, generalized periodontitis	AD	Not known	Not known
IX	Soft, somewhat extensible skin; bladder diverticula; bladder rupture; rhizomelic shortening of the arms with limitation of supination; occipital horns; broad clavicles	XR	Abnormal copper utilization with multiple enzymopathy	Variable fibril diameter
X Fibronectin platelet defect	Soft, mildly hyperextensible skin; mild joint hypermobility; easy bruising	AR	Fibronectin defect	Fibrils similar to EDS II

*From Byers PH, Holbrook KA: Molecular basis of clinical heterogeneity in the Ehlers-Danlos syndrome. *Ann. N.Y. Acad. Sci.* 460:298, 1985. Used by permission.
†EDS = Ehlers-Danlos syndrome; AD = autosomal dominant; AR = autosomal recessive; XR = X-linked recessive.

cle, lateral ventricles and supracerebellar cistern, herniated intervertebral disk; (11) miscellaneous: eventration of the diaphragm, external abdominal hernias, amniotic band, painful pedal papules, postoperative bleeding, etc.

Notes: (a) Ehlers-Danlos syndrome, type X, represents a mild familial form of the syndrome that is associated with a defect in platelet aggregation in response to collagen; (b) familial joint instability—recurrent dislocation of joints has been considered a form of Ehlers-Danlos syndrome (McKusick); (c) occipital horn syndrome (occipital bony projections, short broad clavicles, chronic diarrhea, unusual facial appearance, etc.), which at one time was labeled as type IX Ehlers-Danlos syndrome, is now considered to be due to a defective metab-

olism of copper that is associated with deficiency of lysyl oxidase (Figs SY–E–5 to SY–E–8).

REFERENCES

Arneson MA, et al.: A new form of Ehlers-Danlos syndrome: Fibronectin corrects defective platelet function. *J.A.M.A.* 244:144, 1980.

Baumer JH, et al.: Transient pulmonary cysts in an infant with the Ehlers-Danlos syndrome. *Br. J. Radiol.* 53:598, 1980.

Beasley RP, et al.: A new presumably autosomal recessive form of the Ehlers-Danlos syndrome. *Clin. Genet.* 16:19, 1979.

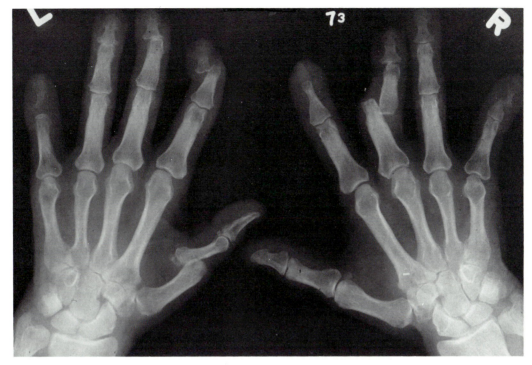

FIG SY—E—5.
Ehlers-Danlos syndrome in a 59-year-old man with dislocations of several joints of the hands. (Courtesy of Dr. C.A. Gooding, San Francisco.)

Beighton P, et al.: The radiology of the Ehlers-Danlos syndrome. *Clin. Radiol.* 20:354, 1969.

Carter C, et al.: Recurrent dislocation of the patella and the shoulder. Their association with familial joint laxity. *J. Bone Joint Surg. [Br.]* 42:721, 1960.

Cavanaugh MJ, et al.: Chronic pulmonary disease in a child with the Ehlers-Danlos syndrome. *Acta Paediatr. Scand.* 65:679, 1976.

Danlos H: Un cas de cutis laxa avec tumeurs par contusion chronique des coudes et des genoux. *Bull. Soc. Fr. Dermatol. Syph.* 19:70, 1908.

Driscoll SHM, et al.: Perforation of the superior vena cava: A complication of digital angiography in Ehlers-Danlos syndrome. *A.J.R.* 142:1021, 1984.

Ehlers E: Cutis laxa, Neigung zu Hämorrhagien in der Haut, Lockerung mehrerer Artikulationen. *Dermatol. Wochenschr.* 8:173, 1901.

Friedman JM, et al.: An unusual connective tissue disease in mother and son: A "new" type of Ehlers-Danlos syndrome? *Clin. Genet.* 21:168, 1982.

Hagino H, et al.: Computed tomography in patients with Ehlers-Danlos syndrome. *Neuroradiology* 27:443, 1985.

Hammeschmidt DE, et al.: Maternal Ehlers-Danlos syndrome type X: Successful management of pregnancy and parturition. *J.A.M.A.* 248:2487, 1982.

Harris RD: Small-bowel dilatation in Ehlers-Danlos syndrome—an unreported gastrointestinal manifestation. *Br. J. Radiol.* 47:623, 1974.

Hollister DW: Heritable disorders of connective tissues: Ehlers-Danlos syndrome. *Pediatr. Clin. North Am.* 25:575, 1978.

Kahana M, et al.: Painful piezogenic pedal papules on a child with Ehlers-Danlos syndrome. *Pediatr. Dermatol.* 3:45, 1985.

Kozlova SI, et al.: Presumed homozygous Ehlers-Danlos syndrome type I in a highly inbred kindred. *Am. J. Med. Genet.* 18:763, 1984.

Kuivaniemi H, et al.: Abnormal copper metabolism and deficient lysyl oxidase activity in a heritable connective tissue disorder. *J. Clin. Invest.* 69:730, 1982.

Kuivaniemi H, et al.: Type IX Ehlers-Danlos syndrome and Menkes syndrome: The decrease in lysyl oxidase activity is associated with a corresponding deficiency in the enzyme protein. *Am. J. Hum. Genet.* 27:798–808, 1985.

Lees MH, et al.: Ehlers-Danlos syndrome associated with multiple pulmonary stenoses and tortuous systemic arteries. *J. Pediatr.* 75:1031, 1969.

Lüscher TF, et al.: Renovascular hypertension: A rare cardiovascular manifestation of the Ehlers-Danlos syndrome. *Mayo Clin. Proc.* 62:223, 1987.

Mabille J-P, et al.: Un cas de syndrome d'Ehlers-Danlos avec acro-ostéolyse. *Ann. Radiol. (Paris)* 15:781, 1972.

Mahour GH, et al.: α_2-Macroglobulin deficiency in a patient with Ehlers-Danlos syndrome. *Pediatrics* 61:894, 1978.

Mauseth R, et al.: Infantile polycystic disease of the kidneys and Ehlers-Danlos syndrome in an 11-year-old patient. *J. Pediatr.* 90:81, 1977.

McEntyre RL, et al.: Surgical complications of Ehlers-Danlos syndrome in children. *J. Pediatr. Surg.* 12:531, 1977.

McKusick VA: *Mendelian Inheritance in Man.* Baltimore, Johns Hopkins University Press, 1988, pp 217–220.

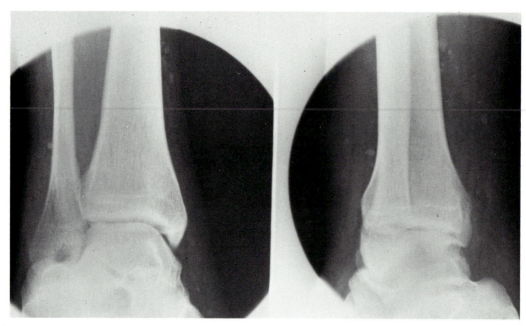

FIG SY—E—6.
Ehlers-Danlos syndrome in a 35-year-old man with hyperflexibility of the joints, multiple "cigarette paper" scars over the extremities, and ankle swelling. Note the multiple small calcific densities within the soft tissue. (From Lapayowker MS: Cutis hyperelastica, the Ehlers-Danlos syndrome. *A.J.R.* 84:232, 1960. Used by permission.)

Nardone DA, et al.: Gastrointestinal complications of Ehlers-Danlos syndrome. *N. Engl. J. Med.* 300:863, 1979.
Pope FM, et al.: Clinical presentations of Ehlers Danlos syndrome type IV. *Arch. Dis. Child.* 63:1016, 1988.

Pretorius ME, et al.: Neurologic manifestations of Ehlers-Danlos syndrome. *Neurology* 33:1087, 1983.
Rizzo R, et al.: Familial Ehlers-Danlos syndrome type II: Abnormal fibrillogenesis of dermal collagen. *Pediatr. Dermatol.* 4:197, 1987.

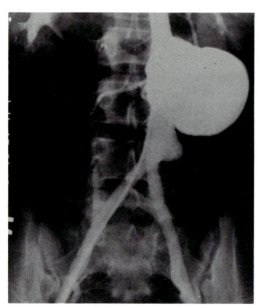

FIG SY—E—7.
Ehlers-Danlos syndrome in a 17-year-old girl. A retrograde percutaneous femoral aortogram reveals two saccular aortic aneurysms, 7 cm and 3 cm in diameter, just above the aortic bifurcation. (From Burnett HF, Bledsoe JH, Char F, et al.: Abdominal aortic aneurysmectomy in a 17-year-old patient with Ehlers-Danlos syndrome: Case report and review of the literature, *Surgery* 74:617, 1973. Used by permission.)

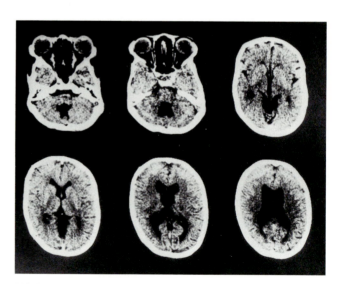

FIG SY—E—8.
Ehlers-Danlos syndrome, type III: Computed tomography of the brain in a 16-year-old female. The fourth ventricle is markedly dilated. The supracerebellar cistern is also enlarged. The quadrigeminal cistern can be seen to be irregular. The configuration of the posterior horn is angular rather than round. The posterior fossa has a short anteroposterior diameter but extends unusually far inferiorly. (From Hagino H, Eda I, Takashima S, et al.: Computed tomography in patients with Ehlers-Danlos syndrome. *Neuroradiology* 27:443, 1985. Used by permission.)

Rudd NL, et al.: Pregnancy complications in type IV Ehlers-Danlos syndrome. *Lancet* 1:50, 1983.

Sartoris DJ, et al.: Type IX Ehlers-Danlos syndrome. A new variant with pathognomonic radiographic features. *Radiology* 152:665, 1984.

Shohet I, et al.: Cardiovascular complications in the Ehlers-Danlos syndrome with minimal external findings. *Clin. Genet.* 31:148, 1987.

Sykes EM: Colon perforation in Ehlers-Danlos syndrome. Report of two cases and review of the literature. *Am. J. Surg.* 147:410, 1984.

Young ID, et al.: Amniotic bands in connective tissue disorders. *Arch. Dis. Child.* 60:1061, 1985.

EISENMENGER SYNDROME

Clinical Manifestations: (a) *pulmonary hypertension with a bidirectional or reversed cardiovascular shunt,* most often with a ventricular septal defect; (b) failure to thrive, cyanosis, exertional dyspnea, recurrent pulmonary infection, right ventricular hypertrophy; (c) mild defect of pulmonary ventilatory function with a raised residual volume and closing capacity and a reduction of other lung volumes and maximal expiratory flows.

Radiologic Manifestations: (a) *heart size normal to moderately enlarged, mild to severely dilated pulmonary artery segment, dilatation of the central portion of the pulmonary arteries with abrupt tapering in the middle zone of the lung;* (b) calcification in the wall of the pulmonary artery (in some); (c) small aortic knob in an atrial septal defect, normal or small aortic knob in a ventricular septal defect, enlarged aortic knob in patent ductus arteriosus; (d) calcification of a patent ductus (rarely); (e) *cardioangiography: reversed or bidirectional shunt;* (f) ultrasonography: (1) pulmonary valve: attenuation of the a wave, delayed opening, steep systolic opening slope and a complete midsystolic closure of the posterior leaflet followed by a complete reopening of the valve in late systole; (2) aortic valve: sudden partial closure of the right coronary cusp in late systole.

REFERENCES

Anderson RE, et al.: Eisenmenger's complex mimicking pulmonary stenosis on plain films. *Radiology* 98:381, 1971.

Cohen BA, et al.: Computer tomography demonstration of pulmonary artery calcification in Eisenmenger's syndrome. *J. Comput. Tomogr.* 9:153, 1985.

Eisenmenger V: Die angeborenen Defekte der Kommerscheidewand des Herzens. *Z. Klin. Med. [Suppl.]* 32:1, 1897.

Haugland H, et al.: Echocardiographic characteristics of pulmonary and aortic valve motion in the Eisenmenger's syndrome from ventricular septal defect. *Am. J. Cardiol.* 54:927, 1984.

MacArthur CGC, et al.: Ventilatory function in the Eisenmenger syndrome. *Thorax* 34:348, 1979.

Rees RSO, et al.: The Eisenmenger syndrome. *Clin. Radiol.* 18:366, 1967.

Spitz HB: Eisenmenger's syndrome. *Semin. Roentgenol.* 3:373, 1968.

ELASTOSIS SYNDROMES

Classification: (a) cutis laxa: (1) inherited: autosomal recessive, autosomal dominant; (2) transient neonatal (fetal penicillamine syndrome); (3) acquired: type 1 (generalized acquired elastosis), type 2 (Marshall syndrome); (b) anetodermia (macular atrophy): (1) primary: Jadassohn type, Schweninger-Buzzi type; (2) secondary; (c) perifollicular elastolysis.

REFERENCE

Koch SE, Williams ML: Acquired cutis laxa: Case report and review of disorders of elastolysis. *Pediatr. Dermatol.* 2:282, 1985.

EMPTY SELLA SYNDROME

Definition: An extension of the subarachnoid space into the pituitary fossa with enlargement of the pituitary fossa associated with compression and/or atrophy of the pituitary gland.

Etiology: (a) *idiopathic:* (1) discovered at postmortem examination in presumably normal people with space above pituitary gland remnant filled by cerebrospinal fluid (CSF) as an extension of the subarachnoid space; (2) most commonly reported in middle-aged obese women complaining of headaches; associated with diabetes mellitus, hypertension, normal pituitary function, or very rarely mild hypopituitarism, etc.; (b) *secondary:* Sheehan syndrome, necrotic pituitary adenoma, microadenoma of the pituitary gland, postsurgical, postirradiation, communicating hydrocephalus, mucopolysaccharidosis, panhypopituitarism, polycystic intrasellar dilatation of the infundibular recess, pseudotumor cerebri, syphilitic arachnoiditis, sarcoidosis; (c) *familial:* very rare familial cases have been reported, very infrequent in children; (d) association with endocrine disorders (hyperprolactinemia, hypothyroidism, Cushing syndrome, inappropriate thyroid-stimulating hormonal secretion, hyperparathyroidism, adrenocorticotropic hormone hypersecretion, hypothalmic-pituitary dysfunction, etc.), local skull dysplasia, Rieger anomaly of the anterior chamber of the eye (prominent Schwalbe ring with attached strands of iris, hypoplasia of the iris stroma, predisposition to the development of juvenile glaucoma), pulmonary emphysema, etc.

Clinical Manifestations: (a) headaches, difficulty in walking, light-headedness, weakness, numbness; (b) visual disorders: blurred vision, diminished acuity, diplopia, optic atrophy, visual field constriction; (c) precocious puberty, amenorrhea, laboratory tests may show one or more defects in anterior pituitary hormone secretion; (d) CSF rhinorrhea.

Radiologic Manifestations: (a) *skull: normal or enlarged sella with various configurations (normal, cuplike, quadran-*

gular, omega-shaped, balloonlike deep sella), erosion of the cortical margin of the sella, thin cranial vault, increased digital marking of the calvaria; (b) computed tomography, contrast study, magnetic resonance imaging: normal course of the pituitary stalk traversing the cistern to the pituitary gland and inserting in the midline of a flattened pituitary gland located posteroinferiorly; (c) γ-cisternography: convexity CSF block combined with widened CSF transport pathways and enlarged basal cisterns; (d) other reported abnormalities: intrasellar herniation of the optic chiasm, coexistence of an empty sella and a pituitary adenoma, normal-sized sella in most cases of Sheehan syndrome, rarely enlarged sella in this syndrome.

REFERENCES

Al-Mefty O, et al.: The empty sella: Air-enhanced CT. *Radiology* 155:253, 1985.

Applebaum EL, et al.: Primary empty sella syndrome with CSF rhinorrhea. *J.A.M.A.* 244:1606, 1980.

Bajraktari Xh: Skull changes with intrasellar cisternal herniation (empty sella). *Neuroradiology* 13:89, 1977.

Baker BA, et al.: Association of empty sella syndrome and primary hyperparathyroidism. *Mayo Clin. Proc.* 57:259, 1982.

Brismar K, et al.: CSF circulation in subjects with the empty sella syndrome. *Neuroradiology* 21:167, 1981.

Bursztyn EN, et al.: Empty sella syndrome with intrasellar herniation of the optic chiasm. *A.J.N.R.* 4:167, 1983.

Busch W: Die Morphologie der Sella turcica und ihre Beziehungen zur Hypophyse. *Arch. Pathol. Anat.* 320:437, 1951.

Chiang R, et al.: Empty sella turcica in intracranial sarcoidosis. *Arch. Neurol.* 41:662, 1984.

Costigan DC, et al.: The "empty sella" in childhood. *Clin. Pediatr. (Phila.)* 23:437, 1983.

Ellenbogen KA: Empty sella syndrome caused by syphilitic arachnoiditis. *J.A.M.A.* 255:1882, 1986.

Gharib H, et al.: Coexistent primary empty sella syndrome and hyperprolactinemia. Report of 11 cases. *Arch. Intern. Med.* 143:1383, 1983.

Fleckman M, et al.: Empty sella of normal size in Sheehan's syndrome. *Am. J. Med.* 75:585, 1983.

Haughton VM, et al.: Recognizing the empty sella by CT: The infundibulum sign. *A.J.R.* 136:293, 1981.

Hoffman WH, et al.: Empty sella associated with inappropriate TSH secretion. *Neuropediatrics* 18:37, 1987.

Kleinmann RE, et al.: Primary empty sella and Rieger's anomaly of the anterior chamber of the eye. A familial syndrome. *N. Engl. J. Med.* 304:90, 1981.

Lipkin EW, et al.: Cushing's syndrome in a patient with suppressible hypercortisolism and an empty sella. *West J. Med.* 140:613, 1984.

McVie R: Abnormal TSH regulation, pseudotumor cerebri, and empty sella after replacement therapy in juvenile hypothyroidism. *J. Pediatr.* 105:768, 1984.

Mühlendahl KEV, et al.: Empty sella syndrome in a boy with mucopolysaccharidosis type VI (Maroteaux-Lamy). *Helv. Paediatr. Acta* 30:185, 1975.

Nass R, et al.: Empty sella syndrome in childhood. *Pediatr. Neurol.* 2:224, 1986.

Pompili A, et al.: CT Iopamidol cisternographic diagnosis of coexisting partial empty sella and pituitary adenoma. Report of two cases. *Neuroradiology* 29:93, 1987.

Querci F, et al.: Empty sella syndrome and growth deficiency in childhood. *Helv. Paediatr. Acta* 42:49, 1987.

Scirè G, et al.: Primary empty sella and endocrinopathies in childhood: High prevalence among children with precocious puberty. *Eur. J. Pediatr.* 147:665, 1988.

Shulman DI, et al.: Hypothalamic-pituitary dysfunction in primary empty sella syndrome in childhood. *J. Pediatr.* 108:540, 1986.

Sindler BH, et al.: Primary empty sella syndrome, ACTH hypersecretion, and normal adrenocortical function. *Am. J. Med.* 73:449, 1982.

Stacpoole PW, et al.: Primary empty sella, hyperprolactinemia, and isolated ACTH deficiency after postpartum hemorrhage. *Am. J. Med.* 74:905, 1983.

Surtees R, et al.: Empty sella syndrome and growth failure. *Helv. Paediatr. Acta* 42:335, 1987.

Turner RM, et al.: Erosion and enlargement of the sella turcica: Uncommon signs of pulmonary emphysema. *A.J.R.* 141:1235, 1983.

Turpin G, et al.: Panhipopituitarism et nanisme chez un homme ayant une selle turcique vide primitive. *Nouv. Presse Med.* 8:847, 1979.

Wolpert SM: Empty sella and Rieger anomaly. *N. Engl. J. Med.* 304:1177, 1981.

ENCEPHALO-CRANIO-CUTANEOUS LIPOMATOSIS

Synonym: Fishman syndrome.

Frequency: Rare.

Pathology: A neurocutaneous syndrome: (a) unilateral temporofrontal lipomatosis of the scalp and neck; (b) homolateral multiple intracranial lipomas and cervical spinal cord lipoma; (c) leptomeningeal lipogranulomatosis, congenital malformations, cortical calcifications in the homolateral cerebral hemisphere; (d) lipomatosis of the skull, eye, and heart.

Clinical Manifestations: (a) seizures with onset in infancy; (b) mental retardation; (c) skin lesions: usually unilateral frontoparietal lesions, large hairless soft-tissue masses; (d) choriostomas on the sclerae.

Radiologic Manifestation: (a) *ipsilateral cerebral atrophy and ventricular dilatation, defective opercularization of the insula, large porencephalic cyst in the posterior part of the brain, superficial and deep brain calcification*, etc.; (b) localized area of widening of the diploic space; (c) angiography: vascular malformations.

Differential Diagnosis: Linear nevus sebaceous syndrome (Fig SY–E–9).

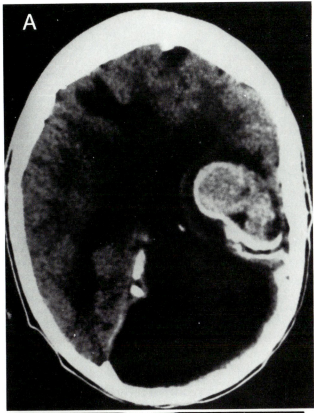

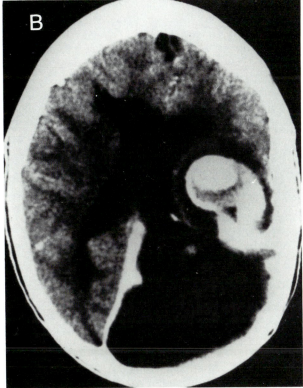

FIG SY–E–9.
Encephalocraniocutaneous lipomatosis in a 14-year-old boy. **A,** nonenhanced computed tomography of the brain demonstrates two spherical lesions with a surrounding wall. **B,** partial enhancement of the lesions is present. Note the large parencephalic cyst communicating with the lateral ventricle and calcification adjacent to the medial aspect of the cyst. (From Fishman MA: Encephalocraniocutaneous lipomatosis. *J. Child Neurol.* 2:186, 1987. Used by permission.)

REFERENCES

Bitoun P, et al.: Encephalocraniocutaneous lipomatosis. *Am. J. Dis. Child.* 136:1086, 1982.

Brumback RA, et al.: Fishman's syndrome (Encephalocraniocutaneous lipomatosis): A field defect of ectomesoderm. *J. Child Neurol.* 2:168, 1987.

Fishman MA: Encephalocraniocutaneous lipomatosis. *J. Child Neurol.* 2:186, 1987.

Fishman MA, et al.: Encephalocraniocutaneous lipomatosis. *Pediatrics* 61:580, 1978.

Haberland C, et al.: Encephalocraniocutaneous lipomatosis. A new example of ectodermomesodermal dysgenesis. *Arch. Neurol.* 22:144, 1970.

Miyao M, et al.: Encephalocraniocutaneous lipomatosis: A recently described neurocutaneous syndrome. *Child Brain* 11:280, 1984.

EPIDERMAL NEVUS SYNDROME

Synonyms: Solomon syndrome; Feuerstein-Mims syndrome; linear sebaceous nevus sequence; organoid nevus syndrome.

Frequency: Uncommon.

Clinical Manifestations: (a) variants of the *skin lesions* (alone or in combination): nevus unius lateris, ichthyosis hystrix, linear nevus sebaceus, congenital acanthosis nigricans; (b) *adnexal tumors*: syringocystadenoma papilliferum, nevus sebaceus of Jadassohn, endocrine gland and duct tumor; (c) *pigmentary skin changes*: hypopigmentation, café au lait spots, junction nevi, intradermal nevi; (d) *vascular lesions*: extranuchal nevus flammeus, cavernous hemangiomas, sclerosing hemangiomas; (e) *cutaneous malignancies*: keratoacanthoma, basal cell carcinoma, squamous cell carcinoma; (f) *neurological manifestations*: seizures, mental retardation, hyperkinesia, cerebrovascular accidents, hemiparesis, quadriplegia, cranial nerve and cranial nuclei abnormalities, neoplasms, unilateral hypsarrhythmia, Lennox-Gastraut electroencephalographic pattern; (g) *ocular abnormalities*: epidermal nevus extension to the eyelid conjunctiva; lipodermoid tumors of the subconjunctiva; ectopic lacrimal glands; coloboma of the lid, iris, choroid, and retina; corneal opacity and pannus formation; oculomotor dysfunction; nystagmus; cortical blindness; (h) *predilection for hamartomas and systemic malignancies* (Wilms tumor, glioma, astrocytoma, rhabdomyosarcoma, leukemia), leptomeningeal hemangioma, cystic adenoma of the liver; (i) other reported abnormalities: limb deformity, short limbs, skull asymmetry, kyphoscoliosis, vitamin D–resistant rickets, hemihypertrophy.

Radiologic Manifestations: (a) *skeletal anomalies*: asymmetry of the facial bones and orbits, premature closure of the sphenofrontal suture, sphenoid bone malformations, abnormalities of the sella turcica, limb abnormalities (hypoplasia, localized gigantism, etc.), bone cysts, ankylosis, scoliosis, kyphoscoliosis, pelvic deformities, lytic defects of the ribs, bowing of the tubular bones, bone sclerosis, monostotic fi-

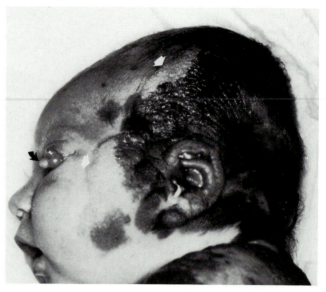

FIG SY–E–10.

Linear sebaceous nevus on the left side of the face *(white arrows)*. The posterior part of it is pigmented. A *black arrow* indicates the epibulbar lipodermoid of the left upper eyelid. (From Mimouni F, Han BB, Barnes L, et al.: Multiple hamartomas associated with intracranial malformation. *Pediatr. Dermatol.* 3:219, 1986. Used by permission.)

brous dysplasia, finger and toe deformities, soft-tissue thickening and calcification; (b) *central nervous system*: cerebral atrophy, porencephaly, hydrocephalus, widening of the subarachnoid space, hemiacrocephaly, aneurysm, widened insula, low computed tomographic density of the white matter, brain calcification, coarctation of the lateral ventricle, heterotopic gray matter, spinal cord compression, etc.; (c) other reported abnormalities: cardiac malformations, renal malformations, hypoplastic teeth, hypophosphatemic rickets/osteomalacia, intrascleral bone formation, etc. (Figs SY–E–10 to SY–E–12).

REFERENCES

Baker RS, et al.: Neurologic complications of the epidermal nevus syndrome. *Arch. Neurol.* 44:227, 1987.

Besser FS: Linear sebaceous naevi with convulsions and mental retardation (Feuerstein-Mims' syndrome), vitamin-D–resistant rickets. *Proc. R. Soc. Med.* 69:519, 1976.

Carey DE, et al.: Hypophosphatemic rickets/osteomalacia in linear sebaceous nevus syndrome: A variant of tumor-induced osteomalacia. *J. Pediatr.* 109:994, 1986.

Clancy RR, et al.: Neurologic manifestations of the organoid nevus syndrome. *Arch. Neurol.* 42:236, 1985.

Feuerstein R, Mims LC: Linear naevus sebaceus with convulsions and mental retardation. *Am. J. Dis. Child.* 104:675, 1962.

Goldberg LH, et al.: The epidermal nevus syndrome: Case report and review. *Pediatr. Dermatol.* 4:27, 1987.

Hornstein L, et al.: Linear nevi, hemihypertrophy, connective tissue hamartomas, and unusual neoplasms in children. *J. Pediatr.* 110:404, 1987.

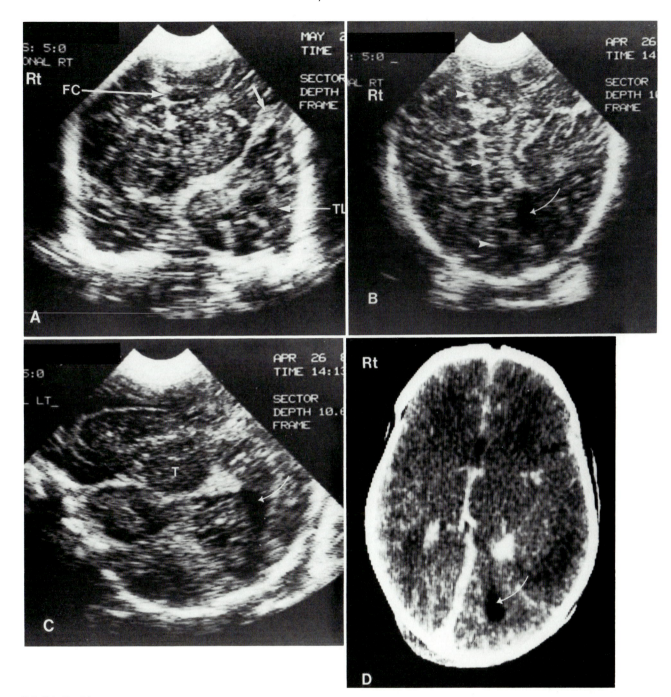

FIG SY–E–11.

Multiple hamartomas, including an epidermal nevus syndrome (linear sebaceous nevus on the left side of face, epibulbar lipodermoid of the left upper eyelid, etc.) in a newborn. Head sonography: coronal **(A),** more posterior coronal **(B),** and left parasagittal **(C)** scans show diffuse enlargement of the left hemisphere with a shift of the midline to the right *(arrowheads).* Echogenicity of the left hemisphere is abnormal, and there is disruption of normal anatomy. The temporal lobe *(TL)* is most markedly involved, with elevation of the sylvian fissure *(arrow).* The small echolucent area seen in the posterior left portion of the brain *(curved arrow)* is thought to be a dysmorphic occipital horn of the left lateral ventricle. The right hemisphere appears grossly normal *(FC = falx cerebri; T = thalamus).* **D,** postcontrast computed tomographic scan shows a midline shift to the right, numerous low-density areas, and irregularly enhancing areas mostly in the left hemisphere. No discrete mass is seen. (From Mimouni F, Han BB, Barnes L, et al.: Multiple hamartomas associated with intracranial malformations. *Pediatr. Dermatol.* 3:219, 1986. Used by permission.)

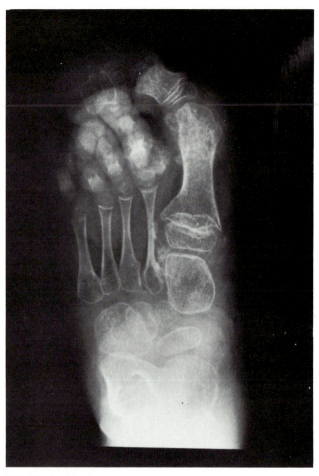

FIG SY–E–12.
Linear nevi, hemihypertrophy, and connective soft-tissue hamarto-mas. A radiograph of the left foot of a 6-year-old patient shows marked deformity of the first digit, soft-tissue thickening, and calci-fication. The examination of the cutaneous lesions revealed a mi-croscopic appearance typical of epidermal nevi. (From Hornstein L, Bove KE, Towbin RB: Linear nevi, hemihypertrophy, connective tis-sue hamartomas, and unusual neoplasms in children. *J. Pediatr.* 110:404, 1987. Used by permission.)

Leiber B: Schimmelpenning-Feurerstein-Mims-Syndrom. *Monatsschr. Kinderheilkd.* 127:585, 1979.

Leonidas JC, et al.: Radiographic features of the linear nevus sebaceus syndrome. *A.J.R.* 132:277, 1979.

Levin S, et al.: Computed tomography appearances in the linear sebaceous naevus syndrome. *Neuroradiology* 26:469, 1984.

Mimouni F, et al.: Multiple hamartomas associated with in-tracranial malformation. *Pediatr. Dermatol.* 3:219, 1986.

Moorjani R, et al.: Feuerstein and Mims syndrome with re-sistant rickets. *Pediatr. Radiol.* 5:120, 1976.

Moynahan EJ, et al.: A new neuro-cutaneous syndrome (skin-eye and brain) consisting of linear naevus, bilateral lipo-dermoid of the connectiva, cranial thickening, cere-bral cortical atrophy and mental retardation. *Br. J. Derma-tol.* 79:651, 1967.

Raynaud F, et al.: Le syndrome de Solomon (syndrome du naevus épidermique). *Ann. Pediat. (Paris)* 29:46, 1982.

Sarwar M, et al.: Brain malformations in linear nevus seba-ceous syndrome: An MR study. *J. Comput. Assist. Tomogr.* 12:338, 1988.

Schimmelpenning GW: Klinischer Beitrag zur Symptomatol-ogie der Phakomatosen. *Fortschr. Rontgenstr.* 87:716, 1957.

Solomon LM: The epidermal nevus syndrome. *Arch. Derma-tol.* 97:273, 1968.

Solomon LM, et al.: Epidermal and other congenital orga-noid nevi. *Curr. Probl. Pediatr.* 6:3, 1975.

Vles JSH, et al.: Neuroradiological findings in Jadassohn ne-vus phakomatosis: A report of four cases. *Eur. J. Pediatr.* 144:290, 1985.

Wilkes SR, et al.: Ocular malformation in association with ipsilateral facial nevus of Jadassohn. *Am. J. Ophthalmol.* 92:344, 1981.

EPIDERMOLYSIS BULLOSA DYSTROPHICA

Mode of Inheritance: Autosomal dominant (Cockayne-Touraine type, Pasini type, Bart type) and autosomal reces-sive forms.

Frequency: Rare.

Clinical Manifestations: Heterogenous group of mecha-nobullous disorders often classified by the level of blistering of the skin: (a) minimal trauma causing disruption of cohe-sion between the dermis and epidermis and the formation of *ulcers, vesicles, and bullae;* (b) *ulceration of the mucosa, healing with marked scar formation,* laryngeal obstruction; (c) deformed or absent nails; (d) dental caries, periapical abscess formation; (e) other reported abnormalities: renal amyloido-sis, squamous cell carcinoma of the skin.

Radiologic Manifestations: (a) *osteoporosis,* slender long bones, deformed hands and feet with *flexion contracture and webbing of the fingers and toes, wedge-shaped or hooklike appearance of the terminal phalanges,* subluxations in se-verely involved extremities, soft-tissue calcification adjacent to the terminal phalangeal tufts, superficial fascial calcifica-tion; (b) hypoplastic upper maxilla, increased mandibular an-gle and prognathism; (c) loss of teeth, dental caries, periapi-cal abscesses, jagged contours of the crowns, retained roots; (d) stenosis of the pharynx, *esophageal involvement* (diffuse inflammatory changes, nodular filling defects due to blisters of bullae, motility disorders, ulcers, scars, webs, pseudodi-verticula, shortening of the esophagus, esophageal rupture, hiatal hernia, gastroesophageal reflux, stricture, complete ob-struction of the lumen, membraneous congenital esophageal atresia), pyloric atresia (epidermolysis bullosa hereditaria le-talis), fecal impaction; (e) mucosal pseudopolyp of the blad-der, ulceration of the glans tip with scarring producing ob-struction and secondary ureterectasia and hydronephrosis, vaginal stenosis, chronic vaginal urinary reflux, urinary reten-tion.

Note: The autosomal recessive form is most often associ-ated with mucosal lesions and is severely mutilating; the

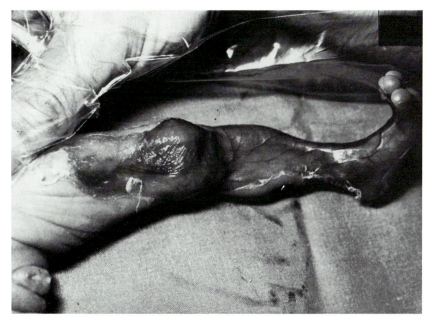

FIG SY−E−13.
Epidermolysis bullosa: blisters and erosions involving the lower extremities. (From Orens M, Garcia Hernández JB, Celorio C, et al.: Pyloric atresia associated with epidermolysis bullosa. *Pediatr. Radiol.* 17:435, 1987. Used by permission.)

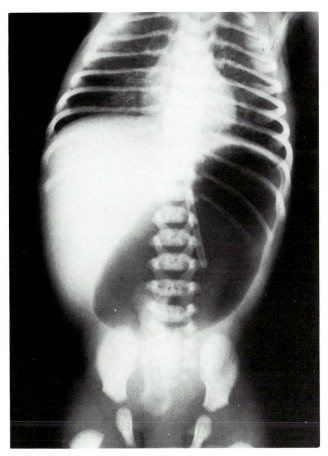

FIG SY−E−14.
Pyloric atresia associated with epidermolysis bullosa. Note the single gastric bubble. (From Orens M, Garcia Hernández JB, Celorio C, et al.: Pyloric atresia associated with epidermolysis bullosa. *Pediatr. Radiol.* 17:435, 1987. Used by permission.)

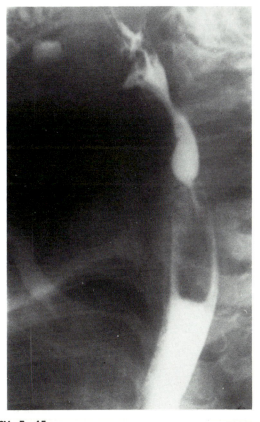

FIG SY−E−15.
Epidermolysis bullosa dystrophica in a 9-year-old female with epidermolysis bullosa involving the skin and mucous membranes of the oral cavity and dysphagia. Note the annular stenosis of the esophagus just above the thoracic inlet. (From Becker MH, Swinyard CA: Epidermolysis bullosa dystrophica in children. *Radiology* 90:124, 1968. Used by permission.)

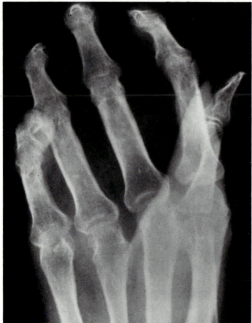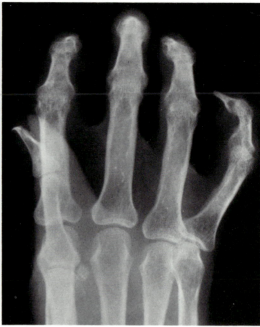

FIG SY—E—16.
Epidermolysis bullosa dystrophica in a 49-year-old female who had had the dystrophic type of epidermolysis bullosa for 25 years. Bilateral contracture deformities with a clawhand appearance, soft-tissue webbing between the fingers, and a hooklike appear-ance of the distal phalanges can be seen. (From Brinn LB, Khilnani MT: Epidermolysis bullosa with characteristic hand deformities. *Radiology* 89:272, 1967. Used by permission.)

Cockayne-Touraine variant (autosomal dominant) is usually limited to the extremities; the Pasini form (autosomal dominant) usually has both mucosal and skin manifestations (Figs SY—E—13 to SY—E—16).

REFERENCES

Agha EP, et al.: Esophageal involvement in epidermolysis bullosa dystrophica: Clinical and roentgenographic manifestations. *Gastrointest. Radiol.* 8:111, 1983.

Becker MH, Surnyard, CA: Epidermolysis bullosa dystrophica in children. *Radiology* 90:124, 1968.

Bouwes Bavinck JN, et al.: Autosomal dominant epidermolysis bullosa dystrophica: Are the Cockayne-Touraine, the Pasini and the Bart-types different expressions of the same mutant gene? *Clin. Genet.* 31:416, 1987.

Brinn LB, Khilnani MT: Epidermolysis bullosa with characteristic hand deformities. *Radiology* 89:272, 1967.

Cooper TW, et al.: Epidermolysis bullosa: A review. *Pediatr. Dermatol.* 3:181, 1984.

Davies H, et al.: Acute laryngeal obstruction in junctional epidermolysis bullosa. *Pediatr. Dermatol.* 4:98, 1987.

Doi O, et al.: A case of epidermolysis bullosa dystrophicans with congenital esophageal atresia. *J. Pediatr. Surg.* 21:943, 1986.

Eklöf O, et al.: Epidermolysis bullosa dystrophica with urinary tract involvement. *J. Pediatr. Surg.* 19:215, 1984.

Goldschneider A: Hereditäre Neigung zur Blasenbildung. *Monatsch. Prakt. Dermatol.* 1:163, 1882.

Honig PJ, et al.: Acquired pyloric obstruction in a patient with epidermolysis bullosa letalis. *J. Pediatr.* 102:598, 1983.

Kübler W: Knochenbefall durch ein Plattenephithelkarzinom der Haut bei Epidermolysis hereditaria dystrophica. *Radiologe* 22:566, 1982.

Málaga S, et al.: Renal amyloidosis complicating a recessive epidermolysis bullosa in childhood. *Helv. Paediatr. Acta* 38:167, 1983.

Mauro MA, et al.: Epidermolysis bullosa: Radiographic findings in 16 cases. *A.J.R.* 149:925, 1987.

Panicek DM, et al.: Superficial fascial calcification in epidermolysis bullosa. *A.J.R.* 148:577, 1987.

Rosenberg D, et al.: Alleinte du tractus urinaire au cours du syndrome épidermolyse bulleuse congénitale-atrésie du pylore. *Arch. Fr. Pediatr.* 44:867, 1987.

Rosenbloom MS, et al.: Congenital pyloric atresia and epidermolysis bullosa letalis in premature siblings. *J. Pediatr. Surg.* 22:374, 1987.

Spraker MK: Report on the first national epidermolysis bullosa conference November 29 to December 1, 1984. *Pediatr. Dermatol.* 3:79, 1985.

Tishler JM, et al.: Esophageal involvement in epidermolysis bullosa dystrophica. *A.J.R.* 141:1283, 1983.

F

F SYNDROME

Mode of Inheritance: Autosomal dominant.

Clinical Manifestations: (a) syndactyly, polydactyly; (b) prominence of the sternum with or without pectus excavatum.

Radiologic Manifestations: (a) *carpal and tarsal synostoses,* deformity of the first and second fingers with frequent *syndactyly* between these digits; (b) *hypoplasia, deformity, and proximal synostosis of the metatarsals;* proximal polydactyly of the toes and extensive webbing of adjacent toes; (c) spina bifida occulta.

REFERENCE

Grosse FR, et al.: The F-form of acro-pectoro-vertebral dysplasia: The F-syndrome. *Birth Defects* 5(3):48, 1969.

FACIO-AUDIO-SYMPHALANGISM SYNDROME

Synonyms: Symphalangism-surdity syndrome; multiple synostoses with conductive hearing impairment; symphalangism-brachydactyly syndrome; WL syndrome; deafness-symphalangism syndrome of Herrmann.

Mode of Inheritance: Autosomal dominant.

Frequency: Very rare.

Clinical Manifestations: (a) *progressive conduction deafness with onset in childhood,* fixation of the foot plate of the stapes in the oval window; (b) *distinct facial features: long and narrow face, broad and hemicylindrical nose, lack of alar flare, broad nasal bridge, thin upper lip,* low-set ears, asymmetrical mouth, internal strabismus; (c) *proximal symphalangia of the fingers (2, 3, 4) and toes (2, 3, 4),* brachydactyly, clinodactyly, hypoplasia or aplasia of the distal segments of the fingers and/or toes and corresponding nails, hypoplasia of the thenar and hypothenar muscles, cutaneous syndactyly of the fingers (2, 3, 4) and toes (2, 3).

Radiologic Manifestations: (a) *proximal symphalangism:* progressive narrowing of the interphalangeal joints resulting in fusion of the phalanges, proximal interphalangeal joints of the fingers and distal interphalangeal joints of the toes usually involved, thumbs and great toes not affected; (b) brachydactyly; (c) other reported abnormalities: short arm, dislocated head of the radius, carpal and tarsal fusion, clinodactyly, hypoplastic/aplastic middle phalanx, hypoplastic/dysplastic distal phalanx, cubitus valgus, short legs, genus valgus, pes planovalgus, short foot, short hallux, pectus excavatum, short sternum, humeroradial fusion (Fig SY–F–1).

REFERENCES

Cushing H: Hereditary anchylosis of proximal phalangeal joints (symphalangism). *Genetics* 1:90, 1916.
Gorlin RJ, et al.: Stapes fixation and proximal symphalangism. *Z. Kinderheilkd.* 108:12, 1970.
Herrmann J: Symphalangism and brachydactyly syndrome; report of WL symphalangism-brachydactyly syndrome. Review of literature and classification. *Birth Defects* 10:23, 1974.
Higashi K, et al.: Conductive deafness, symphalangism, and facial abnormalities: The WL syndrome in a Japanese family. *Am. J. Med. Genet.* 16:105, 1983.
Hurvitz SA, et al.: The facio-audio-symphalangism syndrome: Report of a case and review of the literature. *Clin. Genet.* 28:61, 1985.
Maroteaux JP, et al.: La maladie des synostoses multiples. *Nouv. Presse Med.* 1:3041, 1972.
Strasburger AK, et al.: Symphalangism: Genetic and clinical aspects. *Bull. Johns Hopkins Hosp.* 117:108, 1965.
Vesell ES: Symphalangism, strabismus and hearing loss in mother and daughter. *N. Engl. J. Med.* 263:839, 1960.

FACIO-AURICULO-RADIAL DYSPLASIA

Mode of Inheritance: Autosomal dominant, very variable expression.

Frequency: Reported in two families (Harding et al.).

Clinical and Radiological Manifestations: (a) *dysmorphic facies;* (b) *conductive deafness;* (c) *deformity of the pinna* (primitively formed); (d) *asymmetrical radial dysplasia;* (e) other reported abnormalities: hooked-shaped clavicles, hypoplasia of the humerus, carpal and metacarpal anomalies, hypoplastic fibula, synostosis of the radius and ulna, vertebral fusion, etc.

Differential Diagnosis: Nager syndrome; LARD syndrome (lacrimo-auriculo-radiodental syndrome); Juberg-Hayward syndrome.

REFERENCES

Harding AE, et al.: Autosomal dominant asymmetrical radial dysplasia, dysmorphic facies, and conductive hearing loss

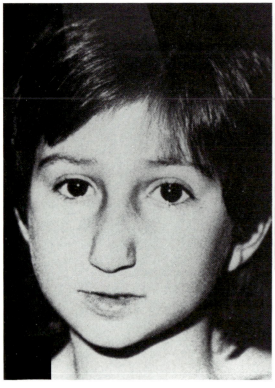

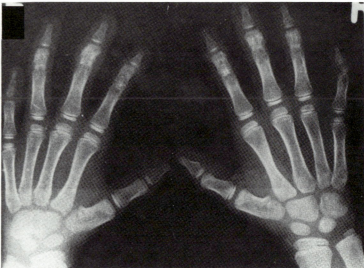

FIG SY—F—1.
Facio-audio-symphalangism in a 5-year-old girl. **A,** broad, hemicylindrical nose without an alar flare and an asymmetrical mouth with a thin upper lip. **B,** symphalangia, short first metacarpal, fusion of the carpal bones, and clinodactyly of the fifth digits. (From Hurvitz SA, Goodman RM, Hertz M, et al.: The facio-audio-symphalangism syndrome: Report of a case and review of the literature. *Clin. Genet.* 28:61, 1985. Used by permission.)

(facioauriculoradial dysplasia). *J. Med. Genet.* 19:110, 1982.

Stoll C, et al.: L'association phocomelie-ectrodactylie, malformations des oreilles avec surdité, arythmie sinusale. *Arch. Fr. Pediatr.* 31:669, 1974.

FANCONI ANEMIA

Synonyms: Fanconi pancytopenia; Fanconi syndrome.

Mode of Inheritance: Autosomal recessive; genetic heterogeneity; clinical and cytogenetic diversity.

Frequency: Uncommon.

Clinical Manifestations: (a) hematologic disorders usually appearing between 5 and 10 years of age: bleeding tendency, *pancytopenia* (macrocytic hyperchromic anemia, granulocytopenia, thrombocytopenia), increased levels of fetal hemoglobin, hypocellular bone marrow; (b) brown *pigmentation* of the skin; (c) radial ray deformity, radial ray reduction deformities, supernumerary thumbs; (d) small stature; (e) microcephaly; (f) chromosomal abnormalities: (1) spontaneous chromosomal instability (breaks, ring or cross chromosomes, chromosome exchanges, endoreduplications); (2) high mitomycin C sensitivity of peripheral lymphocytes in culture; (3) postnatal and prenatal diagnosis and carrier detection by exposure of blood lymphocytes or amniotic fluid cells to diepoxybutane (increase in chromosomal breakage); (g) increased incidence of malignancies: leukemia, squamous cell carcinoma, and hepatic tumor (adenoma, hepatocellular carcinoma, hepatoma); hepatosplenic peliosis (steroid treat-

ment related); (h) growth hormone deficiency, isolated or combined with other hypothalamopituitary defects; primary testicular failure associated with cryptorchidism; (i) other reported abnormalities: anomalies of the genitourinary organs, heart, ears, eyes; mental retardation, deficient T-cell function, association with hemophilia A, intracranial bleeding, deafness, liver abscess.

Radiologic Manifestations: (a) *limb anomalies: absent, hypoplastic, or supernumerary thumb; hypoplasia or absence of the first metacarpal;* greater multangular and navicular bones; hypoplasia or absence of the radius, digitalized thumb, bifid thumb; (b) retarded skeletal maturation; (c) microcephaly, thickened calvaria; (d) *renal anomalies:* absent kidney, horseshoe kidney, hydronephrosis, etc.; (e) ⁹⁹ᵐTc sulfur colloid bone marrow scans: irregular tracer distribution; (f) other reported abnormalities: osteoporosis, syndactyly, hip dislocation, clubfoot, flatfoot, Klippel-Feil deformity, moyamoya, nonossifying fibroma-related osteomalacia (healing of osteomalacia after removal of the bone tumor), etc.

Differential Diagnosis: TAR syndrome; WT limb-blood syndrome (radial and ulnar hypoplasia, transient or permanent bone marrow failure, and in some cases leukemia; autosomal dominant transmission) (Fig SY—F—2).

REFERENCES

Abbondanzo SL, et al.: Hepatocellular carcinoma in an 11-year-old girl with Fanconi's anemia. Report of a case and

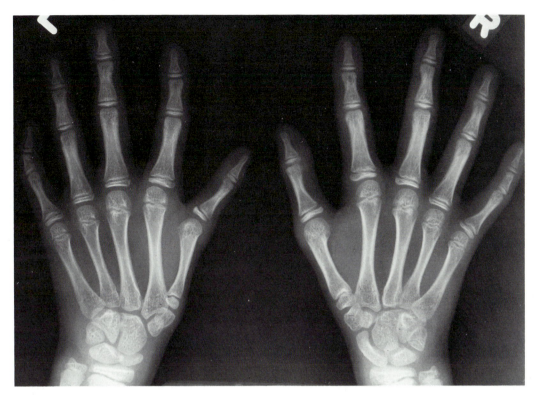

FIG SY–F–2.
Fanconi anemia in a 13-year-old female. The phalanges of the left thumb are hypoplastic, and the first metacarpal is deficient proximally. Clinodactyly of the fifth fingers is present. The right navicular bone is unusually long. (From Minagi H, Steinbach HL: Roent-gen appearance of anomalies associated with hypoplastic anemias of childhood: Fanconi's anemia and congenital hypoplastic anemia (erythrogenesis imperfecta). *A.J.R.* 97:100, 1966. Used by permission.)

review of the literature. *Am. J. Pediatr. Hematol. Oncol.* 8:334, 1986.

Ahuja HG, et al.: Acute nonlymphoblastic leukemia in the first of three siblings affected with Fanconi's syndrome. *Am. J. Pediatr. Hematol. Oncol.* 8:347, 1986.

Auerbach AD, et al.: Fanconi anemia: Prenatal diagnosis in 30 fetuses at risk. *Pediatrics* 76:794, 1985.

Aynsley-Green A, et al.: Endocrine studies in Fanconi's anemia. *Arch. Dis. Child.* 53:126, 1978.

Cervenka J, et al.: Mitomycin C test for diagnostic differentiation of idiopathic aplastic anemia and Fanconi anemia. *Pediatrics* 67:119, 1981.

Cohen N, et al.: Moya moya and Fanconi's anemia. *Pediatrics* 65:804, 1980.

Despert F, et al.: Maladie de Fanconi avec péliose hépato-splénique. *Arch. Fr. Pediatr.* 38:29, 1981.

Duckworth-Rysiecki G, et al.: Clinical and cytogenetic diversity in Fanconi's anaemia. *J. Med. Genet.* 21:197, 1984.

Fanconi G: Familiäre, infantile periciosaähnliche Anämie (Pernizioses Blutbild und Konstitution). *J. Kinderheilkd.* 117:257, 1927.

Garel L, et al.: Adénomes multiple du foie et anémie de Fanconi. *Ann. Radiol. (Paris)* 24:53, 1981.

Gastearena J, et al.: Fanconi's anemia. Clinical study of six cases. *Am. J. Pediatr. Hematol. Oncol.* 8:173, 1986.

Glanz A, et al.: Spectrum of anomalies in Fanconi anaemia. *J. Med. Genet.* 19:412, 1982.

Gonzalez CH, et al.: The WT syndrome—a "new" autosomal dominant pleiotropic trait of radial-ulnar hypoplasia with high risk of bone marrow failure and/or leukemia. *Birth Defects* 8:31, 1977.

Kennedy AW, et al.: Multiple squamous-cell carcinomas in Fanconi's anemia. *Cancer* 50:811, 1982.

Leehey DJ, et al.: Fanconi syndrome associated with a non-ossifying fibroma of bone. *Am. J. Med.* 78:708, 1985.

Ljung R, et al.: Fanconi's anemia associated with haemophilia A. *Clin. Genet.* 16:364, 1979.

Mera CL, et al.: P clostridium liver abscess and massive hemolysis. *Clin. Pediatr. (Phila.)* 23:126, 1984.

Minagi H, Steinbach HL: Roentgen appearance of anomalies associated with hypoplastic anemias of childhood: Fanconi's anemia and congenital hypoplastic anemia (erythrogenesis imperfecta). *A.J.R.* 97:100, 1966.

Nordan UZ, et al.: Fanconi's anemia with growth hormone deficiency. *Am. J. Dis. Child.* 133:291, 1979.

Pedersen FK, et al.: Indication of primary immune deficiency in Fanconi's anemia. *Acta Paediatr. Scand.* 66:745, 1977.

Shindler D, et al.: Confirmation of Fanconi's anemia and detection of a chromosomal aberration (1Q12-32 triplication) via BRDU/Hoechst flow cytometry. *Am. J. Pediatr. Hematol. Oncol.* 9:172, 1987.

FAT EMBOLISM SYNDROME

Etiology: Acute respiratory failure following *skeletal injuries due to deposition of marrow fat within pulmonary capil-*

laries that results in a capillary leak within the lung, pulmonary edema, hemorrhage, and microatelectasis.

Clinical Manifestations: Signs and symptoms evident within 12 to 72 hours after injury: (a) *fever, tachypnea, hyperpnea, dyspnea, tachycardia, cyanosis,* hemoptysis; (b) altered sensorium; (c) petechiae; (d) fat in the retinal vessels; (e) lipuria; fat in a cryostat-frozen section of clotted blood; increase in platelet adhesiveness; decrease in platelets, hemoglobin, and hematocrit; normal or reduced fibrinogen levels in initial phase followed in some cases by a delayed rise above normal levels; hypercalcemia.

Radiologic Manifestations: (a) *widespread increase in lung density (alveolar and interstitial),* more marked in the perihilar region initially, followed by extension to the periphery and generalized pulmonary involvement; (b) normal heart and pulmonary vasculature; (c) perfusion imaging: diffuse, subsegmental ("mottled") appearance of the lungs; normal ventilation images.

Note: Proposed criteria for a positive diagnosis of the syndrome based on respiratory insufficiency (Lindeque et al): (a) a sustained Pa_{O_2} of less than 60 mm Hg; (b) a sustained Pa_{CO_2} of more than 55 mm Hg or a pH of less than 7.3; (c) a sustained respiratory rate of more than 35 breaths per minute even after adequate sedation; (d) increased work of breathing dyspnea, the use of accessory respiratory muscles, and tachycardia-combined with anxiety; a patient showing at least one of the above criteria is considered to have developed the fat emboli syndrome.

REFERENCES

Feldman F, et al.: The fat embolism syndrome. *Radiology* 114:535, 1975.
Guenter CA, et al.: Fat embolism syndrome: Changing prognosis. *Chest* 79:143, 1981.
Lindeque BGP, et al.: Fat embolism and the fat embolism syndrome. A double-blind therapeutic study. *J. Bone Joint Surg. [Br.]* 69:128, 1987.
Peltier LF: The diagnosis of fat embolism. *Surg. Gynecol. Obstet.* 121:371, 1965.
Pollak R, et al.: Early diagnosis of the fat embolism syndrome. *J. Trauma* 18:121, 1978.
Williams AG, et al.: Fat embolism syndrome. *Clin. Nucl. Med.* 11:495, 1986.

FELTY SYNDROME

Clinical Manifestations: Triad (a to c): (a) *rheumatoid arthritis;* (b) *splenomegaly;* (c) *hypersplenism* (anemia, leukopenia, granulocytopenia); (d) generalized lymphadenopathy; (e) liver disease: hepatomegaly, nodular regenerative hyperplasia, portal fibrosis, abnormal lobular arrangement, portal hypertension, esophageal varices; (f) IgG antibodies against white blood cells; (g) other reported abnormalities: leg ulcers, recurrent infections.

Radiologic Manifestations: (a) *rheumatoid arthritis;* (b) *splenomegaly;* (c) scintigraphy (^{99m}Tc sulfur colloid): a reversal of the liver-to-spleen uptake ratio despite normal liver function test results; virtually no visualization of the bone marrow of the sternum, vertebrae, and ribs.

Notes: (a) familial cases have been reported; (b) low frequency in blacks.

REFERENCES

Blendis LM, et al.: Familial Felty's syndrome. *Ann. Rheum. Dis.* 35:279, 1976.
Editorial: Felty's syndrome. *Lancet* 1:540, 662, 1978.
Felty AR: Chronic arthritis in the adult, associated with splenomegaly and leucopenia: A report of five cases of an unusual clinical syndrome. *Bull. Johns Hopkins Hosp.* 35:16, 1924.
Lewis RB: Felty's syndrome in blacks (letter). *Arthritis Rheum.* 23:377, 1980.
Logue GL, et al.: Felty's syndrome without splenomegaly. *Am. J. Med.* 66:703, 1979.
Louie JS, et al.: Felty's syndrome. *Semin. Hematol.* 8:216, 1971.
Rosenthal FD, et al.: White-cell antibodies and the aetiology of Felty's syndrome. *Q. J. Med.* 43:187, 1974.
Shih WJ, et al.: Radiocolloid scintigraphy in Felty's syndrome. *A.J.R.* 146:181, 1986.
Thorne C, et al.: Liver disease in Felty's syndrome. *Am. J. Med.* 73:35, 1982.
Toomey K, et al.: Felty syndrome in juvenile arthritis. *J. Pediatr.* 106:254, 1985.

FEMORAL-FACIAL SYNDROME

Synonym: Femoral hypoplasia–unusual facies syndrome.

Mode of Inheritance: Multifactorial pathogenesis most likely; an affected father and daughter have been reported.

Frequency: Rare.

Clinical Manifestations: (a) *facial features:* short nose with broadened tip, elongated philtrum, thin upper lip, *micrognathia,* upslanting palpebral fissure, cleft palate, ear deformities (overfolded helices; posterior rotation; cupped, microtic, hypoplastic cartilage); (b) *short thighs;* (c) other reported abnormalities: restricted motion of the elbows, clubfoot deformity, infant of a diabetic mother with genitourinary system anomalies and femoral-facial syndrome, Sprengel deformity, limited motion of the shoulder or elbow.

Radiologic Manifestations: (a) *short or absent femora;* (b) short or absent fibulas; (c) other reported abnormalities: mild shortness of the humeri, constricted ilial base, vertical ischial axis, acetabular hypoplasia, large obturator foramina, Sprengel deformity, radiohumeral synostosis, radio-ulnar synostosis, rib anomalies (tapered, missing, fused), vertebral anomalies (missing, hemivertebrae, sacralization of the lower lumbar vertebrae, scoliosis, sacral dysplasia), foot deformities (clubfoot, polydactyly, oligodactyly, syndactyly), genitourinary anomalies (polycystic kidneys, renal malposition, absent kidney(s), abnormal renal collecting system, septated bladder, hypoplastic penis), cardiovascular anomalies (truncus arteriosus, pulmonary stenosis), alimentary tract abnormalities (anorectal agenesis, gastroesophageal reflux), polysplenia, superiorly placed adrenals.

Differential Diagnosis: kyphomelic dysplasia (Maclean) (Figs SY−F−3 and SY−F−4).

REFERENCES

Daentl DL, et al.: Femoral hypoplasia−unusual facies syndrome. *J. Pediatr.* 86:107, 1975.

DePalma L, et al.: Femoral hypoplasia−unusual facies syndrome: Autopsy findings in an unusual case. *Pediatr. Pathol.* 5:1, 1986.

Johnson JP, et al.: Femoral hypoplasia−unusual facies syndrome in infants of diabetic mothers. *J. Pediatr.* 102:866, 1983.

Lampert RP: Dominant inheritance of femoral hypoplasia−unusual facies syndrome. *Clin. Genet.* 17:255, 1980.

Lord J, et al.: The femoral hypoplasia−unusual facies syndrome: A genetic entity? *Clin. Genet.* 20:267, 1981.

Maclean RN: Reply to Dr. Pitt (letter). *Am. J. Med. Genet.* 24:367, 1986.

Maclean RN, et al.: Brief clinical report: Skeletal dysplasia

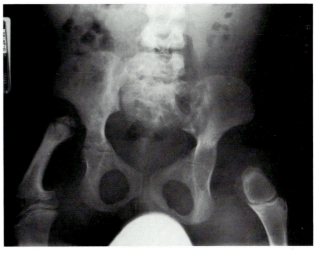

FIG SY−F−4.
Femoral-facial syndrome. Absence of the left femur, hypoplasia of the right femur and acetabula bilaterally, and a dysplastic sacrum are present. (From Johnson JP, Carey JC, Gooch M, et al.: Femoral hypoplasia−unusual facies syndrome in infants of diabetic mothers. *J. Pediatr.* 102:866, 1983. Used by permission.)

with short, angulated femora (kyphomelic dysplasia). *Am. J. Med. Genet.* 14:373, 1983.

Pitt D: Kyphomelic dysplasia versus femoral hypoplasia−unusual facies syndrome (letter). *Am. J. Med. Genet.* 24:365, 1986.

Pitt DB, et al.: Femoral hypoplasia−unusual facies syndrome. *Aust. Paediatr. J.* 18:63, 1982.

FEMUR-FIBULA-ULNA SYNDROME

Synonym: FFU syndrome.

Frequency: Rare.

Clinical and Radiologic Manifestations: (a) femoral anomalies ranging from hypoplasia to absence; (b) absent fibula; (c) anomalies of the upper limbs: amelia, peromelia at the lower end of the humerus, defects of the ulna and ulnar rays, humeroradial synostosis (Fig SY−F−5).

REFERENCES

Hirose K, et al.: Antenatal ultrasound diagnosis of the femur-fibula-ulna syndrome. *J. Clin. Ultrasound* 16:199, 1988.

Kühne D, et al: Defekt von Femur und Fibula mit Amelie, Peromelie oder ulnaren Strahldefekten der Arme. Ein Syndrome. *Humangenetik* 3:244, 1967.

FETAL ALCOHOL SYNDROME

Synonym: Alcohol fetopathy.

Etiology: Chronic heavy alcoholic intake by the mother during pregnancy.

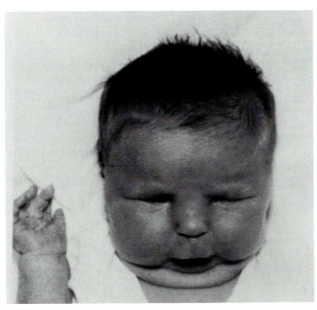

FIG SY−F−3.
Femoral-facial syndrome. Note the extreme micrognathia, thin upper lip, and unusual appearance of the nose. (From Johnson JP, Carey JC, Gooch M, et al.: Femoral hypoplasia−unusual facies syndrome in infants of diabetic mothers. *J. Pediatr.* 102:866, 1983. Used by permission.)

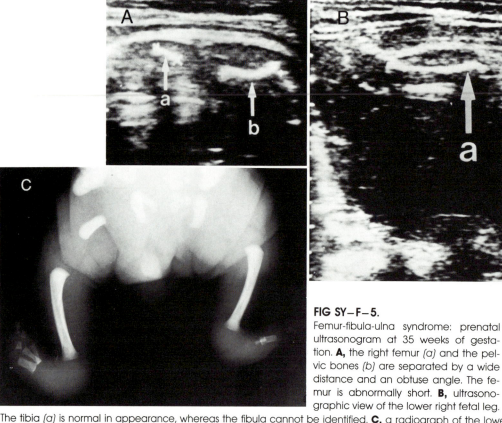

FIG SY—F—5.
Femur-fibula-ulna syndrome: prenatal ultrasonogram at 35 weeks of gestation. **A,** the right femur *(a)* and the pelvic bones *(b)* are separated by a wide distance and an obtuse angle. The femur is abnormally short. **B,** ultrasonographic view of the lower right fetal leg.

The tibia *(a)* is normal in appearance, whereas the fibula cannot be identified. **C,** a radiograph of the lower limbs shows that the femur on the right side is short and on the left side it is absent. Two toes on the right side and three toes on the left side are missing. (From Hirose K, Koyanagia T, Hara K, et al.: Antenatal ultrasound diagnosis of the femur-fibula-ulna syndrome. *J. Clin. Ultrasound* 16:199, 1988. Used by permission.)

Clinical Manifestations: (a) *prenatal and postnatal growth retardation;* (b) *mental retardation, poor coordination, hypotonia, irritability in infancy, hyperactivity in childhood;* (c) *craniofacial manifestations: microcephaly, midfacial hypoplasia, retrognathia in infancy, micrognathia or relative prognathism in adolescence, posterior rotation of the ears, poorly formed concha, hypoplastic philtrum, small vermilion border of the lips, cleft lip or palate, high-arched palate, short palpebral fissures, ptosis, strabismus, epicanthal folds, myopia, microphthalmos, blepharomiosis, abnormal fundi (tortuosity of the retinal vessels, optic nerve hypoplasia or atrophy, pallor of the optic disk), reduced visual acuity;* (d) *cutaneous anomalies:* hemangiomas, hirsutism in infancy, absence or dysplasia of the nails; (e) *cardiovascular anomalies:* atrial septal defect, ventricular septal defect, aberrant great vessels, tetrology of Fallot, mitral stenosis, hypoplastic pulmonary arteries, patent ductus arteriosus, aortic arch interruption, single umbilical artery, etc.; (f) urinary system abnormalities: oligomeganephronic hypoplasia, nephrotic syndrome, etc.; (g) association with tumors: neuroblastoma, adrenal carcinoma, hepatoblastoma, ganglioneuroblastoma, sacrococcygeal teratoma, rhabdomyosarcoma, nephroblastoma, endodermal sinus tumor, medulloblastoma, Hodgkin disease, acute lymphocytic leukemia; (h) hepatobiliary abnormalities: hepatic dysfunction, bile duct proliferation, hepatic fibrosis, biliary atresia; (i) other reported abnormalities: diaphragmatic hernia, abdominal hernias, abnormal palmar creases, accessory nipple, combined fetal alcohol and hydantoin syndromes, association with celiac disease, upper airway obstruction (small nasopharyngeal space, choanal stenosis, laryngeal web), hearing disorders, etc.

Radiologic Manifestations: (a) *skeletal anomalies:* scoliosis, hemivertebrae, Klippel-Feil syndrome, pectus excavatum, pectus carinatum, clubfoot, flexion contracture, radio-ulnar synostosis, camptodactyly, clinodactyly, tetradactyly, short metatarsals, punctate epiphyseal calcification, congenital hip dislocation, a distinctive hand pattern profile (shortness of the metacarpals and phalanges of about 2 SD below the mean, in particular, at the fifth terminal phalanx, narrowness of the terminal phalanges), etc.; (b) *nervous system anomalies:* malformation of neuronal and glial migration, *microcephaly,* hydrocephaly, anencephaly, porencephaly, agenesis of the corpus callosum, meningomyelocele, lumbosacral lipoma, Dandy-Walker deformity, etc.; (c) *urogenital anomalies:* renal anomalies (hypoplasia, aplasia, hydronephrosis, hamartoma, caliceal cyst, fused kidneys, duplication, cystic kidneys), bladder diverticula, vesicovaginal fistula, urogenital sinus, hypospadias, labial hypoplasia, etc. (Fig SY—F—6).

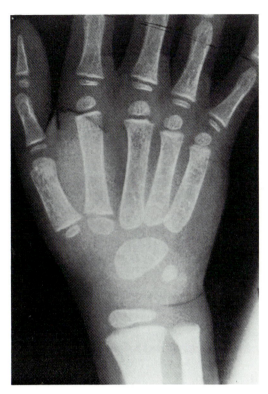

FIG SY—F—6.
Fetal alcohol syndrome in an 8-year-old boy: capitate-hamate carpal fusion and metacarpal pseudoepiphysis. (From Cremin BJ, Jaffer Z: Radiological aspects of the fetal alcohol syndrome. *Pediatr. Radiol.* 11:151, 1981. Used by permission.)

REFERENCES

Badois C, et al.: Maladie des épiphyses ponctuées (MEP) associée a une Foetopathie éthylique (FE). Trois premiers cas rapportés. *Ann. Radiol. (Paris)* 26:244, 1983.

Christoffel KK, et al.: Fetal alcohol syndrome in dizygotic twins. *J. Pediatr.* 87:963, 1975.

Church MW, et al: Hearing disorders in children with fetal alcohol syndrome: Findings from case reports. *Pediatrics* 82:147, 1988.

Clarren SK, et al.: Facial effects of fetal alcohol exposure: Assessment by photographs and morphometric analysis. *Am. J. Med. Genet.* 26:651, 1987.

Crain LS, et al.: Nail dysplasia and fetal alcohol syndrome. *Am. J. Dis. Child.* 137:1069, 1983.

Cremin BJ, et al.: Radiological aspects of the fetal alcohol syndrome. *Pediatr. Radiol.* 11:151, 1981.

Fanconi A, et al.: Oligomeganephronic hypoplasia in a child with fetal alcohol syndrome (FAS). *Helv. Paediatr. Acta* 41:142, 1986.

Ferrer I, et al.: Dendritic spine anomalies in fetal alcohol syndrome. *Neuropediatrics* 18:161, 1987.

Frias JL, et al.: A cephalometric study of fetal alcohol syndrome. *J. Pediatr.* 101:870, 1982.

Goldstein G, et al.: Neural tube defect and renal anomalies in a child with fetal alcohol syndrome. *J. Pediatr.* 93:636, 1978.

Graham JM, et al: Independent dysmorphology evaluations at birth and 4 years of age for children exposed to varying amounts of alcohol in utero. *Pediatrics* 81:772, 1988.

Habbick BF, et al.: Liver abnormalities in three patients with fetal alcohol syndrome. *Lancet* 1:580, 1979.

Havers W, et al.: Anomalies of the kidneys and genitourinary tract in alcohol embryopathy. *J. Urol.* 124:108, 1980.

Herrmann J, et al.: Tetraectrodactyly and other skeletal manifestations in the fetal alcohol syndrome. *Eur. J. Pediatr.* 133:221, 1980.

Houston CS: Hand pattern profile in fetal alcohol syndrome. Presented at the 26th Annual Meeting of the Society for Pediatric Radiology, Atlanta, 1983.

Jaffer Z, et al.: Bone fusion in the fetal alcohol syndrome. *J. Bone Joint Surg. [Br.]* 63:569, 1981.

Johnson CAC, et al.: Fetal alcohol syndrome with hydrocephalus. *S. Afr. Med. J.* 65:738, 1984.

Kiess W, et al.: Fetal alcohol syndrome and malignant disease. *Eur. J. Pediatr.* 143:160, 1984.

Lefkowitch JH, et al.: Hepatic fibrosis in fetal alcohol syndrome. Pathologic similarities to adult alcoholic liver disease. *Gasteroenterology* 85:951, 1983.

Neidengard L, et al.: Klippel-Feil malformation complex in fetal alcohol syndrome. *Am. J. Dis. Child.* 132:929, 1978.

Neri G, et al.: Facial midline defect in the fetal alcohol syndrome: Embryogenetic considerations in two clinical cases. *Am. J. Med. Genet.* 29:477, 1988.

Newman SL, et al.: Simultaneous occurrence of extrahepatic biliary atresia and fetal alcohol syndrome. *Am. J. Dis. Child.* 133:101, 1979.

Paditz E, et al.: Alkoholembryopathie mit symptomatischer chondrodysplasia punctata. *Helv. Paediatr. Acta* 40:61, 1985.

Qazi Q, et al.: Renal anomalies in fetal alcohol syndrome. *Pediatrics* 63:886, 1979.

Rabinowicz IM: New ophthalmic findings in fetal alcohol syndrome. *J.A.M.A.* 245:108, 1981.

Salcedo JR: Idiopathic nephrotic syndrome in fetal alcohol syndrome. *Clin. Pediatr. (Phila.)* 25:365, 1986.

Sandor GGS, et al.: Cardiac malformations in the fetal alcohol syndrome. *J. Pediatr.* 98:771, 1981.

Steeg CN, et al.: Cardiovascular malformations in the fetal alcohol syndrome. *Am. Heart J.* 98:635, 1979.

Streissguth AP, et al.: Natural history of the fetal alcohol syndrome: A 10-year follow-up of eleven patients. *Lancet* 2:85, 1985.

Ulleland CW: The offspring of alcoholic mothers. *Ann. N.Y. Acad. Sci.* 197:167, 1972.

Usowicz AG, et al.: Upper airway obstruction in infants with fetal alcohol syndrome. *Am. J. Dis. Child.* 140:1039, 1986.

Wilker R, et al.: Combined fetal alcohol and hydantoin syndromes. *Clin. Pediatr. (Phila.)* 21:331, 1982.

FETAL CYTOMEGALOVIRUS INFECTION

Synonym: Congenital cytomegalovirus infection.

Clinical Manifestations: (a) *intrauterine growth retardation;* (b) *microcephaly,* hydrocephaly; (c) *mental and motor retardation;* neurological deficits; seizure disorders; disorders of language, learning, and hearing; (d) *chorioretinitis;* optic atrophy; (e) *hepatosplenomegaly*, prolonged jaundice; (f) *purpura*; (g) *thrombocytopenia*, erythroblastemia, *inclusion bodies in epithelial cells in the urine, cytomegalovirus cultured from the urine, pathognomonic cells in various organs with intranuclear inclusion bodies,* specific IgM and IgG antibodies, DNA spot hybridization and restriction endonuclease analysis of the virus isolate; (h) other reported abnormalities: cleft palate, high-arched palate, micrognathia, facial weakness, congenital cardiovascular diseases, ascites, antenatal pericardial effusion, hydrops fetalis with supraventricular tachycardia, nephrotic syndrome, pancreatic cystadenoma, infected enteric ganglion cells with hypoganglionosis and colonic dysmotility, etc.

Radiologic Manifestations: (a) *central nervous system calcification of various form and severity* (periventricular, cerebrum, cerebellum, spinal cord), brain atrophy, microgyria, cysts of the subependymal germinal matrix, intraventricular strands, ventriculomegaly, periventricular necrotic inflammatory foci presenting as echo-dense periventricular collections mimicking cerebral hemorrhage; (b) skeletal changes in newborns: *irregularity of the provisional zone of calcification of long bones, streaky linear or ovoid lucent regions between zones of sclerosis in the metaphyses of long bones* ("rubella-like" bone changes) with extension into the diaphyses; (c) other reported abnormalities: calcification in the sclera and choroid of the eye, failure of normal rib development, small-caliber colon, intestinal pseudo-obstruction—associated hypoganglionosis, marked renal cortical echogenicity related to renal parenchymal disease, etc. (Figs SY—F—7 and SY—F—8).

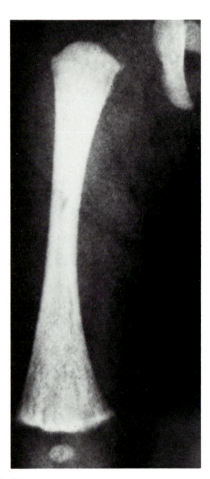

FIG SY—F—7.
Fetal cytomegalovirus infection in a female newborn with classic clinical manifestations of congenital cytomegalovirus inclusion disease: the right femur on first day of life with ovoid and linear lucent regions between zones of sclerosis; this is most marked in the distal metaphysis. The zone of provisional calcification is finely irregular and serrated. There are no periosteal changes. (From Graham CB, Thal A, Wassum CS: Rubella-like bone changes in congenital cytomegalic inclusion disease. *Radiology* 94:39, 1970. Used by permission.)

REFERENCES

Amir G, et al.: Neonatal cytomegalovirus infection with pancreatic cystadenoma and nephrotic syndrome. *Pediatr. Pathol.* 6:393, 1986.

Binder ND, et al.: Outcome for fetus with ascites and cytomegalovirus infection. *Pediatrics* 82:100, 1988.

Butt W, et al.: Intracranial lesions of congenital cytomegalovirus infection detected by ultrasound scanning. *Pediatrics* 73:611, 1984.

Cramer BC, et al.: Sonographic appearance of cytomegalovirus nephritis in a neonate. *Pediatr. Radiol.* 15:56, 1985.

Dias MJM, et al.: Prenatal cytomegalovirus disease and cerebral microgyria: Evidence for perfusion failure, not disturbance of histogenesis, as the major cause of fetal cytomegalovirus encephalopathy. *Neuropediatrics* 15:18, 1984.

Dimmick JE, et al.: Cytomegalovirus infection of the bowel in infancy: Pathogenetic and diagnostic significance. *Pediatr. Pathol.* 2:95, 1984.

Filloux F, et al.: Hydrops fetalis with supraventicular tachycardia and cytomegalovirus infection. *Clin. Pediatr. (Phila.)* 24:534, 1985.

Foucaud P, et al.: Pseudo-obstruction intestinale et infection à cytomégalovirus des plexus myentériques. *Arch. Fr. Pediatr.* 42:713, 1985.

Graham CB, Thal A, Wassum CS: Rubella-like bone changes in congenital cytomegalic inclusion disease. *Radiology* 94:39, 1970.

Jenson HB, et al.: Congenital cytomegalovirus infection with osteolytic lesions: Use of DNA hybridization in diagnosis: *Clin. Pediatr. (Phila.)* 26:448, 1987.

Romanet P, et al.: Epanchement péricardique anté-natal témoin d'une maladie des inclusions cytomégaliques mortelle chez un nouveau-né. *Presse Med.* 13:1748, 1984.

Shakelford GD, et al.: Cysts of the subependymal germinal matrix: Sonographic demonstration with pathologic correlation. *Radiology* 149:117, 1983.

Silverman FN: Virus diseases of bone: Do they exist? (the Neuhauser lecture). *A.J.R.* 126:677, 1976.

Sofer S, et al.: Cytomegalic virus periventriculitis: A sonographic picture mimicking ventricular hemorrhage. *J. Clin. Ultrasound* 13:574, 1985.

Williamson WD, et al.: Symptomatic congenital cytomegalovirus. Disorders of language, learning, and hearing. *Am. J. Dis. Child.* 136:902, 1982.

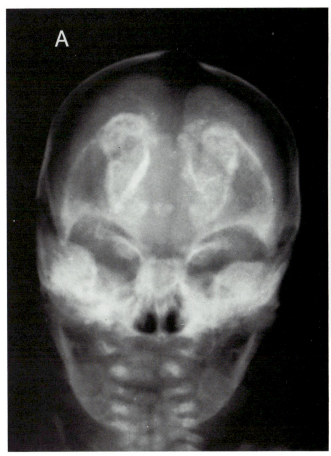

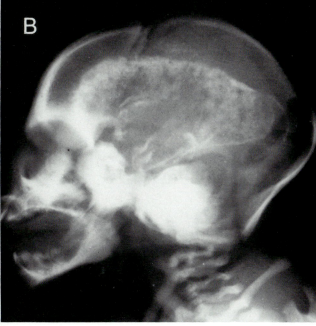

FIG SY–F–8.
A and **B,** fetal cytomegalovirus infection: microcephaly and ventricular subependymal calcification. (From Roach ES, Sumner TE, Volberg FM, et al.: Radiological case of the month. *Am. J. Dis. Child.* 137:799, 1983. Used by permission.)

FETAL HERPES SIMPLEX INFECTION

Clinical Manifestations: (a) *intrauterine growth retardation*; (b) *microcephaly, mental retardation,* deafness, *neurological deficits*; (c) *microphthalmos, chorioretinitis, retinal dysplasia,* (d) *hepatosplenomegaly, jaundice*; (e) *mucocutaneous vesicular lesions*; (f) *thrombocytopenia, positive specific serologic tests, isolation of virus (cerebrospinal fluid, urine).*

Radiologic Manifestations: (a) *cerebral calcification* (periventricular, hippocampal); (b) *hepatic calcification,* adrenal calcification; (c) *slight irregularity of the provisional zone of calcification, transverse bands of metaphyseal rarefaction in the long bones at birth.*

REFERENCES

Burkett G: Perinatal infections: *J. Fla. Med. Assoc.* 70:749, 1983.
Florman AL, et al.: Intrauterine infection with herpes simplex virus: Resultant congenital malformations. *J.A.M.A.* 225:129, 1973.
Morrison SC, et al: Calcification in the adrenal glands associated with disseminated herpes simplex infection. *Pediatr. Radiol.* 18:240, 1988.
Shackelford GD, et al.: Neonatal hepatic calcification secondary to transplacental infection. *Radiology* 122:753, 1977.

FETAL HYDANTOIN SYNDROME

Etiology: Maternal ingestion of a hydantoin anticonvulsant drug (diphenylhydantoin, mephenytoin, ethotoin) in the early stage of pregnancy; full syndrome in about 11% of exposed infants, partial expression of the teratogenic effects in 31%; discordant expression of the syndrome in heteropaternal dizygotic twins; partial expression (elongated fingers and hyperphalangia) in siblings and triplets.

Clinical Manifestations: (a) *prenatal and postnatal growth deficiency, psychomotor development retardation;* (b) *head: microcephaly, ridging of metopic suture, large anterior and posterior fontanelles, short and broad nose, depressed nasal bridge, mild hypertelorism, inner epicanthal folds, strabismus, ptosis of the eyelids, low-set ears, wide mouth, relative prognathism, prominent lips, cleft lip and/or palate, low posterior hairline, short neck;* (c) *limb anomalies: hypoplasia of the nails, fingerlike thumb, hypoplasia of the distal phalanges of the hands and feet, pes cavus, clubfoot, polydactyly, congenital hip dislocation, scoliosis, adactyly, etc.;* (d) *car-*

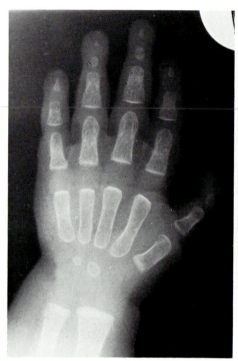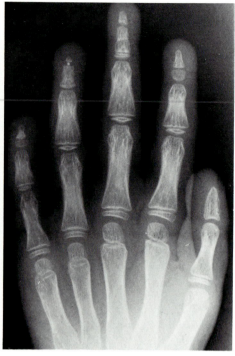

FIG SY−F−9.

Fetal hydantoin syndrome. Radiograms of the hand of a child at 8 months *(left)* and 6 years of age *(right)* show hyperphalangia of the third and fourth fingers. The second finger exhibits either an unusual hypertrophied epiphysis or hyperphalangia of the termi-

nal phalanx. (From Wood BP, Young LW: Pseudohyperphalangism in fetal Dilantin syndrome. *Radiology* 131:371, 1979. Used by permission.)

diovascular anomalies (atrial septal defect, ventricular septal defect, pulmonary stenosis, coarctation of the aorta etc.); (e) other reported abnormalities: umbilical hernia, inguinal hernia, hypospadias, bifid or shawl scrotum, tumor (neuroblastoma, ganglioneuroblastoma, melanotic neuroectodermal tumor), total absence of a phalanx or finger, deep pilonidal dimple, meningomyelocele, anencephaly, pyloric stenosis, intestinal atresia, dermatoglyphic abnormalities, large eyes, cupped ears, undescended testes, coarse hair, widely spaced nipples, Hodgkin lymphoma in fetal alcohol−hydantoin syndrome, diaphragmatic hernia, cardiovascular anomalies, cystic hygroma, cutaneous telangiectasis, capillary phlebectasis, etc.

Radiologic Manifestations: (a) *skeletal abnormalities;* apparent distal hyperphalangia due to the division of an otherwise normal phalanx, extra phalanx located between the metacarpal and proximal phalanx, poor skeletal mineralization, slenderness of the diaphysis of long bones, transverse radiolucent metaphyseal band, clinodactyly, distal digital hypoplasia (30%), adactyly, digital hypoplasia, triphalangeal thumbs, syndactyly, polydactyly, clubfeet, congenital scoliosis, rib anomalies, etc.; (b) other reported abnormalities: medullary sponge kidneys; diaphragmatic hernia; various anomalies of the ribs, sternum, spine, etc. (Fig SY−F−9).

REFERENCES

Allen RW, et al.: Fetal hydantoin syndrome, neuroblastoma and hemorrhagic disease in a neonate. *J.A.M.A.* 244:1464, 1980.

Anderson RC: Cardiac defects in children of mothers receiving anticonvulsant therapy during pregnancy. *J. Pediatr.* 89:318, 1976.

Bostrom B, et al.: Hodgkin disease in a child with fetal alcohol−hydantoin syndrome. *J. Pediatr.* 103:760, 1983.

Chodirker BN, et al.: Possible prenatal hydantoin effect in a child born to a nonepileptic mother. *Am. J. Med. Genet.* 27:373, 1987.

Ehrenbard LT, et al.: Cancer in the fetal hydantoin syndrome. *Lancet* 2:97, 1981.

Frederich A: Lésions osseuses des nouveau nés des mères prenant des anteconvulsants. *Arch. Fr. Pediatr.* 38:221, 1981.

Hampton GR, et al.: Ocular manifestations of the fetal hydantoin syndrome. *Clin. Pediatr. (Phila.)* 20:475, 1981.

Holmes LB, et al: Teratogenic effects of anticonvulsant drugs. *J. Pediatr.* 112:579, 1988.

Johnson JP: Acquired craniofacial features associated with chronic phenytoin therapy. *Clin. Pediatr. (Phila.)* 23:671, 1984.

Kelly TE: Teratogenicity of anticonvulsant drugs. I: Review of the literature. *Am. J. Med. Genet.* 19:413, 1984.

Kelly TE: Teratogenicity of anticonvulsant drugs. III: Radiographic hand analysis of children exposed in utero to diphenylhydantoin. *Am. J. Med. Genet.* 19:445, 1984.

Kelly TE, et al.: Teratogenicity of anticonvulsant drugs. II: A prospective study. *Am. J. Med. Genet.* 13:435, 1984.

Kogutt MS, et al.: Fetal hydantoin syndrome. *Am. J. Dis. Child.* 138:405, 1984.

Kousseff B: Subcutaneous vascular abnormalities in fetal hydantoin syndrome. Presented at a *Birth Defect Conference,* San Diego, 1981.

Kousseff BG, et al.: Expanding phenotype of fetal hydantoin syndrome. *Pediatrics* 70:328, 1982.

Phelan MC, et al.: Discordant expression of fetal hydantoin syndrome in heteropaternal dizygotic twins. *N. Engl. J. Med.* 307:99, 1982.

Pinto W Jr, et al.: Abnormal genitalia as a presenting sign in two male infants with hydantoin embryopathy syndrome. *Am. J. Dis. Child.* 131:452, 1977.

Sherman S, et al.: Fetal hydantoin syndrome and neuroblastoma. *Lancet* 2:517, 1976.

Verdeguer JM, et al: Onychopathy in a patient with fetal hydantoin syndrome. *Pediatr. Dermatol.* 5:56, 1988.

Waziri M, et al.: Teratogenic effect of anticonvulsant drugs. *Am. J. Dis. Child.* 130:1022, 1976.

Wood BP, et al: Pseudohyperphalangism in fetal Dilantin syndrome. *Radiology* 131:371, 1979.

FETAL ISOTRETINOIN SYNDROME

Synonyms: Isotretinoin embryopathy; retinoic acid embryopathy; isotretinoin teratogen syndrome.

Pathology: (a) hydrocephalus (communicating or obstruction with a fourth ventricle cyst), holoprosencephaly, architecture-distorting brain malformation associated with ventriculomegaly, cerebellar hypoplasia, agenesis of the vermis, cerebellar microdysgenesis, megacisterna magna, focal cortical agenesis, focal agyria, heterotopias, brain calcification, accessory parietal sutures; (b) congenital heart defects; (c) thymic abnormalities: ectopia, hypoplasia, aplasia.

Clinical Manifestations: (a) *craniofacial malformations*: narrow forehead relative to the parietal-occipital size, flat and depressed nasal bridge, hypertelorism, micrognathia, U-shaped cleft palate, *microtia or anotia* (low-set, agenesis, or marked stenosis of the external ear canal), microphthalmos; (b) immune disorders, recurrent pneumonias.

Radiologic Manifestations: Craniofacial and central nervous system anomalies (Fig SY—F—10).

REFERENCES

Benke PJ: The isotretinoin teratogen syndrome. *J.A.M.A.* 251:3267, 1984.

Cohen M, et al.: Thymic hypoplasia associated with isotretinoin embryopathy. *Am. J. Dis. Child.* 141:263, 1987.

Kawashima H, et al.: Syndrome of microtia and aortic arch anomalies resembling isotretinoin embryopathy. *J. Pediatr.* 111:738, 1987.

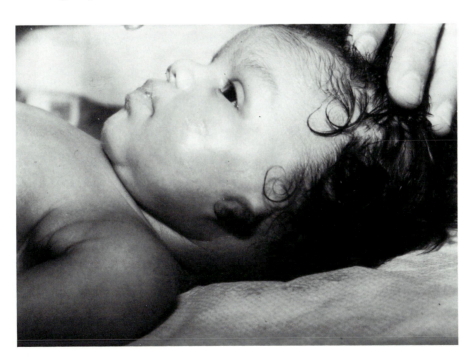

FIG SY—F—10.
Fetal isotretinoin syndrome: abnormal facial features showing a supraorbital ridge, a flattened nasal bridge, and anteverted nares. (From Cohen M, Rubinstein A, Li JK, et al.: Thymic hypoplasia associated with isotretinoin embryopathy. *Am. J. Dis. Child.* 141:263, 1987. Used by permission.)

Lammer EJ, et al.: Retinoic acid embryopathy. *N. Engl. J. Med.* 313:837, 1985.

Lott IT, et al.: Fetal hydrocephalus and ear anomalies associated with maternal use of isotretinoin. *J. Pediatr.* 105:597, 1984.

FETAL PRIMIDONE SYNDROME

Clinical and Radiologic Manifestations: (a) *growth deficiency;* (b) *head and neck:* depressed nasal bridge, hypertelorism, epicanthal folds, ptosis of the eyelids, down-slanted palpebral fissures, low-set and posteriorly rotated ears, wide anterior fontanelle, widely spaced sutures, webbed neck; (c) other reported abnormalities: nail hypoplasia, pectus excavatum, congenital heart defects, hypospadias, strabismus, etc. (Fig SY−F−11).

REFERENCES

Krauss CM, et al.: Four siblings with similar malformations after exposure to phenytoin and primidone. *J. Pediatr.* 105:750, 1984.

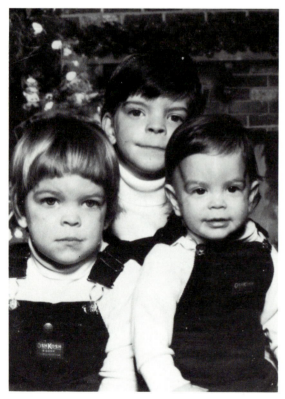

FIG SY−F−11.
Exposure either to phenytoin and primidone or to primidone alone: three brothers at ages 3½ years, 5½ years, and 14 months, respectively. Note the short nose, depressed bridge of the nose, and long upper lip. (From Krauss CM, Holmes LB, Van Lang QN, et al.: Four siblings with similar malformations after exposure to phenytoin and primidone. *J. Pediatr.* 105:750, 1984. Used by permission.)

Myhre SA, et al.: Teratogenic effects associated with maternal primidone therapy. *J. Pediatr.* 99:160, 1981.

Thomas D, et al.: Teratogenic effects of anticonvulsants. *J. Pediatr.* 99:163, 1981.

FETAL RUBELLA SYNDROME

Synonyms: Congenital rubella syndrome; rubella syndrome.

Clinical Manifestations: (a) *low birth weight;* (b) *thrombocytopenic purpura;* (c) *hepatosplenomegaly;* (d) *congenital cataract,* microphthalmos, retinopathy; (e) *deafness;* (f) cardiac defects; (g) psychomotor retardation; (h) isolation of rubella virus from cerebrospinal fluid, pharyngeal secretions, etc.; (i) specific rubella IgM antibody, persistence of rubella; antibody after 8 to 12 months of age; (j) other reported abnormalities: cryptorchidism, endocrine disorders (growth hormone deficiency, hypothyroidism, hyperthyroidism, thyroiditis, diabetes mellitus), extra chromosome fragments, arthritis, microcephaly, late onset of progressive mental and motor deterioration (second decade of life), desquamative interstitial pneumonia, etc.

Radiologic Manifestations: (a) *linear or ovoid areas of radiolucency and sclerosis (celery stalk) in the metaphyses of long bones,* irregularity and poor mineralization of the provisional zone of calcification, coarse trabeculae, transverse metaphyseal radiolucent bands, fracture (rare); (b) *large anterior fontanelle;* (c) chronic pneumonia; (d) cardiovascular disorders: *patent ductus arteriosus, pulmonary artery branch stenosis,* foreshortened main pulmonary, vertically tilted pulmonary valve, pulmonary valvular insufficiency, ventricular septal defect, aortic luminal occlusion, aortic hypoplasia, hypoplasia of the aortic branches, left ventricular aneurysm; (e) cerebral abnormalities: computed tomographic demonstration of low density in the white matter of the centrum ovale, low density in the periventricular white matter, calcification in the white matter and in the basal ganglia; cysts of the subependymal germinal matrix; (f) other reported abnormalities: pathological fracture, premature craniosynostosis associated with hyperthyroidism, delayed diaphyseal modeling of long bones (within 2 months after birth), delayed appearance of secondary ossification centers in the knee in neonates, esophageal atresia, aqueductal occlusion (Figs SY−F−12 and SY−F−13).

REFERENCES

Ansari BM, et al: Chromosomal abnormality in congenital rubella. *Pediatrics* 59:13, 1977.

Boner A, et al.: Desquamative interstitial pneumonia and antigen-antibody complexes in two infants with congenital rubella. *Pediatrics* 72:835, 1983.

Celers J, et al.: Rubéole et cataractes congenitales. *Arch. Fr. Pediatr.* 40:391, 1983.

Elliott LP, et al.: Angiocardiographic observation in the post-rubella syndrome. *A.J.R.* 97:164, 1966.

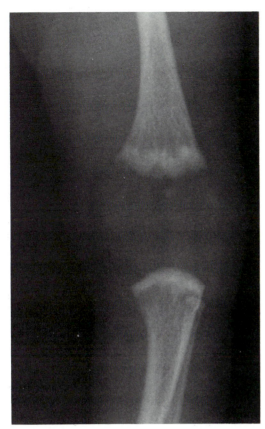

FIG SY−F−12.
Fetal rubella syndrome in a 2-day-old female. Microcephaly and bilateral cataracts were present at birth. Linear radiolucency and sclerotic changes (celery stalk appearance) are present in the distal segment of the femur and the proximal tibia.

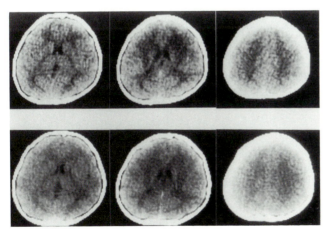

FIG SY−F−13.
Fetal rubella syndrome: computed tomographic scans obtained at 1 year, 7 months of age *(top)* and at 3 years, 7 months of age *(bottom)*. Low density in the white matter is present. Some reduction of the low density is observed in the latter scan. (From Ishikawa A, Murayama T, Sakuma N, et al.: Computed cranial tomography in congenital rubella syndrome. *Arch. Neurol.* 39:420, 1982. Used by permission.)

Floret D, et al.: Hyperthyroidism, diabetes mellitus and the congenital rubella syndrome. *Acta Paediatr. Scand.* 69:259, 1980.

Fortuin AG, et al.: Late vascular manifestations of rubella syndrome. *Am. J. Med.* 51:134, 1971.

Hanid TK: Hypothyroidism in congenital rubella. *Lancet* 2:854, 1976.

Harpey J-P, et al.: Congenital rubella with pneumonitis. *Lancet* 1:1104, 1985.

Ishikawa A, et al.: Computed cranial tomography in congenital rubella syndrome. *Arch. Neurol.* 39:420, 1982.

Kuhns LR, et al.: Knee maturation as a differentiating sign between congenital rubella and cytomegalic infections. *Pediatr. Radiol.* 6:36, 1977.

Munro ND, et al.: Temporal relations between maternal rubella and congenital defects. *Lancet* 2:201, 1987.

Preece MA, et al.: Growth-hormone deficiency in congenital rubella. *Lancet* 2:842, 1977.

Priebe CJ, et al.: Abnormalities of the vas deferens and epididymis in cryptorchid boys with congenital rubella. *J. Pediatr. Surg.* 14:834, 1979.

Rudolph AJ, et al.: Transplacental rubella infection in newly born infants. *J.A.M.A.* 191:843, 1965.

Sacks R, et al.: Pathological fracture in congenital rubella. *J. Bone Joint Surg. [Am.]* 59:557, 1977.

Shakelford GD, et al.: Cysts of the subependymal germinal matrix: Sonographic demonstration with pathologic correlation. *Radiology* 149:117, 1983.

Siassi B, et al.: Hypoplasia of the abdominal aorta associated with the rubella syndrome. *Am. J. Dis. Child.* 120:476, 1970.

Singleton EB, et al.: The roentgenographic manifestations of the rubella syndrome in newborn infants. *A.J.R.* 97:82, 1966.

Tang JS, et al.: Hypoplasia of the pulmonary arteries in infants with congenital rubella. *Am. J. Cardiol.* 27:491, 1971.

Townsend JJ, et al.: Progressive rubella panencephalitis. Late onset after congenital rubella. *N. Engl. J. Med.* 292:990, 1975.

van der Horst RL, et al.: Left ventricular aneurysm in rubella heart disease. *Am. J. Dis. Child.* 120:248, 1970.

Weil ML, et al.: Chronic progressive panencephalitis due to rubella virus simulating subacute sclerosing panencephalitis. *N. Engl. J. Med.* 292:994, 1975.

Whalen JP, et al.: Neonatal transplacental rubella syndrome. Its effect on normal maturation of the diaphysis. *A.J.R.* 121:166, 1974.

FETAL TOXOPLASMOSIS INFECTION

Synonym: Congenital toxoplasmosis.

Clinical Manifestations: (a) *psychomotor retardation, seizures, hydrocephaly, microcephaly;* (b) *chorioretinopathy;* (c) prenatal diagnosis: isolating the parasite in amniotic fluid, fetal blood samples showing nonspecific laboratory signs of fetal infection, specific antibodies of fetal origin (IgM), and parasitemia; ultrasonography of the fetus; (d) Sabin-Feldman test, complement fixation test; (e) other reported abnormalities: postnatal continuation of the development of new lesions, nephrotic syndrome, neonatal ascites, concomitant cytomegalovirus infection and congenital toxoplasmosis.

Radiologic Manifestations: (a) cerebritis, multicystic encephalomalacia, porencephalic cysts, hydrocephalus (aqueductal stenosis), hydranencephaly, calcification (often multiple, predilection for the periventricular and basal ganglia), calcification surrounded by a thin area of edematous density, focal destruction of cerebral tissue associated with enlargement of the neighboring cistern or ventricle, ocular calcification, microphthalmos; (b) hepatic and splenic calcifications; (c) metaphyseal bands and irregularity of the metaphyseal border of the growth plates.

REFERENCES

Couvreur J et al.: Etude d'une série homogène de 210 cas de toxoplasmose congénitale chez des nourrissons âgés de o à 11 mois et dépistés de façon prospective. *Ann. Pediatr. (Paris)* 31:815, 1984.

Couvreur J, et al.: Rein et toxoplasmose. *Ann. Pediatr. (Paris)* 31:847, 1984.

Desmonts G, et al.: Histoire naturelle de la toxoplasmose congénitale. *Ann. Pediatr. (Paris)* 31:799, 1984.

Desmonts G, et al.: Prenatal diagnosis of congenital toxoplasmosis. *Lancet* 1:500, 1985.

deZegher F, et al.: Concomitant cytomegalovirus infection and congenital toxoplasmosis in a newborn. *Eur. J. Pediatr.* 147:424, 1988.

Diebler C, et al.: Congenital toxoplasmosis. Clinical and neuroradiological evaluation of the cerebral lesions. *Neuroradiology* 27:125, 1985.

Gouyon JB, et al.: Toxoplasmose congénitale et hydranencéphalie. *Ann. Pediatr. (Paris)* 28:427, 1981.

Koppe JG, et al.: Results of 20-year follow-up of congenital toxoplasmosis. *Lancet* 1:254, 1986.

Milgram JW: Osseous changes in congenital toxoplasmosis. *Arch. Pathol.* 97:150, 1974.

Neuenschwander S, et al.: Toxoplasmose congénitale: Apport de l'échotomographie transfontanellaire et de la tomodensitométrie. *Ann. Pediatr. (Paris)* 31:837, 1984.

Roussel B, et al.: Syndrome nephrotique congénital associé à une toxoplasmose congénitale. *Arch. Fr. Pediatr.* 44:795, 1987.

Sauerbrei EE, et al.: Neonatal brain: Sonography of congenital abnormalities. *A.J.R.* 136:1167, 1981.

Sever JL, et al.: Toxoplasmosis: Maternal and pediatric findings in 23,000 pregnancies. *Pediatrics* 82:181, 1988.

Shackelford GD, et al.: Neonatal hepatic calcification secondary to transplacental infection. *Radiology* 122:753, 1977.

Vanhaesebrouck P, et al: Congenital toxoplasmosis presenting as massive neonatal ascites. *Helv. Paediatr. Acta* 43:97, 1988.

FETAL TRIMETHADIONE SYNDROME

Clinical and Radiologic Manifestations: (a) prenatal growth failure, *mental deficiency*, speech disorders, visual and hearing deficits; (b) *craniofacial dysmorphism*; microcephaly, brachycephaly, midfacial hypoplasia, short nose, malformed and/or low-set ears, mild micrognathia, cleft lip and/or palate, high-arched palate, irregularities of the teeth, strabismus, myopia, V-shaped eyebrows, epicanthus, (c) cardiovascular anomalies; (d) urogenital anomalies: renal anomalies, hypospadias, etc.; (e) skeletal anomalies: congenital hip dislocation, clinodactyly, etc.; (f) other reported abnormalities: inguinal or umbilical hernia, webbed neck, short neck with a low hairline, widely spaced nipples, branchial cleft, common laryngoesophagus, tracheoesophageal defects, imperforate anus, simian creases, scoliosis, clubhand, meningomyelocele.

REFERENCES

Feldman GL, et al.: The fetal trimethadione syndrome. *Am. J. Dis. Child.* 131:1389, 1977.

German J, et al.: Trimethadione and human teratogenesis. *Teratology* 3:349, 1970.

Goldman AS, et al.: Fetal trimethadione syndrome. *Teratology* 17:103, 1978.

Zackai EH, et al.: The fetal trimethadione syndrome. *J. Pediatr.* 87:280, 1975.

FETAL VALPROATE SYNDROME

Clinical and Radiologic Manifestations: (a) *craniofacial anomalies:* midface hypoplasia, short nose with a broad and/or flat bridge, anteverted nostrils, shallow philtrum, thin upper lip, thick lower lip, epicanthic folds, minor abnormalities of the ear, micrognathia, ridging of the metopic suture, outer orbital ridge deficiency, bifrontal narrowing; (b) *developmental delay, neurological abnormalities;* (c) other reported abnormalities: tracheomalacia, talipes equinovarus, lumbosacral meningocele, urogenital anomalies, inguinal hernia, umbilical hernia, minor digital anomalies, heart defects (Fig SY—F—14).

REFERENCES

Ardinger HH, et al.: Verification of the fetal valproate syndrome phenotype. *Am. J. Med. Genet.* 29:171, 1988.

Chitayat D, et al: Congenital abnormalities in two sibs exposed to valproic acid in utero. *Am. J. Med. Genet.* 31:369, 1988.

DiLiberti JH, et al.: The fetal valproate syndrome. *Am. J. Med. Genet.* 19:473, 1984.

Winter RM, et al.: Fetal valproate syndrome: Is there a recognizable phenotype? *J. Med. Genet.* 24:692, 1987.

FETAL VARICELLA SYNDROME

Clinical Manifestations: (a) small for dates; (b) *cicatricial skin areas that correspond to dermatome distribution;* (c) *neurological anomalies:* limb paresis, seizures, Horner syndrome, bulbar dysphagia, mental retardation, optic nerve atrophy, anal sphincter malfunction, microcephaly, phrenic nerve palsy, auditory nerve palsy; (d) *eye anomalies:* chori-

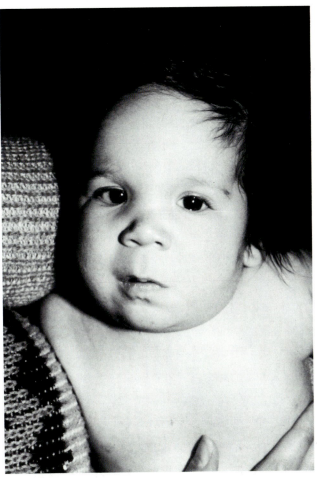

FIG SY–F–14.
Fetal valproate syndrome in a 2-month-old male having a tall, hirsute forehead with a depressed nasal bridge, hypertelorism, epicanthic folds, a long shallow philtrum, and a small mouth with a thin upper and a full lower lip. (From Winter RM, Donnai D, Burn J, et al.: Fetal valproate syndrome: Is there a recognisable phenotype? *J. Med. Genet.* 24:692, 1987. Used by permission.)

oretinitis, anisocoria, nystagmus, microphthalmos, cataract, coneal opacity, heterochromia; (e) hypoplasia of the limbs, hypoplasia of the digits, equinovarus, calcaneovalgus, hypoplasia of the mandible.

Radiologic Manifestations: (a) hydrocephalus, cortical brain atrophy, cerebral hypoplasia, basal ganglia and brain stem calcification; (b) hypoplasia of the scapulae and clavicles, hypoplasia of the ribs, scoliosis, lacunar skull; (c) alimentary tract anomalies; (d) genitourinary anomalies (Fig SY–F–15).

REFERENCES

Alkalay AL, et al.: Fetal varicella syndrome. *J. Pediatr.* 111:320, 1987.
Cuthbertson G, et al.: Prenatal diagnosis of second-trimester congenital varicella syndrome by virus-specific immunoglobulin M. *J. Pediatr.* 111:592, 1987.
Greenspoon JS, et al.: Fetal varicella syndrome. *J. Pediatr.* 112:505, 1988.
Palmer CGS, et al.: Intrauterine varicella infection. *J. Pediatr.* 112:506, 1988.

FG SYNDROME

Synonym: Opitz-Kaveggia syndrome.

Mode of Inheritance: X-linked, incompletely recessive.

Frequency: About 30 published cases (Thompson et al.).

Clinical and Radiologic Manifestations: (a) *mental retardation, congenital hypotonia,* seizures, short stature, sloping shoulders, brain dysgenesis (megalencephaly, heterotopia of neuroglial tissue, pachygyria, cortical dysgenesis); (b) *head: high and broad forehead, prominent nose, hypertelorism, frontal hair upsweep, medial eyebrow flare, small ears with a simple structure, micrognathia, inverted V-shaped upper lip, large mouth, protruding tongue, malocclusion;* (c) spinal anomalies, lumbar hyperlordosis, clubfoot, hyperextensible joints, broad thumbs and big toes, minimal cutaneous syndactyly; (d) other reported abnormalities: facial skin wrinkling, constipation, simian creases, recurrent episodes of pneumonia, cryptorchidism, agenesis of the corpus callosum, sensorineural deafness, *anal anomaly* (stenosis, imperforate anus), pyloric stenosis, hernia (umbilical, inguinal), high fin-

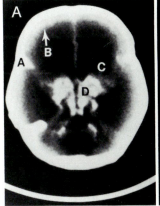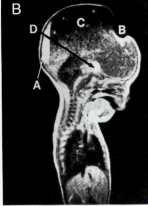

FIG SY–F–15.
Fetal varicella syndrome. **A,** postnatal computed tomography shows marked hydrocephalus *(C)* with only a thin mantle of cerebrum *(B)* persisting around enlarged ventricles and the underlying skull *(A)*. Also noted are extensive calcification in the basal ganglia *(D)* and brain stem (not shown). **B,** magnetic resonance imaging confirms presence of hydrocephalus *(C)*, with fluid-fluid level of different intensity in dependent occiput *(A)*. Calcifications were again seen in basal ganglia *(D)*. Also visible is cranial artifact secondary to metallic intravenous catheter in scalp vein *(B)*. (From Cuthbertson G, Weiner CP, Giller RH, et al.: Prenatal diagnosis of second-trimester congenital varicella syndrome by virus-specific immunoglobulin M. *J. Pediatr.* 111:592, 1987. Used by permission.)

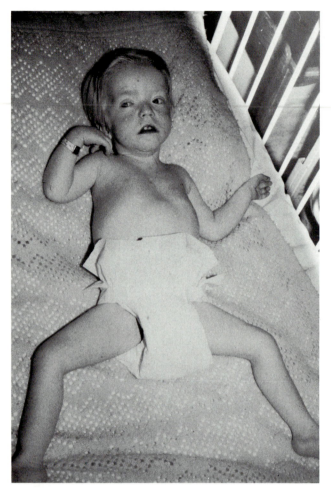

FIG SY–F–16.
The FG syndrome in 5⁸/₁₂-year-old male. Note the hypotonic posture, relative macrocephaly, broad forehead and "cowlicks" on the hairline, hypertelorism, and long philtrum. (From Thompson EM, Baraitser M, Lindenbaum RH, et al.: The FG syndrome: 7 new cases. *Clin. Genet.* 27:582, 1985. Used by permission.)

gertip whorl count and/or persistent fetal pads, "cystic" cavum septum pellucidi, etc. (Fig SY–F–16).

Note: F and G represent the initials of the families (Opitz et al.).

REFERENCES

Keller MA, et al.: A new syndrome of mental deficiency with craniofacial, limb, and anal anomalies. *J. Pediatr.* 88:589, 1976.
Neri G, et al.: Sensorineural deafness in the FG syndrome: Report on four new cases. *Am. J. Med. Genet.* 19:369, 1984.
Opitz JM, et al.: FG syndrome update 1988: Note of 5 new patients and bibliography. *Am. J. Med. Genet.* 30:309, 1988.
Opitz JM, et al.: Studies of malformation syndromes of man

XXXIII: The F G syndrome. An X-linked recessive syndrome of multiple congenital anomalies and mental retardation. *Z. Kinderheilkd.* 117:1, 1974.
Thompson EM, et al.: The FG syndrome: 7 new cases. *Clin. Genet.* 27:582, 1985.

FIBRODYSPLASIA OSSIFICANS PROGRESSIVA

Synonym: Myositis ossificans progressiva.

Mode of Inheritance: Autosomal dominant; complete penetrance; variable expressivity.

Frequency: Approximately 360 published cases (Thickman et al.).

Pathology: A mesodermal disorder, *progressive swelling and ossification of the fascia, aponeuroses, ligaments, tendons and connective tissue of skeletal muscle.*

Clinical Manifestations: (a) heat, muscle pain, inflammatory swelling, induration; (b) torticollis; (c) *microdactyly* (thumbs, hallux), webbed toes; (d) other reported abnormalities: fever, reduction defects of all digits, deafness, baldness of the scalp, mental retardation, progressive disability, restrictive movement of the spine and shoulder, exacerbation related to various factors (trauma, operation to excise ectopic bone, biopsy of the lumps, intramuscular injections and venipuncture, dental treatment), abnormal electrocardiogram, restrictive spirometry because of chest wall fixation.

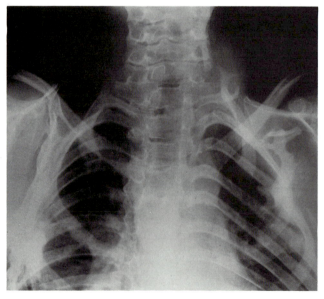

FIG SY–F–17.
Fibrodysplasia ossificans progressiva: ossification within soft tissues of the chest wall and neck. (From Wiedemann HR: Clinical syndromes associated with skeletal dysplasia. *Klin. Paediatr.* 184:165, 1972. Used by permission.)

Radiologic Manifestations: (a) *fibrous dysplasia with progressive ossification in muscles and subcutaneous tissues* in an apicocaudal direction with the neck involved in an early stage; (b) computed tomographic appearance: swelling of the muscular fascial planes prior to the development of ectopic ossification, ossification with a multifocal site pattern adjacent to and extending around muscles; magnetic resonance imaging: high signal intensity of the soft tissues, especially with T_2 weighting, nuclear medicine (technetium phosphate): enhanced uptake; (c) *ankylosis of interphalangeal, carpometacarpal, and metatarsophalangeal joints;* (d) *microdactyly (of the great toes and thumbs)* caused by shortness of the metatarsals and metacarpals, monophalangic great toe resulting from synostosis; (e) miscellaneous abnormalities of the extremities (hallux valgus, webbed toes, polydactyly, phalangeal synostosis, clinodactyly of the fifth fingers); (f) small vertebral bodies and enlarged pedicles in early childhood, variable degree of vertebral fusion in late childhood and in adults (neural arches first, followed by fusion of the vertebral bodies), narrow spinal canal; (g) exostoses commonly located in the proximal tibias, broad and short femoral neck, acetabular dysplasia, subluxation of the femoral head, delay in skeletal maturation, dysharmonious bone maturation, medial cortical thickening of the proximal tibia, accessory epiphysis of the second phalanx of the fifth finger, decreased humeral/epicondylar angle; (i) abnormal teeth (absence of the upper incisors).

Differential Diagnosis: Initial clinical presentation may be mistaken for skin, muscle, or bone infection; cervical vertebral changes may be confused with those of Klippel-Feil syndrome or rheumatoid arthritis; traumatic myositis ossificans; multiple exostoses; extraskeletal osteosarcoma; etc. (Figs SY−F−17 to SY−F−20).

REFERENCES

Connor JM, et al.: Cardiopulmonary function in fibrodysplasia ossificans progressiva. *Thorax* 36:419, 1981.

Connor JM, et al.: Fibrodysplasia ossificans progressiva. The clinical features and natural history of 34 patients. *J. Bone Joint Surg. [Br.]* 64:76, 1982.

Connor JM, et al.: Genetic aspects of fibrodysplasia ossificans progressiva. *J. Med. Genet.* 19:35, 1982.

Connor JM, et al.: The cervical spine in fibrodysplasia ossificans progressiva. *Br. J. Radiol.* 55:492, 1982.

Cremin B, et al.: The radiological spectrum of fibrodysplasia ossificans progressiva. *Clin. Radiol.* 33:499, 1982.

DiPietro MA: MRI of evolving fibrodysplasia ossificans progressiva (abstract). Presented at an International Pediatric Radiology Conference, Toronto, 1987.

Hall CM, et al.: Fibrodysplasie ossifiante progressive. *Ann. Radiol. (Paris)* 22:119, 1979.

Hentzer B, et al.: Fibrodysplasia (myositis) ossificans progressiva treated with disodium etidronate. *Clin. Radiol.* 29:69, 1978.

Reinig JW, et al.: Fibrodysplasia ossificans progressiva: CT appearance. *Radiology* 159:153, 1986.

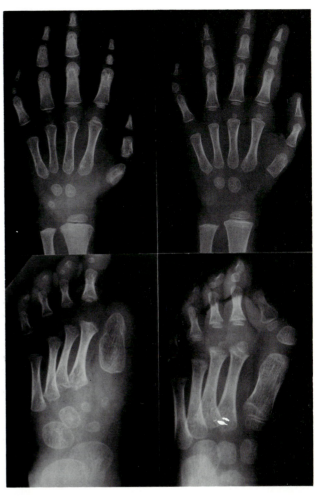

FIG SY−F−18.

Fibrodysplasia ossificans progressiva with microdactyly, shortness, and deformity of some of the metacarpals, metatarsals, and phalanges and hallux valgus. (From Wiedemann HR: Clinical syndromes associated with skeletal dysplasia. *Klin. Paediatr.* 184:165, 1972. Used by permission.)

Resnick D: Diagnosis: Fibrodysplasia ossificans progressiva (FOP): Radiological and gross pathological abnormalities in a macerated cadaver. *Skeletal Radiol.* 10:131, 1983.

Riley HD Jr, et al.: Myositis ossificans progressiva. *Pediatrics* 8:753, 1951.

Rogers JG, et al.: Fibrodysplasia ossificans progressiva: A survey of forty-two cases. *J. Bone Joint Surg. [Am.]* 61:909, 1979.

Smith R, et al.: Myositis ossificans progressiva. *J. Bone Joint Surg. [Br.]* 58:48, 1976.

Stizmann FC, et al.: Beitrag zum Krankheitsbild der Myositis ossificans progressiva. *Klin. Paediatr.* 186:384, 1974.

Thickman D, et al.: Fibrodysplasia ossificans progressiva. *A.J.R.* 139:935, 1982.

Voynow JA, et al.: Fibrodysplasia ossificans progressiva presenting as osteomyelitis-like syndrome. *Clin. Pediatr. (Phila.)* 25:373, 1986.

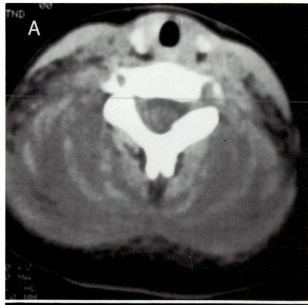

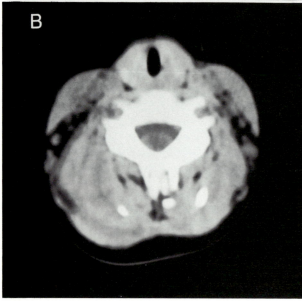

FIG SY–F–19.
Fibrodysplasia ossificans progressiva. **A,** muscles in the posterior part of the neck are separated by edema, which is present diffusely in the fascial plane in this computed tomographic scan. **B,** 6 months later, most of the edema has resolved in the left side of neck posteriorly; some residual edema is present in the right side of the neck. Small areas of ossification are present along the fascial planes in both sides of the neck. (From Reinig JW, Hill SC, Fang M, et al.: Fibrodysplasia ossificans progressiva: CT appearance. *Radiology* 159:153, 1986. Used by permission.)

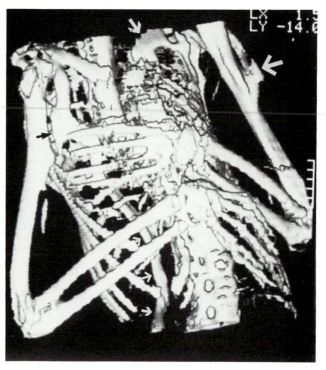

FIG SY–F–20.
Fibrodysplasia ossificans progressiva: three-dimensional reconstruction with extensive soft-tissue ossification *(arrows).* (Courtesy of Professor B.J. Cremin, Cape Town, South Africa.)

Wiedemann HR: Clinical syndromes associated with skeletal dysplasia. *Klin. Paediatr.* 184:165, 1972.
Wood BJ, et al.: Drug induced bone changes in myositis ossificans progressiva. *Pediatr. Radiol.* 5:40, 1976.

FIBROGENESIS IMPERFECTA OSSIUM

Mode of Inheritance: No apparent hereditary factor; one case report of a father and daughter affected by the disease.

Frequency: Rare.

Pathology: Replacement of the lamellar bone with abnormally thick and poorly calcified osteoid, absent lamellar collagen on polarized light microscopy; thin randomly distributed collagen fibrils with amorphous areas seen on electron microscopy.

Clinical Manifestations: (a) *progressive skeletal pain with onset in adult life;* (b) bone tenderness; (c) weakness; (d) muscular atrophy; (e) contractures; (f) *very high level of serum alkaline phosphatase,* benign paraproteinuria; (g) death within 3 years of diagnosis in about 40% of the cases.

Radiologic Manifestations: (a) *enlarged outer diameter of the bones of the appendicular skeleton;* (b) *coarse, thick, amorphous, and indistinct bone trabeculae;* (c) spotty in-

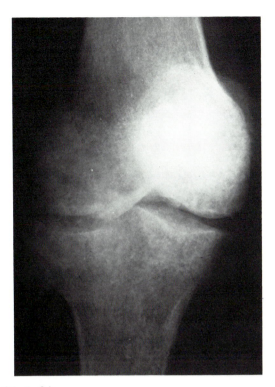

FIG SY—F—21.
Fibrogenesis imperfecta ossium: radiogram of a knee of a 51-year-old man with progressive pain in legs and pelvis. Coarsened, indistinct trabeculae with mottled areas of increased bone density and indistinct cortical margins are seen in the knee region. (From Frame B, Frost HM, Pack CY, et al.: Fibrogenesis imperfecta ossium: A collagen defect causing osteomalacia. *N. Engl. J. Med.* 285:769, 1971. Used by permission.)

creased bone density; (d) *thinning of the cortex;* (e) superimposed degenerative joint changes.

Differential Diagnosis: Paget disease; osteomalacia; osteoporosis (Fig SY-F-21).

REFERENCES

Baker SL, Turnbull HM: Two cases of hitherto undescribed disease characterized by a gross defect in the collagen of the bone matrix. *J. Pathol. Bacteriol.* 62:132, 1950.

Camus JP: Fibrogenesis imperfecta ossium. Study of two cases in one family. *Ann. Med. Interne (Paris)* 126:583, 1975.

Connor R: Fibrogenesis imperfecta ossium: Case of the season. *Semin. Roentgenol.* 20:325, 1985.

Frame B, et al.: Fibrogenesis imperfecta ossium: A collagen defect causing osteomalacia. *N. Engl. J. Med.* 285:769, 1971.

Stamp TCB, et al.: Fibrogenesis imperfecta ossium: Remission with melphalan. *Lancet* 1:582, 1985.

Stoddart PGP, et al.: Fibrogenesis imperfecta ossium. *Br. J. Radiol.* 57:744, 1984.

Swan CHJ, et al.: Fibrogenesis imperfecta ossium. *Q. J. Med.* 45:178, 1976.

FIBROUS DYSPLASIA CLASSIFICATION

1. Monostotic fibrous dysplasia, sporadic
2. Monostotic fibrous dysplasia, congenital
3. Polyostotic fibrous dysplasia (Jaffe-Lichtenstein)
4. Polyostotic fibrous dysplasia with pigmentary skin changes and precocious puberty (McCune-Albright syndrome)
5. Cherubism
6. Congenital fibromatosis (of bone and soft tissues)
7. Fibrous cortical defect and nonossifying fibroma
8. Ossifying fibroma
9. Fibrogenesis imperfecta ossium
10. Focal fibrocartilaginous dysplasia causing tibia vara
11. Panostotic fibrous dysplasia: a congenital disorder of bone with unusual facial appearance, bone fragility, hyperphosphatasemia, and hypophosphatemia
12. Jaffe-Campanacci syndrome

FIBROUS DYSPLASIA (CONGENITAL MONOSTOTIC)

Synonym: Congenital monostotic fibrous dysplasia.

Mode of Inheritance: Autosomal recessive.

Frequency: Two reported cases.

Clinical Manifestations: Presentation in infancy: mandibular swelling, bulging alveolar ridge, secondary dental abnormalities.

Radiologic Manifestations: Expanding lytic lesion of the mandible involving the symphyseal region; tooth displacement.

Differential Diagnosis: Cherubism.

REFERENCE

El Deeb M, et al.: Congenital monostotic fibrous dysplasia—a new possibly autosomal recessive disorder. *J. Oral Surg.* 37:520, 1979.

FIBROUS DYSPLASIA (JAFFE-LICHTENSTEIN)

Synonym: Polyostotic fibrous dysplasia.

Mode of Inheritance: Sporadic.

Frequency: Uncommon, underreported.

Pathology: Excessive proliferation of spindle cell fibrous tissues in bones.

Clinical Manifestations: Symptoms appear in childhood or adolescence: (a) pain; (b) limp; (c) *limb deformity, discrepancy of leg length, pathological fracture;* (d) *skull asymmetry,* leontiasis appearance; (e) scoliosis, lordosis, spinal cord compression, chest deformity; (f) other reported abnormalities: hypophosphatemic osteomalacia, osseous sarcoma, pituitary gigantism and hyperthyroidism, familial occurrence of hyperparathyroidism and fibrous dysplasia (mother and daughter), fibrodysplasia ossificans progressiva, arteriovenous malformations, platelet trapping (Kasabach-Merritt syndrome); (g) malignant transformation usually osteosarcoma (0.5%).

Radiologic Manifestations: Tendency to unilateral skeletal involvement: (a) *lacunar or mixed, somewhat opaque lesions;* (b) *thinning and expansion of the cortex;* (c) *bowing of long bones;* (d) pathological fracture with abundant periosteal new bone formation; (e) epiphyseal involvement (rare); (f) *hyperostosis of the skull,* in particular, at the base; *obliteration of paranasal sinuses, decrease in size of the involved orbit.*

REFERENCES

Dent CE, et al.: Hypophosphataemic osteomalacia in fibrous dysplasia. *Q. J. Med.* 45:411, 1976.
Firat D, et al.: Fibrous dysplasia of the bone. Review of twenty-four cases. *Am. J. Med.* 44:421, 1968.
Frame B, et al.: Polyostotic fibrous dysplasia and myositis ossificans progressiva. *Am. J. Dis. Child.* 124:120, 1972.
Gibson MJ, et al.: Fibrous dysplasia of bone. *Br. J. Radiol.* 44:1, 1971.
Grabias SL, et al.: Fibrous dysplasia. *Orthop. Clin. North Am.* 8:771, 1977.
Lemli L, et al.: Fibrous dysplasia of bone. Report of female monozygotic twins with and without the McCune-Albright syndrome. *J. Pediatr.* 91:947, 1977.
Lichtenstein L: Polyostotic fibrous dysplasia. *Arch. Surg.* 36:874, 1938.
Lichtenstein L, Jaffe HL: Fibrous dysplasia of bone. *Arch. Pathol.* 33:777, 1942.
Mouterde P, et al.: Les problèmes orthopédiques de la dysplasie fibreuse des os chez l'enfant: À propos de 23 observations. *Chir. Pediatr.* 19:169, 1978.
Nixon GW, et al.: Epiphyseal involvement in polyostotic fibrous dysplasia: A report of two cases. *Radiology* 106:167, 1973.
Pons A, et al.: La dégénérescence maligne de la dysplasie fibreuse des os: Revue générale à propos de deux observations. *Ann. Radiol. (Paris)* 17:713, 1974.
Saito A, et al.: Pre and post operative management of Kasabach-Merrit syndrome. *Masui* 33:423, 1984.
Taconis WK: Osteosarcoma in fibrous dysplasia. *Skeletal Radiol.* 17:163, 1988.
Tchang SPK: The small orbit sign in supraorbital fibrous dysplasia. *J. Can. Assoc. Radiol.* 24:65, 1973.

FILIPPI SYNDROME

Mode of Inheritance: Three of eight siblings affected.

Clinical and Radiological Manifestations: (a) low birth weight, growth retardation; (b) unusual facial appearance (protuding forehead, broad and prominent nasal root, diminished alar flare); (c) syndactyly of the third and fourth fingers, clinodactyly of the fifth fingers, syndactyly of the toes (2, 3, 4); (d) mental retardation.

REFERENCE

Filippi G: Unusual facial appearance, microcephaly, growth and mental retardation, and syndactyly. A new syndrome? *Am. J. Med. Genet.* 22:821, 1985.

FITZ-HUGH–CURTIS SYNDROME

Synonym: Venereal perihepatitis.

Pathology and Etiology: Anterior perihepatitis; (b) genitourinary infection (gonococcus, *Chlamydia trachomatis).*

Clinical Manifestations: (a) *acute right upper quadrant abdominal pain* that may be referred to the right shoulder and back; (b) guarding, positive Murphy sign; (c) laparoscopy: *perihepatitis,* salpingitis (not in all cases).

Radiologic Manifestations: (a) ultrasonography: perihepatic effusion, thickening of the Glisson capsule; (b) salpingitis; (c) absence of right renal, hepatic, or biliary system abnormalities.

REFERENCES

Curtis H: A cause of adhesions in the right upper quadrant. *J.A.M.A.* 94:1221, 1930.
Fitz-Hugh T Jr: Acute gonococcic perihepatitis of the right upper quadrant in women. *J.A.M.A.* 102:2094, 1934.
Katzman DK, et al.: *Chlamydia trachomatis* Fitz-Hugh–Curtis syndrome without salpingitis in female adolescents. *Am. J. Dis. Child.* 142:996, 1988.
Paavonen J, et al.: Association of infection with *Chlamydia trachomatis* with Fitz-Hugh–Curtis syndrome. *J. Infect. Dis.* 144:176, 1981.
Saint D, et al.: Le syndrome de Fitz-Hugh Curtis. A propos d'un aspect ultrasonore hépatique particulier. *J. Radiol.* 65:477, 1984.
Shanahan D, et al.: Chlamydial Fitz-Hugh/Curtis syndrome. *Lancet* 1:1216, 1986.

FLOPPY VALVE SYNDROME

Synonym: Multiple floppy valve syndrome.

Pathology: *Disruption and loss of normal valvular architecture and an increase in ground substance* (aortic and mitral valves primarily involved).

Clinical Manifestations: (a) dyspnea, chest pain; (b) cardiomegaly, *cardiac murmur,* congestive heart failure (in some), *left ventricular hypertrophy;* (c) echocardiography: fluttering and large excursion of valves, cardiac chamber enlargement.

Radiologic Manifestations: (a) cardiomegaly; (b) cardio-angiographic demonstration of cardiac chamber enlargement, left ventricular hypertrophy, *valvular insufficiency, prolapsing valvular cusps.*

Note: Aortic valve prolapse may occur in 4% to 22% of patients with mitral valve prolapse; isolated aortic valve prolapse has rarely been reported.

REFERENCES

Arvan S: Aortic valve prolapse in congenital and acquired systemic disease. *Arch. Intern. Med.* 145:1601, 1985.
Barlow JB, et al.: Billowing, floppy, prolapsed or flail mitral valves? *Am. J. Cardiol.* 55:501, 1985.
Chandraratna AN, et al.: Echocardiography of the "floppy" aortic valve. *Circulation* 52:959, 1975.
Read RC, et al.: Symptomatic valvular myxomatous transformation (the floppy valve syndrome): A possible forme fruste of the Marfan syndrome. *Circulation* 32:897, 1965.
Rippe JM, et al.: Multiple floppy valves: An echocardiographic syndrome. *Am. J. Med.* 66:817, 1979.
Tutassaura H, et al.: Mucoid degeneration of the mitral valve. *Am. J. Surg.* 132:276, 1976.

FLYNN-AIRD SYNDROME

Mode of Inheritance: Autosomal dominant.

Clinical and Radiologic Manifestations: (a) *premature senility;* (b) *myopia, cataract, retinitis pigmentosa;* (c) *peripheral neuropathy, ataxia, seizures, dementia,* sensorineural hearing loss, elevated cerebrospinal fluid protein levels; (d) *cutaneous atrophy,* chronic ulceration, baldness; (e) other abnormalities: joint stiffness, dental caries, osteoporosis, kyphoscoliosis, cystic changes in the pelvic bones, muscular atrophy.

REFERENCE

Flynn P, Aird RB: A neuroectodermal syndrome of dominant inheritance. *J. Neurol. Sci.* 2:161, 1965.

FOCAL SCLERODERMA

Clinical Manifestations: (a) skin lesions on the face, trunk, and limbs of different size and shape, often unilateral; scalp and facial lesions have a coup de sabre appearance; *erythema and edema in the early phase followed by a waxy color and finally skin atrophy and hypopigmentation;* (b) other reported abnormalities: contracture; arthralgia; nerve compression; central nervous system changes; impaired esophageal peristalsis; secondary changes in subcutaneous tissue, muscle, tendon, and synovial tissue (atrophy, growth

arrest, contracture); nodules in the tendons; carpal tunnel syndrome, Raynaud phenomenon.

Radiologic Manifestations: (a) *skeletal demineralization* and muscular atrophy underlying the skin lesions; (b) *soft-tissue calcification.*

Note: The terms *cutaneous* and *subcutaneous inflammatory sclerotic syndromes* are used for systemic scleroderma, morphea profunda, eosinophilic fasciitis, and focal scleroderma.

REFERENCES

Chazen EM, et al.: Focal scleroderma: Report of 19 cases in children. *J. Pediatr.* 60:385, 1962.
Christianson HB, et al.: Localized scleroderma: Clinical study of 235 cases. *Arch. Dermatol.* 74:629, 1956.
Doyle JA, et al.: Cutaneous and subcutaneous inflammatory sclerosis syndromes. *Arch. Dermatol.* 118:886, 1982.
Fagge CH: On keloid, scleriasis, morphea, and some allied affections. *Guy's Hosp. Rep.* 13:255, 1867.
Floyd WE, et al.: Focal scleroderma affecting the hand. *J. Bone Joint Surg. [Am.]* 67:637, 1985.
Kornreich HK, et al.: Scleroderma in childhood. *Arthritis Rheum.* 20:343, 1977.
Sussman SJ, et al.: Picture of month: Focal scleroderma. *Am. J. Dis. Child.* 123:486, 1972.

FOSTER KENNEDY SYNDROME

Clinical and Radiologic Manifestations: (a) retrobulbar neuritis with the formation of a central scotoma and primary optic atrophy on the side of the lesion; (b) papilledema in the opposite eye; (c) depression or a loss of the sense of smell on the side of retrobulbar neuritis; (d) intracranial basofrontal lesion.

REFERENCES

Frenkel RE, et al.: Visual loss and intoxication. *Surv. Ophthalmol.* 30:391, 1986.
Gupta SR, et al.: Foster-Kennedy syndrome due to optochiasmatic arachnoiditis. *Surg. Neurol.* 20:216, 1983.
Jarus GD, et al.: Clinical and computed tomographic findings in the Foster Kennedy syndrome. *Am. J. Ophthalmol.* 93:317, 1982.
Kennedy F: Retrobulbar neuritis as an exact diagnostic sign of certain tumors and abscesses in the frontal lobe. *Am. J. Med. Sci.* 142:355, 1911.
Massey EW, et al.: Foster Kennedy syndrome. *Arch. Neurol.* 41:658, 1984.

FOUNTAIN SYNDROME

Mode of Inheritance: Autosomal recessive.

Frequency: Seven published cases (Fryns et al.).

Clinical Manifestations: (a) mental retardation; (b) deaf mutism; (c) coarse face, full lips, swelling of the face with "edematous" infiltration of the subcutaneous tissue; (d) short, stubby hand.

Radiologic Manifestations: (a) anomalies of the turns of the cochlea; (b) marked thickness of the calvarium; (c) short metacarpals and phalanges with a thick cortex.

REFERENCES

Fountain RB: Familial bone abnormalities, deaf mutism, mental retardation, and skin granulomas. *Proc. R. Soc. Med.* 67:878, 1974.
Fryns J-P, et al.: Mental retardation, deafness, skeletal abnormalities, and coarse face with full lips: Confirmation of the Fountain syndrome. *Am. J. Med. Genet.* 26:551, 1987.

FRASER SYNDROME

Synonyms: Cryptophthalmos-syndactyly syndrome; cryptophthalmia syndrome.

Frequency: 68 published cases to 1987 (Gattuso et al.).

Clinical Manifestations: (a) craniofacial abnormalities: *unilateral or bilateral cryptophthalmos* (93%), extended hair growth on the forehead (34%), ear abnormalities (cupped, low-set, underdeveloped, fused, atresia or stenosis of the external auditory canals, defect of the middle ear) (44%), hypertelorism, nose abnormalities (37%), midline fissure (nose, upper lip, tongue), dental abnormalities, lacrimal duct defects, coloboma of the upper eyelid, cleft lip/palate, tongue tie, Potter facies; (b) *syndactyly of the fingers* (54%); (c) urinary system abnormalities (37%): renal hypoplasia or agenesis, ureteral anomalies, bladder anomalies, cystic dysplastic kidneys; (d) genital anomalies (49%): clitoral hypertrophy, bicornuate uterus, vaginal atresia, cystic ovaries, rudimentary uterus, undifferentiated genital tubercle, cryptorchidism, underdeveloped penis, hypospadias, indeterminate sex; (e) other reported abnormalities: laryngeal stenosis/atresia, umbilical hernia, exomphalos, pulmonary hypoplasia, anal atresia, anal stenosis, hypoplasia or an absent thumb, clubfoot, microcephaly, congenital heart defect, umbilical displacement, gonadoblastoma in situ, etc.

Radiologic Manifestations: (a) *ocular abnormalities*: calcified lens, absence of the lens, abnormal size and contour of the globe, abnormalities of the rectus muscles (thin), cystic structure within the orbit, absence of lacrimal glands, etc.; (b) skull abnormalities: parietal lacunae, flattening of the frontal eminence or temple, microcephaly, meningoencephalocele; (c) urogenital anomalies: renal dysplasia, renal agenesis; (d) *syndactyly*; (e) other reported abnormalities: wide separation of the pubic symphysis, bowel malrotation (Fig SY–F–22).

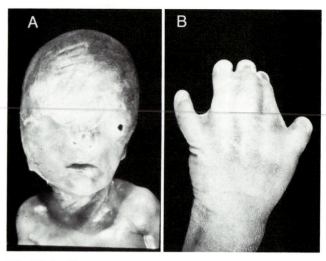

FIG SY–F–22.
Fraser syndrome (cryptophthalmos-syndactyly syndrome) in a 24-week-old fetus. **A,** cryptophthalmos, complete on the right and partial on the left. **B,** syndactyly of the fingers. (From Boyd PA, Keeling JW, Lindenbaum RH: Fraser syndrome (cryptophthalmos-syndactyly syndrome): A review of eleven cases with postmortem findings. *Am. J. Med. Genet.* 31:159, 1988. Used by permission.)

REFERENCES

Bïaler MG, et al.: Syndromic cryptophthalmos. *Am. J. Med. Genet.* 30:835, 1988.
Brodsky I, et al.: Cryptophthalmos or ablepharia: A survey of the condition with a review of the literature and the presentation of a case. *Med. J. Aust.* 1:894, 1940.
Burn J, et al.: Fraser syndrome presenting as bilateral renal agenesis in three sibs. *J. Med. Genet.* 19:360, 1982.
Dinno ND, et al.: The cryptophthalmos-syndactyly syndrome. *Clin. Pediatr. (Phila.)* 13:219, 1974.
Fraser GR: Malformation syndromes with eye or ear involvement. *Birth Defects* 5:130, 1969.
Gattuso J, et al.: The clinical spectrum of the Fraser syndrome: Report of three new cases and review. *J. Med. Genet.* 24:549, 1987.
Greenberg F, et al.: Gonadal dysgenesis and gonadoblastoma in situ in a female with Fraser (cryptophthalmos) syndrome. *J. Pediatr.* 108:952, 1986.
Koenig R, et al.: Cryptophthalmos-syndactyly syndrome without cryptophthalmos. *Clin. Genet.* 29:413, 1986.
Levine RS, et al.: The cryptophthalmos syndrome. *A.J.R.* 143:375, 1984.
Lurie IW, et al.: Renal agenesis as a diagnostic feature of the cryptophthalmos-syndactyly syndrome. *Clin. Genet.* 25:528, 1984.
Thomas IT, et al.: Isolated and syndromic cryptophthalmos. *Am. J. Med. Genet.* 25:85, 1986.

FREEMAN-SHELDON SYNDROME

Synonyms: Whistling face syndrome; craniocarpotarsal dystrophy; craniocarpotarsal dysplasia.

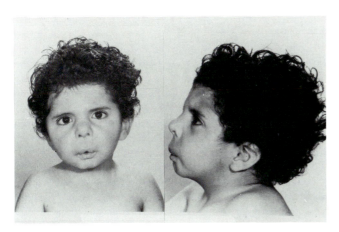

FIG SY–F–23.
Freeman-Sheldon syndrome. A masklike rigid face, a low fore-head, pseudoconvergent strabismus, hypertelorism, a broad nasal bridge, a long flat philtrum, protruding lips (whistling face), receding chin, low hairlines, a short neck, and low-set ears are present. (Courtesy of Dr. H. Malkawi, Amman, Jordan.)

Mode of Inheritance: Genetic heterogeneity: autosomal dominant; sporadic (usually more sererely affected); autosomal recessive in some families.

Frequency: More than 60 published cases to 1987 (Wang et al.).

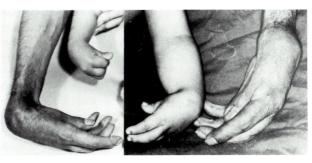

FIG SY–F–24.
Freeman-Sheldon syndrome; hand deformities of a father and son: contracture of the wrists and thumb-in-hand deformity. (From Malkawi H, Tarawneh M: The whistling face syndrome, or cranio-carpo-tarsal dysplasia. Report of two cases in a father and son and review of the literature. *J. Pediatr. Orthop.* 3:364, 1983. Used by permission.)

Clinical Manifestations: (a) *characteristic facies: microstomia, lip protrusion held as in whistling, H-shaped groove of the chin, flatness of the midface,* small nose, sunken eyes, high-arched palate, small tongue, ocular hypertelorism, long philtrum, epicanthus; (b) short and broad neck, mild pterygium coli; (c) *ulnar deviation of the hands, finger contractures,* nonopposable thumbs, camptodactyly; (d) *clubfoot deformity;* (e) small stature; (f) other reported abnormalities: strabismus, ptosis, blepharophimosis, low birth weight,

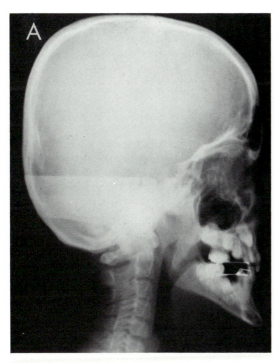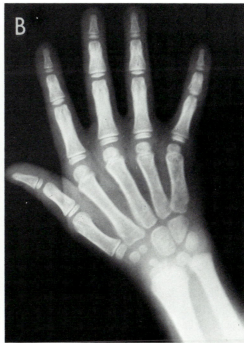

FIG SY–F–25.
Freeman-Sheldon syndrome in a 10-year-old female. **A,** the skull in lateral projection has a square form, and the anterior cranial base is short and steep; facial height is reduced, and the midface is flattened. The chin has a pointed appearance. **B,** note the ulnar deviation of the fingers without evidence of bony deformities. (From Weinstein S, Gorlin RJ: Cranio-carpo-tarsal dystrophy. *Am. J. Dis. Child.* 117:427, 1969. Used by permission.)

Syndromes

walking difficulties, feeding difficulties, mental retardation, microcephaly, brachycephaly, muscle wasting, global increase in muscle tone, an adducted and palm-clutched thumb, inguinal hernia, undescended testes, rocker-bottom appearance of the feet.

Radiologic Manifestations: (a) *craniofacial disproportion,* dolichocephaly, steep anterior fossa, small malar bones, small mandible; (b) *ulnar deviation of the hands, flexed thumbs, contracture of the fingers and toes, equinovarus feet;* (c) retarded skeletal maturation, disharmonious maturation with retarded development of the carpal centers when compared with those in the phalanges; (d) other reported abnormalities: tall vertebrae with a narrow anteroposterior diameter, flattened vertebrae, kyphosis or kyphoscoliosis, spina bifida occulta, spatulate ("canoe paddle") ribs, increase in the width of the long bones, hip contracture, hip dislocation, long and vertically oriented ischia, genu valgum deformity, vertical talus deformity, renal anomalies (atrophy, hydronephrosis), etc. (Figs SY−F−23 to SY−F−25).

REFERENCES

Freeman EA, Sheldon JH: Cranio-carpo-tarsal dystrophy: An undescribed congenital malformation. *Arch. Dis. Child.* 13:277, 1938.

Hashemi G: The whistling-face syndrome: Report of a case with a renal anomaly. *Indian J. Pediatr.* 40:23, 1973.

Malkawi H, et al.: The whistling face syndrome, or cranio-carpotarsal dysplasia. Report of two cases in a father and son and review of the literature. *J. Pediatr. Orthop.* 3:364, 1983.

O'Connell DJ, et al.: Cranio-carpo-tarsal dysplasia: A report of seven cases. *Radiology* 123:719, 1977.

Patel M, et al.: A case of Freeman-Sheldon syndrome (cranio-carpotarsal dysplasia) with spatulate ("canoe paddle") ribs. *Br. J. Radiol.* 56:50, 1983.

Sánchez JM, et al.: New evidence for genetic heterogeneity of the Freeman-Sheldon syndrome. *Am. J. Med. Genet.* 25:507, 1986.

Sheldon (syndrome du siffleur). *Arch. Fr. Pediatr.* 30:218, 1973.

Vaněk J, et al.: Freeman-Sheldon syndrome: A disorder of congenital myopathic origin? *J. Med. Genet.* 23:231, 1986.

Wang TR, et al.: Further evidence for genetic heterogeneity of whistling face or Freeman-Sheldon syndrome in a Chinese family. *Am. J. Med. Genet.* 28:471, 1987.

FRIEDREICH ATAXIA

Synonyms: Friedreich disease; ataxia hereditaria; spinal hereditary ataxia; hereditary ataxia.

Mode of Inheritance: Autosomal recessive.

Clinical Manifestations: *Progressive spinocerebellar degeneration with an onset of symptoms in the preadolescent period:* (a) incoordination, dysarthria, Babinsky sign, *dimin-ished or absent tendon reflexes,* impairment of vibratory and position senses, convulsions, eye movement abnormalities (fixation instability, inaccurate saccades with normal peak velocity, impaired smooth pursuit and optokinetic slow phases, decreased vestibulo-ocular reflex gain, impaired visual-vestibular interaction), auditory dysfunction (brain stem origin), normal motor conduction; (b) *kyphoscoliosis, pes cavus, hammer toe;* (c) cardiomyopathy: palpitation, dyspnea, pain, syncope, cardiac murmurs; left ventricular hypertrophy; echocardiographic demonstration of muscular hypertrophy with or without evidence of outflow tract obstruction, normal or small left ventricular chamber, abnormal systolic movement of the mitral valve, cardiopathy as the presenting manifestation of the disease in childhood (echocardiographic concentric left ventricular hypertrophy preceding the neurological syndrome), heart failure; (d) glucose metabolism alterations.

Radiologic Manifestations: (a) *generalized cardiac enlargement or left ventricular enlargement;* cardioangiographic demonstration of septal hypertrophy, outflow obstruction and large coronary arteries; (b) kyphoscoliosis; (c) foot deformities.

REFERENCES

Ackroyd RS, et al.: Friedreich's ataxia. A clinical review with neurophysiological and echocardiographic findings. *Arch. Dis. Child.* 59:217, 1984.

Alboliras ET, et al.: Spectrum of cardiac involvement in Friedreich's ataxia: Clinical, electrocardiographic and echocardiographic observations. *Am. J. Cardiol.* 58:518, 1986.

Berg RA, et al.: Friedreich's ataxia with acute cardiomyopathy. *Am. J. Dis. Child.* 134:390, 1980.

Daher YH, et al.: Spinal deformities in patients with Friedreich ataxia: A review of 19 patients. *J. Pediatr. Orthop.* 5:553, 1985.

Finocchiaro G, et al.: Glucose metabolism alterations in Friedreich's ataxia. *Neurology* 38:1292, 1988.

Friedreich N: Ueber degenerative Atrophie der spinalen Hinterstränge. *Arch. Pathol. Anat.* 26:391, 433, 1863.

Furman JM, et al.: Eye movements in Friedreich's ataxia. *Arch. Neurol.* 40:343, 1983.

Jabbari B, et al.: Early abnormalities of brainstem auditory evoked potentials in Friedreich's ataxia: Evidence of primary brainstem dysfunction. *Neurology* 33:1071, 1983.

James TN, et al.: Coronary disease, cardioneuropathy, and conduction system abnormalities in the cardiomyopathy of Friedreich's ataxia. *Br. Heart J.* 57:446, 1987.

Palagi B, et al.: Biventricular function in Friedreich's ataxia: A radionuclide angiographic study. *Br. Heart J.* 59:692, 1988.

Sharratt GP, et al.: Friedreich's ataxia presenting as cardiac disease. *Pediatr. Cardiol.* 6:41, 1985.

FRONTO-FACIO-NASAL DYSPLASIA

Mode of Inheritance: Autosomal recessive.

Frequency: Two siblings and one sporadic case (Gallop et al.).

Clinical and Radiologic Manifestations: (a) craniofacial anomalies: blepharophimosis; lagophthalmos; primary telecanthus; S-shaped palpebral fissures; eyelid coloboma; facial hypoplasia; widow's peak; cranium bifidum occultum defect; frontal lipoma; nasal hypoplasia; bifid nose; deformed nostrils; cleft lip, premaxilla, palate, and uvula; (b) other reported abnormalities: encephalocele, cataract, absent eyelashes, microphthalmos, microcornea, coloboma of the iris.

REFERENCES

Gollop TR: Fronto-facio-nasal dysostosis—a new autosomal recessive syndrome (letter). *Am. J. Med. Genet.* 10:409, 1981.
Gollop TR, et al.: Frontofacionasal dysplasia: Evidence for autosomal recessive inheritance. *Am. J. Med. Genet.* 19:301, 1984.

FRYNS SYNDROME

Mode of Inheritance: Autosomal recessive most likely.

Frequency: Seven published cases (Schwyzer et al.).

Clinical and Radiologic Manifestations: A lethal (prenatal or postnatal) syndrome, corneal clouding, diaphragmatic defect, anteverted nares, abnormal helices/lobules, micrognathia, short/thick neck, camptodactyly, hypoplastic lung, renal anomalies, genital anomalies, central nervous system anomalies, cleft palate, hypoplastic nails (Fig SY–F–26).

REFERENCES

Fryns JP: Fryns syndrome: A variable MCA syndrome with diaphragmatic defects, coarse face, and distal limb hypoplasia. *J. Med. Genet.* 24:271, 1987.
Fryns JP, et al.: A new lethal syndrome with cloudy corneae, diaphragmatic defects and distal limb deformities. *Hum. Genet.* 50:65, 1979.

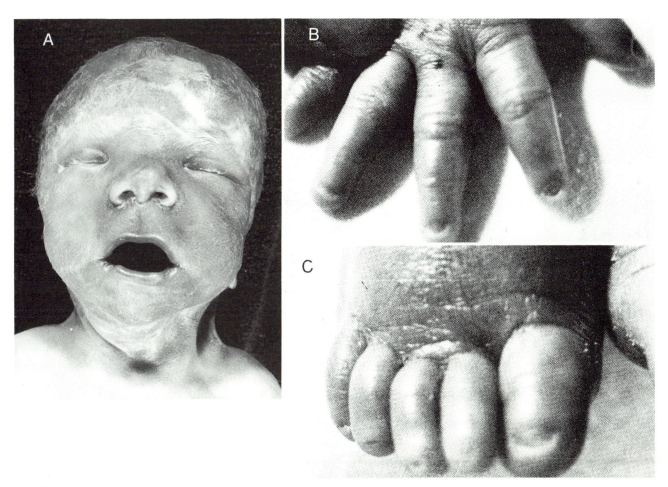

FIG SY–F–26.
Fryns syndrome. **A,** coarse face, broad flat nasal bridge, and micrognathia. **B** and **C,** hypoplastic terminal phalanges of all fingers and toes with small nails. (From Fryns JP: Fryns syndrome: A variable MCA syndrome with diaphragmatic defects, coarse face, and distal limb hypoplasia. *J. Med. Genet.* 24:271, 1987. Used by permission.)

Schwyzer U, et al.: Fryns syndrome in a girl born to consanguineous parents. *Acta. Paediatr. Scand.* 76:167, 1987.

FUKUYAMA-TYPE MUSCULAR DYSTROPHY

Synonym: Muscular dystrophy, Fukuyama type.

Mode of Inheritance: Autosomal recessive, most prevalent in Japanese.

Pathology: Brain dysgenesis: cerebral and cerebellar micropolygyria, fibroglial proliferation in the leptomeninges, hydrocephalus, focal interhemispheric fusion, hypoplasia of the corticospinal tracts, etc.

Clinical Manifestations: Onset of symptoms in early infancy: (a) *hypotonia, muscular weakness;* (b) *mental retardation;* (c) *seizures;* (d) *abnormal electroencephalographic findings.*

Radiologic Manifestations: *Micropolygyria;* hydrocephalus.

REFERENCES

Fukuyama Y, et al.: A peculiar form of congenital progressive muscular dystrophy. Report of fifteen cases. *Paediatr. Universit (Tokyo)* 4:5, 1960.

Fukuyama Y, et al.: Congenital progressive muscular dystrophy of the Fukuyama type: Clinical, genetic and pathologic considerations. *Brain Dev.* 3:1, 1981.

McMenamin JB, et al.: Fujuyama-type congenital muscular dystrophy. *J. Pediatr.* 101:580, 1982.

Mitsuishi Y, et al.: X-ray CT and MRI findings in Fukuyama type congenital muscular dystrophy (abstract). *Neuroradiology* 29:591, 1987.

Takada K, et al.: Cortical dysplasia in congenital muscular dystrophy with central nervous system involvement (Fukuyama type). *J. Neuropathol. Exp. Neurol.* 43:395, 1984.

Wakayama Y, et al.: Freeze-fracture studies of muscle plasma membrane in Fukuyama-type congenital muscular dystrophy. *Neurology* 35:1587, 1985.

G SYNDROME

Synonyms: Opitz-Frias syndrome; Opitz-G syndrome.

Mode of Inheritance: Autosomal dominant sex-limited transmission.

Frequency: Over 100 cases (Opitz, 1987).

Clinical Manifestations: (a) *cephalofacial features:* dolichocephalic skull, prominent parietal eminences and occiput, large anterior fontanelle, hypertelorism, flattened nasal bridge, anteversion of nostrils, narrow palpebral fissures, epicanthic folds, strabismus, micrognathia, auricular abnormalities; (b) *hoarse cry;* (c) swallowing/respiratory difficulties; (d) *hypospadias,* chordee; (e) other reported abnormalities: congenital heart disease, imperforate anus, rectourethral fistula, cleft lip, cleft palate, laryngotracheoesophageal cleft, hypoplasia of the larynx, mental retardation in surviving children, high-arched palate, hypotonia, neurological abnormalities, umbilical hernia, inguinal hernia, lacrimal duct obstruction, congenital lymphedema, simian crease(s), crowded toes, brachycephaly, pectus carinatum, pectus excavatum, cryptorchidism, deep sacral dimple, short lingual frenulum, abnormal tooth position, long fingers/toes, clinodactyly, Sandifer syndrome, sudden death.

Radiologic Manifestations: (a) neuromuscular disorder with *incoordination in swallowing and esophageal function,* gastroesophageal regurgitation; (b) aspiration pneumonia; (c) other reported abnormalities: hiatal hernia, small stomach, gastrointestinal anomalies, bowel malrotation, agenesis of the gallbladder, large anterior fontanelle, wide cranial sutures, absent corpus callosum, etc.

Note: "G" represents the initial of the first family reported with this syndrome.

REFERENCES

Allanson JE: G syndrome: An unusual family. *Am. J. Med. Genet.* 31:637, 1988.

Côté GB, et al.: The G syndrome of dysphagia, ocular hypertelorism and hypospadias. *Clin. Genet.* 19:473, 1981.

Einfeld SL, et al.: Sudden death in childhood in a case of the G syndrome. *Am. J. Med. Genet.* 28:293, 1987.

Little JR, et al.: The G syndrome. *Am. J. Dis. Child.* 121:505, 1971.

Neri G, et al.: A girl with G syndrome and agenesis of the corpus callosum. *Am. J. Med. Genet.* 28:287, 1987.

Opitz JM: G syndrome (hypertelorism with esophageal abnormality and hypospadias, or hypospadias-dysphagia, or "Opitz-Frias" or "Opitz-G" syndrome)—Perspective in 1987 and bibliography (editorial). *Am. J. Med. Genet.* 28:275, 1987.

Opitz JM, Frias JL, Gutenberger JE, et al.: The G syndrome of multiple congenital anomalies. *Birth Defects* 5(2):95, 1969.

Tolmie JL, et al.: Congenital anal anomalies in two families with the Opitz G syndrome. *J. Med. Genet.* 24:688, 1987.

Williams CA, et al.: Apparent G syndrome presenting as neck and upper limb dystonia and severe gastroesophageal reflux. *Am. J. Med. Genet.* 28:297, 1987.

Wilson GN, et al.: Further delineation of the G syndrome: A manageable genetic cause of infantile dysphagia. *J. Med. Genet.* 25:157, 1988.

Young ID, et al.: Discordant expression of the G syndrome in monozygotic twins. *Am. J. Med. Genet.* 29:863, 1988.

GAPO SYNDROME

Synonym: Growth retardation-alopecia-pseudoanodontia-optic atrophy.

Mode of Inheritance: Autosomal recessive.

Frequency: Six published cases (Tipton et al.).

Clinical Manifestations: (a) *growth retardation,* normal mental development; (b) *alopecia;* (c) *pseudoanodentia* (failure of tooth eruption); (d) *optic atrophy (not present in all cases);* (e) craniofacial features: high and bossing forehead, wide anterior fontanelle, midface hypoplasia, thick lips, protruding eyes, micrognathia; (f) other reported abnormalities: umbilical hernia, prominent scalp veins, hypoplasia of the breasts, hyperconvex nails, etc.

Radiologic Manifestations: (a) unerupted dentition; (b) skeletal maturation retardation; (c) mandibular hypoplasia, shallow orbits, protruding eyes, thickening of the lateral orbital walls, hypertelorism; (d) dilatation of the intracranial and scalp veins (venous obstruction).

Differential Diagnosis: Progeria (Fig SY–G–1).

REFERENCES

Andersen TH, Pindborg JJ: Et tilfaelde at total "pseudo-anodonti" inforbindelse med Kraniedeformitet, dvaergvaekst og ektodermal displasi. *Odont. T.* 55:484, 1947.

Manouvrier-Hanu S, et al.: The GAPO syndrome. *Am. J. Med. Genet.* 26:683, 1987.

191

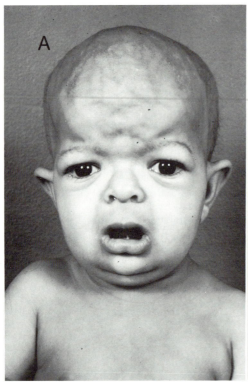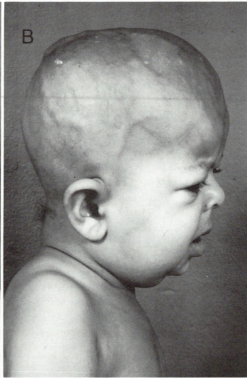

FIG SY—G—1.
A and **B,** GAPO syndrome. Note the hypertelorism, depressed nasal bridge, high and bossing forehead, prominent lips, microretrognathia, and prominent ears. (From Manouvrier-Hanu S,

Tipton RE, et al.: Growth retardation, alopecia, pseudoanodontia, and optic atrophy—the GAPO syndrome: Report of a patient and review of the literature. *Am. J. Med. Genet.* 19:209, 1984.

GARCIN SYNDROME

Synonym: Hemibasis syndrome.

Clinical Manifestations: *Unilateral paralysis of all cranial nerves, absence of cerebral signs and symptoms such as motor or sensory disturbances, no signs of increased intracranial pressure.*

Radiologic Manifestations: Tumor with invasion of the basal bones of the skull.

REFERENCES

Chouza C, et al.: Jugular chemodectoma with Garcin syndrome. *Acta Neurol. Latinoam.* 27:155, 1981.
Harada S, et al.: Basal skull metastasis of stomach cancer presenting with Garcin's syndrome—a case report. *No Shinkei Geka* 15:765, 1987.
Massey EW, et al: Cylindroma causing Garcin's syndrome (letter). *Arch. Neurol.* 37:786, 1980.

Largilliere C, Benalioua M, et al.: The GAPO syndrome. *Am. J. Med. Genet.* 26:683, 1987. Used by permission.)

Takahashi T, et al.: Rhabdomyosarcoma presenting as Garcin's syndrome. *Surg. Neurol.* 17:269, 1982.

GARDNER SYNDROME

Mode of Inheritance: Autosomal dominant, incompletely penetrant.

Frequency: Uncommon.

Clinical Manifestations: (a) *soft-tissue tumors:* epidermoid inclusion cysts of the skin, dermoid tumors, fibroma, lipoma, lipofibroma, leiomyoma, intra-abdominal tumors (desmoids and peritoneal fibromas); (b) *osteomatosis;* (c) *gastrointestinal polyposis;* (d) other reported abnormalities: abnormal dentition, increased incidence of periampullary malignancy, possible association of Gardner syndrome and chromosome deletion (questionable), keloids, hypertrophic scars, mammary fibrosis, hypertrophy of the retinal pigment epithelium, etc.

Radiologic Manifestations: (a) benign *osteomatosis* (skull, trunk, and limbs, in particular, lobulated osteomas of the mandibular angle most characteristic); (b) dental abnormalities (supernumerary teeth, unerupted teeth, numerous dental caries, odontomas); (c) *gastrointestinal polyposis,* co-

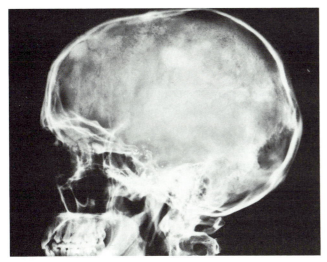

FIG SY–G–2.
Gardner syndrome. A lateral roentgenogram of the skull shows numerous well-defined bony opacities of varying size affecting the calvaria and mandible. These features are typical of the osteomas of Gardner syndrome. (From Bessler W, Egloff B, Sulser H: Gardner syndrome with aggressive fibromatosis. *Skeletal Radiol.* 11:56, 1984. Used by permission.)

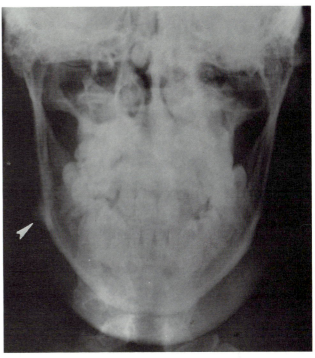

FIG SY–G–3.
Gardner syndrome in a 21-year-old male with multiple polyps throughout the colon. Note the small protuberant osteoma *(arrowhead)* arising from the cortex of the mandibular angle. (From Chang CH, Piatt ED, Thomas KE, et al.: Bone abnormalities in Gardner's syndrome. *A.J.R.* 103:645, 1968. Used by permission.)

lon the most common site; polypoid lymphoid hyperplasia of the small bowel, carcinoma of the colon, gastric adenocarcinoma; (d) *desmoid tumor* with involvement of the mesenteric root causing vascular obstruction; spiculation of the small-bowel pattern and mural changes; small-bowel obstruction; (e) hydronephrosis and hydroureter due to obstruction by desmoid tumor; (f) other reported abnormalities: cancer of the thyroid, cancer of the adrenal gland, leontiasis ossea (skull and facial bones) (Figs SY–G–2 to SY–G–4).

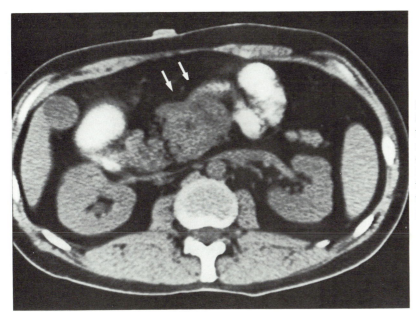

FIG SY–G–4.
Desmoid tumor in Gardner syndrome. CT scan at the level of the middle of the kidneys: soft-tissue mass at the midline *(arrows)*. Jejunal loops are displaced but not obstructed by the mass. (From Magid D, Fishman EK, Jones B, et al.: Desmoid tumors in Gardner syndrome: Use of computed tomography. *A.J.R.* 142:1141, 1984. Used by permission.)

REFERENCES

Bessler W, et al.: Case report 253. *Skeletal Radiol.* 11:56, 1984.

Blair NP, et al.: Hypertrophy of the retinal pigment epithelium associated with Gardner's syndrome. *Am. J. Ophthalmol.* 90:661, 1980.

Coffey RJ Jr, et al.: Gastric adenocarcinoma complicating Gardner's syndrome in a North American woman. *Gastroenterology* 88:1263, 1985.

Endo A, et al.: Gardner syndrome and interstitial chromosome deletion (letter). *Am. J. Med. Genet.* 28:511, 1987.

Gardner EJ, et al.: Cancer of the lower digestive tract in one family group. *Am. J. Hum. Genet.* 2:41, 1950.

Krush AJ, et al.: Hepatoblastoma, pigmented ocular fundus lesions and jaw lesions in Gardner syndrome. *Am. J. Med. Genet.* 29:323, 1988.

Lattimer JK, et al.: The treatment of ureteral obstruction in Gardner's syndrome: Renal autotransplantation. *J. Urol.* 138:133, 1987.

Lyons LA, et al: A genetic study of Gardner syndrome and congenital hypertrophy of the retinal pigment epithelium. *Am. J. Hum. Genet.* 42:290, 1988.

Magid D, et al.: Desmoid tumors in Gardner syndrome: Use of computed tomography. *A.J.R.* 142:1141, 1984.

Naylor EW, et al.: Adrenal adenomas in a patient with Gardner's syndrome. *Clin. Genet.* 20:67, 1981.

Palmer TH: Gardner's syndrome: Six generations. *Am. J. Surg.* 143:405, 1982.

Peters PE, et al.: Röntgendiagnostik und Klinik des Gardner-Syndroms. *Fortschr. Rontgenstr.* 136:133, 1982.

Ushio K, et al.: Lesions associated with familial polyposis coli: Studies of lesions of the stomach, duodenum, bones, and teeth. *Gastrointest. Radiol.* 1:67, 1976.

Vanhoutte JJ: Polypoid lymphoid hyperplasia of the terminal ileum in patients with familial polyposis coli and with Gardner's syndrome. *A.J.R.* 110:340, 1970.

GARDNER-SILENGO-WACHTEL SYNDROME

Synonym: Genito-palato-cardiac syndrome.

Mode of Inheritance: Either autosomal recessive or X-linked recessive.

Frequency: 13 published cases (Greenberg et al.).

Clinical and Radiologic Manifestations: (a) craniofacial: micrognathia, low-set ears, cleft palate, cleft alveolar ridge, prominent occiput, depressed nasal bridge, anteverted nares, "carp" mouth; (b) congenital heart disease; (c) limb anomalies: clubfeet, prominent heels, flexion deformity of the thumbs; (d) 46,XY, female internal genitalia; hypospadias; gonadal dysgenesis.

REFERENCES

Gardner LI, et al.: 46,XY female: Anti-androgenic effect of oral contraceptive? *Lancet* 2:667, 1970.

Greenberg F, et al.: The Gardner-Silengo-Wachtel or genito-palato-cardiac syndrome: Male pseudohermaphroditism with micrognathia, cleft palate, and conotruncal cardiac defect. *Am. J. Med. Genet.* 26:59, 1987.

Silengo M, et al.: A 46,XY infant with uterus, dysgenetic gonads, and multiple anomalies. *Humangenetik* 25:65, 1974.

Wachtel SS: *H-Y Antigen and the Biology of Sex Determination.* New York, Grane & Stratton, 1983, p. 224.

GASTROCUTANEOUS SYNDROME

Synonym: Ulcer–multiple lentigines syndrome.

Mode of Inheritance: Reported in a French Canadian family; autosomal dominant with high penetrance and variable expressivity.

Clinical and Radiologic Manifestations: (a) *peptic ulcer,* hiatal hernia; (b) *multiple lentigenes/café au lait spots;* (c) apparent hypertelorism; (d) myopia; (e) other reported abnormalities: ischemic heart disease, congenital heart disease, maturity-onset diabetes, abnormal dermatoglyphics.

REFERENCES

Halal F, et al.: Gastro-cutaneous syndrome: Peptic ulcer/hiatal hernia, multiple lentigines/café-au-lait spots, hypertelorism, and myopia. *Am. J. Med. Genet.* 11:161, 1982.

Rotter JL, et al.: Additional comments on the ulcer–multiple lentigines syndrome (letter). *Am. J. Med. Genet.* 11:251, 1982.

GERMAN SYNDROME

Frequency: Four published cases (Lewin et al.).

Clinical and Radiologic Manifestations: (a) prenatal growth retardation; (b) head: dolichocephaly, micrognathia, wide interorbital distance, epicanthal folds, low-set ears, carplike mouth, high-arched palate, small tongue; (c) hypotonia, weak cry; (d) pectus excavatum, flexion contracture of the knees and digits, subluxation of the hip, vertical talus, etc.

REFERENCES

German J, et al.: Generalized dysmorphia of a similar type in two unrelated babies. *Birth Defects* 11:34, 1975.

Lewin SO, et al.: German syndrome in sibs. *Am. J. Med. Genet.* 26:385, 1987.

GERODERMA OSTEODYSPLASTICA HEREDITARIA

Synonyms: Gerodermia osteodysplastica; geroderma osteodysplasticum, Walt Disney dwarfism, Bamatter syndrome.

Mode of Inheritance: Autosomal recessive.

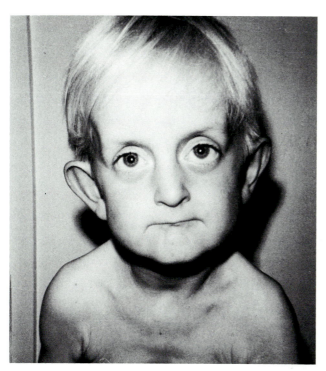

FIG SY–G–5.
Geroderma osteodysplastica in a 3⅓-year-old male with a droopy, jowly, older-than-age appearance; broad forehead; malar flatness; downward angulation of the ears; downturned lower lip; and relative mandibular prognathism. (From Hunter AGW, Martsolf JT, Baker CG, et al.: Geroderma osteodysplastica. A report of two affected families. *Hum. Genet.* 40:311, 1978. Used by permission.)

Frequency: Rare.

Clinical Manifestations: Symptoms with onset in infancy: (a) *short stature;* (b) *senile facial features* (Walt Disney dwarf appearance), sagging cheeks, sunken eyes, tendency to microcornea; (c) *thin skin with poor turgor and elasticity, easily wrinkled, prominent veins;* (d) defects in dental implantation; (e) muscular hypotonia; (f) *hyperlaxity of joints;* (g) severe flatfoot deformity; (h) other reported abnormalities: brachycephaly, prominent forehead, ptosis of the upper eyelids, jutting fleshy nose, malar flattening, downturned lower lip, dental malocclusion, high palate, mandibular hypoplasia, large ears, span more than height, malar flush, narrow chest, microcornea, inguinal hernia, simian crease, exophthalmos, winged scapulae, etc.

Radiologic Manifestations: (a) *generalized osteoporosis;* (b) *predisposition to fractures;* (c) *platyspondyly,* biconcave vertebral bodies, bone-within-bone appearance, multiple parallel lines in the vertebral bodies, scoliosis; (d) *dislocated hips,* knee subluxation, flatfoot; (e) other reported abnormalities: sternal abnormalities, minor hand anomalies, multiple wormian bones, posterior displacement of the maxilla with relative mandibular prognathism.

Differential Diagnosis: Progeria; Ehlers-Danlos syndrome; cutis laxa; acrogeria; osteogenesis imperfecta; etc. (Figs SY–G–5 and SY–G–6.)

REFERENCES

Bamatter F, Franceschetti A, Klein D, et al.: Gérodermie ostéodysplastique héréditaire (un nouveau biotype de la "progeria"). *Ann. Pediatr. (Paris)* 174:126, 1950.
Hall BD: Geroderma osteodysplastica: A rare autosomal re-

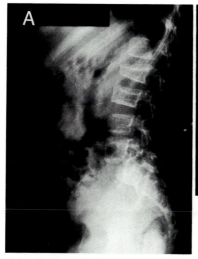
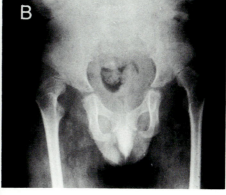

FIG SY–G–6.
Geroderma osteodysplastica hereditaria. **A,** osteoporosis, compression fractures of the vertebrae. **B,** hypoplasia of the iliac bones, hip dislocation, and coxa valga. (From Lisker R, Hernández A, Martínez-Lavin M, et al.: Gerodermia osteodysplastica hereditaria: Report of three affected brothers and literature review. *Am. J. Med. Genet.* 3:389, 1979. Used by permission.)

cessive connective tissue disorder with either variability or heterogeneity or both (abstract). *Proc. Greenwood Genet. Center* 2:101, 1983.

Hunter AGW, et al.: Geroderma osteodysplastica: A report of two affected families. *Hum. Genet.* 40:311, 1978.

Lisker R, et al.: Geroderma osteodysplastica hereditaria: Report of three affected brothers and literature review. *Am. J. Med. Genet.* 3:389, 1979.

Suter H, et al.: Geroderma osteoplastica hereditaria (GOH) in a girl, in Papadatos CJ, Bartsocas CS (eds.): *Skeletal Dysplasias.* New York, Alan R Liss Inc, 1982, pp. 327–329.

Wiedemann H-R: Geroderma osteodysplastica *(Hum. Genet.* 40:311–324)—What would Virchow have thought about it?! *Hum. Genet.* 43:245, 1978.

GILLES DE LA TOURETTE SYNDROME

Clinical Manifestations: (a) *muscular tics* (face, head-shoulders, arms, legs, trunk); (b) *vocal tics* (grunting, barking sounds, throat clearing, screaming, coprolalia); (c) suggestive organic basis of the disorder: organic traits by psychiatric testing, soft neurological signs (abnormal voluntary movements, nonspecific electroencephalographic abnormalities, etc.).

Radiologic Manifestations: Porencephalic cyst and a unilateral weak enhancement of the basal ganglia after contrast injection (computed tomographic examination) reported in one case (causal relation to the syndrome questionable).

REFERENCE

Kjaer M, et al.: Abnormal CT scan in a patient with Gilles de la Tourette syndrome. *Neuroradiology* 28:362, 1986.

GLENOID HYPOPLASIA

Synonyms: Glenoid dysplasia; dysplasia of the scapular neck; dentated glenoid anomaly.

Mode of Inheritance: Majority sporadic; a dominant gene in some familial cases.

Clinical Manifestations: Usually asymptomatic in children, often discovered on chest radiographs as an incidental finding; (a) shoulder pain; (b) limitation of motion; (c) recurrent dislocation (uncommon).

Radiologic Manifestations: (a) bilateral hypoplasia of the scapular neck, widened glenohumeral joint space, irregular glenoid surface, dentated or notched articular surface; (b) other reported shoulder region abnormalities: hypoplasia of the humeral head and neck, varus deformity of the proximal portion of the humerus, enlargement and bowing of the acromion and clavicle; (c) premature development of osteoarthritis; (d) other reported abnormalities: spina bifida, cervical ribs, hemivertebrae, webbing of the axillae.

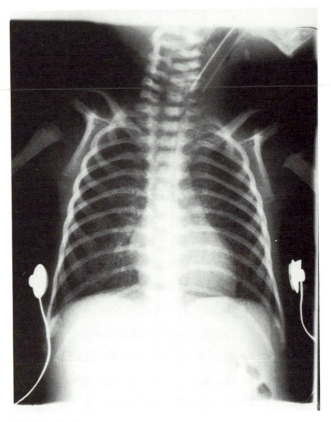

FIG SY–G–7.
Hypoplasia of the glenoid fossae in a newborn male who also has the amniotic band syndrome.

Differential Diagnosis: Brachial plexus injury at birth; mucopolysaccharidoses; trauma; hemophilia; etc. (Fig SY-G-7).

REFERENCES

Kozlowski K, et al.: Congenital bilateral glenoid hypoplasia: A report of four cases. *Br. J. Radiol.* 60:705, 1987.

Pettersson H: Bilateral dysplasia of the neck of scapula and associated anomalies. *Acta. Radiol.* 22:81, 1981.

Resnick D, et al.: Bilateral dysplasia of the scapular neck. *A.J.R.* 139:387, 1982.

Valentin B: Die kongenitale Schulterluxation. *Z. Orthop. Chir.* 55:229, 1931.

GOLDENHAR SYNDROME

Synonyms: Goldenhar-Gorlin syndrome; Goldenhar spectrum; hemifacial microsomia syndrome; facio-auriculovertebral anomalad; oculo-auriculo-vertebral dysplasia; first and second branchial arch syndrome.

Mode of Inheritance: Usually sporadic; familial cases rare; genetic heterogeneity.

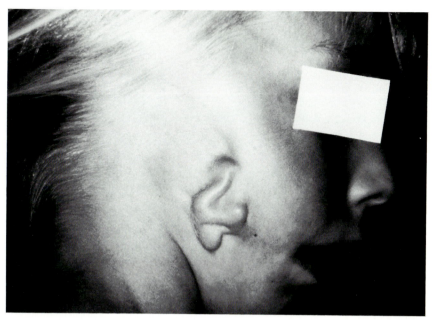

FIG SY—G—8.
Goldenhar syndrome. A lateral photograph of the face shows a deformed ear and hypoplasia of the mandible. (From Avon SW, Shively JL: Orthopedic manifestations of Goldenhar syndrome. *J. Pediatr. Orthop.* 8:683, 1988. Used by permission.)

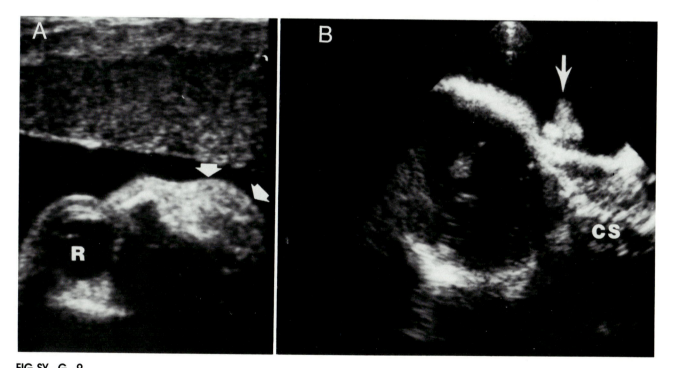

FIG SY—G—9.
Goldenhar syndrome. **A,** a prenatal axial sonogram at the midorbital level of the fetal face at 30 weeks' gestation demonstrates an absence of the left orbit *(arrows)* (R = right eye). **B,** an oblique parasagittal sonogram of the left side of the fetal head and neck displays the low-set malformed left external ear *(arrow)* (CS = cervical spine). (From Tamas DE, Mahony BS, Bowie JD, et al.: Prenatal sonographic diagnosis of hemifacial microsomia (Goldenhar-Gorlin syndrome). *J. Ultrasound Med.* 5:461, 1986. Used by permission.)

Frequency: Uncommon.

Clinical Manifestations: (a) *maxillary and/or mandibular hypoplasia* (usually unilateral), insufficient closure of the jaw, temporomandibular joint anomalies, macrostomia associated with a lateral facial cleft, facial muscular hypoplasia; (b) *ocular anomalies:* antimongoloid slant of the palpebral fissures, *epibulbar dermoid and/or lipodermoid, coloboma of the upper eyelid,* coloboma of the iris and choroid, irregular astigmatism, congenital ophthalmoplegia, microcornea, microphthalmos, anophthalmia, anterior polar cataract; (c) *ear anomalies: hypoplasia or atresia of the external auditory meatus and canal; preauricular tags and/or a blind fistula,* middle-ear and inner-ear anomalies, deafness; (d) *oropharyngolaryngeal anomalies:* parotid gland aplasia, ectopic salivary gland tissue, cleft lip/palate, high-arched palate, tongue deformities, velolaryngeal insufficiency, hypernasal speech; (e) cardiovascular anomalies: ventricular septal defect, tetralogy of Fallot, right aortic arch, coarctation of the aorta, patent ductus arteriosus, etc.; (f) other reported abnormalities: prenatal growth retardation, mental retardation, intracranial dermoid cyst, renal anomalies (absence, duplication, ectopia, etc.), hypoplasia or aplasia of the lung, pulmonary sequestration, occipital encephalocele, dental anomalies, limb anomalies (hypoplastic distal phalanges, polydactyly, etc.), association with other syndromes (Duane, Saethre-Chotzen, Seckel, neurofibromatosis, trisomy 18, cri du chat), imperforate anus, diaphragmatic hernia, duodenal stenosis, radial limb anomalies, chromosome abnormality, etc.

Radiologic Manifestations: (a) *hypoplasia of the mandible, maxilla, and temporal bones* (atresia or narrowing of one or both external auditory canals, narrowing of the middle ear with absent ossicles, underdeveloped internal auditory canal, etc.); (b) *various vertebral anomalies* (hemivertebrae, blocked vertebrae, supernumerary vertebrae, cuneiform vertebrae, spina bifida, occipitalization of the atlas); (c) hypoplasia of the external carotid artery, altered cerebral blood flow; (d) craniocephalic abnormalities: intracranial lipoma (corpus callosum, etc.), intracranial dermoid, calcification of the falx, encephalocele, hydrocephalus, aqueductal stenosis, agenesis of the corpus callosum, agenesis of the vermis, arhinencephalia, porencephalia, cerebral hypoplasia, plagiocephaly, skull defect, cranium bifidum, microcephaly, etc; (e) other reported anomalies: rib anomalies, pulmonary agenesis or hypoplasia, cleft palate, congenital absence of the portal vein, prenatal sonographic diagnosis (anophthalmia and a malformed, low-set ipsilateral ear), etc. (Figs SY–G–8 to SY–G–10).

Note: Hemifacial microsomia with radial defects is considered to be basically the same as "Goldenhar syndrome."

REFERENCES

Aleksic S, et al.: Intracranial lipomas, hydrocephalus and other CNS anomalies in oculoauriculo-vertebral dysplasia (Goldenhar-Gorlin syndrome). *Child Brain* 11:285, 1984.

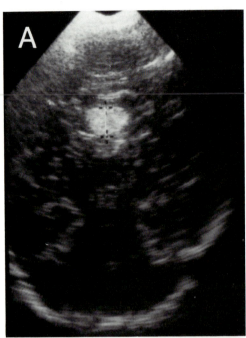
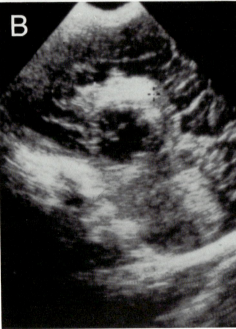

FIG SY–G–10.
Goldenhar syndrome: lipoma of the corpus callosum in a newborn girl. Cranial sonograms (coronal **[A]** and sagittal sections **[B]**) show an echogenic mass within the corpus callosum. Note the increased separation of the central parts of the lateral ventricles. (From Beltinger C, Saule H: Imaging of lipoma of the corpus callosum and intracranial dermoids in the Goldenhar syndrome. *Pediatr. Radiol.* 18:72, 1988. Used by permission.)

Beltinger C, et al.: Imaging of lipoma of the corpus callosum and intracranial dermoids in the Goldenhar syndrome. *Pediatr. Radiol.* 18:72, 1988.
Boles DJ, et al.: Goldenhar complex in discordant monozygotic twins: A case report and review of the literature. *Am. J. Med. Genet.* 28:103, 1987.

Bowen AD III, et al.: Bronchopulmonary foregut malformation in the Goldenhar anomalad. *A.J.R.* 134:186, 1980.

Burck U: Genetic aspects of hemifacial microsomia. *Hum. Genet.* 64:291, 1983.

Feingold M, et al.: Goldenhar's syndrome. *Am. J. Dis. Child.* 132:136, 1978.

Goldenhar M: Associations malformatives de l'oeil et de l'oreille, en particulier le syndrome dermoide épibulbaire-appendices auriculaires-fistula auris congenita et ses relations avec la dysostose mandibulofaciale. *J. Genet. Hum.* 1:243, 1952.

Gorlin RJ, et al.: Oculoauriculovertebral dysplasia. *J. Pediatr.* 63:991, 1963.

Greenwood RD, et al.: Cardiovascular malformations in oculoauriculovertebral dysplasia (Goldenhar syndrome). *J. Pediatr.* 85:816, 1974.

Herman GE, et al: Multiple congenital anomaly/mental retardation (MCA/MR) syndrome with Goldenhar complex due to a terminal del(22q). *Am. J. Med. Genet.* 29:909, 1988.

Moeschler J, et al.: Familial occurrence of hemifacial microsomia with radial limb defects. *Am. J. Med. Genet.* 12:371, 1982.

Morse SS, et al.: Congenital absence of the portal vein in oculoauriculovertebral dysplasia (Goldenhar syndrome). *Pediatr. Radiol.* 16:437, 1986.

Rees DO, et al.: Radiological aspects of oculoauriculovertebral dysplasia. *Br. J. Radiol.* 45:15, 1972.

Robinson LK, et al.: Vascular pathogenesis of unilateral craniofacial defects. *J. Pediatr.* 111:236, 1987.

Rollnick BR, et al.: Hemifacial microsomia and variants: Pedigree data. *Am. J. Med. Genet.* 15:233, 1983.

Rollnick BR, et al.: Oculoauriculovertebral dysplasia and variants: Phenotypic characteristics of 294 patients. *Am. J. Med. Genet.* 26:361, 1987.

Ryan CA, et al.: Discordance of signs in monozygotic twins concordant for the Goldenhar anomaly. *Am. J. Med. Genet.* 29:755, 1988.

Tamas DE, et al.: Prenatal sonographic diagnosis of hemifacial microsomia (Goldenhar-Gorlin syndrome). *J. Ultrasound Med.* 5:461, 1986.

Wilson GN: Cranial defects in the Goldenhar syndrome. *Am. J. Med. Genet.* 14:435, 1983.

GOLDEN-LAKIM SYNDROME

Clinical and Radiologic Manifestations: (a) dolichocephaly, pointed facies, small mandible, bifid uvula; (b) pterygium colli; (c) limb deformities: flexion deformity of the knees without popliteal webs, pes cavus, clubfoot, atrophy of the calf muscles, camptodactyly of the fifth digits; (d) kyphoscoliosis, defective ossification of the lamina of some vertebrae; (e) pectus excavatum.

REFERENCE

Golden RL, Lakim H: The form fruste in Marfan's syndrome. *N. Engl. J. Med.* 260:797, 1959.

GOLTZ SYNDROME

Synonyms: Goltz-Gorlin syndrome; focal dermal hypoplasia.

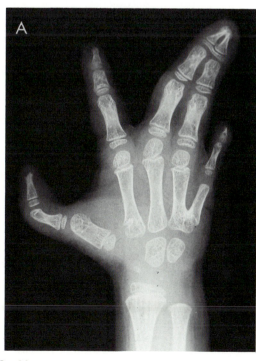 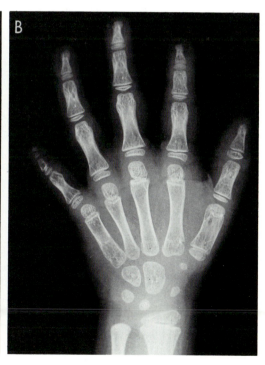

FIG SY–G–11.
Goltz syndrome in a 6-year-old female. **A,** multiple anomalies including syndactyly, brachydactyly, and metacarpal shortening. The thumb is proximally placed. **B,** brachyphalangia of the fifth digit. (From Ginsburg LD, Sedano HO, Gorlin RJ: Focal dermal hypoplasia syndrome. *A.J.R.* 110:561, 1970. Used by permission.)

Mode of Inheritance: X-linked dominant most likely due to predominance in females; lethal in males with full expression of the trait.

Frequency: Approximately 200 published cases (Almeida et al.).

Clinical Manifestations: (a) *poikiloderma with focal dermal hypoplasia* (skin atrophy, linear pigmentations, fat deposit in the superficial layers of the skin), *papillomas of the mucous membranes,* sparse scalp hair, nail dystrophy (grooves, spooned); (b) limb anomalies; (c) other reported abnormalities: absent uvula, split soft palate, single umbilical artery, facial asymmetry, conductive deafness, teeth abnormalities (fragile enamel, dental caries), eye abnormalities (coloboma, cataract), hypogenitalia, small breasts, congenital heart disease, microphthalmos, unilateral anophthalmia, strabismus, nystagmus, obstructed tear ducts, aniridia, irregular pupils, mental and growth retardation, hypoplasia of the external ear.

Radiologic Manifestations: (a) *syndactyly;* (b) *dental anomalies* (microdontia, oligodontia, deformed teeth, retarded eruption, etc.); (c) other reported abnormalities: microcephaly, hypoplasia of the craniofacial skeleton, steep clivus, scoliosis, segmentation errors of the vertebrae, rudimentary tail, hypoplasia of the ribs, bifurcation of the ribs, oligodactyly, polydactyly, adactyly, foot deformities, hypoplasia of the pelvic bones, association with osteopathia striata, generalized osteopenia, multiple bone lesions resembling giant-cell tumors of bone, pelvic hemangioma, renal anomalies, midclavicular aplasia or hypoplasia, etc. (Fig SY—G—11).

REFERENCES

Almeida L, et al: Myelomeningocele, Arnold-Chiari anomaly and hydrocephalus in focal dermal hypoplasia. *Am. J. Med. Genet.* 30:917, 1988.
Barthels W, et al.: Die Osteopathia striata: Ein charakteristischer Röntgenbefund bei der fokalen dermalen Hypoplasie (Goltz-Gorlin-Syndrom). *Radiologe* 22:562, 1982.
Ginsburg LD, Sedano HO, Gorlin RJ: Focal dermal hypoplasia syndrome. *A.J.R.* 110:561, 1970.
Goltz RW, et al.: Focal dermal hypoplasia. *Arch. Dermatol.* 86:708, 1962.
Goltz RW, et al.: Focal dermal hypoplasia syndrome. *Arch. Dermatol.* 101:1, 1970.
Gorlin RJ, et al.: Focal dermal hypoplasia syndrome. *Acta Derm Venereol (Stockh.)* 43:421, 1963.
Joannides T, et al.: Giant cell tumour of bone in focal dermal hypoplasia. *Br. J. Radiol.* 56:684, 1983.
Knockaert D, et al.: Osteopathia striata and focal dermal hypoplasia. *Skeletal Radiol.* 4:223, 1979.
Kunze J, et al.: Diaphragmatic hernia in a female newborn with focal dermal hypoplasia and marked asymmetric malformations (Goltz-Gorlin syndrome). *Eur. J. Pediatr.* 131:213, 1979.
Wechsler MA, et al: Variable expression in focal dermal hypoplasia. An example of differential X-chromosome inactivation. *Am. J. Dis. Child.* 142:297, 1988.

GOODMAN CAMPTODACTYLY SYNDROME A

Mode of Inheritance: Probably autosomal recessive.

Clinical and Radiologic Manifestations: (a) short stature, peculiar facies; (b) camptodactyly, syndactyly, abnormal palmar creases; (c) clubfoot; (d) muscular hypoplasia of the chest, pelvis, and limbs; (e) scoliosis, etc.

REFERENCES

Goodman RM, et al.: Camptodactyly—occurrence in two new genetic syndromes and its relationship to other syndromes. *J. Med. Genet.* 9:203, 1972.
Temtamy S, McKusick VA: Goodman camptodactyly syndrome. A. *Birth Defects* 14:456, 1978.

GOODMAN CAMPTODACTYLY SYNDROME B

Mode of Inheritance: Probably autosomal recessive.

Clinical and Radiologic Manifestations: (a) abnormal facies (broad nose, flaring nostrils, etc.); (b) large hands and feet, arachnodactyly, contracture of the fingers, hammertoes; (c) thoracic scoliosis; (d) low-normal intelligence.

REFERENCES

Goodman RM, et al.: Camptodactyly—occurrence in two new genetic syndromes and its relationship to other syndromes. *J. Med. Genet.* 9:203, 1972.
Temtamy S, McKusick VA: Goodman camptodactyly syndrome B. *Birth Defects* 14:485, 1978.

GOODPASTURE SYNDROME

Etiology: Three groups: (a) anti—glomerular basement membrane antibody—induced disease; (b) systemic vasculitis; (c) idiopathic (no systemic disease, no anti—glomerular basement membrane antibody detectable).

Essential Features: (a) *glomerulonephritis;* (b) *hemoptysis;* (c) *pulmonary infiltrates.*

Clinical Manifestations: (a) weakness, cough, pallor, low-grade fever, tachycardia; (b) *pulmonary hemorrhage, hemoptysis;* (c) *renal disease: hematuria, albuminuria, uremia;* (d) *biopsy: linear immunofluorescent patterns* along the glomerular and pulmonary alveolar basement membranes; (e) *high titers of circulating antibodies to glomerular basement membrane;* (f) *strong association between HLA-DRw2 and antibody-mediated Goodpasture syndrome;* (g) microcytic anemia.

Radiologic Manifestations: (a) *pulmonary infiltration of various types:* patchy, fine, powdery, stippled, linear, nodu-

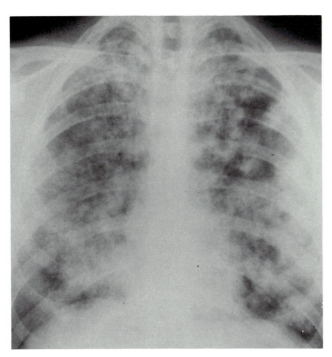

FIG SY–G–12.
Goodpasture syndrome in a 15-year-old male with respiratory difficulty, fever, hemoptysis, and anemia. There are extensive bilateral pulmonary patchy and confluent densities. The heart size is normal.

lar, mottled, and massive consolidation; perihilar pattern with apices and bases being relatively clear; (b) pleural effusion; (c) cardiomegaly (Fig SY–G–12).

REFERENCES

Bergrem H, et al.: Goodpasture's syndrome: A report of seven patients including long-term follow-up of three who received a kidney transplant. *Am. J. Med.* 68:54, 1980.

Bowley NB, et al.: Chest x-ray in antiglomerular basement membrane antibody disease (Goodpasture's syndrome). *Clin. Radiol.* 30:419, 1979.

Curtis JJ, et al.: Goodpasture's syndrome in a patient with the nail-patella syndrome. *Am. J. Med.* 61:401, 1976.

Garnone CF, et al.: Le syndrome de Goodpasture. *J. Radiol.* 60:429, 1979.

Goodpasture EW: The significance of certain pulmonary lesions in relation to etiology of influenza. *Am. J. Med. Sci.* 158:863, 1919.

Herman PG, et al.: The pulmonary-renal syndrome. *A.J.R.* 130:1141, 1978.

Holdsworth S, et al.: The clinical spectrum of acute glomerulonephritis and lung haemorrhage (Goodpasture's syndrome). *Q. J. Med.* 55:75, 1985.

Klasa RJ, et al: Goodpasture's syndrome: Recurrence after a five-year remission. Case report and review of the literature. *Am. J. Med.* 84:751, 1988.

Martini A, et al.: Goodpasture's syndrome in a child. *Acta Paediatr. Scand.* 70:435, 1981.

Mehler PS, et al.: Chronic recurrent Goodpasture's syndrome. *Am. J. Med.* 82:833, 1987.

Ozsoylu S: Goodpasture's syndrome. *Arch. Dis. Child.* 59:189, 1984.

Rees AJ, et al.: Strong association between HLA-DRw2 and antibody-mediated Goodpasture's syndrome. *Lancet* 1:966, 1978.

Schwartz EE, et al.: Pulmonary hemorrhage in renal disease: Goodpasture syndrome and other causes. *Radiology* 122:39, 1977.

Zell SC, et al.: Alveolar hemorrhage associated with a membranoproliferative glomerulonephritis and smooth muscle antibody. *Am. J. Med.* 82:1073, 1987.

GORDON SYNDROME

Mode of Inheritance: Autosomal dominant.

Clinical Manifestations: (a) *camptodactyly, clubfoot* (varus or valgus); (b) *cleft palate;* (c) other reported abnormalities: short stature, nevus flammeus, dermatoglyphic anomalies, omphalocele, undescended testes.

Radiologic Manifestations: (a) *camptodactyly,* pseudoepiphysis of the second metacarpal, atypical carpal ossification sequence; (b) *clubfoot deformities;* (c) stenosis of the spinal canal, narrow intervertebral disks.

REFERENCES

Gordon H, et al.: Camptodactyly, cleft palate, and clubfoot. A syndrome showing the autosomal-dominant pattern of inheritance. *J. Med. Genet.* 6:266, 1969.

Halal F, et al.: Camptodactyly, cleft palate, and clubfoot (the Gordon syndrome). *J. Med. Genet.* 16:149, 1979.

Robinow M, et al.: The Gordon syndrome: Autosomal dominant cleft palate, camptodactyly, and club feet. *Am. J. Med. Genet.* 9:139, 1981.

Say B, et al.: The Gordon syndrome (letter). *J. Med. Genet.* 17:405, 1980.

GORLIN-CHAUDHRY-MOSS SYNDROME

Synonym: Gorlin syndrome.

Clinical Manifestations: (a) "dished-out" appearance of the middle of the face, antimongoloid obliquity of the palpebral fissures, defective eyelid development; (b) hypertrichosis; (c) hypoplasia of the labia majora; (d) patent ductus arteriosus; (e) dental anomalies.

Radiologic Manifestations: (a) craniofacial dysostosis: premature synostosis of the coronal sutures, lordosis of the petrous ridges, clival hypoplasia, elevation of the lesser sphenoidal wings, brachycephaly, relative ocular hypertelorism, underdeveloped maxillary and nasal bones; (b) dental anomalies: wide spread diastemas, congenitally missing teeth, malformed unerupted permanent teeth, cervical constriction of the mandibular incisors, diminution of pulp chambers and canals (Fig SY–G–13).

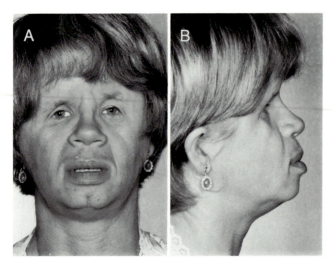

FIG SY–G–13.
A and **B,** Gorlin-Chaudhry-Moss syndrome. "Dished out" appearance of the mid-face and defective eyelid development are present. (Courtesy of Robert J. Gorlin, D.D.S., M.S., Minneapolis.)

REFERENCE

Gorlin RJ, Chaudhry AP, Moss ML: Craniofacial dysostosis, patent ductus arteriosus, hypertrichosis, hypoplasia of labia majora, dental and eye anomalies—a new syndrome? *J. Pediatr.* 56:778, 1960.

GRADENIGO SYNDROME

Synonyms: Petrous apicitis; apical petrositis.

Clinical Manifestations: (a) *chronic purulent otorrhea;* (b) *pain: the ear, face, and retrobulbar region;* (c) *abducens paralysis;* (d) other reported abnormalities: hearing loss; meningitis; facial paralysis; nerve VIII, IX, and X involvement.

Radiologic Manifestations: (a) *mastoiditis;* (b) *petrositis* with osteoporosis in the early phase and bone destruction at the apex in the late phase of the disease; (c) dural involvement, cerebritis, phlebitis, thrombosis.

Note: Noninfectious conditions, in particular, neoplastic invasion of the petrous apex, may result in the clinical manifestations of Gradenigo syndrome.

REFERENCES

Chole RA, et al.: Petrous apicitis. Clinical considerations. *Ann. Otol. Rhinol. Laryngol.* 92:544, 1983.
Gillanders DA: Gradenigo's syndrome revisited. *J. Otolaryngol.* 12:169, 1983.
Gradenigo G: A special syndrome of endocranial otitic complications (paralysis of the motor oculi externus of otitic origin). *Ann. Otol. Rhinol. Laryngol.* 13:637, 1904.
Horowitz S: Gradenigo's syndrome and report of two cases. *J. Laryngol. Otol.* 62:639, 1948.

Woody RC, et al.: The role of computerized tomographic scan in the management of Gradenigo's syndrome. *Pediatr. Infect. Dis.* 3:595, 1984.

GRANT SYNDROME

Mode of Inheritance: Consistent with autosomal dominant.

Frequency: Very rare.

Clinical Manifestations: (a) camptomelia; (b) blue sclerae; (c) mandibular hypoplasia; (d) normal serum calcium, phosphate, and alkaline phosphatase levels; (e) short stature; (f) no tendency to fracture, no dentinogenesis imperfecta.

Radiologic Manifestations: (a) wormian bones persistent beyond childhood, brachycephaly; (b) osteopenia in infancy; (c) bowing of the long bones of the lower limb, improvement after infancy; (d) shallow glenoid fossae, tendency to shoulder dislocation.

Notes: (a) the eponym *Grant* originates from the affected family's surname; (b) this syndrome may belong in the osteogenesis imperfecta spectrum; (c) some similarities to the family reported by Beighton (dentinogenesis imperfecta, blue sclerae, and wormian bones without fractures).

REFERENCES

Beighton P: Familial dentinogenesis imperfecta, blue sclera, and wormian bones without fractures: Another type of osteogenesis imperfecta? *J. Med. Genet.* 18:124, 1981.
Maclean JR, et al: The Grant syndrome. Persistent wormian bones, blue sclerae, mandibular hypoplasia, shallow glenoid fossae and camptomelia—an autosomal dominant trait. *Clin. Genet.* 29:523, 1986.

GREIG CEPHALOPOLYSYNDACTYLY SYNDROME

Synonym: Frontodigital syndrome.

Mode of Inheritance: Autosomal dominant with complete penetrance and variable expressivity.

Frequency: Over 40 reported cases (Baraister et al.; Gollop et al.).

Clinical and Radiologic Manifestations: (a) *craniofacial dysmorphism,* macrocephaly, broad nasal root, frontal bossing, scaphocephaly, brachycephaly, large fontanelle, hypertelorism, ear anomaly, lack of craniosynostosis; (b) hand anomalies: *postaxial* (occasionally preaxial) *polydactyly,* broad thumbs, syndactyly; (c) foot anomalies: *preaxial* (rarely postaxial) *polydactyly,* syndactyly, broad halux; (c) other reported abnormalities: chromosome abnormality: reciprocal

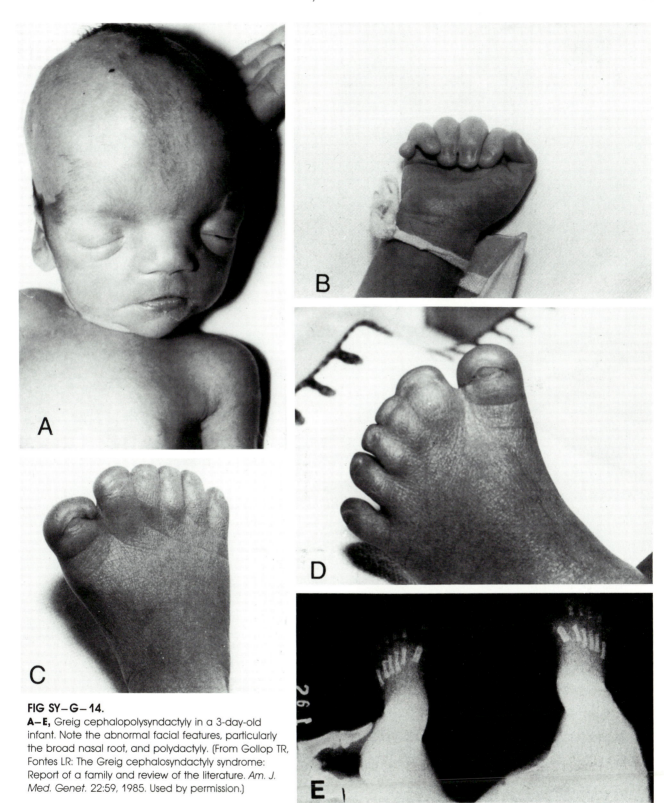

FIG SY–G–14.
A–E, Greig cephalopolysyndactyly in a 3-day-old infant. Note the abnormal facial features, particularly the broad nasal root, and polydactyly. (From Gollop TR, Fontes LR: The Greig cephalosyndactyly syndrome: Report of a family and review of the literature. *Am. J. Med. Genet.* 22:59, 1985. Used by permission.)

translocation t(3;7)(p21.1;p13), advanced bone age in a new-born, camptodactyly of the fingers and toes, inguinal hernia, etc.

Differential Diagnosis: Acrocallosal syndrome (Fig SY–G–14).

REFERENCES

Baraitser M, et al.: Greig cephalopolysyndactyly: Report of 13 affected individuals in three families. *Clin. Genet.* 24:257, 1983.

Chudley AE, et al.: The Greig cephalopolysyndactyly syndrome in a Canadian family. *Am. J. Med. Genet.* 13:269, 1982.

Gollop TR, et al.: The Greig cephalopolysyndactyly syndrome: Report of a family and review of the literature. *Am. J. Med. Genet.* 22:59, 1985.

Greig DM: Oxycephaly. *Edinb. Med. J.* 33:189, 1926.

Marshall RE, et al.: Frontodigital syndrome: A dominantly inherited disorder with normal intelligence. *J. Pediatr.* 77:129, 1970.

Merlob P, et al.: Le syndrome de Greig. Manifestations radiologiques néonatales. *J. Radiol.* 65:187, 1984.

Temtamy S, et al.: Synopsis on hand malformations with particular emphasis on genetic factors. *Birth Defects* 5:125, 1969.

Tommerup N, et al.: A familial reciprocal translocation t(3;7)(p21.1;p13) associated with the Greig polysyndactyly–craniofacial anomalies syndrome. *Am. J. Med. Genet.* 16:313, 1983.

GRISEL SYNDROME

Synonyms: "Torticolis naso-pharyngien"; torticollis atlanto-epistrophealis.

Etiology: Primary rhinopharyngitis; postoperative inflammation of the pharynx.

Clinical Manifestations: rapid onset of torticollis in conjunction with an inflammatory disease of the nasopharynx or in the postoperative period (tonsillectomy).

Radiologic Manifestations: anterior subluxation of the atlas over the axis.

REFERENCES

Grisel P: Enucléation de l'atlas et torticolis naso-pharyngien. *Presse Med.* 38:50, 1930.

Mozziconacci P, et al.: Luxation atloïdo-axoïdienne rheumatoid et syndrome de Grisel. *Ann. Pediatr. (Paris)* 20:405, 1973.

Parke WW, et al.: The pharyngovertebral veins: An anatomical rationale for Grisel's syndrome. *J. Bone Joint Surg. [Am.]* 66:568, 1984.

GROLL-HIRSCHOWITZ SYNDROME

Mode of Inheritance: Autosomal recessive has been suggested.

Frequency: Two families (Postaman et al.).

Clinical Manifestations: Onset in childhood or early adulthood: (a) neurological abnormalities: *nerve deafness,* dysarthria, ptosis, *absent tendon reflexes,* peripheral neuropathy, external ophthalmoplegia; (b) progressive weight loss, *cachexia;* (c) frequent loose stools; (d) *loss of teeth,* dental caries; (e) tachycardia (considered to be an expression of vagal system involvement); (f) other reported abnormalities: steatorrhea, hypoalbuminemia, protein-losing enteropathy, short fifth finger, pes cavus; (g) premature death.

Radiologic Manifestations: (a) *gastric retention* with a marked delay in emptying; (b) multiple duodenal and small-bowel diverticula.

REFERENCES

Groll A, Hirschowitz BJ: Steatorrhea and familial deafness in two siblings (abstract). *Clin. Res.* 14:47, 1966.

Potasman I, et al.: The Groll-Hirschowitz syndrome. *Clin. Genet.* 28:76, 1985.

GUILLAIN-BARRÉ SYNDROME

Pathology: Acute inflammatory demyelinating polyradiculoneuropathy.

Clinical Manifestations: (a) *symmetrical, flaccid, usually incomplete paralysis* that may involve the facial and bulbar nerves; myokymia; ophthalmoplegia; limited regional signs/symptoms (pharyngeal-cervical-brachial weakness with ptosis, paraparesis with normal power and reflexes in the arm, early severe ptosis without other signs of oculomotor weakness, acute severe midline back pain at the onset); abnormal brain stem auditory evoked potentials; dysautonomia; (b) subjective *sensory symptoms* and less often sensory loss, pain preceding weakness (buttock, back, thighs, etc.); (c) *high protein content of the cerebrospinal fluid without a proportional rise in cellular elements;* (d) normal body temperature, sedimentation rate, and leukocyte count (in noncomplicated cases); (e) association with certain viruses (cytomegalovirus, Epstein-Barr virus, smallpox vaccination, influenza vaccination, sporadic non-A, non-B viral hepatitis, etc.), typhoid fever, *Campylobacter jejuni* enteritis, pseudotumor cerebri, sarcoidosis, surgical procedures, epidural anesthesia, treatment with corticosteroids and danazol, membranous glomerulonephritis; (f) complications: immobilization hypercalcemia, voiding dysfunction with large postvoiding residuals or urinary retention, protracted respiratory failure, bilateral vocal cord paralysis and upper airway obstruction, bradycardia and asystole, etc.

Radiologic Manifestations: (a) widening of the nerve roots and obliteration of the root sleeves (edema of the nerves and roots in the acute phase, fibrous thickening and inflammatory exudates in the chronic phase); (b) complications of disease: recurrent atelectasis, pneumonia, pneumothorax, aspiration, peptic ulcer, urinary tract infection; (c) sequelae: scoliosis, deformities of the extremities.

Differential Diagnosis: Miller Fisher syndrome (acute external ophthalmoplegia, ataxia, and hyporeflexia).

REFERENCES

Berger JR, et al.: Guillain-Barré syndrome complicating typhoid fever. *Ann. Neurol.* 20:649, 1986.

Dehaene I, et al.: Guillain-Barré syndrome with ophthalmoplegia: Clinicopathologic study of the central and peripheral nervous systems, including the oculomotor nerves. *Neurology* 36:851, 1986.

Gracey DR, et al.: Respiratory failure in Guillain-Barré syndrome. *Mayo Clin. Proc.* 57:742, 1982.

Guillain G, Barré JA, et al.: Sur un syndrome de radiculonévrite avec hyperalbuminose du liquide céphalorachidien sans réaction cellulaire: Remarques sur les caractères cliniques et graphiques des réflexes tendineux. *Bull. Soc. Med. Hop. (Paris)* 40:1462, 1916.

Hart IK, et al: Guillain-Barré syndrome associated with cytomegalovirus infection. *Q. J. Med.* 67:425, 1988.

Hodson AK, et al.: Dysautonomia in Guillain-Barré syndrome with dorsal root ganglioneuropathy, wallerian degeneration, and fatal myocarditis. *Ann. Neurol.* 15:88, 1984.

Hory B, et al.: Guillain-Barré syndrome following danazol and corticosteroid therapy for hereditary angioedema. *Am. J. Med.* 79:111, 1985.

Hvidsten K, et al.: Myelography in Guillain-Barré syndrome (acute inflammatory polyradiculoneuropathy). *Neuroradiology* 14:235, 1978.

King EG, et al.: "Complications" of the Landry-Guillain-Barré-Strohl syndrome. *Can. Med. Assoc. J.* 104:393, 1971.

Kohler PC, et al.: Guillain-Barré syndrome following *Campylobacter jejuni* enteritis. *Arch. Neurol.* 44:1219, 1987.

Le Luyer B, et al.: Polyradiculonévrite révélatrice d'une sarcoïdose de l'enfant. *Arch. Fr. Pediatr.* 40:175, 1983.

Macleod WN: Sporadic non-A, non-B hepatitis and Epstein-Barr hepatitis associated with the Guillain-Barré syndrome. *Arch. Neurol.* 44:438, 1987.

Marés-Segura R, et al.: Guillain-Barré syndrome associated with hepatitis A. *Ann. Neurol.* 19:100, 1986.

Mateer JE, et al.: Myokymia in Guillain-Barré syndrome. *Neurology (N.Y.)* 33:374, 1983.

Meythaler JM, et al.: Immobilization hypercalcemia associated with Landry-Guillain-Barré syndrome. *Arch. Intern. Med.* 146:1567, 1986.

Najem Al-Din A, et al: Brainstem encephalitis and the syndrome of Miller Fisher: A clinical entity. *Brain* 105:481, 1982.

Narayan D, et al.: Bradycardia and asystole requiring permanent pacemaker in Guillain-Barré syndrome. *Am. Heart J.* 108:426, 1984.

Renlund DG, et al.: Guillain-Barré syndrome following coronary artery bypass surgery. *Am. Heart J.* 113:844, 1987.

Rodrigues JF, et al.: Upper airway obstruction in Guillain-Barré syndrome. *Chest* 86:147, 1984.

Ropper AH: Unusual clinical variants and signs in Guillain-Barré syndrome. *Arch. Neurol.* 43:1150, 1986.

Ropper AH, et al.: Mechanism of pseudotumor in Guillain-Barré syndrome. *Arch. Neurol.* 41:259, 1984.

Ropper AH, et al.: Pain in Guillain-Barré syndrome. *Arch. Neurol.* 41:511, 1984.

Schiff JA, et al.: Brainstem auditory evoked potentials in Guillain-Barré syndrome. *Neurology* 35:771, 1985.

Steiner I, et al.: Guillain-Barré syndrome after epidural anesthesia: Direct nerve root damage may trigger disease. *Neurology* 35:1473, 1985.

Talamo TS, et al.: Membranous glomerulonephritis associated with the Guillain-Barré syndrome. *Am. J. Clin. Pathol.* 78:563, 1982.

Wheeler JS, et al.: The urodynamic aspects of the Guillain-Barré syndrome. *J. Urol.* 131:917, 1984.

Winer JB, et al.: Guillain-Barré syndrome and influenza vaccine. *Lancet* 1:1182, 1984.

HAGLUND SYNDROME

Clinical Manifestations: (a) posterior heel pain; (b) tender soft-tissue swelling at the level of the Achilles tendon insertion.

Radiologic Manifestations: (a) prominent calcaneal bursal projection; (b) retrocalcaneal bursitis; (c) thickening of the Achilles tendon; (d) convexity of the superficial soft tissue at the level of the Achilles tendon insertion ("pump-bump").

Differential Diagnosis: Isolated retrocalcaneal bursitis, superficial bursitis (Achilles tendon), rheumatoid arthritis, Reiter syndrome, etc.

REFERENCES

Haglund P: Beitrag zur Klinik der Achillessehne. *Z. Orthop. Chir.* 49:49, 1927.
Heneghan MA, et al.: The Haglund painful heel syndrome. Experimental investigation of cause and therapeutic implications. *Clin. Orthop.* 187:228, 1984.
Pavlov H, et al.: The Haglund syndrome: Initial and differential diagnosis. *Radiology* 144:83, 1982.
Warren Burhenne LJ, et al.: Xeroradiography in the diagnosis of the Haglund syndrome. *J. Can. Assoc. Radiol.* 37:157, 1986.

HAJDU-CHENEY SYNDROME

Synonyms: Arthrodento-osteo-dysplasia; osteolysis (Hajdu-Cheney type).

Mode of Inheritance: Autosomal dominant and sporadic.

Frequency: Rare.

Clinical Manifestations:

(A) INFANCY AND CHILDHOOD: (a) *craniofacial features:* prominent occiput, synophrys, long lashes, thick eyebrows, low-set ears, high-arched palate, dental maleruption and malocclusion; (b) *short stature,* failure to thrive, retarded puberty; (c) short neck; (d) hernia; (e) hirsutism.

(B) ADULTS: (a) *craniofacial features:* prominent occiput, high-arched palate, prognathism, epicanthal folds, telecanthus, antimongoloid palpebral fissures, early loss of teeth; (b) stenotic ear canal, conductive hearing loss; (c) myopia, loss of vision, disk pallor, constriction of the visual field, nystagmus, abducens palsy, ptosis, exotropia, optic atrophy; (d) low-pitched voice; (e) painful paresthesia of the fingers; (f) progressive clubbing of the fingers; (g) intact fingernails; (h) joint laxity; (i) normal or near-normal intelligence.

Radiologic Manifestations: (a) bathrocephaly, basilar impression, depression at the site of the anterior fontanelle, multiple wormian bones, *persistence of cranial sutures in late adult life;* (b) alveolar resorption of the mandible and maxilla, edentulism in young adults; (c) *osteolysis of the terminal phalanges of the hands and feet;* (d) osteoporosis; (e) minimal failure of remodeling of the long bones, bowing of paired long bones, dislocated radial head, hip dislocation, genu valgum, high incidence of fractures; (f) kyphosis, tall lumbar vertebrae, narrow disk spaces, Schmorl nodes, vertebral collapse; (g) calcified aneurysm of a patent ductus arteriosus that had been surgically closed.

Note: A case with some of the features of Hajdu-Cheney syndrome associated with renal cystic dysplasia has been reported under the name of "arthro-osteo-renal dysplasia" (Zahran) (Figs SY–H–1 and SY–H–2).

REFERENCES

Blery M, et al.: Acro-ostéolyse d'Hajdu-Cheney et anévrysme calcifié sur canal artériel redux. *Ann. Radiol. (Paris)* 27:27, 1984.
Cheney WD: Acro-osteolysis. *A.J.R.* 94:595, 1965.
Dorst JP, et al.: Acro-osteolysis (Cheney syndrome). *Birth Defects* 5:215, 1969.
Elias AN, et al.: Hereditary osteodysplasia with acro-osteolysis (the Hajdu-Cheney syndrome). *Am. J. Med.* 65:627, 1978.
Gibofsky A: Genetics of the Hajdu-Cheney syndrome (letter). *Arthritis Rheum.* 30:718, 1987.
Hajdu N, et al.: Cranio-skeletal dysplasia. *Br. J. Radiol.* 21:42, 1948.
Niijima KH, et al.: Familial osteodysplasia associated with trigeminal neuralgia: Case report. *Neurosurgery* 15:562, 1984.
Rosenmann E, et al.: Sporadic idiopathic acro-osteolysis with cranio-skeletal dysplasia, polycystic kidneys and glomerulonephritis. *Pediatr. Radiol.* 6:116, 1977.
Shaw D: Melnick-Needles or Cheney-Hajdu? *Helv. Paediatr. Acta* 42:195, 1987.
Silverman FN, et al.: Acro-osteolysis (Hajdu-Cheney syndrome), in Bergsma D (ed.): *Skeletal Dysplasias.* Amsterdam, Excerpta Medica 1974, pp. 106–123.
Udell J, et al.: Idiopathic familial acroosteolysis: Histomorphometric study of bone and literature review of the Hajdu-Cheney syndrome. *Arthritis Rheum.* 29:1032, 1986.
Van den Houten BR, et al.: The Hajdu-Cheney syndrome. A

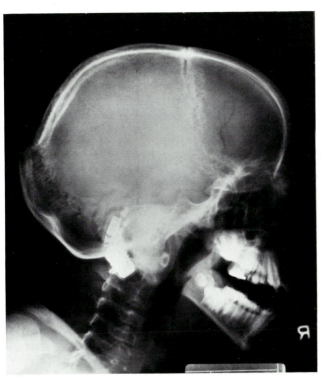

FIG SY–H–1.
Hajdu-Cheney syndrome in a girl aged 11 years, 10 months with persistence of the coronal suture, an elongated sella, a steep clivus, a hypoplastic frontal sinus, and a prominent occiput with thick bone and wormian bones. Note the hearing aid. (From Weleber RG, Beals RK: The Hajdu-Cheney syndrome: Report of two cases and review of the literature. *J. Pediatr.* 88:243, 1976. Used by permission.)

review of the literature and report of 3 cases. *Int. J. Oral Surg.* 14:113, 1985.

Velchik MG: Acro-osteolysis in a patient with Hajdu-Cheney syndrome demonstrated by bone scintigraphy. *Clin. Nucl. Med.* 9:659, 1984.

Weleber RG, Beals RK: The Hajdu-Cheney syndrome. *J. Pediatr.* 88:243, 1976.

Wendel U, et al.: Idiopathische osteolyse vom typ Hajdu-Cheney. *Monatsschr. Kinderheilkd.* 127:581, 1979.

Zahran M, et al.: Arthro-osteo-renal dysplasia. Report of a case. *Acta. Radiol.* 25:39, 1984.

HALLERMANN-STREIFF SYNDROME

Synonyms: Oculo-mandibulo-facial syndrome; François dyscephaly; dyscephaly with hypotrichosis; dyscephaly with congenital cataract and hypotrichosis; Ullrich and Fremerey-Dohna syndrome.

Mode of Inheritance: Not definitely known; familial cases have been reported.

Frequency: Rare.

Clinical Manifestations: (a) *dyscephaly* (scaphocephaly or brachycephaly); (b) *unusual facies* (bird face), small face, *small and pinched nose*, microstomia, thin lips, *micrognathia*, low-set ears, congenital cataracts, *microphthalmos*, blue sclerae, high-arched palate; (c) *hypotrichosis*; (d) *proportionate dwarfism*; (e) absence of teeth, persistence of deciduous teeth, malformation of teeth, natal teeth, supernumerary teeth, crowding of unerupted deciduous teeth and agenesis of all permanent teeth except the first permanent

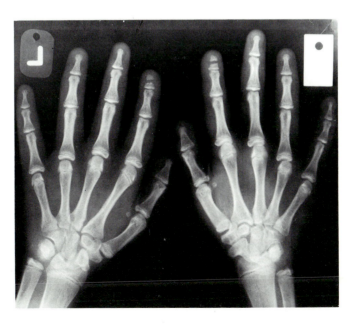

FIG SY–H–2.
Hajdu-Cheney syndrome in a girl aged 11 years and 3 months with a transverse lytic defect in the distal phalanx of the index finger that was associated with mild bulbous swelling of soft tissue.

(From Weleber RG, Beals RK: The Hajdu-Cheney syndrome: Report of two cases and review of the literature. *J. Pediatr.* 88:243, 1976. Used by permission.)

molars, premature and severe caries, etc.; (f) skin atrophy; (g) hyperextensible joints; (h) mental, motor, and speech retardation; (i) other reported abnormalities: syndactyly, clawhand, coxalgia, deficiency of humoral immunity and hypoparathyroidism, congenital heart defects, upper airway obstruction (obstructive sleep apnea, hypoxia, hypercarbia, pulmonary hypertension, etc.).

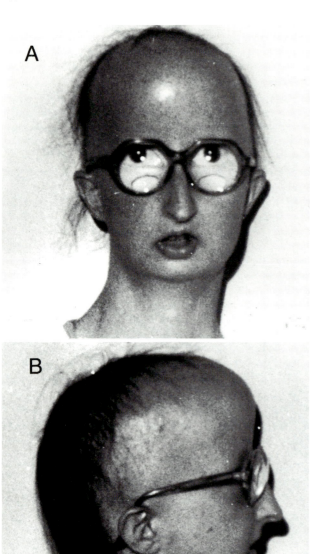

FIG SY–H–3.
Hallermann-Streiff syndrome: frontal **(A)** and lateral **(B)** views of a 19-year-old female. Note the bird face appearance and hypotrichosis. (From Sclaroff A, Eppley BL: Evaluation and surgical correction of the facial skeletal deformity in Hallermann-Streiff syndrome. *Int. J. Oral. Maxillofac. Surg.* 16:738, 1987. Used by permission.)

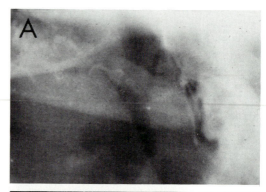

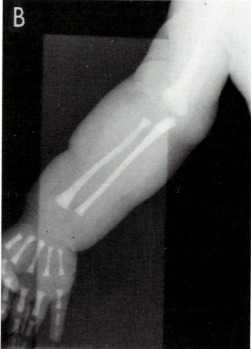

FIG SY–H–4.
Hallermann-Streiff syndrome in an 18-day-old female with an abnormal facial appearance, a small thin nose, a receding double chin, multiple erupted teeth, microphthalmos, and congenital cataract. **A,** an oblique view of the mandible demonstrates marked hypoplasia and deformity of the ramus in form of a bulbous prominence on the posterior aspect of the mandibular body. **B,** the tubular bones are gracile in appearance. (From Kurlander GJ, Lavy NW, Campbell JA: Roentgen differentiation of the oculo-dento-digital syndrome and the Hallermann-Streiff syndrome in infancy. *Radiology* 86:77, 1966. Used by permission.)

Radiologic Manifestations: (a) *brachycephaly, often delayed closure of the fontanelles and persistent wide sutures, frontal and parietal bossing, thin calvaria;* (b) *small face and orbits;* (c) *hypoplasia of the mandibular rami with anterior displacement of temporomandibular joints, abnormally obtuse gonial angle;* (d) *gracile appearance of the tubular bones in infancy;* (e) other reported anomalies: platybasia; calcification of the falx; shallow sella turcica; hypoplasia of nasal, maxillary, and zygomatic bones; osteoporosis; vertebral anomalies; lordosis; scoliosis; platyspondyly; elevated scapulae; dental anomalies (hypoplasia of the teeth; malimplantation; neonatal teeth; partial anodontia); anomalies of the ulna and radius, hip dislocation (Figs SY−H−3 and SY−H−4).

REFERENCES

Chandra RK, et al.: Deficiency of humoral immunity and hypoparathyroidism associated with the Hallermann-Streiff syndrome. *J. Pediatr.* 93:892, 1978.

Dinwiddie R, et al.: Cardiac defects in the Hallermann-Streiff syndrome. *J. Pediatr.* 92:77, 1978.

François J: A new syndrome: Dyscephalia with bird face and dental anomalies, nanism, hypotrichosis, cutaneous atrophy, microphthalmia, and congenital cataract. *Arch. Ophthalmol.* 60:842, 1958.

Friede H, et al.: Cardiorespiratory disease associated with Hallermann-Streiff syndrome: Analysis of craniofacial morphology by cephalometric roentgenograms. *J. Craniofac. Genet. Div. Biol.* [Suppl.] 1:189, 1985.

Hallermann W: Vogelgesicht und Cataracta congenita. *Klin. Monatsbl. Augenheilkd.* 113:315, 1948.

Kurlander GJ, et al.: Roentgen differentiation of the oculo-dento-digital syndrome and the Hallermann-Streiff syndrome in infancy. *Radiology* 86:77, 1966.

Sclaroff A, et al.: Evaluation and surgical correction of the facial skeletal deformity in Hallermann-Streiff syndrome. *Int. J. Oral Maxillofac. Surg.* 16:738, 1987.

Slootweg PJ, et al.: Dento-alveolar abnormalities in oculo-mandibulodyscephaly (Hallermann-Streiff syndrome). *J. Oral Pathol.* 13:147, 1984.

Steel HH, et al.: Bilateral dislocation of the hip in Hallermann-Streiff syndrome. *J. Bone Joint Surg. [Am.]* 57:1002, 1975.

Streiff EB: Dysmorphie mandibulo-faciale (tête d'oiseau) et altération oculaire. *Ophthalmologica* 120:79, 1950.

Ullrich O, Fremerey-Dohna H: Dyskephalie mit Cataracta congenita und Hypotrichose als typischer Merkmalskomplex. *Ophthalmologica* 125:73, 1953.

HAMMAN-RICH SYNDROME

Synonyms: Idiopathic pulmonary fibrosis; familial idiopathic pulmonary fibrosis.

Mode of Inheritance: Autosomal dominant (idiopathic pulmonary fibrosis).

Pathology: (a) *early: edema, cellular infiltration and fibrous deposition in alveolar walls; (b) later: proliferation of fibrous tissue and encroachment of alveolar structures.*

Clinical Manifestations: *Insidious onset with progressive development of dyspnea, tachypnea, dry cough, weight loss, fatigue, sputum, clubbing of the fingers,* cyanosis, signs of pulmonary hypertension, cor pulmonale, cardiac failure.

Radiologic Manifestations: (a) *early: fine reticular mottling pattern of the lung,* most prominent at the base; (b) *later: coarse, reticular, or reticulonodular densities; "honeycomb"-*

type cystic shadows; pneumothorax; bronchial and bronchiolar dilatation; *progressive loss of lung volume;* (c) computed tomography: peripheral rim of reticular and linear densities, peripheral honeycomb cysts, fine irregularity and thickening of the pleural surface.

REFERENCES

Bergin CJ, Müller NL: CT of interstitial lung disease: A diagnostic approach. *A.J.R.* 148:8, 1987.

Bitterman PB, et al.: Familial idiopathic pulmonary fibrosis. Evidence of lung inflammation in unaffected family members. *N. Engl. J. Med.* 314:1343, 1986.

Hamman L, Rich AR: Acute diffuse interstitial fibrosis of lungs. *Bull. Johns Hopkins Hosp.* 74:177, 1944.

Homolka J: Idiopathic pulmonary fibrosis: A historical review. *Can. Med. Assoc. J.* 137:1003, 1987.

Lemire P, et al.: Patterns of desquamative interstitial pneumonia (D.I.P.) and diffuse interstitial pulmonary fibrosis (D.I.P.F.). *A.J.R.* 115:479, 1972.

Ostinelli J, et al: Fibrose pulmonaire interstitielle diffuse primitive familiale avec emphyséme bulleux. *Presse Med.* 15:1285, 1986.

Rubin A, et al.: Diffuse interstitial lung fibrosis from childhood and adolescence to adult life. *Pediatr. Radiol.* 11:125, 1981.

Schwarz MI: Idiopathic pulmonary fibrosis (medical staff conference). *West J. Med.* 149:199, 1988.

Swaye P, et al.: Familial Hamman-Rich syndrome: Report of eight cases. *Dis. Chest* 55:7, 1969.

HAND-FOOT-GENITAL SYNDROME

Synonym: Hand-foot-uterus syndrome.

Mode of Inheritance: Autosomal dominant with full penetrance and variable expression.

Frequency: Rare.

Clinical Manifestations: (a) *small feet, short great toes;* (b) *abnormal thumbs, thenar eminence hypoplasia,* clinodactyly of the fifth fingers; (c) genital anomalies in females: bifid uterus, double uterus, septate vagina, opening of the urethral meatus into the vaginal vault; (d) various degrees of hypospadias in males; (e) association with nevoid basal cell carcinoma syndrome (case report).

Radiologic Manifestations: *Various anomalies of the hands and feet:* (a) *hands:* short first metacarpals, short middle phalanx of the fifth fingers, pseudoepiphyses, pointed distal phalanx of the thumbs, fusion of the trapezium and scaphoid, os centrale, long ulnar styloid, split ulnar epiphysis, a typical "pattern profile" (Poznanski) of the metacarpals and phalanges; (b) *feet:* short first metatarsals, pointed distal phalanx of the great toe, tarsal and phalangeal coalition, absence of most secondary ossification centers of the middle and distal phalanges, short proximal phalanx (middle toe), abnormal navicular bone, short calcaneus, fusion of the cu-

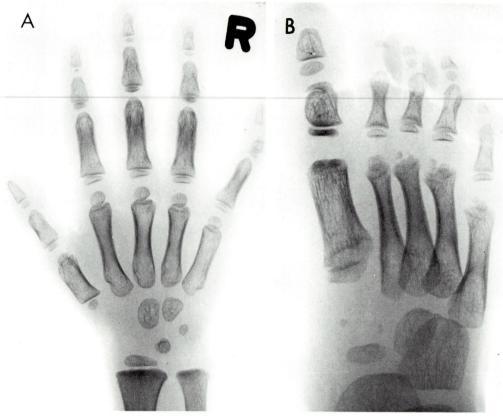

FIG SY—H—5.

Hand-foot-genital syndrome in a 5-year-old boy with hypospadias (one of three brothers with the syndrome). **A,** hand: short first metacarpal, pointed distal phalanx of the thumb, pseudoepiphysis, notch metacarpal, short middle phalanx V, clinodactyly V. **B,** foot: short tuftless distal phalanx of the great toe, broad great toe (soft tissue), dysgenesis of the middle and distal phalanges of the other toes. (From Giedion A, Prader A: Hand-foot-uterus (HFU) syndrome with hypospadias: The hand-foot-genital-(HFG) syndrome. *Pediatr. Radiol.* 4:96, 1976. Used by permission.)

neiform to other bones, delay in appearance or maturation of medial and intermediate cuneiforms (Fig SY—H—5).

REFERENCES

Giedion A, et al.: Hand-foot-uterus-(HFU) syndrome with hypospadias: The hand-foot-genital-(HFG) syndrome. *Pediatr. Radiol.* 4:96, 1976.

Halal F: The hand-foot-genital (hand-foot-uterus) syndrome: Family report and update. *Am. J. Med. Genet.* 30:793, 1988.

Knöbber D, et al.: Stapesanomalie, Gorlin-Goltz-und Hand-Fuss-Uterus-Syndrom als Teilaspekte eines Generalisierten Ektodermal-Mesodermalen Missbildungssyndromes mit wechselnder Expressivität. *Laryngol. Rhinol. Otol.* 65:305, 1986.

Poznanski AK, et al.: A new family with the hand-foot-genital syndrome. A wider spectrum of the hand-foot-uterus syndrome. *Birth Defects* 11:127, 1975.

Poznanski AK, et al.: Radiographic findings in the hand-foot-uterus syndrome (HFUS). *Radiology* 95:129, 1970.

Stern AM, et al: The hand-foot-uterus syndrome. A new hereditary disorder characterized by hand and foot dysplasia, dermatoglyphic abnormalities, and partial duplication of the female genital tract. *J. Pediatr.* 77:109, 1970.

HECHT SYNDROME

Synonym: Trismus-pseudocamptodactyly syndrome.

Mode of Inheritance: Autosomal dominant; more common in females.

Clinical and Radiologic Manifestations: (a) inability to open the mouth fully; (b) pseudocamptodactyly (short finger flexor tendons); (c) short leg muscles producing a foot deformity (talipes equinovarus, metatarsus adductus, etc.); (d) short stature.

REFERENCES

Hecht F, Beals RK: Inability to open the mouth fully. *Birth Defects* 5:96, 1968.

Robertson RD, et al.: Linkage analysis with the trismus-pseudocamptodactyly syndrome. *Am. J. Med. Genet.* 12:115, 1982.

Tsukahara M, et al.: Trismus-pseudocamptodactyly syndrome in a Japanese family. *Clin. Genet.* 28:247, 1985.

HEMIHYPERTROPHY

Synonym: Congenital asymmetry.

Clinical Manifestations: (a) range of asymmetry from *enlargement of one digit to hypertrophy of the entire one half of the body;* (b) spontaneous improvement of the asymmetry (rare); (c) associated reported conditions: mental deficiency, skin lesions (hemangiomas, nevi, telangiectasia, café au lait spots, unilateral folliculitis, acne), unilateral hypertrichosis, precocious development of genital hair, Beckwith-Wiedemann syndrome, hypospadias, Sotos syndrome, phakomatoses, hamartomatous lesions, testicular hypertrophy, etc.

Radiologic Manifestations: (a) *asymmetry,* no difference in bone age between the two sides; (b) genitourinary abnormalities: benign or unilateral nephromegaly, medullary sponge kidney, renal ectopia, cysts, calyceal diverticulum, ovarian cysts; (c) oncogenic potential: liver (hepatoblastoma, hemangioendothelioma), kidney (Wilms tumor, nephroblastomatosis), adrenocortical (adenoma, hyperplasia, carcinoma), gonadoblastoma, carcinoma of an undescended testicle, pheochromocytoma, retroperitoneal sarcoma, cerebellar hemangioblastoma; (d) other reported abnormalities: liver cyst, focal nodular hyperplasia of the liver, cerebral vascular abnormalities (aneurysm, capillary hemangioma, arteriovenous malformation), intestinal lymphangiectasia.

Differential Diagnosis: Hemihypotrophy; hemiatrophy; vascular and lymphatic abnormalities as etiologic factors (Fig SY–H–6).

Notes: (a) the HEMI 3 syndrome refers to a developmental syndrome of (1) hypertrophy involving half or a quadrant of the body and not involving the face, muscle hypertrophy, increased power, increased diameter, length of bone similar to the opposite side; (2) hemihypesthesia; (3) hemiareflexia; (4) progressive scoliosis and foot deformity on the enlarged side; (b) the incidence of the occurrence of tumor (mainly malignant) in the patients with Beckwith-Wiedemann syndrome has been estimated to be 7.5%. In 12.5% of children with this syndrome hemihypertrophy was present; in 40% of the children with Beckwith-Wiedemann syndrome and tumor, hemihypertrophy was present. The following recommendation has been made (Wiedemann): every child with Beckwith-Wiedemann syndrome needs to be examined with renal sonography, first at 3-month intervals and after the third year of life at 6-month intervals.

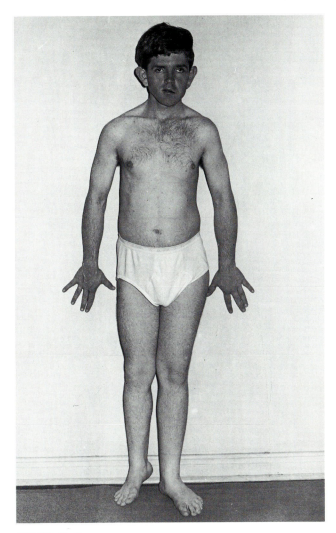

FIG SY–H–6.
Hemihypertrophy (idiopathic) in a 26-year-old patient with facial and body asymmetry. (From Viljoen D, Pearn J, Beighton P: Manifestations and natural history of idiopathic hemihypertrophy: A review of eleven cases. *Clin. Genet.* 26:81, 1984. Used by permission.)

REFERENCES

Beals RK: Hemihypertrophy and hemihypotrophy. *Clin. Orthop.* 166:199, 1982.

Everson RB, et al.: Focal nodular hyperplasia of the liver in a child with hemihypertrophy. *J. Pediatr.* 88:985, 1976.

Ferran J, et al.: Kyste du rein et hémi-hypertrophie corporelle congénitale. *Ann. Radiol. (Paris)* 25:136, 1982.

Fischer EG, et al.: Congenital hemihypertrophy and abnormalities of the cerebral vasculature. Report of two cases. *J. Neurosurg.* 61:163, 1984.

Furukawa T, et al.: Congenital hemihypertrophy: Oncogenic potential of the hypertrophic side. *Ann. Neurol.* 9:199, 1981.

Harris RE, et al.: Medullary sponge kidney and congenital

hemihypertrophy: Case report and literature review. *J. Urol.* 126:676, 1981.

Janik JS, et al.: Delayed onset of hemihypertrophy in Wilms' tumor. *J. Pediatr. Surg.* 11:581, 1976.

Kääpä P, et al.: Hemihypertrophy with unilateral folliculitis and acne. *Acta Paediatr. Scand.* 68:921, 1979.

Kirks DR, et al.: Idiopathic congenital hemihypertrophy with associated ipsilateral benign nephromegaly. *Radiology* 115:145, 1975.

Labrune B, et al: Hyperinsulinisme néonatal, hémihypertrophie corporelle congénitale, tumeur du sein à l'adolescence. *Arch. Fr. Pediatr.* 45:413, 1988.

Nudleman K, et al.: The HEMI 3 syndrome: Hemihypertrophy, hemihypaesthesia, hemiareflexia and scoliosis. *Brain* 107:533, 1984.

Parra G, et al.: Congenital total hemihypertrophy and carcinoma of undescended testicle: A case report. *J. Urol.* 118:343, 1977.

Pavone L, et al.: Lymphangiectasie intestinale chez un enfant atteint d'hémihypertrophie congénitale. *Ann. Pediatr. (Paris)* 30:803, 1983.

Pfister RC, et al.: Congenital asymmetry (hemihypertrophy) and abdominal disease. *Radiology* 116:685, 1975.

Porter FN: Hemihypertrophy associated with a benign congenital liver cyst. *Eur. J. Pediatr.* 139:89, 1982.

Ringrose RE, et al.: Hemihypertrophy: A review. *Pediatrics* 36:434, 1965.

Ritter R, et al.: Hemihypertrophy in a boy with renal polycystic disease: Varied patterns of presentation of renal polycystic disease in his family. *Pediatr. Radiol.* 5:98, 1976.

Roggensack G, et al.: Bilateral nephromegaly in a child with hemihypertrophy. *A.J.R.* 110:546, 1970.

Saypol DC, et al.: Congenital hemihypertrophy with adrenal carcinoma and medullary sponge kidney. *Urology* 21:510, 1983.

Schenck RD: Hemihypertrophie beim Wiedemann-Beckwith Syndrom (Exomphalos-Makroglossie-Gigantismus-Syndrom). *Z. Orthop.* 114:354, 1976.

Schnakenburg KV, et al.: Congenital hemihypertrophy and malignant giant pheochromocytoma—a previously undescribed coincidence. *Eur. J. Pediatr.* 122:263, 1976.

Schneider A, et al.: Hemihypertrophie bei einem Knaben mit polyzystischen Nieren. *Helv. Paediatr. Acta* 42:305, 1987.

See G, et al.: Association d'un gigantisme cérébral type Sotos et d'une hémihypertrophie corporelle totale congénitale. *Ann. Pediatr. (Paris)* 21:223, 1974.

Tank ES, et al.: Neoplasms associated with hemihypertrophy, Beckwith-Wiedemann syndrome and anirida. *J. Urol.* 124:266, 1980.

Tolchin D, et al.: Early detection of Wilms' tumor in a child with hemihypertrophy and ovarian cysts. *Pediatrics* 70:136, 1982.

Tomooka Y, et al.: Congenital hemihypertrophy with adrenal adenoma and medullary sponge kidney. *Br. J. Radiol.* 61:851, 1988.

Viljoen D, et al.: Manifestations and natural history of idiopathic hemihypertrophy: A review of eleven cases. *Clin. Genet.* 26:81, 1984.

Wiedemann H-R: Tumours and hemihypertrophy associated with Wiedemann-Beckwith syndrome. *Eur. J. Pediatr.* 141:129, 1983.

Wood BP, et al.: Infantile hepatic hemangioendotheliomas associated with hemihypertrophy. *Pediatr. Radiol.* 5:242, 1977.

HEMOLYTIC-UREMIC SYNDROME

Classification: (a) the classic form: most common in the first 2 years of life, isolated occurrence or summer outbreaks; (b) the postinfection form (*Escherichia coli, Shigella dysenteriae* 1, *Streptococcus pneumoniae, Salmonella typhi,* certain viruses, immunization, etc.): not limited to infants; (c) the hereditary forms: autosomal dominant and autosomal recessive forms, infants and older age group; recurrence in some cases; (d) immune pathogenesis: may be familial, low plasma C3 levels, evidence of activation of the alternative complement pathway, glomerular C3 deposits, plasma C3 nephritic factor (in some); (e) association with other precipitating factors: illnesses, systemic hypertension, systemic lupus erythematosus, scleroderma, renal radiotherapy, immunosuppressive drugs, etc.; (f) pregnancy or oral contraceptive—related form: microangiopathy mostly arterial.

Pathogenesis: Disseminated intravascular coagulation and microangiopathy resulting in hemolytic anemia and thrombocytopenia.

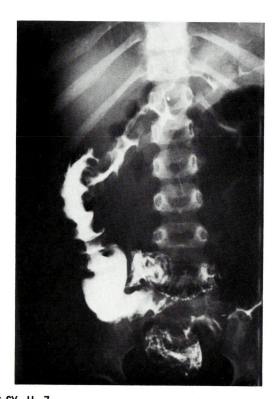

FIG SY—H—7.
Hemolytic-uremic syndrome in a 4-year-old girl with bloody diarrhea. A barium enema shows a prominent filling defect ("thumbprinting").

Clinical Manifestations: (a) upper respiratory tract infection or "flulike" illness as prodromal symptoms; (b) gastrointestinal symptoms: *vomiting; diarrhea, often bloody;* abdominal symptoms that may simulate an acute surgical abdomen or ulcerative colitis; (c) *hematuria, proteinuria,* renal failure; (d) purpura, petechiae; (e) hypertension, congestive heart failure, dilated cardiomyopathy; (f) *central nervous system manifestations:* focal or general seizures, altered consciousness, decerebrate posturing, hemiparesis, eye involvement, ataxia, coma, residual neurological changes (hemiparesis, seizures, cortical visual defect, etc.); (g) *hemolytic anemia, thrombocytopenia, azotemia,* hyponatremia, hyperuricemia, hyperphosphatemia, hyperkalemia, hyperlipidemia, abnormally shaped red blood cells, elevated white blood cell count with a shift to the left, elevated total bilirubin level, intravascular coagulation; (h) pathology: microthrombi (brain, myocardium, kidney, etc.), microangiopathy; (i) other reported abnormalities: acute rhabdomyolysis, decreased plasma fibronectin levels, pancreatic islet cell necrosis, exocrine and endocrine pancreatic insufficiency, insulin-dependent diabetes mellitus, antithrombin III deficiency, association with acquired immunodeficiency syndrome (AIDS), abnormality in prostaglandin I_2 (PGI_2) synthesis, association with Kawasaki disease.

Radiologic Manifestations: (a) cardiomegaly, congestive heart failure, pulmonary edema; (b) digestive tract: *colon changes simulating ulcerative colitis, prominent filling defects, mucosal edema, marginal serrations,* focal or total colonic infarction, gangrene, perforation, stricture; (c) acute renal cortical necrosis: hyperechogenicity of the renal cortex, sonolucent renal pyramids, poor renal function by radionuclide renal scan (anephric pattern not predictive of the development of irreversible renal damage), renal atrophy, cortical calcification; (d) cerebral infarction (cerebral microthrombi, in particular, in the basal ganglia; large-vessel thrombotic strokes less common); (e) other reported abnormalities: bone marrow necrosis in the adult (radionuclide scan), pancreatic calcification, etc.

Differential Diagnosis: Henoch-Schönlein syndrome; thrombotic thrombocytopenia; platelet sequestration (Kasa-

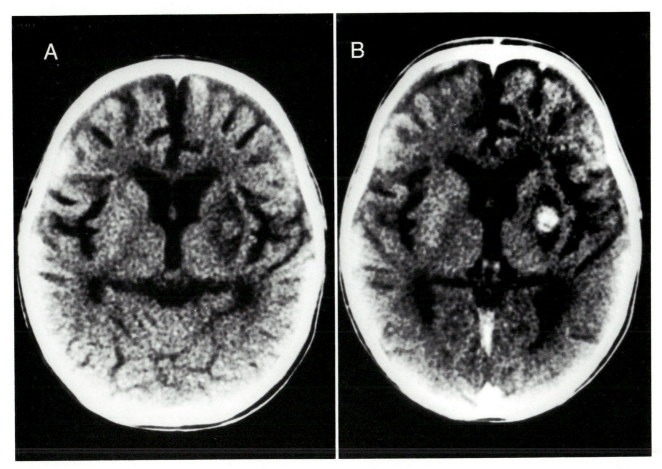

FIG SY—H—8.
Hemolytic-uremic syndrome in a 1-year-old male: computed tomography, precontrast **(A)** scan and postcontrast **(B)** scan about 4 weeks after the onset of symptoms. There is a generalized increase in the ventricular size and subarchnoid space (brain atrophy) and a left basal ganglia infarct. The postcontrast scan shows enhancement in the center of the lesion, which is consistent with neovascularity. (Courtesy of Ronald A. Cohen, M.D., Children's Hospital Medical Center, Oakland, Calif.)

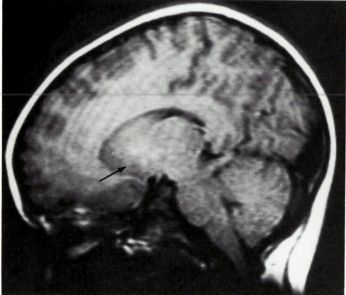
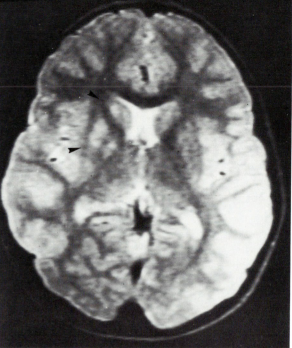

FIG SY–H–9.
Hemolytic-uremic syndrome. **A,** T_1-weighted sagittal image. **B,** T_2-weighted axial image. Both depict punctate foci of increased intensity seen in the region of the right caudate and lentiform nuclei *(arrow, arrowheads).* (From DiMario FJ, Brönte-Stewart H, Sherbotie J, et al.: Lacunar infarction of the basal ganglia as a complication of hemolytic uremic syndrome. *Clin. Pediatr. (Phila.)* 26:586, 1987. Used by permission.)

bach-Merritt syndrome); ulcerative colitis; Crohn disease; pseudomembranous colitis; bacterial colitis; viral gastroenteritis; intussusception; paroxysmal nocturnal hemoglobinuria; etc. (Figs SY–H–7 to SY–H–9).

REFERENCES

Andreoli SP, et al.: Acute rhabdomyolysis associated with hemolytic-uremic syndrome. *J. Pediatr.* 103:78, 1983.

Andreoli SP, et al.: Development of insulin-dependent diabetes mellitus during the hemolytic-uremic syndrome. *J. Pediatr.* 100:541, 1982.

Andreoli SP, et al.: Exocrine and endocrine pancreatic insufficiency and calcinosis after hemolytic uremic syndrome. *J. Pediatr.* 110:816, 1987.

Boccia RV, et al.: A hemolytic-uremic syndrome with the acquired immunodeficiency syndrome. *Ann. Intern. Med.* 101:716, 1984.

Butler T, et al.: Risk factors for development of hemolytic uremic syndrome during shigellosis. *J. Pediatr.* 110:894, 1987.

Campos A, et al.: Radionuclide studies of the kidney in children with hemolytic-uremic syndrome. *Radiology* 145:811, 1982.

Chamovitz BN, et al.: *Campylobacter jejuni*–associated hemolytic-uremic syndrome in a mother and daughter. *Pediatrics* 71:253, 1983.

Choyke PL, et al.: Cortical echogenicity in the hemolytic uremic syndrome: Clinical correlation. *J. Ultrasound Med.* 7:439, 1988.

Cosio FG, et al.: Decreased plasma fibronectin levels in children with hemolytic-uremic syndrome. *Am. J. Med.* 78:549, 1985.

DiMario FJ, et al.: Lacunar infarction of the basal ganglia as a complication of hemolytic-uremic syndrome. *Clin. Pediatr. (Phila.)* 26:586, 1987.

Drummond KN: Hemolytic uremic syndrome—then and now. *N. Engl. J. Med.* 312:116, 1985.

Edelsten AD, et al.: Familial haemolytic uraemic syndrome. *Arch. Dis. Child.* 53:255, 1978.

Ferriero DM, et al.: Hemolytic uremic syndrome associated with Kawaski disease. *Pediatrics* 68:405, 1981.

Gasser von C, et al.: Hämolytisch-urämische Syndrom: Bilaterale Nierenrindennekrosen bei akuten erworbenen hämolytischen Anämien. *Schweiz. Med. Wochenschr.* 85:905, 1955.

Hicks CB, et al.: Adult hemolytic-uremic syndrome and bone marrow necrosis. *West. J. Med.* 141:680, 1984.

Kenney PJ, et al.: Sonography of the kidneys in hemolytic uremic syndrome. *Invest. Radiol.* 21:547, 1986.

Kirks DR: The radiology of enteritis due to hemolytic-uremic syndrome. *Pediatr. Radiol.* 12:179, 1982.

Kletzel M, et al.: Paroxysmal nocturnal hemoglobinuria presenting as recurrent hemolytic uremic syndrome. *Clin. Pediatr. (Phila.)* 26:319, 1987.

Neill MA, et al.: *Escherichia coli* 0157:H7 as the predominant pathogen associated with the hemolytic uremic syndrome: A prospective study in the Pacific Northwest. *Pediatrics* 80:37, 1987.

Poulton J, et al.: Dilated cardiomyopathy associated with haemolytic uraemic syndrome. *Br. Heart J.* 57:181, 1987.

Roth B, et al.: Deficiency of antithrombin III in children with hemolytic-uremic syndrome. *Eur. J. Pediatr.* 142:16, 1984.

Sawaf H, et al.: Ischemic colitis and stricture after hemolytic-uremic syndrome. *Pediatrics* 61:315, 1978.

Sheth KJ, et al.: Neurological involvement in hemolytic-uremic syndrome. *Ann. Neurol.* 19:90, 1986.

Siegler RL, et al.: Ocular involvement in hemolytic-uremic syndrome. *J. Pediatr.* 112:594, 1988.

Steele BT, et al.: Post-partum haemolytic uraemic syndrome and verotoxin-producing *Escherichia coli. Lancet* 1:511, 1984.

Stuart MJ, et al.: Abnormal platelet and vascular prostaglandin synthesis in an infant with hemolytic uremic syndrome. *Pediatrics* 71:120, 1983.

Sty JR, et al.: Acute renal cortical necrosis in hemolytic uremic syndrome. *J. Clin. Ultrasound* 11:175, 1983.

Trevathan E, et al.: Large thrombotic strokes in hemolytic-uremic syndrome. *J. Pediatr.* 111:863, 1987.

HEMORRHAGIC SHOCK—ENCEPHALOPATHY SYNDROME

Clinical Manifestations: Sudden development of symptoms: (a) hyperthermia; (b) encephalopathy; (c) severe shock; (d) diarrhea, intestinal bleeding; (e) renal and hepatic dysfunction; (f) disseminated intravascular coagulation; (g) hemorrhagic foci in the brain, lung parenchyma, etc. (autopsy).

Radiologic Manifestations: Cerebral edema.

REFERENCES

Hervás JA, et al.: Further observations in haemorrhagic shock and encephalopathy syndrome. *Helv. Paediatr. Acta* 41:469, 1986.

Hervé F, et al.: Le syndrome de choc hémorragique avec encéphalopathie. *Arch. Fr. Pediatr.* 44:195, 1987.

Levin M, et al.: Hemorrhagic shock and encephalopathy: A new syndrome with high mortality in young children. *Lancet* 2:64, 1983.

Roth B, et al.: Haemorrhagic shock—encephalopathy syndrome: Plasmapheresis as a therapeutic approach. *Eur. J. Pediatr.* 146:83, 1987.

Sofer S, et al.: Hemorrhagic shock and encephalopathy syndrome. Its association with hypertermia. *Am. J. Dis. Child.* 140:1252, 1986.

HENOCH-SCHÖNLEIN SYNDROME

Synonyms: Schönlein-Henoch syndrome; anaphylactoid purpura; rheumatoid purpura; Henoch-Schömlein purpura.

Pathology: Allergic necrotizing arteritis with submucosal hemorrhage and mucosal ulceration of the bowel.

Etiology: Diffuse vasculitis, often idiopathic, may be induced by drugs, infectious agents, foods, chemicals, or insect bites; probable antigen-antibody reaction causing damage to the vascular epithelium (IgA the main pathogenic antibody).

Clinical Manifestations: (a) *insidious or sudden onset of pain in the abdomen,* vomiting; (b) *painful joints;* (c) *cutaneous purpura,* maculopapular or urticarial rash in some (in addition to the purpura); (d) gastrointestinal hemorrhage, endoscopic demonstration of submucosal hemorrhage, superficial ulcer, erosive gastritis, hemorrhagic-erosive duodenitis, purpuric lesions, ulcers of the rectosigmoid colon; (e) *nephritis,* hematuria, proteinuria, dysuria, leukocyturia, bacteriuria, anuria, hemorrhagic ureteritis associated with colicky flank pain and hematuria; (f) edema; (g) headaches, behavioral changes during acute phase, seizures, intracranial hemorrhage, focal neurological deficits, mononeuropathies, polyradiculoneuropathies, Guillain-Barré syndrome, brachial plexopathy, coma; (h) testicular and scrotal swelling; (i) arrhythmias, cardiac failure; (j) elevated erythrocyte sedimentation rate, leukocytosis, polynucleosis, hypoproteinemia, thrombocytosis; (k) decrease in factor XIII levels during acute phase; increase in IgA-bearing peripheral blood lymphocytes, raised levels of IgA immune complexes, raised levels of IgG immune complexes in those who develop nephritis, characteristic granular deposition of IgA shown by immunofluorescence in clinically involved and uninvolved tissues (skin, kidney, small intestine, lung, heart), development of inhibitors to factors VIII and IX in association with Henoch-Schönlein syndrome; (l) other reported abnormalities: malabsorption syndrome, appendicitis, acute pancreatitis, serosanguineous pleural effusion, selective IgA deficiency associated with mesangial proliferative glomerulonephritis, muscle pain, recurrent acute pulmonary failure, and development of fatal lung disease (pulmonary alveolar edema, interstitial fibrosis, arterial fibrinoid thrombosis).

Radiologic Manifestations: (a) *small bowel: spiking or cobblestone appearance of the bowel wall resulting from mucosal edema, rigidity, and thumbprints resulting from submucosal intestinal hemorrhage;* colonic wall edema; intussusception; spontaneous bowel perforation; massive necrosis of the esophagus; mucosal erosion; intestinal stricture as a late complication; ultrasonography and computed tomography demonstration of gastrointestinal involvement (mural thickening, luminal narrowing, intramural hemorrhage); (b) urinary system: ureteral obstruction at different levels with variable degrees of upper urinary tract dilatation, irregular mural filling defect in the urinary bladder, swelling of the bladder wall; (c) scrotal imaging (^{99m}Tc pertechnetate): increased uptake on affected side; (d) other reported abnormalities: pulmonary infiltrates, pleural effusion, intracranial hemorrhage, hydrops of the gallbladder, etc. (Figs SY—H—10 and SY—H—11).

REFERENCES

Ashkenazi S, et al.: Henoch-Schönlein vasculitis following varicella. *Am. J. Dis. Child.* 139:440, 1985.

Belman AL, et al.: Neurologic manifestations of Schoenlein-Henoch purpura: Report of three cases and review of the literature. *Pediatrics* 75:687, 1985.

Branski D, et al.: Pancreatitis as a complication of Henoch-

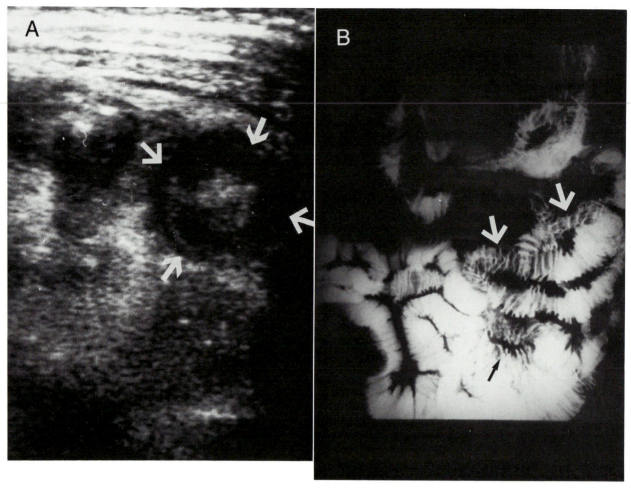

FIG SY–H–10.
Henoch-Schönlein syndrome in a 13-year-old male. **A,** an ultrasonogram shows a markedly thickened bowel wall *(arrows)*. **B,** a contrast study of the bowel following ultrasonography shows swelling of the bowel wall and a spiking appearance *(arrows)*. (Courtesy of Kenneth W. Martin, M.D., and Peter E. Kane, M.D., Children's Hospital Medical Center, Oakland, Calif.)

FIG SY–H–11.
Henoch-Schönlein syndrome: computed tomographic scans of the upper portion of the abdomen. There is a low-attenuation area *(arrowheads)* in the submucosal region that corresponds to either hemorrhage or edema. There is profound mural thickening. Air and contrast material are visible in the lumen *(arrow)*. (From Siskind BN, Burrell MI, Pun H, et al.: CT demonstration of gastrointestinal involvement in Henoch-Schönlein syndrome. *Gastrointest. Radiol.* 10:352, 1985. Used by permission.)

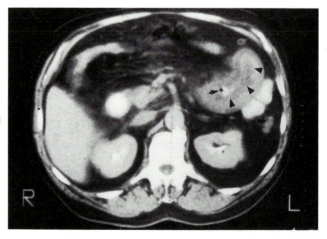

Schönlein purpura. *J. Pediatr. Gastroenterol. Nutr.* 1:275, 1982.

Clark JH, et al.: Hemorrhagic complications of Henoch-Schönlein syndrome. *J. Pediatr. Gastroenterol. Nutr.* 4:311, 1985.

Cooper SG, et al.: Ultrasound diagnosis of acute scrotal hemorrhage in Henoch-Schönlein purpura. *J. Clin. Ultrasound* 16:353, 1988.

Doyle T, et al.: The radiological features of Henoch-Schönlein purpura in the gastrointestinal tract. *Australas. Radiol.* 30:313, 1986.

Duell PB, et al.: Henoch-Schönlein purpura following thiram exposure. *Arch. Intern. Med.* 147:778, 1987.

Glasier CM, et al.: Henoch-Schönlein syndrome in children: Gastrointestinal manifestations. *A.J.R.* 136:1081, 1981.

Gouyon JB, et al.: Inhibitors of factors VIII and IX in a child with Henoch-Schönlein syndrome. *Am. J. Pediatr. Hematol. Oncol.* 7:376, 1985.

Hardoff D, et al.: Recurrent episodes of testicular swelling preceding Henoch-Schönlein purpura by 11 months. *Eur. J. Pediatr.* 146:613, 1987.

Henoch EH: Uber den Zusammenhang von Purpura und Intestinalstörungen. *Berliner Klin. Wochenschr.* 5:517, 1868.

Kathuria S, et al.: Fatal pulmonary Henoch-Schönlein syndrome. *Chest* 82:654, 1982.

Kauffmann RH, et al.: Circulating IgA-immune complex in Henoch-Schönlein purpura. *Am. J. Med.* 69:859, 1980.

Kereiakes DJ, et al.: Endomyocardial biopsy in Henoch-Schönlein purpura. *Am. Heart J.* 107:382, 1984.

Kher KK, et al.: Stenosing ureteritis in Henoch-Schönlein purpura. *J. Urol.* 129:1040, 1983.

Law F, et al.: Ileal perforation: A late surgical complication of Henoch-Schönlein purpura. *Pediatr. Surg. Int.* 2:187, 1987.

Lefrere JJ, et al.: Purpura rhumatoïde et infection par le parvovirus humain. *Ann. Pediatr. (Paris)* 33:415, 1986.

LeLuyer B, et al.: Apport de l'échographie dans le diagnostic des hématomes des parois digestives au cours du purpura rhumatoïde. *Arch. Fr. Pediatr.* 42:379, 1985.

Lombard KA, et al.: Ileal stricture as a late complication of Henoch-Schönlein purpura. *Pediatrics* 77:396, 1986.

Maggiore G, et al.: Hepatitis B virus infection and Schönlein-Henoch purpura. *Am. J. Dis. Child.* 138:681, 1984.

Marandian MH, et al.: Manifestations pulmonaires du purpura rhumatoïde de Schönlein-Henoch chez un enfant de huit ans. *Arch. Fr. Pediatr.* 39:255, 1982.

Martinez-Frontanilla LA, et al.: Intussusception in Henoch-Schönlein purpura: Diagnosis with ultrasound. *J. Pediatr. Surg.* 23:375, 1988.

Martini A, et al.: Henoch-Schönlein syndrome and selective IgA deficiency. *Arch. Dis. Child.* 60:160, 1985.

McCrindle BW, et al.: Henoch-Schönlein syndrome. Unusual manifestations with hydrops of the gallbladder. *Clin. Pediatr. (Phila.)* 27:254, 1988.

Russo M, et al.: Pancréatite aiguë au cours d'un purpura rhumatoïde. *Arch. Fr. Pediatr.* 44:473, 1987.

Saulsbury FT: Henoch-Schönlein purpura. *Pediatr. Dermatol.* 1:195, 1984.

Saulsbury FT: IgA rheumatoid factor in Henoch-Schönlein purpura. *J. Pediatr.* 108:71, 1986.

Saulsbury FT, et al.: Thrombocytosis in Henoch-Schönlein purpura. *Clin. Pediatr. (Phila.)* 22:185, 1983.

Schönlein JL: *Allgemeine und spezielle Pathologie und Therapie.* Würzburg, 1832.

Siskind BN, et al.: CT demonstration of gastrointestinal involvement in Henoch-Schönlein syndrome. *Gastrointest. Radiol.* 10:352, 1985.

Somekh E, et al.: Muscle involvement in Schönlein-Henoch syndrome. *Arch. Dis. Child.* 58:929, 1983.

Stein BS, et al.: Scrotal imaging in the Henoch-Schönlein syndrome. *J. Urol.* 124:568, 1980.

Tomomasa T, et al.: Endoscopic findings in pediatric patients with Henoch-Schönlein purpura and gastrointestinal symptoms. *J. Pediatr. Gastroenterol. Nutr.* 6:725, 1987.

Warter J, et al.: Syndrome de malabsorption à la phase initiale d'un purpura rheumatoïde sévère. *Nouv. Presse Med.* 8:1245, 1979.

Weisgerber G, et al.: Necrose aigüe de l'oesophage thoracique et de l'ileon au cours d'une purpura rheumatoïde. *Arch. Fr. Pediatr.* 36:194, 1979.

HEPATIC FIBROSIS—RENAL CYSTIC DISEASE

Mode of Inheritance: Probably autosomal recessive.

Frequency: Uncommon.

Pathology: Congenital hepatic fibrosis has been reported in heterogenous group of clinically and genetically distinct diseases; wide range of hepatic and renal involvement (severe renal disease associated with mild liver abnormality at one end of the spectrum and minimal kidney disease associated with severe liver involvement at other end): (a) liver: hepatic fibrosis with proliferation and dilatation of the bile ducts; (b) medullary cystic disease of the kidneys, infantile type of polycystic disease, adult type of polycystic disease, renal dysplasia, nephronophthisis.

Clinical Manifestations: Onset in childhood or early adulthood: (a) *portal hypertension* manifested by hematemesis or melena; (b) hepatosplenomegaly; (c) renal failure; (d) other reported abnormalities: liver cell carcinoma, cholangiocarcinoma, protein-losing enteropathy, latent chronic cholangitis, pulmonary fibrosis, intracranial hemorrhage (hemangioma, aneurysm).

Radiologic Manifestations: (a) kidneys: *renal tubular dilatation* similar to that described in medullary sponge kidney with or without calcification, renal cystic disease, nephromegaly, distorted renal echo pattern; (b) high level of echoes in the liver, *dilatation of intrahepatic biliary ducts*; (c) *portal hypertension*, esophageal varices; (d) duplication of intrahepatic venous channels; (e) other reported abnormalities: giant intrahepatic biliary cyst, ascites, cerebellar hemangioma, cerebral aneurysm, etc.

REFERENCES

Alvarez F, et al: Congenital hepatic fibrosis in children. *J. Pediatr.* 99:370, 1981.

Boichis H, et al.: Congenital hepatic fibrosis and nephronophthisis: A family study. *Q. J. Med.* 42:221, 1973.

Caine Y, et al.: Congenital hepatic fibrosis—unusual presentations. *Arch. Dis. Child.* 59:1094, 1984.

Davies CH, et al.: Congenital hepatic fibrosis with saccular dilatation of intrahepatic bile ducts and infantile polycystic kidneys. *Pediatr. Radiol.* 16:302, 1986.

Dewhurst NG, et al.: Severe pulmonary hypertension and multiple left coronary arterial fistulas in association with congenital hepatic fibrosis. *Br. Heart J.* 58:525, 1987.

Kaplan BS, et al.: Variable expression of autosomal recessive polycystic kidney disease and congenital hepatic fibrosis within a family. *Am. J. Med. Genet.* 29:639, 1988.

Kerr DN, et al.: A lesion resembling medullary sponge kidney in patients with congenital hepatic fibrosis. *Clin. Radiol.* 13:85, 1962.

King K, et al.: Congenital hepatic fibrosis and cerebral aneurysm in a 32-year-old woman. *J. Pediatr. Gastroenterol. Nutr.* 5:481, 1986.

Odievre M, et al.: Anomalies of the intrahepatic portal venous system in congenital hepatic fibrosis. *Radiology* 122:427, 1977.

Pedersen PS, et al.: Congenital hepatic fibrosis combined with protein-losing enteropathy and recurrent thrombosis. *Acta Paediatr. Scand.* 69:570, 1980.

Pereira-Lima J, et al.: Congenital hepatic fibrosis: A family study. *J. Pediatr. Gastroenterol. Nutr.* 3:626, 1984.

Rosenfield AT, et al.: Gray scale ultrasonography in medullary cystic disease in the kidney and congenital hepatic fibrosis with tubular ectasia, New observations. *A.J.R.* 129:297, 1977.

Six R, et al.: A spectrum of renal tubular ectasia and hepatic fibrosis. *Radiology* 117:117, 1975.

Stillman AE, et al.: Hepatobiliary scintigraphy for cholestasis in congenital hepatic fibrosis. *Am. J. Dis. Child.* 139:41, 1985.

HEYDE SYNDROME

Clinical and Radiologic Manifestations: (a) aortic stenosis; (b) gastrointestinal bleeding; (c) angiodysplasia of the gastrointestinal tract, in particular, the ascending colon, demonstrable by endoscopy (usually multiple lesions: red, flat, or slightly elevated) and angiography (early venous filling, vascular tufting, slow venous emptying).

REFERENCES

Heyde EC: Gastrointestinal bleeding in aortic stenosis. *N. Engl. J. Med.* 259:196, 1958.

Scheffer SM, et al.: Resolution of Heyde's syndrome of aortic stenosis and gastrointestinal bleeding after aortic valve replacement. *Ann. Thorac. Surg.* 42:477, 1986.

Schwartz BM: Additional note on bleeding in aortic stenosis. *N. Engl. J. Med.* 259:456, 1958.

HHHH SYNDROME (HEREDITARY HEMIHYPOTROPHY, HEMIPARESIS, HEMIATHETOSIS)

Mode of Inheritance: Autosomal dominant, X-linked, and autosomal recessive are the possibilities.

Clinical Manifestations: (a) congenital left hemihypoplasia, hemiparesis, hypertonicity; (b) left-hand athetosis; (c) lack of progression after childhood.

Radiologic Manifestations: Right cerebral atrophy or hypoplasia.

REFERENCES

Haar F, Dyken P: Hereditary nonprogressive athetotic hemiplegia: A new syndrome. *Neurology* 27:849, 1977.

McKusick VA: *Mendelian Inheritance in Man*, ed 8. Baltimore, Johns Hopkins University Press, 1988, p. 1313.

HINMAN SYNDROME

Synonyms: Nonneurogenic neurogenic bladder; NNNB, etc.

Clinical Manifestations: A childhood clinical entity: (a) day and night wetting; (b) infected urine; (c) fecal retention; (d) normal neurological evaluation; (e) good response to medical nonsurgical treatment.

Radiologic Manifestations: (a) large bladder capacity, "neurogenic-type" bladder configuration; (b) secondary upper urinary tract disease in some (hydroureter-hydronephrosis).

REFERENCES

Beer E: Chronic retention of urine in children. *J.A.M.A.* 65:1709, 1915.

Hinman F Jr: Nonneurogenic neurogenic bladder (the Hinman syndrome)—15 years later. *J. Urol.* 136:769, 1986.

HIRSCHSPRUNG DISEASE

Mode of Inheritance: Heterogenous etiologic factors; incidence approximately 1 in 5,000 in the general population; male-to-female ratio of 3:1 to 5:1; two- and three-generation transmission reported; positive family history in 3% to 7% of cases; in aganglionosis of the entire colon (Zuelzer-Wilson syndrome) positive family history in 21%; multifactorial sex-modified inheritance in the nonsyndromic cases; possible autosomal recessive in agangliosis of the entire bowel.

Clinical and Radiologic Manifestations: (a) signs and symptoms of bowel obstruction, constipation, etc.; (b) association with other clinical entities: Down syndrome and some other chromosomal disorders; Waardenburg syndrome; dominant sensorineural deafness and some other forms of deafness (mendelian); Bardet-Biedl syndrome; Ondine curse; neuroblastoma; multifocal ganglioneuroblastoma; pheochromocytoma; rubella embryopathy; cytomegalic infection of the rectum; metaphyseal chondrodysplasia (McKusick type, cartilage hair dysplasia); Aarskog syndrome, syndrome of congenital heart defect, broad halluces, and ulnar polydactyly in siblings; syndrome of microcephaly, hypertelorism, short stature, and submucous cleft palate; colon atresia; internal hyperthermia in the mother in the first trimester of pregnancy; type D brachydactyly; polydactyly; cat-eye syndrome; Hirschsprung disease—macrocephaly—iris coloboma (Hurst, 1988).

REFERENCES

Goldberg RB, et al.: Hirschsprung megacolon and cleft palate in two sibs. *J. Craniofac. Genet. Dev. Biol.* 1:185, 1981.

Hannon RJ, et al.: Discordant Hirschsprung's disease in monozygotic twins: A clue to pathogenesis? *J. Pediatr. Surg.* 23:1034, 1988.

Hassinger DD, et al.: Aarskog's syndrome with Hirschsprung's disease, midgut malrotation, and dental anomalies. *J. Med. Genet.* 17:235, 1980.

Hershlag A, et al.: Cytomegalic inclusion virus and Hirschsprung's disease. *Z. Kinderchir.* 29:253, 1984.

Larsson LT, et al.: Neuropeptide Y, calcitonin gene—related peptide, and galanin in Hirschsprung's disease: An immunocytochemical study. *J. Pediatr. Surg.* 23:342, 1988.

Laurence KM, et al.: Hirschsprung's disease associated with congenital heart malformation, broad big toes, and ulnar polydactyly in sibs: A case for fetoscopy. *J. Med. Genet.* 12:334, 1975.

Lipson A: Hirschsprung disease in the offspring of mothers exposed to hyperthermia during pregnancy. *Am. J. Med. Genet.* 29:117, 1988.

Lipson AH, et al.: Three-generation transmission of Hirschsprung's disease. *Clin. Genet.* 32:175, 1987.

Michna BA, et al.: Multifocal ganglioneuroblastoma coexistent with total colonic aganglionosis. *J. Pediatr. Surg.* 23:57, 1988.

O'Dell K, et al.: Total colonic aganglionosis (Zuelzer-Wilson syndrome) and congenital failure of automatic control of ventilation (Ondine's curse). *J. Pediatr. Surg.* 22:1019, 1987.

Passage E: Hirschsprung's disease and other developmental defects of the gastrointestinal tract, in Emery AE, Rimoin DL (eds.): *Principles and Practice of Medical Genetics.* New York, Churchill Livingston, 1983, p. 886.

Reynolds JF, et al.: Familial Hirschsprung disease and type D brachydactyly: A report of four affected males in two generations. *Pediatrics* 71:246, 1983.

Santos H, et al.: Hirschsprung disease associated with polydactyly, unilateral renal agenesis, hypertelorism, and congenital deafness: A new autosomal recessive syndrome. *J. Med. Genet.* 25:304, 1988.

HISTIOCYTIC SYNDROMES

A. Histiocytosis X and Related Syndromes (Proliferation of Langerhans Cells): Letterer-Siwe disease, Hand-Schüller-Christian disease, and eosinophilic granuloma.

Clinical Manifestations: (a) *general symptoms:* fever, failure to thrive, weight loss, lethargy, irritability, diarrhea, etc.; (b) *bone lesions:* soft-tissue swelling, pain, limitation of motion, loose teeth, draining ears, otitis media, proptosis, optic nerve and muscle involvement; (c) *skin and mucous membrane lesions:* diffuse papular scaling lesions resembling seborrheic eczema, purpura, petechiae, granulomatous ulcerative lesions, xanthomatous lesions, bronzing of skin; (d) *hepatosplenomegaly,* abnormal liver function test results; (e) *hematopoietic disorders:* leukocytosis, normocytic anemia, thrombocytopenia, leukocytopenia with relative lymphocytosis, elevated sedimentation rate; (f) *endocrine disorders:* hypothalamic dysfunction with secondary partial or complete hypopituitarism, diabetes insipidus, growth retardation, delayed sexual maturation, goiter, hypothyroidism, adrenal insufficiency; (g) *abnormal immunity:* presence of circulating lymphocytes spontaneously cytotoxic to cultured human fibroblasts or the presence of antibody to autologous erythrocytes, T-cell histamine H_2 receptor deficiency, hypergammaglobulinemia; (h) *pulmonary symptoms:* dry cough, tachypnea, dyspnea, cyanosis, spontaneous pneumothorax; (i) *other reported abnormalities:* lymphadenopathy, cerebellar and/or bulbar phenomena, nuclear or peripheral nerve palsy, mental retardation, convulsions, hydrocephalus, meningoencephalitis, thymic infiltration, thyroid infiltration, diarrhea, gastrointestinal bleeding, malabsorption, protein-losing enteropathy, bowel ulceration, ulcerative penile lesion, hypercalcemia (eosinophilic granuloma), liver histiocytosis X with catecholamine excess, association of Hodgkin disease and primary pulmonary histiocytosis, etc.

Radiologic Manifestations: (a) *bone; skull* (most common site, "beveled edge," rounded and lytic lesions with sharp and serrated margins and an absence of sclerosis in the calvarial location, occasionally sclerosis present with orbital lesions, greater destruction of outer table, soft-tissue mass not containing calcium or fat as shown by computed tomography, button sequestrum appearance in some cases, orbital involvement, mastoid and petrous ridge involvement with erosion of the cortex of mastoid air cells, tegmen tympani and lateral sinus plate, destruction of the inner and external ears, zygoma, paranasal sinuses, alveolar bone associated with displacement of teeth), *ribs* (second most common site, often multiple lesions, destruction associated with expansion of a rib and in some case pathological fracture), *pelvis and scapulae* (common sites, bone destruction, minimal periosteal reaction, sclerotic border in some lesions located in the supra-acetabular region), *spine* (common site, most often in the thoracic region, lytic destruction of the vertebral body, compression fracture, vertebra plana), *tubular bones* (rare below the knees and elbows, round to oval-shaped bone destruction with expansion of the medullary cavity and scalloping of the inner cortex, periosteal reaction, onion skin appearance, epiphysis very rarely involved), myelosclerosis and myelofibrosis in treated histiocytosis X, radionuclide bone survey less accurate in detecting bone lesions as compared with radiographic bone survey (the sensitivity of radionuclide image varies according to various reports [35% to 94%]); (b) *lung and mediastinum:* alveolar pattern in an early stage; destructive pulmonary changes, hyperexpansion, fibrosis, cystic changes, subpulmonary bleb, and recurrent spontaneous pneumothorax in an advanced stage of disease; endobronchial lesions; mediastinal lymphadenopathy; cavitating mediastinal mass; thymic enlargement; (c) *gastrointestinal tract:* coarse nodular pattern of the duodenum and small-bowel mucosa, motility disorders, dilatation, thickening of mucosal folds, mesenteric lymphadenopathy, ascites due to peritoneal involvement; (d) *urinary system:* obstruction with secondary hydronephrosis and hydroureter, megacystis and dilatation of the upper collecting system that are associated with diabetes insipidus; (e) *central nervous system:* extrinsic involvement with extradural extension of bony lesions and a compression effect, direct brain involvement (mass lesion, meningoencephalitic type of involvement), communicating hydrocephalus, extrinsic cord compression (vertebral lesion), spinal cord lesion; (f) other reported abnormalities: lymph node involvement as the sole manifestation or part of a disseminated process (enlarged foamy nodes on lymphangiography), biliary tract involvement in children (irregularity of the intrahepatic ducts, a pattern resembling that of sclerosing cholangitis), liver lesion (echo dense, hypodense on computed tomography).

B. Syndromes in Which Phagocytic Histiocytes Other Than Langerhans Cells Are Involved: hemophagocytic lymphohistiocytosis ("familial hemophagocytic reticulosis"), infection associated (Epstein-Barr virus, cytomegalovirus, typhoid fever).

C. Malignant Histiocytic Disorders.

REFERENCES

Abramson SJ, et al.: Cavitation of anterior mediastinal masses in children with histiocytosis-X. *Pediatr. Radiol.* 17:10, 1987.

Al-Radhan NRF, et al.: Histiocytosis-X of the spinal cord: A case report. *Neurosurgery* 19:837, 1986.

Baber WW, et al.: Eosinophilic granuloma of the cervical spine without vertebrae plana. *J. Comput. Tomogr.* 11:346, 1987.

Banna M, et al.: Orbital histiocytosis on computed tomography. *J. Comput. Tomogr.* 7:167, 1983.

Bove KE, et al.: Thymus in untreated systemic histiocytosis X. *Pediatr. Pathol.* 4:99, 1985.

Braunstein GD, et al.: Endocrine manifestations of histiocytosis. *Am. J. Pediatr. Hematol. Oncol.* 3:6, 1981.

Broadbent V, et al.: Histiocytosis X—current controversies. *Arch. Dis. Child.* 60:605, 1985.

Christian H: Defects in membranous bones, exophthalmos and diabetes insipidus: An unusual syndrome of dyspituitarism. *Med. Clin. North Am.* 3:849, 1920.

Corbeel L: Histiocytic syndrome. *Eur. J. Pediatr.* 148:9, 1988.

Cunningham MJ, et al.: Histiocytosis X of the temporal bone: CT findings. *J. Comput. Assist. Tomogr.* 12:70, 1988.

Dean HJ, et al.: Growth hormone deficiency in patients with histiocytosis X. *J. Pediatr.* 109:615, 1986.

Deprettere A, et al.: Intractable diarrhea in histiocytosis-X. *Helv. Paediatr. Acta* 38:291, 1983.

Drolshagen LF, et al.: Cervical meningeal histiocytosis demonstrated by magnetic resonance imaging. *Pediatr. Radiol.* 17:63, 1987.

Ganick DJ, et al.: Histiocytosis X with catecholamine excess. *Acta. Paediatr. Scand.* 71:681, 1982.

Graif M, et al.: MR imaging of histiocytosis X in the central nervous system. *A.J.N.R.* 7:21, 1986.

Hand A Jr: Polyuria and tuberculosis. *Arch. Pediatr.* 10:673, 1893.

Hyams JS, et al.: Colonic ulceration in histiocytosis X. *J. Pediatr. Gastroenterol. Nutr.* 4:286, 1985.

Jinkins JR: Histiocytosis-X of the hypothalamus: Case report and literature review. *Comput. Radiol.* 11:181, 1987.

Jurney TH: Hypercalcemia in a patient with eosinophilic granuloma. *Am. J. Med.* 76:527, 1984.

Kirks DR, Taybi H: Histiocytosis X, in Parker BR, Castellino RA (eds.): *Pediatric Oncologic Radiology.* St. Louis, CV Mosby Co, 1977, pp. 209–234.

Lacronique J, et al.: Chest radiological features of pulmonary histiocytosis X: A report based on 50 adult cases. *Thorax* 37:104, 1982.

Lahey ME, et al.: Hypergammaglobulinemia in histiocytosis X. *J. Pediatr.* 107:572, 1985.

Lahey ME, et al.: Involvement of the thyroid in histiocytosis X. *Am. J. Pediatr. Hematol. Oncol.* 8:257, 1986.

Leeson MC, et al.: Eosinophilic granuloma of bone in the growing epiphysis. *J. Pediatr. Orthop.* 5:147, 1985.

Letterer E: Aleukämische Retikulose (ein Beitrag zu den proliferative Erkrankungen des Retikuloendothelialapparates). *Frankf. Z. Pathol.* 30:377, 1924.

Mayer M, et al.: Granulome éosinophile vertébral et compression médullaire. *Arch. Fr. Pediatr.* 42:441, 1985.

McGahan JP, et al.: CT of eosinophilic granuloma of the skull with sonographic correlation. *A.J.N.R.* 1:576, 1980.

Musaji MA, et al.: Lymphographic appearance of histiocytosis X. *Br. J. Radiol.* 56:61, 1983.

Myers DA, et al.: Histiocytosis X presenting as a primary penile lesion. *J. Urol.* 126:268, 1981.

Nauert C, et al.: Eosinophilic granuloma of bone: Diagnosis and management. *Skeletal Radiol.* 10:227, 1983.

Nesbit ME Jr, et al.: The immune system and the histiocytosis syndromes. *Am. J. Pediatr. Hematol. Oncol.* 3:141, 1981.

O'Donnell AE, et al.: Endobronchial eosinophilic granuloma: A rare cause of total lung atelectasis. *Am. Rev. Respir. Dis.* 136:1478, 1987.

Osband ME, et al.: Histiocytosis X: Demonstration of abnormal immunity, T-cell histamine H_2-receptor deficiency, and successful treatment with thymic extract. *N. Engl. J. Med.* 304:146, 1981.

Päivänsalo M, et al.: Liver lesions in histiocytosis X: Findings on sonography and computed tomography. *Br. J. Radiol.* 59:1123, 1986.

Pariente D, et al.: Biliary tract involvement in children with histiocytosis X. *Ann. Radiol. (Paris)* 29:641, 1986.

Sajjad SM, et al.: Primary pulmonary histiocytosis X in two patients with Hodgkin's disease. *Thorax* 37:110, 1982.

Sartoris DJ, et al.: Histiocytosis X: Rate and pattern of resolution of osseous lesions. *Radiology* 152:679, 1984.

Sartoris DJ, et al.: Myelofibrosis arising in treated histiocytosis X. *Eur. J. Pediatr.* 144:200, 1985.

Scart G, et al.: Les syndromes obstructives des voies urinaires au cours de l'histiocytoses X: A propos de 3 observations. *J. Radiol.* 62:19, 1981.

Schaub T, et al.: Radionuclide imaging in histiocytosis X. *Pediatr. Radiol.* 17:397, 1987.

Schüller A: Ueber eigenartige Schädeldefekte im jugendalter. *Fortschr. Rontgenstr.* 23:12, 1915.

Siwe S: Die Retikuloendotheliose—ein neues Krankheitsbild unter den Hepatosplenomegalien. *Z. Kinderheilkd.* 55:212, 1933.

Writing Group of the Histiocytic Society: Histiocytic syndromes in children. *Lancet* 1:208, 1987.

Wroble RR, et al.: Histiocytosis X with scoliosis and osteolysis. *J. Pediatr. Orthop.* 8:213, 1988.

HOLOPROSENCEPHALY

Synonyms: Holotelencephaly; arhinencephaly (defect confined to the olfactory structures).

Mode of Inheritance: Majority sporadic; autosomal recessive and autosomal dominant transmission have been suggested in some cases.

Pathology: (a) alobar type: micrencephaly; monoventricular cavity; fused thalamus and corpus striatum; absence of the corpus callosum, fornix, falx cerebri, optic tracts, and olfactory bulbs; (b) semilobar type: monoventricular cavity, rudimentary occipital horns, rudimentary falx, absence of the olfactory bulbs and corpus callusum, fusion of the thalamus and basal ganglia; (c) lobar type: better separation of ventricles, absent septum pellucidum, partial fusion of the hemisphere in some, absence of the corpus callosum in some, fusion of the thalamus and basal ganglia in some.

Clinical Manifestations: (a) facial dysmorphism: cyclopia (median orbit; single, double, or absent proboscis; absent nasal structures; trigonocephaly), ethmocephaly (separate hypoteloric orbits; single, double, or absent proboscis; absent nasal structures and premaxilla; trigonocephaly), cebocephaly (hypotelorism, small nose with a single nostril above or below the eyes, absent premaxilla and nasal septum), premaxillary agenesis (hypotelorism, small flat nose, absent intermaxillary segment of the face, absent prolabium, absent primary palate); (b) ocular anomalies: microphthalmos, coloboma, retinal dysplasia, etc.; (c) unilateral or bilateral cleft lip, cleft palate; (d) seizures; (e) chromosomal abnormalities: trisomy 13, 13q−, 18p−, trisomy 21, ring chromosome 21, triploidy, etc.; (f) endocrine deficiency: growth, antidiuretic, and adrenocortical hormones; (g) various organ system anomalies: cardiovascular, genitourinary, respiratory, alimentary, skeletal; (h) syndromes associated with arhinencephalia (hypoplasia or absence of the olfactory bulbs and tracts): Kallmann syndrome, Perrin syndrome (anosmia, mental deficiency, hypogonadism, congenital ichthyosis), Varadi syndrome (cleft lip/palate, growth deficiency, mental retardation, duplicated halluces, supernumerary fingers, lingual nodule, etc.), camptomelic dysplasia, radiohumeral synostosis syndrome (anosmia, Robin sequence [Cohen]); (i) other syndromes associated with holoprosencephaly: Hall-Pallister syndrome, aprosencephaly syndrome (aprosencephaly, radial aplasia, genital anomalies), Fitch syndrome (arhinencephalia, absent corpus callosum, hydrocephaly, absent left leaf of the diaphragm, ventricular septal defect, absent fifth fingernails),

Cyclopia without Proboscis

Cyclopia with Proboscis

Ethmocephaly with Single Proboscis

Ethmocephaly with Two Proboscides

Cebocephaly

Cebocephaly with Otocephaly & Microstomia

Premaxillary Agenesis

Less Severe Facial Dysmorphia

FIG SY−H−12.

Facial anomalies in holoprosencephaly. (From Leech RW, Shuman RM: Holoprosencephaly and related midline cerebral anomalies: A review. *J. Child Neurol.* 1:3, 1986. Used by permission.)

COH syndrome (arhinencephalia, polymicrogyria, hydrocephaly, cloverleaf skull, small penis, bifid scrotum, duplication of the thumb), DiGeorge syndrome, etc.; (j) other reported abnormalities: diabetic mother, single central incisor (also reported in the relatives), etc.

Radiologic Manifestations: (a) microcephaly, orbital hypotelorism, absent or marked hypoplasia of the median facial structures and crista galli; (b) brain dysgenesis: (1) alobar holoprosencephalon; horseshoe-shaped single ventricle; absent third ventricle; absence of the interhemispheric fissure, flax, and corpus callosum; absent superior sagittal sinus and internal cerebral veins; hypoplastic middle cerebral arteries; azygous anterior cerebral arteries; (2) semilobar holoprosencephaly: partial differentiation of the ventricle (temporo-occipital horns), rudimentary third ventricles, partial formation of the posterior interhemispheric fissure and falx, rudimentary or absent corpus callosum, partial formation of deep veins and dural sinuses; (3) lobar holoprosencephaly: partial fusion of the frontal lobes with direct continuity of gray and white matter across the midline under the shallow interhemispheric fissure, narrow body of the lateral ventricles, well-formed temporal and occipital horns, absent septum pellucidum; (c) dorsal cyst, extra-axial fluid collection; (d) prenatal ultrasonography: recognition of facial features and brain anomalies (alobar and semilobar).

Differential Diagnosis: Agenesis of the corpus callosum; absent septum pellucidum; hydranencephaly (Figs SY−H−12 and SY−H−13).

REFERENCES

Altman NR, et al.: Holoprosencephaly classified by computed tomography. *A.J.N.R.* 5:433, 1984.

Aronson DC, et al.: A male infant with holoprosencephaly,

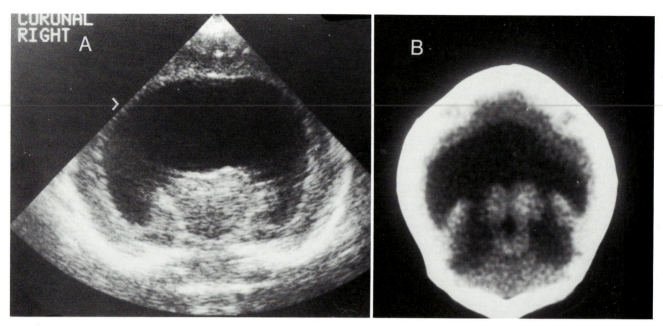

FIG SY–H–13.
Holoprosencephaly (alobar): Ultrasonogram **(A)** and computed tomogram **(B)**. Note the monoventricle and absence of the interhemispheric fissure and septum pellucidum. (Courtesy of Paul A. Nancarrow, M.D., Children's Hospital Medical Center, Oakland, Calif.)

associated with ring chromosome 21. *Clin. Genet.* 31:48, 1987.

Barr M, et al.: Holoprosencephaly in infants of diabetic mothers. *J. Pediatr.* 102:565, 1983.

Benacerraf BR, et al.: The fetal face: Ultrasound examination. *Radiology* 153:495, 1984.

Benke PJ, et al.: Recurrence of holoprosencephaly in families with a positive history. *Clin. Genet.* 24:324, 1983.

Berry SA, et al.: Single central incisor in familial holoprosencephaly. *J. Pediatr.* 104:877, 1984.

Bundy AL, et al.: Antenatal sonographic diagnosis of cebocephaly. *J. Ultrasound Med.* 7:395, 1988.

Burck U: Genetic counselling in holoprosencephaly. *Helv. Paediatr. Acta* 37:231, 1982.

Cohen MM: An update on the holoprosencephalic disorders. *J. Pediatr.* 101:865, 1982.

DeMyer WE, et al.: The face predicts the brain: Diagnostic significance of median facial anomalies for holoprosencephaly (arhinencephaly). *Pediatrics* 34:256, 1964.

Epstein CJ, et al.: Chance vs. causality in the association of Down syndrome and holoprosencephaly. *Am. J. Med. Genet.* 30:939, 1988.

Filly RA, et al.: Alobar holoprosencephaly: Ultrasonographic prenatal diagnosis. *Radiology* 151:455, 1984.

Fitz CR: Holoprosencephaly and related entities. *Neuroradiology* 25:225, 1983.

Fryns JP, et al.: Single central maxillary incisor and holoprosencephaly. *Am. J. Med. Genet.* 30:943, 1988.

Hattori H, et al.: Single central maxillary incisor and holoprosencephaly. *Am. J. Med. Genet.* 28:483, 1987.

Leech RW, et al.: Holoprosencephaly and related midline cerebral anomalies: A review. *J. Child Neurol.* 1:3, 1986.

Moerman P, et al.: Holoprosencephaly and postaxial polydactyly: Another observation. *J. Med. Genet.* 25:501, 1988.

Münke M, et al.: Holoprosencephaly: Association with interstitial deletion of 2p and review of the cytogenetic literature. *Am. J. Med. Genet.* 30:929, 1988.

Nyberg DA, et al.: Holoprosencephaly: Prenatal sonographic diagnosis. *A.J.R.* 149:1051, 1987.

Pauli RM, et al.: Familial agnathia-holoprosencephaly. *Am. J. Med. Genet.* 14:677, 1983.

Schnabel R, et al.: Karyotype 47,XXY,18p− in a newborn child with holoprosencephaly. *Clin. Genet.* 23:186, 1983.

HOLT-ORAM SYNDROME

Synonyms: Heart-hand syndrome; cardiac-limb syndrome; cardiomelic syndrome.

Frequency: Uncommon.

Modes of Inheritance: Autosomal dominant with variable expressivity; patients with skeletal defect alone can transmit full clinical manifestations of syndrome (cardiac and limb defects).

Clinical Manifestations: (a) *congenital cardiovascular diseases* (atrial septal defect, ventricular septal defect, etc.); (b) *fingerlike* or *absent thumb*; (c) limitation of motion of the shoulder and elbow, narrow shoulder; (d) other reported abnormalities: skin tag over the lower part of the sternum, deficiency of immunoglobulins and impaired cellular immunity, association with malignancy, association with Duane syndrome (deficiencies of ocular muscular functions), hypoplasia of the peripheral vessels, aplastic anemia, severe myopia, spotty melanotic pigmentation of the skin, deletion of 14q.

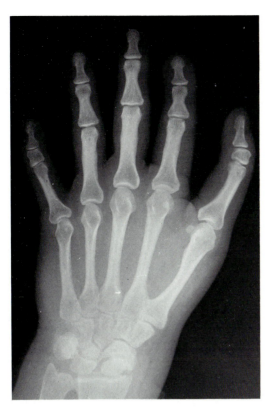

FIG SY−H−14.
Holt-Oram syndrome: triphalangeal curved thumb with a short middle phalanx in both the thumb and fifth finger as well as two accessory carpal bones. (From Poznanski AK, Gall JC, Stern AM: Skeletal manifestations of the Holt-Oram syndrome. *Radiology* 94:45, 1970. Used by permission.)

Radiologic Manifestations: (a) *thumb anomalies:* digitalized, absent, hypoplastic, triphalangeal, bifid; (b) *finger anomalies:* clinodactyly, syndactyly, absent, hypoplastic; (c) *carpal bone anomalies:* delayed ossification/absence, hypoplastic, fused, irregular, extracarpal/os centrale, enlarged, etc.; (d) first metacarpal anomalies: absent, hypoplastic, abnormal plane, etc.; (e) second to fifth metacarpal anomalies; (f) anomalies of the forearm: hypoplasia or absence of the radius, anomalous radial head, hypoplasia, absence of the ulna, radio-ulnar synostosis, humero-ulnar synostosis; (g) anomalies of the humerus: hypoplasia or absence; (h) shoulder anomalies: hypoplasia of the clavicle, broadened clavicle, deformed humeral head, prominent coracoclavicular joint, rotated and small scapula, hypoplastic glenoid fossa, Sprengel deformity, accessory bones; (i) chest wall anomalies: deficiency of pectoral muscles, pectus excavatum, pectus carinatum, rib anomalies (hypoplasia, extra ribs, etc.); (j) vertebral anomalies: scoliosis, fusion, hemivertebrae (Fig SY−H−14).

REFERENCES

Ferrell RL, et al.: Simultaneous occurrence of the Holt-Oram and the Duane syndromes. *J. Pediatr.* 69:630, 1966.

Giraud F, et al.: Syndrome de Holt-Oram (à propos d'une observation familiale portant sur cinq generations. *Arch. Fr. Pediatr.* 31:765, 1974.

Gladstone I, et al.: Holt-Oram syndrome: Penetrance of the gene and lack of maternal effect. *Clin. Genet.* 21:98, 1982.

Hoeffel JC, et al.: Aspects radiologiques des cardiopathies associées à des malformation génétiques des main. *J. Radiol.* 55:177, 1974.

Holt M, Oram S: Familial heart disease with skeletal malformations. *Br. Heart J.* 22:236, 1960.

Kaufman RL, et al.: Variable expression of the Holt-Oram syndrome. *Am. J. Dis. Child.* 127:21, 1974.

Kristoffersson U, et al.: Normal high-resolution karyotypes in three patients with the Holt-Oram syndrome. *Am. J. Med. Genet.* 28:229, 1987.

Miller AB, et al.: Prolapsed mitral valve associated with the Holt-Oram syndrome. *Chest* 67:230, 1975.

Najjar H, et al.: Variability of the Holt-Oram syndrome in Saudi individuals. *Am. J. Med. Genet.* 29:851, 1988.

Nik-Akhtar B, et al.: Association of Holt-Oram syndrome and lymphosarcoma. *Chest* 66:729, 1974.

Oppenheimer BS, et al.: The association of interatrial septal defects and anomalies of the osseous system. *Trans. Assoc. Am. Physicians* 62:284, 1949.

Poznanski A, et al.: Skeletal manifestations of the Holt-Oram syndrome. *Radiology* 94:45, 1970.

Poznanski AK, et al.: Objective evaluation of the hand in the Holt-Oram syndrome. *Birth Defects* 8:125, 1972.

Smith AT, et al.: Holt-Oram syndrome. *J. Pediatr.* 95:538, 1979.

Stratton RF, et al.: An unusual cardiomelic syndrome. *Am. J. Med. Genet.* 29:333, 1988.

Turleau C, et al.: Two patients with interstitial del (14q), one with features of Holt-Oram syndrome. Exclusion mapping of PI (alpha-l-antitrypsin). *Ann. Genet. (Paris)* 27:237, 1984.

Zhang K-Z, et al.: Holt-Oram syndrome in China: A collective review of 18 cases. *Am. Heart J.* 111:572, 1986.

HORNER SYNDROME

Pathophysiology: Interruption of sympathetic pathways in their course from the hypothalamus to the orbit; caused by tumor, central nervous system disease, lymphadenopathy, or vascular lesions (aneurysm, thrombosis, etc.); herniated disk at the T_1-T_2 level, trauma, etc.; association with heterochromia iridis in infants with a cervical or mediastinal neural crest tumor, multinodular goiter, iatrogenic causes (Swan-Ganz catheterization, neck surgery, carotid angiography, catheterization of the internal jugular vein, chest drainage tube with the tip near the first thoracic intervertebral space, hydromediastinum, etc.).

Clinical Manifestations: (a) *homolateral miosis;* (b) *ptosis of the upper lid;* (c) *minimal enophthalmos;* (d) *facial flushing and anhidrosis.*

Radiologic Manifestations: Roentgenographic manifestations of causes: *trauma, neoplasm, thrombosis, aneurysm of innominate artery, substernal thyroid,* etc.

Notes: (a) with lesions located distal to the bifurcation of the common carotid artery, sweating impairment is confined to the medial aspect of the forehead and side of the nose; (b) postganglionic lesions produce little or no anhidrosis.

REFERENCES

Asch A: Turner's syndrome occurring with Horner's syndrome: Seen with coarctation of the aorta and aortic aneurysm. *Am. J. Dis. Child.* 133:827, 1979.

Bernard C: Des phénomènes oculopupillaires produits par la section du nerf sympathique cervical; ils sont indépendants des phénomènes vasculaires caloriques de la tête. *C.R. Acad. Sci. (Paris)* 55:381, 1862.

Bertino RE, et al.: Horner syndrome occurring as a complication of chest tube placement. *Radiology* 164:745, 1987.

Horner F: Ueber eine Form von Ptosis. *Klin. Monatsbl. Augenheilkd.* 7:193, 1869.

Levin R, et al.: Bilateral Horner's syndrome secondary to multinodular goiter. *Ann. Intern. Med.* 105:550, 1986.

Lloyd TV, et al.: Horner's syndrome secondary to herniated disk at T1–T2. *A.J.R.* 134:184, 1980.

McRae D Jr, et al.: Ganglioneuroma, heterochromia iridis and Horner's syndrome. *J. Pediatr. Surg.* 14:612, 1979.

Milam MG, et al.: Horner's syndrome secondary to hydromediastinum. A complication of extravascular migration of a central venous catheter. *Chest* 94:1093, 1988.

Mokri B, et al.: Spontaneous internal carotid dissection, hemicrania, and Horner's syndrome. *Arch. Neurol.* 36:677, 1979.

Morris JGL, et al.: Facial sweating in Horner's syndrome. *Brain* 107:751, 1984.

Ogita S, et al.: Congenital cervical neuroblastoma associated with Horner syndrome. *J. Pediatr. Surg.* 23:991, 1988.

Rosegger H, et al.: Horner's syndrome after treatment of tension pneumothorax with tube thoracostomy in a newborn infant. *Eur. J. Pediatr.* 133:67, 1980.

Sataline LR, et al.: Horner's syndrome occurring with spontaneous pneumothorax. *N. Engl. J. Med.* 287:1098, 1972.

Sauer C, et al.: Horner's syndrome in childhood. *Neurology (N.Y.)* 26:216, 1976.

Spigelblatt L, et al.: Neuroblastoma with heterochromia and Horner syndrome. *J. Pediatr.* 88:1067, 1976.

Stone WM, et al.: Horner's syndrome due to hypothalamic infarction. Clinical, radiologic, and pathologic correlations. *Arch. Neurol.* 43:199, 1986.

Teich SA, et al.: Horner's syndrome secondary to Swan-Ganz catheterization. *Am. J. Med.* 78:168, 1985.

Thompson BM, et al.: Pseudo-Horner's syndrome. *Arch. Neurol.* 39:108, 1982.

Yang PJ, et al.: Horner's syndrome secondary to traumatic pseudoaneurysms. *A.J.N.R.* 7:913, 1986.

HUGHES-STOVIN SYNDROME

Frequency: Rare.

Pathology: *Thromboses* occurring in the legs, vena cava, superior sagittal sinus, jugular vein, or right side of the heart in association with *pulmonary artery aneurysms*.

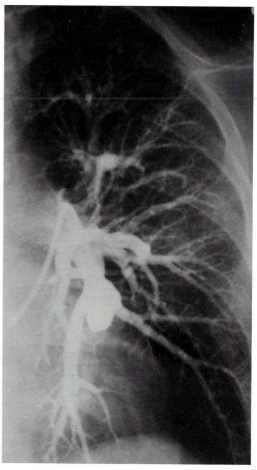

FIG SY—H—15.
Hughes-Stovin syndrome in a 27-year-old male. A selective left pulmonary artery angiogram demonstrates an aneurysm originating from the left lower lobe pulmonary artery with a distal avascular area. (From Wolpert SM, Kahn PC, Farbman K: The radiology of the Hughes-Stovin syndrome. *A.J.R.* 112:383, 1971. Used by permission.)

Clinical Manifestations: (a) *headaches, fever, cough, hemoptysis, papilledema;* (b) associated diseases: Behçet syndrome, pulmonary angiitis, focal glomerulonephritis.

Radiologic Manifestations: (a) plain film: *round densities on a chest film representing aneurysms, diminished vascularity in different section of the lung;* (b) aneurysms of segmental branches of pulmonary arteries (Fig SY—H—15).

REFERENCES

Beattie JM: Multiple embolic aneurysms of pulmonary arteries from veins of leg: Death from rupture of aneurysm into lung. *Proc. R. Soc. Med.* 5:147, 1911.

Grenier Ph, et al.: Syndrome de Hughes-Stovin: A propos d'un cas révélant une maladie de Behçet. *Ann. Radiol. (Paris)* 23:509, 1980.

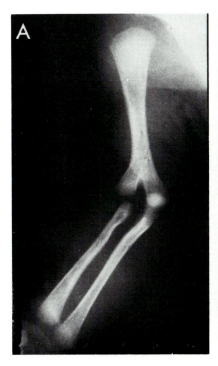
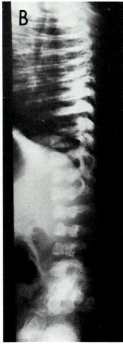

FIG SY–H–16.
Humerospinal dysostosis. **A,** and **B,** infant boy with rhizomelic shortening of the upper limb, a bifid distal humeral end, radial subluxation at the elbow, and midcoronal clefts of the vertebral bodies. (From Kozlowski KS, Clermajer JM, Tink AR: Humero-spinal dysostosis with congenital heart disease. *Am. J. Dis. Child.* 127:407, 1974. Used by permission.)

Hughes JP, Stovin PG: Segmental pulmonary aneurysm with peripheral venous thrombosis. *Br. J. Dis. Chest* 53:19, 1959.

Jeang MK, et al.: Multiple pulmonary artery aneurysms. New use for magnetic resonance imaging. *Am. J. Med.* 81:1001, 1986.

Meireles A, et al.: Hughes-Stovin syndrome with pulmonary angiitis and focal glomerulonephritis. *Chest* 79:598, 1981.

Pons JC, et al.: Syndrome de Hughes-Stovin: A propos d'un nouveau cas. *Ann. Radiol. (Paris)* 24:217, 1981.

Roberts DH, et al.: Multiple pulmonary artery aneurysms and peripheral venous thromboses—The Hughes Stovin syndrome. Report of a case in a 12-year-old boy and a review of the literature. *Pediatr. Radiol.* 12:214, 1982.

Teplick JG, et al.: The Hughes-Stovin syndrome. *Radiology* 113:607, 1974.

Wolpert SM, et al.: The radiology of the Hughes-Stovin syndrome. *A.J.R.* 112:383, 1971.

HUMEROSPINAL DYSOSTOSIS

Frequency: Very rare.

Clinical Manifestations: (a) short arms, elbow deformity, subluxation or dislocation of the knees, clubfoot deformity, lumbar hyperlordosis, narrow thorax; (b) heart murmur, mitral and tricuspid valve disease, pulmonary hypertension.

Radiologic Manifestations: (a) rhizomelic shortening of the limbs, in particular, shortening of the humeri with distal bifurcation; subluxation of the elbow joint, bowing deformity of the proximal ends of the ulnae; undertubulation of the long bones; subluxation of the knees; anterolateral bowing of tibias; talipes equinovarus; (b) coronal cleft of the vertebrae; (c) cardiomegaly (Fig SY–H–16).

Differential Diagnosis: Distal phocomelia with radial ectrodactyly.

REFERENCES

Cortina H, et al.: Humero-spinal dysostosis. *Pediatr. Radiol.* 8:188, 1979.

Kozlowski KS, et al.: Humerospinal dysostosis with congenital heart disease. *Am. J. Dis. Child.* 127:407, 1974.

Leroy JG, et al.: Humeroradioulnar synostosis appearing as distal humeral bifurcation in a patient with distal phocomelia of the upper limbs and radial ectrodactyly. *Am. J. Med. Genet.* 18:465, 1984.

HUNTINGTON DISEASE

Synonym: Huntington chorea.

Frequency: 4 to 7 per 100,000 persons; 195 published cases of juvenile Huntington disease (Van Dijk et al.).

Mode of Inheritance: Autosomal dominant; gene on the short arm of chromosome 4; occurrence in twins; new mutation.

Pathology: Marked atrophy of the caudate nucleus; less severe degeneration in the putamen, globus pallidus, hypothalamus, brain stem, cerebellum, and cerebral cortex; alteration in striatal receptors for γ-aminobutyric acid, benzodiazepines, muscarinic cholinergics, cholecystokinin, and dopamine.

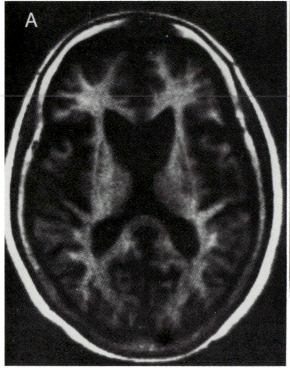
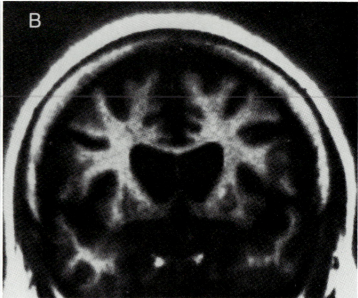

FIG SY–H–17.

Huntington chorea. **A** and **B,** magnetic resonance imaging demonstrates a virtual absence of caudate nuclei with moderate atrophy of the putamina and frontal lobe. (From Simmons JT, Pastakia

B, Chase TN, et al.: Magnetic resonance imaging in Huntington disease. *A.J.N.R.* 7:25, 1986. Used by permission.)

Clinical Manifestations: Onset of symptoms often in midlife: (a) *extrapyramidal involuntary movements* (grimacing, rigidity, akinesia, speech disorders, ataxia), progressive dementia, gait abnormality (wide-based station, lateral swaying, spontaneous knee flexion, variable cadence, and parkinsonian features); (b) abnormal ocular control; (c) sleep disturbance: prolonged sleep-onset latency, interspersed wakefulness, reduced sleep efficiency; (d) first trimester prenatal diagnosis with DNA probes.

Radiologic Manifestations: (a) cerebral atrophy manifested by ventricular dilatation, enlargement of the cerebral sulci, significant relative caudate atrophy, cerebellar atrophy; (b) positron-emission tomography (^{18}F-2-fluoro-2-dexoyglucose): hypometabolism of glucose preceding tissue loss; indices of caudate metabolism highly correlated with the patient's overall functional capacity, indices of putamen metabolism highly correlating with motor functions (chorea, oculomotor abnormalities, fine-motor coordination), indices of the thalamic metabolism correlating with dystonia (Fig SY–H–17).

REFERENCES

Baraitser M, et al.: Huntington's chorea arising as a fresh mutation. *J. Med. Genet.* 20:459, 1983.

Conneally PM: Huntington disease: Genetics and epidemiology. *Am. J. Hum. Genet.* 36:506, 1984.

Frohman EM, et al.: Genetic markers in Huntington's disease. *West J. Med.* 147:486, 1987.

Hansotia P, et al.: Sleep disturbances and severity of Huntington's disease. *Neurology* 35:1672, 1985.

Hattori H, et al.: Cerebellum and brain stem atrophy in a child with Huntington's chorea. *Comput. Radiol.* 8:53, 1984.

Hayden MR, et al.: First-trimester prenatal diagnosis for Huntington's disease with DNA probes. *Lancet* 1:1284, 1987.

Hayden MR, et al.: Positron emission tomography in the early diagnosis of Huntington's disease. *Neurology* 36:888, 1986.

Huntington G: On chorea. *Med. Surg. Reporter* 26:317, 1872.

Koller WC, et al.: The gait abnormality of Huntington's disease. *Neurology* 35:1450, 1985.

Lang C: Is direct CT caudatometry superior to indirect parameters in confirming Huntington's disease? *Neurology* 27:161, 1985.

Leigh RJ, et al.: Abnormal ocular motor control in Huntington's disease. *Neurology* 33:1268, 1983.

Leopold NA, et al.: Dysphagia in Huntington's disease. *Arch. Neurol.* 42:57, 1985.

Martin JB, et al.: Huntington's disease. Pathogenesis and management. *N. Engl. J. Med.* 315:1267, 1986.

Menkes JH: Huntington disease: Finding the gene and after. *Pediatr. Neurol.* 4:73, 1988.

Stober T, et al.: Bicaudate diameter—the most specific and simple CT parameter in the diagnosis of Huntington's disease. *Neuroradiology* 26:25, 1984.

Sudarsky L, et al.: Huntington's disease in monozygotic twins reared apart. *J. Med. Genet.* 20:408, 1983.

Terrence CF, et al.: Computed tomography for Huntington's disease. *Neuroradiology* 13:172, 1977.

Van Dijk JG, et al.: Juvenile Huntington disease. *Hum. Genet.* 73:235, 1986.

Young AB, et al.: PET scan investigations of Huntington's disease: Cerebral metabolic correlates of neurological features and functional decline. *Ann. Neurol.* 20:296, 1986.

HYDROCEPHALUS (X-LINKED)

Synonym: X-linked hydrocephalus.

Mode of Inheritance: X-linked recessive.

Frequency: Reported in more than 30 families (Willems et al., 1987).

Clinical Manifestations: (a) *macrocephaly;* (b) *mental retardation;* (c) thumb deformity (generally adduction deformity) in about half of the cases; (d) *neurological abnormalities:* spasticity, tremor, nystagmus, clumsiness, signs of pyramidal tract lesions, etc.

Radiologic Manifestation: *Hydrocephalus* with or without aqueductal stenosis.

REFERENCES

Bickers DS, et al.: Hereditary stenosis of the aqueduct of Sylvius as a cause of congenital hydrocephalus. *Brain* 72:246, 1949.

Halliday J, et al.: X linked hydrocephalus: A survey of a 20 year period in Victoria, Australia. *J. Med. Genet.* 23:23, 1986.

Teebi AS, et al.: Autosomal recessive nonsyndromal hydrocephalus. *Am. J. Med. Genet.* 31:467, 1988.

Váradi V, et al.: Heterogeneity and recurrence risk for congenital hydrocephalus (ventriculomegaly): A prospective study. *Am. J. Med. Genet.* 29:305, 1988.

Váradi V, et al.: Prenatal diagnosis of X linked hydrocephalus without aqueductal stenosis. *J. Med. Genet.* 24:207, 1987.

Willems PJ: Heterogeneity in familial hydrocephalus. *Am. J. Med. Genet.* 31:471, 1988.

Willems PJ, et al.: X-linked hydrocephalus. *Am. J. Med. Genet.* 27:92, 1987.

HYDROLETHALUS SYNDROME

Synonym: Salonen-Herva-Norio syndrome.

Mode of Inheritance: Autosomal recessive.

Frequency: More than 50 published cases (Aughton et al.).

Clinical Manifestations: (a) *hydrocephalus,* occipitoschisis extending from the foramen magnum; (b) *facial anomalies:* micrognathia, deformed ears, hypoplastic eyes, cleft lip and/or palate, poorly formed nose, tongue anomalies, etc.; (c) *hydramnios;* (d) *limb anomalies:* postaxial polydactyly in the hand and preaxial polydactyly in the feet, hallux duplex, etc.; (e) airway obstruction: laryngotracheal malformation, hypoplasia of the lung, pulmonary agenesis, etc.; (f) other reported abnormalities: genital anomalies, omphalocele, incomplete bowel rotation, congenital heart defects, etc.

Radiologic Manifestations: (a) macrocrania, keyhole-shaped deformity of the base of the skull with a dorsal midline defect of the occipital bone posterior to the foramen magnum, bulging margins of the defect; (b) huge *hydrocephalus, marked brain dysgenesis* (midline defects, cerebral gyral anomalies, absent olfactory lobes, cerebellar heterotopias, brain stem malformation, hypothalamic hamartomas, absent pituitary gland, Dandy-Walker anomaly, etc.; (c) *severe micrognathia;* (d) *limb anomalies:* crossed polydactyly in the hands and feet (hand, postaxial; feet, preaxial), proximal hypoplasia of tibias, short upper limbs, short first metatarsal bone, double hallux varus and short hallux varus, cutaneous syndactyly between the double halluces, etc.; (e) other reported abnormalities: dysplastic adrenal glands, hyperlocation of the liver and spleen, bowing of tubular bones, etc.

Differential Diagnosis: Meckel syndrome (cystic kidneys, oligohydramnios, etc.); trisomy 13; HARD syndrome; Pallister-Hall syndrome; Smith-Lemli-Opitz syndrome (Fig SY−H−18).

REFERENCES

Adetoro OO, et al.: Hydrolethalus syndrome in consecutive African siblings. *Pediatr. Radiol.* 14:422, 1984.

Anyane-Yeboa K, et al.: Hydrolethalus (Salonen-Herva-Norio) syndrome: Further clinicopathological delineation. *Am. J. Med. Genet.* 26:899, 1987.

Aughton DJ, et al.: Hydrolethalus syndrome: Report of an apparent mild case, literature review, and differential diagnosis. *Am. J. Med. Genet.* 27:935, 1987.

Herva R, et al.: Roentgenologic findings of the hydrolethalus syndrome. *Pediatr. Radiol.* 14:41, 1984.

Krassikoff NE, et al.: The hydrolethalus syndrome. *Pediatr. Pathol.* 5:103, 1986.

Salonen R, Herva R, Norio R: The hydrolethalus syndrome: Delineation of a "new" lethal malformation syndrome based on 28 patients. *Clin. Genet.* 19:321, 1981.

Toriello HV, et al.: Bilateral pulmonary agenesis: Association with the hydrolethalus syndrome and review of the literature from a developmental field perspective. *Am. J. Med. Genet.* 21:93, 1985.

HYPEREOSINOPHILIC SYNDROME (IDIOPATHIC)

Synonym: Idiopathic hypereosinophilic syndrome.

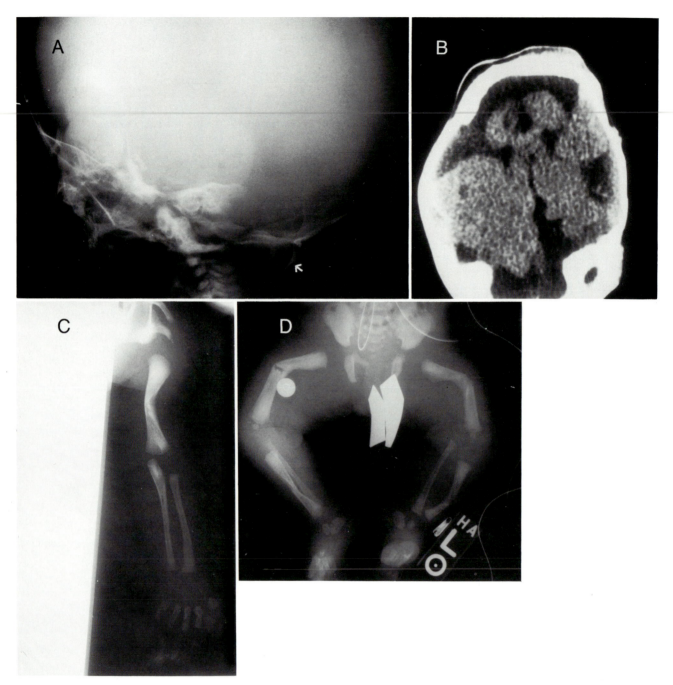

FIG SY—H—18.
Hydrolethalus syndrome in a male neonate with macrocrania, a midline defect of the occipital bone posterior to the foramen magnum, and bulging margins of the defect *(arrow)* **(A).** Note the marked brain dysgenesis on the computed tomographic scan **(B).** Bowing of the tubular bones is present **(C** and **D).** (Courtesy of Kenneth W. Martin, M.D., Children's Hospital Medical Center, Oakland, Calif.)

Criteria for Diagnosis: (a) *eosinophilia of 1,500 cells/mm³; (b) persistence of eosinophilia for at least 6 months or fatal in a short time; (c) eosinophilia-related organ system dysfunction; (d) absence of a recognized cause for the eosinophilia.* Included in this syndrome are fibroplastic endocarditis (Loeffler endocarditis parietalis fibroplastica), disseminated eosinophilic collagen disease, eosinophilic leukemia, eosinophilic gastroenteritis, etc.

Clinical Manifestations: (a) pulmonary symptoms and angioedema; (b) cardiac manifestations: cardiomyopathy, endomyocardial fibrosis, organic heart murmur, congestive heart failure, etc.; (c) nervous system complications: behavioral disturbances, upper neuron signs, peripheral neuropathy, central nervous system abnormalities related to embolic disorders, etc.; (d) other reported abnormalities: fever, weight loss, hepatosplenomegaly, fibrosis and decreased numbers of megakaryocytes in the bone marrow, combined immunodeficiency, hypergammaglobulinemia, elevated levels of serum IgE and circulating immune complexes, cerebrospinal fluid eosinophilia and biochemical evidence for meningitis, positive eosinophil toxicity tests, hypouricemia, transient hypereosinophilia in the infant of a mother with the syndrome, association with polycythemia vera, retinal arteritis, acute lymphoblastic leukemia and an extra C-group chromosome and q14+ marker, granulocytic sarcoma, etc.

Radiologic Manifestations: (a) myocardial disease with both left-sided and right-sided heart failure, mitral regurgitation, cardiac dilatation, mitral regurgitation with echographic demonstration of localized thickening of the posterobasal left ventricular wall behind the posterior mitral leaflet and absent or diminished motion of the posterior mitral leaflet, apical obliteration of one or both ventricles by echogenic material suggestive of fibrosis or thrombosis, computed imaging demonstrating mural thrombosis; (b) patchy parenchymal pulmonary infiltrate; (c) pleural effusion; (d) alimentary system eosinophilic infiltration, in particular, gastric outlet obstruction (Table SY–H–1).

REFERENCES

Acquatella H, et al.: Value of two-dimensional echocardiography in endomyocardial disease with and without eosinophilia. A clinical and pathologic study. *Circulation* 67:1219, 1983.

Alfaham MA, et al.: The idiopathic hypereosinophilic syndrome. *Arch. Dis. Child.* 62:601, 1987.

Carey J, et al.: Transient hypereosinophilia in the infant of a mother with hypereosinophilic syndrome. *Arch. Intern. Med.* 142:1754, 1982.

Chilcote RR, et al.: The hypereosinophilic syndrome and lymphoblastic leukemia with extra C-group chromosome and q14+ marker. *J. Pediatr.* 101:57, 1982.

Churg J, Strauss L: Allergic granulomatosis, allergic angiitis and periarteritis nodosa. *Am. J. Pathol.* 27:277, 1951.

DePace NL, et al.: Dilated cardiomyopathy in the idiopathic hypereosinophilic syndrome. *Am. J. Cardiol.* 52:1359, 1983.

Farcet JP, et al.: A hypereosinophilic syndrome with retinal arteritis and tuberculosis. *Arch. Intern. Med.* 142:625, 1982.

Gottdiener JS, et al.: Two-dimensional echocardiographic assessment of the idiopathic hypereosinophilic syndrome. Anatomic basis of mitral regurgitation and peripheral embolization. *Circulation* 67:572, 1983.

Harley JB, et al.: Atrioventricular valve replacement in the idiopathic hypereosinophilic syndrome. *Am. J. Med.* 73:77, 1982.

TABLE SY–H–1.

Some Recognized Causes of Eosinophilia*

1. Allergic disorders†: asthma, hay fever, allergic rhinitis, urticaria, eczema, pulmonary aspergillosis
2. *Drug reactions*
3. Parasitic infestations: *visceral larva migrans* (toxocariasis), *trichinosis, ascariasis, hookworm disease, stronglyloidiasis,* filariasis (tropical eosinophilia), schistosomiasis, hydatid disease, malaria
4. Skin disorders: eczema, dermatitis herpetiformis, exfoliative dermatitis, psoriasis, pemphigus
5. Infections: brucellosis, scarlet fever, acute infectious lymphocytosis, infections due to mycobacteria, chlamydia, cytomegalovirus, and *Pneumocytis carinii*
6. Hematologic: Fanconi anemia, thrombocytopenia with absent radii, postsplenectomy
7. Neoplastic disorders: *Hodgkin disease,* lymphosarcoma, leukemia, carcinoma of the lung and gut
8. Connective tissue/vasculitis/granulomatous disorders, especially those involving the lungs: *polyarteritis nodosa,* Churg-Strauss syndrome, rheumatoid arthritis, systemic lupus erythematosus, scleroderma, cryptogenic pulmonary eosinophilia
9. Immune deficiency disorders: congenital immune deficiency syndromes, hyper-IgE with infections
10. Miscellaneous: liver cirrhosis, radiation treatment, Crohn disease, ulcerative colitis, peritoneal dialysis, congenital heart disease, familial eosinophilia (?autosomal dominant), *idiopathic hypereosinophilic syndrome (including eosinophilic leukemia)*

*(From Alfaham MA, et al.: The idiopathic hypereosinophilic syndrome. *Arch. Dis. Child.* 62:601, 1987. Used by permission.)

†All disorders mentioned might cause hypereosinophilia. Those that might be associated with a very high eosinophil count are in italics.

Harley JB, et al.: Noncardiovascular findings associated with heart disease in the idiopathic hypereosinophilic syndrome. *Am. J. Cardiol.* 52:321, 1983.

Hidayat AA, et al.: Angiolymphoid hyperplasia with eosinophilia (Kimura's disease) of the orbit and ocular adnexa. *Am. J. Ophthalmol.* 96:176, 1983.

LeDeist F, et al.: Déficit immunitaire mixte et grave avec hyperéosinophilie. Etude immunologique de cinq observations. *Arch. Fr. Pediatr.* 42:11, 1985.

Lugassey G, et al.: Hypouricemia in the hypereosinophilic syndrome. Response to treatment. *J.A.M.A.* 250:937, 1983.

Matzinger MA, et al.: Esophageal involvement in eosinophilic gastroenteritis. *Pediatr. Radiol.* 13:35, 1983.

Moore PM, et al.: Neurologic dysfunction in the idiopathic hypereosinophilic syndrome. *Ann. Intern. Med.* 102:109, 1985.

Olson TA, et al.: Cardiomyopathy in a child with hypereosinophilic syndrome. *Pediatr. Cardiol.* 3:161, 1982.

Patterson NW, et al.: Computed tomography of mural thrombosis in the hypereosinophilic syndrome. *J. Comput. Tomogr.* 8:129, 1984.

Prin L, et al.: Lésions viscérales des hyperéosinophilies. *Presse Med.* 16:945, 1987.

Snyder JD, et al.: Pyloric stenosis and eosinophilic gastroenteritis in infants. *J. Pediatr. Gastroenterol. Nutr.* 6:543, 1987.

Tan AM, et al.: Hypereosinophilia syndrome with pneumonia in acute lymphoblastic leukaemia. *Aust. Paediatr. J.* 23:359, 1987.

Varon D, et al.: Hypereosinophilic syndrome associated with polycythemia vera. *Arch. Intern. Med.* 146:1440, 1986.

Weingarten JS, et al.: Eosinophilic meningitis and the hypereosinophilic syndrome. Case report and review of the literature. *Am. J. Med.* 78:674, 1985.

Whitington PF, et al.: Eosinophilic gastroenteropathy in childhood. *J. Pediatr. Gastroenterol. Nutr.* 7:379, 1988.

Wichman A, et al.: Peripheral neuropathy in hypereosinophilic syndrome. *Neurology* 35:1140, 1985.

Xipell JM, et al.: Granulocytic sarcoma (GS) with hypereosinophilic syndrome (HES). *Skeletal Radiol.* 16:425, 1987.

HYPERMOBILITY SYNDROME

Criteria for Diagnosis: The ability of the patients to perform at least three of the following five maneuvers (Biro et al.): (a) extension of the wrists and metacarpal phalanges so that the fingers are parallel to the dorsum of the forearm; (b) passive apposition of thumbs to the flexor aspect of the forearm; (c) hyperextension of the elbows ($\geq$10 degrees); (d) hyperextension of the knees ($\geq$10 degrees); (e) flexion of the trunk with the knees extended so that the palms rest on the floor.

Clinical and Radiologic Manifestations: (a) pain, most common in the knees, hands, and fingers; (b) other reported abnormalities: joint dislocation (uncommon), ligamentous injury, premature osteoarthritis, joint effusion.

Differential Diagnoses for Hypermotility: Ehlers-Danlos syndrome; Marfan syndrome; osteogenesis imperfecta; homocystinuria; hyperlysinemia; rheumatologic disorders; chromosomal abnormalities (Down syndrome); neuromuscular disorders; familial joint instability syndrome (Ehlers-Danlos syndrome, type XI); etc.

REFERENCES

Biro F, et al.: The hypermobility syndrome. *Pediatrics* 72:701, 1983.

Bulbena A, et al.: Joint hypermobility syndrome and anxiety disorders. *Lancet* 2:694, 1988.

Finsterbush A, et al.: The hypermobility syndrome. Musculoskeletal complaints in 100 consecutive cases of generalized joint hypermobility. *Clin. Orthop.* 168:124, 1982.

Kirk JA, et al.: The hypermobility syndrome. *Ann. Rheum. Dis.* 26:419, 1967.

HYPEROSTOSIS-HYPERPHOSPHATEMIA SYNDROME

Frequency: Rare.

Synonyms: Multifocal recurrent periostitis; cortical hyperostosis with hyperphosphatemia; chronic polyostotic periostitis; idiopathic periosteal hyperostosis with dysproteinemia; transient idiopathic periosteal reaction.

Pathology: Periosteal fibrous thickening and subperiosteal bone formation; nonspecific inflammation.

Clinical Manifestations: Onset of symptoms in childhood: (a) *swelling, pain, tenderness, and heat in the involved extremities; fever;* long periods of well-being between the symptomatic episodes; (b) laboratory findings (not constant in all reported cases): *elevated sedimentation rate,* hyperglobulinemia, *hyperphosphatemia,* anemia, elevated alkaline phosphatase level.

Radiologic Manifestations: *Minimal to extensive subperiosteal bone formation along the shaft of tubular bones of the limbs, healing with slight osteosclerosis of the affected remaining bone,* increased uptake on skeletal scintigraphic examination.

Differential Diagnosis: Caffey disease; pachydermoperiostitis; diaphyseal dysplasia (Camurati-Engelmann); trauma, syphilis; neoplastic diseases; multifocal bacterial osteomyelitis; chronic recurrent multifocal osteomyelitis; hypertrophic osteoarthropathy; vitamin A intoxication; ischemic lesions; sickle cell hemoglobinopathies; pancreatitis (intramedullary fat necrosis).

Notes: Idiopathic periosteal hyperostosis in association with dysproteinemia (marked hypergammaglobulinemia and hypoalbuminemia) has been referred to as the Goldbloom

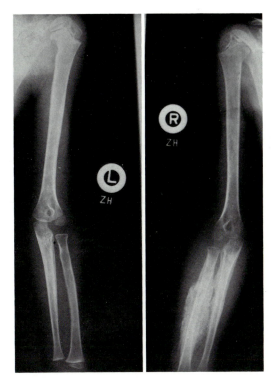

FIG SY–H–19.
Hyperostosis-hyperphosphatemia syndrome: marked periosteal bone formation along the shaft of the radius and ulna in a 5½-year-old boy. The serum alkaline phosphatase value was 6.9 Bodansky units; serum calcium levels were 9.8 and 9.7 mg/100 mL on two occasions; and serum phosphorus levels were 8.7, 8.7, 8.6, and 9.1 mg/100 mL on four occasions. (From Melhem RE, Najjar SS, Khachaturian AK: Cortical hyperostosis with hyperphosphatemia: New syndrome? *J. Pediatr.* 77:986, 1970. Used by permission.)

syndrome; facial bone involvement has been reported in this syndrome; periosteal hyperostosis associated with both hyperphosphatemia and hypergammaglobulinemia has also been reported (Courpotin-Stroh et al.) (Fig SY–H–19).

REFERENCES

Altman HS, et al.: Chronic polyostotic periostitis of unknown etiology. *Pediatrics* 28:719, 1961.

Cameron BJ, et al.: Idiopathic periosteal hyperostosis with dysproteinemia (Goldbloom's syndrome): Case report and review of the literature. *Arthritis Rheum.* 30:1307, 1987.

Courpotin-Stroh A, et al.: Périostose multifocale récurrente de l'enfant. *Ann. Radiol. (Paris)* 22:465, 1979.

Foucaud P, et al.: Periostose multifocale récurrente de l'enfant. *Arch. Fr. Pediatr.* 38:689, 1981.

Goldbloom RB, et al.: Idiopathic periosteal hyperostosis with dysproteinemia: A new entity. *N. Engl. J. Med.* 274:873, 1966.

Grogan DP, et al.: Transient idiopathic periosteal reaction associated with dysproteinemia. *J. Pediatr. Orthop.* 4:491, 1984.

Kozlowski K, et al.: Multifocal recurrent periostitis. Report of two cases. *Fortschr. Rontgenstr.* 135:597, 1981.

Melhem RE, et al.: Cortical hyperostosis with hyperphosphatemia: New syndrome? *J. Pediatr.* 77:986, 1970.

Mikati M, et al.: The syndrome of hyperostosis and hyperphosphatemia. *J. Pediatr.* 99:900, 1981.

Talab YA, et al.: Hyperostosis with hyperphosphatemia: A case report and review of the literature. *J. Pediatr. Orthop.* 8:338, 1988.

HYPERTRICHOSIS-OSTEOCHONDRODYSPLASIA

Mode of Inheritance: Autosomal recessive has been suggested.

Clinical Manifestations: (a) generalized congenital hypertrichosis; (b) macrosomy at birth.

Radiologic Manifestations: (a) narrow thorax, wide ribs, mild platyspondyly, coxa valga, mild "Erlenmeyer flask"–shaped long bones, osteopenia; (b) cardiomegaly.

REFERENCE

Cantú JM, et al.: A distinct osteochondrodysplasia with hypertrichosis—individualization of a probable autosomal recessive entity. *Hum. Genet.* 60:36, 1982.

HYPERTELORISM, MICROTIA, FACIAL CLEFTING SYNDROME

Synonyms: HMC syndrome; Bixler syndrome.

Mode of Inheritance: Probably autosomal recessive.

Clinical and Radiologic Manifestations: (a) Head: *hypertelorism; microtia; meatal atresia; clefting of the lip, palate, and nose; broad nasal tip; bifid nose; microstomia;* hypoplasia of the auditory ossicles, mandibular arch hypoplasia, flattened angle of the mandible; (b) conductive deafness; (c) other reported abnormalities: psychomotor retardation, microcephaly, ectopic kidney, congenital heart malformation, vertebral anomalies, thenar hypoplasia, syndactyly of the second and third toes, shortening of the fifth fingers.

REFERENCES

Baraitser M: The hypertelorism microtia clefting syndrome. *J. Med. Genet.* 19:387, 1982.

Bixler D, Christian JC, Gorlin RJ: Hypertelorism, microtia and facial clefting: A newly described inherited syndrome. *Am. J. Dis. Child.* 118:495, 1969.

Schweckendiek W, et al.: H.M.C. syndrome in identical twins. *Hum. Genet.* 33:315, 1976.

HYPERTROPHIC OSTEOARTHROPATHY (SECONDARY)

Synonyms: Secondary hypertrophic osteoarthropathy; Marie-Bamberger disease.

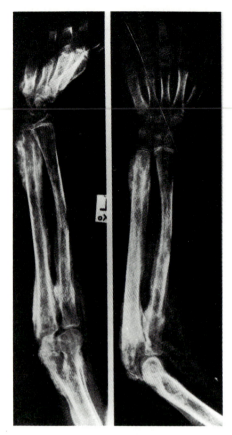

FIG SY—H—20.
Hypertrophic osteoarthropathy: metadiaphyseal periosteal new bone formation in the humerus, radius, ulna, and metacarpals during an acute episode of chronic ulcerative colitis. (From Arlart IP, Maier W, Leupold D, et al.: Massive periosteal new bone formation in ulcerative colitis. _Radiology_ 144:507, 1982. Used by permission.)

Etiology: (a) lung, pleura, and mediastinum: chronic infections, cystic fibrosis, tumors (primary, metastatic), pulmonary fibrosis; (b) congenital cyanotic heart disease; (c) alimentary tract: achalasia, carcinoma of the esophagus, leiomyoma of the esophagus, inflammatory bowel diseases (Crohn disease, ulcerative colitis), nontropical sprue, celiac disease, benign or malignant gastrointestinal tumors, polyposis, etc.; (d) liver diseases, biliary atresia; (e) other etiologic factors: immune disorders associated with lung disease (bare lymphocyte syndrome, agammaglobulinemia), infected axillary-axillary bypass graft with unilateral hypertrophic osteoarthropathy, venous stasis, lower limb osteoarthropathy in association with an infected abdominal aortic bifurcation graft or an aortoenteric fistula, nasopharyngeal tumor.

Clinical Manifestations: (a) _arthralgia, swelling of joints;_ (b) _clubbing of fingers;_ (c) local hyperemia, redness, increased sweating.

Radiologic Manifestations: (a) _periosteal new bone formation of the diaphysis of tubular bones_ with involvement in decreasing order of frequency: radius and ulna, tibia and fibula, humerus and femur, metacarpals, metatarsals, and proximal middle phalanges; the terminal phalanges and the bone of the trunk rarely involved; (b) acro-osteolysis associated with hypertrophic pulmonary osteoarthropathy.

Types of Periosteal Reactions: (a) simple elevation of the periosteum with a radiolucent band between the periosteum and cortex; (b) onion skin appearance; (c) irregular and sporadic periosteal elevation; (d) irregular areas of solid periosteal cloaking having a wavy appearance; (e) completely merged subperiosteal new bone formation with cortex.

Scintigraphic Findings: Increased uptake in various bones: mandible, maxilla, scapulae, clavicle, patellae, long bones (disease more active in the lower limbs), asymptomatic involvement also detectable by scintigraphy (Fig SY—H—20).

REFERENCES

Ali A, et al.: Distribution of hypertrophic pulmonary osteoarthropathy. _A.J.R._ 134:771, 1980.

Arlart IP, et al.: Massive periosteal new bone formation in ulcerative colitis. _Radiology_ 144:507, 1982.

Bamberger E: Ueber Knochenveränderungen bei chronischen Lungen-und Herzkrankheiten. _Z. Klin. Med._ 18:193, 1891.

Beluffi G, et al.: Pulmonary hypertrophic osteoarthropathy in a child with late-onset agammaglobulinemia. _Eur. J. Pediatr._ 139:199, 1982.

Bloom RA, et al.: Hypertrophic osteoarthropathy and primary intestinal lymphoma. _Gastrointest. Radiol._ 11:185, 1986.

Collier DH, et al.: Hypertrophic osteoarthropathy associated with achalasia. _Am. J. Med._ 81:355, 1986.

Doyle L: Hypertrophic osteoarthropathy: Four early reports by British authors (1889—97). _Thorax_ 42:561, 1987.

Draouat S, et al.: À propos d'une maladie de Pierre-Marie-Bomberger chez un enfant. _Ann. Radiol. (Paris)_ 29:539, 1986.

Epstein O, et al.: Hypertrophic hepatic osteoarthropathy. Clinical, roentgenologic, biochemical, hormonal and cardiorespiratory studies, and review of the literature. _Am. J. Med._ 67:88, 1979.

Firooznia H, et al.: Hypertrophic pulmonary osteoarthropathy in pulmonary metastases. _Radiology_ 115:269, 1975.

Galko B, et al.: Hypertrophic pulmonary osteoarthropathy in four patients with interstitial pulmonary disease. _Chest_ 88:94, 1985.

Ho A, et al.: Unilateral hypertrophic osteoarthropathy in a patient with an infected axillary-axillary bypass graft. _Radiology_ 162:573, 1987.

Joseph B, et al.: Acro-osteolysis associated with hypertrophic pulmonary osteoarthropathy and pachydermoperiostosis. _Radiology_ 154:343, 1985.

Katariya S, et al.: Hypertrophic osteoarthropathy in a young child with congenital cyanotic heart disease. _Br. J. Radiol._ 59:75, 1986.

Ladeb MF, et al.: Hypertrophic osteoarthropathy in nasopharyngeal carcinoma of a child. _Pediatr. Radiol._ 18:339, 1988.

Marie P: De l'ostéo-arthropathie hypertrophiante pneumique. *Rev. Med. (Paris)* 10:1, 1890.

Nathanson I, et al.: Pulmonary hypertrophic osteoarthropathy in cystic fibrosis. *Radiology* 135:649, 1980.

Oppenheimer DA, et al.: Hypertrophic osteoarthropathy of chronic inflammatory bowel disease. *Skeletal Radiol.* 9:109, 1982.

Pineda CJ, et al.: Periostitis in hypertrophic osteoarthropathy: Relationship to disease duration. *A.J.R.* 148:773, 1987.

Simpson EL, et al.: Association of hypertrophic osteoarthropathy with gastrointestinal polyposis. *A.J.R.* 144:983, 1985.

Spencer RP: Hepatic hypertrophic osteodystrophy detected on bone imaging. *Clin. Nucl. Med.* 13:611, 1988.

Sty JR, et al.: Bone scintigraphy: Hypertrophic osteoarthropathy in biliary atresia. *Clin. Nucl. Med.* 12:657, 1987.

Taets van Amerongen AHM, et al.: Hypertrophic osteoarthropathy in a young child with cytomegalovirus pneumonia and the bare lymphocyte syndrome. *Pediatr. Radiol.* 16:257, 1986.

HYPOGLOSSIA-HYPODACTYLY SYNDROME

Synonym: Aglossia-adactylia syndrome.

Mode of Inheritance: Not inherited; no sex predilection.

Frequency: Rare.

Clinical Manifestations: (a) *microstomia, micrognathia, syngnathia, hypoglossia of variable degrees;* (b) *absence of development of the distal segments of the limbs* (digits in particular); (c) other reported anomalies: missing lower incisors, cleft or high-arched palate, intraoral bands, hypertrophic enlargement of sublingual and submaxillary glands, mild defect of the lower lip, amelogenesis imperfecta, imperforate anus, fused labia majora.

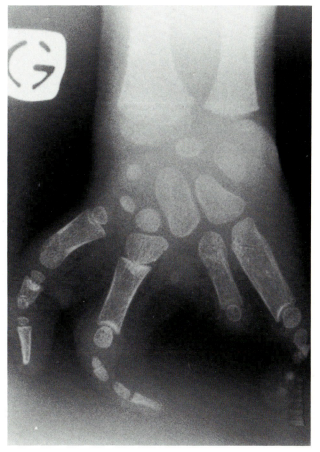

FIG SY–H–22.
Hypoglossia-hypodactyly syndrome. Hypodactyly and deformed metacarpals and phalanges are present. (From Schuhl JF: L'aglossie-adactylie: A propos d'une observation. Revue de la littérature. *Ann. Pediatr. (Paris),* 33:137, 1986. Used by permission.)

Radiologic Manifestations: (a) *micrognathia;* (b) *hypoplasia of the extremities* (peromelia to absence of the distal segments of the digits); (c) dental anomalies (absence of mandibular incisors, natal teeth); (d) other reported associated anomalies: dextrocardia, transposition of abdominal organs, bony fusion of the jaws, jejunal atresia, short bowel, "apple peel" bowel.

Differential Diagnosis: Hanhart syndrome; Möbius syndrome, Charlie M syndrome (Figs SY–H–21 and SY–H–22).

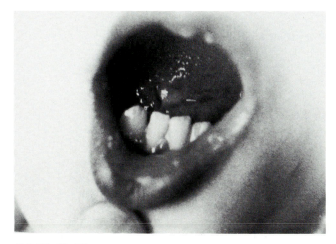

FIG SY–H–21.
Hypoglossia-hypodactyly: absent lingual frenum and facial asymmetry due to left seventh nerve palsy. (From Schuhl JF: L'aglossie-adactylie: A propos d'une observation. Revue de la littérature. *Ann. Pediatr. (Paris)* 33:137, 1986. Used by permission.)

REFERENCES

Bury F, et al.: Aglossie-adactylie avec atrésie jejunale. *Arch. Fr. Pediatr.* 34:604, 1977.

Curvelier B, et al.: L'aglossie-adactylie: Deux nouvelles observations. *Ann. Pediatr. (Paris)* 28:433, 1981.

De Jussieu M: Observation sur la manière dont une fille sans langue s'acquitte des fonctions qui dépendent de cet organe. *Hist. Acad. R. Soc. (Paris)* 6–14, 1718 (quoted in Stallard et al.).

Johnson GF, et al.: Aglossia-adactylia. *Radiology* 128:127, 1978.

Lecannellier J, et al.: Das Aglossie-Adactylie-Syndrom. *Helv. Paediatr. Acta* 31:77, 1976.

Schuhl JF: L'aglossie-adactylie. A propos d'une observation. Revue de la littérature. *Ann. Pediatr. (Paris)* 33:137, 1986.

Stallard MC, et al.: Aglossia-adactylia syndrome: Case reports. *Plast. Reconstr. Surg.* 57:92, 1976.

HYPOMELANOSIS OF ITO

Synonyms: Incontinentia pigmenti achromians; Ito's hypomelanosis.

Mode of Inheritance: Unknown, majority sporadic; familial cases have been reported; autosomal dominant and autosomal recessive transmissions have been suggested.

Frequency: Rare.

Pathology: Nonspecific: (a) reduced number of melanocytes, decreased numbers of pigment granules in melanocytes and keratocytes, increased number of vacuolated cells in the epidermis (occasionally); (b) brain abnormalities: atrophy, gray matter heterotopias within the cerebral white matter and cortical lamination with extensive gliosis, widespread white matter involvement similar to that of the leukodystrophies.

Clinical Manifestations: (a) skin manifestations are present at birth or appear in the first few months after birth: irregular hypopigmented whorls, patches, streaks, or zig-zag pattern often bilateral and asymmetrical (trunk and extremities; not present on the scalp, palms, soles, and mucous membranes); best evaluated by Wood's lamp; (b) central nervous system manifestations (in 40% to 50% of cases): seizures, psychomotor delay, strabismus, hypotonicity, hypertonicity, hemiparesis, speech delay, optic atrophy, ataxia, asymmetrical reflexes, sensory deficits, macrocephaly, microcephaly, focal electroencephalographic abnormalities, etc.; (c) choroidal atrophy, pigmentary retinopathy, myopia, microphthalmos, coloboma; (d) chromosomal rearrangement, mosaicism: mos,45,XY,t(14q21q)/44,XY,t(14q21q), + mar; 46,XX,t(2;8)(q37.2;p21.1); mos,45,X/46,X,+frag; mos,46,XX/46,XX,del(15)(q11 or 13); etc.; (e) other reported abnormalities: diminished capillary resistance, ichthyosis, morphea, alopecia, hypertrichosis, hamartomas, benign tumors, dental anomalies (irregularly spaced teeth, single central deciduous maxillary incisor, hamartomatous dental cusps, etc.), hypertelorism, dystrophy of the nails, coarse facial features, asymmetry of the limbs, retrognathism, dacryostenosis, short stature, undescended testes, etc.

Radiologic Manifestations: (a) macrocephaly, hemispheric asymmetry, low density in cerebral hemispheres on computed tomographic examination, neuronal heterotopias (magnetic resonance imaging), brain atrophy, porencephaly, etc.; (b) extra neurocutaneous reported abnormalities: clinodactyly, syndactyly, triphalangeal thumbs, kyphosis, scoliosis, dental anomalies, etc.

Notes: (a) hypomelanosis of Ito has been considered a neurocutaneous syndrome due to its high incidence of central nervous system abnormalities; (b) the term *incontinentia pig-*

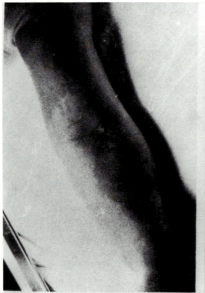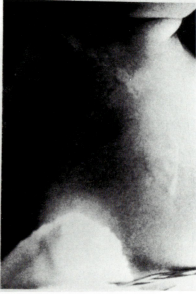

FIG SY—H—23.
Hypomelanosis of Ito. With the use of ultraviolet light, the hypopigmented lesions on the left arm and over the upper portion of the thorax are shown. (From Ardinger HH, Bell WE: Hypomelanosis of Ito. Wood's light and magnetic resonance imaging as diagnostic measures. *Arch. Neurol.* 43:848, 1986. Used by permission.)

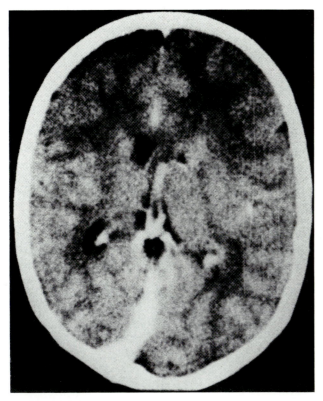

FIG SY–H–24.
Hypomelanosis of Ito: cranial computed tomogram with enhancement. The anterior horn of the left ventricle is collapsed, but no adjacent lesions are seen. The deviation of the straight sinus toward the right is related to enlargement of the entire left cerebral hemisphere, best seen on other computed tomographic sections. (From Ardinger HH, Bell WE: Hypomelanosis of Ito. Wood's light and magnetic resonance imaging as diagnostic measures. *Arch. Neurol.* 43:848, 1986. Used by permission.)

menti achromians refers to a negative image of the skin abnormalities seen in incontinentia pigmenti (Bloch-Sulzberger) (Figs SY–H–23 to SY–H–25).

REFERENCES

Ardinger HH, et al.: Hypomelanosis of Ito. Wood's light and magnetic resonance imaging as diagnostic measures. *Arch. Neurol.* 43:848, 1986.

Bartholomew DW, et al.: Single maxillary central incisor and coloboma in hypomelanosis of Ito. *Clin. Genet.* 32:370, 1987.

David TJ: Hypomelanosis of Ito: A neurocutaneous syndrome. *Arch. Dis. Child.* 56:798, 1981.

Golden SE, et al.: Hypomelanosis of Ito: Neurologic complications. *Pediatr. Neurol.* 2:170, 1986.

Happle R, et al.: Hamartomatous dental cusps in hypomelanosis of Ito. *Clin. Genet.* 21:65, 1982.

Ito M: Studies on melanin. XI. Incontinentia pigmenti achromians. A singular case of nevus depigmentosus systematicus bilateralis. *Tohoku J. Exp. Med.* 55 (suppl):57, 1952.

Moss C, et al.: Genetic counselling in hypomelanosis of Ito: Case report and review. *Clin. Genet.* 34:109, 1988.

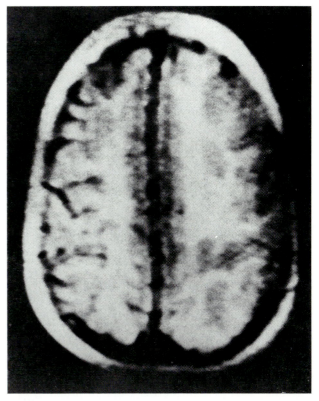

FIG SY–H–25.
Hypomelanosis of Ito: magnetic resonance image, T_1 weighted. The left cerebral hemisphere is to the viewer's right. The left cerebral hemisphere is larger than right is, and the cortical layer is thicker and has fewer sulci than the right does. Neuronal heterotopias giving a signal like that of cortical tissue are present in white matter in the left hemisphere, mainly posteriorly placed in this section. On lower axial sections, large heterotopias were seen adjacent to and collapsing the anterior horn of the left lateral ventricle. (From Ardinger HH, Bell WE: Hypomelanosis of Ito. Wood's light and magnetic resonance imaging as diagnostic measures. *Arch. Neurol.* 43:848, 1986. Used by permission.)

Peserico A, et al.: Unilateral hypomelanosis of Ito with hemimegalencephaly. *Acta Paediatr. Scand.* 77:446, 1988.

Rosemberg S, et al.: Hypomelanosis of Ito. Case report with involvement of the central nervous system and review of the literature. *Neuropediatrics* 15:52, 1984.

Turleau C, et al.: Hypomelanosis of Ito (incontinentia pigmenti achromians) and mosaicism for a microdeletion of 15q1. *Hum. Genet.* 74:185, 1986.

HYPOPLASTIC LEFT-HEART SYNDROME

Mode of Inheritance: Multifactorial inheritance; high recurrence risk in siblings.

Pathology: *Combined aortic and mitral valve obstruction (stenosis or atresia), mild to severe underdevelopment of the left ventricle and left atrium.*

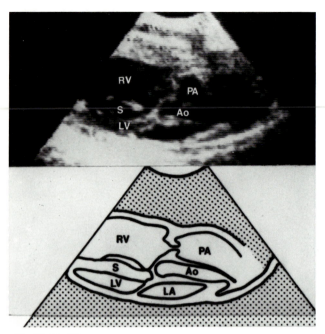

FIG SY–H–26.

Hypoplastic left-heart syndrome: two-dimensional echocardiogram, long-axis view. Note the large right ventricle *(RV)*, hypoplastic left ventricle *(LV)*, left atrium *(LA)*, atretic mitral valve and aortic valve (Ao = aorta; S = septum; PA = pulmonary artery.) (From Kashani IA, Kimmons H, Valdes-Cruz LM, et al.: Congenital right-sided diaphragmatic hernia and hypoplastic left heart syndrome. *Am. Heart J.* 109:177, 1985. Used by permission.)

Clinical Manifestations: (a) *cyanosis, congestive heart failure in the first days of life;* (b) echocardiography: *left ventricular end-diastolic dimension of less than 0.9 cm, aortic root diameter of less than 0.6 cm, ratio of left ventricular end-diastolic to right ventricular end-diastolic dimension less than 0.6, absent or greatly distorted low-amplitude mitral valve echo;* (c) major extracardiac anomalies; (d) chromosomal abnormalities.

Radiologic Manifestations: (a) prenatal diagnosis (ultrasonography): apex of both ventricles not at the same level, difference in ventricular size (subject of measurement error), atresia of the aortic valve, hypoplasia of the proximal portion of the ascending aorta, enlarged right ventricle and right atrium, high-velocity flow of the right-side atrioventricular valve (Doppler); (b) plain film: moderate cardiomegaly with a prominent right atrial border, moderate to marked engorgement of the pulmonary vasculature and pulmonary edema; (c) angiocardiography: in patients with aortic valve atresia, injection of contrast medium into the distal arch reveals a *small ascending aorta and retrograde filling of coronary arteries,* while injection into the left atrium reveals *left-to-right shunt and hypoplasia of the left cardiac chambers;* (d) other reported abnormalities: congenital right-sided diaphragmatic hernia, transposition of the great arteries, dysplastic pulmonic valve, hydrops fetalis, etc. (Figs SY–H–26 and SY–H–27).

REFERENCES

Bharati S, et al.: Hypoplastic left heart syndrome with dysplastic pulmonary valve with stenosis. *Pediatr. Cardiol.* 5:127, 1984.

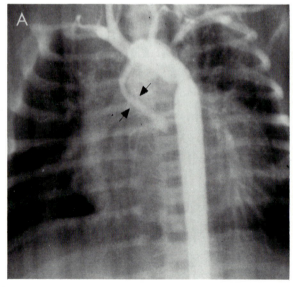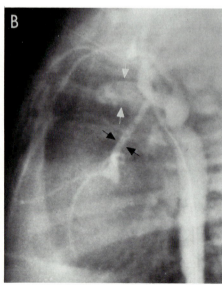

FIG SY–H–27.

Hypoplastic left-heart syndrome in a 2-day-old male with cyanosis and congestive heart failure. **A,** injection of contrast medium into the distal aortic arch shows a very narrow ascending aorta *(black arrows)* and atresia of the aortic valve. **B,** contrast medium also opacifies the pulmonary artery *(white arrows)* via a patent ductus arteriosus. At postmortem study, hypoplasia of the left cardiac chambers and atresia of mitral and aortic valves were found. (From Taybi H: Roentgen evaluation of cardiomegaly in the newborn period and early infancy. *Pediatr. Clin. North Am.* 18:1031, 1971. Used by permission.)

Egmond HV, et al.: Familial hypoplastic left heart syndrome. *Acta Paediatr. Belg.* 29:25, 1976.

Farooki ZQ, et al.: Echocardiographic spectrum of the hypoplastic left heart syndrome. *Am. J. Cardiol.* 38:337, 1976.

Kashani IA, et al.: Congenital right-sided diaphragmatic hernia and hypoplastic left heart syndrome. *Am. Heart J.* 109:177, 1985.

Lang D, et al.: Hypoplastic left heart with complete transposition of the great arteries. *Br. Heart J.* 53:650, 1985.

Lo RNS, et al.: Demonstration of ascending aorta in hypoplastic left heart syndrome with aortic atresia by balloon occlusion aortography. *Pediatr. Radiol.* 17:370, 1987.

Monin P, et al.: Hypoplasie du coeur gauche chez deux frères. *Arch. Fr. Pediatr.* 34:1008, 1977.

Natowicz M, et al.: Genetic disorders and major extracardiac anomalies associated with the hypoplastic left heart syndrome. *Pediatrics* 82:698, 1988.

Noonan JA, Nadas AS: Hypoplastic left heart syndrome. *Pediatr. Clin. North Am.* 5:1029, 1958.

Sahn DJ, et al.: Prenatal ultrasound diagnosis of hypoplastic left heart syndrome in utero associated with hydrops fetalis. *Am. Heart J.* 104:1368, 1982.

Shokeir MHK: Hypoplastic left heart. Evidence for possible autosomal recessive inheritance. *Birth Defects* 10:223, 1974.

Taybi H: Roentgen evaluation of cardiomegaly in the newborn period and early infancy. *Pediatr. Clin. North Am.* 18:1031, 1971.

Unger FM, et al.: Real-time ultrasonic diagnosis of valvular aortic atresia and other hypoplastic left heart syndromes. *RadioGraphics* 3:679, 1983.

VanEgmond H, et al.: Hypoplastic left heart syndrome and 45X karyotype. *Br. Heart J.* 60:69, 1988.

Vincent RN, et al.: Prenatal diagnosis of an unusual form of hypoplastic left heart syndrome. *J. Ultrasound Med.* 6:261, 1987.

HYPOPLASTIC RIGHT-HEART COMPLEX

Synonym: Hypoplastic right-heart syndrome.

Clinical Manifestations: *Congestive heart failure* in early neonatal life.

Radiologic Manifestations: (a) considerable anatomic heterogeneity: (1) isolated right ventricular hypoplasia; (2) pulmonary atresia with an intact ventricular septum; (3) tricuspid atresia; (b) abnormal anatomy shown by various imaging modalities: ultrasonography, cardioangiography, magnetic resonance imaging (Fig SY−H−28).

REFERENCES

Freedom RM, et al.: The hypoplastic right heart complex. *Semin. Roentgenol.* 20:169, 1985.

Jacobstein MD, et al.: Magnetic resonance imaging in patients with hypoplastic right heart syndrome. *Am. Heart J.* 110:154, 1985.

HYPOTHENAR HAMMER SYNDROME

Clinical Manifestations: (a) cold sensation, painful digits, paresthesias, cyanosis, pallor or mottling; (b) aggravation of symptoms with exposure to cold; (c) Raynaud phenomenon;

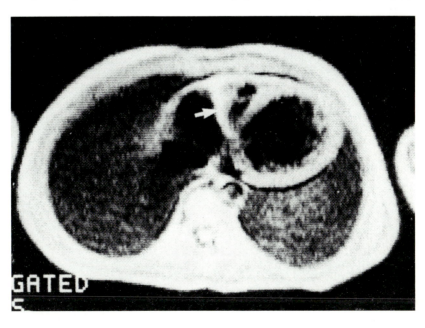

FIG SY−H−28.
Hypoplastic right-heart syndrome in an 11-year-old boy with tricuspid atresia: transverse section. A sausage-shaped hypoplastic right ventricular cavity and a dilated, globular left ventricle are shown. The muscular right atrial floor *(arrow)* produces intense resonance signals. (From Jacobstein MD, Fletcher BD, Goldstein S, et al.: Magnetic resonance imaging in patients with hypoplastic right heart syndrome. *Am. Heart J.* 110:154, 1985. Used by permission.)

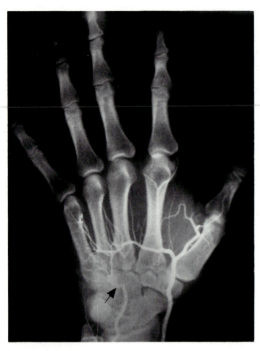

FIG SY–H–29.
Hypothenar hammer syndrome in the hand of a 38-year-old lumberyard foreman who frequently struck stacks of lumber with the palm of his right hand. He developed ischemia of the little finger secondary to occlusion of the distal ulnar artery *(arrow)*. (From Conn J Jr, Bergan JJ, Bell JL: Recognition of hypothenar hammer syndrome. *Surgery* 68:1122, 1970. Used by permission.)

(d) positive Allen test (with clenched fist blood is pressed out from the palm, the radial artery is pressed tightly, and the fist is opened: delay in disappearance of the palmar pallor due to the ulnar artery obstruction), digital coldness, hypotenar callus or mass, atrophy and softening of digital finger pads, tender hypothenar eminence, ischemic ulcer, subungual hemorrhage, gangrene.

Pathology: Occlusion of the distal ulnar artery or superficial volar arch of the hand subjected to repetitive blunt trauma (hammer, push, or pound).

Radiologic Manifestations: Angiographic demonstration of *occlusion of the distal ulnar artery, a superficial volar arch, or a digital artery;* aneurysm with or without occlusion of the palmar arterial system, embolism to the digital arteries from thrombi formed on damaged intima of the distal ulnar artery (Fig SY–H–29).

REFERENCES

Arany L, et al.: Hypothenar hammer syndrome. *Fortschr. Rontgenstr.* 141:702, 1984.
Benedict KT Jr, et al.: The hypothenar hammer syndrome. *Radiology* 111:57, 1974.
Conn J Jr, et al.: Recognition of hypothenar hammer syndrome. *Surgery* 68:1122, 1970.
Foster DR, et al.: Hypothenar hammer syndrome. *Br. J. Radiol.* 54:995, 1981.
Pineda C, et al.: Hypothenar hammer syndrome. Form of reversible Raynaud's phenomenon. *Am. J. Med.* 79:561, 1985.
Pouliadis GP, et al.: Das arteriographische Bild des Hypothenar-Hammer-Syndroms. *Fortschr. Rontgenstr.* 127:345, 1977.
Rosen S von: Ein Fall von Thrombose in der Arteria ulnaris nach Einwirkung von stumpfer Gewalt. *Acta Chir. Scand.* 73:500, 1934.
Vayssairt M, et al.: Hypothenar hammer syndrome: Seventeen cases with long-term follow-up. *J. Vasc. Surg.* 5:838, 1987.

IMMOTILE CILIA SYNDROME

Synonyms: Ciliary dyskinesia; dyskinetic cilia syndrome; primary ciliary dyskinesia.

Mode of Inheritance: Autosomal recessive, no sex predilection.

Histology: *Ciliary abnormalities:* (a) *deficiency of dynein arms* (not all cilia show a complete absence of dynein arms); (b) *spoke defect;* (c) *microtubular transposition abnormality;* (d) assessment of beat pattern, degree of immobility, measurement of ciliary beat frequency (nasal samples observed under light microscope); (e) variants: motile cilia with immotile spermatozoa, motile cilia with abnormal waveforms and structurally defective axonemes.

Clinical Manifestations: Onset of symptoms usually in infancy or childhood: (a) *recurrent pneumonia, recurrent bronchitis, recurrent otitis, recurrent sinusitis,* nasal polyp, episodic and/or persistent wheezes; (b) abnormal pulmonary function test findings indicating airway obstruction, gas trapping, hypoxia; (c) abnormal mucociliary clearance test result (inhalation of technetium-labeled albumin microspheres by aerosol and recording of upward particle movement in the trachea); (d) digital clubbing; (e) *oligospermia, absent or marked decrease in sperm motility;* (f) association with other abnormalities: polycystic kidney disease, hydrocephalus, gastroesophageal reflux, immunodeficiency syndrome, etc.

Radiologic Manifestations: (a) pulmonary consolidations, peribronchial thickening, atelectasis, bronchiectasis, obstructive lung disease with hyperinflation; (b) *sinusitis, mucosal thickening;* (c) Kartagener syndrome in about half of the cases.

Differential Diagnosis: Acquired transient ciliary defect in viral infections (Fig SY–I–1).

REFERENCES

Afzelius BA: "Immotile-cilia" syndrome and ciliary abnormalities induced by infection and injury. *Am. Rev. Respir. Dis.* 124:107, 1981.

Antonelli M, et al.: Leukocyte locomotory function in children with the immotile cilia syndrome. *Helv. Paediatr. Acta* 41:409, 1986.

Bashi S, et al.: Immotile-cilia syndrome with azoospermia: A case report and review of the literature. *Br. J. Dis. Chest* 82:194, 1988.

Buchdahl RM, et al.: Ciliary abnormalities in respiratory disease. *Arch. Dis. Child.* 63:238, 1988.

Caciani M, et al.: The association of supernumerary microtubules and immotile cilia syndrome and defective neutrophil chemotaxis. *Acta Paediatr. Scand.* 77:606, 1988.

Carson JL, et al.: Acquired ciliary defects in nasal epithelium of children with acute viral upper respiratory infections. *N. Engl. J. Med.* 312:463, 1985.

Eliasson R, et al.: The immotile-cilia syndrome. A congenital ciliary abnormality as an etiologic factor in chronic airway infections and male sterility. *N. Engl. J. Med.* 297:1, 1977.

Fauré C, et al.: Syndrome d'immotilité ciliaire congénitale chez l'enfant: Aspect radiologique pulmonaire. *Ann. Radiol. (Paris)* 29:301, 1986.

Greenstone MA, et al.: Hydrocephalus and primary ciliary dyskinesia. *Arch. Dis. Child.* 59:481, 1984.

Greenstone MA, et al.: Primary ciliary dyskinesia. *Arch. Dis. Child.* 59:704, 1984.

Jewett MAS, et al.: Necrospermia or immotile cilia syndrome as a cause of male infertility. *J. Urol.* 124:292, 1980.

Matwijiw I, et al.: Aplasia of nasal cilia with situs inversus, azoospermia and normal sperm flagella: A unique variant of the immotile cilia syndrome. *J. Urol.* 137:522, 1987.

Nadel HR, et al.: The immotile cilia syndrome: Radiological manifestations. *Radiology* 154:651, 1985.

Reyes de la Rocha S, et al.: Dyskinetic cilia syndrome: Clinical, radiographic and scintigraphic findings. *Pediatr. Radiol.* 17:97, 1987.

Rossman CM, et al.: Immotile cilia syndrome in persons with and without Kartagener's syndrome. *Am. Rev. Respir. Dis.* 121:1011, 1980.

Rossman CM, et al.: Nasal ciliary ultrastructure and function in patients with primary ciliary dyskinesia compared with that in normal subjects and in subjects with various respiratory diseases. *Am. Rev. Respir. Dis.* 129:161, 1984.

Saeki H, et al.: Immotile cilia syndrome associated with polycystic kidney. *J. Urol.* 132:1165, 1984.

Sturgess JM, et al.: Genetic aspects of immotile cilia syndrome. *Am. J. Med. Genet.* 25:149, 1986.

Whitelaw A, et al.: Immotile cilia syndrome: A new cause of neonatal respiratory distress. *Arch. Dis. Child.* 56:432, 1981.

Wilton LJ, et al.: Kartagener's syndrome with motile cilia and immotile spermatozoa: Axonemal ultrastructure and function. *Am. Rev. Respir. Dis.* 134:1233, 1986.

INCONTINENTIA PIGMENTI

Synonyms: Bloch-Sulzberger syndrome; Bloch-Siemens syndrome; Siemens-Bloch syndrome.

Mode of Inheritance: Considered X-linked dominant with lethality in the male, variable expression in both sexes.

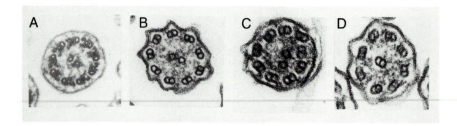

FIG SY−I−1.
Transmission electron micrographs showing genetic abnormalities of cilia that cause the immotile-cilia syndrome (magnification, ×104,000). **A,** normal cilium; **B,** complete dynein defect; **C,** radial spoke defect; **D,** microtubular transposition. (From Nadel HR, et al.: The immotile cilia syndrome: Radiological manifestations. *Radiology* 154:651, 1985. Used by permission.)

Clinical Manifestations: (a) *inflammatory erythematous vesicular lesions followed by verrucous, hyperkeratotic, and pigmentary lesions;* (b) cataract, strabismus, optic atrophy, glioma, retinal detachment, retinal dysplasia, astigmatism, myopia, microphthalmos, blue sclerae; (c) seizures, motor abnormalities, spasticity and hyperreflexia, weakness and flaccidity, anterior horn cell degeneration, cerebellar ataxia; (d) mental deficiency (in one third of cases); (e) dental anomalies: delayed eruption, missing teeth, conical crown; (f) atrophic patchy alopecia (in one fifth of cases), nail dystrophy; (g) other reported abnormalities: single umbilical artery; elevated IgM levels; deformities of ears; neurological changes; encephalitis; recurrent infections (encephalomyelitis, meningitis, etc.); transient loss of suppressor T cells (suggests an immune-mediated disease); hypertrophy of a limb; hypoplasia of the shoulder, arm, and breast; partial sweat gland aplasia; short stature; sacral dimple; clubfeet; eosinophilia (vesicular stage); chromosomal abnormalities (XXY karyotype of Klinefelter syndrome, translocation, 45X/46,X,r(X) mosaicism).

Radiologic Manifestations: (a) microcephaly, brain edema, brain atrophy, hydrocephalus, porencephalic cyst; (b) skeletal abnormalities (in 20%) such as vertebral anomalies, syndactyly, supernumerary ribs, hemiatrophy, shortening of the legs and arms, skeletal maturation retardation, subungual dysplastic nodules associated with dorsal scalloped erosion of the terminal tuft of the phalanx; (c) dental anomalies such as hypodontia, malformed teeth, delayed tooth eruption.

Differential Diagnosis: Epidermolysis bullosa; bullous impetigo; Naegeli syndrome; ectodermal dysplasia; congenital syphilis; etc. (Fig SY−I−2).

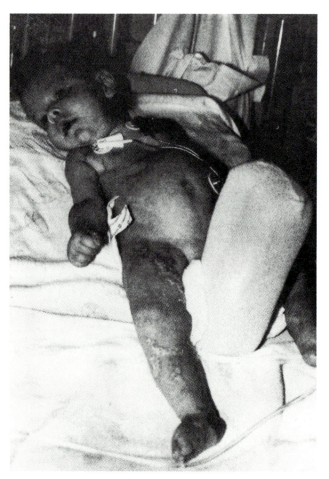

FIG SY−I−2.
Incontinentia pigmenti in a 6-week-old girl. Note the verrucous and vesicular eruption of the lower limb (From Larsen R, Ashwal S, Peckham N: Incontinentia pigmenti: Association with anterior horn cell degeneration. *Neurology* 37:446, 1987. Used by permission.)

REFERENCES

Avrahami E, et al.: Computed tomographic demonstration of brain changes in incontinentia pigmenti. *Am. J. Dis. Child.* 139:372, 1985.

Barson WJ, et al.: Coxsackievirus B2 infection in a neonate with incontinentia pigmenti. *Pediatrics* 77:897, 1986.

Bloch B: Eigentümliche bisher nicht beschriebene Pigmentaffektion (Incontinentia pigmenti). *Schweiz. Med. Wochenschr.* 56:404, 1926.

Brunquell PJ: Recurrent encephalomyelitis associated with incontinentia pigmenti. *Pediatr. Neurol.* 3:174, 1987.

Cannizzaro LA, et al.: Gene for incontinentia pigmenti maps to band Xp11 with an (X;10)(p11;q22) translocation. *Clin. Genet.* 32:66, 1987.

Diamantopoulos N, et al.: Actinomycosis meningitis in a girl with incontinentia pigmenti. *Clin. Pediatr. (Phila.)* 24:651, 1985.

Doyle TCA, et al: Tuft erosion in incontinentia pigmenti. *Australas. Radiol.* 31:304, 1987.

Garrod AE: Peculiar pigmentation of the skin in an infant. *Trans. Clin. Soc. London* 39:216, 1906.

Gilgenkrantz S, et al.: Translocation (X;9)(p11;q34) in a girl with incontinentia pigmenti (IP): Implications for the regional assignment of the IP locus to Xp11? *Ann. Genet. (Paris)* 28:90, 1985.

Grouchy J, et al.: Incontinentia pigmenti (IP) and r(X). Tentative mapping of the IP locus to the X juxtacentromeric region. *Ann. Genet. (Paris)* 28:86, 1985.

Hecht F, et al.: Incontinentia pigmenti in Arizona Indians including transmission from mother to son inconsistent with the half chromatid mutation model. *Clin. Genet.* 21:293, 1982.

Kajii T, et al.: Translocation (X;13)(p11.21;q12.3) in a girl with incontinentia pigmenti and bilateral retinoblastoma. *Ann. Genet. (Paris)* 28:219, 1985.

Kurczynski TW, et al.: Studies of a family with incontinentia pigmenti variably expressed in both sexes. *J. Med. Genet.* 19:447, 1982.

Langenbeck U: Transmission of incontinentia pigmenti from mother to son inconsistent with a half chromatid backmutation (reversion) model. *Clin. Genet.* 22:290, 1982.

Larsen R, et al.: Incontinentia pigmenti: Association with anterior horn cell degeneration. *Neurology* 37:446, 1987.

O'Brien JE, et al.: Incontinentia pigmenti. A longitudinal study. *Am. J. Dis. Child.* 139:711, 1985.

Ormerod AD, et al.: Incontinentia pigmenti in a boy with Klinefelter's syndrome. *J. Med. Genet.* 24:439, 1987.

Pallotta R, et al.: Chromosomal instability in incontinentia pigmenti: Study of four families. *Ann. Genet. (Paris)* 31:27, 1988.

Rott H-D: Partial sweat gland aplasia in incontinentia pigmenti Bloch-Sulzberger. Implications for nosologic classification. *Clin. Genet.* 26:36, 1984.

Sommer A, et al.: Incontinentia pigmenti in a father and his daughter. *Am. J. Med. Genet.* 17:655, 1984.

Sparrow G, et al.: Hyperpigmentation and hypohidrosis (the Naegeli-Franceschetti-Jadassohn syndrome): Report of a family and review of the literature. *Clin. Exp. Dermatol.* 1:127, 1976.

Sulzberger MB: Ueber eine bisher nicht beschriebene congenitale Pigmentanomalie (Incontinentia pigmenti). *Arch. Dermatol. Syph.* 154:19, 1928.

Trabelsi M, et al.: L'incontinentia pigmenti ou syndrome de Bloch-Sulzberger. A propos d'une observation chez un nourrisson de sexe masculin. *Ann. Pediatr. (Paris)* 35:53, 1988.

INDIFFERENCE TO PAIN (CONGENITAL)

Synonyms: Congenital insensitivity to pain; congenital indifference to pain; congenital analgesia; congenital general pure analgesia; insensitivity to pain.

Mode of Inheritance: Autosomal recessive.

Clinical Manifestations: (a) *absence or marked diminution of the sense of pain,* touch perception not affected; (b)

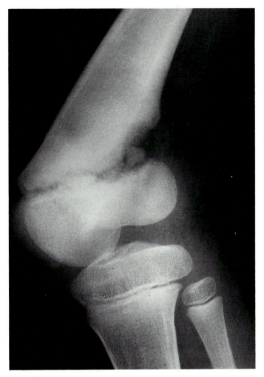

FIG SY–I–3.
Indifference to pain (congenital) in an 8-year-old female: epiphyseal separation and valgus deformity of the femur resulting from an apparent undergrowth of the lateral portion of the metaphysis. Note the gross irregularity of the growth plate and irregular radiolucency extending into the metaphysis laterally. (From Silverman FN, Gilden JJ: Congenital insensitivity to pain: A neurologic syndrome with bizarre skeletal lesions. *Radiology* 72:176, 1959. Used by permission.)

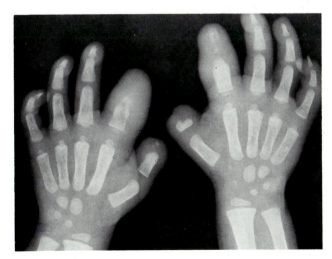

FIG SY–I–4.
Indifference to pain (congenital) in a 2-year-old male with a history of infections of both thumbs and forefingers. An open sore had been present from infancy. Pinprick testing produced no pain. Touch perception was not impaired. There is extensive bone and soft tissue destruction. (From Tucker AS, Johnson C: Congenital indifference to pain. *Am. J. Dis. Child.* 112:584, 1966. Used by permission.)

ulcers of the lips and tongue due to biting; (c) early loss of teeth; (d) corneal opacity; (e) infection of fingers, toes, and the mandible; (f) neglected fractures; (g) multiple bruises.

Radiologic Manifestations: (a) *microfractures and macrofractures, epiphyseal separation;* (b) *osteomyelitis* (mandible, fingers, and toes in particular); (c) aseptic necrosis in the juxta-articular regions of weight-bearing long bones (hips, knees, and ankles); (d) subperiosteal hemorrhage in infancy; (e) degenerative changes and loose bodies in the joints in older cases, neuropathic joints, recurrent dislocation of the hip.

Differential Diagnosis: Congenital insensitivity to pain with anhidrosis (autosomal recessive); hereditary sensory radicular neuropathy (autosomal dominant); congenital sensory neuropathy (sporadic); familial dysautonomia (autosomal recessive); Lesch-Nyhan syndrome (X-linked); autosomal dominant insensitivity to pain (Figs SY–I–3 and SY–I–4).

REFERENCES

Berkley HY: The pathological findings in a case of general cutaneous and sensory anesthaesia without psychical implication. *Brain* 23:111, 1900.

Comings D, et al: Autosomal dominant insensitivity to pain with hyperplastic myelinopathy and autosomal dominant indifference to pain. *Neurology* 24:838, 1974.

Dearborn G: A case of congenital pure analgesia. *J. Nerv. Ment. Dis.* 75:612, 1932.

Drummond RP, et al.: A twenty-one-year review of a case of congenital indifference to pain. *J. Bone Joint Surg. [Br.]* 57:241, 1975.

Ervin FR, et al.: Hereditary insensitivity to pain. *Trans. Am. Neurol. Assoc.* 85:70, 1960.

Fath MA, et al.: Congenital absence of pain. A family study. *J. Bone Joint Surg. [Br.]* 65:186, 1983.

Fauré C, et al.: Lesions ostéo-articulaires des déficits de la perception douloureuse chez l'enfant. *J. Radiol.* 64:667, 1983.

Greider TD: Orthopedic aspects of congenital insensitivity to pain. *Clin. Orthop.* 172:177, 1983.

Itoh Y, et al: Congenital insensitivity to pain with anhidrosis: Morphological and morphometrical studies on the skin and peripheral nerves. *Neuropediatrics* 17:103, 1986.

Lamy J, et al.: L'analgesie generalisée congenitale. *Arch. Fr. Pediatr.* 15:433, 1958.

Manfredi M, et al.: Congenital absence of pain. *Arch. Neurol.* 38:507, 1981.

Matsuo M, et al.: Congenital insensitivity to pain with anhidrosis in a 2-month-old boy. *Neurology* 31:1190, 1981.

Roberts JM, et al.: Recurrent dislocation of the hip in congenital indifference to pain. *J. Bone Joint Surg. [Am.]* 62:829, 1980.

Silverman FN, Gilden JJ: Congenital insensitivity to pain: A neurologic syndrome with bizarre skeletal lesions. *Radiology* 72:176, 1959.

INFANTILE MULTISYSTEM INFLAMMATORY DISEASE

Synonyms: IMID; Prieur-Griscelli syndrome; CINCA syndrome.

Frequency: Over 30 published cases (Prieur et al.).

Clinical Manifestations: Symptoms usually present at birth or during early infancy: (a) *evanescent rash;* (b) *arthritis;* (c) *fever;* (d) *adenopathy;* (e) *persistent open fontanelle;* (f) other reported clinical manifestations: head enlargement, splenomegaly, papilledema, uveitis, convulsions, hepatomegaly, feeding problems, deafness, protruding eyeballs, growth and mental retardation, etc.; (g) laboratory data: *cerebrospinal fluid pleocytosis, anemia, leukocytosis, elevated sedimentation rate, IgG elevation,* elevated antibody titers against *Ixodes ricinus–Borrelia* (Lyme disease) in one case (Lampert).

Radiologic Manifestations: (a) *osteoporosis,* vertebral compression fractures; (b) *swelling at the end of the long bones (bony and cartilaginous overgrowth); minimal joint effusion; joint contracture; muscle and soft-tissue wasting; shortening of the long bones of the limb in association with bowing (varus deformities of the proximal portions of the femora and tibias); widening of the shaft of the long bones in association with a periosteal reaction that cloaks the ends of the long bones (the ulnae and fibulas relatively unaffected); irregularity and cupping of the metaphyses; large, irregular, and fragmented epiphyses; premature fusion of the physes; cone-shaped epiphysis and notching of the corresponding metaphysis of the distal segment of the femur;* (c) relatively tall vertebrae and a short anteroposterior diameter, gibbous deformity at the thoracolumbar junction; (d) hepatosplenomegaly, mild cardiomegaly; (e) macrocrania, frontal bossing, wormian bones, thickened and dense base of the skull, slightly peaked orbits, widened mandibular angle, slight antegonial notching, tooth mineralization adequate, mild cerebral ventricular dilatation (laterals and third), wide extra-axial fluid spaces (Fig SY–I–5).

REFERENCES

Kaufman RA, et al: Infantile-onset multisystem inflammatory disease: Radiologic findings. *Radiology* 160:741, 1986.

Lampert F: Infantile multisystem inflammatory disease: Another case of a new syndrome. *Eur. J. Pediatr.* 144:593, 1986.

Lorber J: Syndrome for diagnosis: Dwarfing, persistently open fontanelle, recurrent meningitis, recurrent subdural effusions with temporary alternate-sided hemiplegia, high-tone deafness, visual defect with pseudopapillaedema, slowing intellectual development, recurrent acute polyarthritis, erythema marginatum, splenomegaly, and iron-resistant hypochromic anemia. *Proc. R. Soc. Med.* 6:1070, 1973.

Prieur AM, Griscelli C: Arthropathy with rash, chronic men-

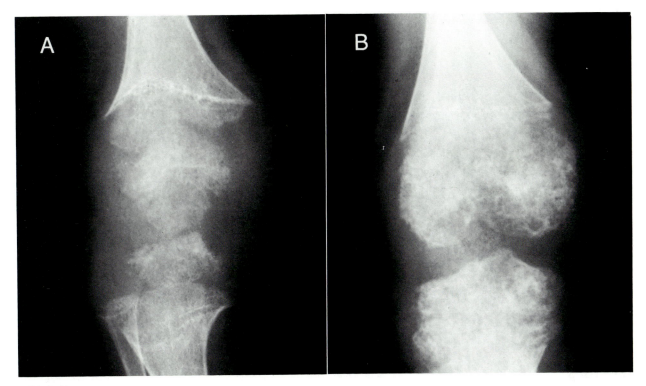

FIG SY–I–5.
Infantile multisystem inflammatory disease. **A,** anteroposterior view of a knee at 2 years of age with grotesque, enlarged epiphyses and fragmented ossification. The metaphyses are flared and concave toward the diaphysis, yet remain well defined. **B,** anteroposterior view of the same patient at 4 years of age. The bizarre ossi-fication pattern continues as the epiphysis is slowly incorporated into the shaft. (From Kaufman RA, Lovell DJ: Infantile-onset multisystem inflammatory disease: Radiologic findings. *Radiology* 160:741, 1986. Used by permission.)

ingitis, eye lesions, and mental retardation. *J. Pediatr.* 99:79, 1981.

Prieur AM, et al.: A chronic, infantile, neurological, cutaneous and articular (CINCA) syndrome. A specific entity analysed in 30 patients. *Scand. J. Rheumatol.* Suppl. 66:57, 1987.

Yarom A, et al: Infantile multisystem inflammatory disease: A specific syndrome? *J. Pediatr.* 106:390, 1985.

INTESTINAL ATRESIAS (FAMILIAL)

Synonym: Multiple intestinal atresias (familial).

Mode of Inheritance: Autosomal recessive.

Pathology: *Multiple atresias that may extend from the stomach to the rectum.*

Clinical and Radiologic Manifestations: (a) *bowel obstruction;* (b) *intraluminal calcification.*

Notes: (a) apple peel jejunal atresia has been reported in siblings (autosomal recessive); (b) familial duodenal atresia has been reported.

REFERENCES

Blackburn WR, et al.: The familial intestinal poly-atresia syndrome (abstract). *Proc. Greenwood Genet. Center* 2:122, 1983.

Blyth HM, et al.: Apple peel syndrome (congenital) intestinal atresia. A family study of seven index patients. *J. Med. Genet.* 6:275, 1969.

Daneman A, et al.: A syndrome of multiple gastrointestinal atresias with intraluminal calcification. A report of a case and a review of the literature. *Pediatr. Radiol.* 8:227, 1979.

Der Kaloustian VM, et al.: Familial congenital duodenal atresia (letter). *Pediatrics* 54:118, 1974.

Guttman FM, et al.: Multiple atresias and a new syndrome of hereditary multiple atresias involving the gastrointestinal tract from stomach to rectum. *J. Pediatr. Surg.* 8:633, 1973.

Mishalany HG, et al.: Familial multiple level intestinal atresia: Report of two siblings. *J. Pediatr.* 79:124, 1971.

Seashore JH, et al.: Familial apple peel jejunal atresia: Surgical, genetic, and radiographic aspects. *Pediatrics* 80:540, 1987.

Stensvold K, et al.: Multiple intestinal atresias in two brothers. *Z. Kinderchir.* 42:388, 1987.

INTESTINAL PSEUDO-OBSTRUCTION (IDIOPATHIC)

Synonyms: Chronic idiopathic intestinal pseudo-obstruction; idiopathic intestinal pseudo-obstruction.

Mode of Inheritance: Autosomal dominant with variable penetrance; sporadic.

Clinical Manifestations: (a) *insidious onset of symptoms in childhood or young adult life,* onset in the neonatal period less common, symptoms lasting a few months to many years, death from starvation; (b) *intermittent episodes of dysphagia, vomiting, abdominal pain, abdominal distension, diarrhea, constipation, steatorrhea; (c) history of repeated laparotomies for suspected intestinal obstruction;* (d) esophageal manometry: absence of primary peristalsis, frequent spontaneous waves; (e) *gastrointestinal dysfunction: hyperactive incoordinated smooth muscle contractions* (manometric studies); disorganized, decreased, or absent motility in segments of the alimentary tract; absent primary peristaltic waves in the esophagus; weak and infrequent jejunal contractions that are not accelerated after feeding.

Radiologic Manifestations: *Small-bowel involvement most common;* dysfunction of the esophagus, stomach, and colon less common; (a) esophagus: air-fluid level, dilatation, abnormal contractions, absent peristaltic waves, progressive peristalsis in the distal two thirds of the esophagus, lack of normal emptying action; (b) *megaduodenum* ("superior mesenteric artery syndrome"); (c) *small bowel: dilatation of various length and location,* delayed transit time; (d) colon: atonia, marked segmentation movement and ineffectual peristalsis, hypomotility, absent haustra, multiple diverticula, megacolon, retention of barium in the colon with barium inspissation and impaction; (e) high incidence of volvulus of the large and small bowels; (f) megalocystis, megaloureters.

Differential Diagnosis: Secondary pseudo-obstruction.

Note: Megaduodenum alone or in association with megalocystis has been reported with autosomal dominant transmission.

REFERENCES

Anuras S, et al.: Chronic intestinal pseudoobstruction in young children. *Gastroenterology* 91:62, 1986.

Anuras S, et al.: The familial syndrome of intestinal pseudoobstruction. *Am. J. Hum. Genet.* 33:584, 1981.

Bryne WJ, et al.: Chronic idiopathic intestinal pseudo-obstruction syndrome. *Diagn. Imaging (Basel)* 50:294, 1981.

Christensen J: The syndromes of intestinal pseudo-obstruction. *J. Pediatr. Gastroenterol. Nutr.* 7:319, 1988.

Cohen NP, et al.: Successful management of idiopathic in-testinal pseudoobstruction with cisapride. *J. Pediatr. Surg.* 23:229, 1988.

Dudley HA, et al.: Intestinal pseudo-obstruction. *J. R. Coll. Surg. Edinb.* 3:206, 1958.

Faulk DL, et al: A familial visceral myopathy. *Ann. Intern. Med.* 89:600, 1978.

Hyman PE, et al.: Antroduodenal motility in children with chronic intestinal pseudo-obstruction. *J. Pediatr.* 112:899, 1988.

Law DH, et al: Familial megaduodenum and megacystis. *Am. J. Med.* 33:911, 1962.

Reinarz S, et al.: Splenic flexure volvulus: A complication of pseudo-obstruction in infancy. *A.J.R.* 145:1303, 1985.

Roy AD, et al.: Idiopathic intestinal pseudo-obstruction: A familial visceral neuropathy. *Clin. Genet.* 18:291, 1980.

Schuffler MD, et al.: Chronic intestinal pseudo-obstruction. A report of 27 cases and review of the literature. *Medicine (Baltimore).* 60:173, 1981.

Schuffler MD, et al.: The radiologic manifestations of idiopathic intestinal pseudoobstruction. *A.J.R.* 127:729, 1976.

Vargas JH, et al.: Chronic intestinal pseudo-obstruction syndrome in pediatrics. Results of a national survey by members of the North American Society of Pediatric Gastroenterology and Nutrition. *J. Pediatr. Gastroenterol. Nutr.* 7:323, 1988.

Weisgerber G, et al.: Le syndrome "intestin non fonctionnel" primitif chez l'enfant. *Chir. Pediatr.* 21:107, 1980.

Weiss W: Zur Aetiologie des Megaduodenum. *Dtsch. Z. Chir.* 251:317, 1938.

IRRITABLE COLON SYNDROME

Synonyms: Irritable bowel syndrome; spastic colon; mucous colon syndrome, etc.

Etiology: Unknown; psychogenic and food sensitivity have been considered as etiologic factors.

Clinical Manifestations: A chronic relapsing condition usually diagnosed after the exclusion of organic bowel diseases: (a) *abdominal distension;* (b) *relief of pain with bowel movement;* (c) *looser and more frequent bowel movements with the onset of pain;* (d) *mucus in stools;* (e) *sensation of incomplete evacuation;* (f) *palpable spastic colon;* (g) *tenderness;* (h) *negative sigmoidoscopy;* (i) colonic myoelectric activity study: abnormally prolonged postprandial increase in both colonic spike and motor activity.

Radiologic Manifestations: (a) *excessive colonic motility, reduced width of the lumen, increased number of haustral markings, segmental spasm;* (b) dynamic ^{99m}Tc bran scan: significantly slow ileocecal clearance; (c) association with mitral valve prolapse.

REFERENCES

Acharya U, et al.: Failure to demonstrate altered gastric emptying in irritable bowel syndrome. *Dig. Dis. Sci.* 28:889, 1983.

Baron JH: Irritable colon, bowel, or gut syndrome. *Lancet* 1:268, 1980.

Kumar D, et al.: The irritable bowel syndrome: A paroxysmal motor disorder. *Lancet* 2:973, 1985.

Lumsden K, et al.: The irritable colon syndrome. *Clin. Radiol.* 14:54, 1963.

Newcomer AD, et al.: Irritable bowel syndrome. Role of lactase deficiency. *Mayo Clin. Proc.* 58:339, 1983.

Sataline L: Irritable bowel syndrome and mitral valve prolapse syndrome. *J.A.M.A.* 253:41, 1985.

Sullivan MA, et al.: Colonic myoelectrical activity in irritable-bowel syndrome: Effect of eating and anticholinergics. *N. Engl. J. Med.* 298:878, 1978.

Treacher DF, et al.: Irritable bowel syndrome: Is a barium enema necessary? *Clin. Radiol.* 37:87, 1986.

Trotman IF, et al.: Bloated irritable bowel syndrome defined by dynamic ^{99m}Tc bran scan. *Lancet* 2:364, 1986.

IRRITABLE HIP SYNDROME

Synonyms: Observation hip syndrome; transient synovitis of the hip; coxitis fugas; coxitis serosa seu simplex; etc.

Clinical Manifestations: A childhood disease usually with an acute onset: (a) pain; (b) limp; (c) limitation of motion; (d) other reported abnormalities: fever, contracture, tenderness over the anterior hip region, palpable soft-tissue swelling, slight leukocytosis, increase in the sedimentation rate; (e) usually a relatively quick and uncomplicated recovery, recurrence rare.

Radiologic Manifestations: (a) periarticular inflammatory signs (blurring and/or displacement of the periarticular medial and lateral fat pads, widening of the joint space, focal demineralization; (b) arthrosonography: joint effusion, hip-joint capsule to femoral neck distance of more than 3 mm (normal, 2.2 mm ± 0.5 mm), and a difference of more than 2 mm between the two sides; increased echogenicity of the articular fluid; (c) nuclear scanning: helpful in the differential diagnosis of Legg-Calvé-Perthes disease with normal bone radiographic findings in the early stage and transient synovitis; (d) complication: focal growth arrest of the proximal femoral metaphysis.

Differential Diagnosis: Legg-Calvé-Perthes disease; rheumatic arthritis; septic arthritis; osteoid osteoma; etc.

REFERENCES

Adam R, et al.: Arthrosonography of the irritable hip in childhood: A review of 1 year's experience. *Br. J. Radiol.* 59:205, 1986.

Carty H, et al.: Isotope scanning in the "irritable hip syndrome." *Skeletal Radiol.* 11:32, 1984.

Egund N, et al.: Conventional radiography in transient synovitis of the hip in children. *Acta Radiol.* 28:193, 1987.

Haueisen DC, et al.: The characterization of "transient synovitis of the hip" in children. *J. Pediatr. Orthop.* 6:11, 1986.

Kallio P, et al.: Transient synovitis and Perthes' disease. Is there an aetiological connection? *J. Bone Joint Surg. [Br.]* 68:808, 1986.

Marchal GJ, et al.: Transient synovitis of the hip in children: Role of US. *Radiology* 162:825, 1987.

Rosenborg M, et al.: The validity of radiographic assessment of childhood transient synovitis of the hip. *Acta Radiol.* 27:85, 1986.

Wolinski AP, et al.: Femoral neck growth deformity following the irritable hip syndrome. *Br. J. Radiol.* 57:773, 1984.

ISO-KIKUCHI SYNDROME

Synonym: Congenital onchodysplasia of the index finger.

Mode of Inheritance: Autosomal dominant with variable expression most likely.

Clinical Manifestations: *Congenital nail dysplasia involving the index fingers and sometimes their neighbors (micronychia, anonychia, etc.).*

Radiologic Manifestations: *Anomaly of the distal phalanx (dorsal spurlike protrusion at the nail bed).*

REFERENCES

Brunzlow H, et al.: Beitrag zum Iso-Kikuchi-syndrom. Kongenitale Onychodysplasie. *Radiol. Diagn.* 28:773, 1987.

Harper KJ, et al.: Pattern of inheritance in Iso and Kikuchi syndrome. *Clin. Exp. Dermatol.* 10:476, 1985.

Iso R: Congenital nail defects of the index finger and reconstructive surgery. *Orthop. Surg. (Tokyo)* 20:1338, 1969.

Kikuchi L, et al.: Congenital onychodysplasia of the index fingers. *Arch. Dermatol.* 110:743, 1974.

IVIC SYNDROME

Mode of Inheritance: Autosomal dominant with complete penetrance; variable expressivity and wide pleiotropy.

Frequency: 22 published cases in two families (Sammito et al.).

Clinical Manifestations: (a) upper-limb anomalies (radial ray); (b) other reported abnormalities: strabismus, hearing loss, imperforate anus, thrombocytopenia, leukocytosis.

Radiologic Manifestations: (a) upper-limb anomalies (frequently asymmetrical): hypoplastic thumb, triphalangeal thumb, thumb attached to the radial border of the index finger, long and slender first metacarpal bone, hypoplastic carpal bones, fusion of the radius and ulna.

Note: IVIC refers to Instituto Venezulano de Investigaciones Cientificas, from where the original paper was published (Arias et al.).

REFERENCES

Arias S, et al.: The IVIC syndrome: A new autosomal dominant complex pleiotropic syndrome with radial ray hypoplasia, hearing impairment, external ophthalmoplegia, and thrombocytopenia. *Am. J. Med. Genet.* 6:25, 1980.

Sammito V, et al.: IVIC syndrome: Report of a second family. *Am. J. Med. Genet.* 29:875, 1988.

J

JACKSON-WEISS SYNDROME

Mode of Inheritance: Autosomal dominant with variable severity (a large midwestern Amish kindred).

Clinical and Radiologic Manifestations: (a) craniosynostosis, midfacial hypoplasia; (b) foot abnormalities: medially deviated toe, tarsal bone fusion, short and broad metatarsals, short and broad phalanx of the toes, etc.

Note: The phenotypic expression in the reported kindred was so variable that the entire spectrum of dominantly inherited craniofacial dysostoses—acrocephalosyndactyly with the exception of typical Apert syndrome was observed by Jackson et al.

REFERENCE

Jackson CE, et al.: Craniosynostosis, midfacial hypoplasia, and foot abnormalities: An autosomal dominant phenotype in a large Amish kindred. *J. Pediatr.* 88:963, 1976.

JADASSOHN-LEWANDOWSKY SYNDROME

Synonym: Pachyonychia congenita syndrome.

Mode of Inheritance: Autosomal dominant.

Clinical Manifestations: (a) *palmoplantar keratosis and hyperhidrosis, follicular keratosis, epidermal cysts; (b) pachyonchia congenita; (c) mucous membrane lesions:* oral leukokeratosis, hoarseness due to laryngeal involvement, etc.; (d) other reported abnormalities: dry and sparse hair, corneal thickening, tympanic membrane thickening, cataracts, mental retardation, propensity for early loss of secondary teeth, marked caries, natal teeth, early adult-onset of mild-to-moderate large-joint arthritis, bushy eyebrows, scalloped tongue in association with leukokeratosis ori, laryngeal cartilage involvement, exophytic lesions in the larynx, etc.

Radiologic Manifestations: (a) narrowing of the esophagus, intestinal diverticula; (b) osteomas (Fig SY—J—1).

REFERENCES

Benjamin B, et al.: Pachyonychia congenita with laryngeal involvement. *Int. J. Pediatr. Otorhinolaryngol.* 13:205, 1987.

Franzot J, et al.: Pachyonychia congenita (Jadassohn-Lewandowsky syndrome). A review of 14 cases in Slovenia. *Dermatologica* 162:462, 1981.

Hagemann J, et al.: Jadassohn-Lewandowsky-Syndrom mit Veränderungen am Öesophagus. *Fortschr. Rontgenstr.* 132:5, 1980.

Jadassohn J, Lewandowsky F: *Pachyonychia congenita, Ikonographia Dermatologica.* Berlin-Wien, Urban Schwarzenberg, 1906.

Stieslitz JB, et al.: Pachyonychia congenita (Jadassohn-Lewandowsky syndrome): A seventeen-member, four-generation pedigree with unusual respiratory and dental involvement. *Am. J. Med. Genet.* 14:21, 1983.

JAFFE-CAMPANACCI SYNDROME

Synonym: Nonossifying fibromata—extraskeletal anomalies.

Frequency: Rare.

Clinical Manifestations: (a) pain, swelling; (b) *café au lait spots;* (c) other reported abnormalities: mental retardation, hypogonadism, cryptorchidism, gonadotropin deficiency, eye anomalies, congenital heart disease, alopecia, precocious puberty.

Radiologic Manifestations: (a) *disseminated "nonossifying fibromas"* of the long bone and pelvis (spindle and giant cells, hemorrhagic foci, hemosiderin pigment); (b) fracture(s); (c) kyphoscoliosis.

Differential Diagnosis: Neurofibromatosis; fibrous dysplasia; hyperparathyroidism; multiple giant-cell tumors; etc.

Notes: (a) the lesions in the long bones have been called nonossifying fibroma and those of mandible, giant-cell reparative granuloma; (b) the name of Campanacci is also associated with osteofibrous dysplasia of the tibia and fibula (Figs SY—J—2 and SY—J—3).

REFERENCES

Campanacci M, et al.: Multiple non-ossifying fibromata with extra—skeletal anomalies: A new syndrome? *J. Bone Joint Surg. [Br.]* 65:627, 1983.

Campanacci M, et al.: Osteofibrous dysplasia of the tibia and fibula. *J. Bone Joint Surg. [Am.]* 63:367, 1981.

Jaffe HL: *Non-ossifying Fibroma. Tumors and Tumorous Conditions of the Bones and Joints.* London, Henry Kimpton, 1958, pp. 83—91.

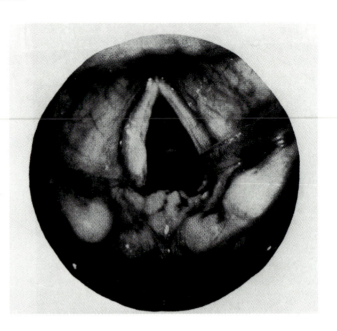

FIG SY—J—1.
Jadassohn-Lewandowsky syndrome in a 15-year-old girl with pachyonychia congenita: direct laryngoscopic photograph under general anesthesia. There is a multilobed midline mass in the posterior commissure. (From Benjamin B, Parson DS, Molloy HF: Pachyonychia congenita with laryngeal involvement. *Int. J. Pediatr. Otorhinolaryngol.* 13:205, 1987. Used by permission.)

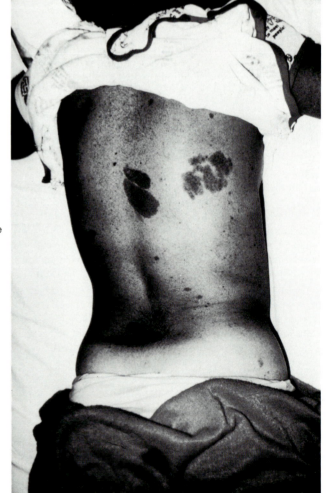

FIG SY—J—2.
Jaffe-Campanacci syndrome. Notice the numerous café au lait—like macules, freckles, and pigmented nevi. (From Mirra JM, Gold RH, Rand F: Disseminated nonossifying fibromas in association with café au lait spots (Jaffe-Campanacci syndrome). *Clin. Orthop.* 168:192, 1982. Used by permission.)

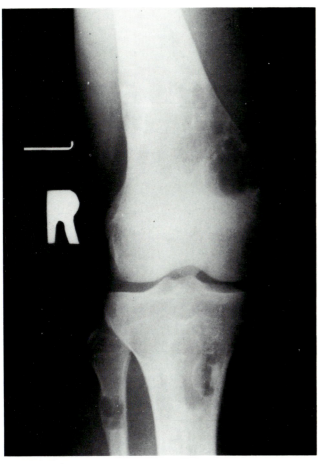

FIG SY−J−3.
Jaffe-Campanacci syndrome with multiple nonossifying fibromas (distal portion of the femur and proximal segments of the tibia and fibula). (From Mirra JM, Gold RH, Rand F: Disseminated nonossifying fibromas in association with café-au-lait spots (Jaffe-Campanacci syndrome). *Clin. Orthop.* 168:192, 1982. Used by permission.)

Mirra JM, et al.: Disseminated nonossifying fibromas in association with café-au-lait spots (Jaffe-Campanacci syndrome). *Clin. Orthop.* 168:192, 1982.
Steinmetz JC, et al.: Jaffe-Campanacci syndrome. *J. Pediatr. Orthop.* 8:602, 1988.

JARCHO-LEVIN SYNDROME

Synonyms: Spondylothoracic dysostosis; costovertebral dysplasia; occipito-facial-cervico-thoracic-abdomino-digital dysplasia.

Mode of Inheritance: Autosomal recessive; consanguinity in some families; predominance in Hispanic families.

Frequency: Rare.

Pathology: (a) skeletal: costovertebral anomalies; (b) associated nonskeletal anomalies: undescended testes, bilobed bladder, hydronephrosis, absent external genitalia, anal atresia, urethral atresia, uterus didelphys, single umbilical artery, cerebral polygyria, hydrocele, inguinal hernia, abdominal wall hernias.

Clinical Manifestations: Deformities present at birth: (a) *marked shortness of the neck and posterior aspect of the chest, increased anteroposterior diameter of the thoracic cage;* (b) protuberant abdomen; (c) long, thin limbs with tapering digits; (d) craniofacial features: prominent occiput, broad forehead, mongoloid slant of the eyes, wide nasal bridge, prominent philtrum, anteverted nares, inverted V-shaped mouth; (e) other reported abnormalities: soft-tissue syndactyly, camptodactyly, hammertoes, difficult delivery due to trunk deformities, etc.; (f) death in infancy from respiratory complications.

Radiologic Manifestations: (a) *serious vertebral anomalies:* hemivertebrae, widely open neural arches, missing vertebral bodies, block vertebrae; (b) *fan-shaped appearance of the ribs* in the posteroanterior direction with posterior convergence of the ribs.

Differential Diagnosis: Spondylocostal dysostosis; COVESDEM (costovertebral segmentation defect with mesomelia) syndrome.

Notes: The distribution of vertebral anomalies does not seem to be helpful in the differential diagnosis of spondylothoracic dysostosis and spondylocostal dysostosis; the dysostosis and deformities are generally more severe in spondylothoracic dysostosis (Jarcho-Levin syndrome) (Fig SY−J−4).

REFERENCES

Aymé S, et al.: Spondylocostal/spondylothoracic dysostosis: The clinical basis for prognosticating and genetic counseling. *Am. J. Med. Genet.* 24:599, 1986.
Heilbronner DM, et al.: Spondylothoracic dysplasia. *J. Bone Joint Surg. [Am.]* 66:302, 1984.
Jarcho S, Levin PM: Hereditary malformation of the vertebral bodies. *Bull. Johns Hopkins Hosp.* 62:216, 1938.
Kozlowski K, et al.: Spondylo-costal dysplasia—Severe and moderate types (report of 8 cases). *Australas. Radiol.* 25:81, 1981.
Manzia S, et al.: La sindrome delle anomalie vertebro-costali di Jarcho-Levin. *Minerva Pediatr.* 28:2141, 1976.
Pérez-Comas A, et al.: Occipito-facial-cervico-thoraco-abdomino-digital dysplasia; Jarcho-Levin syndrome of vertebral anomalies: Report of six cases and review of the literature. *J. Pediatr.* 85:388, 1974.
Poor MA, et al.: Nonskeletal malformations in one of three siblings with Jarcho-Levin syndrome of vertebral anomalies. *J. Pediatr.* 103:270, 1983.
Roberts AP, et al.: Spondylothoracic and spondylocostal dysostosis. Hereditary forms of spinal deformity. *J. Bone Joint Surg. [Br.]* 70:123, 1988.

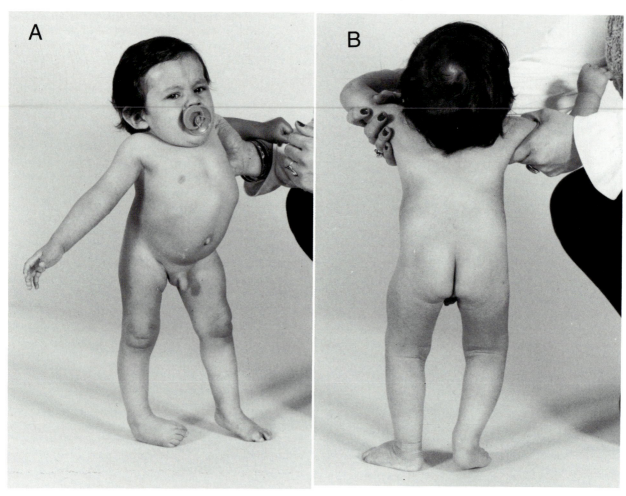

FIG SY—J—4.
A and **B,** Jarcho-Levin syndrome (spondylothoracic dysplasia) in a 10-month-old boy with a short neck, prominent occiput, low hairline, short trunk, bell-shaped chest due to costal flaring, and normal upper and lower limbs. Vertebral anomalies and crablike

Wadia RS, et al.: Recessively inherited costovertebral segmentation defect with mesomelia and peculiar facies (COVESDEM syndrome). A new genetic entity? *J. Med. Genet.* 15:123, 1978.

JERVELL AND LANGE-NIELSEN SYNDROME

Synonyms: Surdo-cardiac syndrome; cardioauditory syndrome of Jervell and Lange-Nielsen.

Mode of Inheritance: Autosomal recessive.

Frequency: 0.3% of congenitally deaf individuals (Wahl et al.).

Clinical Manifestations: (a) *congenital bilateral nerve deafness (deaf mutism)*; (b) *prolonged Q–T interval*; (c) *syncopal attacks*; (d) *hypochromic anemia*; (e) *sudden death*.

bunching of the ribs were seen on the radiographic examination of the trunk. (From Heilbronner DM, Renshaw TS: Spondylothoracic dysplasia. *J. Bone Joint Surg. [Am.]* 66:302, 1984. Used by permission.)

Radiologic Manifestations: No evidence of organic heart disease.

Differential Diagnosis: (a) seizure disorder; (b) Romano-Ward syndrome (prolonged QT interval with normal hearing).

REFERENCES

Behera M: Jervell and Lange-Nielsen syndrome in a middle aged patient. *Postgrad. Med. J.* 63:395, 1987.
Hartzler GO, et al.: Invasive electrophysiological study in the Jervell and Lange-Nielsen syndrome. *Br. Heart J.* 45:225, 1981.
Jervell A, Lange-Nielsen F: Congenital deaf-mutism, functional heart disease with prolongation of the Q–T interval and sudden death. *Am. Heart J.* 54:59, 1957.
Langslet A, et al.: Surdocardiac syndrome of Jervell and Lange-Nielsen, with prolonged QT interval present at

birth, and severe anaemia and syncopal attacks in childhood. *Br. Heart J.* 37:830, 1975.

Sundaram MB, et al.: Cardiac tachyarrhythmias in hereditary long QT syndromes presenting as a seizure disorder. *Can. J. Neurol. Sci.* 13:262, 1986.

Wahl RA, et al.: Congenital deafness with cardiac arrhythmias: The Jervell and Lange-Nielsen syndrome. *Am. Ann. Deaf* 125:34, 1980.

JOHANSON-BLIZZARD SYNDROME

Mode of Inheritance: Probably autosomal recessive.

Frequency: Over 20 published cases (Moeschler et al.)

Clinical and Radiologic Manifestations: (a) *low birth weight; motor, somatic, and mental retardation; hypotonia; hyperextensibility of joints;* (b) craniofacial anomalies: *microcephaly, aplastic alae nasi, skin dimples and defects over the fontanelles,* hair anomalies, eyelid ptosis, strabismus, cutaneolacrimal fistula, *severe oligodontia, small teeth,* micrognathia; (c) sensorineural deafness; (d) hypothyroidism; (e) malabsorption, *exocrine pancreatic insufficiency,* pancreatic lipomatosis; (f) other reported abnormalities: *rectourogenital anomalies,* imperforate anus, hydronephrosis, caliectasis, recurrent urinary tract infections, edema of the hands and feet, hypoplastic nipples, skeletal maturation retardation, anemia, congenital heart defect, maxillary hypoplasia (Fig SY–J–5).

REFERENCES

Bresson JL, et al.: Le syndrome de Johanson-Blizzard. *Arch. Fr. Pediatr.* 37:21, 1980.

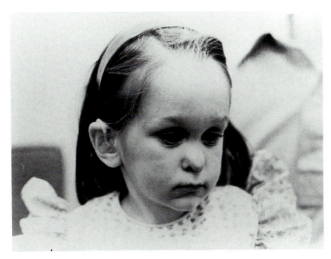

FIG SY–J–5.
Johanson-Blizzard syndrome in a 4¾-year-old patient. Note the hypoplastic nasal alae, frontal hair upsweep, and hearing aid. (From Moeschler JB, Lubinsky MS: Johanson-Blizzard syndrome with normal intelligence. *Am. J. Med. Genet.* 22:69, 1985. Used by permission.)

Johanson A, Blizzard R: A syndrome of congenital aplasia of the alae nasi, deafness, hypothyroidism, dwarfism, absent permanent teeth, and malabsorption. *J. Pediatr.* 79:982, 1971.

Mardini MK, et al.: Johanson-Blizzard syndrome in a large inbred kindred with three involved members. *Clin. Genet.* 14:247, 1978.

Moeschler JB, et al.: Johanson-Blizzard syndrome with normal intelligence. *Am. J. Med. Genet.* 22:69, 1985.

Moeschler JB, et al.: The Johanson-Blizzard syndrome: A second report of full autopsy findings. *Am. J. Med. Genet.* 26:133, 1987.

Morris MD, et al.: Trypsinogen deficiency disease. *Am. J. Dis. Child.* 114:203, 1967.

Townes PL: Proteolytic and lipolytic deficiency of the exocrine pancreas. *J. Pediatr.* 75:221, 1969.

Zerres K, et al.: The Johanson-Blizzard syndrome: Report of a new case with special reference to the dentition and review of the literature. *Clin. Genet.* 30:177, 1986.

JOUBERT SYNDROME

Synonyms: Joubert-Boltschauser syndrome; cerebelloparenchymal disorder IV (CPD IV).

Mode of Inheritance: Autosomal recessive, male preponderance.

Frequency: 33 published cases (King et al.)

Pathology: *Aplasia of the cerebellar vermis;* unsegmented midbrain tectum; occipital meningocele; microcephaly; sacral dermoid sinus.

Clinical Manifestations: (a) low-set ears, high-arched palate, epicanthus, mongoloid slant of the eyes, short neck; (b) *mental retardation, ataxia, episodic hyperpnea, abnormal eye movements, rhythmic protrusion of the tongue;* (c) *bilateral chorioretinal coloboma,* retinal aplasia; (d) other reported abnormalities: polydactyly, contracture of the wrists, high-arched palate, occipital meningoencephalocele, seizures, abnormal electroencephalographic findings, ptosis, facial weakness, clinodactyly, syndactyly, camptodactyly, polydactyly, hemifacial spasms, lingual nodules.

Radiologic Manifestations: (a) absence of the vermis (partial agenesis of the vermis in some), absent corpus callosum, enlarged cisterna magna with abnormally shaped anterior and upper borders, cisterna magna connected with a malformed fourth ventricle via an anomalous channel; (b) cystic kidneys.

Differential Diagnosis: Dandy-Walker syndrome; simple aplasia of the vermis; tectocerebellar dysraphia with an occipital encephalocele; dominantly inherited cerebellar vermis atrophy with early onset in childhood in association with spontaneous upbeating nystagmus and mild gait ataxia (Furman et al., Tomiwa et al.); cerebro-oculo-hepato-renal syndrome—Arima syndrome (Leber amaurosis, agenesis of the cerebellar vermis, infantile polycystic kidneys, fatty liver, hepatic cirrhosis, etc.); Meckel syndrome.

REFERENCES

Aicardi J, et al.: Le syndrome de Joubert. A propos de cinq observations. *Arch. Fr. Pediatr.* 40:625, 1983.
Boltschauser E, et al.: Joubert syndrome: Episodic hyperpnea, abnormal eye movements, retardation and ataxia, associated with dysplasia of the cerebellar vermis. *Neuropaediatrie* 8:57, 1977.
Casaer P, et al.: Variability of outcome in Joubert syndrome. *Neuropediatrics* 16:43, 1985.
De Haene A: Agenesie partielle du vermis du cervelet à caracter familial. *Acta Neurol. Belg.* 55:622, 1955.
Furman JM, et al.: Infantile cerebellar atrophy. *Ann. Neurol.* 17:399, 1985.
Ito J, et al.: Joubert syndrome. Report of a case (abstract). *Neuroradiology* 29:592, 1987.
Joubert M, et al.: Familial agenesis of the cerebellar vermis. A syndrome of episodic hyperpnea, abnormal eye movements, ataxia, and retardation. *Neurology* 19:813, 1969.
King MD, et al.: Joubert's syndrome with retinal dysplasia: Neonatal tachypnoea as the clue to a genetic brain-eye malformation. *Arch. Dis. Child.* 59:709, 1984.
Lindhout D: The Joubert syndrome associated with bilateral chorioretinal coloboma. *Eur. J. Pediatr.* 134:173, 1980.
Lindhout D, et al.: Chorioretinal coloboma and Joubert syndrome (letter). *J. Pediatr.* 107:158, 1985.
Matsuzaka T, et al.: Cerebro-oculo-hepato-renal syndrome (Arima's syndrome): A distinct clinicopathological entity. *J. Child Neurol.* 1:338, 1986.
Tomiwa K, et al.: Dominantly inherited congenital cerebellar ataxia with atrophy of the vermis. *Pediatr. Neurol.* 3:360, 1987.

JUBERG-HAYWARD SYNDROME

Synonym: Orocraniodigital syndrome.

Mode of Inheritance: Autosomal recessive with variable expressivity.

Clinical and Radiologic Manifestations: Five siblings reported with one or more of a specific group of *oral, cranial, and digital anomalies:* (a) cleft lip and palate; (b) microcephaly; (c) hypoplasia (shortening of the metacarpals and phalanges), distal displacement of both thumbs, interphalangeal inflexibility of the thumbs; (d) elbow deformities that limit extension; (e) toe anomalies; (f) other reported abnormalities (following the original description of Juberg and Hayward): bilateral absent thumbs, anomalous carpal bones, deformity of the radial head, short stature, growth hormone deficiency, absence of the pituitary fossa without evidence of endocrine dysfunction (Fig SY–J–6).

REFERENCES

Juberg RC, Hayward JR: A familial syndrome of oral, cranial and digital anomalies. *J. Pediatr.* 74:755, 1969.
Kingston HM, et al.: Orocraniodigital (Juberg-Hayward) syndrome with growth hormone deficiency. *Arch. Dis. Child.* 57:790, 1982.
Nevin NC, et al.: A case of the orocraniodigital (Juberg-Hayward) syndrome. *J. Med. Genet.* 18:478, 1981.

JUGULAR FORAMEN SYNDROME

Clinical and Radiologic Manifestations: Cranial nerve palsies involving more than one of the last four cranial nerves and resulting from tumor, trauma, vascular occlusion, infection, etc., at the basis of the skull and retroparotid space.

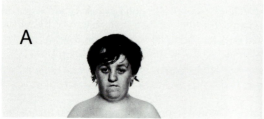

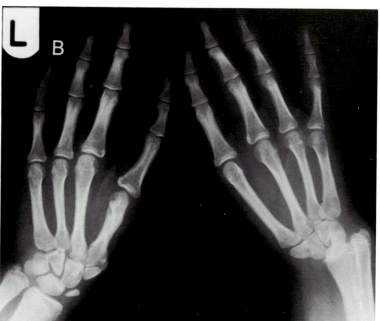

FIG SY–J–6.
Juberg-Hayward syndrome in a 17-year-old (**A** and **B**) boy with a unilateral cleft lip and palate (repaired), bilateral absent thumbs, a prominent forehead, hypoplasia of the midface, micrognathia, a short neck, and a micropenis. (From Kingston HM, Hughes IA, Harper PS: Orocraniodigital (Juberg-Hayward) syndrome with growth hormone deficiency. *Arch. Dis. Child.* 57:790, 1982. Used by permission.)

REFERENCES

Graus F, et al.: Papilledema in the metastatic jugular foramen syndrome. *Arch. Neurol.* 40:816, 1983.

Havelius U, et al.: Carotid fibromuscular dysplasia and paresis of lower cranial nerves (Collet-Sicard syndrome). *J. Neurosurg.* 56:850, 1982.

Wilson H, et al.: Jugular foramen syndrome as a complication of metastatic cancer of the prostate. *South Med. J.* 77:92, 1984.

JUVENILE XANTHOGRANULOMA

Mode of Inheritance: No known familial tendency.

Histology: Nodular infiltrate of histiocytes in the skin with variable numbers of xanthomatous cells, Touton-type giant cells, and eosinophils; visceral involvement rare (lungs, subpleural space, liver, testicle, pericardium, lymph node, kidney).

Clinical Manifestations: A benign, self-limited histiocystosis of infancy and childhood: (a) *skin lesions* (most common on the head and neck, single or multiple): *1-mm to 5-cm macular or nodular reddish brown lesions,* regression of the lesion usually in 6 to 12 months, some may persist to adulthood; (b) hepatosplenomegaly, renal mass.

Radiologic Manifestations: (a) pulmonary well-demarcated nodules; (b) echogenic nodules (liver, kidney), hypodense intrarenal mass (computed tomography).

Differential Diagnosis: Histiocytosis X; visceral fibromatosis; primary or metastatic neoplasms.

REFERENCES

Diard F, et al.: Neonatal juvenile xanthogranulomatosis with pulmonary, extrapleural, and hepatic involvement. One case report. *Ann. Radiol. (Paris)* 25:113, 1982.

Gilbert TJ, et al.: Juvenile xanthogranuloma of the kidney. *Pediatr. Radiol.* 18:169, 1988.

Gupta AK, et al.: Juvenile xanthogranuloma with pulmonary lesions. *Pediatr. Radiol.* 18:70, 1988.

KABUKI MAKE-UP SYNDROME

Synonym: Niikawa-Kuroki syndrome.

Mode of Inheritance: Unknown, autosomal dominant and X-linked possibilities have been suggested, but are highly questionable.

Frequency: Over 60 published cases (Niikawa et al.).

Clinical Manifestations: (a) *facial features (reminiscent of the Kabuki actors' makeup):* arching eyebrows, sparse in the lateral half; long eyelashes; long palpebral fissures; ectropion of the lower eyelids; broad and depressed nasal tip; prominent ears; short nasal septum; (b) mental retardation; (c) postnatal dwarfism; (d) stubby fingers; (e) other reported abnormalities: short fifth fingers, susceptibility to infections, cleft or high-arched palate, widely spaced teeth, low posterior hairline, epicanthus, preauricular dimple, retrognathia, single flexion crease of the fifth fingers, blue sclerae, paralysis of the soft palate, deficient dentition, single flexion of the fourth fingers, finger pad, hearing loss, accessory nipples, imperforate anus, rectovaginal fistula, leukoderma, undescended testes, hirsutism, small penis, cleft uvula, café au lait spots, uveitis, abnormal dermatoglyphics, precocious puberty, etc.

Radiologic Manifestations: (a) clinodactyly, brachymesophalangia of the fifth fingers; (b) vertebral anomalies: scoliosis, butterfly, sagittal cleft, narrow intervertebral disk spaces; (c) pseudoepiphyses; (d) hip dislocation, coxa valga, dislocated hypoplastic patella.

REFERENCES

Koutras A, et al.: Niikawa-Kuroki syndrome: A new malformation syndrome of postnatal dwarfism, mental retardation, unusual face, and protruding ears. *J. Pediatr.* 101:417, 1982.
Kuroki Y, et al.: A new malformation syndrome of long palpebral fissures, large ears, depressed nasal tip, and skeletal anomalies associated with postnatal dwarfism and mental retardation. *J. Pediatr.* 99:570, 1981.
Kuroki Y, et al.: Precocious puberty in kabuki makeup syndrome. *J. Pediatr.* 110:750, 1987.
Niikawa N, et al.: Kabuki make-up syndrome: A syndrome of mental retardation, unusual facies, large and protruding ears, and postnatal growth deficiency. *J. Pediatr.* 99:565, 1981.
Niikawa N, et al.: Kabuki make-up (Niikawa-Kuroki) syndrome: A study of 62 patients. *Am. J. Med. Genet.* 31:656, 1988.

KALLMANN SYNDROME

Synonyms: Hypogonadotropic hypogonadism and anosmia; Kallmann-deMorsier syndrome; anosmia and hypothalamic hypogonadism.

Mode of Inheritance: Possibilities: X-linked recessive or male limited, autosomal dominant, autosomal recessive, X-linked dominant.

Frequency: Not infrequent; 19 patients in 791 hypogonadal males (Pawlowitzki et al.).

Clinical Manifestations: (a) *hypogonadotropic hypogonadism;* (b) *anosmia;* (c) other reported abnormalities: cryptorchidism, neurosensory deafness, color blindness, choanal atresia, X-linked ichthyosis, mild ocular hypotelorism, mild microcephaly, mild mental retardation, brachytelephalangia, unusual facies (square forehead, small nose, telecanthus, thin upper lip), mitral valve prolapse, cardiovascular defects (Ebstein anomaly, atrial septal defect, right-sided aortic arch), gynecomastia, cleft lip/palate, high-arched palate, obesity, diabetes mellitus, shortened frenulum of the tongue.

Radiologic Manifestations: (a) magnetic resonance imaging: *hypoplastic or absent olfactory sulcus* (unilateral or bilateral); (b) other reported anomalies: extensive brain calcification (lentiform and dentate nuclei, thalami, gray and white matter junction), supracellar cyst, choanal atresia, renal abnormalities (unilateral absence, diverticulum), malrotation of the bowel, hand anomalies (short fourth metacarpal, clinodactyly, camptodactyly, etc.) (Fig SY–K–1).

REFERENCES

Ballabio A, et al.: X-linked ichthyosis, due to steroid sulphatase deficiency, associated with Kallmann syndrome (hypogonadotropic hypogonadism and anosmia): Linkage relationships with Xg and cloned DNA sequences from the distal short arm of the X chromosome. *Hum. Genet.* 72:237, 1986.
deMorsier G: Etudes sur les dysraphies cranio-encéphaliques. 1.Agénésie des lobes olfactif (télencéphaloschizis latéral) et des commissures calleuse et antérieure (télencéphaloschizis médian): la dysplasie olfacto-génitale. *Schweiz. Arch. Neurol. Neurochir. Psychiatr.* 74:309, 1954.
Evain-Brion D, et al.: Diagnosis of Kallmann's syndrome in early infancy. *Acta. Paediatr. Scand.* 71:937, 1982.
Hermanussen M, et al.: Heterogeneity of Kallmann's syndrome. *Clin. Genet.* 28:106, 1985.

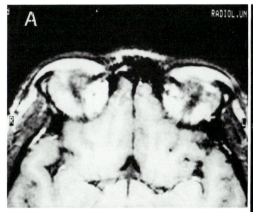 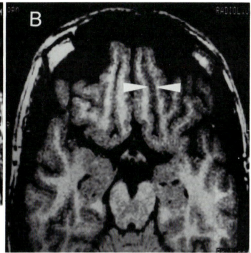

FIG SY–K–1.
Kallmann syndrome. **A,** a transverse magnetic resonance (MR) image through the rhinencephalon of a man with anosmia (Kallman syndrome) shows no olfactory sulci. **B,** a transverse MR image through the rhinencephalon of a normal man shows an approximately 40-mm-long gray band *(arrows)* corresponding to the olfactory sulci (for comparison with **A**). (From Klingmüller D, Dewes W, Krache T, et al.: Magnetic resonance imaging of the brain in patient with anosmia and hypothalamic hypogonadism (Kallmann's syndrome). *J. Clin. Endocrinol. Metab.* 65:581, 1987. Used by permission.)

Hunter AGW, et al.: Characteristic craniofacial appearance and brachytelephalangy in a mother and son with Kallman syndrome in the son. *Am. J. Med. Genet.* 24:527, 1986.

Kallmann FJ, Schoenfeld WA, Barrera SE: The genetic aspects of primary eunuchoidism. *Am. J. Ment. Defic.* 48:203, 1944.

Klein VR, et al.: Kallmann syndrome associated with choanal atresia. *Clin. Genet.* 31:224, 1987.

Klingmüller D, et al.: Magnetic resonance imaging of the brain in patients with anosmia and hypothalamic hypogonadism (Kallmann's syndrome). *J. Clin. Endocrinol. Metab.* 65:581, 1987.

Lieblich JM, et al.: Syndrome of anosmia with hypogonadotropic hypogonadism (Kallmann syndrome). Clinical and laboratory studies in 23 cases. *Am. J. Med.* 73:506, 1982.

Maestre de San Juan A: Teratologia: Falta total de los nervios olfactorios con anosmia en un individuo en quien existia un atrofia congenita de los testiculos y miembro viril. *El Siglo Medico* 3:211, 1856.

Malat J, et al.: Brain calcification in Kallman's syndrome. Computed tomographic appearance. *Pediatr. Neurosci.* 12:257, 1985.

Moorman JR, et al.: Kallman's syndrome with associated cardiovascular and intracranial anomalies. *Am. J. Med.* 77:369, 1984.

Pawlowitzki IH, et al.: Estimating frequency of Kallmann syndrome among hypogonadic and among anosmic patients. *Am. J. Med. Genet.* 26:473, 1987.

Weidenreich F: Über partiellen Riechlappendefect und Eunuchoidismus beim Menschen. *Z. Morphol. Anthropol.* 18:157, 1914.

KARSCH-NEUGEBAUER SYNDROME

Synonyms: Split hand–nystagmus; split foot/split hand and congenital nystagmus.

Mode of Inheritance: A single, pleiotropic dominant gene has been suggested.

Frequency: Reported in three families.

Clinical and Radiologic Manifestations: (a) *nystagmus;* (b) *split foot, split hand,* articulating "cross-bone" in the hand; (c) other reported abnormalities: cataract, strabismus, pigmental changes of the retina.

REFERENCES

Karsch J: Erbliche Augenmissbildung in Verbindung mit Splathand und -Fuss. *Z. Augenheilk.* 89:274, 1936.

Neugebauer H: Splathand und -Fuss mit familiarer Besonderheit. *Z. Orthop.* 95:500, 1962.

Pilarski RT, et al.: Karsch-Neugebauer syndrome: Split foot/split hand and congenital nystagmus. *Clin. Genet.* 27:97, 1985.

KARTAGENER SYNDROME

Mode of Inheritance: Autosomal recessive.

Clinical Manifestations: (a) *situs inversus;* (b) *sinusitis* with mucopurulent nasal discharge from infancy; (c) ciliary dyskinesia (immotile cilia syndrome): about 50% of the patients with ciliary dyskinesia have Kartagener syndrome; (d) other reported abnormalities: bouts of upper and lower respiratory infections, nasal polyposis, conductive hearing loss, recurrent otitis, congenital heart disease; (e) other reported abnormalities: bouts of upper and lower respiratory tract infection, nasal polyposis, conductive hearing loss, recurrent

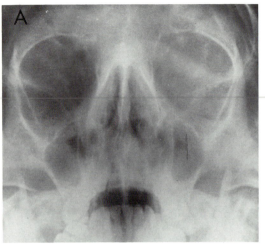
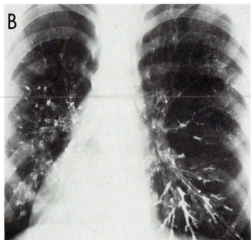

FIG SY–K–2.
Kartagener syndrome in an 18-year-old female who had a right lower lobectomy at the age of 8 years for bronchiectasis. **A,** cloudy paranasal sinuses. **B,** dextrocardia and bronchiectasis. (Courtesy of Dr. Robert S. Arkoff, San Francisco.)

otitis, congenital heart disease; (f) normal spermatozoa and fertility, motile cilia with immotile spermatozoa, motile cilia with abnormal waveforms and structurally defective axonemes, etc. (Fig SY–K–2).

Radiologic Manifestations: (a) *situs inversus* or *isolated dextrocardia;* (b) absent or underdeveloped paranasal sinuses, *sinusitis;* (c) *bronchiectasis.*

Variations: (a) complete situs inversus and congenital heart disease without sinusitis; (b) dextrocardia, congenital heart disease, sinusitis, and bronchiectasis; (c) sinusitis and bronchiectasis without situs inversus.

REFERENCES

Child AH: Kartagener syndrome: A family study. *Clin. Genet.* 17:61, 1980.
Fischer TJ, et al.: Middle ear ciliary defect in Kartagener's syndrome. *Pediatrics* 62:443, 1978.
Greenstone M, et al.: Normal axonemal structure and function in Kartagener's syndrome: An explicable paradox. *Thorax* 40:956, 1985.
Jonsson MS, et al: Kartagener's syndrome with motile spermatozoa. *N. Engl. J. Med.* 307:1131, 1982.
Kartagener M: Zur Pathogenese der Bronchiektasien. *Beitr. Klin. Erforsch. Tuberk. Lungenkr.* 83:489, 1933.
Kartagener M, et al.: Bronchiectasis with situs inversus. *Arch. Pediatr.* 79:193, 1962.
Lake K, et al.: Kartagener's syndrome and deaf-mutism: An unusual association. *Chest* 64:661, 1973.
Newmark H III, et al.: Kartagener's syndrome seen on CT. *Comput. Radiol.* 9:279, 1985.
Samuel I: Kartagener's syndrome with normal spermatozoa. *J.A.M.A.* 258:1329, 1987.
Siewert AK: Ueber einen Fall von Bronchiectasis bei einem: Patienten mit Situs inversus viscerum. *Ber. Munch. Tieraerztl. Wochenschr.* 2:139, 1904.

KASABACH-MERRITT SYNDROME

Synonyms: Hemangioma with thrombocytopenia; platelet-trapping hemangioma; hemangioma with consumptive coagulopathy.

Clinical Manifestations: (a) *hemangioma* or *hemangioendothelioma* of different sizes and locations (skin, viscera, skeleton, central nervous system); (b) sudden growth in hemangioma accompanied by hemorrhagic tendency and *thrombocytopenia* with profuse intratumoral bleeding; (c) progressive increase in the uptake of ^{111}In-labeled platelets within the lesion, concentration of labeled fibrinogen within the lesion, decreased platelet survival time; (d) other reported abnormalities: hypofibrinogenemia, cardiac failure, joint effusion.

Radiologic Manifestations: Findings depend on the involved organs: (a) osteolytic lesions; (b) *visceromegaly;* (c) hydronephrosis; (d) hydrocephalus; (e) lung involvement with pneumothorax; (f) imaging of hemangioma (ultrasound, dynamic computed tomography, magnetic resonance) for evaluation of the lesions and involvement of the organ(s); (g) angiography for demonstration of the vascular mass and transcatheter embolization of the feeding vessels (Figs SY–K–3 and SY–K–4).

REFERENCES

Bowles LJ, et al.: Perinatal hemorrhage associated with the Kasabach-Merritt syndrome. *Clin. Pediatr. (Phila.)* 20:428, 1981.
El-Dessouky M, et al.: Kasabach-Merritt syndrome. *J. Pediatr. Surg.* 23:109, 1988.
Kasabach HH, Merritt KK: Capillary hemangioma with extensive purpura: Report of a case. *Am. J. Dis. Child.* 59:1063, 1940.

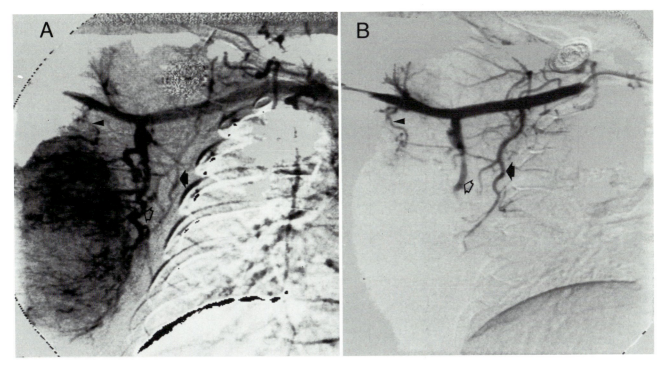

FIG SY–K–3.
Kasabach-Merritt syndrome in a 2-month-old infant with enlarging hemangioma of the right chest wall and thrombocytopenia. **A,** aortography shows a large vascular mass supplied by subscapular *(white arrow),* lateral thoracic *(black arrow),* and circumflex humeral *(arrowhead)* arteries. **B,** postembolization subclavian angiography shows obstruction of the subcapsular *(white arrow)* and lateral thoracic *(black arrow)* arteries. (From Sato Y, Wicklund B, Kisker CT, et al.: Embolization therapy in the management of infantile hemangioma with Kasabach-Merritt syndrome. *Pediatr. Radiol.* 17:503, 1987. Used by permission.)

Larsen EC, et al.: Kasabach-Merritt syndrome: Therapeutic considerations. *Pediatrics* 79:971, 1987.

Lozman J, et al.: Cavernous hemangiomas associated with scoliosis and a localized consumptive coagulopathy. *J. Bone Joint Surg. [Am.]* 58:1021, 1976.

Saadi A, et al.: Hémangiome géant chez l'enfant associé à une thrombopénie (syndrome de Kasabach-Merritt). *Ann. Radiol. (Paris)* 29:553, 1986.

Sato Y, et al.: Embolization therapy in the management of infantile hemangioma with Kasabach Merritt syndrome. *Pediatr. Radiol.* 17:503, 1987.

Schmidt RP, et al.: Hemangioma with consumptive coagulopathy (Kasabach-Merritt syndrome) detection by indium-111 oxine-labeled platelets. *Clin. Nucl. Med.* 9:389, 1984.

Sencer S, et al.: Splenic hemangioma with thrombocytopenia in a newborn. *Pediatrics* 79:960, 1987.

Shah K: Computed tomography and radiotherapy in giant hemangioma with thrombocytopenia. *Comput. Radiol.* 7:319, 1983.

KAUFMAN-McKUSICK SYNDROME

Synonyms: McKusick-Kaufman syndrome.

Mode of Inheritance: Autosomal recessive, phenotypic variability; consanguinity.

Frequency: Approximately 60 published cases (Chitayat et al., Cantani et al.).

Pathology: (a) genital anomalies: *hydrometrocolpos* (vaginal atresia, transverse vaginal septum, vaginal stenosis), duplication of the vagina, cervical atresia, intravaginal displacement of the urethral meatus, persistent urogenital sinus, Müllerian duct anomalies, absent labia minor; (b) urinary system anomalies: *hydronephrosis, hydroureter,* polycystic kidneys; (c) digestive system anomalies: imperforate anus, rectovaginal or vesicovaginal fistulas, Hirschsprung disease, intestinal malrotation; (d) other reported abnormalities: congenital heart disease, lung hypoplasia, subglottic stenosis, bifid epiglottis, pituitary dysplasia, etc.

Clinical Manifestations: (a) *postaxial polydactyly;* (b) *abdominal mass, external genital anomalies:* vaginal anomalies, hypospadias, undescended testes; (c) *urinary retention;* (d) other reported abnormalities: genu recurvatum, micrognathia, edema of the legs, eye abnormalities, developmental delay.

Radiologic Manifestations: (a) *hydrometrocolpos;* (b) *hydronephrosis and hydroureter;* (c) *postaxial polydactyly;* (d) other reported abnormalities: hip dislocation, knee dislocation, vertebral anomalies, oligohydramnios, syndactyly, peritoneal cyst (refluxing vaginal secretion), etc.

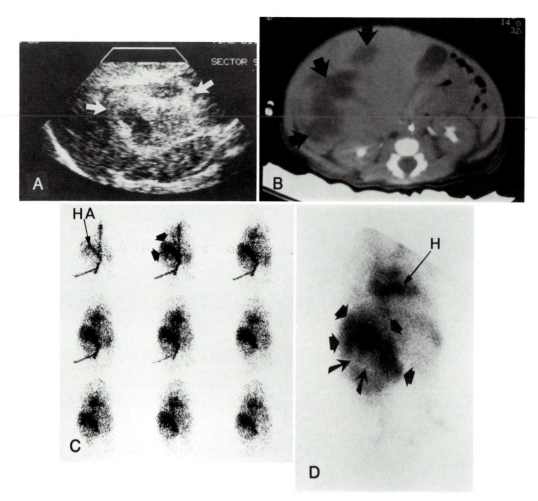

FIG SY–K–4.

Kasabach-Merritt syndrome. **A,** a longitudinal ultrasonographic section of liver reveals an echogenic mass *(arrows)* with internal areas of reduced echogenicity suggesting tumor necrosis within the right lobe of the liver. This ultrasonographic appearance was considered to be compatible with a malignant tumor arising within the liver. **B,** a contrast-enhanced computed tomographic scan of the abdomen reveals marked enlargement of the right lobe of the liver. Multiple low-density areas *(arrows)* are seen in the right lobe of the liver. Several areas suggesting contrast enhancement are seen. The appearance suggests the presence of necrotic hepatic malignancy. **C,** an anterior abdominal flow study performed in a neonatal intensive care unit with a mobile gamma camera on ^{99m}Tc-labeled red blood cells (RBCs) reveals marked hypertrophy of the hepatic artery *(HA)* and an extremely vascular lesion *(arrowheads)* involving a majority of the right lobe of the liver. **D,** a static 300,000-count ^{99m}Tc RBC scintiphotograph of the abdomen obtained after flow study reveals a large lesion *(arrowheads)* involving a majority of the right lobe of the liver with intense blood pool activity equal to that of the heart *(H)*. Centrally located within this mass are "cold" or photopenic areas *(arrows)* indicating clot formation within this liver tumor of vascular origin. (From Loh W Jr, Miller JH, Gomperts D: Imaging with technetium 99m–labeled erythrocytes in evaluation of the Kasabach-Merritt syndrome. *J. Pediatr.* 113:856, 1988. Used by permission.)

Note: Polydactyly and undescended testes reported in male siblings (Figs SY–K–5 and SY–K–6).

REFERENCES

Caillé G, et al.: A propos de deux cas d'hydrocolpos par atrésie vaginale associés a une polydactylie. *Ann. Radiol. (Paris)* 26:477, 1983.

Cantani A, et al.: The Kaufman-McKusick syndrome. A review of the 44 cases reported in the literature. *Ann. Genet. (Paris)* 30:70, 1987.

Chitayat D, et al.: Further delineation of the McKusick-Kaufman hydrometrocolpos-polydactyly syndrome. *Am. J. Dis. Child.* 141:1133, 1987.

Farrell SA, et al.: Abdominal distension in Kaufman-McKusick syndrome. *Am. J. Med. Genet.* 25:205, 1986.

Hofman U, et al.: Clinical aspects, diagnosis, and treatment of the Kaufman syndrome (hydrocolpos, hypospadias and polydactyly). *Prog. Pediatr. Surg.* 17:71, 1984.

Kaufman RL, et al: Family studies in congenital heart disease II: A syndrome of hydrometrocolpos, postaxial polydactyly and congenital heart disease. *Birth Defects* 8:85, 1972.

McKusick VA, et al.: Hydrometrocolpos as a simply inherited malformation. *J.A.M.A.* 189:813, 1964.

Stjimorovic I: Hydrometrokolpos novorodenceta. *Acta Chir. Iugosl.* 3:175, 1956.

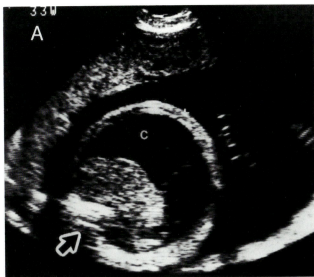

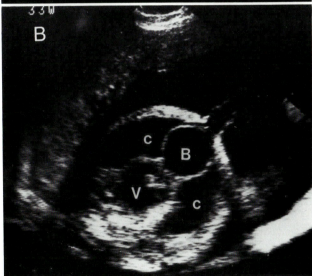

FIG SY–K–5.
Kaufman-McKusick syndrome. **A,** an ultrasonogram shows a cross section of a fetal abdomen at 33 weeks' gestation just below the liver with the loculated peritoneal cysts *(c)* filling the anterior aspect of the peritoneal cavity and displacing the bowel posteriorly. The abdominal wall is slightly thickened. The *arrow* marks the spine for orientation. **B,** a section taken just caudal to **A** at the level of the umbilical vessels shows the distended urinary bladder *(B)* located just anterior to the distended vagina *(V)* and surrounded by peritoneal cysts on either side *(c)*. (From Farrell SA, Davidson RG, De Maria JE, et al.: Abdominal distension in Kaufman-McKusick syndrome. *Am. J. Med. Genet.* 25:205, 1986. Used by permission.)

KAWASAKI SYNDROME

Synonyms: Mucocutaneous lymph node syndrome; Kawasaki disease; "juvenile" periarteritis nodosa.

Clinical Manifestations: Acute multisystem vasculitis; most patients under 5 years of age: (a) *fever* lasting 1 to 2 weeks; (b) *skin rash,* polymorphous (erythematous, urticaria-

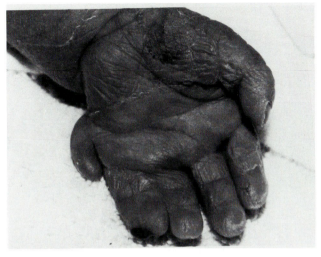

FIG SY–K–6.
Kaufman-McKusick syndrome: postaxial polydactyly. (From Farrell SA, Davidson RG, De Maria JE, et al.: Abdominal distension in Kaufman-McKusick syndrome. *Am. J. Med. Genet.* 25:205, 1986. Used by permission.)

like, etc.) with onset often in the palms and soles and spreading to the trunk, followed by desquamation (peripheral extremities, periungual); (c) *bilateral conjunctival injection;* (d) *mucous membrane changes:* injected pharynx, injected lips, "strawberry" tongue, fissured lips, necrotic pharyngitis; (e) *adenopathy;* (f) other relatively common manifestations: pneumonia, diarrhea, arthralgia/arthritis, meatitis, photophobia, meningitis, electrocardiographic changes; (g) uncommon manifestations: severe abdominal pain, abdominal distension, encephalopathy, facial palsy, hemiparesis, ataxia, febrile convulsions, tonsillar exudate, unusual rashes (vesicular, petechial, purpuric), anterior uveitis, peripheral vasculitis of the extremities causing ischemic necrosis, necrotic pharyngitis, pancreatitis, hepatomegaly, hepatitis, liver necrosis, intrahepatic cholangitis, jaundice, splenomegaly, recurrence of disease (very rare); (h) myocarditis, pericarditis, cardiac tamponade, myocardial infarction, mitral regurgitation, tricuspid regurgitation, aortic valve regurgitation, aortic aneurysm; (i) elevated acute phase reactants (C-reactive protein, sedimentation rate, α_1-antitripsin), thrombocytosis (after day 10), thrombocytopenia, sterile pyuria, negative antistreptolysin O, leukoerythroblastosis, mild normochromic and normocytic anemia, autoimmune hemolytic anemia, impaired granulocyte chemotaxis and increased circulating immune complexes, hyponatremia, low plasma fibronectin concentration in the first and second week of disease; (j) association with hemolytic-uremic syndrome.

Radiologic Manifestations: (a) coronary, peripheral, cerebral, and visceral arterial abnormalities: *thrombosis, stenosis, and aneurysm* (spherical, fusiform), rupture of an aneurysm, arterial wall calcification; (b) *cardiomegaly,* myocardial damage (^{201}T1 scintigraphy), ventricular aneurysm, pericardial effusion, valvular regurgitation (mitral, tricuspid, aortic), left ventricular wall motion abnormalities, myocarditis; (c) pneumonia, pleural effusion; (d) hydrops of the gallbladder,

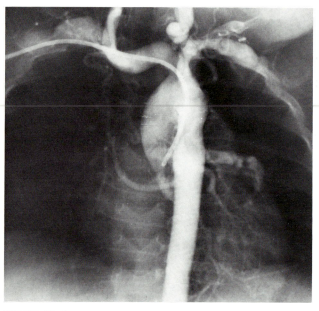

FIG SY–K–7.
Kawasaki syndrome in an 8-month-old boy. A thoracic aortogram shows a completely obstructed right coronary artery and aneurysmal dilatation of the circumflex branch of the left coronary artery with partial thrombosis. Aneurysms also involve both subclavian and axillary arteries. A large bronchial artery anastomosing with intercostal arteries is evident on the right side. (From Cook A, l'Heureux P: Radiographic findings in the mucocutaneous lymph node syndrome. *A.J.R.* 132:107, 1979. Used by permission.)

gallbladder necrosis, gallbladder perforation; (e) intestinal pseudo-obstruction, bowel necrosis, ischemic colitis, bowel obstruction (stricture as a complication of the disease); (f) avascular necrosis of the femoral head, aseptic necrosis of the calcaneous, hip pyarthrosis; (g) parapharyngeal adenopathy, necrotic pharyngitis; (h) renal involvement: increased cortical echogenicity, enhanced corticomedullary differentiation, renomegaly; (i) cerebral vascular disease, aneurysm, cerebral infarction.

Note: To make a clinical diagnosis of Kawasaki syndrome patients should meet five of six criteria listed under clinical manifestations (fever, bilateral conjunctival infection, mucous membrane changes, skin lesions of the palms and soles, polymorphous truncal rash without vesicles or crusts, and cervical adenopathy) and have other diseases excluded (Fig SY–K–7).

REFERENCES

Bligard CA: Kawasaki disease and its diagnosis. *Pediatr. Dermatol.* 4:75, 1987.

Bowler J, et al.: Kawasaki syndrome presenting as pyarthrosis of the hip. *J. Bone Joint Surg. [Am.]* 68:467, 1986.

Bradford BF, et al.: Ultrasonographic evaluation of the gallbladder in mucocutanous lymph node syndrome. *Radiology* 142:381, 1982

Brion L, et al.: Mucocutaneous lymph node syndrome with necrotic pharyngitis. *Eur. J. Pediatr.* 135:111, 1980.

Bunin NJ, et al.: Autoimmune hemolytic anemia in association with Kawasaki disease. *Am. J. Pediatr. Hematol. Oncol.* 8:351, 1986.

Edwards KM, et al.: Intrahepatic cholangitis associated with mucocutaneous lymph node syndrome. *J. Pediatr. Gastroenterol. Nutr.* 4:140, 1985.

Fan ST, et al.: Ischemic colitis in Kawasaki disease. *J. Pediatr. Surg.* 21:964, 1986.

Ferriero DM, et al.: Hemolytic uremic syndrome associated with Kawasaki disease. *Pediatrics* 68:405, 1981.

Freij BJ, et al.: Aortic and mitral regurgitation in an infant with Kawasaki disease. *Pediatr. Cardiol.* 6:95, 1985.

Frey EE, et al: Coronary artery aneurysms due to Kawasaki disease: Diagnosis with ultrafast CT. *Radiology* 167:725, 1988.

Guillou MA, et al: Etiopathogénie du syndrome de Kawasaki. *Arch. Fr. Pediatr.* 45:55, 1988.

Grenadier E, et al.: Left ventricular wall motion abnormalities in Kawasaki's disease. *Am. Heart J.* 107:966, 1984.

Hara T, et al.: Thrombocytopenia: A complication of Kawasaki disease. *Eur. J. Pediatr.* 147:51, 1988.

Hattori T, et al.: Facial palsy in Kawasaki disease. *Eur. J. Pediatr.* 146:601, 1987.

Hicks RV, et al.: Kawasaki syndrome. *Pediatr. Clin. North Am.* 33:1151, 1986.

Kato H, et al.: Myocardial infarction in Kawasaki disease: Clinical analyses in 195 cases. *J. Pediatr.* 108:923, 1986.

Kawasaki T: Acute febrile mucocutaneous syndrome with lymphoid involvement with specific desquamation of the fingers and toes in children: Clinical observations of 50 cases. *Jpn. J. Allergol.* 16:178, 1967.

Lacroix J, et al.: Etude prospective de 64 cas de maladie de Kawasaki. *Arch. Fr. Pediatr.* 42:771, 1985.

Lapointe JS, et al.: Cerebral infarction and regression of widespread aneurysms in Kawasaki's disease. *Pediatr. Radiol.* 14:1, 1984.

Laurent F, et al.: CT appearance of coronary aneurysm in Kawasaki disease. *J. Comput. Assist. Tomogr.* 11:151, 1987.

Laxer RM, et al.: Hyponatremia in Kawasaki disease. *Pediatrics* 70:655, 1982.

Lipson MH: Ruptured hepatic artery aneurysm and coronary artery aneurysms with myocardial infarction in a 14-year-old boy: New manifestations of mucocutaneous lymph node syndrome. *J. Pediatr.* 98:933, 1981.

Matsuura H, et al.: Gallium-67 myocardial imaging for the detection of myocarditis in the acute phase of Kawasaki disease (mucocutaneous lymph node syndrome): The usefulness of single photon emission computed tomography. *Br. Heart J.* 58:385, 1987.

Mercer S, et al.: Surgical complications of Kawasaki disease. *J. Pediatr. Surg.* 16:444, 1981.

Miyake T, et al.: Small bowel pseudo-obstruction in Kawasaki disease. *Pediatr. Radiol.* 17:383, 1987.

Murphy DJ, et al.: Small bowel obstruction as a complication of Kawasaki disease. *Clin. Pediatr. (Phila.)* 26:193, 1987.

Nakano H, et al.: Doppler detection of tricuspid regurgitation following Kawasaki disease. *Pediatr. Radiol.* 16:123, 1986.

Nakano H, et al.: High incidence of aortic regurgitation following Kawasaki disease. *J. Pediatr.* 107:59, 1985.

Nardi PM, et al.: Renal manifestations of Kawasaki's disease. *Pediatr. Radiol.* 15:116, 1985.

Ohshio G, et al.: Hepatomegaly and splenomegaly in Kawasaki disease. *Pediatr. Pathol.* 4:257, 1985.

Ono S, et al.: Impaired granulocyte chemotaxis and increased circulating immune complexes in Kawasaki disease. *J. Pediatr.* 106:567, 1985.

Puczynski M, et al.: Mucocutaneous lymph node syndrome. *J. Comput. Assist. Tomogr.* 8:175, 1984.

Puczynski MD, et al.: Bone involvement in the mucocutaneous lymph node syndrome. *Clin. Pediatr. (Phila.)* 24:657, 1984.

Sasaguri Y, et al.: Regression of aneurysms in Kawasaki disease: A pathological study. *J. Pediatr.* 100:225, 1982.

Shimizu S, et al.: Plasma fibronectin concentrations in mucocutaneous lymph node syndrome. *Arch. Dis. Child.* 61:72, 1986.

Sills RH, et al.: Leukoerythroblastosis in Kawasaki disease. *Am. J. Pediatr. Hematol. Oncol.* 7:193, 1985.

Stoler J, et al.: Pancreatitis in Kawasaki disease. *Am. J. Dis. Child.* 141:306, 1987.

Sty JR, et al.: Gallbladder perforation in a case of Kawasaki disease: Image correlation. *J. Clin. Ultrasound* 11:381, 1983.

Suzuki A, et al.: Coronary arterial lesions of Kawasaki disease: Cardiac catheterization findings of 1100 cases. *Pediatr. Cardiol.* 7:3, 1986.

Tatara K, et al.: Long-term prognosis of giant coronary aneurysm in Kawasaki disease: An angiographic study. *J. Pediatr.* 111:705, 1987.

Trumble T, et al.: Kawasaki disease—A cause of vasculitis in children. *J. Pediatr. Orthop.* 6:92, 1986.

Ueda K, et al.: Thallium-201 scintigraphy in an infant with myocardial infarction following mucocutaneous lymph node syndrome. *Pediatr. Radiol.* 9:183, 1980.

Vargo TA, et al.: Recurrent Kawasaki disease. *Pediatr. Cardiol.* 6:199, 1986.

Williamson MR, et al.: Indium-111 leukocyte scanning localization for detecting early myocarditis in Kawasaki disease. *A.J.R.* 146:255, 1986.

Yanagitani Y, et al.: Avascular necrosis of the femoral head associated with mucocutaneous lymph node syndrome. *J. Pediatr. Orthop.* 6:107, 1986.

KBG SYNDROME

Mode of Inheritance: Probably autosomal dominant with significant variability of expression.

Clinical Manifestations: (a) *craniofacial appearance:* round face, brachycephaly, biparietal prominence, broad eyebrows, telecanthus; (b) dental anomalies: short alveolar ridges, macrodontia, oligodontia, malposition, enamel hypoplasia; (c) *short stature;* (d) *moderate mental retardation;* (e) palmar distal axial triradius and simian creases; (f) hearing deficit.

Radiologic Manifestations: Anomalies of vertebrae, shortness of the tubular bones of the hands, hexadactyly, short neck, syndactyly of toes 2 and 3, skeletal maturation retardation, pectus excavatum, cervical ribs.

REFERENCES

Fryns JP, et al.: Mental retardation, short stature, minor skeletal anomalies, craniofacial dysmorphism and macrodontia in two sisters and their mother. Another variant example of the KBG syndrome? *Clin. Genet.* 26:69, 1984.

Herrmann J, et al.: The KBG syndrome—a syndrome of short stature, characteristic facies, mental retardation, macrodontia, and skeletal abnormalities, *Birth Defects* 11:7, 1975.

KERATODERMA HEREDITARIA MUTILANS

Synonyms: Vohwinkel syndrome; congenital deafness with keratopachydermia and constrictions of the fingers and toes.

Mode of Inheritance: Usually autosomal dominant; autosomal recessive and sporadic also reported.

Clinical and Radiologic Manifestations: Onset usually in infancy: (a) *diffuse honeycombed hyperkeratosis of the palmar and plantar surfaces, star-shaped keratosis located on the dorsa of the digits, linear keratosis on the elbows and knees;* (b) *ainhumlike constriction of the digits, autoamputation;* (c) other reported abnormalities: high-frequency hearing loss, deaf mutism, ichthyosis, cicatricial alopecia.

REFERENCES

Gibbs RC, et al.: Keratoderma hereditaria mutilans (Vohwinkel): Differentiating features of conditions with constriction of digits. *Arch. Dermatol.* 94:619, 1966.

Goldfarb MT, et al.: Keratoderma hereditaria mutilans (Vohwinkel's syndrome): A trial of isotretinoin. *Pediatr. Dermatol.* 2:216, 1985.

Schamroth JM, et al.: Mutilating keratoderma. *Int. J. Dermatol.* 25:249, 1986.

Vohwinkel KH: Keratoderma hereditarium mutilans. *Arch. Dermatol.* 158:354, 1929.

KERATOSIS PALMARIS ET PLANTARIS FAMILIARIS (TYLOSIS)

Mode of Inheritance: Autosomal dominant.

Clinical Manifestations: Onset of symptoms between the age of 3 and 12 months: (a) *diffuse extensive symmetrical cornification of the skin beginning on the palms and soles with extension of the process dorsally in some cases;* (b) *keratoma;* (c) *hyperhidrosis;* (d) *maceration;* (e) *autoamputation in severe cases.*

Radiologic Manifestations: (a) thickening and disorganization of normal soft-tissue planes; (b) osteoporosis; (c) tapering of the distal phalanges; progressive amputation of the phalanges, metacarpals, and metatarsals; (d) luxation of joints; (e) fusion of carpal bones.

REFERENCES

Chung HL: Keratoma palmare et plantare hereditarium, with special reference to its mode of inheritance as traced in six and seven generations, respectively, in two Chinese families. *Arch. Dermatol. Syph.* 36:303, 1937.
Hermel MB, et al.: Keratoderma palmaris et plantaris, roentgenologic aspects. *Radiology* 92:1101, 1969.
Presley NL, et al.: The roentgen appearance of mutilating palmoplantar keratosis. *A.J.R.* 86:944, 1961.

KEUTEL SYNDROME

Mode of Inheritance: Probably autosomal recessive.

Frequency: Six published cases (Cormode et al.).

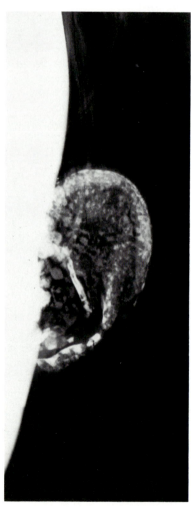

FIG SY—K—8.
Keutel syndrome in a 13-year-old girl with cartilage calcification of the ear. (From Fryns JP, Fleteren A, Mattelaer P, et al.: Calcification of cartilages, brachytelephalangy and peripheral pulmonary stenosis. Confirmation of the Keutel syndrome. *Eur. J. Pediatr.* 142:201, 1984. Used by permission.)

Clinical Manifestations: (a) *brachytelephalangia;* (b) *hearing loss* (mixed, conductive); (c) *characteristic facies:* midfacial hypoplasia, depressed nasal bridge, small alae nasi; (d) other reported abnormalities: peripheral pulmonary stenosis, ventricular septal defect, respiratory symptoms (recurrent upper respiratory infection, wheezing, bronchiectasis, asthma), mental retardation, short stature.

Radiologic Manifestations: (a) *widespread cartilage calcification/ossification:* external ears, nose, larynx, tracheobronchial tree, ribs; (b) *stippled epiphyses;* (c) *peripheral pulmonary stenosis* (in half of the cases), ventricular septal defect (Fig SY—K—8).

REFERENCES

Cormode EJ, et al.: Keutel syndrome: Clinical report and literature review. *Am. J. Med. Genet.* 24:289, 1986.
Keutel J, et al.: A new autosomal recessive syndrome: Peripheral pulmonary stenoses, brachytelephalangism, neural hearing loss and abnormal cartilage calcification/ossification. *Birth Defects* 8:60, 1972.

KIRGHIZIAN DERMATO-OSTEOLYSIS

Synonym: Dermato-osteolysis, Kirghizian type.

Mode of Inheritance: Autosomal recessive has been suggested.

Frequency: Five siblings (Kozlova et al.).

Clinical and Radiologic Manifestations: Onset in infancy; progressive course for several years: (a) recurrent skin ulceration, nail dystrophy; (b) fever; (c) arthralgia, fistulous osteolysis around the joints; (d) oligodontia; (e) keratitis with visual impairment or blindness; (f) pseudoacromegalic appearance of the hands and feet, clawed fingers; (g) shortness of the lower-limb long bones due to the growth plate involvement.

Note: The family affected with the disease resided in the Kirghiz Republic of Soviet Central Asia.

REFERENCE

Kozlova SI, et al.: Self-limited autosomal recessive syndrome of skin ulceration, arthroosteolysis with pseudoacromegaly, keratitis, and oligodontia in a Kirghizian family. *Am. J. Med. Genet.* 15:205, 1983.

KIRNER DEFORMITY

Synonyms: Dystelephalangia; incurving of the terminal phalanges of the fifth fingers; familial symmetrical bowing of the terminal phalanges of the fifth fingers.

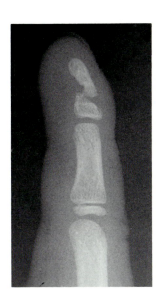

FIG SY–K–9.
Kirner deformity in an 11-year-old male with incurving of the distal phalanx of the fifth digit. Note the oblique defect at the metaphyseo-epiphyseal region, some sclerosis of the border of the proximal segment, and angulation at the site of the defect. (From Taybi H: Bilateral incurving of terminal phalanges of fifth fingers. *J. Pediatr.* 62:431, 1963. Used by permission.)

Mode of Inheritance: Sporadic; autosomal dominant with incomplete penetrance.

Frequency: Underreported; 23 published cases to 1986 (Kerboul et al., Beluffi et al.).

Clinical Manifestations: *Painless soft-tissue swelling beginning in childhood* followed by progressive volar-radial curving of the distal phalanx of the fifth fingers.

Radiologic Manifestations: *Angulation of the distal phalanx at the metaphysis, shaft bent, fusion of the epiphysis and shaft at an abnormal angle* resulting in permanent deformity, normal or slight retardation of closure of the physis (Fig SY–K–9).

REFERENCES

Beluffi G, et al.: Anomalie de Kirner (cas radiologique du mois). *Arch. Fr. Pediatr.* 41:737, 1984.

Blank E, et al.: Symmetric bowing of the terminal phalanges of the fifth fingers in a family (Kirner's deformity). *A.J.R.* 93:367, 1965.

Dykes RG: Kirner's deformity of the little finger. *J. Bone Joint Surg. [Br.]* 60:58, 1978.

Kerboul B, et al.: La déformation de Kirner. A propos de 3 nouveaux cas. Revue de la littérature. *J. Radiol.* 67:523, 1986.

Kirner J: Doppelseitge Verkrümmungen des Kleinfingerendgliedes als selbständiges Krankheitsbild. *Fortschr. Rontgenstr.* 36:804, 1927.

Taybi H: Bilateral incurving of terminal phalanges of fifth fingers (osteochondrosis?). *J. Pediatr.* 62:431, 1963.

KLEIN-WAARDENBURG SYNDROME

Synonyms: Klein syndrome; Waardenburg-Klein syndrome.

Mode of Inheritance: Some evidence for autosomal dominant inheritance.

Frequency: Six published cases (Goodman et al.).

Clinical Manifestations: (a) *lateral displacement of the medial canthi, heterochromia of the iris, blepharophimosis, heavy eyebrows (medial portion), large root of the nose, hy-*

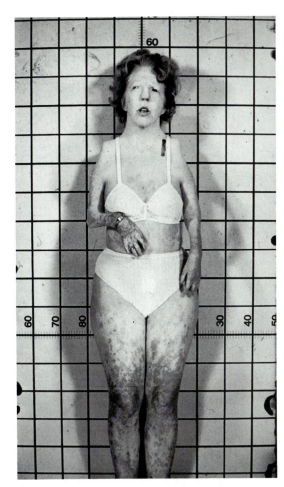

FIG SY–K–10.
Klein-Waardenburg syndrome in a 34-year-old female with an abnormally large inner canthal diameter; partial albinism of the hair, eyebrows, and skin (scalp hair tinted); a high nasal root; hypoplastic alae nasi; and depigmented skin patches on the trunk and limbs. (From Klein D: Historical background and evidence for dominant inheritance of the Klein-Waardenburg syndrome (type III). *Am. J. Med. Genet.* 14:231, 1983. Used by permission.)

poplastic alae, cupid bow-shaped upper lip, prognathism, white forelock; (b) deafness, unilateral or bilateral; (c) albinotic skin patches; (d) *thin upper limbs, with hypoplasia of musculoskeletal structures;* (e) *flexion deformity* (elbow, wrist, fingers).

Radiologic Manifestations: (a) syndactyly of the hands; (b) *carpal bone fusion* (Fig SY−K−10).

REFERENCES

Goodman RM, et al.: Upper limb involvement in the Klein-Waardenburg syndrome. *Am. J. Med. Genet.* 11:425, 1982.

Klein D: Historical background and evidence for dominant inheritance of the Klein-Waardenburg syndrome (type III). *Am. J. Med. Genet.* 14:231, 1983.

Klein PD: Albinisme partiel (leucisme) avec surdi-mutité, blépharophimosis et dysplasie myo-ostéo-articulaire. *Helv. Paediatr. Acta* 5:38, 1950.

Marx P, et al.: Un cas de syndrome de Waardenburg-Klein. *Bull. Soc. Ophtalmol. Fr.* 68:444, 1963.

KLIPPEL-FEIL SYNDROME

Synonym: Congenital brevicollis.

Mode of Inheritance: Autosomal recessive and autosomal dominant modes of inheritance have been suggested; sporadic.

Classification: Type I: extensive cervical and upper thoracic spinal fusion; type II: the most common type, one or two interspace fusion, usually associated with hemivertebrae and occipitoatlantal fusion, C_2–C_3 and C_5–C_6 most often fused; type III: combined cervical and lower thoracic or lumbar fusion.

Frequency: Approximately 1 in 42,000 births (DaSilva)

Clinical Manifestations: (a) *short or "absent" neck, decreased mobility of the head;* (b) *low occipital hairline;* (c) deafness (in about 30%): usually sensorineural hearing impairment, rarely conductive or mixed hearing loss; (d) other reported abnormalities: webbing of the neck, cardiovascular anomalies, facial asymmetry, torticollis, scoliosis, synkinesia, Mayer-Rokitansky-Küster syndrome, fetal alcohol syndrome, Duane syndrome, Klippel-Feil deformity with conductive deafness and absent vagina, mirror motions (involuntary paired movements of the hands and the arms), etc.

Radiologic Manifestations: (a) *fused cervical or cervicothoracic vertebrae, hemivertebrae deformities;* (b) ear anomalies: absent auditory canal, microtia, deformed ossicles, underdevelopment of the bony labyrinth, Mondini defect, small or absent internal auditory canal, etc.; (c) genitourinary anomalies: renal agenesis, malrotation, duplication, ectopia, dysgenesis; (d) other reported abnormalities: atlanto-occipital fusion, Sprengel deformity, micrognathia, spina bifida, rib fusion, spinal canal stenosis, intraspinal tumor, frontonasal dysplasia and postaxial polydactyly, recurrent vertebrobasilar embolism, atlantoaxial instability and spinal cord compression, syringomyelia, isolation of the right subclavian artery with subclavian steal (subclavian artery supply disruption sequence), etc.

Differential Diagnosis: Wildervank syndrome, acquired vertebral fusion (juvenile rheumatoid arthritis, rheumatoid spondylitis, infection, etc.).

Note: The classical triad of low posterior hairline, short neck, and limitation of head and neck motion is not present in all cases.

REFERENCES

Born CT, et al.: Cerebrovascular accident complicating Klippel-Feil syndrome. A case report. *J. Bone Joint Surg. [Am.]* 70:1412, 1988.

Brill CB, et al.: Isolation of the right subclavian artery with subclavian steal in a child with Klippel-Feil anomaly: An example of the subclavian artery supply disruption sequence. *Am. J. Med. Genet.* 26:933, 1987.

Da Silva EO: Autosomal recessive Klippel-Feil syndrome. *J. Med. Genet.* 19:130, 1982.

Elster AD: Quadriplegia after minor trauma in the Klippel-Feil syndrome. A case report and review of the literature. *J. Bone Joint Surg. [Am.]* 66:1473, 1984.

Falk RH, et al.: Klippel-Feil syndrome associated with aortic coarctation. *Br. Heart J.* 38:1220, 1976.

Fragoso R, et al.: Frontonasal dysplasia in the Klippel-Feil syndrome: A new associated malformation. *Clin. Genet.* 22:270, 1982.

Holliday PO, et al.: Multiple meningiomas of the cervical spinal cord associated with Klippel-Feil malformation and atlantooccipital assimilation. *Neurosurgery* 14:353, 1984.

Klippel M, Feil A: Anomalie de la colonne vértebrale par absence des vértebres cervicales: Cage thoracic remonant jusqu' à la base du crâne. *Bull. Mem. Soc. Ant. (Paris)* 87:185, 1912.

Moore WB, et al.: Genitourinary anomalies associated with Klippel-Feil syndrome. *J. Bone Joint Surg. [Am.]* 57:355, 1975.

Morrison SG, et al.: Congenital brevicollis (Klippel-Feil syndrome) and cardiovascular anomalies. *Am. J. Dis. Child.* 115:614, 1968.

Nagib MG, et al.: Identification and management of high-risk patients with Klippel-Feil syndrome. *J. Neurosurg.* 61:523, 1984.

Neidengard L: Klippel-Feil malformation complex in fetal alcohol syndrome. *Am. J. Dis. Child.* 132:929, 1978.

Park IJ, et al.: A new syndrome in two unrelated females: Klippel-Feil deformity, conductive deafness and absent vagina. *Birth Defects* 7:311, 1971.

Roach JW, et al.: Atlanto-axial instability and spinal cord compression in children—Diagnosis by computerized tomography. *J. Bone Joint Surg. [Am.]* 66:708, 1984.

Ross CA, et al.: Recurrent vertebrobasilar embolism in an

infant with Klippel-Feil anomaly. *Pediatr. Neurol.* 3:181, 1987.

Sakai M, et al.: Klippel-Feil syndrome with conductive deafness and histological findings of removed stapes. *Ann. Otol. Rhinol. Laryngol.* 92:202, 1983.

Vaquero J, et al.: Klippel-Feil syndrome with epidural fibroblastoma in the area of vertebral fusion. *Arch. Neurol.* 39:318, 1982.

Windle-Taylor PC, et al.: Ear deformities associated with the Klippel-Feil syndrome. *Ann. Otol. Rhinol. Laryngol.* 90:210, 1981.

KLIPPEL-TRENAUNAY SYNDROME

Synonyms: Angio-osteohypertrophy syndrome; Klippel-Trenaunay-Weber syndrome.

Frequency: Uncommon.

Clinical Manifestations: Usually monomelic: (a) *superficial varices*; (b) *port-wine telangiectatic nevi*; (c) *soft-tissue and bone hypertrophy*; (d) other reported abnormalities: protein-losing enteropathy, thrombocytopenia (platelet sequestration), hematuria, rectal bleeding, systemic hypertension, chronic renal failure.

Radiologic Manifestations:

(A) PRENATAL: Ultrasonographic demonstration of hemihypertrophy, visceral and peripheral vascular anomalies.

(B) POSTNATAL: Diagnosis using various imaging modalities including angiography, computed tomography, ultrasonography, and scintigraphy: (a) elongation and widening of the bones of a limb *(hypertrophy)*, cortical thickening; (b) *hy-*

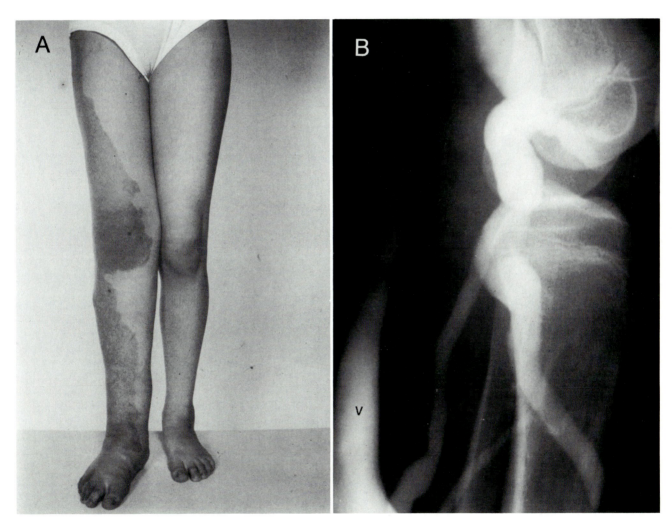

FIG SY–K–11.

Klippel-Trenaunay syndrome. **A,** 11-year-old girl with diffuse hemangioma of the right lower limb, superficial varicosities, and a small angiokeratoma around the knee. **B,** a right lower limb venogram shows abnormally enlarged veins around the knee. Most of the veins were tortuous but one *(v)* was almost straight vertical and extended from the calf to the upper portion of the thigh in a posterolateral location. (From Azouz EM: Hematuria, rectal bleeding and pelvic phleboliths in children with the Klippel-Trenaunay syndrome. *Pediatr. Radiol.* 13:82, 1983. Used by permission.)

poplasia or atresia of some major deep veins, abnormal venous channels connecting deep veins to dilated superficial veins, nonvisualization of valves in some veins, decompensation of superficial veins; (c) other associated vascular abnormalities: abdominal hemangiomas (intestine, urinary system, spleen, etc.), varicose pulmonary veins, spinal cord arteriovenous malformation, cutaneous lymphangiomas, Sturge-Weber syndrome, aplasia of the cervical internal carotid artery and malformation of the circle of Willis, duplication of the inferior vena cava; (d) other reported abnormalities: macrodactyly, dental abnormalities, atrophy of involved areas, nephroblastomatosis, hemihypertrophy of the face, syndactyly, polydactyly, dislocation of the hip, scoliosis, kyphosis, phleboliths, cerebral and cerebellar hemihypertrophy, etc.

Differential Diagnosis: Parkes-Weber syndrome; neurofibromatosis; dystrophia lipomatosa; Beckwith-Wiedemann syndrome; Maffucci syndrome; lymphedema; etc.

Notes: The Parkes-Weber syndrome should be differentiated from the Klippel-Trenaunay syndrome by the presence of arteriovenous ectasia; some have considered the two syndromes a single entity and used the eponym Klippel-Trenaunay-Weber syndrome (Fig SY—K—11).

REFERENCES

Anlar B, et al.: Klippel-Trenaunay-Weber syndrome: A case with cerebral and cerebellar hemihypertrophy. *Neuroradiology* 30:360, 1988.

Azouz EM: Hematuria, rectal bleeding and pelvic phleboliths in children with the Klippel-Trenaunay syndrome. *Pediatr. Radiol.* 13:82, 1983.

Campistol JM, et al.: Renal hemangioma and renal artery aneurysm in the Klippel-Trenaunay syndrome. *J. Urol.* 140:134, 1987.

Caplan DB, et al.: Angioosteohypertrophy syndrome with protein-losing enteropathy. *J. Pediatr.* 74:119, 1969.

Djindjian M, et al.: Spinal cord arteriovenous malformations and the Klippel-Trenaunay-Weber syndrome. *Surg. Neurol.* 8:229, 1977.

Ghahremani GG, et al.: Diffuse cavernous hemangioma of the colon in the Klippel-Trenaunay syndrome. *Radiology* 118:673, 1978.

Goldstein SJ, et al.: Aplasia of the cervical internal carotid artery and malformation of the circle of Willis associated with Klippel-Trenaunay syndrome. *J. Neurosurg.* 61:786, 1984.

Gorenstein A, et al.: Congenital aplasia of the deep veins of lower extremities in children: The role of ascending functional phlebography. *Surgery* 99:414, 1986.

Jafri SZH, et al.: Computed tomography and ultrasound findings in Klippel-Trenaunay syndrome. *J. Comput. Assist. Tomogr.* 7:457, 1983.

Klippel M, Trenaunay P: Du naevus variqueux ostéo-hypertrophique. *Arch. Gen. Med. (Paris)* 3:641, 1900.

Kloiber R, et al.: Platelet sequestration in a vascular malformation of Klippel-Trenaunay syndrome. *A.J.R.* 149:1275, 1987.

Lewis BD, et al.: Cutaneous and visceral hemangiomata in

the Klippel-Trenaunay-Weber syndrome: Antenatal sonographic detection. *A.J.R.* 147:598, 1986.

Mankad VN, et al.: Bilateral nephroblastomatosis and Klippel-Trenaunay syndrome. *Cancer* 33:1462, 1974.

Pakter RL, et al.: CT findings in splenic hemangiomas in the Klippel-Trenaunay-Weber syndrome. *J. Comput. Assist. Tomogr.* 11:88, 1987.

Proesmans W, et al.: Syndrome de Klippel-Trenaunay avec hypertension artérielle et insuffisance rénale chronique. *Ann. Pediat. (Paris)* 29:671, 1982.

Schmitt B, et al.: Severe hemorrhage from intestinal hemangiomatosis in Klippel-Trenaunay syndrome: Pitfalls in diagnosis and management. *J. Pediatr. Gastroenterol. Nutr.* 5:155, 1986.

Schofield D, et al.: Klippel-Trenaunay and Sturge-Weber syndromes with renal hemangioma and double inferior vena cava. *J. Urol.* 136:442, 1986.

Servelle M: Klippel and Trénaunay's syndrome. 768 operated cases. *Ann. Surg.* 201:365, 1985.

Shalev E, et al.: Klippel-Trenaunay syndrome: Ultrasonic prenatal diagnosis. *J. Clin. Ultrasound* 16:268, 1988.

Viljoen DL: Klippel-Trenaunay-Weber syndrome (angio-osteohypertrophy syndrome). *J. Med. Genet.* 25:250, 1988.

Warhit JM, et al.: Klippel-Trenaunay-Weber syndrome: Appearance in utero. *J. Ultrasound Med.* 2:515, 1983.

Weber FP: Angioma formation in connection with hypertrophy of limbs and hemihypertrophy. *Br. J. Dermatol.* 19:231, 1907.

Yousem DM, et al.: Case report 440: Klippel-Trenaunay of the right lower extremity. *Skeletal Radiol.* 16:652, 1987.

KLÜVER-BUCY SYNDROME

Etiology: *Temporal lobe damage* from degenerative disorders; adrenoleukodystrophy; encephalitis; surgery; arteriosclerosis; epilepsy; hypoglycemic cerebral damage; toxoplasmic encephalitis; Alzheimer disease; Pick disease; trauma (may be transient); hypoxia (may be transient).

Clinical Manifestations: *Severe behavior problems, hyperactivity, rage reaction, marked emotional liability, urge to place all objects into the mouth,* visual agnosia, hypersexuality, alteration in dietary habits, problems in intermediate memory, partial expression in some cases.

Radiologic Manifestations: (a) *hydrocephalus ex vacuo in the temporal lobe region (temporal hydrocephalus);* (b) computed tomographic changes in the etiologic factor: surgical removal, encephalitis, degenerative disorders, etc.

REFERENCES

Cummings JL, et al.: Klüver-Bucy syndrome in Pick disease: Clinical and pathologic correlations. *Neurology* 31:1415, 1981.

Dickson DW, et al.: Klüver-Bucy syndrome and amyotrophic lateral sclerosis: A case report with biochemistry, morphometrics, and Golgi study. *Neurology* 36:1323, 1986.

Hooshmand J, et al.: Klüver-Bucy syndrome. *J.A.M.A.* 229:1782, 1974.

Klüver H, Bucy PC: "Psychic blindness" and other symptoms following bilateral temporal lobectomy in rhesus monkeys. *Am. J. Physiol.* 119:352, 1937.

Lilly R, et al.: The human Klüver-Bucy syndrome. *Neurology* 33:1141, 1983.

Powers JM, et al.: Klüver-Bucy syndrome caused by andreno-leukodystrophy. *Neurology* 30:1231, 1980.

Tonsgard JH, et al.: Klüver-Bucy syndrome in children. *Pediatr. Neurol.* 3:162, 1987.

KOLLER SYNDROME

Mode of Inheritance: Autosomal dominant (a family from northern Norway).

Clinical Manifestations: (a) waddling gait, muscle weakness, leg pain; (b) ichthyosis of slight to severe degree.

Radiologic Manifestations: (a) endosteal cortical thickening of long tubular bones; (b) bowing of weight-bearing bones; (c) tendency to fracture.

REFERENCE

Koller ME, et al.: A familial syndrome of diaphyseal cortical thickening of the long bones, bowed legs, tendency to fracture and ichthyosis. *Pediatr. Radiol.* 8:179, 1979.

KOUSSEFF SYNDROME

Mode of Inheritance: Autosomal recessive.

Frequency: Four published cases (Toriello et al.).

Clinical and Radiologic Manifestations: (a) sacral meningocele; (b) conotruncal cardiac defects; (c) other reported abnormalities: low-set posteriorly angulated ears, retrognathia, short neck with a low posterior hairline, unilateral renal agenesis.

REFERENCES

Kousseff BG: Sacral meningocele with conotruncal heart defects: A possible autosomal recessive trait. *Pediatrics* 74:395, 1984.

Toriello HV, et al.: Autosomal recessive syndrome of sacral and conotruncal developmental field defects (Kousseff syndrome). *Am. J. Med. Genet.* 22:357, 1985.

KUGELBERG-WELANDER SYNDROME

Synonyms: Proximal spinal muscular atrophy; muscular atrophy (juvenile); spinal muscular atrophy; Wohlfart-Kugelberg-Welander disease.

Mode of Inheritance: Autosomal recessive; autosomal dominant in some families has been suggested.

Clinical Manifestations: A degenerating disease of the anterior horn cells of the spinal cord; onset usually between 3 and 18 years of age: (a) *atrophy and weakness of proximal limb muscles followed by involvement of the distal muscles;* (b) *occurrence of fasciculation and electromyographic and muscle biopsy findings of a lower motor neuron lesion;* (c) cardiomyopathy associated with arrhythmias.

Radiologic Manifestations: (a) computed tomography: development of patches of low-density tissue in the muscles; progressive spread and enlargement of the low-density areas all over the surface of the muscles, with the muscles developing a ragged outline; progressive submergence of muscles into the adipose tissue; (b) cardiomegaly and echocardiographic manifestations of cardiac chamber enlargement and arrhythmias; (c) esophageal dilatation with absence of peristalsis, small-bowel dilation, loss of colonic haustrations.

REFERENCES

Bulcke JAL, Baert AL: Spinal muscular atrophies (s.m.a.), in *Clinical and Radiological Aspects of Myopathies*. Berlin, Springer-Verlag, 1982, pp. 114–120.

Hausmanowa-Petrusewicz I, et al.: Chronic proximal spinal muscular atrophy of childhood and adolescence: Problems of classification and genetic counselling. *J. Med. Genet.* 22:350, 1985.

Karasick D, et al.: Gastrointestinal radiologic manifestations of proximal spinal muscular atrophy (Kugelberg-Welander syndrome). *J. Natl. Med. Assoc.* 74:475, 1982.

Kugelberg E, Welander L: Heredofamilial juvenile muscular atrophy simulating muscular dystrophy. *Arch. Neurol. Psychiatr.* 75:500, 1956.

Plo JK, et al.: Amyotrophie spinale infantile pseudo-myopathique (maladie de Wohlfart-Kugelberg-Welander). A propos d'un cas et revue de la littérature. *Ann. Pediatr. (Paris)* 34:329, 1987.

Tanaka H, et al.: Cardiac involvement in the Kugelberg-Welander syndrome. *Am. J. Cardiol.* 38:528, 1976.

Tanaka H, et al.: Myocardial ultrastructural changes in Kugelberg-Welander syndrome. *Br. Heart J.* 39:1390, 1977.

Wohlfart G, et al.: Hereditary proximal spinal muscular atrophy: A clinical entity simulating progressive muscular dystrophy. *Acta Pyschiatr. Neurol. Scand.* 30:395, 1955.

Zerres K, et al.: Genetic counseling in families with spinal muscular atrophy type Kugelberg-Welander. *Hum. Genet.* 65:74, 1983.

KUSKOKWIM SYNDROME

Mode of Inheritance: Autosomal recessive.

Clinical Manifestations: (a) *multiple congenital joint contractures* (ankles and knees in particular); (b) kyphosis in infants; (c) atrophy or compensatory hypertrophy of associated muscle groups; (d) other reported abnormalities: pigmented nevi, diminished corneal reflexes; (e) normal intelligence.

Radiologic Manifestations: (a) *hypoplasia of the first or second vertebral body,* progressive elongation of the pedicles of the fifth lumbar vertebra with *spondylolisthesis;* (b) *osteolytic areas in the outer one third of the clavicles in childhood;* (c) *osteolytic lesions of the proximal humeral metaphysis* in infancy and childhood; (d) *hypoplasia of patellae;* (e) other reported abnormalities: pelvic deformity, loss of vertebral height in the midthoracic region, clubfoot, pseudoarthrosis of the clavicle.

REFERENCES

Petajan JH, et al.: Arthrogryposis syndrome (Kuskokwim disease) in the Eskimo. *J.A.M.A.* 209:1481, 1969.
Wright DG: The unusual skeletal findings of the Kuskokwim syndrome. *Birth Defects* 6:16, 1970.

L

LAMBERT-EATON SYNDROME

Synonyms: Eaton-Lambert syndrome; Lambert-Eaton myasthenic syndrome.

Etiology: Association with other conditions: (a) bronchial carcinoma (often small-cell carcinoma) in about two thirds of cases; (b) autoimmune disorders: rheumatoid arthritis, Sjögren syndrome, pernicious anemia, celliac disease, thyrotoxicosis, hypothyroidism, systemic lupus erythematosus, congenital, etc.

Clinical and Radiologic Manifestations: (a) weakness, easy fatigability of the legs secondary to proximal muscle weakness, especially the pelvic girdle and proximal limb muscles, usually sparing cranial muscles; (b) paradoxical potentiation in electromyographic studies (progressive reduction in size of the muscle action potential evoked by nerve stimuli at low stimuli frequencies and an increase in response at higher frequencies of nerve stimulation); (c) strong evidence of autoimmune pathophysiology; (d) respiratory failure, either as a result of the administration of a muscle relaxant drug or spontaneously, requiring mechanical ventilation.

REFERENCES

Bady B, et al.: Congenital Lambert-Eaton myasthenic syndrome. *J. Neurol. Neurosurg. Psychiatry* 50:476, 1987.

Dell'Osso LF, et al.: Edrophonium test in Eaton-Lambert syndrome: Quantitative oculography. *Neurology* 33:1157, 1983.

Fukuoka T, et al.: Lambert-Eaton myasthenic syndrome: I. Early morphological effects of IgG on the presynaptic membrane active zones. *Ann. Neurol.* 22:193, 1987.

Gracey DR, et al.: Respiratory failure in Lambert-Eaton myasthenic syndrome. *Chest* 91:716, 1987.

Hughes RL, et al.: The Eaton-Lambert (myasthenic) syndrome in association with systemic lupus erythematosus. *Arch. Neurol.* 43:1186, 1986.

Lambert EH, Eaton LM, Rooke ED: Defect of neuromuscular conduction associated with malignant neoplasm. *Am. J. Physiol.* 187:612, 1956.

Lang B, et al.: Autoimmune aetiology for myasthenic (Eaton-Lambert) syndrome. *Lancet* 2:224, 1981.

O'Neill JH: The Lambert-Eaton myasthenic syndrome. A review of 50 cases. *Brain* 111:577, 1988.

Ramos-Yeo YL, et al.: Myasthenic syndrome (Eaton-Lambert syndrome) associated with pulmonary adenocarcinoma. *J. Surg. Oncol.* 34:239, 1987.

LARSEN SYNDROME

Mode of Inheritance: Sporadic, autosomal recessive, and dominant transmissions have been reported.

Frequency: Rare; probably underdiagnosed and underpublished.

Clinical Manifestations: Anomalies present at birth: (a) *distinctive facies*: flat face, hypertelorism, depressed nasal bridge, prominent forehead, cleft palate, cleft uvula; (b) laxity of the joints; *dislocated elbows, hips, and knees* (genu recurvatum), etc.; (c) cylindric fingers, spatula-like thumbs, short and broad fingertips; (d) resistant clubfoot deformity; (e) other reported abnormalities: cleft palate, broad thumbs, and anti-mongoloid slant, long philtrum, subependymal glial proliferation of the lateral ventricle that resembles tuberous sclerosis, prenatal growth deficiency, congenital heart defects, aortic dilatation and valvular insufficiency, aneurysm of the ductus arteriosus, undescended testes, collapsing thorax, neurological impairment (cord compression), mixed hearing loss, etc.

Radiologic Manifestations: (a) *joint dislocations,* usually the large joints, less commonly metacarpophalangeal and interphalangeal joints; (b) abnormal skeletal mineralization; (c) accessory ossicles of the hands, wrists, knees, elbows, feet; (d) double or triple calcaneal ossification center; (e) *short metacarpals, metatarsals, and distal phalanges; spatulate thumbs;* (f) *flattened frontal bone, small base of the skull and facial bones, shallow orbits, hypertelorism, micrognathia;* (g) abnormal segmentation of the vertebrae, flat vertebrae, cervical kyphosis, scoliosis, cervicothoracic lordosis, hypoplasia of the cervical vertebrae, dislocation of the upper cervical vertebrae in association with congenital defects; (h) other reported abnormalities: laxity of the trachea, larynx, and costochondral cartilages; short humerus with hypoplasia of the distal end; short fibulas, congenital heart disease, increased anterior bowing of tibias, foot deformities (adductus, valgus, cavus, equinovarus), toe deformities, "square" tubular bones, skeletal maturation retardation, finger clubbing, thin ribs, long clavicles, deficiency of pubic bone ossification, aortic root dilatation.

Differential Diagnosis: Arthrogryposis, multiplex congenita; otopalatodigital syndrome; "lethal, Larsen-like multiple joint dislocation syndrome" (Chen et al.); Ehler-Danlos syndrome; Marfan syndrome; the syndrome of short stature, joint laxity, and developmental delay (Anderson et al.) (Figs SY−L−1 and SY−L−2).

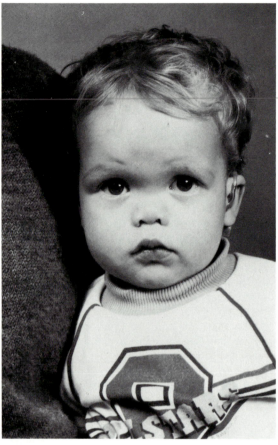

FIG SY—L—1.
Larsen syndrome. Note the flat facial appearance and depressed nasal bridge. (From Stanley CS, Thelin JW, Miles JH: Mixed hearing loss in Larsen syndrome. *Clin. Genet.* 33:395, 1988. Used by permission.)

REFERENCES

Anderson CE, et al.: A syndrome of short stature, joint laxity and developmental delay. *Clin. Genet.* 22:40, 1982.

Bowen JR, et al.: Spinal deformities in Larsen's syndrome. *Clin. Orthop.* 197:159, 1985.

Chen H, et al.: A lethal, Larsen-like multiple joint dislocation syndrome. *Am. J. Med. Genet.* 13:149, 1982.

Fauré C, et al.: Le syndrome de Larsen: A propos de trois observations nouvelles. *Ann. Radiol (Paris)* 19:629, 1976.

Henriksson P, et al.: Larsen syndrome and glial proliferation in the brain. *Acta Paediatr. Scand.* 66:653, 1977.

Houston CS, et al.: Separating Larsen syndrome from the "Arthrogryposis basket". *J. Can. Assoc. Radiol.* 32:206, 1981.

Kiel EA, et al.: Cardiovascular manifestations in the Larsen syndrome. *Pediatrics* 71:942, 1983.

Kozlowski K, et al.: Radiographic findings in Larsen's syndrome. *Australas. Radiol.* 18:336, 1974.

Larsen LJ, Schottstaedt ER, Bost FC: Multiple congenital dislocations associated with characteristic facial abnormality. *J. Pediatr.* 37:574, 1950.

Lefort G, et al.: Dislocation du rachis cervical supérieur dans le syndrome de Larsen. *Chir. Pediatr.* 24:211, 1983.

Maroteaux P: L'hétérogénéité du syndrome de Larsen. *Arch. Fr. Pediatr.* 32:597, 1975.

Renault F, et al.: Le syndrome de Larsen. Aspects cliniques et génétiques. *Arch. Fr. Pediatr.* 39:35, 1982.

Silverman FN: Larsen's syndrome: Congenital dislocation of the knees and other joints, distinctive facies, and frequently, cleft palate. *Ann. Radiol. (Paris)* 15:297, 1972.

Stanley CS, et al.: Mixed hearing loss in Larsen syndrome. *Clin. Genet.* 33:395, 1988.

Stanley D, et al.: The Larsen syndrome occurring in four generations of one family. *Int. Orthop.* 8:267, 1985.

Strisciuglio P, et al.: Severe cardiac anomalies in sibs with Larsen syndrome. *J. Med. Genet.* 20:422, 1983.

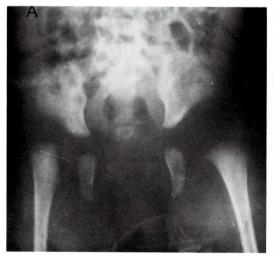
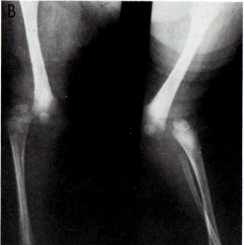

FIG SY—L—2.
Larsen syndrome in a 3-day-old female. **A,** bilateral dislocation of the hips and delayed mineralization of the os pubis and ischial rami. **B,** bilateral dislocation of tibias on femora with genu recurvatum. (From Silverman FN: Larsen's syndrome. *Ann. Radiol. (Paris)* 15:297, 1972. Used by permission.)

LEIGH DISEASE

Synonym: Subacute necrotizing encephalomyelopathy.

Mode of Inheritance: Autosomal recessive.

Pathology: Focal symmetrical necrosis of the thalamus, hypothalamus, putamen, dentate nuclei, cerebellum, optic chiasm, spinal cord; demyelination, vascular proliferation, astrocytosis.

Clinical Manifestations: Progressive neurodegenerative disease with an onset of symptoms usually in infancy or early childhood (juvenile and adult onset rare): (a) regressive psychomotor development, feeding difficulties, somnolence, hypotonia, ataxia, bulbar paresis, nystagmus, blindness, deafness, abnormal eye movements, vegetative state, autonomic respiratory failure, etc.; (b) pyruvate dehydrogenase complex deficiency; (c) cytochrome c oxidase deficiency; (d) alaninuria, pyruvic acidemia, lactic acidemia, fumaric aciduria.

Radiologic Manifestations: Variable and widespread distribution of lesions of the gray and white matter in the brain and spinal cord: (a) computed tomography: focal, symmetrical, nonenhancing, and low-attenuation lesions in the basal ganglia, periventricular regions, and cortex; atrophy; (b) magnetic resonance imaging: increased signal on T_2-weighted sequence, hypointense on T_1-weighted spin-echo sequence.

Note: Benke et al. suggested the existence of an X-linked recessive form of Leigh disease (Fig SY−L−3).

REFERENCES

Benke PJ, et al.: X-linked Leigh's syndrome. *Hum. Genet.* 62:52, 1982.

Cummiskey J, et al.: Automatic respiratory failure: Sleep studies and Leigh's disease (case report). *Neurology* 37:1876, 1987.

Davis PC, et al.: MR of Leigh's disease (subacute necrotizing encephalomyelopathy). *A.J.N.R.* 8:71, 1987.

DiMauro S, et al.: Cytochrome c oxidase deficiency in Leigh syndrome. *Ann. Neurol.* 22:498, 1987.

Geyer CA, et al.: Leigh disease (subacute necrotizing encephalomyelopathy): CT and MR in five cases. *J. Comput. Assist. Tomogr.* 12:40, 1988.

Kissel JT, et al.: Magnetic resonance imaging in a case of autopsy-proved adult subacute necrotizing encephalomyelopathy (Leigh's disease). *Arch. Neurol.* 44:563, 1987.

Kretzschmar HA, et al.: Pyruvate dehydrogenase complex deficiency as a cause of subacute necrotizing encephalopathy (Leigh disease). *Pediatrics* 79:370, 1987.

Paltiel HJ, et al.: Subacute necrotizing encephalomyelopathy (Leigh disease): CT study. *Radiology* 162:115, 1987.

LENNOX-GASTAUT SYNDROME

Synonym: Childhood epileptic encephalopathy.

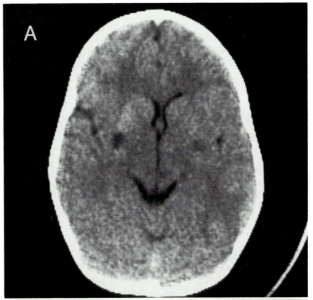

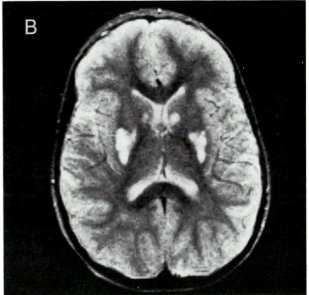

FIG SY−L−3.
Leigh disease in a 3½-year-old girl. **A,** an unenhanced computed tomographic scan shows characteristic focal bilateral, symmetrical lucencies in the basal ganglia and questionable focal lucency in the periaqueductal region. **B,** a T_2-weighted magnetic resonance study shows characteristic focal lesions of the globus pallidus, putamen, and caudate. (From Davis PC, Hoffman JC, Braun IF, et al.: MR of Leigh's disease (subacute necrotizing encephalomyopathy. *A.J.N.R.* 8:71, 1987. Used by permission.)

Clinical Manifestations: Onset of symptoms usually before the age of 5 years: (a) *mixed seizure disorder:* minor motor, tonic-clonic, atypical absence, partial seizures; (b) *electroencephalography: generalized 1.5 to 2.5 per second spike-wave discharges,* etc.; (c) *intellectual impairment.*

Radiologic Manifestations: (a) computed tomography: nonspecific: mild ventricular dilatation, cerebral atrophy; (b)

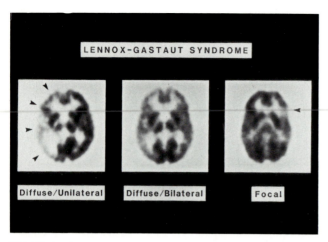

FIG SY–L–4.
Lennox-Gestaut syndrome: Three interictal abnormalities in patterns of cerebral glucose utilization seen in children with the Lennox-Gestaut syndrome by FDG-PET. The child with left diffuse hypometabolism is an 8-year-old boy with normal results of x-ray computed tomography (CT) and predominantly right tonic seizures followed by transient right hemiparesis. X-ray CT of a 5-year-old boy with right posterior frontal hypometabolism revealed a small calcified lesion just lateral to the head of the right caudate nucleus, but not all patients with focal hypometabolism had corresponding structural lesions on CT or magnetic resonance imaging. Bilateral diffuse hypometabolism is illustrated in a 6-year-old child whose CT demonstrated only diffuse cortical atrophy. (From Chugani HT, Phelps ME: PET in children with seizures. *Appl. Radiol.* 17:37, 1988. Used by permission.)

positron-emission tomographic scan: hypometabolism: (1) unilateral focal; (2) unilateral diffuse, bilateral diffuse (Fig SY–L–4).

REFERENCES

Chugani HT, et al.: The Lennox-Gastaut syndrome: Metabolic subtypes determined by 2-deoxy-2[^{18}F] fluoro-D-glucose positron emission tomography. *Ann. Neurol.* 21:4, 1987.
Gastaut H, et al.: Childhood epileptic encephalopathy with diffuse slow spike-waves (otherwise known as "petit mal variant") or Lennox syndrome. *Epilepsia* 7:139, 1966.
Lennox WG, et al.: Clinical correlates of the fast and slow spikewave electroencephalogram. *Pediatrics* 5:626, 1950.
Iinuma K, et al.: Cerebral glucose metabolism in five patients with Lennox-Gastaut syndrome. *Pediatr. Neurol.* 3:12, 1987.
Theodore WH, et al.: Cerebral glucose metabolism in the Lennox-Gastaut syndrome. *Ann. Neurol.* 21:14, 1987.

LENZ MICROPHTHALMOS SYNDROME

Synonym: Lenz dysplasia.

Mode of Inheritance: X-linked recessive.

Clinical Manifestations: (a) *microphthalmos or anophthalmia;* (b) mental retardation; (c) microcephaly; (d) malformations of the pinnae (tags, pits, etc.); (e) dental anomalies: peglike teeth, diastemas, irregular tooth eruption; (f) other reported abnormalities: strabismus, short stature, speech defect, urogenital anomalies (cryptorchidism, hypospadias, etc.), high-arched palate, cleft lip, cleft palate, simian crease(s), congenital heart defect, hirsutism, webbed neck, sacral pits.

Radiologic Manifestations: (a) renal anomalies (horseshoe kidneys, ectopic kidney, duplication; (b) kyphoscoliosis, lordosis; (c) thin clavicles, clinodactyly, camptodactyly, syndactyly, webbed toes; (d) intestinal anomalies.

REFERENCES

Baraitser M, et al.: Lenz microphthalmia—a case report. *Clin. Genet.* 22:99, 1982.
Glanz A, et al.: Lenz microphthalmia: A malformation syndrome with variable expression of multiple congenital anomalies. *Can. J. Ophthalmol.* 18:41, 1983.
Herrmann J, et al.: The Lenz microphthalmia syndrome. *Birth Defects* 5:138, 1969.
Lenz W: Rezessiv-geschlechtsgebundene Mikrophthalmie mit multiplen Missbildungen. *Z. Kinderheilkd.* 77:384, 1955.

LEOPARD SYNDROME

Synonyms: Cardiomyopathic lentiginosis; lentiginosis syndrome; multiple lentigines syndrome.

Mode of Inheritance: Autosomal dominant.

Frequency: Rare.

Clinical Manifestations: (a) lentigines (invariably present): skin lesions most common on the neck and the upper part of the trunk, less common on the face, scalp, genitalia, palms, and soles; (b) cardiac conduction defect: complete heart block, complete bundle-branch block, etc.; (c) cardiomyopathy involving the interventricular septum, subaortic and subpulmonary stenosis; (d) pulmonary valvular stenosis; (e) genital anomalies: hypospadias, cryptorchidism, gonadal hypoplasia, late puberty; (f) retardation of growth; (g) deafness (sensorineural); (h) other reported abnormalities: pterygium colli, cutaneous abnormalities (axillary "freckling," café au lait spots, localized hypopigmentation, dermatoglyphic abnormalities, interdigital webs, onychodystrophy, multiple granular cell myoblastomas, hyperelasticity), endocrine disorders, neurological defects (mild mental retardation, oculomotor defects, seizures, etc.), craniofacial dysmorphism (ocular hypertelorism, mandibular prognathism, broad nasal root, dysmorphic skull, low-set ears, dental abnormalities, high-arched palate, ptosis of the upper lids, epicanthal folds).

Radiologic Manifestations: (a) cardiovascular abnormalities; (b) skeletal abnormalities: skeletal maturation retardation, pectus carinatum or excavatum, kyphoscoliosis, winging scapulae, hypermobile joints, cubitus valgus, rib anomalies, hypoplastic fifth digit, syndactyly, zygodactyly, cervical spine fusion, spina bifida occulta, Madelung deformity of the wrist, delayed healing of fractures, severe scoliosis with posterior spinal fusion.

Differential Diagnosis: Noonan syndrome; fetal rubella syndrome; etc.

Note: LEOPARD is an acronym: *L*entigines, *E*lectrocardiographic conduction abnormalities, *O*cular hypertelorism, *P*ulmonary stenosis, *A*bnormal genitalia, *R*etardation of growth, *D*eafness.

REFERENCES

Balducci R, et al.: Etude endocrinologique chez une enfant atteinte de syndrome léopard. *Arch. Fr. Pediatr.* 39:23, 1982.

Blieden LC, et al.: Unifying link between Noonan's and Leopard syndromes? *Pediatr. Cardiol.* 4:168, 1983.

Gorlin RJ, et al.: Leopard (multiple lentigines) syndrome revisited. *Laryngoscope* 81:1674, 1971.

Malpuech G, et al.: Syndrome léopard et insuffisance hypophysaire. *Arch. Fr. Pediatr.* 36:413, 1979.

Senn M, et al.: Hypertrophe Kardiomyopathie und Lentiginose. *Schweiz. Med. Wochenschr.* 114:838, 1984.

Sutton MG St J, et al.: Hypertrophic obstructive cardiomyopathy and lentiginosis: A little known neural ectodermal syndrome. *Am. J. Cardiol.* 47:214, 1981.

Voron DA: Multiple lentigines syndrome: Case report and review of the literature. *Am. J. Med.* 60:447, 1976.

Watson GH: Pulmonary stenosis, café-au-lait spots, and dull intelligence. *Arch. Dis. Child.* 42:303, 1967.

LERICHE SYNDROME

Pathology: Complete thrombotic obliteration of the aortic bifurcation, often in young adult males.

Clinical Manifestations: Intermittent claudication; weakness of lower limbs; soft-tissue atrophy of both lower limbs; *pallor of the legs and feet on standing; absence of trophic changes of the skin or nails;* slow wound healing; *inability to maintain erection; absent or very poor pulse over the aorta and iliac arteries and in the periphery.*

Radiologic Manifestations: (a) calcification at the aortic bifurcation; (b) *aortic occlusion at the bifurcation, collateral circulation;* (c) contrast computed tomography with bolus injection demonstrating a sclerotic, normal-calibered aorta with a hypodense center below the level of the renal arteries; ultrasonography less sensitive in detecting the obstruction at this level.

REFERENCES

Bean WJ, et al.: Leriche syndrome: Treatment with streptokinase and angioplasty. *A.J.R.* 144:1285, 1985.

Beckwith R, et al.: Chronic aortoiliac thrombosis: A review of sixty-five cases. *N. Engl. J. Med.* 258:721, 1958.

Goldwasser B, et al.: Impotence due to the pelvic steal syndrome: Treatment by iliac transluminal angioplasty. *J. Urol.* 133:860, 1985.

Landtman M, et al.: The Leriche syndrome. A comparative investigation using angiography, computed tomography and ultrasonography. *Acta. Radiol.* 26:265, 1985.

Leriche R: De la résection du carrefour aortoiliaque avec double sympathectomie lombaire pour thrombose artéritique de l'aorte: Le syndrome de l'oblitération termino-aortique par artérite. *Presse. Med.* 48:33, 1940.

Velasquez G, et al.: Nonsurgical aortoplasty in Leriche syndrome. *Radiology* 134:359, 1980.

LEVY-HOLLISTER SYNDROME

Synonyms: Lacrimo-auriculo-dento-digital syndrome; LADD syndrome.

Mode of Inheritance: Autosomal dominant.

Frequency: 12 published cases (Kreutz et al.).

Clinical and Radiologic Manifestations: (a) lacrimal anomalies (unilateral, bilateral): absent or hypoplastic lacrimal glands or puncta and/or nasolacrimal ducts and/or tear sac, diminished or absent tears or recurrent or chronic tearing; (b) malformed ear(s), hearing disorder; (c) dental anomalies: delayed tooth eruption, peg-shaped teeth, enamel dysplasia, anodontia; (d) digital anomalies: thumb anomalies (fingerlike, bifid, hypoplastic), finger anomalies, polydactyly, abnormal metacarpophalangeal profile pattern; (e) salivary gland anomalies: absent gland (parotid, submaxillary); (f) other reported abnormalities: synostosis of the radius and ulna, renal anomalies, high narrow palate, beaklike nose, hip dislocation, hypospadias, downward palpebral fissures, hiatal hernia, broad sunken nose, nasolacrimal duct fistula, radial aplasia, unusual dermal ridge patterns.

REFERENCES

Calabro A, et al.: Lacrimo-auriculo-dento-digital (LADD) syndrome. *Eur. J. Pediatr.* 146:536, 1987.

Hollister DW, et al.: The lacrimo-auriculo-dento-digital syndrome. *Pediatrics* 59:927, 1977.

Kreutz JM, et al.: Levy-Hollister syndrome. *Pediatrics* 82:96, 1988.

Levy WJ: Mesoectodermal dysplasia. *Am. J. Ophthalmol.* 63:978, 1967.

Wiedemann H-R, et al.: LADD syndrome: Report of new cases and review of the clinical spectrum. *Eur. J. Pediatr.* 144:579, 1986.

LICHTENSTEIN SYNDROME

Mode of Inheritance: Reported in a pair of monozygotic twins.

Clinical and Radiologic Manifestations: (a) peculiar facies: carp mouth, anteverted nostrils, synophrys; (b) immune disorders: neutropenia, IgA deficiency; (c) skeletal abnormalities: peripheral osteoporosis, fractures, subluxation at C_1–C_2 level, spondylolysis L_5, large foramen magnum, camptodactyly; (d) lung cyst.

REFERENCE

Lichtenstein JR: A "new" syndrome with neutropenia, immunoglobulin deficiency, peculiar facies and bony abnormalities. *Birth Defects* 8:178, 1972.

LIMB DUPLICATION—RENAL AGENESIS

Clinical and Radiologic Manifestations: (a) partial duplication of a lower limb; (b) aplasia of ipsilateral kidney; (c) other reported abnormalities: talipes equinovarus, dislocated tabus, hyperflexibility of joint, ectopic anus, rectovestibular fistula, prolapse of rectum, hyperelasticity of skin, hypotonia.

REFERENCE

Weisselberg B, et al.: Partial duplication of the lower limb with agenesis of ipsilateral kidney—a new syndrome: Report of a case and review of the literature. *Clin. Genet.* 33:234, 1988.

LIPOID DERMATOARTHRITIS

Synonym: Multicenteric reticulohistiocytosis.

Pathology: Lipid-laden giant histiocytes in the skin and synovial lesions.

Clinical Manifestations: Onset of symptoms between adolescence and senescence: (a) *cutaneous papules, cutaneous and subcutaneous nodular lesions* (ears, bridge of the nose, scalp, dorsum of the hands, and nail beds the most common sites); (b) polyarthritis usually preceding the cutaneous eruptions by an average of 3 years, progressive crippling deformities of the hands; (c) leonine facies in advanced stage of disease.

Radiologic Manifestations: (a) *juxta-articular erosions at insertion of synovia;* (b) *destruction of articular cartilage and subchondral bones of the phalanges,* which may in progressive cases result in telescoping of soft tissues; destruction of odontoid process and atlas; (c) thinning of distal phalanges; (d) other reported abnormalities: marginal erosion in the feet, shoulders, wrists, hips, knees, and sternomanubrial joints, noncalcified soft-tissue masses.

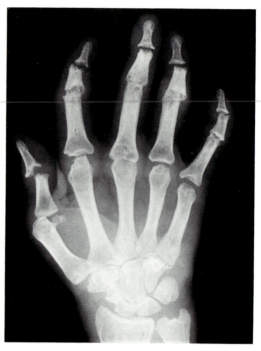

FIG SY–L–5.
Lipoid dermatoarthritis in a 31-year-old man. All joints are severely eroded, but destruction of subchondral bone predominates at the interphalangeal joints. Subperiosteal new bone is absent, and osteoporosis is disproportionately mild. (From Gold RH, Metzger AL, Mirra JM, et al.: Multicenteric reticulohistiocytosis (lipoid dermatoarthritis). *A.J.R.* 124:610, 1975. Used by permission.)

Differential Diagnosis: Psoriatic arthritis; Reiter syndrome; etc. (Fig SY–L–5).

REFERENCES

Barrow MV, et al.: Multicenteric reticulohistiocytosis: A review of 33 patients. *Medicine (Baltimore)* 48:287, 1969.
Gold RH, et al.: Multicenteric reticulohistiocytosis (lipoid dermatoarthritis). *A.J.R.* 124:610, 1975.
Gold RH, et al.: Radiologic comparison of erosive polyarthritides with prominent interphalangeal involvement. *Skeletal Radiol.* 8:89, 1982.
Stögmann W, et al.: Lipoiddermatoarthritis (multizentrische reticulohisticytose). *Eur. J. Pediatr.* 121:71, 1975.

LISSENCEPHALY SYNDROMES

Classification: Type I (Miller-Dieker syndrome, Norman-Roberts syndrome, isolated lissencephaly): microcephaly and a thickened cortex with four rather than six layers, smooth brain surface, pachygyria in some areas, wide sylvian fossa, thin white matter, hetertopic rests scattered throughout with a nodular appearance of the ventrical walls, ventriculomegaly, colpocephaly, absent or hypoplastic corpus callosum, small brain stem, small inferior olives and dentate nuclei, small cerebellar hemispheres, cerebellar sclerosis, etc.; type II or

TABLE SY–L–1.

Classification of Lissencephaly Syndromes*

Syndrome	Type	Grade	Cause†
Miller-Dieker syndrome (MDS)	I	2	del 17p13.3
Norman-Roberts syndrome (NRS)	I	1	AR
Isolated lissencephaly (ILS)	I	1–3	Unknown or AR
Walker-Warburg syndrome (WWS)	II	1–2	AR
Cerebro-oculo-muscular syndrome (COMS)	II	1–2	AR
Neu-Laxova syndrome (NLS)	?	1?	AR
Cerebrocerebellar lissencephaly (CCL)	CCL	1	Unknown or AR
XK aprosencephaly syndrome	a/at	1	Unknown
Isotretinoin embryopathy	I?	?	In utero exposure

*Modified from Dobyns WB, et al.: Further comments on the lissencephaly syndromes (letter). *Am. J. Med. Genet.* 22:197, 1985.
†AR = autosomal recessive; a/a = aprosencephaly/atelencephaly.

hydrocephalic type of lissencephaly (Walker-Warburg syndrome, cerebro-oculo-muscular syndrome, etc): hydrocephalus, absent septum pellucidum and corpus callosum, vermis hypoplasia with or without Dandy-Walker malformation, posterior encephalocele (in some) (Table SY–L–1).

REFERENCES

Dobyns WB, et al.: Further comments on the lissencephaly syndromes (letter). *Am. J. Med. Genet.* 22:197, 1985.

Dobyns WB, et al.: Syndromes with lissencephaly. I: Miller-Dieker and Norman-Roberts syndromes and isolated lissencephaly. *Am. J. Med. Genet.* 18:509, 1984.

Dobyns WB, et al.: Syndromes with lissencephaly. II: Walker-Warburg and cerebro-oculo-muscular syndromes and a new syndrome with type II lissencephaly. *Am. J. Med. Genet.* 22:157, 1985.

Kotagal P, et al.: Norman-Roberts syndrome (letter). *Am. J. Med. Genet.* 29:681, 1988.

Mielke R, et al.: Zerebro-okulo-muskuläres Syndrom. *Helv. Paediatr. Acta* 41:369, 1986.

Pavone L, et al.: Hydrocephalus, lissencephaly, ocular abnormalities and congenital muscular dystrophy. A Warburg syndrome variant? *Neuropediatrics* 17:206, 1986.

LISSENCEPHALY (MILLER-DIEKER)

Synonyms: Lissencephaly, type I; Miller-Dieker syndrome.

Mode of Inheritance: Familial cases have been reported: balanced reciprocal translocation in a carrier parent and unbalanced translocations in the affected offspring, deletion 17 p 13.3.

Frequency: Uncommon.

Pathology: Microencephaly, colpocephaly, cavum septi pellucidi, absent claustrum, pachygyria, ectopic olivary nuclei, abnormalities of dentate nuclei, cerebellar sclerosis, inverted pyramidal cells in the superficial part of the cortical layer.

Clinical Manifestations: (a) *craniofacial dysmorphism*: microcephaly, hollow temples, dolichocephaly, micrognathia, anteversion of the nostrils; (b) *seizures* (generalized, infantile spasms—hypsarrhythmia); (c) *poor reflexes*; (d) *hypotonia, failure to thrive, poor motor development*; (e) *inability to swallow, frequent pulmonary infections*; (f) other reported abnormalities: hirsutism, polyhydramnios, circumlimbal corneal clouding, duodenal atresia, polydactyly, camptodactyly, simian crease, congenital heart disease, renal anomaly, undescended testes, hepatosplenomegaly, prolonged neonatal jaundice, abnormal electroencephalographic findings (two prominent and abnormally rapid rhythms, either alternating with each other or mixed together); (g) death in infancy or early childhood.

Radiologic Manifestations: *Microcephaly; round midline calcification in the septum pellucidum or genu of the corpus callosum; absence or hypoplasia of the corpus callosum; prominent subarachnoid space; smooth cortical surface; wide sylvian fissures; absence of insular opercularization, generalized dilatation of the ventricular system (colpocephaly), enlarged basal cisterns, etc.* (Figs SY–L–6 and SY–L–7).

REFERENCES

Bordarier C, et al.: Inverted neurons in agyria. A Golgi study of a case with abnormal chromosome 17. *Hum. Genet.* 73:374, 1986.

Burn J, et al: A syndrome with intracranial calcification and microcephaly in two sibs, resembling intrauterine infection. *Clin. Genet.* 30:112, 1986.

Dieker H, et al.: The lissencephaly syndrome. *Birth Defects* 5:53, 1969.

Dobyns WB, et al.: Computed tomographic appearance of lissencephaly syndromes. *A.J.N.R.* 6:545, 1985.

Dobyns WB, et al.: Syndromes with lissencephaly. 1: Miller-Dieker and Norman-Roberts syndromes and isolated lissencephaly. *Am. J. Med. Genet.* 18:509, 1984.

Gastaut H, et al.: Lissencephaly (agyria-pachygyria): Clinical findings and serial EEG studies. *Dev. Med. Child Neurol.* 29:167, 1987.

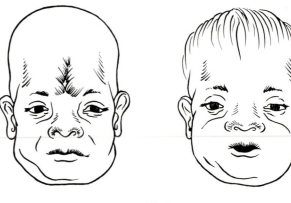

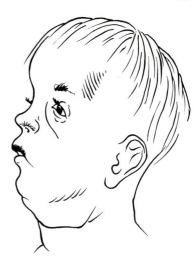

FIG SY–L–6.
Lissencephaly (Miller-Dieker syndrome): composite drawings of the classic facial features of Miller-Dieker syndrome. Microcephaly with bitemporal grooving, vertical midline wrinkling of the forehead, anteverted nares, ear anomalies with low-set ears, and micrognathia. (From Byrd SE, Bohan TP, Osborn RE: Computed tomography in the evaluation of migrational disorders of the brain. Part I: Lissencephaly. *J. Med. Imag.* 2:222, 1988. Used by permission.)

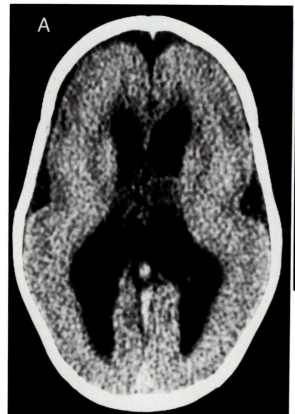

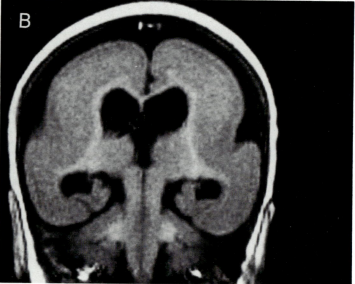

FIG SY–L–7.
Lissencephaly: axial enhanced computed tomographic scan **(A)** and a coronal magnetic resonance image, 500/30 **(B).** A completely agyric brain with an oval configuration, shallow sylvian grooves, increased cortical gray matter and a relatively small amount of white matter, and an absence of normal cortical white matter interdigitations is present. (From Byrd SE, Bohan TP, Osborn RE, et al.: The CT and MR evaluation of lissencephaly. *A.J.N.R.* 9:923, 1988. Used by permission.)

Goutières F, et al.: Syndrome de Miller-Dieker familial et translocation chromosomique (15;17). *Arch. Fr. Pediatr.* 44:501, 1987.

Greenberg F, et al.: Familial Miller-Dieker syndrome associated with pericentric inversion of chromosome 17. *Am. J. Med. Genet.* 23:853, 1986.

Jones KL, et al.: The Miller-Dieker syndrome. *Pediatrics* 66:277, 1980.

Krawinkel M, et al.: Magnetic resonance imaging in lissencephaly. *Eur. J. Pediatr.* 146:205, 1987.

Lee BCP: MR of lissencephaly. *A.J.N.R.* 9:804, 1988.

Miller JQ: Lissencephaly in two siblings. *Neurology* 13:841, 1963.

Motte J, et al.: Sonographic diagnosis of lissencephaly. *Pediatr. Radiol.* 17:362, 1987.

Noorani PA, et al: Colpocephaly: Frequency and associated findings. *Neurology* 38:100, 1988.

Selypes A, et al: Miller-Dieker syndrome and monosomy 17p13: A new case. *Hum. Genet.* 80:103, 1988.

Stratton RF, et al.: New chromosomal syndrome: Miller-Dieker syndrome and monosomy 17p13. *Hum. Genet.* 67:193, 1984.

LÖFFLER SYNDROME

Synonyms: Löffler pneumonia; Loeffler pneumonia.

Classification: (a) true pulmonary eosinophilia (blood eosinophil count >400/mm^3, eosinophilic lung infiltrate) with known cause (fungi, drugs, parasites) or unknown cause (cryptogenic-vasculitis-granuloma spectrum, hypereosinophilic syndrome); (b) secondary pulmonary eosinophilia (blood eosinophil count >400/mm^3); increased lung density on radiographs without eosinophilic infiltrate (lavage/biopsy); caused by infections, neoplasm (Hodgkin lymphoma, bronchial carcinoma), sarcoidosis, etc.

Clinical Manifestations: Symptoms usually mild and of short duration: (a) *chest pain, dyspnea, slight fever, cough, wheezing*; (b) *peripheral eosinophilia*; (c) other reported abnormalities: cryptogenic pulmonary eosinophilia in identical twins at different times, eosinophilic pneumonia without radiographic pulmonary infiltrates, etc.

Radiologic Manifestations: *Transient and migratory patchy pulmonary infiltrations*: single or multiple peripheral areas of consolidation, often homogeneous, ill-defined, and nonsegmental.

REFERENCES

Bahk YW: Pulmonary paragonimiasis as a cause of Loeffler's syndrome. *Radiology* 78:598, 1962.

Bailey CC, et al.: Lymphosarcoma presenting as Löffler's syndrome. *Br. Med. J.* 1:460, 1973.

Barnes N, et al.: Pulmonary eosinophilia in identical twins. *Thorax* 38:318, 1983.

Bray DA, et al.: Löffler's syndrome as a complication of bipedal lymphangiography. *J.A.M.A.* 214:369, 1970.

Citro LA, et al.: Eosinophilic lung disease (or how to slice P.I.E.). *A.J.R.* 117:787, 1973.

Dejaegher P, et al.: Eosinophilic pneumonia without radiographic pulmonary infiltrates. *Chest* 84:637, 1983.

Geddes DM: Pulmonary eosinophilia. *J. R. Coll. Physicians Lond.* 20:139, 1986.

Löffler W: Zur Differential-Diagnose der Lungeninfiltrierungen, Ueber flüchtige Succendan-Infiltrate (mit Eosinophilie). *Beitr. Klin. Tuberk.* 79:368, 1932.

Paty E, et al: Le poumon éosinophile chez l'enfant. *Arch. Fr. Pediatr.* 43:243, 1986.

LOW BACK PAIN SYNDROME

Classification (McNab, Schellinger): (a) viscerogenic (intra-abdominal) disorders; (b) vascular diseases (aortic aneurysm, peripheral vascular disease); (c) psychogenic; (d) neurogenic (central nervous system or peripheral nerve lesion); (e) spondylogenic back pain (disk diseases, lateral spinal stenosis, central spinal stenosis, osteoarthritis of facet joints, etc.).

REFERENCES

Buirski G: The investigation of sciatica and low back pain syndromes: Current trends. *Clin. Radiol.* 38:151, 1987.

McNab I: *Backache.* Baltimore, Williams & Wilkins, 1977.

Schellinger D: The low back pain syndrome. Diagnostic impact of high-resolution computed tomography. *Med. Clin. North Am.* 68:1631, 1984.

Verbiest H: Neurogenic intermittent claudication in cases with absolute and relative stenosis of the lumbar vertebral canal (ASLC and RSLC), in cases with narrow lumbar intervertebral foramina, and in cases with both entities. *Clin. Neurosurg.* 20:204, 1973.

LUMBO-COSTO-VERTEBRAL SEQUENCE

Clinical Manifestations: (a) *lumbar hernia;* (b) *congenital rib cage deformity;* (c) *scoliosis.*

Radiologic Manifestations: (a) *rib anomalies:* agenesis, hypoplasia; (b) *vertebral anomalies:* hemivertebrae, anterior meningocele.

REFERENCE

Touloukian RJ: The lumbocostovertebral syndrome: A single somatic defect. *Surgery* 71:174, 1972.

LUTEMBACHER SYNDROME

Clinical Manifestations: *Atrial septal defect associated with mitral valve stenosis.*

Radiologic Manifestations: (a) varying degrees of *cardiomegaly,* marked *right atrial enlargement,* normal or slightly enlarged left atrial and ventricular chambers; (b) *dilated pul-*

monary artery and branches; (c) echocardiography: *diminished rate of mitral valve closure, thickened mitral leaflet, abnormal diastolic anterior motion of the posterior mitral valve leaflet, paradoxical motion of the interventricular septum.*

REFERENCES

Alvarez H, et al.: Two-dimensional echocardiography of Lutembacher's syndrome. *J. Clin. Ultrasound* 9:455, 1981.

Forman HR, et al.: Lutembacher's syndrome: Recognition by echocardiography. *J. Clin. Ultrasound* 7:53, 1979.

Gueron M, et al.: Lutembacher syndrome obsolete? A new modified concept of mitral valve disease and left-to-right shunt at the atrial level. *Am. Heart J.* 91:535, 1976.

Lutembacher R: De la sténose mitrale avec communication interauriculaire. *Arch. Mal. Coeur.* 9:237, 1916.

LYMPHEDEMA (CLASSIFICATION)

    I. Genetic lymphedema syndromes.

   II. Primary lymphatic dysplasia: (a) association with chylothorax, chylous ascites; (b) other reported abnormalities: splenomegaly, thrombocytopenia, afibrinogenemia, hemangioma, lymphangioma, hydrops fetalis, congenital heart disease.

  III. Acquired lymphedema.

Note: The familial case reported by Kääriäinen had distichiasis (double row of eyelashes), yellow dystrophic nails, and recurrent severe attacks of lymphangitis (overlapping of some of the types shown in Table SY−L−2).

REFERENCES

Corbett CRR, et al.: Congenital heart disease in patients with primary lymphedemas. *Lymphology* 15:85, 1982.

Crowe CA, et al.: A genetic association between microcephaly and lymphedema. *Am. J. Med. Genet.* 24:131, 1986.

Kääriäinen H: Hereditary lymphedema: A new combination of symptoms not fitting into present classifications. *Clin. Genet.* 26:254, 1984.

Leung AKC: Dominantly inherited syndrome of microcephaly and congenital lymphedema. *Clin. Genet.* 27:611, 1985.

Lewis JM, et al.: Lymphedema praecox. *J. Pediatr.* 104:641, 1984.

Smeltzer DM, et al.: Primary lymphatic dysplasia in children: Chylothorax, chylous ascites, and generalized lymphatic dysplasia. *Eur. J. Pediatr.* 145:286, 1986.

Vajro P, et al.: Aagenaes's syndrome in an Italian child. *Acta Paediatr. Scand.* 73:695, 1984.

Windebank KP, et al.: Hydrops fetalis due to abnormal lymphatics. *Arch. Dis. Child.* 62:198, 1987.

LYMPHEDEMA-HYPOPARATHYROIDISM SYNDROME

    Mode of Inheritance: Autosomal recessive or X-linked recessive (two adult brothers).

    Clinical and Radiologic Manifestations: (a) congenital lymphedema; (b) hypoparathyroidism; (c) other abnormalities: nephropathy, prolapsing mitral valve, brachydactyly, short nail beds, Kerley B lines in lungs (possible pulmonary lymphangiectasia), pleural thickening, etc.

REFERENCE

Dahlberg PJ, et al: Autosomal or X-linked recessive syndrome of congenital lymphedema, hypoparathyroidism, nephropathy, prolapsing mitral valve, and brachytelephalangy. *Am. J. Med. Genet.* 16:99, 1983.

TABLE SY−L−2.

Hereditary Lymphedema Syndromes*

Type	Inheritance	Age at Onset of L†	Associated Features
Milroy disease	AD†	At birth	Pleural effusion
Meige disease	AD	Puberty	
L + intestinal lymphangiectasia	AD	Infancy	Diarrhea, growth failure
L + yellow nails	AD	Adulthood	Pleural effusion
L + distichiasis	AD	Puberty or later	Ectropion of lower lid, spinal anomalies
L + recurrent lymphangitis	AD	Childhood or puberty	
L + recurrent cholestasis (Aagenae syndrome)	AR	At birth or childhood	May develop into cirrhosis of the liver
L + cerebrovascular anomaly	AD	Puberty or later	Pulmonary hypertension
L + ptosis	AD	Puberty	
L + microcephaly	AD	At birth	
Noonan syndrome	AD	Puberty	
Turner syndrome	"XO"	At birth	

*Modified after Kääriänen H: Hereditary lymphedema: A new combination of symptoms not fitting into present classifications. *Clin. Genet.* 26:254, 1984.
†L = lymphedema; AD = autosomal dominant.

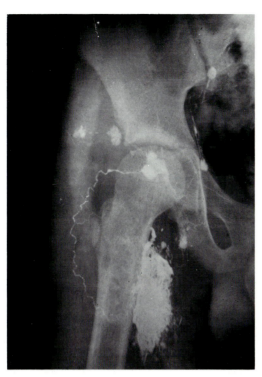

FIG SY—L—8.

Lymphedema (Nonne-Milroy type): lymphangiogram of lymphangiomatous malformation. In a film obtained at the end of the injection, some contrast medium extravasated. One large afferent vessel is present laterally, and a few small afferent vessels are seen medially. (From Gough MH: Primary lymphedema: Clinical and lymphangiographic studies. *Br. J. Surg.* 53:917, 1966. Used by permission.)

LYMPHEDEMA (NONNE-MILROY TYPE)

Synonyms: Milroy disease; Nonne-Milroy—type hereditary lymphedema.

Mode of Inheritance: Autosomal dominant.

Clinical Manifestations: (a) *lymphedema*, often of the lower limbs; (b) associated reported findings: congenital chylous ascites, protein-losing lymphangiectasia of the bowel, pleural effusion; (c) susceptibility of affected tissues to infection, acute nephritis (Fig SY—L—8).

Radiologic Manifestations: (a) *hypoplasia* (decreased number and/or size of subcutaneous lymphatics) *or absence of lymphatic channels;* (b) dermal lymphatic filling in feet on visual and roentgenographic lymphangiograms; (c) weakness of the lymphatic wall resulting in *extravasation;* (d) absence of lymphatic valves.

REFERENCES

Buonocore E, et al.: Lymphangiographic evaluation of lymphedema and lymphatic flow. *A.J.R.* 95:751, 1965.
Feldman MA, et al.: Acute nephritis complicating Milroy's disease. *Lancet* 1:336, 1987.

Gough MH: Primary lymphedema: Clinical and lymphangiographic studies. *Br. J. Surg.* 53:917, 1966.
Hurwitz PA, et al.: Pleural effusion in chronic hereditary lymphedema (Nonne-Milroy-Meige's disease): Report of two cases. *Radiology* 82:246, 1964.
Kinmonth JB, et al.: Primary lymphoedema: Clinical and lymphangiographic studies of a series of 107 patients in which the lower limbs were affected. *Br. J. Surg.* 45:1, 1957.
Meige H: Le trophoedème chronique héréditaire. *Nouv. Iconogr. (Salpêtrière)* 12:453, 1889.
Milroy WF: An undescribed variety of hereditary edema. *N.Y. Med. J.* 56:505, 1892.
Nonne M: Vier Fälle von Elephantiasis congenita hereditaria. *Arch. Pathol. Anat. (Berlin)* 125:189, 1891.
Schroeder E, et al.: Chronic hereditary lymphedema (Nonne-Milroy-Meige's syndrome). *Acta Med. Scand.* 137:198, 1950.

LYMPHOPROLIFERATIVE SYNDROME

Synonyms: Duncan syndrome; lymphoproliferative disease; X-linked lymphoproliferative syndrome.

Mode of Inheritance: X-linked recessive.

Clinical and Radiologic Manifestations: (a) immunodeficiency (hypogammaglobulinemia or agammaglobulinemia); (b) marked susceptibility to the disease induced by the Epstein-Barr virus; (c) fatal infectious mononucleosis; (d) malignancies: malignant lymphoma (in the bowel in particular), sarcoma; (e) aplastic anemia.

REFERENCES

Grierson H, et al.: Epstein-Barr virus infections in males with the X-linked lymphoproliferative syndrome. *Ann. Intern. Med.* 106:538, 1987.
Hamilton JK, et al.: X-linked lymphoproliferative syndrome registry report. *J. Pediatr.* 96:669, 1980.
Harrington DS, et al.: Malignant lymphoma in the X-linked lymphoproliferative syndrome. *Cancer* 59:1419, 1987.
Harris A, et al.: X-linked lymphoproliferative disease: Linkage studies using DNA probes. *Clin. Genet.* 33:162, 1988.
Hayoz D, et al.: X-linked lymphoproliferative syndrome. Identification of a large family in Switzerland. *Am. J. Med.* 84:529, 1988.
Purtilo DT, et al: X-linked recessive progressive combined variable immunodeficiency (Duncan disease). *Lancet* 1:935, 1975.
Purtilo DT: Pathogenesis and phenotypes of an X-linked recessive lymphoproliferative syndrome. *Lancet* 2:882, 1976.

LYNCH SYNDROMES I AND II

A. Lynch Syndrome I ("Site-Specific Familial Colonic Cancer"): Colonic mucinous or colloid-type malignancies (without polyposis) occurring usually at early ages and often located in the proximal segment of the colon; multiple primary carcinomas may be present at the time of initial investigation; high likelihood of cancer recurrence if part of the colon is not removed; autosomal dominant inheritance.

B. Lynch Syndrome II ("Cancer Family Syndrome"): Features of Lynch syndrome I associated with cancer in the female genital tract and other sites, in particular, carcinoma of the endometrium and ovary; also reported are carcinoma of the pancreas, gastric carcinoma, complete intestinal metaplasia, chronic atrophic gastritis restricted to the antrum, etc.

REFERENCES

Abusamra H, et al.: Cancer family syndrome of Lynch. *Am. J. Med.* 83:981, 1987.

Cristofaro G, et al.: New phenotypic aspects in a family with Lynch syndrome II. *Cancer* 60:51, 1987.

Fitzgibbons R, et al.: Recognition and treatment of patients with hereditary nonpolyposis colon cancer (Lynch syndromes I and II). *Ann. Surg.* 206:289, 1987.

Lynch HT, et al.: Hereditary nonpolyposis colorectal cancer (Lynch syndromes I and II). I. Clinical description of resource. *Cancer* 56:934, 1985.

Lynch HT, et al: Hereditary nonpolyposis colorectal cancer (Lynch syndromes I and II). II. Biomarker studies. *Cancer* 56:939, 1985.

M

MACROCEPHALY AND MESODERMAL HAMARTOMAS

TABLE SY−M−1.
Clinical Features and Genetic Transmission in Syndromes With Macrocephaly and Mesodermal Hamartomas*

Source	Macrocephaly	Mesodermal Hamartoma	Pigmentary Changes	Pseudo-papilledema	Respiratory Involvement	Mental Retardation	Genetic Transmission
Riley and Smith	+†	+	+	+	+	−†	Autosomal dominant
Bannayan	+	+	+	−	+	−	Sporadic
Zonana et al.	+	+	−	−	−	−	Autosomal dominant
Ruvalcaba et al.	+	+	+	−	−	+	Sporadic
Higginbottom et al.	+	+	−	−	−	−‡	Autosomal dominant
Saul et al.	+	+	−§	−	−	+	Autosomal dominant
Halal	+	+	+	−	−	+	Autosomal dominant
Diliberti et al.	+	+	+	−	−	+	Autosomal dominant
Miles et al.	+	+	−	−	+	+	Autosomal dominant

*From Dvir M, et al.: Heredofamilial syndrome of mesodermal hamartomas, macrocephaly, and pseudopapilledema. *Pediatrics* 81:287, 1988. Used by permission.
†+ = present; − = absent.
‡Mental retardation appeared later (M.C. Higginbottom, personal communication, 1982).
§Pigmentary changes were reported in 1986.

MACRODYSTROPHIA LIPOMATOSA

Synonym: Macrolipodystrophy.

Pathology: A form of localized gigantism due to progressive hypertrophy of all the mesenchymal elements (fibroadipose, vessels, nerves, tendons, and bone) with a disproportionate increase in the fibroadipose tissue; usually one or more digits of the hand or foot is involved (macrodactyly), rarely a forearm or an entire limb may be involved.

Clinical Manifestations: Onset since birth: (a) slowly progressive unilateral focal gigantism; (b) progressive arthropathy; (c) psoriasiform rash.

Radiologic Manifestations: (a) *marked proliferation of subcutaneous fat; (b) enlargement of bones, marginal erosions, exostoses, joint destruction, irregular periosteal reaction, ankylosis* by bands of dense bone; (c) absence of angioma or arteriovenous fistula.

Differential Diagnosis: Neurofibromatosis; lymphangiomatosis; Klippel-Trenaunay syndrome; Ollier disease; idiopathic hemihypertrophy; Proteus syndrome (Fig SY−M−1).

REFERENCES

Bidat E, et al.: Macrolipodystrophie. Intérêt de la radiographie des parties molles. *Arch. Fr. Pediatr.* 43:337, 1986.
Goldman AB, et al.: Macrodystrophia lipomatosa: Radiographic diagnosis. *A.J.R.* 128:101, 1977.
Laval-Jeantet M, et al.: Macrodystrophie lipomateuse: Aspect artériographique. *J. Radiol.* 60:653, 1979.
Moran V, et al.: X-ray diagnosis of macrodystrophia lipomatosa. *Br. J. Radiol.* 57:523, 1984.
Oosthwizen SF, et al.: Two cases of lipomatosis involving bone. *Br. J. Radiol.* 20:426, 1947.

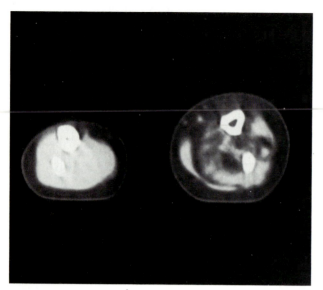

FIG SY—M—1.
Macrodystrophia lipomatosa in a 15-month-old girl. Computed tomography shows the fatty infiltration of the left leg. (From Bidat E, Hervé F, Raynaud-Delage C, et al.: Macrolipodystrophie: Intérêt de la radiographie des parties molles. *Arch. Fr. Pediatr.* 43:337, 1986. Used by permission.)

MADELUNG DISEASE

Synonyms: Launois-Bensaude disease; Buschke disease; cervical lipomatosis; Madelung neck; multiple symmetrical lipomatosis.

Mode of Inheritance: Most commonly noted in the countries around the Mediterranean Sea; male predominance; familial occurrence, autosomal dominant mode of inheritance has been postulated.

Frequency: Over 200 published cases; estimated incidence of 1:25,000 males for an Italian population (Enzi).

Clinical Manifestations: Onset in adulthood: (a) *massive lipomatosis (normal fat that often begins on the back of the neck* and extends anteriorly to the submental region and to the thorax in a symmetrical fashion) may spread to the scrotal region; (b) respiratory system symptoms related to tracheal compression and recurrent palsy; (c) venous stasis of the chest wall in association with mediastinal involvement; (d) neuropathy (sensory, motor, autonomic): muscular weakness, tendon areflexia, muscle atrophy, tremor, cramps, loss of viratory sensation, hypoesthesia, sciatica-like pain, trophic changes, segmental hyperhidrosis, gustatory sweating, impotence, tachycardia at rest, etc; (e) metabolic abnormalities: marked increase in adipose tissue lipoprotein lipase activity, plasma hyperalphalipoproteinemia, defect in the adrenergic-stimulated lipolysis in lipomatous tissue, hyperuricemia, reduced glucose tolerance, renal tubular acidosis; (f) red blood cell macrocytosis, macrocytic anemia; (g) abnormal liver function test results related to elevated alcohol intake; (h) no signs of abdominal or pelvic involvement; (i) sudden death.

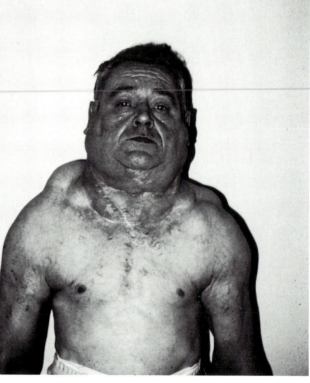

FIG SY—M—2.
Madelung syndrome: mediastinal fat accumulation causing venous stasis of the thoracic wall. Fatty tumors of the neck are seen. (From Enzi G, Biondetti PR, Fiore D, et al.: Computed tomography of deep fat masses in multiple symmetrical lipomatosis. *Radiology* 144:121, 1982. Used by permission.)

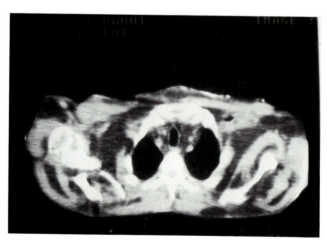

FIG SY—M—3.
Madelung syndrome. A computed tomographic scan at the level of the thoracic inlet shows superior mediastinal lipomatosis, tracheal narrowing, tissue calcification, and symmetrical deep fat deposits between the upper back muscles. (From Enzi G, Biondetti PR, Fiore D, et al.: Computed tomography of deep fat masses in multiple symmetrical lipomatosis. *Radiology* 144:121, 1982. Used by permission.)

Radiologic Manifestations: (a) lipomatosis (neck, mediastinum, below the trapezius muscle); (b) calcification/ossification within the lipomatous masses; (c) tracheal narrowing and deformity; (d) venous stasis; (e) absence of pericardial, intra-abdominal, retroperitoneal, and pelvic lipomatosis (Figs SY—M—2 and SY—M—3).

REFERENCES

Bonnichon Ph, et al.: Maladie de Launois-Bensaude. Traitement par large cervicotomie transversale. *Presse Med.* 15:2247, 1986.

Buschke A, et al.: Die traumatische Ätiologie und die Begutachtung der symmetrischen Lipomatose. *Klin. Wochenschr.* 8:880, 1929.

Enzi G: Multiple symmetric lipomatosis: An updated clinical report. *Medicine (Baltimore)* 63:56, 1984.

Enzi G, et al.: Computed tomography of deep fat masses in multiple symmetrical lipomatosis. *Radiology* 144:121, 1982.

Enzi G, et al.: Sensory, motor, and autonomic neuropathy in patients with multiple symmetric lipomatosis. *Medicine (Baltimore)* 64:388, 1986.

Gate A, et al.: Le syndrome de Launois-Bensaude: A propos de 12 cas cliniques. *Ann. Chir. Plast.* 11:193, 1966.

Madelung O: Ueber den Fetthals (diffuses Lipom des Halses). *Arch. Klin. Chir. (Berlin)* 37:106, 1888.

MALABSORPTION SYNDROME

Classification: (a) primary: celiac disease, nontropical sprue, tropical sprue; (b) constitutional diseases, small-bowel diseases, postsurgical etc.

Clinical Manifestations: (a) *bulky, fatty, and foul-smelling stools;* (b) weight loss; (c) growth retardation; (d) abdominal distension; (e) skin pigmentation; (f) jejunal biopsy: atrophy of intestinal villi; (g) development of intestinal lymphoma or carcinoma in long-standing sprue.

Radiologic Manifestations: (a) *dilatation of the small bowel with abnormal contractility, segmentation, hypersecretion, decrease in prominence of mucosal folds, prolonged transit time, moulage sign,* duodenal changes, (dilatation, decrease in the number of mucosal folds, thickening and asymmetry of the mucosal folds), nonhomogeneous appearance of barium granules throughout colon (less common with modern barium suspension), adaptation of the ileum in nontropical sprue (increase in the ileal fold pattern and a decrease in the jejunal fold pattern, reversed pattern representing chronic inflammation and atrophy of the jejunum and compensatory hypertrophy of the ileum), floating feces (horizontal beam, double-contrast enema); (b) small-bowel ulcers; (c) intramural hematoma; (d) angiography: dilatation of the superior mesenteric artery and its small-bowel branches selectively, increased capillary blush, early drainage into the dilated vein; (e) thick mesentery (sprue).

Note: The "malabsorption pattern" (flocculation and segmentation of barium, thickening of mucosal folds, and dilation of intestinal loops) is a nonspecific finding in children, and in the absence of the clinical features suggestive of malabsorption or growth failure, further investigations may not be justified (Weizman et al.).

REFERENCES

Baer AN, et al.: Intestinal ulceration and malabsorption syndromes. *Gastroenterology* 79:754, 1980.

Bova JG, et al.: Adaptation of the ileum in nontropical sprue: Reversal of the jejunoileal fold pattern. *A.J.R.* 144:299, 1985.

Brandborg LL: Histologic diagnosis of diseases of malabsorption. *Am. J. Med.* 67:999, 1979.

Carroll JE, et al.: Inflammatory myopathy, IgA deficiency, and intestinal malabsorption. *J. Pediatr.* 89:216, 1976.

Cynn WS, et al.: Mesenteric angiography of nontropical sprue. *A.J.R.* 125:442, 1975.

Gerson DE, et al.: Intramural small bowel hemorrhage: Complication of sprue. *Radiology* 108:521, 1973.

Hornsby VPL: Case report: Floating faeces in statorrhea—a new sign. *Clin. Radiol.* 39:454, 1988.

McLean AM, et al.: The relationship between hypoalbuminaemia and the radiological appearances of the jejunum in tropical sprue. *Br. J. Radiol.* 55:725, 1982.

Smith DS: Roentgenology and malabsorption syndromes (letter). *Pediatrics* 76:140, 1985.

Weizman Z, et al.: Radiologic manifestations of malabsorption: A nonspecific finding. *Pediatrics* 74:530, 1984.

MALLORY-WEISS SYNDROME

Pathology: Tears of the gastric mucosa and submucosa with or without extension across the gastroesophageal junction; limited to the lower portion of the esophagus in 5% to 10% of cases.

Etiology: The tear is considered to be the result of a transient transmural pressure gradient between the intrathoracic pressure and the intragastric pressure at the gastroesophageal junction; causes: forced emesis or wretching (alcohol debauchery, cancer chemotherapy, travel sickness, uremia, ipecac therapy, migraine, pancreatitis, etc.), increased intra-abdominal pressure (pregnancy, blunt trauma, closed chest massage, forced Valsalva maneuver, hiccups, coughing seizures), endoscopy, etc.

Clinical Manifestations: (a) *painless hematemesis,* usually following straining or vomiting; (b) *pallor and tachycardia;* (c) endoscopic visualization of the *laceration* site; (d) subserosal staining of blood on the lesser curvature and anterior wall of the stomach at the gastroesophageal junction (laparotomy).

Radiologic Manifestations: (a) barium outlining the laceration in the form of a *streaky collection of media in the wall* (roentgenographic detection uncommon); (b) *arterio-*

graphic demonstration of the site of laceration in patients with active bleeding (extravasation of contrast medium); (c) esophageal obstruction secondary to an intraluminal thrombus; (d) serendipitous detection on hepatic nuclear medicine imaging.

REFERENCES

Baptist EC, et al.: Mallory-Weiss syndrome in a 16-week-old infant. *Clin. Pediatr. (Phila.)* 20:59, 1981.

Brinberg DE, et al.: Mallory-Weiss tear with colonic lavage. *Ann. Intern. Med.* 104:894, 1986.

Cannon RA, et al.: Gastrointestinal hemorrhage due to Mallory-Weiss syndrome in an infant. *J. Pediatr. Gastroenterol. Nutr.* 4:323, 1985.

Fisher RG, et al.: Angiotherapy with Mallory-Weiss tear. *A.J.R.* 134:679, 1980.

Fishman ML, et al.: Mallory-Weiss tear. A complication of cancer chemotherapy. *Cancer* 52:2031, 1983.

Hastings PR: Mallory-Weiss syndrome. Review of 69 cases. *Am. J. Surg.* 142:560, 1981.

Mallory GK, Weiss S: Hemorrhage from lacerations of the cardiac orifice of the stomach due to vomiting. *Am. J. Med. Sci.* 178:506, 1929.

Powell TW, et al.: Mallory-Weiss syndrome in a 10-month-old infant requiring surgery. *J. Pediatr. Surg.* 19:596, 1984.

Ross LA: Mallory-Weiss syndrome in a 10-month-old infant. *Am. J. Dis. Child.* 133:1069, 1979.

Sugawa C, et al.: Mallory-Weiss syndrome. A study of 224 patients. *Am. J. Surg.* 145:30, 1983.

Swayne LC, et al.: Serendipitous detection of a Mallory-Weiss tear on hepatic imaging. *Clin. Nucl. Med.* 11:597, 1986.

MANDIBULOACRAL DYSPLASIA

Synonym: Craniomandibular dermatodysostosis.

Mode of Inheritance: Autosomal recessive.

Frequency: Nine families (Tenconi et al.).

Clinical Manifestations: (a) *hypoplasia of the mandible, beaked nose, facial hypoplasia (Andy Gump appearance); (b) dental crowding, premature loss of teeth; (c) stiff joints; (d) localized areas of skin atrophy, alopecia, hair anomaly, nail dysplasia; (e) short stature.*

Radiologic Manifestations: (a) *delayed cranial suture closure, wormian bones, mandibular hypoplasia; (b) acro-osteolysis; (c) clavicular hypoplasia, rib hypoplasia; (d) soft-tissue calcification.*

Differential Diagnosis: Acrogeria; progeria; cleidocranial dysplasia; Werner syndrome; pyknodysostosis; Hallermann-Streiff syndrome; "absent eyebrows and eyelashes with mental retardation"; Cockayne syndrome.

REFERENCES

Hall BD, et al.: Mandibuloacral dysplasia: A rare progressive disorder with postnatal onset (abstract). *Proc. Greenwood Genet. Center* 4:125, 1985.

Pallotta R, et al.: Mandibuloacral dysplasia: A rare progeroid syndrome. Two brothers confirm autosomal recessive inheritance. *Clin. Genet.* 26:133, 1984.

Tenconi R, et al.: Another Italian family with mandibuloacral dysplasia: Why does it seem more frequent in Italy? *Am. J. Med. Genet.* 24:357, 1986.

Young LW, et al.: New syndrome manifested by mandibular hypoplasia, acroosteolysis, stiff joints and cutaneous atrophy (mandibuloacral dysplasia) in two unrelated boys. *Birth Defects* 7:291, 1971.

MAN-IN-THE-BARREL SYNDROME

Clinical Manifestations: Acute cerebral hypoperfusion associated with severe hypotension, brachial diplegia without motor disturbance of the legs, facial grimacing, coma.

Radiologic Manifestations: Bilateral watershed infarction in the temporo-occipital area and in the frontal white matter between the supply territories of the anterior and middle cerebral arteries.

REFERENCES

Delavelle J, et al.: Man-in-the-barrel syndrome: First CT images. *Neuroradiology* 29:501, 1987.

Mohr JP: Distal field infarction. *Neurology* 12:279, 1969.

Sage JI, et al.: Man-in-the-barrel syndrome. *Neurology* 36:1102, 1986.

MARDEN-WALKER SYNDROME

Mode of Inheritance: Probably autosomal recessive.

Frequency: 16 cases (Gossage et al.).

Clinical and Radiologic Manifestations: (a) *psychomotor retardation, failure to thrive; (b) craniofacial abnormalities:* fixed facial expression, blepharophimosis, low-set ears, micrognathia, hypertelorism, epicanthic folds, strabismus, cleft palate, small mouth, everted lower lips, long philtrum, upturned nose tip, etc.; (c) *multiple congenital joint contractures* (elbows, hips, knees), decreased muscle masses of the limbs, hypotonia; (d) other reported abnormalities: microcystic renal disease, dextrocardia, congenital heart disease, kyphoscoliosis, pectus carinatum, high-arched palate, deep-set eyes, preauricular tag, dolichocephaly, arachnodactyly, hirsutism, low hairlines, equinovarus foot deformity, association with Zollinger-Ellison syndrome, enlarged cisterna magna and fourth ventricle, microcephaly, camptodactyly, pectus excavatum, simian crease, pyloric stenosis, etc. (Fig SY—M—4).

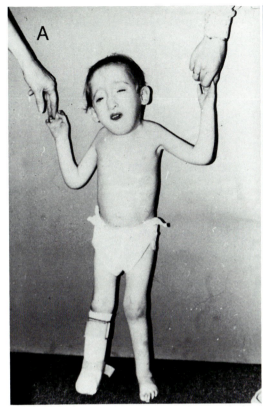

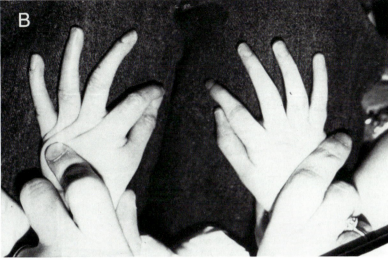

FIG SY—M—4.
Marden-Walker syndrome: abnormal facies, blepharophimosis, hypertelorism, apparently low-set ears, micrognathia **(A)**, arachnodactyly **(B)**. (From Gossage D, et al.: Brief clinical report and review: A 26-month-old child with Marden-Walker syndrome and pyloric stenosis. *Am. J. Med. Genet.* 26:915, 1987. Used by permission.)

REFERENCES

Abe K, et al.: Zollinger-Ellison syndrome with Marden-Walker syndrome. *Am. J. Dis. Child.* 133:735, 1979.

Fitch N, et al.: Congenital blepharophimosis, joint contractures, and muscular hypotonia. *Neurology* 21:1214, 1971.

Gossage D, et al.: Brief clinical report and review: A 26-month-old child with Marden-Walker syndrome and pyloric stenosis. *Am. J. Med. Genet.* 26:915, 1987.

Howard FM, et al.: Two brothers with Marden-Walker syndrome: Case report and review. *J. Med. Genet.* 18:50, 1981.

Kubryk N, et al.: Dysmorphie crânio-faciale avec flexion des doigts. Syndrome de Marden-Walker? *Ann. Pediatr. (Paris)* 29:208, 1982.

Marden PM, Walker WA: A new generalized connective tissue syndrome. *Am. J. Dis. Child.* 112:225, 1966.

Passarge E: Marden-Walker syndrome. *Birth Defects* 11:470, 1975.

MARFAN SYNDROME

Mode of Inheritance: Autosomal dominant with variable degree of expression; new mutation.

Frequency: About 5 per 100,000 births; 15% spontaneous mutations (Chemke et al.).

Clinical Manifestations: (a) *dolichocephaly, long limbs, arachnodactyly,* thumb sign (ability to protrude the thumb beyond the palm of the closed hand), wrist sign (positive if the distal phalanges of the first and fifth digits of one hand overlap when wrapped around the opposite wrist), hyperextensible joint, ligament laxity; (b) *ocular abnormalities* (ectopia lentis, myopia, etc.); (c) cardiovascular abnormalities: (1) midsystolic click, midsystolic click and late systolic murmur, aortic regurgitation murmur, mitral regurgitation murmur, ventricular dysrhythmia; (2) echocardiography: aortic enlargement, abnormal compliance of the aortic wall, prolapse of the posterior leaflet of the mitral valve, appearance of shaggy echoes on the anterior mitral leaflet, abnormal echogram in a high percentage of first-degree relatives of patients with Marfan syndrome, triple-valve prolapse (mitral, tricuspid, aortic), calcification of an incompetent foramen ovale, atrial septal aneurysm, massive calcification of the mitral valve annulus in young adults; (d) mild emphysema, forced vital capacity less than that predicted, cor pulmonale due to severe kyphoscoliosis, spontaneous pneumothorax, pneumonia, excessively frequent respiratory infections; (e) other reported abnormalities: precocious puberty, deviated nasal septum, narrow and high-arched palate, temporomandibular joint pain and arthritis, pes planus, striae distensae, inguinal hernia, histadinemia, rapid statural growth in infancy and childhood and slow weight gain resulting in thinness, intrapartum death associated with mitral and tricuspid valve anomalies, Wilms tumor of a solitary kidney, bacterial endocarditis and hepatic peliosis, hyperthyroidism, asymmetrical Marfan syndrome (left side), neuropsychological deficits (learning disability, attention deficit disorder, hyperactivity, a performance IQ score different from the verbal score by more than 20 points); (f) death causes: aortic and mitral valve incompetence, aortic dissection, aneurysmal rupture, mural complications of an ascending aortic aneurysm, subacute bacterial endocarditis; etc.

Radiologic Manifestations: (a) skeletal: (1) long, tall, and thick skull; (2) enlarged paranasal sinuses; (3) atlantoaxial instability, kyphoscoliosis, laxity of lumbar vertebral joints, spondylolisthesis, increased interpediculate space and wide spinal canal, thoracic meningocele, sacral abnormalities (expansion of the central sacral spinal canal, enlargement of sacral foramina in association with extensive bony erosion, sacral meningocele); (4) high metacarpal index (ratio of length to width of the second to fifth metacarpals is normally 5.5 to 8; the ratio is 8.5 to 10.5 in Marfan syndrome); (5) elongated fingers (the length of the phalanges of the third finger exceeds 1.5 times the length of its metacarpal); (6) dislocation of the sternoclavicular joint, hip dislocation, perilunate dislocation unrelated to trauma; (7) protrusio acetabuli (90% associated with scoliosis); (8) bone maturity in childhood between chronological and statural age; (b) *chest*: (1) pectus carinatum or pectus excavatum; (2) rib notching; (3) congenital malformations of the bronchi; (4) bronchiectasis; (5) *pulmonary dysaeration* (pulmonary emphysema, bullae), spontaneous pneumothorax, cystic disease, diffuse reticular interstitial densities; (c) *cardiovascular:* (1) *mitral abnormalities* with insufficiency (an irregular and unusually large mitral annulus and prolapse of

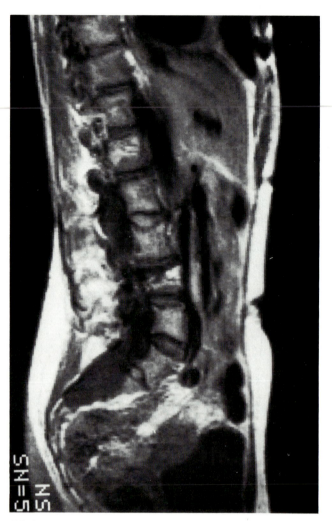

FIG SY—M—6.
Marfan syndrome. Widened spinal canal and dural eclasia are present. (From Soulen RL, Fishman EK, Pyeritz RE, et al.: Marfan syndrome: Evaluation with MR imaging versus CT. *Radiology* 165:697, 1987. Used by permission.)

the mitral valve into the left atrium during ventricular systole); (2) *aortic sinus dilatation, aortic insufficiency;* (3) aortic and pulmonary arterial aneurysm, aneurysm of the ductus arteriosus, isolated aneurysm of the abdominal aorta; (4) *cystic medial necrosis of the aorta* and occasionally of peripheral vessels, aortic dissection, multiple small intimal flaps, coarctation of the aorta, dissecting aneurysm of the ductus arteriosus; (5) other reported abnormalities: side-to-side mobility of the abdominal aorta (ultrasonography), absent right coronary artery, etc. (Figs SY—M—5 and SY—M—6).

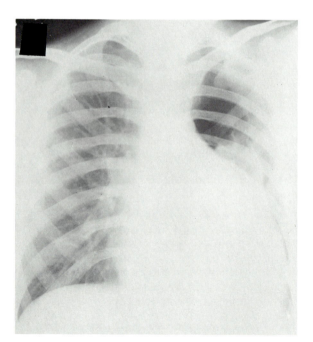

FIG SY—M—5.
Marfan syndrome in a 15-year-old male who had a sudden onset of dyspnea. A chest roentgenogram at admission shows cardiomegaly, left pneumothorax, and a bulla in the apical region of the right lung. A heart murmur was noted at admission. Cardiac catheterization and cardioangiography revealed mitral insufficiency, marked dilatation of aortic sinuses, and moderate dilatation of the ascending aorta.

REFERENCES

Becker AE, et al.: The coronary arteries in Marfan's syndrome. *Am. J. Cardiol.* 36:315, 1975.

Beals RK, et al.: The Marfan skull. *Radiology* 140:723, 1981.

Birch JG, et al.: Spinal deformity in Marfan syndrome. *J. Pediatr. Orthop.* 7:546, 1987.

Boucek RJ, et al.: The Marfan syndrome: A deficiency in chemically stable collagen cross-link. *N. Engl. J. Med.* 305:988, 1981.

Bruno L, et al.: Cardiac, skeletal, and ocular abnormalities in patients with Marfan's syndrome and in their relatives. Comparison with the cardiac abnormalities in patients with kyphoscoliosis. *Br. Heart J.* 51:220, 1984.

Buchanan R, et al.: Marfan's syndrome presenting as an intrapartum death. *Arch. Dis. Child.* 60:1074, 1985.

Burgio RG, et al.: Asymmetric Marfan syndrome. *Am. J. Med. Genet.* 30:905, 1988.

Chemke J, et al.: Homozygosity for autosomal dominant Marfan syndrome. *J. Med. Genet.* 21:173, 1984.

Chen S-C, et al.: Ventricular dysrhythmias in children with Marfan's syndrome. *Am. J. Dis. Child.* 139:273, 1985.

Come PC, et al.: Echocardiographic assessment of cardiovascular abnormalities in the Marfan syndrome. Comparison with clinical findings and with roentgenographic estimation of aortic root size. *Am. J. Med.* 74:465, 1983.

Day DL, et al.: Pulmonary emphysema in a neonate with Marfan syndrome. *Pediatr. Radiol.* 16:518, 1986.

Dominguez R, et al.: Pulmonary hyperinflation and emphysema in infants with the Marfan syndrome. *Pediatr. Radiol.* 17:365, 1987.

Eldridge R: The metacarpal index: A useful aid in the diagnosis of the Marfan syndrome. *Arch. Intern. Med.* 113:248, 1964.

Fishman EK, et al.: Sacral abnormalities in Marfan syndrome. *J. Comput. Assist. Tomogr.* 7:851, 1983.

Geva T, et al.: The clinical course and echocardiographic features of Marfan's syndrome in childhood. *Am. J. Dis. Child.* 141:1179, 1987.

Gillan JE, et al.: Spontaneous dissecting aneurysm of the ductus arteriosus in an infant with Marfan syndrome. *J. Pediatr.* 105:952, 1984.

Goodman A, et al.: Occult thoraco-abdominal dissecting aneurysm in a patient with Marfan's syndrome—Diagnosis by real-time ultrasound. *J. Clin. Ultrasound* 12:115, 1984.

Goodman HB, et al.: Marfan's syndrome with massive calcification of the mitral annulus at age twenty-six. *Am. J. Cardiol.* 24:426, 1969.

Hofman KJ, et al.: Marfan syndrome: Neuropsychological aspects. *Am. J. Med. Genet.* 31:331, 1988.

Hollister DW, et al.: Marfan syndrome: Abnormalities of the microfibrillar fiber array detected by immunohistopathologic studies. Presented at the Birth Defect Meeting, Baltimore, 1988.

Jugdutt BI, et al.: The Marfan syndrome, coarctation of the aorta, and precocious puberty. *Chest* 71:797, 1977.

Kerstin-Sommerhoff BA, et al.: MR imaging of the thoracic aorta in Marfan patients. *J. Comput. Assist. Tomogr.* 11:633, 1987.

Kuhlman JE, et al.: Acetabular protrusion in the Marfan syndrome. *Radiology* 164:415, 1987.

Leak D: Rib notching in Marfan's syndrome. *Am. Heart J.* 71:387, 1966.

Leitch AG, et al.: A case of Marfan's syndrome with absent right coronary artery complicated by aortic dissection and right ventricular infarction. *Thorax* 30:352, 1975.

Levander B, et al.: Atlantoaxial instability in Marfan's syndrome. Diagnosis and treatment: A case report. *Neuroradiology* 21:43, 1981.

Magherini A, et al.: Atrial septal aneurysm, ectasia of a sinus of valsalva and mitral valve prolapse in Marfan's syndrome. *Am. J. Cardiol.* 58:172, 1986.

Marfan AB: Un cas de déformation congénitale des quatre membres, plus prononcée aux extremités caracterisée par l'alongement des os avec un certain degré d'amincissement. *Bull. Mem. Soc. Med. Hop. (Paris)* 13:220, 1896.

Müller NL, et al.: Ductus arteriosus aneurysm in Marfan syndrome. *J. Can. Assoc. Radiol.* 37:195, 1986.

Newbold SG, et al.: Stage III Wilms' tumor of a solitary kidney in a patient with Marfan's syndrome: A 5-yr survival. *J. Pediatr. Surg.* 17:841, 1982.

Paling MR, et al.: The roving aorta of Marfan's syndrome: A case report. *Cardiovasc. Intervent. Radiol.* 4:249, 1981.

Pautard JCl, et al.: Peliose hepatique au cours d'une endocardite bacterienne chez une enfant atteinte de maladie de Marfan. *Presse Med.* 18:1973, 1986.

Payvandi MN, et al.: Cardiac, skeletal and ophthalmologic abnormalities in relatives of patients with Marfan syndrome. *Circulation* 55:797, 1977.

Pennes DR, et al.: Carpal ligamentous laxity with bilateral perilunate dislocation in Marfan syndrome. *Skeletal Radiol.* 13:62, 1985.

Petitalot JP, et al.: Echocardiographic follow-up in Marfan's syndrome: Mitral, tricuspid, and aortic valve prolapse with calcification of patent foramen ovale. *J. Clin. Ultrasound* 14:707, 1986.

Prockop DJ, et al.: Heritable diseases of collagen. *N. Engl. J. Med.* 311:376, 1984.

Pyeritz RE: Maternal and fetal complications of pregnancy in the Marfan syndrome. *Am. J. Med.* 71:784, 1981.

Pyeritz RE, et al.: Mitral valve dysfunction in the Marfan syndrome. Clinical and echocardiographic study of prevalence and natural history. *Am. J. Med.* 74:797, 1983.

Roy C, et al.: Étude longitudinale de la croissance dans le syndrome de Marfan pendant la première enfance. *Ann. Pediatr. (Paris)* 30:665, 1983.

Sablayrolles B, et al.: Maladie de Basedow, maladie de Marfan et prolapsus de la valve mitrale. *Presse Med.* 14:598, 1985.

Schollin J, et al: Probable homozygotic form of the Marfan syndrome in a newborn child. *Acta Paediatr. Scand.* 77:452, 1988.

Shapiro LR, et al.: The diagnosis of Marfan syndrome in children: The value of echocardiography. Presented at the Birth Defect Meeting, Baltimore, 1988.

Sisk HE, et al.: The Marfan syndrome in early childhood: Analysis of 15 patients diagnosed at less than 4 years of age. *Am. J. Cardiol.* 52:353, 1983.

Soulen RL, et al.: Marfan syndrome: Evaluation with MR imaging versus CT. *Radiology* 165:697, 1987.

Steiner RM, et al.: Renal arteriovenous fistula: Unique finding in the Marfan syndrome. *J. Urol.* 106:631, 1971.

Van Ooijen B: Marfan's syndrome and isolated aneurysm of the abdominal aorta. *Br. Heart J.* 59:81, 1988.

Wanderman KL, et al.: Cor pulmonale secondary to severe kyphoscoliosis in Marfan's syndrome. *Chest* 67:250, 1975.

Wilner HI, et al.: Skeletal manifestations in the Marfan syndrome. *J.A.M.A.* 187:490, 1964.

Wood JR, et al.: Pulmonary disease in patients with Marfan syndrome. *Thorax* 39:780, 1984.

MARFANOID HYPERMOBILITY SYNDROME

Clinical and Radiologic Manifestations: (a) *marfanoid habitus;* (b) *generalized hypermobility of the joints;* (c) *hyperextensibility of the skin;* (d) cardiovascular abnormalities: floppy mitral valve, aortic aneurysm, aortic regurgitation, dissecting aortic aneurysm, coarctation of the aorta; (e) skeletal abnormalities: pectus excavatum, genu recurvatum, scoliosis; (f) association with Duane retraction syndrome (Fig SY–M–7).

REFERENCES

Cotton DJ, et al.: Cardiovascular abnormalities in the marfanoid hypermobility syndrome. *Arthritis Rheum.* 19:763, 1976.
Daneshwar A, et al.: Marfanoid hypermobility syndrome

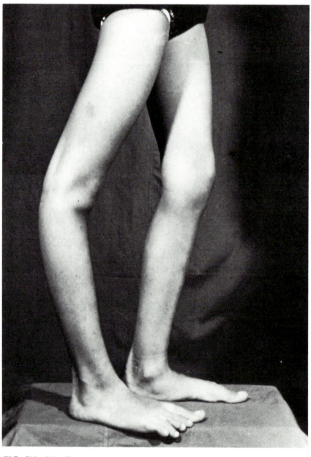

FIG SY–M–7.
Marfanoid hypermobility syndrome in a 6-year-old girl. Note the genu recurvatum and flatfeet. (From Ronen S, Rozenman Y, Arnon N, et al.: Marfanoid hypermobility syndrome associated with Duane's retraction syndrome. *Ann. Ophthalmol.* 15:862, 1983. Used by permission.)

associated with coarctation of the aorta. *Br. Heart J.* 41:621, 1979.
Ronen S, et al.: Marfanoid hypermobility syndrome associated with Duane's retraction syndrome. *Ann. Ophthalmol.* 15:862, 1983.
Verma KC, et al.: Marfanoid hypermobility syndrome associated with flail mitral valve. *Indian Heart J.* 34:108, 1982.
Walker BA, et al.: The marfanoid hypermobility syndrome. *Ann. Intern. Med.* 71:349, 1969.

MARINESCO-SJÖGREN SYNDROME

Mode of Inheritance: Autosomal recessive.

Clinical Manifestations: (a) mild to moderate *dwarfism;* (b) *cerebellar ataxia;* (c) moderate to severe *mental retardation;* (d) weakness; (e) *congenital cataract;* (f) lysosomal storage disorder has been suggested (abnormally enlarged lysosomes containing whorled lamellar or amorphous inclusion bodies seen on electron microscopic studies); (g) other reported abnormalities: pyramidal signs, sensory changes, alopecia, fine hair, hypogonadism, pectus carinatum, etc.

Radiologic Manifestations: (a) *various limb anomalies* common: talipes equinovarus, pes planus, short digits; (b) kyphosis; (c) irregularities of the teeth; (d) microcrania; (e) skeletal maturation retardation.

REFERENCES

Mahloudji M, et al.: Marinesco-Sjögren syndrome: Report of an autopsy. *Brain* 95:675, 1972.
Marinesco G, et al.: Nouvelle maladie familiale caracterisée par une cataracte congénitale et an arrêt du developpement somatoneuro-psychique. *Encephale* 26:97, 1931.
Sjögren T: Hereditary congenital spinocerebellar ataxia combined with congenital cataract and oligophrenia. *Acta Psychiatr. Scand.* 46(suppl.):286, 1947.
Superneau D, et al.: The Marinesco-Sjögren syndrome described a quarter of a century before Marinesco (letter). *Am. J. Med. Genet.* 22:647, 1985.
Walker PD, et al.: Marinesco-Sjögren syndrome: Evidence for a lysosomal storage disorder. *Neurology* 35:415, 1985.

MARSHALL SYNDROME

Mode of Inheritance: Autosomal dominant.

Frequency: Approximately 30 published cases (Nguyen et al.).

Clinical Manifestations: (a) *short nose, anteverted nostrils, flat malar bones;* (b) *myopia,* congenital cataract; (c) *deafness;* (d) prominent upper incisors; (e) other reported abnormalities: mental retardation, retinal detachment, cleft palate, hypohidrotic ectodermal dysplasia, short stature, etc.

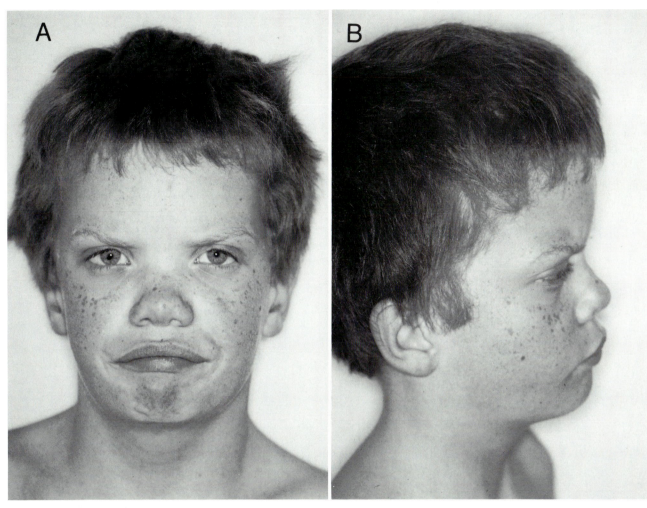

FIG SY—M—8.
Marshall syndrome in a 12-year-old patient with facial dysmorphism: short nose, flat nasal root, anteverted nostrils, flat malar bones, hypertelorism, and mild retrognathia. (From Taillard F, Des-bois J-Cl, Delepine N, et al.: Syndrome de Marshall ou syndrome de Stickler? Discussion à propos d'une famille. *Ann. Pediatr. (Paris)* 34:279, 1987. Used by permission.)

Radiologic Manifestations: (a) *osseous abnormalities:* thickened calvaria, beaked or bullet-shaped vertebra in the younger patient, platyspondyly with irregular ossification of end plates, small iliac bones with irregular lateral border, mild bowing of the radius and ulna, coxa valga, poorly formed and irregular epiphyses; (b) dural calcification.

Differential Diagnosis: Stickler syndrome: some have suggested that the Marshall and Stickler syndromes represent the same entity and recommended the term Marshall-Stickler syndrome be used; this recommendation has been rejected by others (Fig SY—M—8).

REFERENCES

Aymé S, et al.: The Marshall and Stickler syndromes: Objective rejection of lumping. *J. Med. Genet.* 21:34, 1984.
Baraitser M: Marshall/Stickler syndrome. *J. Med. Genet.* 19:139, 1982.

Marshall D: Ectodermal dysplasia: Report of kindred with ocular abnormalities and hearing defect. *Am. J. Ophthalmol.* 45:143, 1958.
Miny P, et al.: Autosomal recessive deafness with skeletal dysplasia and facial appearance of Marshall syndrome. *Am. J. Med. Genet.* 21:317, 1985.
Nguyen J, et al.: Syndrome de Marshall. Deux nouveaux cas. *Arch. Fr. Pediatr.* 45:49, 1988.
O'Donnell JJ, et al.: Generalized osseous abnormalities in the Marshall syndrome. *Birth Defects* 12:299, 1976.
Taillard F, et al.: Syndrome de Marshall au syndrome de Stickler? Discussion à propos d'une famille. *Ann. Pediatr. (Paris)* 34:279, 1987.
Zellweger H, et al.: The Marshall syndrome—Report of a new family. *J. Pediatr.* 84:868, 1974.

MARSHALL-SMITH SYNDROME

Clinical Manifestations: (a) *craniofacial features: long cranium, prominent forehead, prominent eyes associated* *with shallow orbits, underdeveloped and upturned nose, bluish sclerae, coarse eyebrows;* (b) *failure to thrive;* (c) *motor and mental retardation;* (d) *underweight for length, accelerated linear growth;* (e) other reported abnormalities: choanal atresia, microstomia, micrognathia, rudimentary epiglottis, omphalocele, hypertrichosis, widening of the middle phalanges or the proximal and middle phalanges, respiratory difficulties, immunologic abnormalities, deep crease between the hallux and second toe, pulmonary hypertension, laryngomalacia, stridor, pneumonia, atelectasis, apneic spells; (f) death in infancy (respiratory problems).

Radiologic Manifestations: (a) *marked early acceleration of skeletal maturation;* (b) *shallow orbits;* (c) *prominent forehead;* (d) *hypoplastic mandibular rami;* (e) *tubular thinning of long bones;* (f) *relatively broad middle phalanges of the finger and narrowness of the distal phalanges.*

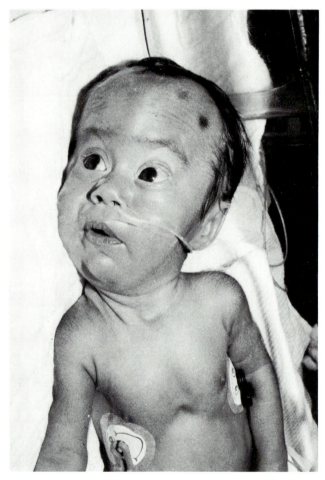

FIG SY—M—9.
Marshall-Smith syndrome. Note the ridging of the forehead, dysplastic ears, prominent eyes, upturned nose, long philtrum, micrognathia, hypertrichosis, neck hyperextension, and short sternum with retractions. (From Johnson JP, Carey JC, Glassy FJ, et al.: Marshall-Smith syndrome: Two case reports and a review of pulmonary manifestations. *Pediatrics* 71:219, 1983. Used by permission.)

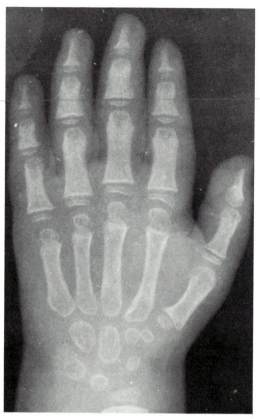

FIG SY—M—10.
Marshall-Smith syndrome. At 10 months of age, osseous development of this infant boy compares with atlas standards for ages 6 to 7 years. (From Marshall RE, Graham B, Scott CR, et al.: Syndrome of accelerated skeletal maturation and relative failure to thrive: A newly recognized clinical growth disorder. *J. Pediatr.* 78:95, 1971. Used by permission.)

Differential Diagnosis: Weaver-Smith (Weaver) syndrome (Figs SY—M—9 and SY—M—10).

REFERENCES

Fitch N: Update on the Marshall-Smith-Weaver controversy (letter). *Am. J. Med. Genet.* 20:559, 1985.
Hassan M, et al.: The syndrome of accelerated bone maturation in the newborn infant with dysmorphism and congenital malformations (the so-called Marshall-Smith syndrome). *Pediatr. Radiol.* 5:53, 1976.
Johnson JP, et al.: Marshall-Smith syndrome: Two case reports and a review of pulmonary manifestations. *Pediatrics* 71:219, 1983.
Marshall RE, Graham B, Scott CR, et al.: Syndrome of accelerated skeletal maturation and relative failure to thrive: A newly recognized clinical growth disorder. *J. Pediatr.* 78:95, 1971.
Menguy C, et al.: Le syndrome de Marshall. *Ann. Pediatr. (Paris)* 33:339, 1986.
Perrin JCS, et al.: Accelerated skeletal maturation syndrome with pulmonary hypertension. *Birth Defects* 12:209, 1976.

Shimura T, et al.: Marshall-Smith syndrome with large bifrontal diameter, broad distal femora, camptodactyly, and without broad middle phalanges. *J. Pediatr.* 94:93, 1979.

MARTSOLF SYNDROME

Mode of Inheritance: Probably autosomal recessive.

Frequency: Seven cases to 1988.

Clinical and Radiologic Manifestations: (a) mental retardation; (b) short stature; (c) cataract; (d) craniofacial anomalies: microcephaly, maxillary retrusion, pouting mouth, mal-aligned teeth, mildly dysplastic pinnae; (e) hypogonadism; (f) short metacarpals and phalanges (Fig SY–M–11).

REFERENCES

Hennekam RCM, et al.: Martsolf syndrome in a brother and sister: Clinical features and pattern of inheritance. *Eur. J. Pediatr.* 147:539, 1988.
Martsolf JT, et al: Severe mental retardation, cataracts, short stature, and primary hypogonadism in two brothers. *Am. J. Med. Genet.* 1:291, 1978.

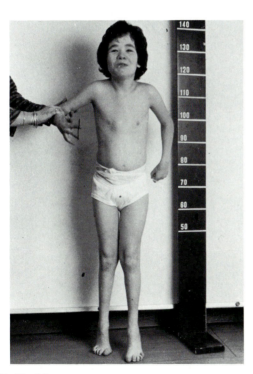

FIG SY–M–11.
Martsolf syndrome. Note the antimongoloid slant of the palpebral fissures, bilateral epicanthus, low nasal bridge, mildly hypoplastic maxilla, broad nasal tip, short philtrum, pectus carinatum, and thin lower legs. (From Hennekam RCM, van de Meeberg AG, van Doorne JM, et al.: Martsolf syndrome in a brother and sister: Clinical features and pattern of inheritance. *Eur. J. Pediatr.* 147:539, 1988. Used by permission.)

Strisciuglio P, et al: Martsolf's syndrome in a non-Jewish boy. *J. Med. Genet.* 25:267, 1988.

MASA SYNDROME

Mode of Inheritance: Not definitely known; possibilities: X-linked recessive, sex-influenced autosomal dominant, etc.; reported in a Mexican American family (six males in four sibships of three generations and one female).

Frequency: Seven members of a family (Bianchine and Lewis).

Clinical and Radiologic Manifestations: (a) mental retardation; (b) aphasia; (c) shuffling gait; (d) adducted thumbs.

Note: The acronym MASA refers to the above manifestations of the syndrome.

REFERENCE

Bianchine JW, Lewis RC Jr: The MASA syndrome: A new heritable mental retardation syndrome. *Clin. Genet.* 5:298, 1974.

MAYER-ROKITANSKY-KÜSTER SYNDROME

Synonyms: Mayer-Rokitansky-Küster-Hauser syndrome; Mayer-Rokitansky syndrome; Rokitansky-Küster-Hauser syndrome.

Pathology: (a) vaginal atresia/agenesis; (b) variable müllerian duct abnormalities: bicornuate or septated uterus, rudimentary uterus, ectopic position of the uterine bud in the inguinal region, solid duplication of the uterus, fibromatous lesions from the uterine bud (fibromyoma), etc; (c) usually normal fallopian tubes and ovaries, broad and round ligaments; (d) renal anomalies (in about 35% to 50% of cases): unilateral agenesis, pelvic kidney, etc; (e) endometriosis.

Clinical Manifestations: (a) cyclical cramping lower abdominal pain; (b) abdominal mass; (c) amenorrhea; (d) vaginal atresia; (e) normal genotype, phenotype, and endocrine status; (f) other reported abnormalities: congenital deafness, facial abnormalities, Turner syndrome.

Radiologic Manifestations: (a) ultrasonographic demonstration of the genitourinary anomalies: absence of vagina, thin uncanalized vaginal plate, uterus anomalies, renal anomalies; (b) skeletal anomalies (in about 10% of cases): brachymesophalangia of digits 2 to 5, long proximal phalanx of digits 3 and 4, long metacarpals of digits 1 to 4, radial dysplasia, carpal abnormalities, phocomelia, vertebral anomalies (fusion, wedge shaped, Klippel-Feil syndrome), etc. (Fig SY–M–12).

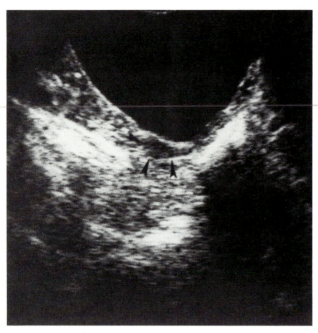

FIG SY–M–12.
Mayer-Rokitansky-Küster syndrome in an 18-year-old woman with primary amenorrhea and the absence of cyclical cramping lower abdominal pain. A longitudinal midline scan of the pelvis shows a thin vaginal plate with an absence of the usual bright midline vaginal echo. The uterus is severely atretic *(arrowheads)* with nonvisualization of the endometrial echos. (From Swayne LC, Rubenstein JB, Mitchell B: The Mayer-Rokitansky-Küster-Hauser syndrome: Sonographic aid to diagnosis. *J. Ultrasound Med.* 5:287, 1986. Used by permission.)

REFERENCES

Griffin JE, et al.: Congenital absence of the vagina—the Mayer-Rokitansky-Küster-Hauser syndrome. *Ann. Intern. Med.* 85:224, 1976.

Hauser GA, et al.: Das Mayer-Rokitansky-Küster-Syndrom. *Schweiz. Med. Wochenschr.* 91:381, 1961.

Küster H: Uterus bipartitus solidus rudimentarius cum vagina solida. *Z. Geb. Gyn.* 67:692, 1910 (cited in Griffin et al.).

Mahboubi S, et al.: Computed tomography finding in Mayer-Rokitansky-Küster-Hauser syndrome associated with endometriosis: A case report. *J. Comput. Tomogr.* 11:301, 1987.

Mayer CAJ: Uber Verdoppelungen des Uterus und ihre Arten, nebst Bemerkungen über Hasenscharte und Wolfsrachen. *J. Chir. Auger* 13:525, 1829.

Opitz JM: Editorial comment: Vaginal atresia (von Mayer-Rokitansky-Küster or MRK anomaly) in hereditary renal adysplasia (HRA). *Am. J. Med. Genet.* 26:873, 1987.

Pavanello Rde C, et al.: Relationship between Mayer-Rokitansky-Küster (MRK) anomaly and hereditary renal adysplasia (HRA). *Am. J. Med. Genet.* 29:845, 1988.

Rokitansky K: Ueber sog. Verdoppelung des Uterus. *Med. Jb. Osterreich Staates* 26:39, 1838.

Rosenberg HK, et al.: Mayer-Rokitansky-Küster-Hauser syndrome: US aid to diagnosis. *Radiology* 161:815, 1986.

Stephens FD: The Mayer-Rokitansky syndrome. *J. Urol.* 135:106, 1986.

Strübbe EH, et al.: Evaluation of radiographic abnormalities of the hand in patients with the Mayer-Rokitansky-Küster-Hauser syndrome. *Skeletal Radiol.* 16:227, 1987.

Swayne LC, et al.: The Mayer-Rokitansky-Küster-Hauser syndrome: Sonographic aid to diagnosis. *J. Ultrasound Med.* 5:287, 1986.

Toublanc JE, et al.: Syndrome de Turner et syndrome de Rokitansky-Küster-Hauser. Association chez une patiente à caryotype 45,X/46,XX. *Ann. Pediatr. (Paris)* 34:43, 1987.

Vainright JR Jr, et al.: MR imaging of vaginal agenesis with hematocolpos. *J. Comput. Assist. Tomogr.* 12:891, 1988.

MAY-THURNER SYNDROME

Pathology: "Spur" (medial, lateral, diaphragm) of the left common iliac vein at the level of the crossover position of the right common iliac artery; marked hypertrophy of the intima of the left common iliac vein.

Clinical Manifestations: (a) long-standing edema of the left leg; (b) hemodynamic study: significant difference of pressure between the lower inferior cava and the external iliac vein.

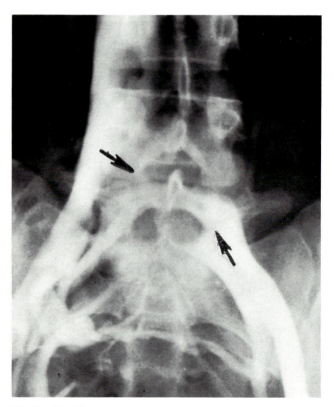

FIG SY–M–13.
May-Thurner syndrome. A left femoral venogram illustrates the defect (between the *arrows*) that causes the partial obstruction. Note the collateral flow across the midline to opacify the right internal and common iliac veins. (From Ferris EJ, Lim WN, Smith PL, et al.: May-Thurner syndrome. *Radiology* 147:29, 1983. Used by permission.)

Radiologic Manifestations: Venous obstruction shown by venography or computed tomography.

Note: Variant of the syndrome: left-leg edema associated with venous obstruction due to compression by a tortuous left common iliac artery (Fig SY–M–13).

REFERENCES

Ferris EJ, et al.: May-Thurner syndrome. *Radiology* 147:29, 1983.
Hassell DR, et al.: Unilateral left leg edema: A variation of the May-Thurner syndrome. *Cardiovasc. Intervent. Radiol.* 10:89, 1987.
May R, Thurner J: Ein Gefßspornin der v. iliaca com. sin. als wahrscheinliche Ursache der uberwiegend liknsseitigen Beckenvenenthrombose. *Z. Kreislforsch.* 45:912, 1956.

MAXILLOFACIAL DYSOSTOSIS

Mode of Inheritance: Autosomal dominant.

Frequency: Rare.

Clinical and Radiologic Manifestations: (a) maxillary hypoplasia (anteroposterior shortening of the maxilla); (b) delayed onset of speech, poor development of language skills without associated hearing loss; (c) other reported abnormalities: downslanting of the palpebral fissures, minor auricle abnormalities.

Differential Diagnosis: Treacher Collins syndrome; Binder syndrome.

REFERENCES

Escobar V, et al.: Maxillofacial dysostosis. *J. Med. Genet.* 14:355, 1977.
Villaret M, et al.: L'hypoplasie primitive familiale due maxillaire superieur. *Ann. Med.* 32:378, 1932.

McCUNE-ALBRIGHT SYNDROME

Synonym: Albright syndrome; Weil-Albright syndrome.

Mode of Inheritance: Usually sporadic; some autosomal dominant pedigrees.

Frequency: Uncommon, but probably underreported; predominantly female, about 13 males reported.

The Triad: (a) *patchy cutaneous pigmentation;* (b) *sexual precocity;* (c) *polyostotic fibrous dysplasia.*

Clinical Manifestations: Onset of symptoms in childhood: (a) *precocious puberty;* (b) *café au lait spots,* often unilateral on the same side as the bone manifestation; (c) *various endocrinopathies:* hyperthyroidism, goiter, hyperadrenocorticism, gigantism, acromegaly, luteinized follicular cysts of the ovaries, gynecomastia, accelerated growth without precocious puberty, hyperparathyroidism, hyperplasia of target organs, pituitary adenoma, hyperprolactinemia; (d) other reported abnormalities: height and weight greater than 95th percentile for age, hypophosphatemic rickets/osteomalacia, high-output cardiac failure, kyphoscoliosis, soft-tissue myxoma, etc.

Radiologic Manifestations: (a) *advanced skeletal maturation,* premature closure of growth plates resulting in short stature; (b) *polyostotic fibrous dysplasia,* often unilateral, with the pelvis and upper portion of the femur the most common sites; dense skull lesions; bone scintigraphy valuable in early detection of the lesions; (c) pathological fractures; (d) upward convexity of the intrasellar contents, focal area of abnormal attenuation of the pituitary, increase in the height (>7 mm) of the pituitary; (e) pelvic ultrasonography: *enlarged ovaries,* asymmetrical enlargement of the ovaries, ovarian cysts, postpubertal uterine size.

Notes: (a) sexual precocity may be gonadotropin dependent (true precocious puberty) or gonadotropin independent (precocious pseudopuberty) due to autonomous ovarian hyperactivity; (b) autonomous multiendocrine hyperfunction in some cases; (c) an autosomal "dominant" lethal gene surviving by mosaicism has been postulated, with endocrinopathy being either of central or peripheral origin according to the

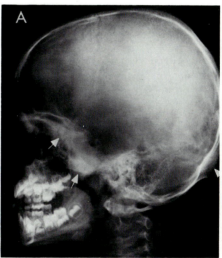
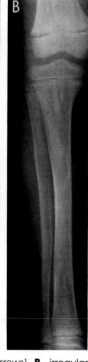
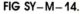

FIG SY–M–14.
McCune-Albright syndrome in a 6-year-old female who was first evaluated at 3 years of age for precocious puberty and café au lait spots. A skeletal survey showed generalized fibrous dysplasia, more marked on right side. **A,** increased density at the base of the skull *(arrows)*. **B,** irregular opaque lesions of the femur, tibia, and fibula. Note the widening of the proximal two thirds of the fibula and a segment of the shaft of the tibia.

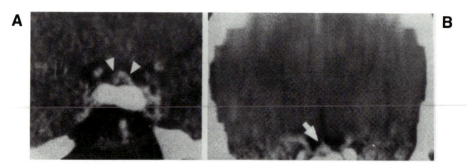

FIG SY—M—15.

McCune-Albright syndrome: Transverse axial **(A)** and coronal **(B)** computed tomographic scans through the pituitary gland after contrast material administration shows an enlarged, upward convex pituitary *(arrowheads).* (From Rieth KG, Comite F, Shawker TH, et al.: Pituitary and ovarian abnormalities demonstrated by CT and ultrasound in children with features of McCune-Albright syndrome. *Radiology* 153:389, 1984. Used by permission.)

random distribution of the mutant population of cells (Happle) (Figs SY—M—14 and SY—M—15).

REFERENCES

Albright F, et al.: Syndrome characterized by osteitis fibrosa disseminata, areas of pigmentation and endocrine dysfunction with precocious puberty in females: Report of five cases. *N. Engl. J. Med.* 216:727, 1937.

Chung KF, et al.: Acromegaly and hyperprolactinemia in McCune-Albright syndrome. Evidence of hypothalamic dysfunction. *Am. J. Dis. Child.* 137:134, 1983.

D'Armiento M, et al.: McCune-Albright syndrome: Evidence for autonomous multiendocrine hyperfunction. *J. Pediatr.* 102:584, 1983.

Dohler JR, et al.: Fibrous dysplasia of bone and the Weil-Albright syndrome. *Int. Orthop.* 10:53, 1986.

Edeburn GF, et al.: Value of bone scan in the McCune-Albright syndrome. *Acta Radiol.* 27:719, 1986.

Foster CM, et al.: Absence of pubertal gonadotropin secretion in girls with McCune-Albright syndrome. *J. Clin. Endocrinol. Metab.* 58:1161, 1984.

Friedel VB, et al.: Verlauf und Differentialdiagnostik des McCune-Albright-Syndroms. *Fortschr. Rontgenstr.* 144:552, 1986.

Happle R: The McCune-Albright syndrome: A lethal gene surviving by mosaicism. *Clin. Genet.* 29:321, 1986.

Joishy SK, et al.: McCune-Albright syndrome associated with a functioning pituitary chromophobe adenoma. *J. Pediatr.* 89:73, 1976.

Kaplan FS, et al.: Estrogen receptors in bone in a patient with polyostotic fibrous dysplasia (McCune-Albright syndrome). *N. Engl. J. Med.* 319:421, 1988.

Lever EG, et al.: Albright's syndrome associated with a soft-tissue myxoma and hypophosphataemic osteomalacia. *J. Bone Joint Surg. [Br.]* 65:621, 1983.

Lightner ES, et al.: Pituitary adenoma in McCune-Albright syndrome (letter). *J. Pediatr.* 89:159, 1976.

McArthur RG, et al.: Albright's syndrome with rickets. *Mayo Clin. Proc.* 54:313, 1979.

McCune DJ: Osteitis fibrosa cystica: The case of a nine-year-old girl who also exhibits precocious puberty, multiple pigmentations of the skin and hyperthyroidism. *Am. J. Dis. Child.* 52:743, 1936.

Pasquino AM, et al.: Precocious puberty in the McCune-Albright syndrome. *Acta Paediatr. Scand.* 76:841, 1987.

Pasquino AM, et al.: Precocious puberty in the McCune-Albright syndrome. Progression from gonadotrophin-independent to gonadotrophin-dependent puberty in a girl. *Acta Paediatr. Scand.* 76:841, 1987.

Probst FP: The Albright-McCune syndrome. *Radiologe* 21:186, 1981.

Rieth KG, et al.: Pituitary and ovarian abnormalities demonstrated by CT and ultrasound in children with features of the McCune-Albright syndrome. *Radiology* 153:389, 1984.

Tanaka T, et al.: A case of McCune-Albright syndrome with hyperthyroidism and vitamin D—resistant rickets. *Helv. Paediatr. Acta* 32:263, 1977.

Weil H: Pubertas praecox und knochenbruchigkeit. *Klin. Wochenschr.* 1:2114, 1922.

MECKEL SYNDROME

Synonyms: Dysencephalia splanchnocystica; Gruber syndrome.

Mode of Inheritance: Autosomal recessive.

Frequency: Approximately 100 reported cases to 1984; 67 cases in 48 Finnish families (Salonen).

Pathology: (a) *microcephaly/anencephaly, occipital encephalocele, hydrocephaly;* (b) *cystic dysplasia of the kidneys;* (c) *fibrotic liver changes, proliferation and dilatation of the bile ducts;* (d) other reported abnormalities: congenital heart defects; urinary system anomalies; alimentary system anomalies; microcystic hamartomatous malformations of the liver, pancreas, and lung; cleft or hypoplastic epiglottis; ear anomalies; absent olfactory lobes; Arnold-Chiari malformation; situs anomalies; M-anisosplenia syndrome.

Clinical Manifestations: Phenotypic variability: (a) *microcephaly, occipital encephalocele;* (b) *cleft lip and palate;* (c) *polydactyly (hands, feet),* clubfeet; (d) microphthalmos/anophthalmia; (e) α-fetoprotein assay in midtrimester: ele-

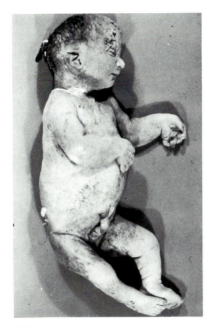

FIG SY—M—16.
Meckel syndrome: Postmortem photograph. Note the microcephaly, small encephalocele, bulging abdomen, and polydactyly. (From Seppänen U, Herva R: Roentgenologic features of the Meckel syndrome. *Pediatr. Radiol.* 13:329, 1983. Used by permission.)

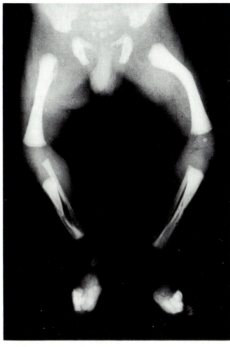

FIG SY—M—18.
Meckel syndrome: bowing of the long tubular bones of the lower limbs. The patient had an occipital encephalocele, preaxial and postaxial polysyndactyly of the hands, and duplication of the big toes. (From Majewski F, Stöss H, Goecke T, et al.: Are bowing of long tubular bone and preaxial polydactyly signs of the Meckel syndrome? *Hum. Genet.* 65:125, 1983. Used by permission.)

vated; (f) other reported abnormalities: micrognathia, lobulated tongue, small or ambiguous genitalia, short neck, webbed neck, short limbs, syndactyly, clinodactyly, abdominal distension, narrow thorax, polysplenia, etc.

Radiologic Manifestations: (a) *brain dysgenesis* (encephalocele, hydrocephalus, etc.); (b) short limbs; (c) prenatal sonography: oligohydramnios, small head diameter, cystic mass at the occiput, large kidneys, absent bladder (Figs SY—M—16 to SY—M—18).

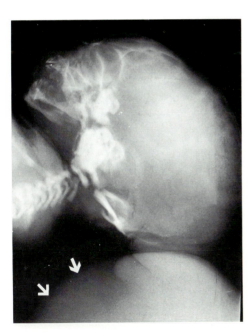

FIG SY—M—17.
Meckel syndrome. A lateral view of the head shows an occipital defect and a retrocranial "mass" *(arrows)*. (From Seppänen U, Herva R: Roentgenologic features of the Meckel syndrome. *Pediatr. Radiol.* 13:329, 1983. Used by permission.)

REFERENCES

Fraser FC, et al.: Spectrum of anomalies in the Meckel syndrome, or: "Maybe there is a malformation syndrome with at least one constant anomaly." *Am. J. Med. Genet.* 9:67, 1981.

Gruber GB: Beiträge zur Frage "gekoppelter" Missbildungen (Akrocephalo-Syndactylie und Dysencephalia splanchnocystica). *Beitr. Pathol. Anat.* 93:459, 1934.

Johnson VP, et al.: Prenatal diagnosis of Meckel syndrome: Case reports and literature review. *Am. J. Med. Genet.* 18:699, 1984.

Lawry RB, et al.: Survival and spectrum of anomalies in the Meckel syndrome. *Am. J. Med. Genet.* 14:417, 1983.

Majewski F, et al.: Are bowing of long tubular bones and

preaxial polydactyly signs of the Meckel syndrome? *Hum. Genet.* 65:125, 1983.

Meckel JF: Beschreibung zweier durch sehr ähnliche Bildungsabweichungen entstellter Geschwister. *Dtsch. Arch. Physiol.* 7:99, 1822.

Moerman Ph, et al.: Association of Meckel syndrome with M-anisosplenia in one patient. *Clin. Genet.* 22:143, 1982.

Salonen R: The Meckel syndrome: Clinicopathological findings in 67 patients. *Am. J. Med. Genet.* 18:671, 1984.

Seller MJ: Phenotypic variations in Meckel syndrome. *Clin. Genet.* 20:74, 1981.

Seppänen U, et al.: Roentgenologic features of the Meckel syndrome. *Pediatr. Radiol.* 13:329, 1983.

Shen-Schwarz S, et al.: Meckel syndrome with polysplenia: Case report and review of the literature. *Am. J. Med. Genet.* 31:349, 1988.

MECONIUM PLUG SYNDROME

Clinical Manifestations: (a) abdominal distension; (b) vomiting of green-stained material; (c) *passage of meconium plug* followed usually by clinical improvement; (d) ileal meconium plug (white plug) associated with a high incidence of complications; (e) association with other diseases: cystic fibrosis, Hirschsprung disease, exocrine pancreatic insufficiency, intussusception (ileal meconium plug), small left colon syndrome.

Radiologic Manifestations: (a) *small- and large-bowel distension, mottled or bulky intraluminal colonic meconium masses,* presacral "mass" on a lateral radiogram of the abdomen (intraluminal rectal plug), air-fluid levels in the bowel uncommon; (b) contrast enema: *meconium cast in the colon,* long narrow segment of bowel (small left colon); (c) prenatal ultrasound: progressive dilatation of intestines, relief of obstruction by intrauterine therapy (swallowed contrast material used for amniography) (Fig SY–M–19).

REFERENCES

Berdon WE, et al.: Neonatal small left colon syndrome: Its relationship to aganglionosis and meconium plug syndrome. *Radiology* 125:457, 1977.

Campbell JB, et al.: Hirschsprung disease presenting as the meconium plug syndrome (abstract). Presented at the International Pediatric Radiology Meeting, Toronto, 1987.

Clatworthy HW Jr, et al.: Meconium plug syndrome. *Surgery* 39:131, 1956.

Cooney DR, et al.: Maternal and postnatal hypermagnesemia and the meconium plug syndrome. *J. Pediatr. Surg.* 11:167, 1976.

Hen J Jr, et al.: Meconium plug syndrome associated with cystic fibrosis and Hirschsprung's disease. *Pediatrics* 66:466, 1980.

Pochaczevsky R, et al.: The meconium plug syndrome: Roentgen evaluation and differentiation from Hirschsprung's disease and other pathologic states. *A.J.R.* 120:342, 1974.

Rosenstein BJ, et al.: Incidence of meconium abnormalities in newborn infants with cystic fibrosis. *Am. J. Dis. Child.* 134:72, 1980.

Samuel N, et al.: Early diagnosis and intrauterine therapy of meconium plug syndrome in the fetus: Risks and benefits. *J. Ultrasound Med.* 5:425, 1986.

Starshak RJ, et al.: Meconium plug syndrome associated with neonatal intussusception. *Gastrointest. Radiol.* 6:75, 1981.

Talwalker V, et al.: Ileal meconium plugs. *Arch. Dis. Child.* 55:288, 1980.

Taybi H, Patterson J: Plain film diagnosis of meconium plug syndrome: Presacral "mass." *Radiology* 104:113, 1972.

Townes PL, et al.: Meconium plug syndrome, cystic fibrosis and exocrine pancreatic deficiency. *Am. J. Dis. Child.* 132:1043, 1978.

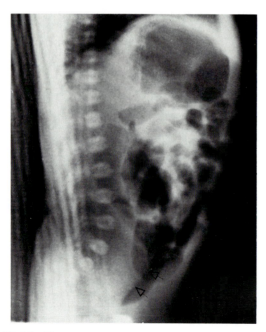

FIG SY–M–19.
Meconium plug syndrome. A meconium plug in the rectum *(arrows)* is outlined anteriorly by gas. (From Taybi H, Patterson J: Plain film diagnosis of meconium plug syndrome: Presacral mass. *Radiology* 104:113, 1972. Used by permission.)

MEDIAN CLEFT FACE SYNDROME

Synonym: Frontonasal dysplasia.

Mode of Inheritance: Most cases sporadic; few familial cases (autosomal recessive or dominant).

Frequency: Uncommon.

Classification: Four types according to the severity of the congenital anomalies: (a) cranium bifidum occultum frontalis; orbital hypertelorism; a complete cleft between the orbits, maxillary bones, and ethmoid elements; absence of the corpus callosum in some; (b) orbital hypertelorism, median cleft of the nose, cranium bifidum occultum frontalis; (c) orbital hypertelorism, median cleft nose, median cleft prolabium; (d) orbital hypertelorism, median cleft nose.

Clinical Manifestations: (a) *unilateral or bilateral notching of the nose or the alae nasi, ocular hypertelorism, broad nasal bridge, absence of the tip of the nose, anterior cranium bifidum,* V-shaped frontal hairline, primary telecanthus, median cleft upper lip, median cleft palate; (b) ocular abnormalities: epicanthal folds, accessory nasal eyelid tissue with secondary displacement of the inferior puncti laterally, uveal colobomas, epibulbar dermoid tumors, coloboma of the upper lids, unilateral microphthalmos, vitreoretinal degeneration with retinal detachment, congenital cataracts; (c) other reported abnormalities: brachydactyly, clinodactyly, camptodactyly, preauricular skin tags, encephalocele associated with cranium bifidum frontalis, meningocele, meningoencephalocele, cryptorchidism, tetralogy of Fallot, mental retardation in association with an absent corpus callosum, etc.

Radiologic Manifestations: (a) cranium bifidum frontalis, orbital hypertelorism, midline cleft involving various bony structures, maxillary hypoplasia, hypoplastic frontal sinuses; (b) deformed anterior portion of the lateral ventricles and anterior cerebral arteries, agenesis/hypogenesis of the corpus callosum, lipoma of the corpus callosum, vertical bony bar in the intracranial midline; (c) other reported abnormalities: hydrocephalus, holoprosencephaly, choanal atresia.

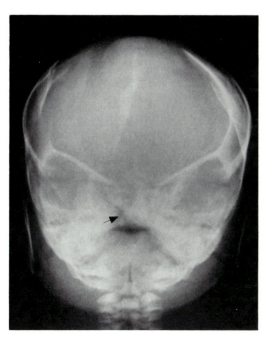

FIG SY—M—20.
Median cleft face syndrome (type 1) in a 1-day-old male with marked hypertelorism. Maxillary bones are separated by "ethmoid filler." Note the cleft in the palatine processes of the maxillary bones *(arrow).* A median bony bar is present in the frontal region, with large defects in ossification on either side. (From Kurlander GJ, De Myer W, Campbell JA: Roentgenology of the median cleft face syndrome. *Radiology* 88:473, 1967. Used by permission.)

Differential Diagnosis: deMorsier syndrome (septo-optic dysplasia); cranio-fronto-nasal dysplasia; bifid nose (dominantly inherited) without apparent hypertelorism; median cleft of the upper lip associated with lipomas of the central nervous system and cutaneous polyps (Fig SY—M—20).

REFERENCES

Anyane-Yeboa K, et al.: Dominant inheritance of bifid nose. *Am. J. Med. Genet.* 17:561, 1984.

Bömelburg T, et al.: Median cleft face syndrome in association with hydrocephalus, agenesis of the corpus callosum, holoprosencephaly and choanal atresia. *Eur. J. Pediatr.* 146:301, 1987.

De Moor MMA, et al.: Frontonasal dysplasia associated with tetralogy of Fallot. *J. Med. Genet.* 24:107, 1987.

DeMyer W: Median facial malformations and their implications for brain malformation. *Birth Defects* 11:155, 1975.

Fontaine G, et al.: La dysplasie fronto-nasale (A propos de quatre observations). *J. Genet. Hum.* 31:351, 1983.

Fuenmayor HM: The spectrum of frontonasal dysplasia in an inbred pedigree. *Clin. Genet.* 17:137, 1980.

Gollop TR: Fronto-facio-nasal dysostosis—A new autosomal recessive syndrome (letter). *Am. J. Med. Genet.* 10:409, 1981.

Kinsey JA, et al.: Ocular abnormalities in the median cleft face syndrome. *Am. J. Ophthalmol.* 83:261, 1977.

Kurlander GJ, DeMyer W, Campbell JA: Roentgenology of the median cleft face syndrome. *Radiology* 88:473, 1967.

Kwee ML, et al.: Frontonasal dysplasia, coronal craniosynostosis, pre- and postaxial polydactyly and split nails: A new autosomal dominant mutant with reduced penetrance and variable expression? *Clin. Genet.* 24:200, 1983.

LaRoche GR, et al.: Septo-optic dysplasia and median cleft face syndrome. *Am. J. Dis. Child.* 138:795, 1984.

Naidich TP, et al.: Median cleft face syndrome: MR and CT data from 11 children. *J. Comput. Assist. Tomogr.* 12:57, 1988.

Pai GS, et al.: Median cleft of the upper lip associated with lipomas of the central nervous system and cutaneous polyps. *Am. J. Med. Genet.* 26:921, 1987.

Pascual-Castroviejo I, et al.: Fronto-nasal dysplasia and lipoma of the corpus callosum. *Eur. J. Pediatr.* 144:66, 1985.

MEDITERRANEAN FEVER

Synonyms: Paroxysmal syndrome; familial recurrent polyserositis; periodic disease; Siegal-Cattan-Mamou disease; Armenian disease; periodic abdominalgia; benign paroxysmal peritonitis; Reimann periodic disease.

Mode of Inheritance: Autosomal recessive, principally affecting Armenians, Turks, Arabs, Jews.

Clinical Manifestations: (a) *episodes of abdominal, chest, or joint pain; (b) fever; (c) serositis (pleuritis, peritonitis, pericarditis, and meningitis); (d) erysipelas-like erythema, purpura, panniculitis; (e) secondary amyloidosis, nephrotic syndrome and kidney failure, renal vein thrombosis, glomer-*

ulonephritis, hypersensitivity angiitis, spontaneous perirenal hematoma; (f) leukocytosis; elevated erythrocyte sedimentation rate; elevated values of C-reactive protein, seromucoid, plasma fibrinogen, lipoproteins, and haptoglobins; appearance of cryofibrinogenemia during attacks; C5a inhibitor deficiency in peritoneal and synovial fluids; (g) positive metaraminol provocative test (10-mg dose of metaraminol infusion resulting in a typical diseaselike attack within 48 hours, preventable by colchicine therapy).

Radiologic Manifestations: (a) pleural effusion, peritoneal effusion, pericardial effusion and/or thickening, high and almost immobile diaphragm; (b) joint effusion, periarticular swelling (sacroiliac, hip, knee, and temporomandibular joints in particular), joint narrowing, progressive joint destruction, bone sclerosis adjacent to joint cartilage with or without bone erosions; (c) aseptic necrosis of the femoral head; (d) osteoporosis; (e) bowel obstruction due to peritoneal adhesions, adynamic ileus, discontinuity of a barium column with dilatation and a delay in transit time of the contrast medium.

REFERENCES

Barakat MH, et al.: Metaraminol provocative test: A specific diagnostic test for familial Mediterranean fever. *Lancet* 1:656, 1984.
Bradey PA, et al.: Radiographic changes in the sacroiliac joints in familial Mediterranean fever. *Radiology* 114:331, 1975.
Dabestani A, et al.: Pericardial disease in familial Mediterranean fever. *Chest* 81:592, 1982.
Danar DA, et al.: Panniculitis in familial Mediterranean fever. *Am. J. Med.* 82:829, 1987.
Dor J-F, et al.: Hématome péri-rénal spontané au cours d'une maladie périodique. *Nouv. Presse Med.* 8:1927, 1979.
Gilsanz V, et al.: Familial Mediterranean fever. *A.J.R.* 134:1293, 1980.
Lachaux A, et al.: Les manifestations cutanées de la maladie périodique. *Arch. Fr. Pediatr.* 43:711, 1986.
Matzner Y, et al.: C5a-inhibitor deficiency in peritoneal fluids from patients with familial Mediterranean fever. *N. Engl. J. Med.* 311:287, 1984.
Méry J-Ph: L'amylose de la maladie périodique. *Presse Med.* 13:475, 1984.
Reuben A, et al.: Renal vein thrombosis as the major cause of renal failure in familial Mediterranean fever. *Q. J. Med.* 46:243, 1977.
Shamir H, et al.: Cryofibrinogen in familial Mediterranean fever. *Arch. Intern. Med.* 134:125, 1974.
Siegal S: Benign paroxysmal peritonitis. *Ann. Intern. Med.* 23:1, 1945.
Simon G, et al.: Familial Mediterranean fever with temporomandibular joint arthritis. *Pediatrics* 57:810, 1976.
Sneh E, et al.: Protracted arthritis in familial Mediterranean fever. *Rheumatol. Rehabil.* 16:102, 1979.
Tal Y, et al.: Intestinal obstruction caused by primary adhesions due to familial Mediterranean fever. *J. Pediatr. Surg.* 15:186, 1980.
Yagil Y, et al.: Case report 195: Inflammatory synovitis due to familial Mediterranean feve (FMF) of left third metatarso-phalangeal joint. *Skeletal Radiol.* 8:157, 1982.
Zemer D, et al.: Colchicine in the prevention and treatment of the amyloidosis of familial Mediterranean fever. *N. Engl. J. Med.* 314:1001, 1986.

MEGACYSTIS-MEGAURETER SYNDROME

Synonym: Megaureter-megacystis syndrome.

Clinical Manifestations: (a) fever, abdominal pain, failure to thrive; (b) infrequent voiding, urinary retention, enuresis, weak urinary stream; (c) urinary tract infection in about three fourths of cases.

Pathophysiology: Vesicoureteral reflux; constant recycling of large volumes of refluxed urine.

Radiologic Manifestations: (a) large-capacity, smooth, thin-walled bladder; (b) massive vesicoureteral reflux; (c) no bladder outlet or urethral obstruction.

Differential Diagnosis: Hinman syndrome.

REFERENCES

Burbige KA, et al.: The megacystis-megaureter syndrome. *J. Urol.* 131:1133, 1984.
Koefoot RB Jr, et al.: The primary megacystis syndrome. *J. Urol.* 125:232, 1981.
Willi UV, et al.: The so-called megaureter-megacystis syndrome. *A.J.R.* 133:409, 1979.
Williams DI: The chronically dilated ureter: Hunterian lecture. *Ann. R. Coll. Surg.* 14:107, 1954.

MEGACYSTIS-MICROCOLON-INTESTINAL HYPOPERISTALSIS SYNDROME

Synonym: Berdon syndrome.

Mode of Inheritance: Autosomal recessive; female preponderance of 4:1.

Frequency: More than 30 published cases (Vintzileos et al., and others).

Pathology: Abundant intestinal ganglion cells in early biopsies and normal or even decreased numbers of ganglion cells in later biopsies (probably due to bowel dilatation), ischemic changes of bowel wall, elastosis of the urinary bladder, electron microscopic examination of the ileum and urinary bladder: vacuolar degenerative changes in the smooth muscle cells with an abundant amount of connective tissue between the muscle cells ("visceral myopathy").

Clinical Manifestations: Onset of symptoms in the neonatal period: (a) *abdominal distension, decreased or absent bowel movements,* bilious vomiting, absent or decreased

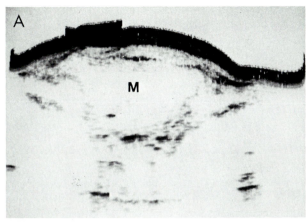

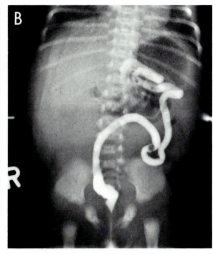

FIG SY-M-21.
Megacystis-microcolon-intestinal hypoperistalsis syndrome in a newborn girl with abdominal distension and bilious vomiting. **A,** abdominal sonography shows a cystic abdominal mass (huge bladder, *M*). **B,** a contrast enema shows a microcolon. (From Sumner TE, Crowe JE, Klein A, et al.: Radiological case of the month. *Am. J. Dis. Child.* 135:67, 1981. Used by permission.)

bowel sounds; (b) external appearance of a "prune belly," thin abdominal muscles but always present, bilateral flank masses (kidneys), large midline abdominal mass (bladder); (c) manometric study of the stomach and duodenum: low frequency and low amplitude of the contractions; (d) intrauterine death.

Radiologic Manifestations: (a) *microcolon,* malrotation/malfixation of the bowel, *intestinal hypoperistalsis, dilated small bowel,* volvulus of the bowel; (b) *megalocystis,* hydronephrosis, hydroureter, absence of bladder outlet obstruction, vesicoureteral reflux; (c) antenatal ultrasound: polyhydramnios, markedly enlarged bladder, thick-walled fetal bladder, hydroureter, hydronephrosis.

Differential Diagnosis: Vesical gigantism without obstruction in the bladder neck or urethra; idiopathic intestinal pseudo-obstruction; etc.

Notes: (a) a newborn girl has been reported whose brother had prune-belly syndrome; (b) a newborn girl with this syndrome was born to a mother who ingested clomiphene during pregnancy (Fig SY-M-21).

REFERENCES

Bagwell CE, et al.: Neonatal intestinal pseudoobstruction. *J. Pediatr. Surg.* 19:732, 1984.

Berdon WE, et al.: Megacystis-microcolon-intestinal hypoperistalsis syndrome: A new cause of intestinal obstruction in the newborn. Report of radiologic findings in five newborn girls. *A.J.R.* 126:957, 1976.

Doğruyol H, et al.: Megacystis-microcolon-intestinal hypoperistalsis syndrome in a newborn after clomiphene ingestion during pregnancy. *Z. Kinderchir.* 42:321, 1987.

Farrell SA: Intrauterine death in megacystis-microcolon-intestinal hypoperistalsis syndrome. *J. Med. Genet.* 25:350, 1988.

Hurwitz A, et al.: Hydramnios caused by pure megacystis. *J. Clin. Ultrasound* 12:110, 1984.

Inamdar S, et al.: Vesical gigantism or congenital megacystis. *Urology* 24:601, 1984.

Leonidas JC, et al.: Berdon Syndrome. *A.J.R.* 139:1236, 1982.

Oliveira G, et al.: Megacystis-microcolon-intestinal hypoperistalsis syndrome in a newborn girl whose brother had prune belly syndrome: Common pathogenesis? *Pediatr. Radiol.* 13:294, 1983.

Puri P, et al.: Megacystis-microcolon-intestinal hypoperistalsis syndrome: A visceral myopathy. *J. Pediatr. Surg.* 18:64, 1983.

Sumner TE, Crowe JE, Klein A, et al.: Radiological case of the month. *Am. J. Dis. Child.* 135:67, 1981.

Tomomasa T, et al.: Manometric study on the intestinal motility in a case of megacystis-microcolon-intestinal hypoperistalsis syndrome. *J. Pediatr. Gastroenterol. Nutr.* 4:307, 1985.

Vintzileos AM, et al.: Megacystis-microcolon-intestinal hypoperistalsis syndrome. Prenatal sonographic findings and review of the literature. *Am. J. Perinatol.* 3:297, 1986.

Winter RM, et al.: Megacystis-microcolon-intestinal hypoperistalsis syndrome: Confirmation of autosomal recessive inheritance. *J. Med. Genet.* 23:360, 1986.

MEIGS SYNDROME

Clinical Manifestations: (a) *benign or malignant ovarian tumor;* (b) *pleural effusion,* spontaneously disappearing after removal of ovarian tumor.

Radiologic Manifestations: *Pelvic tumor, pleural effusion, ascites.*

Note: The association of tumors other than benign ovarian neoplasms of fibrous tissue origin (thecoma, granulosa cell tumors, Brenner tumor) with hydrothorax and ascites has been called pseudo-Meigs syndrome by some.

REFERENCES

Demons A: Epanchements pleurétiques compliquant des kystes de l'ovaire. *Bull. Soc. Chir. (Paris)* 13:771, 1887.

Faber HK: Meigs' syndrome with thecomas of both ovaries in a 4-year-old girl. *J. Pediatr.* 61:769, 1962.

Handler CE, et al.: Atypical Meigs's syndrome. *Thorax* 37:396, 1982.

Loung KC: Pseudo-Meigs' syndrome associated with a pseudomucinous cystadenoma. *Postgrad. Med. J.* 46:631, 1970.

Makrohisky JF: So-called "Meigs' syndrome" associated with benign and malignant ovarian tumors. *Radiology* 70:578, 1958.

Meigs JV: Pelvic tumors other than fibromas of the ovary with ascites and hydrothorax. *Obstet. Gynecol.* 3:471, 1954.

Meigs JV, Cass JW: Fibroma of ovary with ascites and hydrothorax. *Am. J. Obstet. Gynecol.* 33:249, 1937.

Salmon UJ: Benign pelvic tumors associated with ascites and pleural effusion. *J. M. Sinai Hosp. N.Y.* 1:169, 1934.

Solomon S, et al.: Fibromyomata of the uterus with hemothorax-Meigs' syndrome? *Arch. Intern. Med.* 127:307, 1971.

MENDELSON SYNDROME

Etiology: Often postsurgical occurrence of pneumonitis caused by silent aspiration of acidic gastric fluid.

Clinical Manifestations: Sudden postoperative appearance of pulmonary symptoms in patients with previously normal respiratory system, (a) *tachypnea, tachycardia, wheezes, rhonchi, crepitant rales;* (b) fall in arterial oxygen tension; (c) pulmonary edema and shock may develop.

Radiologic Manifestations: Irregular *patchy or confluent lung densities,* frequently bilateral.

REFERENCES

Bynum LJ, et al.: Pulmonary aspiration of gastric contents. *Am. Rev. Respir. Dis.* 114:1129, 1976.

Esquirol E, et al.: Le syndrome de Mendelson: Etude radiologique. *Ann. Radiol. (Paris)* 17:523, 1974.

Landay ML, et al.: Pulmonary manifestations of acute aspiration of gastric contents. *A.J.R.* 131:587, 1978.

MacLennan FM: Maternal mortality from Mendelson's syndrome: An explanation. *Lancet* 1:587, 1986.

Mendelson CL: The aspiration of stomach contents into the lung during obstetrics anesthesia. *Am. J. Obstet. Gynecol.* 52:191, 1946.

Wilkins RA, et al.: Radiology in Mendelson's syndrome. *Clin. Radiol.* 27:81, 1976.

MÉNÉTRIER DISEASE

Synonyms: Hyperplastic gastropathy; hypoproteinemic hypertrophic gastropathy.

Clinical Manifestations: (a) *epigastric pain,* ulcerlike symptoms; (b) *hypoproteinemia;* (c) *edema, ascites;* (d) gastroscopy: *large rugae, sometimes present throughout the*

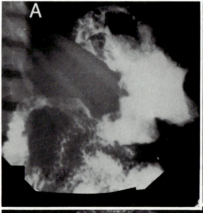
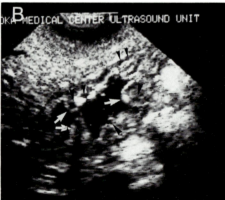
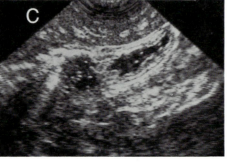

FIG SY–M–22.
Ménétrier disease (transient protein-losing gastropathy) in a 3.5-year-old boy. **A,** a contrast study of the stomach shows irregularity of the gastric contour due to hypertrophied gastric rugae. **B,** gastric ultrasound demonstrates markedly thickened gastric walls and a polypoid tortuosity of the mucosal folds *(arrows).* Note the submucosal echo-free structures *(arrowheads)* representing possibly glandular hypertrophy and basilar cysts. **C,** gastric ultrasound performed 3 months later than **B.** There is complete reversal of mucosal changes. (From Bar-Ziv J, Barki Y, Weizman Z, et al.: Transient protein-losing gastropathy (Ménétrier's disease in childhood). *Pediatr. Radiol.* 18:82, 1988. Used by permission.)

stomach, others limited to various segments of the stomach, most prominent along the greater curvature; (e) other reported abnormalities: anemia, eosinophilia, protein-losing enteropathy, association with gastric ulcer, development of gastric carcinoma, recurrent infections, occlusive thromboembolic and other vascular disorders, pulmonary edema.

Radiologic Manifestations: (a) *enlargement of gastric rugae;* (b) *thick gastric wall;* (c) *mucus mixed with barium;* (d) ultrasonography, computed tomography: thick gastric wall, mucus cysts; (e) ascites, pleural effusion, bowel wall edema.

Differential Diagnosis: Lymphoma; eosinophilic gastroenteritis; multiple gastric polyps; gastric varices; lymphangiectasia; Zollinger-Ellison syndrome.

Note: (a) the prognosis in the childhood form of the disease is generally very good (benign, self-limited, transient), association with cytomegalovirus infection reported in some of the pediatric cases; (b) chronic course in adult form common, with remission in some cases (Fig SY−M−22).

REFERENCES

Baker A, et al.: Childhood Ménétrier's disease: Four new cases and discussion of the literature. *Gastrointest. Radiol.* 11:131, 1986.

Bar-Ziv J, et al.: Transient protein-losing gastropathy (Ménétrier's disease) in childhood. *Pediatr. Radiol.* 18:82, 1988.

Eisenscher A, et al.: Aspect échographique de la gastrite hypertrophique géante ou la maladie de Ménétrier. *J. Radiol.* 61:527, 1980.

Fishman EK, et al.: Ménétrièr Disease. *J. Comput. Assist. Tomogr.* 7:143, 1983.

Marandian MH, et al.: Gastropathie hypertrophique et hémorrhagique de l'enfant, avec une évolution de quinze ans. *Arch. Fr. Pediatr.* 38:513, 1981.

Ménétrier P: Des polyadénomes gastriques et leurs rapports avec le cancer de l'estomac. *Arch. Physiol. Norm. Pathol.* 1:32, 236, 1888.

Searcy RM, et al.: Ménétrièr's disease and idiopathic hypertrophic gastropathy. *Ann. Intern. Med.* 100:565, 1984.

Zenkl B, et al.: Ménétrier disease in a child of 18 months: Diagnosis by ultrasonography. *Eur. J. Pediatr.* 147:330, 1988.

MERMAID SYNDROME

Synonyms: Sirenomelia; sympus apus.

Frequency: 1:60,000 births (Honda et al.).

Clinical and Radiologic Manifestations: (a) *rotation and fusion of the lower limbs;* medial position, fusion, or absence of the fibulas; (b) pelvic bone anomalies; (c) *renal agenesis;* (d) *absence of an anus and external genitalia, blind-ending colon;* (e) oligohydramnios; (f) single umbilical artery; (g) vascular steal has been proposed as the pathogenic mecha-

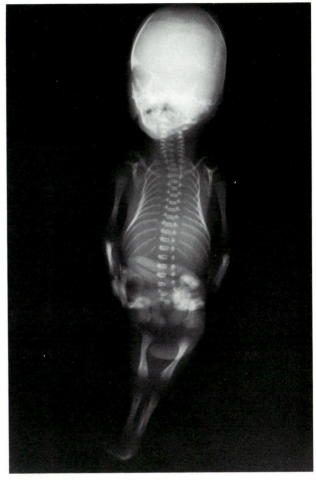

FIG SY−M−23.
Mermaid syndrome: Note fusion of the lower limbs and pelvic anomalies. (From Raabe RD, Harnsberger HR, Lee TG, et al.: Ultrasonographic antenatal diagnosis of "mermaid syndrome." Fusion of fetal lower extremities. *J. Ultrasound Med.* 2:463, 1983. Used by permission.)

nism producing sirenomelia and associate visceral and soft-tissue defects (Fig SY−M−23).

REFERENCES

Honda N, et al.: Antenatal diagnosis of sirenomelia (sympus apus). *J. Clin. Ultrasound* 16:675, 1988.

Raabe. RD, et al.: Ultrasonographic antenatal diagnosis of "mermaid syndrome": Fusion of fetal lower extremities. *J. Ultrasound Med.* 2:463, 1983.

Stevenson RE, et al.: Vascular steal: The pathogenetic mechanism producing sirenomelia and associated defects of the viscera and soft tissues. *Pediatrics* 78:451, 1986.

MEYER DYSPLASIA OF THE FEMORAL HEAD

Synonym: Dysplasia epiphysealis capitis femoris.

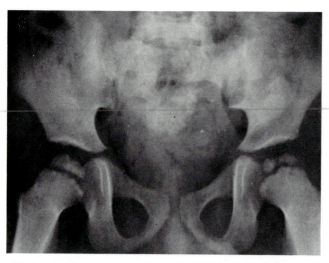

FIG SY—M—24.
Meyer dysplasia of the femoral head in a 3-year, 10-month-old male. Marked delay in development of epiphyseal ossification and irregularity of the ossification center were noted at 2½ years of age on radiograms obtained during excretory urographic examination. As shown, the delay in development and irregularity of ossification persist.

Clinical Manifestations: May be asymptomatic, or there may be limp and hip pain; males more often involved, usually younger than 4 to 5 years of age.

Radiologic Manifestations: (a) *marked delay in development of the epiphyseal ossification center of the femoral heads* (about 2 years); (b) *diffuse granular pattern of ossification* (blackberry type); (c) progression in ossification development, the ossification center becoming normal or near normal at about 6 years of age in most cases; (d) development of aseptic necrosis of the femoral head in some cases (Fig SY—M—24).

REFERENCES

Karup Pedersen E: Dysplasia epiphysealis capitis femoris. *J. Bone Joint Surg. [Br.]* 42:663, 1960.
Maroteaux P, et al.: Dysplasies bilatérales isolées de la hanche chez le jeune enfant. *Ann. Radiol. (Paris)* 24:181, 1981.
Meyer J: Dysplasia epiphysealis capitis femoris: A clinical-radiological syndrome and its relationship to Legg-Calvé Perthès disease. *Acta Orthop. Scand.* 34:183, 1964.

MICROANGIOPATHIC SYNDROME OF ENCEPHALOPATHY-HEARING LOSS-RETINAL ARTERIOLAR OCCLUSION

Clinical and Radiologic Manifestations: (a) subacute encephalopathy (sclerosis of the media and adventitia of small pial and cortical vessels): personality changes, memory loss, unsteady gait, nystagmus, seizures, slurred speech, sensorineural hearing loss, tinnitus, dementia, etc.; (b) retinal branch occlusions; (c) elevated cerebrospinal fluid protein levels; (d) diffuse electroencephalographic slowing; (e) magnetic resonance imaging: several small discrete foci of abnormally high signal intensity throughout the supratentorial white matter in both hemispheres compatible with small infarcts; (f) reported cases have been women in the third or fourth decade of life.

REFERENCE

Monteiro MLR, et al.: A microangiopathic syndrome of encephalopathy, hearing loss, and retinal arteriolar occlusions. *Neurology* 35:1113, 1985.

MIDLINE CERVICAL WEBBING/CLEFT-MICROGNATHIA-SYMPHYSEAL SPUR

Clinical Manifestations: (a) *midline cervical cleft (poorly developed skin, fibrous thickening in the subcutaneous layer and platysma); midline cervical webbing;* (b) *bony prominence in the mental region;* (c) other reported abnormalities: clefting of the lower lip, mandible, and sternum.

Radiologic Manifestations: *Midline bony spur* (exostosis) in the mental region.

Notes: (a) the deformity is considered to be within the spectrum of branchial arch development abnormalities; (b) the deformity related to the subcutaneous fibrous band becomes more conspicuous from childhood to adulthood (Fig SY—M—25).

REFERENCES

Breton P, et al.: Un syndrome malformatif cervical rare: La fissure mentosternale. A propos de 4 observations. *Chir. Pediatr.* 28:170, 1987.
Gargan TJ, et al.: Midline cervical cleft. *Plast. Reconstr. Surg.* 76:225, 1985.
Wood GA, et al.: Anterior midline neck webbing with microgenia and symphyseal exostosis. *Oral Surg.* 56:128, 1983.

MIETENS-WEBER SYNDROME

Mode of Inheritance: Autosomal recessive or incompletely dominant.

Clinical Manifestations: (a) *mental retardation;* (b) *growth failure;* (c) small, narrow, and pointed nose with a depressed root; (d) *bilateral opacity of the corneas, horizontal and rotational nystagmus, strabismus;* (e) *flexion contracture of elbows;* (f) *atrophic calf muscles.*

Radiologic Manifestations: (a) *dislocation of the head of the radius* and absence of its epiphysis; (b) abnormally short ulna and radius; (c) clinodactyly; (d) other reported abnor-

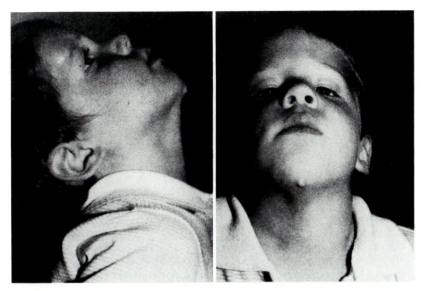

FIG SY–M–25.
Midline cervical webbing and a symphyseal spur are seen. (From Gargan TJ, McKinnon M, Mulliken JB: Midline cervical cleft. *Plast. Reconstr. Surg.* 76:225, 1985. Used by permission.)

malities: absent radii with radial deviation of the hands and flexed thumbs, absent fibula, clubfoot, pes valgus planus.

REFERENCES

Carnevale A, et al.: Mietens-Weber syndrome. A case report. *Rev. Invest. Clin.* 28:347, 1976.
Mietens C, Weber H: A syndrome characterized by corneal opacity, nystagmus, flexion contracture of the elbows, growth failure and mental retardation. *J. Pediatr.* 69:624, 1966.
Nasano A, et al.: Meitens' syndrome. *Arch. Orthop. Unfallchir.* 29:89, 1977.
Waring GO, et al.: Ultrastructure and successful keratoplasty of sclerocornea in Mietens' syndrome. *Am. J. Ophthalmol.* 90:469, 1980.

MIKULICZ SYNDROME

Definition: Any bilateral chronic enlargement of the salivary and lacrimal glands due to disease entities other than Mikulicz disease (benign lymphoepithelial lesion).

Etiology: (a) leukemia; (b) chronic granulomatous diseases (tuberculosis, sarcoidosis, syphilis); (c) lymphoid tissue diseases: malignant lymphoma, Hodgkin disease, lymphoid hyperplasia, Warthin tumor; (d) others: gout, Graves disease, etc.

Clinical Manifestations: (a) *sialadenitis* (periodic episodes of parotid swelling associated with pain, tenderness, and a milky-to-purulent discharge from the Stensen duct), *sialosis* (nontender enlargement of the parotid glands), *multi-nodular enlargement of the gland*; (b) *xerostomia*; (c) *absence or reduction of lacrimation*.

Radiologic Manifestations: (a) sialographic findings of *ectasia of the ducts (sialadenitis), enlarged gland with sparse peripheral ducts (sialosis), decrease in the number of visualized duct radicles and displacement of ducts by granulomatous lesions*; destruction of the duct system in advanced stages; (b) avid tracer accumulation of Ga-67 citrate in the lacrimal and salivary glands and periorbital tissue (in a patient with non-Hodgkin lymphoma; (c) ultrasonography: enlarged lacrimal and salivary glands.

REFERENCES

Mikulicz J: Ueber eine eigenartige symmetrische Erkrankumg der Tränen und Mundspeicheldrüsen. *Beitr. Chir. Fortschr. Gewidmet.* 610, 1892.
Morgan WS, et al.: A clinicopathologic study of "Mikulicz's disease." *Am. J. Pathol.* 29:471, 1953.
Penfold CN: Mikulicz syndrome. *J. Oral Maxillofac. Surg.* 43:900, 1985.
Rubin P, et al.: The sialographic differentiation of Mikulicz's disease and Mikulicz's syndrome. *Radiology* 68:477, 1957.
Singer I, et al: Appearance of Ga-67 citrate scanning in a patient with Mikulicz syndrome associated with non-Hodgkin's lymphoma. *Clin. Nucl. Med.* 9:283, 1984.
Som P, et al.: Manifestations of parotid gland enlargement: Radiographic, pathologic, and clinical correlations. Part II: The diseases of Mikulicz syndrome. *Radiology* 141:421, 1981.
Suzuki S, et al.: Sialographic study of diseases of the major salivary glands. *Acta Radiol.* 8:465, 1969.

MINAMATA DISEASE

Etiology: Ingestion of a large amount of fish and shellfish from Minamata bay contaminated by methylmercury from an adjacent chemical factory.

Clinical Manifestations: (a) sensory disturbances of the extremities, sometimes of the tongue and lips; a concentric constriction of visual fields; cerebellar ataxia; dysarthria; hearing loss; mental disturbances; (b) children born between 1955 and 1959: mental retardation, disturbances of motility, etc.

Radiologic Manifestations: Cortical cerebral atrophy; ventricular enlargement; cerebellar atrophy (hemispheres, vermis).

REFERENCE

Matsumoto SC, et al.: Minamata disease demonstrated by computed tomography. *Neuroradiology* 30:42, 1988.

MIRIZZI SYNDROME

Synonym: Hepatic duct obstruction syndrome.

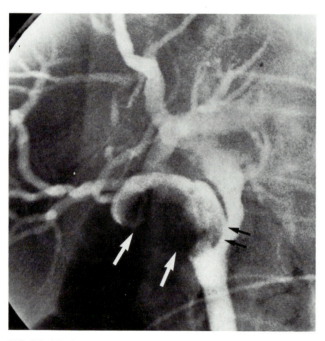

FIG SY–M–26.
Mirrizi syndrome: endoscopic retrograde cholangiogram. A stone *(white arrows)* has penetrated into the common hepatic duct and caused obstruction and stenosis. The shrunken gallbladder is opacified by a cholecystobiliary fistula *(black arrows)*. The cystic duct was not identified at surgery. (From Becker CD, et al.: Preoperative diagnosis of the Mirizzi syndrome: Limitation of sonography and computed tomography. *A.J.R.* 143:591, 1984. Used by permission.)

Definition: Obstruction of the common hepatic duct secondary to stone(s) within or extruded from the cystic duct, from a cystic duct remnant, or in the neck of the gallbladder.

Clinical Manifestations: (a) *obstructive jaundice;* (b) cholecystitis, recurrent cholangitis; (c) ultimately cholangitic cirrhosis.

Radiologic Manifestations: Computed tomography, ultrasonography, endoscopic retrograde cholangiography, or percutaneous transhepatic cholangiography: *dilated intrahepatic duct associated with a normal-caliber distal duct, stone in the area of obstruction* (Fig SY–M–26).

REFERENCES

Becker CD, et al.: Preoperative diagnosis of the Mirizzi syndrome: Limitations of sonography and computed tomography. *A.J.R.* 143:591, 1984.
Cornud F, et al.: Mirizzi syndrome and biliobiliary fistulas: Roentgenologic appearance. *Gastrointest. Radiol.* 6:265, 1981.
Cruz FO, et al.: Radiology of the Mirizzi syndrome: Diagnostic importance of the transhepatic cholangiogram. *Gastrointest. Radiol.* 8:249, 1983.
Hilger DJ, et al.: Mirizzi syndrome with common septum: Ultrasound and computed tomography findings. *J. Ultrasound Med.* 7:409, 1988.
Mirizzi PL: Sindrome del conducto hepatico. *G. Intern. Chir.* 8:731, 1948.
Pedrosa CS, et al.: CT findings in Mirizzi syndrome. *J. Comput. Assist. Tomogr.* 7:419, 1983.
Prober A, et al.: A variant of the Mirizzi syndrome. *Br. J. Radiol.* 61:331, 1988.
Tscholakoff VD, et al.: Mirizzi-Syndrom: Eine songraphische Diagnose? *Fortschr. Rontgenstr.* 141:695, 1984.

MITRAL VALVE INSUFFICIENCY-DEAFNESS-SKELETAL MALFORMATIONS

Mode of Inheritance: Possible autosomal dominant with incomplete penetrance.

Clinical Manifestations: (a) *conductive hearing loss;* (b) *mitral insufficiency;* (c) short stature.

Radiologic Manifestations: *Skeletal anomalies:* cervical vertebral fusion, carpal and tarsal bone fusions, short phalanges.

REFERENCE

Forney WR, et al.: Congenital heart disease, deafness and skeletal malformations: A new syndrome. *J. Pediatr.* 68:14, 1976.

MITRAL VALVE PROLAPSE SYNDROME

Synonyms: Click-murmur syndrome; Barlow syndrome; floppy mitral valve syndrome.

Mode of Inheritance: Estimated prevalence varying from 5% to more than 15% in the general population; autosomal dominant, female preponderance.

Clinical Manifestations: (a) chest pain, dyspnea, fatigue, palpitation, etc.; (b) mid to late systolic clicks, late systolic murmur at the apex of the heart, mobile mid to late systolic clicks at the cardiac apex; (c) apical holosystolic murmur of mitral regurgitation associated with echographic findings of mitral valve prolapse; (d) tall slender body habitus, narrow anteroposterior diameter of the chest, pectus excavatum, straight back, hypomastia; (e) dysrhythmias, low blood pressure, bacterial endocarditis, myxomatous degeneration, tricuspid valve prolapse, aortic valve prolapse, atrial septal an-

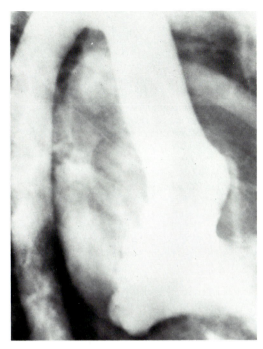

FIG SY—M—28.
Mitral valve prolapse syndrome in a 20-year-old female with systolic thrill accompanying a moderately loud late systolic murmur. A midsystolic click preceded the late systolic murmur. Left ventriculography during systole shows abnormal indentation of the inferior border of the ventricle, mitral regurgitation, and bulging of the posterior leaflet of the mitral valve. (From Grossman H, Fleming RJ, Engle MA, et al.: Angiocardiography in the apical systolic click syndrome. *Radiology* 91:898, 1968. Used by permission.)

eurysm; (f) cerebral ischemia; (g) joint hypermobility; (h) association with hyperthyroidism; (i) association with various syndromes (Marfan, Ehlers-Danlos, Stickler, joint hypermobility, Takayasu, etc.); sudden death.

Radiologic Manifestations: (a) slight to moderate cardiomegaly; (b) minimal left atrial enlargement; (c) *ballooning of the posterior leaflet of the mitral valve, scalloped appearance*

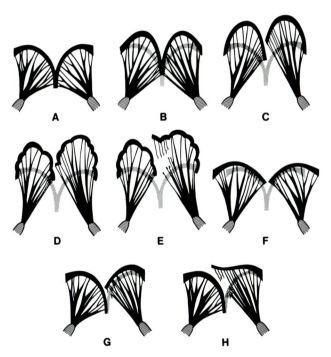

FIG SY—M—27.
Mitral valve abnormalities: billowing (BML), floppy, prolapsed (MVP), and flail mitral valves. **A,** normal mitral valve showing papillary muscles, chordae tendineae, and apposed leaflet edges. **B,** BML; the chordae are lengthened, and the voluminous leaflets "billow" into the left atrium. In this and subsequent drawings, the positions of normal leaflets are superimposed with a stippled pattern. **C,** BML with MVP; the valve is incompetent. **D,** floppy valve with MVP. **E,** floppy valve and flail leaflet. Marked regurgitation is present. **F,** recent-onset anular dilatation causes MVP with minimal BML due to a loss of the "keystone" effect. **G,** a ruptured minor chorda allows MVP without detectable BML. **H,** flail leaflet with mild BML. (From Barlow JB, Pocock WA: Billowing, floppy, prolapsed or flail mitral valves? *Am. J. Cardiol.* 55:501, 1985. Used by permission.)

TABLE SY—M—2.

Conditions Reportedly Associated With Mitral Valve Prolapse*

I. Connective tissue disorders
   Marfan syndrome
   Ehlers-Danlos syndrome
   Pseudoxanthoma elasticum
   Osteogenesis imperfecta
   Idiopathic scoliosis
   Lentiginosis profusa
   Mixed connective tissue disease
   Rheumatoid arthritis
   Raynaud disease

Continued

TABLE SY–M–2 (CONT.).

II. Cardiac disorders
    Congenital heart disease
        Atrial septal defect (secundum)
        Atrial septal aneurysm
        Bicuspid aortic valve
        Ebstein anomaly
        Ventricular septal defect
        Patent ductus arteriosus
        Tetralogy of Fallot
        Tricuspid valve prolapse
        Aortic valve prolapse
        Coronary fistula
        Coronary ectasia
    ECG and conduction abnormalities
        Atrioventricular nodal dysfunction
        Wolff-Parkinson-White syndrome
        Lown-Ganong Levine syndrome
        Idiopathic QT prolongation
    Endomyocardial fibrosis
    Cardiomyopathy
    Hypertrophic cardiomyopathy
    Mitral anular calcification
    Coronary artery spasm
    Atherosclerotic coronary disease
III. Hematologic disorders
    Platelet hypercoagulability
    von Willebrand syndrome
    Sickle cell disease
IV. Neuroendocrine and metabolic disorders
    Migraine
    Thyroid disorders
        Hyperthyroidism
        Chronic thyroiditis
    Autonomic regulatory disorders
        Dysautonomia
        Hypercatecholamines
V. Psychiatric disorders
    Agoraphobia
    Panic attacks
VI. Miscellaneous disorders
    Muscular dystrophy
    Myotonic dystrophy
    Irritable bowel syndrome
    Primary pulmonary hypertension
    Genetic disorders
        Klinefelter syndrome
        Klippel-Feil syndrome
        Fragile chromosome X syndrome
        Turner syndrome
        Noonan syndrome
        Uhl disease

From Levy D, Savage D: Prevalence and clinical features of mitral valve prolapse. Am. Heart J. 113:1281, 1987. Used by permission.

moderate systolic displacement of the leaflets with at least moderate mitral regurgitation, chordal rupture, and annular dilatation; (e) two-dimensional targeted M-mode echocardiography: marked ($\geq$3 mm) late systolic buckling posterior to the C-D line; (f) associated skeletal abnormalities in some: high-arched palate, kyphoscoliosis, incurved fifth fingers, high arch or flatfoot, rib deformities, significantly higher than normal mean metacarpal indices; (g) spontaneous pneumothorax (Figs SY–M–27 and SY–M–28; Table SY–M–2).

REFERENCES

Barlow JB, et al.: Billowing, floppy, prolapsed or flail mitral valves? *Am. J. Cardiol.* 55:50, 1985.

Barlow JB, et al.: The significance of late systolic murmur. *Am. Heart J.* 66:443, 1963.

Chan FL, et al.: Skeletal abnormalities in mitral-valve prolapse. *Clin. Radiol.* 34:207, 1983.

Devereux RB, et al.: Association of mitral-valve prolapse with low body-weight and low blood pressure. *Lancet* 2:792, 1982.

Devereux RB, et al.: Diagnosis and classification of severity of mitral valve prolapse: Methodologic, biologic, and prognostic considerations. *Am. Heart J.* 113:1265, 1987.

Handler CE, et al.: Mitral valve prolapse, aortic compliance, and skin collagen in joint hypermobility syndrome. *Br. Heart J.* 54:501, 1985.

Hirschfeld SS, et al.: Incidence of mitral valve prolapse in adolescent scoliosis and thoracic hypokyphosis. *Pediatrics* 70:451, 1982.

Kubryk N, et al.: Maladie de Takayasu associée a une maladie de Barlow. *Ann. Pediatr. (Paris)* 30:134, 1983.

Levy D, et al.: Prevalence and clinical features of mitral valve prolapse. *Am. Heart J.* 113:1281, 1987.

Liberfarb RM, et al.: Prevalence of mitral-valve prolapse in the Stickler syndrome. *Am. J. Med. Genet.* 24:387, 1986.

Malcolm AD: Mitral valve prolapse associated with other disorders. Casual coincidence, common link, or fundamental genetic disturbance? *Br. Heart J.* 53:353, 1985.

Margaliot SZ, et al.: Spontaneous pneumothorax and mitral valve prolapse. *Chest* 89:93, 1986.

Perloff JK, et al.: Clinical and epidemiologic issues in mitral valve prolapse: Overview and perspective. *Am. Heart J.* 113:1324, 1987.

Pocock WA, et al.: Sudden death in primary mitral valve prolapse. *Am. Heart J.* 107:378, 1984.

Rosenberg CA, et al.: Hypomastia and mitral-valve prolapse. Evidence of a linked embryologic and mesenchymal dysplasia. *N. Engl. J. Med.* 309:1230, 1983.

Savage DD, et al.: Mitral valve prolapse in the general population. I. Epidemiologic features: The Framingham study. *Am. Heart J.* 106:571, 1983.

Wolf PA, et al.: Cerebral ischemia with mitral valve prolapse. *Am. Heart J.* 113:1308, 1987.

MIXED CONNECTIVE TISSUE DISEASE

Synonyms: MCTD; Sharp syndrome.

Clinical Manifestations: (a) *fever, fatigue, weight loss, dyspnea, synovitis, swelling of the hands, polyarthralgia, der-*

of the posterior mitral leaflet, abnormal convex deformity of the inferior aspect of the left ventricle during systole, mitral insufficiency; (d) two-dimensional/Doppler echocardiography: marked systolic displacement of the mitral leaflets with a coaptation point at or on the atrial side of the annulus or

matomyositis, myositis, Raynaud phenomenon, systemic lupus erythematosus—like rash, rheumatoid-type nodules; (b) *high titer of IgM rheumatoid factors and antinuclear antibodies (directed against ribonuclear-sensitive nuclear antigens),* elevated sedimentation rate, anemia, leukopenia, thrombocytopenia; (c) pericarditis, asymmetrical septal hypertrophy, left ventricular dilatation, echocardiographic abnormalities; (d) progressive pulmonary deterioration, abnormal pulmonary function test results before becoming symptomatic and developing positive radiological manifestations, pulmonary hypertension; (e) other reported abnormalities: diarrhea, polyserositis, neurological manifestations, renal manifestations, diminished esophageal motility, dysphagia, hepatitis, etc.

Radiologic Manifestations: (a) diffuse or periarticular *osteoporosis;* (b) *joint manifestations* (metacarpophalangeal, carpal, radiocarpal, metatarsophalangeal, and interphalangeal joints of the hands and feet the most common sites): narrowing of joint spaces, erosion, bony ankylosis, subluxation, osteonecrosis; (c) *resorption of the terminal tufts of the phalanges,* "penciling" of phalangeal tips; (d) *soft-tissue involvement:* periarticular soft-tissue swelling, soft-tissue atrophy, soft-tissue calcification (knee, elbow, hip, digital tips); (e) esophageal dysfunction, gastroesophageal reflux; (f) pulmonary infiltrates (fine, medium, coarse), pleural thickening, mediastinal adenopathy.

REFERENCES

Allen RC, et al.: Overlap connective tissue syndromes. *Arch. Dis. Child.* 61:284, 1986.

Derderian SS, et al: Pulmonary involvement in mixed connective tissue disease. *Chest* 88:45, 1985.

Flick JA, et al.: Esophageal motor abnormalities in children and adolescents with scleroderma and mixed connective tissue disease. *Pediatrics* 82:107, 1988.

Guit GL, et al.: Mediastinal lymphadenopathy and pulmonary arterial hypertension in mixed connective tissue disease. *Radiology* 154:305, 1985.

Gutierrez F, et al.: Esophageal dysfunction in patients with mixed connective tissue diseases and systemic lupus erythematosus. *Dig. Dis. Sci.* 27:592, 1982.

Kahn MF: Connectivite mixte ou syndrome de Sharp. Conceptions actuelles. *Presse Med.* 12:2975, 1983.

Lawson JP: The joint manifestations of the connective tissue diseases. *Semin. Roentgenol.* 17:25, 1982.

Marshall JB, et al: Liver disease in mixed connective tissue disease. *Arch. Intern. Med.* 143:1817, 1983.

Oetgen WJ, et al.: Cardiac abnormalities in mixed connective tissue disease. *Chest* 83:185, 1983.

Rosenthal M: Sharp-Syndrom (mixed connective tissue disease bei Kindern). *Helv. Paediatr. Acta* 33:251, 1978.

Sallière D, et al.: Connectives mixtes de l'enfant. *Arch. Fr. Pediatr.* 38:125, 1981.

Savouret JF, et al.: Clinical and laboratory findings in childhood mixed connective tissue disease: Presence of antibody to ribonucleoprotein containing the small nuclear ribonucleic acid Ul. *J. Pediatr.* 102:841, 1983.

Sharp GC, et al.: Association of antibodies to ribonucleoprotein and Sm antigens with mixed connective-tissue disease, systemic lupus erythematosus and other rheumatic diseases. *N. Engl. J. Med.* 295:1149, 1976.

Sullivan WD, et al.: A prospective evaluation emphasizing pulmonary involvement in patients with mixed connective tissue disease. *Medicine (Baltimore)* 63:92, 1984.

Szántó D: MCTD-Syndrom (mixed connective tissue disease). *Fortschr. Rontgenstr.* 133:445, 1980.

MOBILE CECUM SYNDROME

Pathology: Absent or incomplete fixation of the cecum and ascending colon to the posterior abdominal wall.

Clinical Manifestations: Temporary and recurrent *cramplike abdominal pain* in the periumbilical region or in the right lower quadrant, tenderness over the McBurney point; hyperactive and high-pitched bowel sounds during the attack.

Radiologic Manifestations: *An excessive mobility of the cecum and ascending colon* during fluoroscopy that is demonstrable by compression with examiner's hand lateromedially on the cecum and ascending colon.

Note: In a report on 35 symptomatic patients, subsistence of symptoms occurred in over 90% of cases after surgical fixation of the right colon (Schütter).

REFERENCES

Bruns H-A, et al.: The mobile cecum. *Prog. Pediatr. Radiol.* 2:352, 1969.

Nicole R: Ueber das Coecum-mobile syndrom bei Kindern. *Ann. Pediatr. (Paris)* 183:346, 1954.

Printen KJ: Mobile cecal syndrome in the adult. *Am. Surg.* 42:204, 1976.

Schütter FW, et al.: Mobile caecum—disease pattern and surgery. *Z. Kinderchir.* 37:6, 1982.

Von Scheidt W, et al.: Bridenileus bei Coecum mobile. *Fortschr. Rontgenstr.* 142:230, 1985.

MÖBIUS SYNDROME

Synonyms: Moebius syndrome; congenital facial diplegia; congenital oculofacial paralysis; congenital abducens-facial paralysis.

Mode of Inheritance: Considerable genetic heterogeneity and pleiotropism (sporadic, autosomal dominant, autosomal recessive).

Frequency: Rare.

Clinical Manifestations: (a) *congenital facial diplegia involving cranial nerves VI and VII,* resulting in facial diplegia and bilateral external rectus muscle paralysis; (b) involvement of cranial nerves IX and X (in some); (c) speech, language, and hearing problems; external ear deformity; (d) clubfoot in one third of patients, digital anomalies; (e) arthrogryposis; (f)

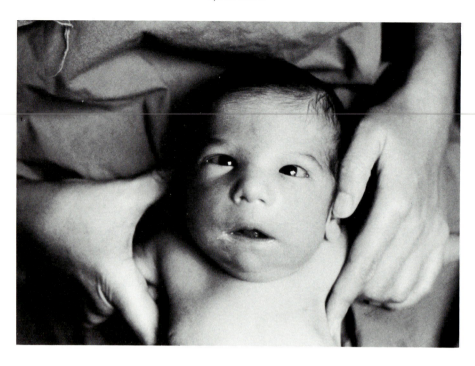

FIG SY−M−29.
Möbius syndrome. Note the bilateral convergent strabismus and expressionless facies (facial diplegia). The infant also has hypoplasia of the left pectoralis major muscle, absence of the left areola, hypoplasia of the left forearm and hand, etc. (Poland syndrome).

(From Bosch-Banyeras JM, Zuasnabar A, Puig A, et al.: Poland-Möbius syndrome associated with dextrocardia. *J. Med. Genet.* 21:70, 1984. Used by permission.)

mental retardation in 10%, developmental delay, seizures, hypotonia, abnormal brainstem auditory evoked potentials, abnormal sensory evoked potentials, childhood psychosis; (g) muscular involvement (pectoralis, trapezius, quadriceps, serratus magnus and semimembranosus), abnormal electromyographic findings; (h) coincidence of infantile liver disease due to α_1-antrypsin deficiency with Möbius syndrome.

Radiologic Manifestations: (a) *motor disturbance of swallowing function* resulting in tracheal aspiration; (b) chronic pneumonia; (c) *anomalies of limbs in one fourth of cases* including clubfoot deformity, digital anomalies (syndactyly, agenesis, polydactyly, brachydactyly), congenital hip dislocation, fibrous ankylosis of the interphalangeal joints; (d) pectoral muscle deficiency; (e) small brain stem; (f) other reported abnormalities: polyhydramnios, dextrocardia.

Note: (a) the term *Poland-Möbius syndrome* is used when the Möbius syndrome is associated with the absence of the pectoral major muscle and ipsilateral upper limb anomalies (Poland syndrome); (b) the term *subclavian artery supply disruption sequence* has been suggested for Möbius, Poland, and Klippel-Feil syndromes based on the theory that these conditions are the result of an interruption of the early embryonic blood supply in the subclavian arteries, the vertebral arteries, and/or their branches. (c) Möbius syndrome 1 refers to oculomotor recurrent paralysis, and Möbius syndrome 2 refers to the entity presented in this section (Fig SY−M−29).

REFERENCES

Beren R, et al.: Möbius syndrome in a patient with α_1-antitrypsin deficiency. *Aust. Paediatr. J.* 17:64, 1981.

Bosch-Banyeras JM, et al.: Poland-Möbius syndrome associated with dextrocardia. *J. Med. Genet.* 21:70, 1984.

Bouwes Bavinck JN, et al.: Subclavian artery supply disruption sequence: Hypothesis of a vascular etiology for Poland, Klippel-Feil, and Möbius anomalies. *Am. J. Med. Genet.* 23:903, 1986.

Collins DL, et al.: Moebius syndrome in a child and extremity defect in her father. *Clin. Genet.* 22:312, 1982.

Fontaine G, et al.: Le syndrome de Poland-Möbius. A propos de 2 observations. *Arch. Fr. Pediatr.* 41:351, 1984.

Gillberg Ch, et al.: Childhood psychosis in a case of Moebius syndrome. *Neuropediatrics* 15:147, 1984.

Goldblatt D, et al.: "I an sniling!": Möbius' syndrome inside and out. *J. Child. Neurol.* 1:71, 1986.

Legum C, et al.: Heterogeneity and pleiotropism in the Moebius syndrome. *Clin. Genet.* 20:254, 1981.

Mitter NS, et al.: Facial weakness and oligosyndactyly:? Independent variable features of familial type of the Möbius syndrome. *Clin. Genet.* 24:350, 1983.

Möbius PJ: Ueber angeborenen doppelseitige Abducensfacialis Lähmung. *Munch. Med. Wochenschr.* 35:91, 108, 1888.

Stabile M, et al.: Abnormal B.A.E.P. in a family with Moebius syndrome: Evidence for supranuclear lesion. *Clin. Genet.* 25:459, 1984.

Sudarshan A, et al.: The spectrum of congenital facial diplegia (Moebius syndrome). *Pediatr. Neurol.* 1:180, 1985.

MOLDED BABY SYNDROME

Synonym: Moulded baby syndrome.

Clinical and Radiologic Manifestations: (a) *plagiocephaly* (intrauterine molding); (b) *pelvic obliquity associated with a unilateral (on the same side as the plagiocephaly) restriction of hip abduction in flexion;* (c) other reported abnormalities: scoliosis, torticollis, bat ears.

REFERENCES

Good C, et al.: The hip in the moulded baby syndrome. *J. Bone Joint Surg. [Br.]* 66:491, 1984.
Watson GH: Relation between the side of plagiocephaly, dislocation of hip, scoliosis, bat ear and sternomastoid tumours. *Arch. Dis. Child.* 46:203, 1971.

MOORE-FEDERMAN SYNDROME

Mode of Inheritance: Autosomal dominant (one family).

Clinical Manifestations: Dwarfism, stiff joints and limitation of articular motions, hepatomegaly, hoarseness, asthma or asthmatic bronchitis, ocular abnormalities (glaucoma, cataract), etc.

Radiologic Manifestations: Broad metacarpals, short phalanges.

REFERENCE

Moore WT, Federman D: Familial dwarfism and "stiff joints." *Arch. Intern. Med.* 115:398, 1965.

MORGAGNI-STEWART-MOREL SYNDROME

Synonyms: Hyperostosis frontalis interna; Stewart-Morel syndrome; "metabolic craniopathy."

Mode of Inheritance: Familial cases have been reported; dominant (sex-limited autosomal or X-linked) transmission also suggested.

Clinical Manifestations: Often occurring in women in the fifth decade of life; may have various associated clinical manifestations: (a) menstrual disorders; (b) *hirsutism;* (c) *obesity;* (d) headaches, vertigo, fatigue; (e) decrease in glucose tolerance, galactorrhea/hyperprolactinemia; (f) poor manual dexterity in obese women with hyperostosis frontalis interna.

Radiologic Manifestations: (a) gradual development of *symmetrical internal hyperostosis of the calvaria,* most prominent in frontal region; (b) transient diminution of activity on early radionuclide images of brain with subsequent filling; (c) bone scintigraphy: symmetrical bifrontal high uptake spreading laterally from and sparing the midline; (d) indium III leukocyte imaging: uptake in the anterior portion of the calvarium.

REFERENCES

Calamé A: *Le syndrome de Morgagni-Morel.* Paris, Masson & Cie, 1941.
Jacobsson H, et al.: Hyperostosis cranii. Radiography and scintigraphy compared. *Acta Radiol.* 29:223, 1988.
Moore S: *Hyperostosis Cranii.* Springfield, IL, Charles C Thomas Publishers, 1955.
Morel F: *L'Hyperostose Frontale Interne. Syndrome de l'Hyperostose Frontale Interne avec Adipose et Troubles Cérébraux.* Paris, Gaston, Doin & Cie, 1930.
Morgagni GB: *De Sedibus et Causis Morborum.* Book II, 1761.
Novetsky GJ, et al.: Bone scintigraphy in hyperostosis frontalis interna. *Clin. Nucl. Med.* 7:265, 1982.
Paulson E, et al.: False-positive calvarial uptake on indium-III leukocytes in a patient with hyperostosis frontalis interna. *Clin. Nucl. Med.* 13:68, 1988.
Pawlikowski M, et al.: Hyperostosis frontalis, galactorrhoea/hyperprolactinaemia, and Morgagni-Stewart-Morel syndrome. *Lancet* 1:474, 1983.
Salmi A, et al.: Hyperostosis cranii in a normal population. *A.J.R.* 87:1032, 1962.
Stewart RM: Localized cranial hyperostosis in the insane. *J. Neurol. Psychopathol. (London)* 8:321, 1928.

MORNING GLORY SYNDROME

Synonyms: Optic nerve coloboma; axial coloboma; peripapillary scleral staphyloma with posterior ectasia of the papilla; papilla "en fleur de liseron."

Pathology: Congenital ocular anomaly (unilateral or bilateral): enlarged and excavated papilla, central bouquet of glial hyperplasia, radially oriented exit of the retinal vessels from the disk periphery.

Clinical Manifestations: (a) *strabismus, amblyopia, loss of visual acuity, refraction anomalies;* (b) *enlarged, funnel-shaped, distorted, excavated optic disk surrounded by an elevated annulus of chorioretinal atrophy and pigmentary changes;* (c) fluorescein angiography: *radially oriented exit of retinal vessels from the periphery of the disk;* (d) other reported abnormalities: retinal detachment, retinoschisis, congenital cataract, chronic glomerulonephritis, cleft lip/palate.

Radiologic Manifestations: (a) ultrasound, computed tomography (CT), magnetic resonance imaging: *colobomatous area,* retinal detachment, cataract, thickened intraocular optic nerve and increased radiodensity in the postcontrast CT, *normal retrobulbar optic nerve;* (b) other reported abnormalities: agenesis of the corpus callosum, sphenoidal encephalocele and other midline defects, renal dysplasia/hypoplasia (Fig SY−M−30).

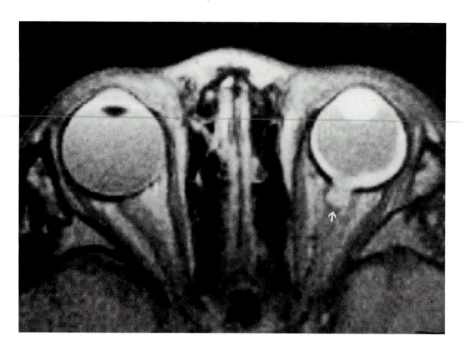

FIG SY—M—30.
Morning glory syndrome: Spin-echo 1,600/70 image showing a cataract, retinal detachment, and a colobomatous area *(arrow)* of the left eye. (From Tonami H, Nakagawa T, Yamamoto I, et al.: MR imaging of morning glory syndrome. *J. Comput. Assist. Tomogr.* 11:529, 1987. Used by permission.)

REFERENCES

Adam P, et al.: Morning glory syndrome: CT findings. *J. Comput. Assist. Tomogr.* 8:134, 1984.
Tonami H, et al.: MR imaging of morning glory syndrome. *J. Comput. Assist. Tomogr.* 11:529, 1987.

Dunne MG, et al: CT features of tracheobronchomegaly. *J. Comput. Assist. Tomogr.* 12:388, 1988.
Gay S, et al.: Tracheobronchomegaly—the Mounier-Kuhn syndrome. *Br. J. Radiol.* 57:640, 1984.
Hunter TB, et al.: Tracheobronchomegaly in an 18-month-old child. *A.J.R.* 123:687, 1975.

MOUNIER-KUHN SYNDROME

Synonyms: Tracheomegaly; tracheobronchomegaly.

Mode of Inheritance: Familial cases have been reported; autosomal recessive inheritance has been suggested.

Clinical Manifestations: (a) *recurrent lower respiratory tract infection;* (b) loud cough; (c) hoarseness; (d) dyspnea; (e) copious purulent sputum production.

Radiologic Manifestations: (a) *tracheobronchomegaly (trachea equal to or greater than the width of the thoracic vertebral body),* increase in lumen of the trachea with the Valsalva maneuver and narrowing with the Müller maneuver; (b) *saclike recesses;* (c) emphysema; (d) pulmonary fibrosis; (e) bullae (Figs SY—M—31 and SY—M—32).

REFERENCES

Czyhlarz ER: Ueber in Pulsionsdivertikel der Trachea mit Bemerkungen über das Verhalten der elastischen Fasern an normalen Tracheen und Bronchien. *Centralblatt Allg. Pathologie Pathol. Anat.* 18:721, 1897.

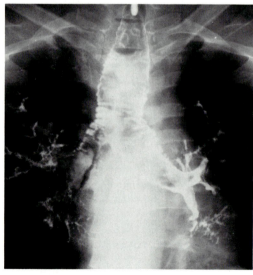

FIG SY—M—31.
Mounier-Kuhn syndrome. A bronchogram in an adult male shows a marked increase in caliber of the trachea and major bronchi. Note the bulging redundant segments of atrophic pars membranacea. (From Katz I, Levine M, Herman P: Tracheobronchomegaly: The Mounier-Kuhn syndrome. *A.J.R.* 88:1084, 1962. Used by permission.)

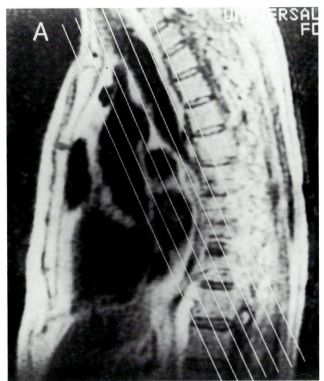

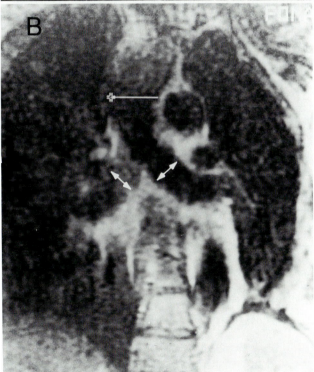

FIG SY–M–32.
Mounier-Kuhn syndrome in a 57-year-old man. **A,** The magnetic resonance sagittal scan that served as the scout for the coronal oblique scan *(lines)* shows marked dilatation of the trachea. **B,** the marked dilatation of the trachea and left and right bronchi *(arrows)* is noted. (From Rindsberg S, Friedman AC, Fiel SB, et al.: MRI of tracheobronchomegaly. *J. Can. Assoc. Radiol.* 38:126, 1987. Used by permission.)

Johnston RF, et al.: Tracheobronchomegaly: Report of five cases and demonstration of familial occurrence. *Am. Rev. Respir. Dis.* 91:35, 1965.

Katz I, LeVine M, Herman P: Tracheobronchiomegaly: The Mounier-Kuhn syndrome. *A.J.R.* 88:1084, 1962.

Lallemand D, et al.: Tracheomégalie et déficit immunitaire chez l'enfant. *Ann. Radiol. (Paris)* 24:67, 1981.

Mildenberger P, et al.: Tracheobronchomegalie. *Radiologe* 28:236, 1988.

Mounier-Kuhn P: Dilatation de la trachée: Constations radio-graphiques et bronchoscopiques. *Lyon Med.* 150:106, 1932.

Rindsberg S, et al.: MRI of tracheobronchomegaly. *J. Can. Assoc. Radiol.* 38:126, 1987.

MOYAMOYA

Mode of Inheritance: Familial incidence of 7% in 600 cases from Japan; most in females, particularly of Japanese origin; reported in identical twins.

Pathology: *Progressive occlusion of the intracranial portions of both internal carotid arteries, both middle and both anterior cerebral arteries, and sometimes the basilar and trunk of the posterior cerebral arteries.*

Clinical Manifestations: Onset of disease in children and young adults; recurring hemispheric ischemic attacks: (a) *headache, paresis, paralysis,* convulsions, twitching movements, speech disturbance, unsteady gait, hemianopia; (b) electroencephalography: prominent high-voltage delta bursts following hyperventilation and slowness of return to a normal pattern; (c) spontaneous intracranial hemorrhage; (d) association with other diseases: peripheral vascular occlusive disease, neurocutaneous syndromes, bacterial meningitis, periarteritis nodosa, head trauma, tuberculosis, sickle cell disease, Fanconi anemia, intracranial aneurysm, brain irradiation, Wilms tumor, Down syndrome, neurofibromatosis, autonomic dysfunction, etc.

Radiologic Manifestations: (a) *occlusion of major arteries, usually without involvement of the distal branches* of the anterior, middle, and posterior cerebral arteries; (b) *collateral channels feeding distal branches* through (1) end-to-end anastomoses over the surface of the brain, (2) dilated vessels in the basal ganglia, and (3) rete mirabile; (c) computed tomography: multiple low-density areas in the brain; cerebral cortical atrophic changes, often most marked in frontal lobe; tortuous and curvilinear vessels in the basal ganglia that correspond to leptomeningeal and parenchymal collateral vessels seen on angiography; poor opacification of the proximal segment of the anterior and middle cerebral arteries; high-density zones in the basal ganglia or brain hemisphere; (d) radionuclide cerebral angiography: increased perfusion at the surface and base of the brain; (e) magnetic resonance imaging: occlusion or stenosis of the internal carotid artery at the fork level and the proximal position of the anterior and middle cerebral arteries, characteristic collateral from the suprasellar cistern to the basal ganglia (moyamoya vessels), ischemia of the brain, infarction, ventricular dilatation, brain atrophy; (f)

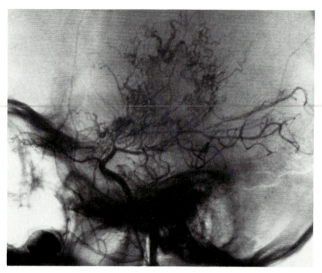

FIG SY–M–33.
Moyamoya in an 8-year-old female with myoclonic movements of her right arm and seizures of the right extremities. Note the "hemangiomatous" network at the base of the brain. (From Nishimoto A, Takeuchi S: Abnormal cerebrovascular network related to the internal carotid arteries. *J. Neurosurg.* 29:255, 1968. Used by permission.)

other reported abnormalities: intracranial hemorrhage (intracerebral and intraventrical most common, subarachnoid less common), aneurysm (within the moyamoya vessels, within the circle of Willis), arteriovenous malformation, aneurysm of the vein of Galen, enlargement of the middle meningeal artery groove, bilateral narrowing of the internal carotid artery in the neck, etc.

Note: In Japanese *moyamoya* refers to "something hazy, like a puff of cigarette smoke drifting in the air" (Fig SY–M–33).

REFERENCES

Aoki N, et al.: Does moyamoya disease cause subarachnoid hemorrhage? Review of 54 cases with intracranial hemorrhage confirmed by computerized tomography. *J. Neurosurg.* 60:348, 1984.

Asari S, et al.: The advantage of coronal scanning in cerebral computed angiotomography for diagnosis of moyamoya disease. *Radiology* 145:709, 1982.

Beyer RA, et al.: Moyamoya pattern of vascular occlusion after radiotherapy for glioma of the optic chiasm. *Neurology* 36:1173, 1986.

Brooks BS, et al.: MR imaging of moyamoya in neurofibromatosis. *A.J.N.R.* 8:178, 1987.

Cohen N, et al.: Moyamoya and Fanconi's anemia. *Pediatrics* 65:804, 1980.

Ellison PH, et al.: Moya-moya disease associated with renal artery stenosis. *Arch. Neurol.* 38:467, 1981.

Erickson RP, et al.: Familial occurrence of intracranial arterial occlusive disease (moyamoya) in neurofibromatosis. *Clin. Genet.* 18:191, 1980.

Fujisawa E, et al.: Moyamoya disease: MR imaging. *Radiology* 164:103, 1987.

Goldberg HJ: "Moyamoya" associated with peripheral vascular occlusive disease. *Arch. Dis. Child.* 49:964, 1974.

Hasuo K, et al.: Moyamoya disease: Use of digital subtraction angiography in its diagnosis. *Radiology* 157:107, 1985.

Inugami A, et al.: Moyamoya disease of twins (abstract). *Neuroradiology* 29:107, 1987.

Ito J, et al.: Aneurysm of the vein of Galen associated with moyamoya disease. Case report (abstract). *Neuroradiology* 29:107, 1987.

Kitahara T, et al.: Familial occurrence of moyamoya disease: Report of three Japanese families. *J. Neurol. Neurosurg. Psychiatr.* 42:208, 1979.

Konishi Y, et al.: Aneurysms associated with moyamoya disease. *Neurosurgery* 16:484, 1985.

Lichtor T, et al.: Arteriovenous malformation in moyamoya syndrome. Report of three cases. *J. Neurosurg.* 67:603, 1987.

Maeda T, et al.: Radionuclide cerebral angiography in moyamoya disease. *Clin. Nucl. Med.* 4:513, 1979.

Miyamoto S, et al.: Study of the posterior circulation in moyamoya disease. Clinical and neuroradiological evaluation. *J. Neurosurg.* 61:1032, 1984.

Morisako T, et al.: Two cases of moyamoya disease associated with bilateral narrowing of the internal carotid artery in the neck (abstract). *Neuroradiology* 29:108, 1987.

Nishimoto A, Takeuchi S: Abnormal cerebrovascular network related to the internal carotid arteries. *J. Neurosurg.* 29:255, 1968.

Pearson E, et al.: Moyamoya and other causes of stroke in patients with Down syndrome. *Pediatr. Neurol.* 1:174, 1985.

Satoh S, et al.: Analysis of the angiographic findings in cases of childhood moyamoya disease. *Neuroradiology* 30:111, 1988.

Tsuchiya K, et al.: Enlargement of the middle meningeal artery groove in moyamoya disease (abstract). *Neuroradiology* 29:598, 1987.

Watanabe Y, et al.: Wilms' tumor associated with moyamoya disease: A case report. *Z. Kinderchir.* 40:114, 1985.

Welch WC, et al.: Moyamoya disease in an infant with autonomic dysfunction: Angiographic and MRI findings. *J. Child Neurol.* 3:110, 1988.

Yamashiro Y, et al.: Cerebrovascular moyamoya disease. *Eur. J. Pediatr.* 142:44, 1984.

MULIBREY NANISM

Mode of Inheritance: Autosomal recessive.

Clinical Manifestations: (a) *progressive growth failure*, growth deficiency evident at birth; (b) hydrocephaloid head, *triangular face*; (c) slenderness and *muscular hypotonia*; (d) *peculiar voice*; (e) ocular abnormalities: yellowish dots *and pigment dispersion in the fundi*; hypoplasia of the choroid, strabismus, astigmatism, atrophy of the corneal epithelium, thickening of the Bowman membrane; (f) *hepatomegaly*; (g) *raised venous pressure*, cardiac lesions often associated with *pericardial constriction*, abnormal electrocardiographic findings; (h) cutaneous nevi flammei; (i) other reported abnormalities: Wilms tumor, slight dysarthria, slight decrease in capacity for maintaining blood sugar level while fasting, frequent episodes of pneumonia.

Radiologic Manifestations: (a) dolichocephaly, *J-shaped sella turcica*, slightly increased basilar angle, *abnormally large cerebral ventricles and cisternae*; (b) cardiomegaly, pulmonary congestion; (c) ascites; (d) skeletal abnormalities; fibrous dysplasia of the tibia with progressive changes, fractures and pseudoarthrosis, thinness of long bones with a relative thickness of the cortex and very narrow or almost obstructed medullary channels.

Differential Diagnosis: Silver-Russell syndrome.

Note: The acronym MULIBREY takes its origin from the names of the organs most prominently involved: MU (muscle), LI (liver), BR (brain), and EY (eyes).

REFERENCES

Cumming GR, et al.: Constrictive pericarditis with dwarfism in two siblings. *J. Pediatr.* 88:569, 1976.
Marttinen E, et al.: Metacarpophalangeal pattern profile (MCPP) in mulibrey nanism and in Russell-Silver dwarfism (abstract). *Pediatr. Radiol.* 15:273, 1985.
Perheentupa J, et al.: Mulibrey nanism, an autosomal recessive syndrome with pericardial constriction. *Lancet* 2:351, 1973.
Perheentupa J, et al.: Mulibrey-nanism: Dwarfism with muscle, liver, brain and eye involvement. *Acta Paediatr. Scand.* 59(suppl. 206):74, 1970.
Similä S, et al.: A case of Mulibrey nanism with associated Wilms' tumor. *Clin. Genet.* 17:29, 1980.
Tarkkanen A, et al.: Mulibrey nanism, an autosomal recessive syndrome with ocular involvement. *Acta Ophthalmol. (Copenh.)* 60:628, 1982.
Tuuteri L, et al.: The cardiopathy of Mulibrey nanism, a new inherited syndrome. *Chest* 65:628, 1974.
Voorhess ML, et al.: Growth failure with pericardial constriction (the syndrome of mulibrey nanism). *Am. J. Dis. Child.* 130:1146, 1976.

MULTIPLE ENDOCRINE NEOPLASIA SYNDROMES

TABLE SY–M–3.
Types and Incidence of the Major Lesions in the Multiple Endocrine Neoplasia Syndromes*

Syndrome	Lesions	Incidence (%)
MEN I† (Wermer syndrome)	Parathyroid adenomas and/ or hyperplasia	90
	Pancreatic islet tumors	80
	Pituitary tumors	65
	Adrenal cortical adenomas	38
	Thyroid adenomas	19

Continued

TABLE SY–M–3. (cont.)

Syndrome	Lesions	Incidence (%)
MEN II or IIa (Sipple syndrome)	Medullary thyroid carcinoma	100
	Pheochromocytoma	>50
	Parathyroid adenomas and/ or hyperplasia	25–50
MEN III or IIb (Froboese syndrome, mucosal neuroma syndrome)	Medullary thyroid carcinoma	100
	Pheochromocytoma	50
	Parathyroid adenoma or hyperplasia	0
	Mucosal neuromas	100
	Intestinal ganglioneuromatosis	100

*Adapted from Fryns JP, Chrzanowska K: Mucosal neuroma syndrome (MEN type IIb (III). *J. Med. Genet.* 25:703, 1988.
†MEN = multiple endocrine neoplasia.

MULTIPLE ENDOCRINE NEOPLASIA, TYPE 1

Synonyms: Wermer syndrome; MEN, type 1; multiple endocrine adenomatosis, type 1 (MEA 1); familial multiple endocrine neoplasia, type I.

Mode of Inheritance: Autosomal dominant; complete penetrance with variable expressivity; equal sex frequency.

Primary Features: (a) parathyroid hyperplasia; (b) *pituitary adenomas*; (c) *islet cell tumors of the pancreas*.

Pathology: (a) *multiple tumors or hyperplasia of several endocrine glands*: parathyroid hyperplasia, islet cell tumor, pituitary adenoma, adrenal adenoma or carcinoma, thyroid abnormalities (follicular adenomas, colloid goiter, Hashimoto thyroiditis), glucagon-secreting tumors, thymoma, prolactinoma; (b) *other tumors*: multiple lipomas, schwannoma, bronchial or abdominal carcinoid.

Clinical Manifestations: Most patients present by the third or fourth decade of life: (a) gastrinoma: severe peptic ulcer disease; (b) insulinoma: hypoglycemia; (c) VIPoma: watery diarrhea, hypokalemia, with achlorhydria (WDHA, Verner-Morrison syndrome, pancreatic cholera); (d) glucagonoma: diabetes mellitus, dermititis, necrolytic migratory erythema, anemia, hypoaminoacidemia, weight loss; (e) pancreatic polypeptide (PP) tumors: usually clinical silent, diagnosed by serum PP levels and immunohistochemical demonstration of the peptid in resected tumors; (f) pituitary adenomas: headaches, visual disturbances, hormonal abnormalities (prolactin, growth hormone, adrenocorticotropic hormone; (g) Zollinger-Ellison syndrome as a frequent component of MEN, type I; (h) other reported abnormalities: association with marfanoid habitus, optic atrophy, mitral valve prolapse, and mental retardation (case report); increased frequency of chromosomal breakage.

Radiologic Manifestations: (a) *roentgenologic findings of endocrinopathy*; (b) alimentary tract *ulcers in unusual loca-*

tions (duodenum and jejunum); (c) marked enlargement of the mucosal folds of the stomach, duodenum, and jejunum; (d) nodular defects of the intestinal wall; (e) megaduodenum; (f) *gastrointestinal dilatation and hypersecretion* (see Table SY−M−3).

REFERENCES

Brunt LM, et al.: The multiple endocrine neoplasia syndrome. *Invest. Radiol.* 20:916, 1985.

Dodds WJ, et al.: MEN I syndrome and islet cell lesions of the pancreas. *Semin. Roentgenol.* 20:17, 1985.

Doppman JL: Multiple endocrine syndromes—a nightmare for the endocrinologic radiologist. *Semin. Roentgenol.* 20:7, 1985.

Duh Q-Y, et al.: Carcinoids associated with multiple endocrine neoplasia syndromes. *Am. J. Surg.* 154:142, 1987.

Erdheim J: Zur normalen und pathologischen histologie der glandula thyroidea, parathyroidea und hypophysis. *Beitr. Pathol. Anat. Allg. Pathol.* 33:158, 1903.

Gustavson K-H, et al.: Chromosomal breakage in multiple endocrine adenomatosis (types I and II). *Clin. Genet.* 23:143, 1983.

Manning GS, et al.: Multiple endocrine neoplasia, type I. Association with marfanoid habitus, optic atrophy, and other abnormalities. *Arch. Intern. Med.* 143:2315, 1983.

Marx SJ, et al.: Multiple endocrine neoplasia type I: Assessment of laboratory tests to screen for the gene in a large kindred. *Medicine (Baltimore)* 65:226, 1986.

Schnall AM, et al.: Multiple endocrine adenomas in a patient with the Maffucci syndrome. *Am. J. Med.* 61:952, 1976.

Underdahl LO, et al.: Multiple endocrine adenomas: Report of 8 cases in which parathyroid, pituitary and pancreatic islets were involved. *J. Clin. Endocrinol.* 13:20, 1953.

Wermer P: Genetic aspects of adenomatosis of endocrine glands. *Am. J. Med.* 16:363, 1954.

MULTIPLE ENDOCRINE NEOPLASIA, TYPE 2A

Synonyms: Sipple syndrome; MEN 2a; MEN, type 2; multiple endocrine adenomatosis, type 2a; MEA 2a.

Mode of Inheritance: Autosomal dominant; reported in twins.

Primary Features: (a) *medullary thyroid carcinoma present in 100%;* (b) *pheochromocytoma;* (c) *multiglandular parathyroid hyperplasia;* (b) and (c) occurrence in 50% or fewer of the patients.

Pathology: (a) medullary thyroid carcinoma; (b) pheochromocytoma; (c) multiglandular parathyroid hyperplasia; (d) other reported abnormalities: hyperplasia of adrenal medullary tissue, parathyroid adenoma, neuroma, neurofibroma, intestinal neurogangliomatosis, breast cancer, carcinoid tumor, thyroid tumor metastases (mediastinum, lung, liver, bone).

Clinical Manifestations: (a) *thyroid related:* neck mass, hoarseness, cough, dysphagia, cervical adenopathy, diarrhea, elevated basal or stimulated levels of the polypeptide hormone calcitonin; (b) *pheochromocytoma related* (in 10% as the initial presenting feature): headaches; palpitation; sweating; hypertension; elevated urinary vanillylmandelic acid (VMA), metanephrine, and catecholamine levels; (c) *parathyroid related:* usually mild and asymptomatic, nephropathy or life-threatening hypercalcemia rare; (d) other reported abnormalities: Cushing syndrome, carcinoid syndrome, Zollinger-Ellison syndrome, lymphoblastic leukemia, presentation with cardiac failure (pheochromocytoma), association with Hirschsprung disease, chromosome 20 deletion, malignant melanoma.

Radiologic Manifestations: (a) *thyroid tumor: calcification in the primary tumor and its metastases,* lack of concentration of ^{131}I by medullary thyroid carcinoma; (b) *pheochromocytoma:* egg shell calcification, demonstration of tumor by various modalities (magnetic resonance imaging probably the most accurate method), ^{131}I-metaiodobenzlguanidine (^{131}I-MIBG) scanning; (c) parathyroid hyperplasia: radiological imaging techniques (ultrasound, etc.), venous catheterization with parathormone level determination; (d) other reported abnormalities: bone metastases, chondrocalcinosis, abnormal haustral pattern, thickened mucosal folds and colonic diverticula in patients with ganglioneuromatosis, rapid transit of barium through the gastrointestinal tract, gastrointestinal ulceration, partial bowel obstruction by the ulcerating mass related to the metastatic lymph nodes (see Table SY−M−3).

REFERENCES

Babu VR, et al.: Chromosome 20 deletion in multiple endocrine neoplasia type 2: Expanded double-blind studies. *Am. J. Med. Genet.* 27:739, 1987.

Bergevin PR, et al.: Sipple syndrome and acute lymphoblastic leukemia. *J.A.M.A.* 231:390, 1975.

Brunt LM, et al.: The multiple endocrine neoplasia syndromes. *Invest. Radiol.* 20:916, 1985.

Dodd GD: The radiologic features of multiple endocrine neoplasia types IIA and IIB. *Semin. Roentgenol.* 20:64, 1985.

Doppman JL: Multiple endocrine syndromes—A nightmare for the endocrinologic radiologist. *Semin. Roentgenol.* 20:7, 1985.

Gagel RF, et al.: The clinical outcome of prospective screening for multiple endocrine neoplasia type 2a. An 18-year experience. *N. Engl. J. Med.* 318:478, 1988.

Gibson RK, et al.: Malignant melanoma in multiple endocrine neoplasia. *Cancer* 58:1779, 1986.

Girvan DP, et al.: Pediatric implications of multiple endocrine neoplasia. *J. Pediatr. Surg.* 22:806, 1987.

Khan AH, et al.: Gastrointestinal manifestations of Sipple syndrome in children. *J. Pediatr. Surg.* 22:719, 1987.

Mathieu E, et al.: MR imaging of the adrenal gland in Sipple disease. *J. Comput. Assist. Tomogr.* 11:790, 1987.

Radin DR, et al.: Computed tomography of Sipple syndrome. *J. Comput. Assist. Tomogr.* 8:169, 1984.

Sipple JH: The association of pheochromocytoma with carcinoma of the thyroid gland. *Am. J. Med.* 31:163, 1961.

Steiner AL, et al.: Study of a kindred with pheochromocytoma, medullary thyroid carcinoma, hyperparathyroidism and Cushing's disease: Multiple endocrine neoplasia, type 2. *Medicine (Baltimore)* 47:371, 1968.

MULTIPLE ENDOCRINE NEOPLASIA, TYPE 2B

Synonyms: Mucosal neuroma syndrome; MEN 2b; MEN, type 3; multiple endocrine adenomatosis, type 2b; MEA 2b; neuromata, mucosal with endocrine tumors; mucosal neuroma syndrome.

Mode of Inheritance: Autosomal dominant and sporadic.

Pathology: (a) medullary thyroid carcinoma (present in 100% of the patients); (b) pheochromocytoma (present in over 90% of the patients); (c) multiple mucosal neuromas: tongue, eyelids, pharynx, larynx; (d) ganglioneuromatosis, hypertrophy of the submucosal and myenteric plexuses; (e) lipoma and other soft-tissue tumors, adenomatous colonic polyp, etc.

Clinical Manifestations: (a) *marfanoid body habitus,* muscle wasting, kyphosis, pectus excavatum, pes planus, pes cavus; (b) coarse facial features; pseudoprognathism; *neuromas of the eyelids, lips (thick), and tongue (thick, nodular, "bumpy");* (c) constipation and/or diarrhea; (d) delayed maturation.

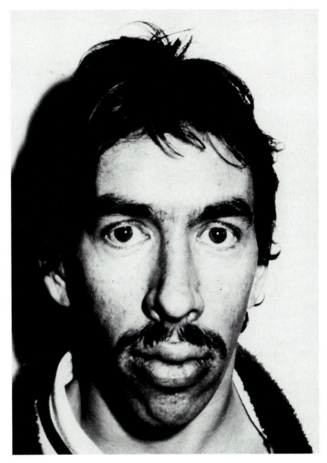

FIG SY–M–35.
Multiple endocrine neoplasia syndrome, type 2b, with an elongated face; large, bumpy, patulous lips; and infiltration of the eyelids. (From Fryns JP, Chrzanowska K: Mucosal neuromata syndrome (MEN type IIb) (III). *J. Med. Genet.* 25:703, 1988. Used by permission.)

Radiologic Manifestations: (a) *thyroid tumor;* (b) *pheochromocytoma;* (c) *alimentary tract manifestations* (ganglioneuromas): disturbed motility of the esophagus (segmental dilatation, tertiary contractions, gastroesophageal reflux, distended stomach with a delayed emptying time, segmental dilatation of the small bowel with an increased or decreased transit time, abnormal colonic haustral pattern, "cornflake" mucosal pattern, megacolon, abnormal mucosal folds of the colon, diverticula of the colon in young patients); (d) musculoskeletal system: pes cavus, slipped capital femoral epiphysis, joint laxity, poor muscle development.

Differential Diagnosis: Hirschsprung disease (constipation, megacolon).

Note: In some publications MEN 2b has been given the synonym "Sipple syndrome" (Figs SY–M–34 to SY–M–37; see Table SY-M-3).

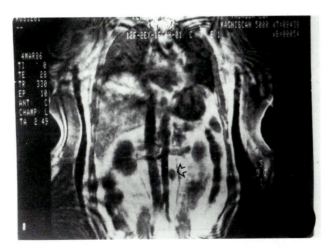

FIG SY–M–34.
Multiple endocrine neoplasia syndrome, type 2b. A coronal section of the abdomen shows a paraaortic mass representing an ectopic pheochromocytoma. The patient also had an enlarged adrenal gland shown by computed tomography and magnetic resonance imaging. (From Mathieu E, Despres E, Delepine N, et al.: MR imaging of the adrenal gland in Sipple disease. *J. Comput. Assist. Tomogr.* 11:790, 1987. Used by permission.)

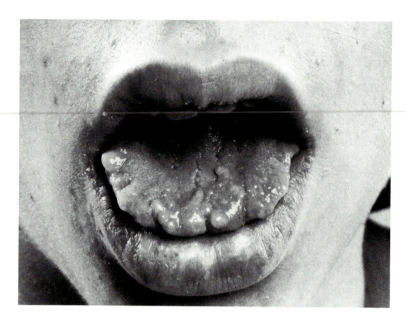

FIG SY–M–36.
Multiple endocrine neoplasia syndrome, type 2b. Multiple mucosal neuromas of the tongue and thick patulous lips are present. (From Saltzman CL, Herzenberg JE, Phillips WA, et al.: Thick lips, bumpy tongue, and slipped capital femoral epiphysis—A deadly combination. *J. Pediatr. Orthop.* 8:219, 1988. Used by permission.)

REFERENCES

Alberts WM, et al.: Mixed multiple endocrine neoplasia syndromes. *J.A.M.A.* 244:1236, 1980.

Brunt LM, et al.: The multiple endocrine neoplasia syndromes. *Invest. Radiol.* 20:916, 1985.

Demos TC, et al.: Multiple endocrine neoplasia (MEN) syndrome. Type IIB: Gastrointestinal manifestations. *A.J.R.* 140:73, 1983.

Dodd GD: The radiologic features of multiple endocrine neoplasia types IIA and IIB. *Semin. Roentgenol.* 20:64, 1985.

Doppman JL: Multiple endocrine syndromes—A nightmare for the endocrinologic radiologist. *Semin. Roentgenol.* 20:7, 1985.

Frank K, et al.: Importance of early diagnosis and follow-up in multiple endocrine neoplasia (MEN IIB). *Eur. J. Pediatr.* 143:112, 1984.

Khan AH, et al.: Gastrointestinal manifestations of Sipple syndrome in children. *J. Pediatr. Surg.* 22:719, 1987.

Lucaya J, et al.: Syndrome of multiple mucosal neuromas, medullary thyroid carcinoma, and pheochromocytoma: Cause of colon diverticula in children. *A.J.R.* 133:1186, 1979.

Perkins JT, et al.: Adenomatous polyposis coli and multiple endocrine neoplasia type 2b. A pathogenetic relationship. *Cancer* 55:375, 1985.

Saltzman CL, et al.: Thick lips, bumpy tongue, and slipped capital femoral epiphysis—A deadly combination. *J. Pediatr. Orthop.* 8:219, 1988.

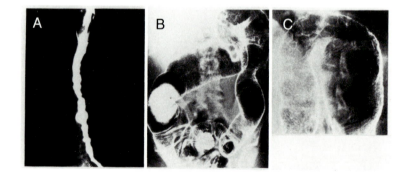

FIG SY–M–37.
Multiple endocrine neoplasia syndrome, type 2b, in an adult male. **A,** tertiary esophageal contractions. **B,** air-contrast enema: dilated colon with prominent transverse mucosal folds. **C,** hepatic flexure with plaquelike mucosal folds. (From Demos TC, Blander J, Shey WL, et al.: Multiple endocrine neoplasia (MEN) syndrome type IIB: Gastrointestinal manifestations. *A.J.R.* 140:73, 1983. Used by permission.)

Williams ED, et al.: Multiple mucosal neuromata with endocrine tumours: A syndrome allied to von Recklinghausen's disease. *J. Pathol. Bacteriol.* 91:71, 1966.

MULTIPLE SYNOSTOSIS SYNDROME

Mode of Inheritance: Autosomal dominant.

Clinical Manifestations: (a) *facial features:* low frontal hair implantation, wide nasal root, beaked nasal tip, alar hypoplasia, hemicylindrical nose, thin upper lip, short philtrum, microstomia, strabismus; (b) *limitation of joint motions* (elbows, hands and wrists, ankles and feet, temporomandibular joints); (c) *conductive hearing deficit* with an onset after adolescence; (d) short stature, failure to thrive; (e) other reported abnormalities: syndactyly, reduction of the tip of the phalanges and associated nail abnormalities, mental retardation, dermatoglyphic abnormalities, low-set ears, an asymmetrical mouth, hypoplasia of the thenar and hypothenar muscles, genu valgus, mild pectus excavatum, broad halluces.

Radiologic Manifestations: (a) *progressive symphalangia;* narrow distance between the proximal and middle phalanges in infancy followed by *progressive bony fusion;* deformity of the distal end of the metacarpals; partial or total absence of the distal phalanges; bony fusion at the elbow and carpal, tibiotarsal, and tarsal joints; radiohumeral fusion; radio-ulnar fusion; radial head subluxation; abnormal configuration of the carpal bones; shortness of the first metatarsals; normal or short middle phalanges; pseudoepiphyses of the proximal phalanges; agenesis of the middle or distal phalanges of the hands and feet; disturbance in bone modeling of the phalanges; (b) *vertebral fusion,* vertebral deformities, Scheuermann disease; (c) *fusion of middle-ear ossicles;* (d) other reported abnormalities: clinodactyly, syndactyly, pes planovalgus with a prominent lateral border.

Notes: (a) WL symphalangia–brachydactyly syndrome (Herrmann) may represent a variant of the multiple synostosis syndrome; (b) the term *polysynostosis* (Gordon) has been used in relation to craniosynostosis in association with radio-ulnar synostosis.

REFERENCES

da-Silva EO, et al.: Multiple synostosis syndrome: Study of a large Brazilian kindred. *Am. J. Med. Genet.* 18:237, 1984.

Gordon IRS, et al.: Polysynostosis: The association of extracranial synostosis and craniostenosis. *Clin. Radiol.* 25:253, 1974.

Herrmann J: Symphalangism and brachydactyly syndrome: Report of WL symphalangism–brachydactyly syndrome: Review of literature and classification. *Birth Defects* 10:23, 1974.

Hurvitz SA, et al.: The facio-audio-symphalangism

syndrome: Report of a case and review of the literature. *Clin. Genet.* 28:61, 1985.

Maroteaux P, et al.: La maladie des synostoses multiples. *Nouv. Presse Med.* 1:3041, 1972.

Pedersen JC: Multiple synostosis syndrome. *Eur. J. Pediatr.* 134:273, 1980.

Poisson D, et al.: Maladie des synostoses multiples. Etude de la variation des symptômes dans une même famille. *Arch. Fr. Pediatr.* 40:35, 1983.

Vessel ES: Symphalangism, strabismus and hearing loss in mother and daughter. *N. Engl. J. Med.* 236:839, 1960.

MYASTHENIC SYNDROMES

Classification: (a) acquired autoimmune diseases: (1) myasthenia gravis; (2) Lambert-Eaton myasthenia syndrome; (b) congenital myasthenic syndromes (nonautoimmune disorders): (1) defect in acetylcholine synthesis or mobilization (autosomal recessive); (2) end-plate acetylcholinesterase deficiency (sporadic); (3) slow-channel syndrome (autosomal dominant and sporadic); (4) end-plate acetylcholine receptor deficiency (autosomal recessive).

Clinical Manifestations: (a) *fatiguability;* (b) *weakness of voluntary muscles: drooping eyelid(s), double vision, alteration in voice, nasal regurgitation, choking, dysphagea, chewing difficulty, weakness of limbs,* etc; (c) associated disorders: thymic hyperplasia, thymoma, hyperthyroidism, hypothyroidism, thyroiditis, rheumatoid arthritis, systemic lupus erythematosus, blood disorders (hemolytic anemia, pernicious anemia, red cell aplasia, idiopathic thrombocytopenic purpura), vitiligo, pemphigus, sarcoidosis, ulcerative colitis, leukemia, lymphoma, polymyositis, Sjögren syndrome, multiple sclerosis, scleroderma, convulsive disorders; (d) anti–acetylcholine receptor antibodies in the sera.

Radiologic Manifestations: *Thymoma; thymic hyperplasia;* radiological manifestations of other associated disorders enumerated under Clinical Manifestations.

Note: Familial infantile myasthenia gravis is characterized by the absence of myasthenia in the mother, absence of severe ophthalmoplegia, occurrence in siblings, severe respiratory problems and feeding difficulties at birth, weakness of the diaphragm, congenital contracture, and absence of anti–acetylcholine receptors.

REFERENCES

Batra P, et al.: Mediastinal imaging in myasthenia gravis: Correlation of chest radiography, CT, MR, and surgical findings. *A.J.R.* 148:515, 1987.

Engel AG: Myasthenia gravis and myasthenic syndromes. *Ann. Neurol.* 16:519, 1984.

Gieron MA, et al.: Familial infantile myasthenia gravis. Report of three cases with follow-up until adult life. *Arch. Neurol.* 42:143, 1985.

Goldberg RE, et al.: Serial CT scans in thymic hyperplasia. *J. Comput. Assist. Tomogr.* 11:539, 1987.

Goulon M, et al.: La myasthénie, modèle de maladie par auto-anticorps. *Ann. Med. Interne (Paris)* 138:444, 1987.

Hageman G, et al.: Muscle weakness and congenital contractures in a case of congenital myasthenia. *J. Pediatr. Orthop.* 6:227, 1986.

Herrmann C Jr: Myasthenia gravis—current concepts. *West J. Med.* 142:797, 1985.

Kerzin-Storrar L, et al.: Genetic factors in myasthenia gravis: A family study. *Neurology* 38:38, 1988.

Morel E, et al.: Neonatal myasthenia gravis: A new clinical and immunologic appraisal on 30 cases. *Neurology* 38:138, 1988.

Thorvinger B, et al.: Computed tomography of the thymus gland in myasthenia gravis. *Acta Radiol.* 28:399, 1987.

MYHRE SYNDROME

Clinical manifestations: (a) prenatal and postnatal growth deficiency; (b) maxillary hypoplasia, prognathism, short palpebral fissures, short philtrum; (c) mental deficiency; (d) generalized muscular hypertrophy, decreased joint mobility; (e) other abnormalities: cardiac anomalies, cryptorchidism, severe mixed hearing loss.

Radiologic Manifestations: (a) thickened calvarium, prominent broad mandible; (b) broad ribs, large and flattened vertebrae with large pedicles, hypoplastic iliac wings; (c) shortness of the long and short tubular bones.

REFERENCES

Myhre SA, Ruvalcaba RHA, Graham CB: A new growth deficiency syndrome. *Clin. Genet.* 20:1, 1981.

Soljak MA, et al.: A new syndrome of short stature, joint limitation and muscle hypertrophy. *Clin. Genet.* 23:441, 1983.

MYOTONIC DYSTROPHY

Synonyms: Dystrophia myotonica; Steinert disease.

Mode of Inheritance: Autosomal dominant; variable expressivity, neonatal form almost exclusively maternally transmitted.

Clinical Manifestations: (a) Neonatal: (1) reduced fetal movement during pregnancy, hydrops, hydramnios; (2) hypotonia, generalized muscle atrophy, tented upper lip, facial diplegia, ptosis, anal sphincter insufficiency; (3) respiratory difficulties after birth, feeding difficulties, pleural effusion; (4) edema; (5) unexplained hematomas (skin, brain, liver); (6) high incidence of foot deformities, joint deformities; (7) confirmation of the suspected diagnosis in a floppy infant: examination of the mother (including myotonic hand grip noted during a routine handshake, ptosis, etc.); (8) high neonatal mortality; (b) children and adults: (1) *myotonia* (prolonged contraction of a voluntary muscle that diminishes with re-peated use of the muscle), muscle wasting, myopathic facies; (2) *cataract*; (3) *frontal baldness*; (4) *cardiovascular manifestations*: left ventricular dysfunction, slowing throughout the conduction system (electrophysiological studies), abnormalities of electrocardiographic findings, arrhythmias, mitral valve prolapse, low blood pressure, congestive heart failure, sudden death (heterogenous replacement of the myocardium and conducting system by fatty and fibrous tissue); (5) endocrinopathy: gonadal atrophy, hypergonadotropic hypogonadism, hyperparathyroidism (adenoma), insulin resistance and hyperinsulinism, hyperthyroidism, Addison disease, hypothyroidism; (6) jejunal manometric study: low-amplitude contractions, abnormal higher-frequency contractions, abnormal retrograde-wave propagation, interruption of contractions; esophageal manometry: anomalous motility, depressed pressure in the lower segment; (7) other reported abnormalities: low serum concentration of IgG and IgA, mental retardation, increased incidence of cholelithiasis, pneumonias (infection, aspiration), association with cystinuria in two brothers, talipes equinovarus, coexistence with myasthenia gravis,

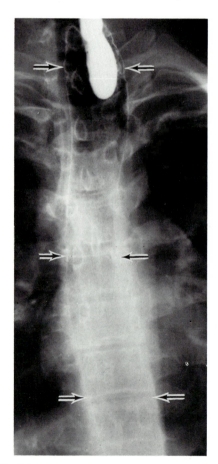

FIG SY–M–38.

Myotonic dystrophy: dilated esophagus *(arrows)* in a 21-year-old male. No peristalsis was seen anywhere in the esophagus at the fluoroscopic examination. The patient also had a megacolon. (From Goldberg HI, Sheft DJ: Esophageal and colon changes in myotonia dystrophica. *Gastroenterology* 63:134, 1972. Used by permission.)

alveolar hypoventilation, atrophy of the distal parts of extremities.

Radiologic Manifestations: (a) neonatal: (1) thin ribs in contrast to the normal appearance of the rest of the skeleton; (2) elevated leaf of diaphragm; (3) aspiration pneumonia; (4) ventricular dilatation; (b) adult: (1) *thick calvaria,* large frontal sinuses, *small sella turcica,* craniokyphosis, small nasal angle, hypotelorism, enlarged mandible, subluxation of temporomandibular joints; (2) *atrophy of skeletal muscles* (loss of muscle mass, increase in fat and connective tissues), sternocleidomastoid muscle atrophy as an earliest manifestation, muscle hypertrophy (abdominal wall and spinal muscles) coexisting with atrophy of limb muscles in the early stage; (3) *alimentary tract dysfunction:* abnormal swallowing with pooling of material within valleculae and pyriform fossae, tracheal aspiration, dilatation of the esophagus, small bowel and colon, deficient haustral pattern of the colon, segmental hypertonicity, decrease in contractility of the biliary tract; (4) unilateral or bilateral elevation of the diaphragm; (5) *urinary tract dysfunction* in the form of poor contractility and poor emptying; (6) other reported abnormalities: pectus excavatum, short fourth metacarpal, arachnodactyly.

Differential Diagnosis: Cerebral hypotonia; Werdnig-Hoffman disease; myotubular myopathy (newborn); nemaline myopathy; etc.

Note: The disease is detectable in childhood; electrical myotonia is demonstrable by electromyography before the appearance of the usual clinical manifestations (Fig SY−M−38).

REFERENCES

Bundey S: Clinical evidence for heterogeneity in myotonic dystrophy. *J. Med. Genet.* 19:341, 1982.
Chassevent J, et al.: Myotonic dystrophy (Steinert's disease) in the neonate. *Radiology* 127:747, 1978.
Chudley AE, et al.: Diaphragmatic elevation in neonatal myotonic dystrophy. *Am. J. Dis. Child.* 133:1182, 1979.
Curry CJR, et al.: Hydrops and pleural effusions in congenital myotonic dystrophy. *J. Pediatr.* 113:555, 1988.
Glantz RH, et al.: Central nervous system magnetic resonance imaging findings in myotonic dystrophy. *Arch. Neurol.* 45:36, 1988.
Harada S-I, et al.: Association of primary hyperparathyroidism with myotonic dystrophy in two patients. *Arch. Intern. Med.* 147:777, 1987.
Kimura S, et al.: Cystinuria with congenital myotonic dystrophy. *Pediatr. Neurol.* 3:233, 1987.
Koh THHG: Do you shake hands with mothers of floppy babies? *Br. Med. J.* 289:485, 1984.
Mabille JP, et al.: Esophageal involvement in a case of congenital myotonic dystrophy. *Pediatr. Radiol.* 12:89, 1982.
Maytal J, et al.: The coexistence of myasthenia gravis and myotonic dystrophy in one family. *Neuropediatrics* 18:8, 1987.
Moorman JR, et al.: Cardiac involvement in myotonic muscular dystrophy. *Medicine (Baltimore)* 64:371, 1985.
Nowak TV, et al.: Small intestinal motility in myotonic dystrophy patients. *Gastroenterology* 86:808, 1984.
Pagliara S, et al.: Hyperthyroidism and Addison's disease in a patient with myotonic dystrophy. *Arch. Intern. Med.* 145:919, 1985.
Perloff JK, et al.: Cardiac involvement in myotonic muscular dystrophy (Steinert's disease): A prospective study of 25 patients. *Am. J. Cardiol.* 54:1074, 1984.
Regev R, et al.: Cerebral ventricular dilation in congenital myotonic dystrophy. *J. Pediatr.* 111:372, 1987.
Rickards D, et al.: Computed tomography in dystrophia myotonica. *Neuroradiology* 24:27, 1982.
Siegel IM, et al.: Contributory etiologic factor for talipes equinovarus in congenital myotonic dystrophy: Comparative biopsy study on intrinsic foot musculature and vastus lateralis in two cases. *J. Pediatr. Orthop.* 4:327, 1984.
Steinert H: Myopathologische Beiträge: Ueber das klinische und anatomische Bild des Muskelschwunds der Myotoniker. *Dtsch. Z. Nervenheilkd.* 37:58, 1909.
Weiner MJ: Myotonic megacolon in myotonic dystrophy. *A.J.R.* 130:177, 1978.
Wesström G, et al.: Congenital myotonic dystrophy. *Acta Paediatr. Scand.* 75:849, 1986.
Yoshida H, et al: Hyperparathyroidism in patients with myotonic dystrophy. *J. Clin. Endocrinol. Metab.* 67:488, 1988.

MYOTUBULAR MYOPATHY

Mode of Inheritance: X-linked, sporadic.

Clinical Manifestations: (a) prenatal: decreased fetal movement, hydramnios; (b) postnatal: respiratory distress due to severe respiratory muscle impairment, asphyxia, height over the 90th percentile (discrepancy between height and weight).

Radiologic Manifestations: Thin ribs; elevated diaphragm.

Note: The muscle biopsy in definite female carriers shows abnormalities including myotubes.

REFERENCES

Barth PG, et al.: X-linked myotubular myopathy with fatal neonatal asphyxia. *Neurology* 25:531, 1975.
LeGuennec J-C, et al.: High stature in neonatal myotubular myopathy. *Acta Paediatr. Scand.* 77:610, 1988.
van Wijngaarden GK, et al.: Familial "myotubular" myopathy. *Neurology (Minneap.)* 19:908, 1969.

MYXOMA-SPOTTY PIGMENTATION-ENDOCRINE OVERACTIVITY

Synonyms: Syndrome myxoma; NAME syndrome; Carney syndrome; myxoma syndrome.

Frequency: Rare.

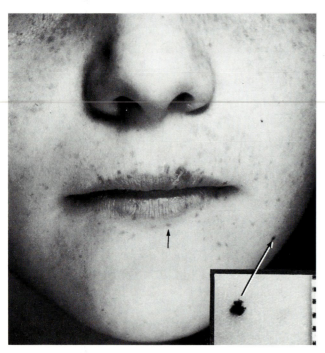

FIG SY–M–39.
"LAMB" syndrome. Brown *(small arrow)* and black *(large arrow)* macules are scattered about the face and lips. The inset is an enlargement of a black macule (scale in millimeters). (From Rhodes AR, Silverman RA, Harrist TJ, et al.: Mucocutaneous lentigines, cardiocutaneous myxomas, and multiple blue nevi: The "LAMB" syndrome. *J. Am. Acad. Dermatol.* 10:72, 1984. Used by permission.)

Clinical and Radiologic Manifestations: (a) *cardiac myxoma,* single or multiple located in atria and/or ventricles; (b) *pigmented skin lesions* ("freckling"), 68%: centrofacial distribution of lesions (simple freckles, lentigines, multiple superficial nevi, "cutaneous pigmented macules," blue nevi; (c) hy- perpigmented macules of the mucous membranes; (d) peripheral tumors (57%): myxoid tumors or neurofibromas (trunk, face, limbs, vocal cords); (e) endocrine neoplasms, Cushing syndrome, pheochromocytoma, testicular tumor (large cell calcifying Sertoli cell, interstitial cell tumor), thyroid, etc.

Notes: (a) NAME syndrome (nevi, atrial myxoma, myxoid neurofibroma, ephelides); (b) the mean age of the patients with this syndrome is 25 years as compared with sporadic cases of cardiac myxoma—56 years; (c) the following abnormalities have been reported in the first-degree relatives of the patients with this syndrome: familial cardiac myxoma, familial noncardiac myxoid tumors, familial endocrine neoplasm, freckling; (d) LAMB syndrome (lentigines, atrial myxoma, mucocutaneous myxoma, blue nevi) is considered to represent a variant of this syndrome (Fig SY–M–39).

REFERENCES

Atherton DJ, et al.: A syndrome of various cutaneous pigmented lesions, myxoid neurofibromata and atrial myxoma: the NAME syndrome. *Br. J. Dermatol.* 103:421, 1980.

Carney JA, et al.: The complex of myxomas, spotty pigmentation, and endocrine overactivity. *Medicine (Baltimore)* 64:270, 1985.

Frankenfeld RH, et al.: Bilateral myxomas of the heart. *Ann. Intern. Med.* 53:827, 1960.

Rhodes AR, et al.: Mucocutaneous lentigines, cardiomucocutaneous myxomas, and multiple blue nevi: The "LAMB" syndrome. *J. Am. Acad. Dermatol.* 10:72, 1984.

Vatterott PJ, et al.: Syndrome cardiac myxoma: More than just a sporadic event. *Am. Heart J.* 114:886, 1987.

Vidaillet H Jr, et al.: "Syndrome myxoma": A subset of patients with cardiac myxoma associated with pigmented skin lesions and peripheral and endocrine neoplasms. *Br. Heart J.* 57:247, 1987.

N SYNDROME

Mode of Inheritance: Either autosomal recessive or X-linked recessive.

Frequency: Two brothers (Hess et al.).

Clinical Manifestations: (a) severe mental and growth retardation, visual impairment, deafness; (b) dolichocephaly, hypotelorism, "scalloped" laterally overlapping upper eyelid, large cornea, abnormal auricles, dental dysplasia; (c) leukemia in the two reported brothers; (d) other reported abnormalities: high fingerprint ridge counts, cryptorchidism, hypospadias, spasticity.

Radiologic Manifestations: Overtubulation of the long bones, distal long bones being relatively shorter than the proximal long bones.

REFERENCES

Hess RO, et al.: The N syndrome, a "new" multiple congenital anomaly–mental retardation syndrome. *Clin. Genet.* 6:237, 1974.

Hess RO, et al.: Update on the N-syndrome: Occurrence of lymphoid malignancy and possible association with a balanced 4;6 translocation. *Pediatr. Pathol.* 5:98, 1986.

NAGER SYNDROME

Synonyms: Acrofacial dysostosis; Nager anomaly.

Mode of Inheritance: Most cases sporadic; autosomal recessive; genetic heterogeneity.

Frequency: Approximately 25 published cases; underreported (Chemke et al., Goldstein et al.).

Clinical Manifestations: (a) *mandibulofacial dysostosis:* hypoplasia of the zygomatic arches, hypoplasia of the mandible, deformed external ear, antimongoloid slant of the palpebral fissures, coloboma of eyelids, Robin anomaly, preauricular fistula, macrostomia; (b) *upper limb anomalies:* short and deformed forearm, thumb aplasia/hypoplasia, limitation of elbow extension; (c) other reported abnormalities: short stature, mild mental retardation, language delay, hearing loss, genital malformations, gastroschisis, simian creases, pigmented nevi, lower-limb anomalies (limitation of knee motion, overlapping toes, absent distal flexion creases in all toes, second toe longer than the great toe), laryngeal and epiglottic hypoplasia, etc.

Radiologic Manifestations: (a) *mandibulofacial dysostosis;* (b) *limb anomalies* (preaxial): radial hypoplasia or aplasia, radio-ulnar synostosis, hypoplasia or aplasia of the thumb, syndactyly of the first and second digital rays, hip dysplasia; (c) vertebral anomalies, rib anomalies; (d) in utero ultrasonographic diagnosis (mandibulofacial deformities and limb anomalies).

Differential Diagnosis: (a) Treacher Collins syndrome (mandibulofacial dysostosis); (b) conditions with mandibulofacial dysostosis associated with acral anomalies: postaxial acrofacial dysostosis, Fountain syndrome (hypoplastic mandible, cleft palate, high nasal bridge, cup-shaped ears, syndactyly, autosomal dominant), distal 2q duplication (Halal et al.), hemifacial microsomia/Goldenhar radial defect syndrome (Halal et al.) (Figs SY–N–1 and SY–N–2).

REFERENCES

Benson CB, et al.: Sonography of Nager acrofacial dysostosis syndrome in utero. *J. Ultrasound Med.* 7:163, 1988.

Chemke J, et al.: Autosomal recessive inheritance of Nager acrofacial dysostosis. *J. Med. Genet.* 25:230, 1988.

Giugiani R, et al.: Nager's acrofacial dysostosis with thumb duplication: report of a case. *Clin. Genet.* 26:228, 1984.

Goldstein DJ, et al.: Nager acrofacial dysostosis: Evidence for apparent heterogeneity. *Am. J. Med. Genet.* 30:741, 1988.

Halal F, et al.: Differential diagnosis of Nager acrofacial dysostosis syndrome: Report of four patients with Nager syndrome and discussion of other related syndromes. *Am. J. Med. Genet.* 14:209, 1983.

Hecht JT, et al.: The Nager syndrome. *Am. J. Med. Genet.* 27:965, 1987.

Kawira EL, et al.: Acrofacial dysostosis with severe facial clefting and limb reduction. *Am. J. Med. Genet.* 17:641, 1984.

Krauss CM, et al.: Anomalies in an infant with Nager acrofacial dysostosis. *Am. J. Med. Genet.* 21:761, 1985.

Nager FR, de Reynier JP: Das Gehöorgan bei den angeborenen Köpfmissbildungen. *Pract. Otorhino-laryngol. [Suppl.]* 2:10:1, 1948.

Pfeiffer RA, et al.: Acrofacial dysostosis (Nager syndrome): Synopsis and report of a new case. *Am. J. Med. Genet.* 15:255, 1983.

Poissonnier M, et al.: Dysostose mandibulo-faciale et ulno-fibulaire léthale. *Ann. Pediatr. (Paris)* 30:713, 1983.

NAIL-PATELLA SYNDROME

Synonyms: Onycho-osteodysplasia; osteo-onychodysplasia; iliac horn syndrome; Turner-Fong syndrome; hereditary onycho-osteodysplasia (HOOD syndrome); Turner-Kieser

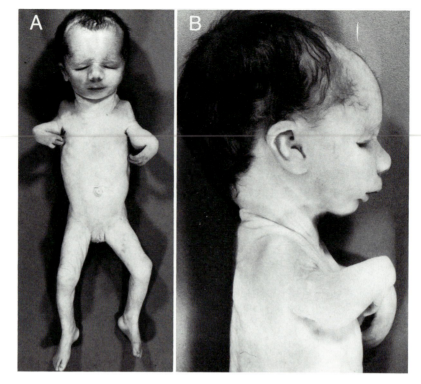

FIG SY–N–1.
A and **B,** Nager syndrome. Stillborn infant with mandibulofacial dysostosis and bilateral radial hemimelia. (From Pfeiffer RA, Stoess

H: Acrofacial dysostosis (Nager syndrome): Synopsis and report of a new case. *Am. J. Med. Genet.* 15:255, 1983. Used by permission.)

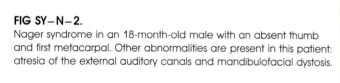

FIG SY–N–2.
Nager syndrome in an 18-month-old male with an absent thumb and first metacarpal. Other abnormalities are present in this patient: atresia of the external auditory canals and mandibulofacial dystosis.

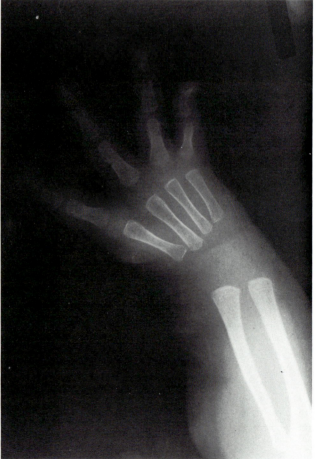

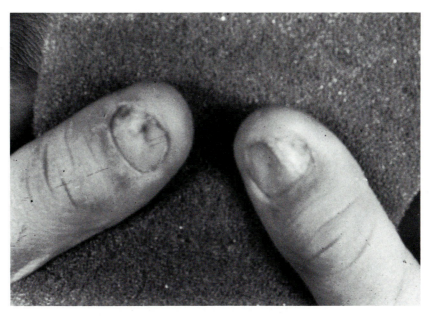

FIG SY−N−3.
Nail-patella syndrome: Nail hypoplasia of the thumbs.

syndrome; Osterreicher-Turner syndrome; elbow-patella syndrome.

Mode of Inheritance: Autosomal dominant.

Frequency: Not very rare (Looij et al.).

Clinical Manifestations: (a) *dysplasia of the nails* (80% to 90%): hypoplasia, absence, ridging, flatness; (b) *hypoplasia or absence of patellae* (60%), palpable iliac horns in some; (c) elbow deformity (60% to 90%) with an inability to fully extend, pronate, or supinate the forearm; flexion and contracture of other joints; (d) nephropathy of various severity and manifestation (30%) (glomerulonephritis or nephrotic syndrome): proteinuria, hematuria, end-stage renal failure in about 20% of patients in 5 to 25 years, electron microscopic demonstration of "pathognomonic changes" in the glomerular basement membrane; (e) short stature; (f) ocular abnor-

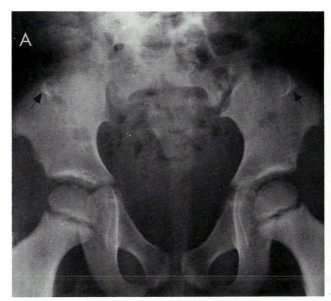
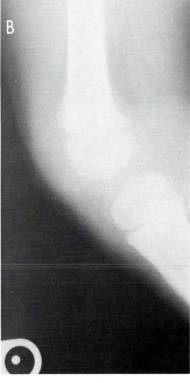

FIG SY−N−4.
Nail-patella syndrome in a 7½-year-old male with clinical features of dysplasia of the nails and absence of patellae. **A,** flaring of the iliac wings and iliac horns *(arrows).* **B,** absence of an ossification center in the patella.

malities: ptosis, abnormal pigmentation of the iris, glaucoma, microcornea, strabismus; (g) other reported abnormalities: webbing of the elbows, scoliosis, foot deformities, familial colon carcinoma, Castleman disease (angiofollicular lymph node hyperplasia causing a neck mass).

Radiologic Manifestations: (a) flaring of the iliac wing and small iliac angle; (b) *iliac horn* arising from the central area of the outer surface of the iliac wing; (c) elongated radius with *hypoplasia of the radial head* and subluxation or dislocation, *hypoplasia of the capitellum;* (d) *disproportionate prominence of the medial condyle of the femur;* (e) other skeletal reported abnormalities: hypoplastic scapula with a shallow glenoid fossa and long acromial process, thickening and convexity of the lateral border of the scapula, clinodactyly, camptodactyly, laxity of finger joints, equinovalgus deformity of the hindfoot and supination of forefoot, asymmetrical development of joints (hypoplasia or hyperplasia), calcaneovalgus deformity of the hind part of the foot, degenerative arthritis, renal osteopathy, pectus carinatum, a ball-and-socket ankle joint, forefoot supination and lateral subluxation of the tarsal-metatarsal joints; (f) renal abnormalities: duplication of the collecting system, asymmetry of kidney size, polycystic kidneys, obstructive uropathy, calculi (Figs SY−N−3 and SY−N−4).

REFERENCES

Fiedler BS, et al.: Foot deformity in hereditary onycho-osteodysplasia. *J. Can. Assoc. Radiol.* 38:305, 1987.

Fong EE: "Iliac horns" (symmetrical bilateral central posterior iliac processes): Case report. *Radiology* 47:517, 1946.

Garces MA, et al.: Hereditary onycho-osteo-dysplasia (HOOD syndrome): Report of two cases. *Skeletal Radiol.* 8:55, 1982.

Gilula LA, et al.: Familial colon carcinoma in nail-patella syndrome. *A.J.R.* 123:783, 1975.

Kieser W: Die Sog. Flughaut beim Menschen. Ihre Beziehung zum Status Dysraphicus und ihre Erblichkeit. *Z. Menschl. Vererb. Konstitutionslehre* 23:594, 1939.

Looij B Jr, et al.: Genetic counselling in hereditary osteo-onychodysplasia (HOOD, nail-patella syndrome) with nephropathy. *J. Med. Genet.* 25:682, 1988.

Neuhold A, et al.: Nail-Patella-Syndrom. *Radiologe* 22:568, 1982.

Österreicher W: Nagel-und Skelettanomalien. *Wien Klin. Wochenschr.* 42:632, 1929.

Reed D, et al.: Computed tomography of "iliac horns" in hereditary osteoonychodysplasia (nail-patella syndrome) *Pediatr. Radiol.* 17:168, 1987.

Salcedo JR: An autosomal recessive disorder with glomerular basement membrane abnormalities similar to those seen in the nail patella syndrome. Report of a kindred. *Am. J. Med. Genet.* 19:579, 1984.

Turner JW: Hereditary arthrodysplasia associated with hereditary dystrophy of nails. *J.A.M.A.* 100:882, 1933.

Williams HJ, et al.: Radiographic diagnosis of osteo-onychodysostosis in infancy. *Radiology* 109:151, 1973.

Wright TE, et al.: Angiofollicular lymph node hyperplasia causing a neck mass in nail-patella syndrome. *Am. J. Dis. Child.* 137:498, 1983.

Yakish SD, et al.: Long-term follow-up of the treatment of a family with nail-patella syndrome. *J. Pediatr. Orthop.* 3:360, 1983.

NANCE-HORAN SYNDROME

Synonyms: Cataract-dental syndrome; mesodens-cataract syndrome.

Mode of Inheritance: X-linked.

Clinical and Radiologic Manifestations: (a) congenital cataract; (b) dental abnormalities: screwdriver-shaped incisors, supernumerary maxillary incisors (mesodens), incisor diastema; (c) large, anteverted pinnae; (d) short fourth metacarpal.

REFERENCES

Bixler D, et al.: The Nance-Horan syndrome: A rare X-linked ocular-dental trait with expression in heterozygous females. *Clin. Genet.* 26:30, 1984.

Horan MB, et al.: X-linked cataract and Hutchinsonian teeth. *Aust. Paediatr. J.* 10:98, 1974.

Nance WE, et al.: Congenital X-linked cataracts, dental anomalies and brachymetacarpalia. *Birth Defects* 10:285, 1974.

NASO-DIGITO-ACOUSTIC SYNDROME

Mode of Inheritance: Reported in two brothers.

Clinical and Radiologic Manifestations: (a) large nose, high and broad nasal bridge, protuberant upper lip with cupid's bow configuration, large mouth, apparent hypertelorism; (b) broad and short distal phalanges, clinodactyly of the fifth fingers, tufting of several phalanges, slender limb bones, coxa valga; (c) sensorineural deafness.

Differential Diagnosis: Rubinstein-Taybi syndrome

REFERENCES

Keipert JA, et al.: A new syndrome of broad terminal phalanges and facial abnormalities. *Aust. Paediat. J.* 9:10, 1973.

McKusick VA: *Mendelian Inheritance in Man*, ed 8. Baltimore, Johns Hopkins University Press, 1988, p. 1096.

NASOPALPEBRAL LIPOMA-COLOBOMA SYNDROME

Synonym: Palpebral coloboma-lipoma syndrome.

Mode of Inheritance: Autosomal dominant.

Frequency: Eight persons in three generations of a Venezuelan family.

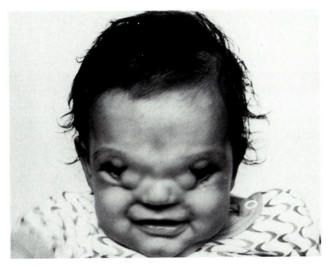

FIG SY—N—5.
Nasopharyngeal lipoma-coloboma syndrome in a 6-week-old male with bilateral symmetrical V-shaped colobomas of both upper and lower lids, sparse eyebrows, absent eyelashes medial to the colobomas, a broad and depressed nasal bridge, and subcutaneous nasopalpebral masses. (From Penchaszadeh VB, Velasquez D, Ramon A: The nasopalpebral lipoma-coloboma syndrome: A new autosomal dominant dysplasia-malformation syndrome with congenital nasopalpebral lipomas, eyelid colobomas, telecanthus, and maxillary hypoplasia. *Am. J. Med. Genet.* 11:397, 1982. Used by permission.)

Clinical Manifestations: (a) congenital symmetrical upper lid and nasopalpebral lipomas; (b) bilateral symmetrical upper and lower palpebral colobomas located at the junction of the inner and middle third of the lids; (c) telecanthus; (d) other reported abnormalities: broad forehead, widow's peak, abnormal pattern of eyebrows and eyelashes, maldevelopment of the lacrimal punctae, increased interpupillary distance (divergent strabismus), persistent epiphora, conjunctival hyperemia, corneal opacities, etc.

Radiologic Manifestations: Normal interorbital distance; abnormal cephalometric measurements (shortness of the anterior cranial base, hypoplasia of the midface, particularly the maxillae) (Fig SY—N—5).

REFERENCE

Penchaszadeh VB, et al.: The nasopalpebral lipoma-coloboma syndrome: A new autosomal dominant dysplasia-malformation syndrome with congenital nasopalpebral lipomas, eyelid colobomas, telecanthus, and maxillary hypoplasia. *Am. J. Med. Genet.* 11:397, 1982.

NELSON SYNDROME

Definition: Development of an adrenocorticotropic hormone (ACTH)-secreting pituitary tumor following total adrenalectomy for Cushing syndrome associated with adrenal hyperplasia (pituitary-dependent Cushing syndrome).

Clinical Manifestations: (a) development or worsening of skin and mucosal hyperpigmentation after adrenalectomy for Cushing syndrome; (b) clinical manifestation of pituitary tumor: assay for hormonal abnormalities (in particular, very important in microadenomas), headaches, bitemporal hemianopia, etc.

Radiologic Manifestations: (a) sellar enlargement and deformity; (b) pituitary tumor.

Note: Baseline imaging of the pituitary gland and regular follow-up examination for hyperpigmentation, visual field changes, and ACTH levels are recommended.

REFERENCES

Aronin N, et al.: Sustained remission of Nelson's syndrome after stopping cyproheptadine treatment. *N. Engl. J. Med.* 302:453, 1980.
Bitton RN, et al.: Development of Nelson's syndrome in a patient with recurrent Cushing's disease. Analysis of secretory behavior of the pituitary tumor. *Am. J. Med.* 84:319, 1988.
Nelson DH, et al.: ACTH-producing pituitary tumors following adrenalectomy for Cushing's syndrome. *Ann. Intern. Med.* 52:560, 1960.
Oldfield EH, et al.: Corticotropin-releasing hormone (CRH) stimulation in Nelson's syndrome: Response of adrenocorticotropin secretion to pulse injection and continuous infusion of CRH. *J. Clin. Endocrinol. Metab.* 62:1020, 1986.
Sheeler LR, et al.: Nelson's syndrome; a new look. *Cleve. Clin. Q.* 47:299, 1980.
Weinstein M, et al.: The sella turcica in Nelson's syndrome. *Radiology* 118:363, 1976.
Wislawski J, et al.: Results of neurosurgical treatment by a transphenoidal approach in 10 patients with Nelson's syndrome. *J. Neurosurg.* 62:68, 1985.
Young LW, et al.: Postadrenalectomy pituitary adenoma (Nelson's syndrome) in childhood: Clinical and roentgenologic detection. *A.J.R.* 126:550, 1976.

NEMALINE MYOPATHY

Synonym: Rod myopathy.

Mode of Inheritance: Autosomal dominant.

Pathology: Rodlike (or threadlike) structures within skeletal muscle cells (light microscopic examination) with close relationship to Z bands shown by ultrastructural studies.

Clinical Manifestations: Onset of symptoms in the neonatal period or later infancy: (a) muscle weakness, hypotonia (floppy infant); (b) persistent vomiting, poor weight gain; (d) recurrent pneumonias; (e) esophageal manometry: decreased lower esophageal sphincter pressure and low-amplitude peristalsis, significant gastroesophageal reflux; (f) progression of the disease through late childhood; (g) narrow, high-arched palate; (h) cardiomyopathy.

Radiologic Manifestations: (a) gastroesophageal reflux; (b) skeletal deformities related to muscular disease: kyphoscoliosis, hyperlordosis, pectus excavatum, limb deformities; (c) recurrent pneumonias, aspiration, atelectasis.

REFERENCES

Berezin S, et al.: Gastroesophageal reflux associated with nemaline myopathy of infancy. *Pediatrics* 81:111, 1988.

Cantani A, et al.: La myopathie á bâtonnets: syndrome à révélation néonatale sévère. *Arch. Fr. Pediatr.* 44:813, 1987.

Kondo K, et al.: Genetics of congenital nemaline myopathy. *Muscle Nerve* 3:308, 1980.

Meier C, et al.: Nemaline myopathy presenting as cardiomyopathy (letter). *N. Engl. J. Med.* 308:1536, 1983.

Shy GM, et al.: Nemaline myopathy. A new congenital myopathy. *Brain* 86:793, 1963.

Van Antwerpen C, et al.: Nemaline myopathy associated with hypertrophic cardiomyopathy. *Pediatr. Neurol.* 4:306, 1988.

NEPHROGENIC HEPATIC DYSFUNCTION SYNDROME

Clinical Manifestations: (a) *hypernephroma;* (b) *abnormal liver function test values, hepatomegaly,* regression of liver enlargement and abnormal liver function test results after nephrectomy (in some cases); (c) nonspecific constitutional symptoms.

Radiologic Manifestations: (a) *renal tumor;* (b) *hepatic arteriographic abnormalities:* pronounced hypervascularity, marked granularity during the capillary phase; (c) *absence of liver metastases.*

REFERENCES

Mena E, et al.: Angiography of the nephrogenic hepatic dysfunction syndrome. *Radiology* 111:65, 1974.

Stauffer MH: Nephrogenic hepatosplenomegaly, abstracted. *Gastroenterology* 40:694, 1961.

NEPHRONOPHTHISIS (FANCONI)

Synonym: Juvenile nephronophthisis.

Mode of Inheritance: Autosomal recessive.

Clinical Manifestations: Onset of symptoms in childhood and early adulthood: (a) growth retardation; (b) *polyuria and polydipsia;* (c) salt-wasting and *progressive uremia;* (d) hypocalcemic tetany; (e) hypertension; (f) *fixed low specific gravity of urine;* (g) anemia; (h) light microscopy: variable numbers of cysts at corticomedullary junction (present in 70% of cases); electron microscopy of tubular basement membrane: homogeneous thickening, splitting, reticulation,

thinning, complete loss, granular disintegration, and collapse.

Radiologic Manifestations: (a) *small kidneys;* (b) *nonvisualization or poor opacification of collecting systems* by excretory urography; (c) ultrasonography: disappearance of corticomedullary differentiation with renal parenchyma either isoechoic or hyperechoic as compared with the liver or spleen, small medullary cysts.

Differential Diagnosis: Autosomal dominant type of medullary cystic kidney with onset usually in adulthood.

Note: Nephronophthisis may be associated with other abnormalities and appear as distinct syndromes: retinitis pigmentosa (Senior syndrome—renal-retinal dystrophy, acrodysplasia with retinitis pigmentosa and nephropathy), liver fibrosis, neurocutaneous dysplasia.

REFERENCES

Dieterich E, et al.: Familial juvenile nephronophthisis with hepatic fibrosis and neurocutaneous dysplasia. *Helv. Paediatr. Acta* 35:261, 1980.

Fanconi G, et al.: Die familiäre juvenile Nephronophthise (die idiopathische parenchymatöse Schrumpfnier). *Helv. Paediatr. Acta* 6:1, 1951.

Garel LA, et al.: Juvenile nephronophthisis: Sonographic appearance in children with severe uremia. *Radiology* 151:93, 1984.

Gruppuso PA, et al.: Juvenile nephronophthisis with blindness in a three-month-old infant. Senior's syndrome associated with relative parathyroid insufficiency. *Clin. Pediatr. (Phila.)* 22:114, 1983.

Valdez RA, et al.: Renal transplantation in children with oculorenal syndrome. *Urology* 30:130, 1987.

Zollinger HU, et al.: Nephronophthisis (medullary cystic disease of the kidney). *Helv. Paediatr. Acta* 35:509, 1980.

NEPHROTIC SYNDROME

Mode of Inheritance: Autosomal recessive in the congenital type (3% to 6% of nephrotic syndrome in children is of the familial type); reported in identical twins.

Etiology: (a) congenital, mesangial sclerosis in infants; (b) idiopathic; (c) associated with neoplasms (Hodgkin lymphoma, lymphocytic lymphoma, leukemia, carcinomas), malaria and other parasitic diseases, collagen disease, membranous glomerulonephropathy, lupus nephritis, toxic nephropathy, amyloidosis, pyelonephritis, congenital toxoplasmosis, nerve deafness, hypoparathyroidism, fetal alcohol syndrome, Hurler syndrome, microcephaly (Galloway syndrome or microcephaly, hiatus hernia, and nephrotic syndrome), varicella infection, mumps virus infection, radiation nephritis, hypothyroidism in the congenital nephrotic syndrome.

Clinical Manifestations: (a) anorexia; (b) diarrhea; (c) *edema;* (d) *albuminuria;* (e) *hypoalbuminemia;* (f) increase in serum concentrations of cholesterol, triglycerides, and low- and very low density lipoproteins; low, normal, or elevated high-density lipoprotein concentrations; (g) *lipiduria;* (h) deficiency of prothrombin, elevated platelet counts and plasma fibrinogen levels, prolonged reptilase and thrombin times, thrombotic complications (arterial, venous).

Radiologic Manifestations: (a) *ascites;* (b) *pleural effusion* (in particular, infrapulmonary); (c) intermittent mediastinal widening; (d) renal enlargement; (d) changing ultrasonic pattern: large diffusely hyperechoic kidneys in the early stage, small kidneys with marked echogenicity of the deep cortex in the late phase of the disease; (e) stretching and narrowness of the intrarenal collecting system due to renal edema; (f) normal or small kidneys in patients with chronic renal disease; (g) pulmonary artery thrombosis (complication); (h) pericardial effusion, pulmonary edema; (i) edema of the bowel wall as seen on contrast studies; (j) renal vein thrombosis: widened renal vein(s) containing thrombi, thrombus in the inferior vena cava, renal enlargement, thickened Gerota fascia and the formation of pericapsular venous collaterals, abnormal renal parenchymal postcontrast enhancement [prolonged corticomedullary discrimination, delayed and/or persistent parenchymal opacification, delayed or absent opacification of the excretory collecting system], association with arterial and other venous thromboses (inferior vena cava, hepatic vein, pulmonary artery, femoral vein, femoral artery, mesenteric artery, cerebral vessels, dural sinus), pulmonary emboli (Fig SY–N–6).

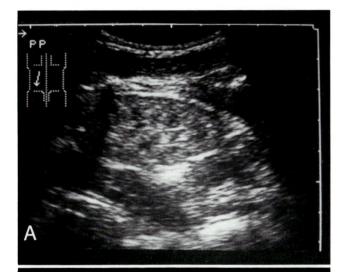

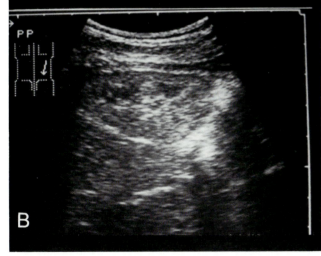

FIG SY–N–6.
Congenital nephrotic syndrome: prone longitudinal ultrasound scans of the left **(A)** and right kidneys **(B)** of a child aged 4 years and 6 months with small hyperechoic kidneys with sinusal echoes and medulla partially recognizable; narrow hypoechoic subcapsular band. (From Perale R, Talenti E, Lubrano G, et al.: Late ultrasonographic pattern in congenital nephrotic syndrome of Finnish type. *Pediatr. Radiol.* 18:71, 1988. Used by permission.)

REFERENCES

Aviad I, et al.: Intermittent mediastinal widening in the nephrotic syndrome. *Br. J. Radiol.* 32:488, 1959.

Barakat AY, et al.: Familial nephrosis, nerve deafness, and hypoparathyroidism. *J. Pediatr.* 91:61, 1977.

Bensman A, et al.: Manifestations frustes des thromboses artérielles pulmonaires au cours du syndrome néphrotique. *Arch. Fr. Pediatr.* 40:335, 1983.

Dunbar JS, et al.: Infrapulmonary pleural effusion with particular reference to its occurrence in nephrosis. *J. Can. Assoc. Radiol.* 10:24, 1959.

Elzouki AY, et al.: Primary nephrotic syndrome in Arab children. *Arch. Dis. Child.* 59:253, 1984.

Epstein AA: Concerning the causation of edema in chronic parenchymal nephritis: Method for its alleviation. *Am. J. Med. Sci.* 154:638, 1917.

Gagliano RG, et al.: The nephrotic syndrome associated with neoplasia: An unusual paraneoplastic syndrome. *Am. J. Med.* 60:1026, 1976.

Gatewood OMB, et al.: Renal vein thrombosis in patients with nephrotic syndrome: CT diagnosis. *Radiology* 159:117, 1986.

Gaudelus J et al.: Association d'un syndrome néphrotique à début précoce et d'une microcéphalie. A propos de 4 observations dans deux familles. *Arch. Fr. Pediatr.* 41:409, 1984.

Helin I, et al.: Nephrotic syndrome after mumps virus infection. *Am. J. Dis. Child.* 137:1126, 1983.

Hoyer PF, et al.: Thromboembolic complications in children with nephrotic syndrome. *Acta Paediatr. Scand.* 75:804, 1986.

Jennette JC, et al.: Radiation nephritis causing nephrotic syndrome. *Urology* 22:631, 1983.

Kher KK, et al.: Nephrotic syndrome in children. *Curr. Probl. Pediatr.* 18:203, 1988.

Kibuta Y, et al.: Nephrotic syndrome with diffuse mesangial sclerosis in identical twins. *J. Pediatr.* 102:586, 1983.

Kleinknecht C, et al.: Coexistence of antenatal infantile and juvenile nephrotic syndrome in a single family. *J. Pediatr.* 98:938, 1981.

Lau SO, et al.: Sagittal sinus thrombosis in the nephrotic syndrome. *J. Pediatr.* 97:948, 1980.

Lewy PR, et al.: Nephrotic syndrome in association with renal vein thrombosis in infancy. *J. Pediatr.* 85:359, 1974.

Lin CY, et al.: Nephrotic syndrome associated with varicella infection. *Pediatrics* 75:1127, 1985.

Martin EC, et al.: Selective renal venography in patients with primary renal disease and the nephrotic syndrome. *Cardiovasc. Intervent. Radiol.* 3:175, 1980.

Moorthy AV, et al.: Nephrotic syndrome in Hodgkin's disease. *Am. J. Med.* 61:471, 1976.

McLean RH, et al.: Hypothyroidism in the congenital nephrotic syndrome. *J. Pediatr.* 101:72, 1982.

Mehls O, et al.: Hemostasis and thromboembolism in children with nephrotic syndrome: Differences from adults. *J. Pediatr.* 110:862, 1987.

Perale R, et al.: Late ultrasonographic pattern in congenital nephrotic syndrome of Finnish type. *Pediatr. Radiol.* 18:71, 1988.

Roos RAC, et al.: Congenital microcephaly, infantile spasms, psychomotor retardation, and nephrotic syndrome in two sibs. *Eur. J. Pediatr.* 146:532, 1987.

Salcedo JR, et al.: Idiopathic nephrotic syndrome in fetal alcohol syndrome. *Clin. Pediatr. (Phila.)* 25:365, 1986.

Shahin B, et al.: Congenital nephrotic syndrome associated with congenital toxoplasmosis. *J. Pediatr.* 85:366, 1974.

Shapiro CM, et al.: Nephrotic syndrome in two patients with cured Hodgkin's disease. *Cancer* 55:1799, 1985.

Taylor J, et al.: Nephrotic syndrome and hypertension in two children with Hurler syndrome. *J. Pediatr.* 108:726, 1986.

Vaziri ND, et al.: Urinary excretion and deficiency of prothrombin in nephrotic syndrome. *Am. J. Med.* 77:433, 1984.

Wagoner RD, et al.: Renal vein thrombosis in idiopathic membranous glomerulopathy and nephrotic syndrome: Incidence and significance. *Kidney Int.* 23:368, 1983.

Zilleruelo G, et al.: Persistence of serum lipid abnormalities in children with idiopathic nephrotic syndrome. *J. Pediatr.* 104:61, 1984.

NEU-LAXOVA SYNDROME

Mode of Inheritance: Autosomal recessive.

Frequency: Over 20 published cases (Tolmie, et al.).

Pathology: (a) brain anomalies: microcephaly, lissencephaly, hypoplastic cerebellum, agenesis of the corpus callosum, ventricular dilatation, hypoplasia of the spinal cord,

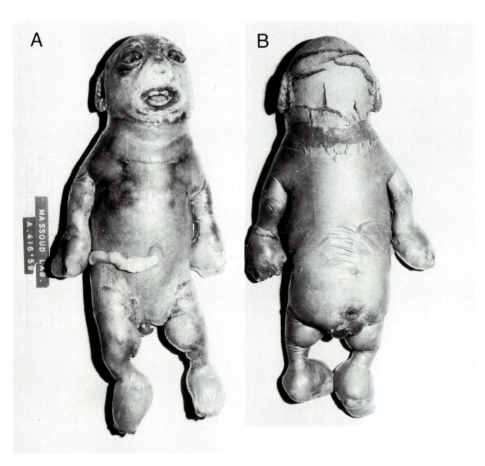

FIG SY–N–7.
Neu-Laxova syndrome. **A,** massive edema of the limbs and facial deformities are striking; **B,** the cracks on the back of the head are characteristic of ichthyotic lesions. Note the location of the anus and external genitalia, which are abnormally dorsal. (From Karimi-

Nejad MH, Khajavi H, Gharavi MJ, et al.: Neu-Laxova syndrome: Report of a case and comments. *Am. J. Med. Genet.* 28:17, 1987. Used by permission.)

etc.; (b) increased subcutaneous fat, atrophic muscles; (c) ichthyosis, edema; (c) hypoplasia of the placenta, short umbilical cord; (d) lung hypoplasia/atelectasis.

Clinical Manifestations: (a) *craniofacial anomalies:* slanted forehead, apparent hypertelorism, flat nose and nasal bridge, deformed ears, protuberant eyes, microphthalmos, cleft lips, micrognathia; (b) *limb anomalies:* hypoplastic fingers, syndactyly of the fingers and toes, rocker-bottom feet; (c) short neck; (d) other reported abnormalities: intrauterine growth retardation, short neck, edema, ichthyosis, hypoplasia of the external genitalia, yellow skin, etc.; (e) *perinatal death.*

Radiologic Manifestations: (a) prenatal ultrasonography: intrauterine growth retardation, hypoechoic skeletal structures, kyphosis, feeble fetal activity, restricted limb movement, microcephaly with a receding forehead and prominent eyes, generalized edema, flexion deformities of the limbs, swollen hands and feet causing the apparent absent digits, hydramnios/oligohydramnios; (b) skeletal system: short limbs,

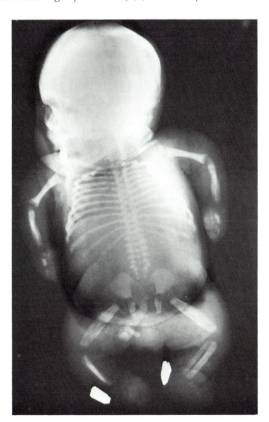

FIG SY—N—8.
Neu-Laxova syndrome in a newborn female: short limbs, poor modeling of the long bones with undertubulation and a "sticklike" appearance, severely underossified tubular bones of the hands and feet, dysplastic ilia with marked hypoplasia of acetabula and poorly ossified pubic bones, and a lack of ossification of the sacrum and coccyx. (From Scott CI, Louro JM, Laurence KM, et al.: Comments on the Neu-Laxova syndrome and CAD complex (letter). *Am. J. Med. Genet.* 9:165, 1981. Used by permission.)

"sticklike" long bones (Scott et al.), poor long bone cortex formation, undermineralization, thick calvaria, etc.

Differential Diagnosis: Cerebro-oculo-facio-skeletal (COFS) syndrome.

Note: Classification of the syndrome into three groups has been suggested (Curry): (a) group I: thin, lemon-colored, scaly skin; joint contractures; partial syndactyly; undermineralized bones; (b) group II: ichthyosis, massive swelling of the hands and feet; undermineralized bones, intrauterine fracture; (c) group III: ichthyosis, "harlequin fetus" appearance, hypoplastic digits, short limbs, "sticklike" long bones. There has been objection to this classification (Fitch) (Figs SY–N–7 and SY–N–8).

REFERENCES

Curry CJR: Further comments on the Neu-Laxova syndrome (letter). *Am. J. Med. Genet.* 13:441, 1982.

Ejeckam GG, et al.: Neu-Laxova syndrome: Report of two cases. *Pediatr. Pathol.* 5:295, 1986.

Fitch N: Comments on Dr. Curry's classification of the Neu-Laxova syndrome (letter). *Am. J. Med. Genet.* 15:515, 1983.

Karimi-Nejad MH, et al.: Neu-Laxova syndrome: Report of a case and comments. *Am. J. Med. Genet.* 28:17, 1987.

Laxova R, et al.: A further example of a lethal autosomal recessive condition in sibs. *J. Ment. Defic. Res.* 16:139, 1972.

Muller LM, et al.: A case of the Neu-Laxova syndrome: Prenatal ultrasonographic monitoring in the third trimester and the histopathological findings. *Am. J. Med. Genet.* 26:421, 1987.

Neu RL, et al.: A lethal syndrome of microcephaly with multiple congenital anomalies in three siblings. *Pediatrics* 47:610, 1971.

Ostrovskaya TI, et al.: Cerebral abnormalities in the Neu-Loxova syndrome. *Am. J. Med. Genet.* 30:747, 1988.

Scott CI, Louro JM, Laurence KM, et al.: Comments on the Neu-Laxova syndrome and CAD complex. *Am. J. Med. Genet.* 9:165, 1981.

Silengo MC, et al.: The Neu-COFS (cerebro-oculo-facio-skeletal) syndrome: Report of a case. *Clin. Genet.* 25:201, 1984.

Tolmie JL, et al.: The Neu-Laxova syndrome in female sibs: Clinical and pathological features with prenatal diagnosis in the second sib. *Am. J. Med. Genet.* 27:175, 1987.

NEUROCUTANEOUS MELANOSIS SEQUENCE

Synonyms: Rokitansky–van Bogaert syndrome; neurocutaneous syndrome.

Pathology: (a) excessive proliferation of melanin-producing cells in the skin and leptomeninges; (b) intracerebral melanotic pigmentation; (c) truncal nevi association with intraspinal melanosis.

Clinical Manifestations: (a) pigmented cutaneous nevi, hairy nevi, rarely diffuse pigmentation without discrete nevi; (b) seizures, chronic meningeal irritation, cranial nerve palsies, increased intracranial pressure, myelopathy; (c) association with malignant neoplasms: malignant melanoma, liposarcoma, rhabdomyosarcoma; (d) other reported abnormalities: psychiatric disturbance, intracranial hemorrhage

Radiologic Manifestations: (a) hydrocephalus (considered to be due to obstruction of cerebrospinal fluid circulation either at the fourth ventricle outlets or within the basal cisterns; (b) calcification in the suprasellar cistern, sylvian fissure, and occipital lobe (Leaney et al.); (c) spinal cord distortion, intraspinal mass, syringomyelia.

Differential Diagnosis: (a) melanotic neuroectomal tumor of the cranium (often in the anterior fontanelle region); (b) melanotic nerve sheath tumor; (c) epidermal nevus syndrome with a central nervous system lesion.

REFERENCES

Faillace WJ, et al.: Neurocutaneous melanosis with extensive intracerebral and spinal cord involvement. *J. Neurosurg.* 61:782, 1984.

Kudel TA, et al.: Computed tomographic findings of primarily malignant leptomeningeal melanoma in neurocutaneous melanosis. *A.J.R.* 133:950, 1979.

Leaney BJ, et al.: Neurocutaneous melanosis with hydrocephalus and syringomyelia. *J. Neurosurg.* 62:148, 1985.

Rokitansky J: Ein ausgezeichneter Fall von Pigmentmal mit ausgebreiteter Pigmentirung der inneren Hirn- und Rückenmarkshäute. *Allg. Wien Med. Ztg.* 6:113, 1861.

Van Bogaert L: La mélanose neurocutanée diffuse hérédofamiliale. *Bull. Acad. R. Med. Belg.* 13:397, 1948.

Zúñiga S, et al.: Rhabdomyosarcoma arising in a congenital giant nevus associated with neurocutaneous melanosis in a neonate. *J. Pediatr. Surg.* 22:1036, 1987.

NEUROFIBROMATOSIS

Synonym: von Recklinghausen disease.

Mode of Inheritance: Autosomal dominant; high rate of new mutation; gene responsible for neurofibromatosis located near the centromere on chromosome 17.

Frequency: Estimated to be 1 case in about 3000 births (Sørensen et al.).

Clinical Manifestations: A hamartomatous disorder (neurocristopathy, neuroectodermal and mesodermal dysplasia); *widespread multiple organ system involvement:* (a) *cutaneous:* café au lait spots, subcutaneous neurofibromas, elephantoid overgrowth of skin and soft tissues, breast enlargement, other skin lesion (hemangioma, red-blue macules, pseudoatrophic lesions, hypomelanotic macules, giant hairy nevi, xanthogranulomas); (b) *gastrointestinal:* pain, hemor-

rhage, nausea, vomiting, distension, constipation, diarrhea, perforation of the bowel, jaundice; (c) *cardiovascular system:* systemic arterial hypertension, idiopathic hypertrophic subaortic stenosis, congenital heart defects (pulmonary stenosis, aortic stenosis, ventricular septal defect, atrial septal defect, etc.), complete heart block, hypotension, aortic coarctation, coronary lesion associated with vasospasm and myocardial infarction, abdominal angina due to compression of the celiac and superior mesenteric arteries by plexiform neurofibromatosis, regressive hypertrophic cardiomyopathy in infancy; (d) *skeletal system:* bowing of the limbs, kyphoscoliosis, skull defects and deformities (temporal or frontal mass, pulsating or nonpulsating exophthalmos, displacement of the globe, edema of the eyelids and ptosis, disturbed vision), macrodactyly, pectus excavatum, pectus carinatum; (e) *neurofibromas of peripheral nerves,* optic nerve involvement; (f) macrocrania, learning disabilities, behavior disturbances, mental retardation, seizures, childhood hypertensive stroke; (g) endocrine and metabolic disorders: hyperparathyroidism, sexual precocity, gigantism, osteomalacia, rickets, multiple endocrine adenomatosis, hypoglycemia, hyperprolactinemia; (h) associated neoplastic lesions: central nervous system (glioma, meningioma, malignant neurilemoma, etc), peripheral nervous system (neurosarcoma, neuromyxoma, acoustic neuroma, etc), others (sarcomas, carcinomas, leukemia, lymphoma, etc), sarcomatous degeneration of neurofibromas, etc.; (i) ocular abnormalities: Lisch nodules (hamartomatous lesions of the iris), eyelid neurofibroma, S-shaped ptosis of the lid, congenital glaucoma, buphthalmos, retinal detachment, retinal phakoma, hypertelorism; (j) other reported abnormalities: abnormal congenital dermatoglyphic patterns, overgrowth or undergrowth, hypertrophy of the clitoris and labia, enlargement of the penis, juvenile xanthogranuloma, fragile X syndrome, postaxial polydactyly, sleep apnea, osteomalacia (vitamin resistant, hypophosphoremic), neurofibromatosis-Noonan syndrome (neurofibromatosis associated with a facial appearance resembling that of patients with Noonan syndrome), sporadic cases of multiple intestinal neurofibromatosis without cutaneous features of von Recklinghausen disease, association with multiple endocrine neoplasia.

Radiologic Manifestations: (a) *skull:* erosions and enlargement of foramina; bone defects, in particular, in the posterior and superior orbital wall and along lambdoid sutures; enlarged orbit; mandibular abnormalities (hypoplasia with flattening of the external contour, thinning of the body and the ramus, widening of the medial and lateral coronoid spaces, bilateral coronoid hyperplasia); (b) cranial contents: macroencephaly, nonneoplastic cerebral and cerebellar calcification, hydrocephalus, tumors (cranial nerve schwannomas, especially acoustic neuromas, optochiasmal gliomas, brain stem and supratentorial gliomas), arachnoid cysts, arterial occlusive disease, moyamoya, signal hyperintensity on T_2-weighted images of optic pathways (optic nerves, optic chiasm, optic tracts, lateral geniculate body, optic radiations, basal ganglia, periventricular white matter, cerebellar white matter, dentate nucleus of the cerebellum), plexiform neurofibromatosis of the orbit, buphthalmos, enlarged internal auditory canals secondary to dural ectasia without associated acoustic neuromas; (c) spine: kyphoscoliosis, enlargement of intervertebral foramina, scalloping of vertebral bodies (anterior, posterior, lateral), prominent "erosive" changes at the apex of the kyphotic curve, agenesis or hypoplasia of pedicle(s), spondylolisthesis, spindling of transverse processes, widening of the gap between the zygapophyseal joints and the transverse processes of adjacent vertebrae (anteroposterior projections of the spine), increased distance between adjacent transverse processes, instability of spinal segments leading to subluxation or dislocation; (d) spinal contents: dural ectasia, meningocele (cervical, thoracic, lumbar), intramedullary neurofibromatosis, stenosis of the neurocanal, cord compression and displacement; (e) limb bones: erosion of bones, S-shaped tortuosity of long bones, irregular periosteal thickening, hyperplasia or hypoplasia, intraosseous radiolucent defects, congenital bowing, pseudarthrosis (tibia most common with anterolateral bowing, other bones: ulna, femur, clavicle, radius, humerus), bone sclerosis, subperiosteal or cortical cysts, intramedullary neurofibromatosis, absence of a patella, dislocation of the radius and ulna, local overgrowth, subperiosteal hemorrhage, calcified hematoma, pathological dislocation of the hip, association of nonossifying fibromas and neurofibromatosis; (f) peripheral soft-tissue neurofibromatosis: computed tomography of masses in the distribution of peripheral nerves (fusiform enlargement of the nerve, central areas of low attenuation, calcification); solid masses (paravertebral, laryngeal, mediastinal, abdominal, pelvis, and ischiorectal fossae): rounded, clearly outlined masses with attenuation values of 30 to 40 Hounsfield units or widespread sheets of nodular tissues; (g) *alimentary tract:* single or multiple tumors, submucosal or intraluminal filling defects, intestinal obstruction, volvulus, intussusception, ulcerations, pseudo-Hirschsprung disease; (h) *chest:* "dumbbell neurofibroma," intercostal neurofibroma, fibrosing alveolitis (diffuse mottled densities changing to a strandy appearance and finally the formation of bullae), rib penciling, twisted ribbon rib deformity, rib notching, mediastinal neurofibroma, spontaneous pneumothorax, hemothorax interstitial fibrosis—associated pulmonary hypertension, pulmonary neurofibroma associated with arteriovenous shunting and hypoxemia; (i) *cardiovascular:* acquired right ventricular outflow obstruction, aneurysm of the superior vena cava, renovascular hypertension resulting from neurofibromatosis of renal arteries, spontaneous rupture of an artery (intercostal, renal, subclavian), abnormalities of the aorta and branches (stenosis, aneurysm) at various sites (renal, celiac, mesenteric, iliac, pulmonary, cerebral, etc.), lymphatic abnormalities (dilatation and tortuosity of lymphatic vessels and filling defects in nodes), left atrial wall aneurysm, arteriovenous fistula, superior vena caval obstruction; (j) *urinary tract:* bladder involvement; intrinsic mass or diffuse infiltrative process; involvement of the prostate, seminal vesicles, scrotum, penis, and ureter; hydronephrosis; hydroureter; displacement of the upper collecting system and bladder by the extrinsic mass(es); (k) accumulation of technetium 99m diethylenetriamine pentaacetic acid (^{99m}Tc=DTPA) in the benign soft-tissue neurofi-

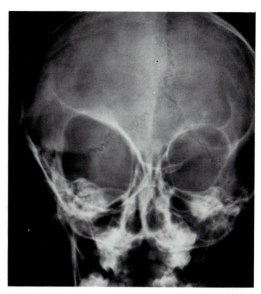

FIG SY–N–9.
Neurofibromatosis in a 2½-year-old male with right exophthalmos, cranial asymmetry, an enlarged right orbit, and a defect in the orbital wall. A triangular defect in the lateral aspect of the right lambdoid suture is projected through the right orbit. (From Taybi H, Silverman FN: Congenital defect of the bony orbit and pulsating exophthalmos. *Am. J. Dis. Child.* 92:138, 1956. Used by permission.)

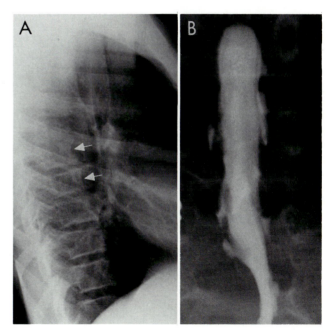

FIG SY–N–10.
Neurofibromatosis. **A,** a 13-year-old male with a known history of neurofibromatosis and a recent history of increasing difficulty in walking on the right lower extremity because of pain and some weakness involving the leg. There is marked concavity of the anterior vertebral margins in the midthoracic region *(arrows).* **B,** in the same patient a myelogram demonstrates an extradural filling defect at the lumbosacral junction. The tumor (neurofibroma) was surgically removed from nerve roots extending from the fourth lumbar level to the second sacral level.

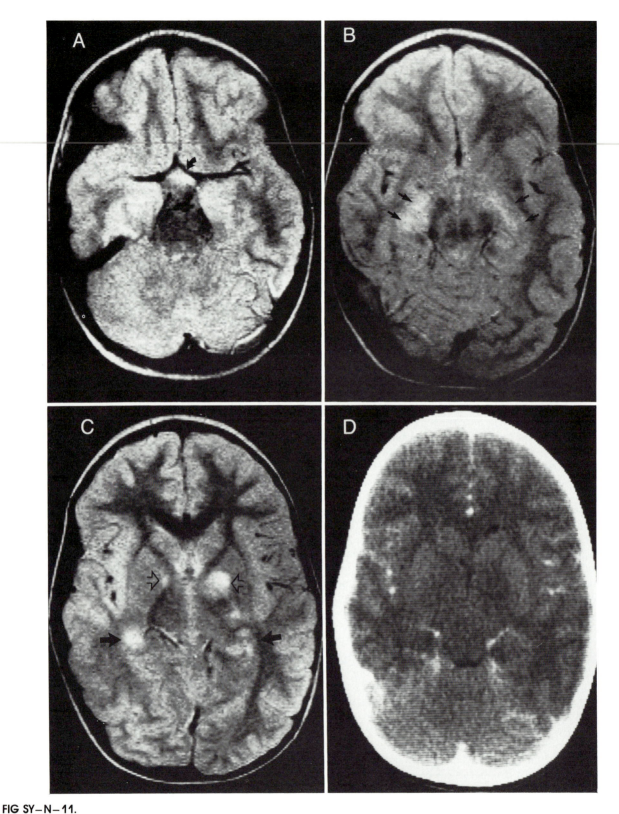

FIG SY−N−11.

Neurofibromatosis, optic-pathway involvement. **A−C,** T$_2$-weighted magnetic resonance images show an optic pathway glioma involving the chiasm **(A)** with extension into the optic tracts **(B)** and lateral geniculate body **C.** There is an abnormal signal intensity bilaterally in the basal ganglia **(C). D,** a contrast-enhanced com-puted tomographic scan at approximately the level of **C** shows no definite abnormality. (From Brown EW, et al.: MR imaging of op-tic pathways in patients with neurofibromatosis. *A.J.N.R.* 8:1031, 1987. Used by permission.)

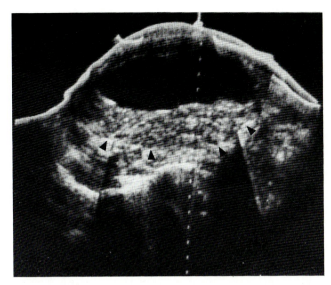

FIG SY–N–12.
Neurofibromatosis of the bladder. A transverse sonogram of the bladder reveals marked thickening of the bladder wall *(arrowheads)*. (From Miller WB, Boal DK, Teele R: Neurofibromatosis of the bladder: sonographic findings. *J. Clin. Ultrasound* 11:460, 1983. Used by permission.)

bromatosis tumors; (l) other reported abnormalities: osteomalacia (vitamin resistant, hypophosphoremic).

Notes: (a) there are two distinct forms of neurofibromatosis: von Recklinghausen (neurofibromatosis 1, peripheral form, 90% of all cases) and the central form (acoustic neurofibromatosis, neurofibromatosis 2); there are at least six other provisional categories of neurofibromatosis (Wertelecki et al.); (b) neurofibromatosis-Noonan syndrome (NF-NS) is considered to be a distinct entity that can be inherited, with variable manifestations of the Noonan phenotype within a family (Figs SY–N–9 to SY–N–12).

REFERENCES

Abuelo DN, et al.: Neurofibromatosis with fully expressed Noonan syndrome. *Am. J. Med. Genet.* 29:937, 1988.

Afifi AK, et al.: Aqueductal stenosis and neurofibromatosis: A rare association. *J. Child Neurol.* 3:125, 1988.

Atlas SW, et al.: Neurofibromatosis and agenesis of the corpus callosum in identical twins: MR diagnosis. *A.J.N.R.* 9:598, 1988.

Barker D, et al.: Gene for von Recklinghausen neurofibromatosis is in the pericentromeric region of chromosome 17. *Science* 236:1100, 1987.

Biondetti PR, et al.: CT appearance of generalized von Recklinghausen neurofibromatosis. *J. Comput. Assist. Tomogr.* 7:866, 1983.

Blatt J, et al.: Neurofibromatosis and childhood tumors. *Cancer* 57:1225, 1986.

Blum MD, et al.: Urologic manifestations of von Recklinghausen neurofibromatosis. *Urology* 26:209, 1985.

Bognanno JR, et al.: Cranial MR imaging in neurofibromatosis. *A.J.R.* 151:381, 1988.

Brooks BS, et al.: MR imaging of moyamoya in neurofibromatosis. *A.J.N.R.* 8:178, 1987.

Brown EW, et al.: MR imaging of optic pathways in patients with neurofibromatosis. *A.J.N.R.* 8:1031, 1987.

Burk DL, et al.: Spinal and paraspinal neurofibromatosis: Surface coil MR imaging at 1.5T. *Radiology* 162:797, 1987.

Butchart EG, et al.: Spontaneous rupture of an intercostal artery in a patient with neurofibromatosis and scoliosis. *J. Thorac. Cardiovasc. Surg.* 69:919, 1974.

Cameron AJ, et al.: Abdominal angina and neurofibromatosis. *Mayo Clin. Proc.* 57:125, 1982.

Carswell H: 'Elephant Man' had more than neurofibromatosis. *J.A.M.A.* 248:1032, 1982.

Chakrabarti S, et al.: The association of neurofibromatosis and hyperparathyroidism. *Am. J. Surg.* 137:417, 1979.

Cohen MM: Further diagnostic thoughts about the elephant man. *Am. J. Med. Genet.* 29:777, 1988.

Coleman BG, et al.: CT of sarcomatous degeneration in neurofibromatosis. *A.J.R.* 140:383, 1983.

Crawford AH Jr, et al.: Osseous manifestations of neurofibromatosis in childhood. *J. Pediatr. Orthop.* 6:72, 1986.

Daneman A, et al.: CT appearance of thickened nerves in neurofibromatosis. *A.J.R.* 141:899, 1983.

D'Aprile P, et al.: Congenital dislocation of dens of the axis in a case of neurofibromatosis. *Neuroradiology* 26:405, 1984.

Deans WR, et al.: Arteriovenous fistula in patients with neurofibromatosis. *Radiology* 144:103, 1982.

Debure C, et al.: Lésions artérielles multiples au cours de la maladie de von Recklinghausen. *Presse Med.* 13:1776, 1984.

Desprechins YM: Bilateral coronoid hyperplasia: Report of a case (abstract). Presented at the Meeting of International Pediatric Radiology, Toronto, 1987.

Donaldson MC, et al.: Hypertension from isolated thoracic aortic coarctation associated with neurofibromatosis. *J. Pediatr. Surg.* 20:169, 1985.

Ducatman BS, et al.: Malignant bone tumors associated with neurofibromatosis. *Mayo Clin. Proc.* 58:578, 1983.

Dunn DW: Neurofibromatosis in childhood. *Curr. Probl. Pediatr.* 17:451, 1987.

Egelhoff JC, et al.: Dural ectasia as a cause of widening of the internal auditory canals in neurofibromatosis. *Pediatr. Radiol.* 17:7, 1987.

Elliott CM, et al.: Idiopathic hypertrophic subaortic stenosis associated with cutaneous neurofibromatosis. *Am. Heart J.* 92:368, 1976.

Fasanelli S, et al.: A case of a thoracic vertebral body dislocation without neurological signs in a child with neurofibromatosis. *Pediatr. Radiol.* 16:262, 1986.

Fauré C, et al.: Multiple and large non-ossifying fibromas in children with neurofibromatosis. *Ann. Radiol. (Paris)* 29:369, 1986.

Floyd A, et al.: The elephant woman. *J. Bone Joint Surg. [Br.]* 69:121, 1987.

Flüeler U, et al.: Iris hamartomata as diagnostic criterion in neurofibromatosis. *Neuropediatrics* 17:183, 1986.

Francis IR, et al.: Peripheral neurofibromatosis. *J. Comput. Assist. Tomogr.* 7:373, 1983.

Griffiths DFR, et al: Multiple endocrine neoplasia associated with von Recklinghausen's disease. *Br. Med. J.* 287:1341, 1983.

Gupta SK, et al.: Craniofacial neurofibromatosis: A roentgen profile. *Australas. Radiol.* 28:97, 1984.

Halper J, et al.: Coronary lesions in neurofibromatosis associated with vasospasm and myocardial infarction. *Am. Heart J.* 108:420, 1984.

Hassell P: Gastrointestinal manifestations of neurofibromatosis in children: A report of two cases. *J. Can. Assoc. Radiol.* 33:202, 1982.

Heitzmann A, et al.: Hyperprolactinémie et neurofibromatose de von Recklinghausen. *Presse Med.* 16:967, 1987.

Holt JF: Neurofibromatosis in children. *A.J.R.* 130:615, 1978.

Holt JF, et al.: Macrocranium and macroencephaly in neurofibromatosis. *Skeletal Radiol.* 1:25, 1976.

Hurst RW, et al.: Multifocal intracranial MR abnormalities in neurofibromatosis. *A.J.N.R.* 9:293, 1988.

Huson SM: The different forms of neurofibromatosis. *Br. Med. J.* 294:1113, 1987.

Ichikawa K, et al.: Coincidence of neurofibromatosis and myotonic dystrophy in a kindred. *J. Med. Genet.* 18:134, 1981.

Joubert MJ: Neurofibromas of the spine—A pathognomonic sign. *S. Afr. Med. J.* 60:509, 1981.

Kaiser MC, et al.: Anterior cervical meningoceles in neurofibromatosis. *A.J.N.R.* 7:1105, 1986.

Kandarpa K, et al.: A case of neurofibromatosis associated with a coronary artery aneurysm and myocardial infarction. *Cardiovasc. Intervent. Radiol.* 11:143, 1988.

Kaneti J, et al.: A case of ambiguous genitalia owing to neurofibromatosis—Review of the literature. *J. Urol.* 140:584, 1988.

Kaplan P, et al.: A distinctive facial appearance in neurofibromatosis von Recklinghausen. *Am. J. Med. Genet.* 21:463, 1985.

Klatte EC, et al.: The radiographic spectrum in neurofibromatosis. *Semin. Roentgenol.* 11:17, 1976.

Lachiewicz PF, et al.: Pathological dislocation of the hip in neurofibromatosis. *J. Bone Joint Surg. [Am.]* 65:414, 1983.

Larrieu AJ, et al.: Spontaneous massive haemothorax in von Recklinghausen's disease. *Thorax* 37:151, 1982.

Laue L, et al.: Precocious puberty associated with neurofibromatosis and optic gliomas. *Am. J. Dis. Child.* 139:1097, 1985.

Levine E, et al.: Malignant nerve-sheath neoplasms in neurofibromatosis: Distinction from benign tumors by using imaging techniques. *A.J.R.* 149:1059, 1987.

Lewis TT, et al.: Magnetic resonance imaging of multiple spinal neurofibromata-neurofibromatosis. *Neuroradiology* 29:562, 1987.

Lipton S, et al.: Familial enteric neurofibromatosis. *Med. Times* 94:544, 1966.

Mandell GA, et al.: Neurofibromas: Location by scanning with Tc-99m DTPA. *Radiology* 157:803, 1985.

Martuza RL, et al.: Neurofibromatosis 2. (Bilateral acoustic neurofibromatosis). *N. Engl. J. Med.* 318:684, 1988.

Mayer JS, et al.: Craniocervical manifestations of neurofibromatosis: MR versus CT studies. *J. Comput. Assist. Tomogr.* 11:839, 1987.

Mendez HMM: The Neurofibromatosis-Noonan syndrome. *Am. J. Med. Genet.* 21:471, 1985.

Merlob P, et al.: Postaxial polydactyly in association with neurofibromatosis. *Clin. Genet.* 32:202, 1987.

Miller WB, et al: Neurofibromatosis of the bladder: Sonographic findings. *J. Clin. Ultrasound* 11:460, 1983.

Mitchell JA, et al.: Neurofibromatosis and fragile-X syndrome in the same patient. *Am. J. Med. Genet.* 22:571, 1985.

Neiman HL, et al.: Neurofibromatosis and congenital heart disease. *A.J.R.* 122:146, 1974.

O'Donohue WJ, et al.: Multiple pulmonary neurofibromas with hypoxemia. Occurrence due to pulmonary arteriovenous shunts within the tumors. *Arch. Intern. Med.* 146:1618, 1986.

O'Neill P, et al: Spinal meningoceles in association with neurofibromatosis. *Neurosurgery* 13:82, 1983.

Paling MR: Plexiform neurofibroma of the pelvis in neurofibromatosis: CT findings. *J. Comput. Assist. Tomogr.* 8:476, 1984.

Patronas NJ, et al.: Ventricular dilatation in neurofibromatosis. *J. Comput. Assist. Tomogr.* 6:598, 1982.

Pentecost M, et al.: Aneurysms of the aorta and subclavian and vertebral arteries in neurofibromatosis. *Am. J. Dis. Child.* 135:475, 1981.

Porterfield JK, et al.: Pulmonary hypertension and interstitial fibrosis in von Recklinghausen neurofibromatosis. *Am. J. Med. Genet.* 25:531, 1986.

Preston JM, et al.: Neurofibromatosis: Unusual lymphangiographic findings. *A.J.R.* 132:474, 1979.

Recklinghausen F, von: *Ueber die multiplen Fibromen der Haut und ihre Beziehung zu den multiplen Neuromen.* Berlin, A. Hirschwald, 1882.

Reed D, et al.: Plexiform neurofibromatosis of the orbit: CT evaluation. *A.J.N.R.* 7:259, 1986.

Rosenquist GC, et al.: Acquired right ventricular outflow obstruction in a child with neurofibromatosis. *Am. Heart J.* 79:103, 1970.

Rowen M, et al.: Thoracic coarctation associated with neurofibromatosis. *Am. J. Dis. Child.* 129:113, 1975.

Satran L, et al.: Neurofibromatosis with congenital glaucoma and buphthalmos in a newborn. *Am. J. Dis. Child.* 134:182, 1980.

Sava P, et al.: A propos d'un cas de neurofibromatose avec hypertrophie segmentaire d'un membre. *Ann. Pediatr. (Paris)* 22:355, 1975.

Schwartz AM, et al.: Neurofibromatosis and multiple nonossifying fibromas. *A.J.R.* 135:617, 1980.

Shuper A, et al.: Noonan's syndrome and neurofibromatosis. *Arch. Dis. Child.* 62:196, 1987.

Sørensen SA, et al.: Long-term follow-up of von Recklinghausen neurofibromatosis. Survival and malignant neoplasms. *N. Engl. J. Med.* 314:1010, 1986.

Stines J, et al.: CT findings of laryngeal involvement in von Recklinghausen disease. *J. Comput. Assist. Tomogr.* 11:141, 1987.

Stone JW, et al.: Dural ectasia associated with spontaneous dislocation of the upper part of the thoracic spine in neurofibromatosis. A case report and review of the literature. *J. Bone Joint Surg. [Am.]* 69:1079, 1987.

Stone MM, et al.: Colonic obstruction in a child with von Recklinghausen's neurofibromatosis. *J. Pediatr. Surg.* 21:741, 1986.

Stradling JR, et al.: Sleep apnoea syndrome caused by neurofibromatosis and superior vena caval obstruction. *Thorax* 36:634, 1981.

Taillan B, et al.: Neurofibromatose de Von Recklinghausen associee à une ostéomalacie vitamino-résistante hypophosphorémique. *Presse Med.* 15:2120, 1986.

Taybi H, Silverman FN: Congenital defect of the bony orbit and pulsating exophthalmos. *Am. J. Dis. Child.* 92:138, 1956.

Tillous-Borde I, et al.: Myocardiopathie hypertrophique régressive chez un nourrisson atteint d'une neurofibromatose de Recklinghausen. *Arch. Fr. Pediatr.* 43:197, 1986.

Tishler JM, et al.: Neurogenic tumors of the duodenum in patients with neurofibromatosis. *Radiology* 149:51, 1983.

Torrington KG, et al.: Recklinghausen's disease. Occurrence with intrathoracic vagal neurofibroma and contralateral spontaneous pneumothorax. *Arch. Intern. Med.* 143:568, 1983.

Turra S, et al.: Macrodactyly of the foot associated with plexiform neurofibroma of the medial plantar nerve. *J. Pediatr. Orthop.* 6:489, 1986.

Uren N, et al.: Congenital left atrial wall aneurysm in a patient with neurofibromatosis. *Br. Heart J.* 59:391, 1988.

Vancoillie P, et al.: Cervical neurofibroma and generalized spinal stenosis in von Recklinghausen disease. *Lancet* 2:1246, 1979.

Van Tassel P, et al.: Cerebellar calcification in central neurofibromatosis: CT in two cases. *A.J.N.R.* 8:913, 1987.

Vormittag W, et al.: Dermatoglyphics and creases in patients with neurofibromatosis von Recklinghausen. *Am. J. Med. Genet.* 25:389, 1986.

Webb WR, et al.: Fibrosing alveolitis in patients with neurofibromatosis. *Radiology* 122:289, 1977.

Wertelecki W, et al.: Neurofibromatosis 2: Clinical and DNA linkage studies of a large kindred. *N. Engl. J. Med.* 319:278, 1988.

Winter RB, et al.: Spine deformity in neurofibromatosis: A review of one hundred and two patients. *J. Bone Joint Surg. [Am.]* 61:677, 1979.

Wolters ECh: Hypertelorism in neurofibromatosis. *Neuropediatrics* 17:175, 1986.

Yaghmai I, et al.: Massive subperiosteal hemorrhage in neurofibromatosis. *Radiology* 122:439, 1977.

Zatz LM: Atypical choroid plexus calcifications associated with neurofibromatosis. *Radiology* 91:1135, 1968.

Zimmerman RA, et al.: Computed tomography of orbital-facial neurofibromatosis. *Radiology* 146:113, 1983.

NEVOID BASAL CELL CARCINOMA SYNDROME

Synonyms: Basal cell–nevus syndrome; Gorlin syndrome; Gorlin-Goltz syndrome; multiple nevoid basal cell carcinoma syndrome.

Mode of Inheritance: Autosomal dominant.

Frequency: Not too uncommon; 53 cases reviewed by Gorlin (1987).

Clinical Manifestations: Onset of symptoms in childhood: (a) *characteristic craniofacial features* (70% of patients): large calvaria with frontal and biparietal bulging, low position of the occiput, prominent supraorbital ridges, heavy eyebrows, wide nasal root, mild hypertelorism, exotropia, pouting lower lips, exaggerated mandibular length; (b)

cutaneous manifestations: *multiple nevoid basal cell carcinomas*, milia and cysts, palmar and plantar pits, comedones, café au lait pigmentations; (c) oral lesions: *odontogenic keratocysts*, defective dentition, prognathism, fibrosarcoma of the jaws, ameloblastoma, cleft lip/palate; (d) ocular abnormalities: hypertelorism, congenital blindness, dystopia canthorum, cataracts, coloboma of the choroid and optic nerve, strabismus, medullated nerve fibers, corneal leukoma, glaucoma, chalazions, enophthalmic appearance, retinitis pigmentosa, falciform folds of the retina with detachment, retinal hamartoma; (e) central nervous system abnormalities: mental retardation, facial nerve palsy, nerve deafness, congenital hemiparesis (absent internal carotid artery), seizures; (f) genital abnormalities: male (hypogonadism, cryptorchidism, female pubic escutcheon, gynecomastia, scanty facial/body hair), female (ovarian cyst, uterine fibroid, fibroma); (g) benign and malignant tumors: medulloblastoma, meningioma, craniopharyngioma, lymphangioma, mesenteric chylous or lymphatic cyst, renal fibroma, melanoma, isolated neurofibroma, leiomyoma, benign mesenchymoma, fetal rhabdomyoma, rhabdomyosarcoma, bronchogenic cyst, adrenal cortical adenoma, gastrointestinal polyposis, ovarian

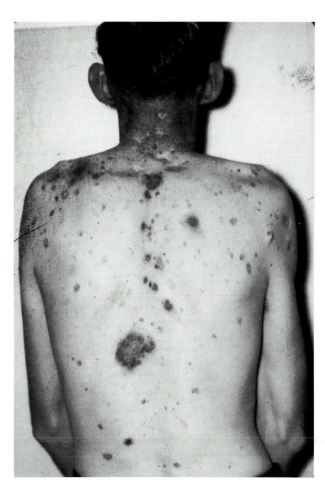

FIG SY–N–13.
Skin lesions in nevoid basal cell carcinoma syndrome. (Courtesy of Dr. Robert A. Gorlin, Minneapolis.)

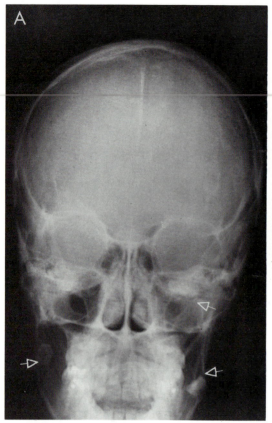

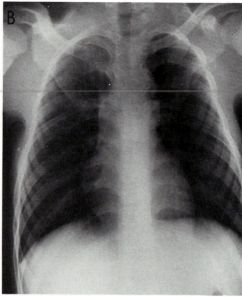

FIG SY—N—14.
Nevoid basal cell carcinoma syndrome in a 13-year-old male who has multiple basal cell nevi and swelling in the mandibular region. **A,** lamellar calcification of falx and odontogenic cysts of mandible and maxilla *(arrows).* **B,** marked deformity and high position of left scapula. Spina bifida of C₆ and C₇, the fusion of some vertebrae in the upper thoracic region, and partial fusion of the upper ribs are seen.

cyst, ovarian fibroma, ovarian fibrosarcoma, seminoma, ameloblastoma, renal cyst, cardiac fibrous histiocytoma, cardiac fibroma; (h) other reported abnormalities: tall stature, marfanoid appearance, anosmia, anomalies of the stapes and incus, elevated serum alkaline phosphatase values, increased calcitonin levels, increased parathormone levels, coexistence with Sotos syndrome, inguinal hernia, facial mutilation, supernumerary nipples, hyperhidrosis, etc.

Radiologic Manifestations: (a) *odotogenic cysts of the maxilla and mandible,* hypoplastic mandible; (b) chest anomalies: *rib anomalies* (bifid, splayed, agenesis, fused, cervical ribs, rudimentary ribs), pectus excavatum or carinatum, Sprengel deformity of the scapula, notching of the medial surface of the scapulae, defective medial clavicle; (c) *vertebral anomalies:* scoliosis, kyphoscoliosis, spina bifida occulta, fusion of spinous processes, narrowed intervertebral disk space, square-shaped vertebrae, osteoporosis of the vertebrae, occipitovertebral junction anomalies (short C₁ or foramen arculale, odontoid agenesis, third occipital condyle, platybasia, cervical spondylolisthesis), lumbarization of the sacrum, etc; (d) frontal and temporoparietal bossing, *lamellar calcification of the falx,* bridging of the sella, other calcified structures (di-

aphragma sellae, tentorium cerebelli, petroclinoid ligaments, dura, pia, choroid plexus), cerebellar atrophy, absent corpus callosum, cyst of the septum pellucidum, hydrocephalus, hyperpneumatized sinuses, small sella turcica; (e) limb abnormalities: supracondylar humeral spurs; widening of the distal segments of the radii; spotty osteoblastic deposits in the phalanges; syndactyly, oligodactyly; brachymetacarpal, tarsal, and carpal fusions; extrametatarsal bone; cysts in the bones and the hands and feet; defective medial segment of the clavicle; (f) widespread cystlike osteolytic bone lesions, osteoblastic spotty "osteopoikilotic" lesions; (g) other reported abnormalities: soft-tissue calcification, renal anomalies (horseshoe kidneys, L-shaped kidney, unilateral renal agenesis, duplication of the collecting system) (Figs SY—N—13 and SY—N—14).

REFERENCES

Aumaitre O, et al.: Manifestations neurologiques de la naevomatose basocellulaire. *Presse Med.* 15:2105, 1986.

Barnes DA, et al.: Cervical spondylolisthesis associated with the multiple nevoid basal cell carcinoma syndrome. *Clin. Orthop.* 162:26, 1982.

Binkley GW, et al.: Epithelioma adenoides cysticum: Basal cell nevi, agenesis of corpus callosum and dental cysts. *Arch. Dermatol. Syph.* 63:73, 1951.

Blinder G, et al.: Widespread osteolytic lesions of the long bones in basal cell nevus syndrome. *Skeletal Radiol.* 12:196, 1984.

Gorlin RJ: Nevoid basal-cell carcinoma syndrome. *Medicine (Baltimore)* 66:98, 1987.

Gorlin RJ, Goltz RN: Multiple nevoid basal-cell epithelioma, jaw cysts and bifid ribs: Syndrome. *N. Engl. J. Med.* 262:908, 1960.

Jones KL, et al.: The Gorlin syndrome: A genetically determined disorder associated with cardiac tumor. *Am. Heart J.* 111:1013, 1986.

Knöbber D, et al.: Stapesanomalie, Gorlin-Goltz- und Hand-Fuss-Uterus-Syndrom als Teilaspekte eines Generalisierten Ektodermal-Mesodermalen Missbildungs-Syndromes mit wechselnder Expressivität. *Laryngol. Rhinol. Otol.* 65:305, 1986.

Murphy KJ: Subcutaneous bone formation in the naevoid basal-cell carcinoma syndrome: Normal urinary cyclic AMP response to parathyroid hormone infusion. *Clin. Radiol.* 26:37, 1974.

Murphy MJ, et al.: Nevoid basal cell carcinoma syndrome and epilepsy. *Ann. Neurol.* 11:372, 1982.

Peracha HU, et al.: Detection of osseous lesions in Gorlin's syndrome by Technetium-99m MDP. *Clin. Nucl. Med.* 13:549, 1988.

Schultz SM, et al.: Ameloblastoma associated with basal cell nevus (Gorlin) syndrome: CT findings. *J. Comput. Assist. Tomogr.* 11:901, 1987.

Springate JE: The nevoid basal cell carcinoma syndrome. *J. Pediatr. Surg.* 21:908, 1986.

Stoll P, et al.: Das Basalzellnaevussyndrom in der Röntgendiagnostik des Schädels. *Radiologe* 26:442, 1986.

NONERUPTING TEETH–MAXILLOZYGOMATIC HYPOPLASIA

Mode of Inheritance: Autosomal recessive (four persons in one family).

Clinical and Radiologic Manifestations: (a) multiple nonerupting teeth with cementum defects; (b) hypoplasia of the alveolar process and the maxillozygomatic region; (c) ear deformities; (d) genu valgum.

REFERENCE

Stoelinga PJW, et al.: Multiple non-erupting teeth, maxillozygomatical hypoplasia and other congenital defects: An autosomal recessive disorder. *Clin. Genet.* 10:222, 1976.

NOONAN SYNDROME

Synonyms: Male Turner syndrome; female pseudo-Turner syndrome; Turner phenotype with normal karyotype.

Mode of Inheritance: Genetic heterogeneity; autosomal dominant, variable expressivity.

Frequency: Approximately 1:8,000 live births (Kitchens et al.).

Clinical Manifestations: (a) short stature (53%); (b) eye abnormalities (95%): epicanthal folds, ptosis, hypertelorism, downward-slanting palpebral fissures, strabismus, myopia, proptosis, nystagmus; (c) ear abnormalities (44%): low set, excessively folded auricular helices, fleshy; (d) high-arched palate (34%), micrognathia (22%); (e) low posterior hairline (32%); (f) neck abnormalities (69%): short neck; (g) thorax abnormalities (53%): flat, shieldlike, funnel chest deformity, pectus excavatum and/or carinatum; (h) cardiovascular anomalies (50%): pulmonary stenosis, hypertrophic cardiomyopathy, atrial septal defect, ventricular septal defect, patent ductus arteriosus, coarctation of the aorta, peripheral pulmonary stenosis, aortic stenosis, tetralogy of Fallot, anomalous pulmonary venous return, absence of the ductus venosus, prolapse of the mitral valve; (i) testicular abnormalities (69%): small, undescended; penis abnormalities (22%): small, large, hypospadias; (j) cubitus valgus (47%); (k) abnormalities of skin and appendages (27%): hyperelastic skin, nevi, moles, "dystrophic" nails, curly hair; (l) mental retardation (24%); (n) other reported abnormalities: limb anomalies, large or asymmetrical head, downy hirsutism, widely spaced

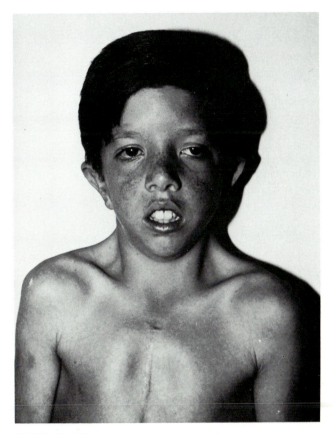

FIG SY–N–15.
Noonan syndrome. Coarse facial features, a triangular face, and shortness and webbing of the neck are present. (From Allanson JE: Noonan syndrome. *J. Med. Genet.* 24:9, 1987. Used by permission.)

and small nipples, dental anomalies and malocclusion, epilepsy, splenomegaly, deafness, cleft palate, deficiency of coagulation factor XI, coincidental occurrence of chromosome abnormalities, association with neurofibromatosis (the neurofibromatosis-Noonan syndrome), aortic dissection; (m) lymphatic system abnormalities: lymphedema, pulmonary lymphangiectasis, intestinal lymphangiectasis, testicular lymphangiectasis, cystic hygroma, nonimmune hydrops fetalis, chylothorax; (n) bleeding diathesis.

Radiologic Manifestations: (a) various anomalies of the skull: hypertelorism, biparietal foramina, dolichocephaly, microcephaly, macrocephaly, bitemporal bulging, steep inclination of the anterior fossa, micrognathia; (b) retardation of skeletal maturation; (c) dental malocclusion; (d) anterior bowing of the sternum at various levels, elongation of the manubrium and shortness of the body of the sternum, premature fusion of ossification centers of the body of the sternum; (e) limb anomalies (25%): genu valga, pes planus, short or long fingers, syndactyly, camptodactyly, clinodactyly of the fifth fingers, congenital dislocation of the radial head, scapula alata; (f) vertebral and rib anomalies (28%): kyphosis, scoliosis, Klippel-Feil syndrome, fusion of vertebrae, caudal slope of the ribs, cervical ribs; (g) lymphatic abnormalities: peripheral lymphedema, hypoplastic peripheral lymph vessels, hypoplastic lymph nodes, chylothorax, pulmonary lymphangiectasis (obstructive changes and collateral formation in the retroperitoneal, mediastinal, pulmonary, and cervical lymphatics and extensive opacification of the pulmonary and visceral pleural lymphatics); (h) urinary system: obstructive uropathy, duplication of the collecting system, renal hypoplasia, polycystic renal disease; (i) gastrointestinal tract: lymphangiectasis, diverticulosis of the small intestine and incomplete rotation of the bowel.

Differential Diagnosis: Williams syndrome; 45, O Turner syndrome; King syndrome (short stature, facial dysmorphism, myopathy, etc.) (Fig SY−N−15).

REFERENCES

Allanson JE: Noonan syndrome. *J. Med. Genet.* 24:9, 1987.

Bawle EV, et al.: Nonimmune hydrops fetalis in Noonan's syndrome. *Am. J. Dis. Child.* 140:758, 1986.

Baltaxe HA, et al.: Pulmonary lymphangiectasia demonstrated by lymphangiography in 2 patients with Noonan's syndrome. *Radiology* 115:149, 1975.

Cumming WA, et al.: Intestinal diverticulosis in Noonan's syndrome. *Br. J. Radiol.* 50:64, 1977.

de Haan M, et al.: Noonan syndrome: Partial factor XI deficiency. *Am. J. Med. Genet.* 29:277, 1988.

Finegan JAK, et al.: Very superior intelligence in a child with Noonan syndrome. *Am. J. Med. Genet.* 31:385, 1988.

Fisher E, et al.: Spontaneous chylothorax in Noonan's syndrome. *Eur. J. Pediatr.* 138:282, 1982.

Gardner TW, et al.: Congenital pulmonary lymphangiectasis. A case complicated by chylothorax. *Clin. Pediatr. (Phila.)* 22:75, 1983.

Hernandez RJ, et al.: Pulmonary lymphangiectasis in Noonan syndrome. *A.J.R.* 134:75, 1980.

Hoeffel JC, et al.: Lymphatic vessels dysplasia in Noonan's syndrome. *A.J.R.* 134:401, 1980.

Hoeffel JC, et al.: Radiologic pattern of the sternum in Noonan's syndrome with congenital heart defect. *Am. J. Dis. Child.* 135:1044, 1981.

Kitchens CS, et al.: Partial deficiency of coagulation factor XI as a newly recognized feature of Noonan syndrome. *J. Pediatr.* 102:224, 1983.

Leonidas JC, et al.: Congenital absence of the ductus venosus: With direct connection between the umbilical vein and the distal inferior vena cava. *A.J.R.* 126:892, 1976.

Mendez HMM, et al.: Noonan syndrome: A review. *Am. J. Med. Genet.* 21:493, 1985.

Nistal M, et al.: Testicular lymphangiectasis in Noonan's syndrome. *J. Urol.* 131:759, 1984.

Noonan JA, et al.: Associated non cardiac malformations in children with congenital heart disease (abstract). *J. Pediatr.* 63:468, 1963.

Opitz JM: Editorial comment: The Noonan syndrome. *Am. J. Med. Genet.* 21:515, 1985.

Opitz JM, et al.: Evidence that the "neurofibromatosis-Noonan syndrome" is a variant of von Recklinghausen neurofibromatosis (letter). *Am. J. Med. Genet.* 26:741, 1987.

Preus M: Differential diagnosis of the Williams and the Noonan syndromes. *Clin. Genet.* 25:429, 1984.

Quattrin T, et al.: Vertical transmission of the neurofibromatosis/Noonan syndrome. *Am. J. Med. Genet.* 26:645, 1987.

Saul RA: Noonan syndrome in a patient with hyperplasia of the myenteric plexuses and neurofibromatosis. *Am. J. Med. Genet.* 21:491, 1985.

Shachter N, et al.: Aortic dissection in Noonan's syndrome (46 XY Turner). *Am. J. Cardiol.* 54:464, 1984.

Steenson AJ, et al.: King's syndrome with malignant hyperthermia. Potential outpatient risks. *Am. J. Dis. Child.* 141:271, 1987.

Tejani A, et al.: Noonan's syndrome associated with polycystic renal disease. *J. Urol.* 115:209, 1976.

Towne WD, et al.: Systolic prolapse of the mitral valve in Noonan's syndrome. *Am. Heart J.* 90:499, 1975.

Traisman ES, et al.: Noonan syndrome. A report of male-to-male transmission. *Clin. Pediatr. (Phila.)* 21:51, 1982.

Witt DR, et al.: Bleeding diathesis in Noonan syndrome: A common association. *Am. J. Med. Genet.* 31:305, 1988.

Witt DR, et al.: Growth curves for height in Noonan syndrome. *Clin. Genet.* 30:150, 1986.

Witt DR, et al.: Lymphedema in Noonan syndrome: Clues to pathogenesis and prenatal diagnosis and review of the literature. *Am. J. Med. Genet.* 27:841, 1987.

Zarabi M, et al.: Cystic hygroma associated with Noonan's syndrome. *J. Clin. Ultrasound* 11:398, 1983.

OBUI-HIMO SYNDROME

Clinical Manifestation: *Cyanosis of the upper extremities* in infants and children carried on the back in an "obui-himo" (a device used in Japan for carrying infants and young children).

Radiologic Manifestation: *Congenital absence of the cephalic vein* demonstrated by venography.

REFERENCE

Osano M, et al.: Cyanosis of the arms associated with anomalies of the veins: Obui-himo syndrome. *Am. J. Dis. Child.* 118:479, 1969.

OCULO-CEREBRO-CUTANEOUS SYNDROME

Frequency: Very rare.

Clinical Manifestations: (a) *ocular anomalies: orbital cyst* (unilateral or bilateral), microphthalmos, eyelid coloboma, hamartoma, persistent hyaloid artery; (b) *psychomotor retardation*, convulsions; (c) *skin anomalies:* appendages (periorbital, postauricular), aplasia, hypoplasia, punch-out defects; (d) other reported abnormalities: generalized asymmetry, cleft lip/palate.

Radiologic Manifestations: (a) *orbital cyst*, microphthalmos, hamartoma; (b) *agenesis of the corpus collosum*, partial absence of the right cerebellar hemisphere, ectopic gray matter; (c) other reported abnormalities: *skull defects*, rib dysplasia, vertebral anomalies (Fig SY–O–1).

REFERENCES

Delleman JW, et al.: Orbital cyst in addition to congenital cerebral and focal dermal malformations. A new entity?. *Clin. Genet.* 19:191, 1981.

Wilson RD, et al.: Oculocerebrocutaneous syndrome. *Am. J. Ophthalmol.* 99:142, 1985.

OCULO-DENTO-OSSEOUS DYSPLASIA

Synonyms: Oculodentodigital dysplasia; ODOD; ODDD; ODD.

Mode of Inheritance: Autosomal dominant with variable expressivity.

Frequency: 50 to 70 published cases.

Clinical Manifestations: (a) *characteristic facial features:* microphthalmos, thin nose with a long prominent nasal bridge, anteverted nostrils, hypoplastic alae nasi; (b) small teeth, generalized enamel hypoplasia, gross dental caries; (c) *syndactyly;* camptodactyly; clinodactyly; phalanx aplasia, hypoplasia, or dysplasia; (d) other reported abnormalities: small palpebral fissures; epicanthal folds; glaucoma; cleft lip/palate; fine, dry, and/or sparse hair; conductive hearing loss; blindness; neurological complications due to spinal cord compression; mental retardation; almost complete aplasia of the foot; mental retardation (very rare); delayed gastric emptying; chronic diarrhea.

Radiologic Manifestations: (a) *bilateral syndactyly and camptodactyly of the fourth and fifth fingers;* (b) clinodactyly of the fifth finger, hypoplasia of the middle phalanx of the index finger or other fingers; *hypoplasia or absence of the middle phalanges of some toes;* (b) small orbits, orbital hypotelorism; (c) wide mandible, thickening and subperiosteal new bone formation of the mandible; (d) *undertubulation of the long bones*, especially the femur; widening of the ribs and clavicles; (e) *amelogenesis imperfecta and microdontia;* (f) other reported abnormalities: cubitus valgus, hip dislocation, cases with severe changes (marked cranial hyperostosis, massive mandibular overgrowth, clavicular widening, basal ganglia calcification, small orbits, calcification in the cornea) (Fig SY–O–2).

REFERENCES

Barnard A, et al.: Intracranial calcification on oculodentoosseous dysplasia. *S. Afr. Med. J.* 16:758, 1981.

Beighton P, et al.: Oculodento-osseous dysplasia: Heterogeneity or variable expressions? *Clin. Genet.* 16:169, 1979.

Dean JA, et al.: Dental management of oculodentodigital dysplasia: Report of case. *J. Dent. Child.* 53:131, 1986.

Fará M, et al.: The question of hypertelorism in oculodento-osseous dysplasia. *Am. J. Med. Genet.* 10:101, 1981.

Gorlin RJ: Oculo-dento-osseous dysplasia. *Semin. Roentgenol.* 8:180, 1973.

Levine DS: Delayed gastric emptying and chronic diarrhea in a patient with oculodentodigital dysplasia syndrome. *J Pediatr. Gastroenterol. Nutr.* 5:329, 1986.

Reisner SH, Kott E, Bornstein B, et al.: Oculodentodigital dysplasia. *Am. J. Dis. Child.* 118:600, 1969.

Schuller MG, et al.: Oculodentodigital dysplasia. *Oral Surg.* 61:418, 1986.

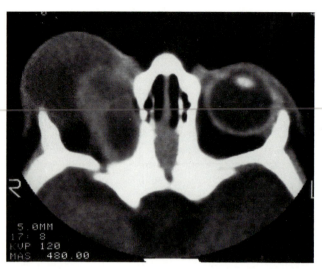

FIG SY–O–1.
Oculo-cerebro-cutaneous syndrome. Computed tomography of the orbits shows an absence of the globe on the right side, a large right orbit, and a partially cystic mass. (From Wilson RD, Traverse L, Hall JG, et al.: Oculocerebrocutaneous syndrome. *Am. J. Ophthalmol.* 99:142, 1985. Used by permission.)

OCULO-GASTRO-INTESTINAL MUSCULAR DYSTROPHY

Mode of Inheritance: Autosomal recessive; consanguinity.

Clinical Manifestations: Onset in childhood: (a) ptosis, ophthalmoplegia, impaired pupillary light reaction; (b) primary myopathy of the gastrointestinal muscles, intact myen-teric plexus and vagus nerves; (c) peripheral neuropathy: distal weakness, hypoesthesia, decreased deep tendon reflexes; (d) malnutrition and death of a young adult age.

Radiologic Manifestations: Intestinal pseudo-obstruction with delayed gastric emptying; jejunal dilatation; diverticula.

Differential Diagnosis: Kearns-Sayre syndrome; oculo-pharyngeal muscular dystrophy (difficulty in swallowing, distal limb weakness, etc.).

REFERENCES

Ionasescu V: Oculogastrointestinal muscular dystrophy. *Am. J. Med. Genet.* 15:103, 1983.

OCULO-PALATO-SKELETAL SYNDROME

Mode of Inheritance: Reported in four siblings (Mexican American).

Frequency: Four siblings (Michels et al.).

Clinical and Radiologic Manifestations: (a) height, weight, and fronto-occipital circumference below the 3rd percentile, mental retardation; (b) blepharoptosis, blepharo-phimosis, epicanthus inversus, telecanthus, anterior chamber defect, abnormal eye motility; (c) hearing deficit; (d) other abnormalities: cleft lip and palate, short fifth finger, spina bifida occulta, premature closure of the lambdoidal suture, thickening of the occipital bone, radio-ulnar synostosis, etc.

REFERENCES

McKusick VA: *Mendelian Inheritance in Man,* ed 8. Baltimore, Johns Hopkins University Press, 1988, p. 1113.
Michels VV, et al.: A clefting syndrome with ocular anterior chamber defect and lid anomalies. *J. Pediatr.* 93:444, 1978.

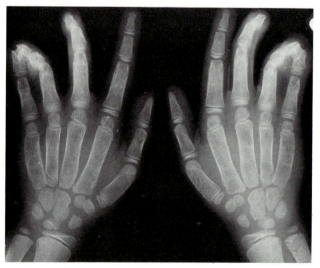

FIG SY–O–2.
Oculo-dento-osseous dysplasia. The hand of a 14-year-old boy demonstrates a lack of modeling of the metacarpals, only two bones in the fifth digit, a cube-shaped middle phalanx in the fourth finger, and terminal syndactyly of the fourth and fifth fingers. (From Reisner SH, Kott E, Bornstein B, et al.: Oculodentodigital dysplasia. *Am. J. Dis. Child.* 118:600, 1969. Used by permission.)

ODONTOMAS-ESOPHAGEAL STENOSIS-LIVER CIRRHOSIS SYNDROME

Mode of Inheritance: Probably autosomal dominant.

Clinical and Radiologic Manifestations: (a) *multiple odontomas;* (b) *esophageal stenosis,* leiomyomatosis of the esophagus; (c) *chronic interstitial liver cirrhosis;* (d) other reported abnormalities: pulmonary stenosis, calcified aortic stenosis, bronchiectasis, hyperplasia of the myenteric plexus, bowel malrotation, anal stenosis, iris colobomas.

REFERENCES

Hermann M: Ueber von Zahnsystem ausgenhende Tumoren bei Kindern. *Fortschr. Kiefer Gesichtschir.* 4:226, 1958.

Schmidseder R, et al.: Multiple odontogenic tumors and other anomalies. *Oral Surg.* 39:249, 1975.

ODONTO-TRICHO-MELIC HYPOHIDROTIC DYSPLASIA

Synonym: Tetramelic ectodermal dysplasia.

Mode of Inheritance: Autosomal recessive.

Clinical and Radiologic Manifestations: (a) *extensive tetramelic reductions;* (b) *oligodentia, conical crowns;* (c) *reduced body hair, hypoplastic or absent areolae;* (d) *cleft lip/palate, deformed pinnae, large nose, protruding lips;* (e) *mental retardation;* (f) *endocrine and metabolic abnormalities (hypogonadism, excess of tyrosine and/or tryptophan in the urine).*

REFERENCES

Freire-Maia N: A newly recognized genetic syndrome of tetramelic deficiencies, ectodermal dysplasia, deformed ears and other abnormalities. *Am. J. Hum. Genet.* 22:370, 1970.
Pinheiro M, et al.: EEC and odontotrichomelic syndrome. *Clin. Genet.* 17:363, 1980.

OGILVIE SYNDROME

Synonyms: Idiopathic pseudo-obstruction of the colon; acute pseudo-obstruction of the colon; spinal ileus; ileus of the colon; etc.

Clinical Manifestations: Most common in geriatric patients: (a) *atypical signs and symptoms of acute large-bowel obstruction;* (b) may be associated with spinal injury, intra-abdominal infection, trauma, respiratory or cardiac failure, pregnancy and Cesarean section, urologic procedures, orthopedic procedures; (c) usually self-limited, mortality greater than 30% reported (cecal perforation, bowel gangrene, etc.).

Radiologic Manifestations: *A pattern of colonic dilatation in the absence of an obstructing lesion* (colonic dilatation may involve the cecum and varying lengths of the colon distal to the cecum), few air-fluid levels, a gradual transition to the collapsed bowel, normal gas and fecal pattern in the rectum.

REFERENCES

Crass JR, et al.: Percutaneous decompression of the colon using CT guidance in Ogilvie syndrome. *A.J.R.* 144:475, 1985.
Fausel CS, et al.: Nonoperative management of acute idiopathic colonic pseudo-obstruction (Ogilvie's syndrome). *West J. Med.* 143:50, 1985.
Geelhoed GW: Colonic pseudo-obstruction in surgical patients. *Am. J. Surg.* 149:258, 1985.

Gilchrist AM, et al.: Acute large-bowel pseudo-obstruction. *Clin. Radiol.* 36:401, 1985.
Ogilvie H: Large-intestine colic due to sympathetic deprivation: A new clinical syndrome. *Br. Med. J.* 2:67, 1948.
Terhune DW, et al.: Ogilvie's syndrome developing after ethanol ablation of renal cell carcinoma. *J. Urol.* 133:838, 1985.
Walker JL, et al.: Ogilvie's syndrome in orthopaedic patients. *Orthop. Rev.* 14:493, 1985.

ONYCHONYCHIA AND THE ABSENCE AND/OR HYPOPLASIA OF THE DISTAL PHALANGES

Mode of Inheritance: Probably autosomal dominant.

Clinical and Radiologic Manifestations: (a) onychodystrophy, anonychia; (b) brachydactyly of the fifth fingers, digitalization of the thumbs; (c) absence and/or hypoplasia of the distal phalanges of the hands and feet.

REFERENCE

Cooks RG, et al.: A new nail dysplasia syndrome with onychonychia and absence and/or hypoplasia of distal phalanges. *Clin. Genet.* 27:85, 1985.

OPERCULUM SYNDROME

Pathology and Etiology: Lesions (usually cerebrovascular accident of thrombotic or embolic origin) in the operculum region: the telencephalic mantle covering the island of Reil (frontal, temporal, and parietal gyri).

Clinical Manifestations: Similar to the pseudobulbar palsy; abscence of mental changes and sphincter dysfunction.

Radiologic Manifestation: Computed tomographic changes of a vascular accident in the region of the sylvian fissure that involves the opercula.

REFERENCE

Sandyk R, et al.: The operculum syndrome. *J. Comput. Assist. Tomogr.* 7:130, 1983.

OPHTHALMO-MANDIBULO-MELIC DYSPLASIA

Synonym: Pillay syndrome.

Mode of Inheritance: Autosomal dominant.

Clinical Manifestations: (a) *corneal opacities;* (b) *mandibular deformity leading to difficulty in mastication;* (c) *short and bowed forearm, flexion deformity of the fingers.*

Radiologic Manifestations: (a) *absence of the coronoid process, obtuse mandibular angle, temporomandibular ankylosis;* (b) *upper-limb anomalies:* shallow glenoid fossa, aplasia of the lateral condyle of the humerus, abnormal trochlea, absent olecranon and coronoid processes of the ulna, absent radial head, dislocation of the radius at the elbow, bowed radial shaft, absent distal segment of the ulna, hypoplasia of the carpal bones; (c) *lower-limb anomalies:* coxa valga, hypoplasia of the lateral femoral condyle, shortness of the proximal portion of the fibula.

REFERENCE

Pillay VK: Ophthalmo-mandibulo-melic dysplasia: An hereditary syndrome. *J. Bone Joint Surg. [Am.]* 46:858, 1964.

OPITZ SYNDROME (BBB)

Synonyms: Hypertelorism-hypospadias syndrome; telecanthus-hypospadias syndrome; hypospadias-hypertelorism syndrome; Opitz oculo-genital-laryngeal syndrome (Opitz BBB/G compound syndrome); BBB syndrome.

Mode of Inheritance: Possibly X-linked.

Frequency: Approximately 40 published cases (Stevens et al.).

Clinical Manifestations: (a) *telecanthus or apparent hypertelorism;* (b) *strabismus;* (c) *cranial asymmetry;* (d) *hypospadias,* cryptorchidism; (e) *mental retardation;* (f) other reported associated abnormalities: flame nevi, cleft lip and palate, lipomatosis, ear anomalies, cranial asymmetry, bifid uvula, diastasis recti, hernias, minor urethral abnormalities in females, strabismus, mental retardation.

Radiologic Manifestations: (a) *hypospadias;* (b) reported associated anomalies: congenital heart defect, imperforate anus, prognathism, maxillary hypoplasia, dentigerous cysts, vertebral anomalies, bony projection in the region of the external occipital protuberance, urinary system abnormalities (ureteral duplication, ureteral stenosis, vesicoureteral reflux).

Note: Due to similarities between BBB syndrome (Opitz syndrome) and G syndrome (Opitz G syndrome), the term *Opitz oculo-genital-laryngeal syndrome* has been suggested.

REFERENCES

Cappa M, et al.: The Opitz syndrome: A new designation for the clinically indistinguishable BBB and G syndromes. *Am. J. Med. Genet.* 28:303, 1987.

Cavallo L, et al.: Endocrinological studies in the hypertelorism-hypospadias (BBB) syndrome. *Eur. J. Pediatr.* 148:89, 1988.

Christian JC, et al.: Familial telecanthus with associated congenital anomalies. *Birth Defects* 5:82, 1969.

Neri G, et al.: The Opitz syndrome. *Am. J. Med. Genet.* 30:851, 1988.

Noe NH, et al.: Hypertelorism-hypospadias syndrome. *J. Urol.* 132:951, 1984.

Opitz JM, et al.: The BBB syndrome—familial telecanthus with associated congenital anomalies. *Birth Defects* 5:86, 1969.

Reed MH, et al.: The hypertelorism-hypospadias syndrome. *J. Can. Assoc. Radiol.* 26:240, 1975.

Sedano HO, et al.: Opitz oculo-genital-laryngeal syndrome (Opitz BBB/G compound syndrome). *Am. J. Med. Genet.* 30:847, 1988.

Stevens CA, et al.: The telecanthus-hypospadias syndrome. *J. Med. Genet.* 25:536, 1988.

Stoll C, et al.: Male-to-male transmission of the hypertelorism-hypospadias (BBB) syndrome. *Am. J. Med. Genet.* 20:221, 1985.

OPSOCLONUS-MYOCLONUS SYNDROME

Synonyms: Oculo-cerebello-myoclonic syndrome; "dancing eyes, dancing feet" syndrome; myoclonic encephalopathy; "opsoclonus-myoclonus-ataxia."

Etiology: (a) almost half of the published cases of infantile myoclonic encephalopathy have been associated with neuroblastoma, ganglioneuroblastoma, or ganglioneuroma; presenting manifestation of neuroblastoma in 2% of the cases; (b) paraneoplastic opsoclonus-myoclonus in adults: adenocarcinoma of the breast and the uterus; bronchogenic carcinoma (small cells, epidermoid, anaplastic, and "undifferentiated"), medullary thyroid carcinoma; (c) central nervous system infection (viral, bacterial); (d) other reported etiologies: intracranial tumor, hydrocephalus, thalamic hemorrhage, multiple sclerosis, toxic encephalopathies (thallium, amitriptyline hydrochloride, the combination of lithium and haloperidol lactate).

Clinical Manifestations: (a) *ataxia;* (b) *somatic myoclonus;* (c) *opsoclonus:* continual, irregular, rapid, chaotic, conjugate, and jerking ocular movements ("dancing eyes"); (d) good prognosis for children with neuroblastoma presenting with opsoclonus-myoclonus.

Radiologic Manifestations: Plain radiography, ultrasonography, and MDP (^{99m}Tc methylene diphosphate) bone scans and if necessary to be followed by body computed tomography (CT) (abdominal CT first without the use of oral or intravenous contrast materials since the calcification in the small tumor may resemble contrast material) or magnetic resonance imaging.

REFERENCES

Altman AJ, et al.: Favorable prognosis for survival in children with coincident opso-myoclonus and neuroblastoma. *Cancer* 37:846, 1976.

Baker ME, et al.: The association of neuroblastoma and my-oclonic encephalopathy: An imaging approach. *Pediatr. Radiol.* 15:185, 1985.

Bowen A'D, et al.: Ultrasonic delineation of left adrenal neuroblastoma in a child with opsoclonus. *J. Clin. Ultrasound* 11:31, 1983.

Donaldson JS, et al.: CT scanning in patients with opsomyo-clonus: Importance of nonenhanced scan. *A.J.R.* 146:781, 1986.

Dropcho E, et al.: Paraneoplastic opsoclonus-myoclonus. Association with medullary thyroid carcinoma and review of the literature. *Arch. Neurol.* 43:410, 1986.

Farrelly C, et al.: Occult neuroblastoma presenting with op-somyoclonus: Utility of computed tomography. *A.J.R.* 142:807, 1984.

Kinsbourne M: Myoclonic encephalopathy of infants. *J. Neurol. Neurosurg. Psychiatr.* 25:271, 1962.

Kuban KC, et al.: Syndrome of opsoclonus-myoclonus caused by coxsackie B3 infection. *Ann. Neurol.* 13:69, 1983.

Nausieda PA, et al.: Opsoclonic cerebellopathy. A paraneo-plastic syndrome responsive to thiamine. *Arch. Neurol.* 38:780, 1981.

Solomon GE, et al.: Opsoclonus and occult neuroblastoma. *N. Engl. J. Med.* 279:475, 1968.

Stephenson JBP, et al.: Reactivity to neuroblastoma extracts in childhood cerebellar encephalopathy ("dancing eye" syndrome). *Lancet* 2:975, 1976.

Willis J, et al.: Cerebellar lesion in myoclonic encephalopa-thy of infants. *Arch. Neurol.* 40:818, 1983.

Ziegelbaum MM, et al.: The association of neuroblastoma with myoclonic encephalopathy of infants: The use of magnetic resonance as an imaging modality. *J. Urol.* 139:81, 1988.

OPTIC ATROPHY–SPASTIC PARAPLEGIA SYNDROME

Mode of Inheritance: Possible sex-linked; cytoplasmic inheritance.

Clinical Manifestation: A degenerative disorder of the central nervous system: (a) *Leber optic atrophy;* (b) *dystonia, rigidity, mental retardation;* (c) other reported abnormalities: abnormal oral glucose tolerance test findings, mild red cell macrocytosis.

Radiologic Manifestations: Striated degeneration: (a) computed tomography: symmetrical low-density lesions in the putamen, occasional caudate lesions; (b) magnetic resonance imaging: high signal intensity on T_2-weighted images and low signal intensity on T_1-weighted images; (c) absence of hemispheric, brain stem, or cerebellar atrophy.

Differential Diagnosis: Wilson disease; Leigh disease; hereditary spastic paraplegia (Strumpell-Lorrain); Hallervor-den-Spatz disease.

REFERENCES

Bruyn GW, Wendt LN: A sex linked heredodegenerative disorder associated with Leber's optic atrophy. *J. Neurol. Sci.* 1:59, 1964.

Seidenwurm D, et al.: MR and CT in cytoplasmically inher-ited striatal degeneration. *A.J.N.R.* 7:629, 1986.

Went LN: A sex-linked heredo-degenerative neurological disorder associated with Leber's optic atrophy II. Labora-tory investigation. *J. Neurol. Sci.* 1:81, 1964.

ORO-FACIO-DIGITAL SYNDROMES

Classifications: *Type I* (Papillon-Leage and Psaume): tongue nodules, bifid tongue, midline lip cleft, cleft palate, frenular hypertrophy, thick alveolar bands, absent lateral in-cisor, aplasia of nasal alae, facial milia, coarse thin hair, alopecia in some cases, mental retardation (almost half), etc; *type II* (Mohr): tongue nodules, bifid tongue, midline lip cleft, cleft palate, absent central incisors, preaxial bilateral poly-dactyly of the big toes, etc; *type III* (Sugarman): lobulated ha-martomatous tongue, bifid uvula, extra small teeth with mal-occlusion, bulbous nose, bilateral postaxial polydactyly of the hands and feet, seesaw winking of the eyelids, mental re-tardation; *type IV* (Temtamy-McKusick) "Mohr-Majewski compound" with some features of the two syndromes, i.e., orofaciodigital syndrome, type 1 (tongue tumors, multiple frenula, broad flat nose, hypertelorism) and short-rib–poly-dactyly syndrome, i.e., the Majewski type with tibial dyspla-sia.

REFERENCES

Baraitser M: The orofaciodigital (OFD) syndromes. *J. Med. Genet.* 23:116, 1986.

Sugarman GI, et al.: See-saw winking in a familial oral-facial-digital syndrome. *Clin. Genet.* 2:248, 1971.

Temtamy S, McKusick VA: The genetics of hand malforma-tions. *Birth Defects* 16:429, 1978.

ORO-FACIO-DIGITAL SYNDROME I

Synonyms: Papillon-Leage and Psaume syndrome; OFD I syndrome; dysplasia linguofacialis.

Mode of Inheritance: X-linked dominant; lethal in an XY male.

Frequency: Rare.

Clinical Manifestations: (a) unusual facial features: prominent forehead, hypoplasia of the mandible, zygomatic hypoplasia, *lateral displacement of the inner canthi, hypopla-sia of the alae nasi, short philtrum;* (b) oral anomalies: *alveo-lar ridges, cleft upper lip, cleft palate, cleft tongue,* lobulated tongue with hypertrophic frenula, *webs* and fibrous bands ex-tending from the buccal mucous membrane to the alveolar clefts, hamartoma of the ventral surface of the tongue, fistula

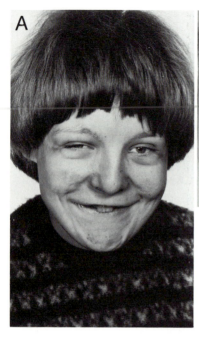
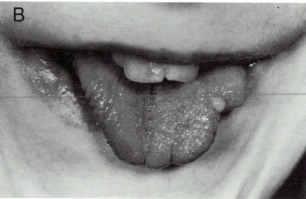

FIG SY—O—3.
Oro-facio-digital syndrome, type I. **A,** characteristic facies with a short upper lip, a broad nasal root, and coarse hair.
B, lobulated tongue with a typical nodule on the left. (From Connacher AA, Forsyth CC, Stewart WK: Orofaciodigital syndrome type I associated with polycystic kidneys and agenesis of the corpus callosum. *J. Med. Genet.* 24:116, 1987. Used by permission.)

in the lower lip; (c) *digital malformations;* (d) mild mental retardation; (e) dry and rough hair, alopecia; (f) dental malformations; (g) evanescent milia of the face in infancy; (h) other reported abnormalities: precocious puberty, chronic renal failure (polycystic kidney disease).

Radiologic Manifestations: (a) *increased nasion-sella-basion angle;* (b) *clinodactyly, syndactyly, brachydactyly,* camptodactyly, adactyly, cone-shaped epiphyses, polydactyly of the halluces; (c) malposition of the teeth, supernumerary cuspids and bicuspids, absent lower lateral incisors; (d) central nervous system anomalies: hydranencephaly, agenesis of the corpus callosum, cortical hypoplasia, ventricular asymmetry, cyst of the septum pellucidum, subdural hygroma, microcephaly, cerebellar encephalocele, microgyria, cerebral cysts, large brain, polygyria, heterotopic gray matter; (e) other reported abnormalities: frontal bossing, short mandible, hydrocephalus, porencephalic cysts, irregular reticulated areas of radiolucency in the shaft of the bones, irregular mottling of metacarpals and phalanges, osteoporosis, metaphyseal rarefaction, shortness of the tubular bones, polycystic kidneys (Fig SY—O—3).

REFERENCES

Annerén G, et al.: Oro-facio-digital syndromes I and II: Radiological methods for diagnosis and the clinical variations. *Clin. Genet.* 26:178, 1984.
Baraitser M: The orofaciodigital (OFD) syndromes. *J. Med. Genet.* 23:116, 1986.
Baraton J: Les malformations cérébrales dans le syndrome oro-facio-digital de Papillon-Leage et Psaume. *J. Radiol. Electrol.* 58:103, 1977.
Connacher AA, et al.: Orofaciodigital syndrome type I associated with polycystic kidneys and agenesis of the corpus callosum. *J. Med. Genet.* 24:116, 1987.
Donnai D, et al.: Familial orofaciodigital syndrome type I presenting as adult polycystic kidney disease. *J. Med. Genet.* 24:84, 1987.
Papillon-Leage Mme, Psaume J: Une malformation héréditaire de la muqueuse buccale: Brides et freins anormaux. *Rev. Stomatol.* 55:209, 1954.
Somer M, et al.: Precocious puberty associated with oral-facial-digital syndrome type I. *Acta Paediatr. Scand.* 75:672, 1986.
Wood BP, et al.: Cerebral abnormalities in the oral-facial-digital syndrome. *Pediatr. Radiol.* 3:130, 1975.

ORO-FACIO-DIGITAL SYNDROME II

Synonyms: Mohr syndrome; OFD II syndrome.

Mode of Inheritance: Autosomal recessive.

Frequency: Rare.

Clinical Manifestations: (a) *lobate tongue with a papilliform protuberance,* high-arched or cleft palate, midline cleft of the lip, hypertrophied frenula; (b) *broad nasal root, broad and bifid tip of the nose;* (c) conductive hearing defect; (d) *anomalies of the extremities;* (e) normal or absent central incisors; (f) episodes of neuromuscular disturbance; (g) other reported abnormalities: moderately short stature, single atrioventricular valve, coarctation of the aorta, mental defect, microcephaly.

Radiologic Manifestations: (a) *high-arched or cleft palate;* (b) *hypoplasia of the body of the mandible;* (c) *digital anomalies:* polydactyly, syndactyly, clinodactyly, brachydactyly; (d) brain abnormalities (in the OFD II "variant"): porencephalia, lipoma, partial agenesis of the corpus callosum, Dandy-Walker anomaly, etc.; (e) other reported abnormali-

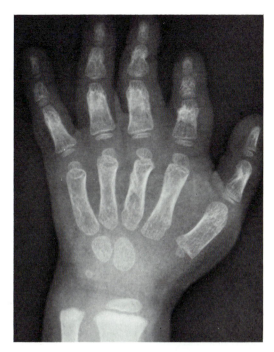

FIG SY—O—4.
Oro-facio-digital syndrome II (Mohr): radiogram of a 4-year-old girl with brachydactyly and irregular mottling of the metacarpals and phalanges. (From Rimoin DL, Edgerton MT: Genetic and clinical heterogeneity in the oral-facial-digital syndrome. *J. Pediatr.* 71:94, 1967. Used by permission.)

ties: supernumerary sutures in the skull, metaphyseal irregularity and flaring (Figs SY—O—4 and SY—O—5).

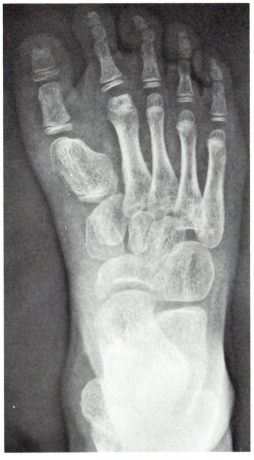

FIG SY—O—5.
Oro-facio-digital syndrome II (Mohr). Note the broad cuboid first metatarsal and extra cuneiform bone in this 6-year-old female. (From Rimoin DL, Edgerton MT: Genetic and clinical heterogeneity in the oral-facial-digital syndrome. *J. Pediatr.* 71:94, 1967. Used by permission.)

REFERENCES

Annerén G, et al.: Oro-facio-digital syndromes I and II: Radiological methods for diagnosis and the clinical variations. *Clin. Genet.* 26:178, 1984.

Baraitser M: The orofaciodigital (OFD) syndromes. *J. Med. Genet.* 23:116, 1986.

Burn J, et al.: Orofaciodigital syndrome with mesomelic limb shortening. *J. Med. Genet.* 21:189, 1984.

Claussen O: Et arvelig syndrom omfattende tungemissdannelse og polydaktyli. *Nord. Med. Tid.* 30:1147, 1946.

Cordero JF, et al.: Heart malformation as a feature of the Mohr syndrome. *J. Pediatr.* 91:683, 1977.

Gillerot Y, et al.: Oro-facial-digital syndrome II. *Clin. Genet.* 33:141, 1988.

Haumont D, et al.: The Mohr syndrome: Are there two variants? *Clin. Genet.* 24:41, 1983.

Levy EP, et al.: Mohr syndrome with subclinical expression of the bifid great toe. *Am. J. Dis. Child.* 128:531, 1974.

Mattel JF, et al.: Syndrome of polydactyly, cleft lip, lingual hamartomas, renal hypoplasia, hearing loss, and psychomotor retardation: Variant of the Mohr syndrome or a new syndrome? *J. Med. Genet.* 20:433, 1983.

Mohr OL: A hereditary sublethal syndrome in man. *Skr. Norske Vidensk. Akad. I. Mat. Naturv. Klasse* 14:3, 1941.

Rimion DL, Edgerton MT: Genetic and clinical heterogeneity in the oral-facial-digital syndrome. *J. Pediatr.* 71:94, 1967.

Silengo MC, et al.: Oro-facial-digital syndrome II. Transitional type between the Mohr and the Majewski syndromes: Report of two new cases. *Clin. Genet.* 31:331, 1987.

Townes PL, et al.: Further heterogeneity of oral-facial-digital syndrome. *Am. J. Dis. Child.* 130:548, 1976.

OROMANDIBULAR-LIMB HYPOGENESIS

Classification: Syndromes and anomalies of mandible, tongue and maxilla associated with reductive limb anomalies (Table SY—O—1).

Description

1. *Charlie M. syndrome:* Ocular hypertelorism, facial paralysis (in some), cleft palate, absent or conically crowned incisors, hypodactyly of the hands and feet.

2. *Glossopalatine ankylosis syndrome:* Linguopalatine adhesion, high-arched palate, cleft palate, hypoplastic man-

TABLE SY—O—1.

Oromandibular-Limb Hypogenesis Syndromes
(Proposed Classification)*

Type I: Micrognathia (mandibular)
Pierre Robin syndrome
Hanhart syndrome
Type II: Microglossia
Hypoglossia
Hypoglossia-hypodactyly
Type III: Dysgnathia (maxillomandibular)
Glossopalatine ankylosis
Glossopalatine ankylosis—hypodactyly
Type IV: Other
Möbius syndrome
Charlie M syndrome
(Amniotic band syndrome)

*From Chicarilli ZN, Polayes IM: Oromandibular limb
hypogenesis syndromes. *Plast. Reconstr. Surg.* 76:13,
1985. (Used by permission.)

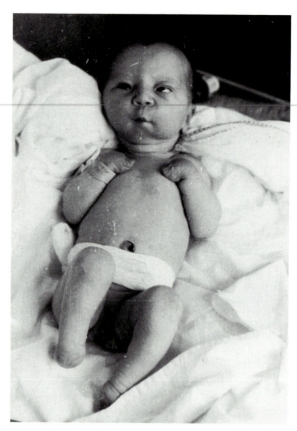

FIG SY—O—6.
Oromandibular-limb hypogenesis/Hanhart syndrome in a new-born infant with abnormal craniofacial features (epicanthus, broad nasal bridge, severe micrognathia, small mouth, receding lower lip, cleft palate, and hypoplastic tongue) and distal limb anomalies. (From Bökesoy I, Aksüzek C, Deniz E: Oromandibular limb hypogenesis/Hanhart's syndrome: Possible drug influence on the malformation. *Clin. Genet.* 24:47, 1983. Used by permission.)

dible, hypodontia, temporomandibular ankylosis, facial paralysis, variable degrees of limb anomalies (oligodactyly, peromelia, polydactyly, syndactyly).

3. *Hanhart syndrome:* Micrognathia, microstomia, hypodontia, delay in appearance of the teeth, deformed teeth, variable limb anomalies (peromelia of the upper limbs or of all four limbs, oligodactyly, short digits) (Fig SY—O—6).

4. *Hypoglossia-hypodactyly syndrome.*

5. *Möbius syndrome.*

REFERENCES

Bökesoy I, et al: Oromandibular limb hypogenesis/Hanhart's syndrome: Possible drug influence on the malformation. *Clin. Genet.* 24:47, 1983.

Chicarilli ZN, et al.: Oromandibular limb hypogenesis syndromes. *Plast. Reconstr. Surg.* 76:13, 1985.

Gorlin RJ, et al.: Oromandibular-limb hypogenesis syndromes, in *Syndromes of the Head and Neck.* New York, McGraw-Hill Book International Co, 1976, pp. 517—580.

Hanhart E: Ueber die Kombination von Peromelie mit Mikrognathie, ein neues Syndrom beim Menschen, entsprechend der Akroteriasis congenita von Wriedt und Mohr beim Rinde. *Arch. Julius Klaus-Stift. Vererbungsforsch.* 25:531, 1950.

Kitamura A, et al.: A case of oromandibular-digital hypogenesis syndrome. *J. Craniomaxillofac. Surg.* 15:291, 1987.

OSTEOARTHROPATHY, FAMILIAL IDIOPATHIC

Synonyms: Hypertrophic osteoarthropathy without pachydermia; familial idiopathic osteoarthropathy; Currarino syndrome.

Mode of Inheritance: Autosomal recessive.

Clinical Manifestations: Onset of symptoms in infancy: (a) *eczematous skin eruption,* increased perspiration of the palms and soles; (b) *clubbing of the fingers;* (c) thickening of the arms and legs, synovial fluid containing few mononuclear cells (noninflammatory joint effusion); (d) chronic periarticular swelling, pain, recurrent joint effusion; (e) low-grade fever; (f) other reported abnormalities: slight increased sweating of the palms and soles, mildly increased serum alkaline phosphatase level.

Radiologic Manifestations: (a) *soft-tissue clubbing;* (b) *periosteal elevation and subperiosteal new bone formation;* (c) joint effusion; (d) *widely open sutures and fontanelles,* wormian bones, *delayed closure of the cranial sutures.*

Differential Diagnosis: Congenital syphilis; Caffey disease; Camarati-Engleman disease; prostaglandin E therapy; hypervitaminosis A; "primary hypertrophic osteoarthropathy" (Diren) (Fig SY—O—7).

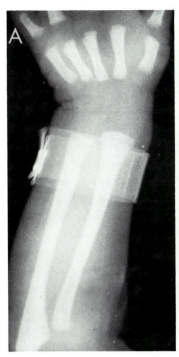

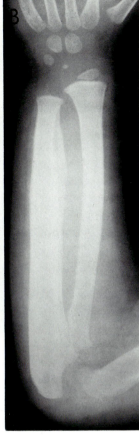

FIG SY−O−7.
Osteoarthropathy, familial idiopathic: normal bones in the neonatal period, **(A)** and periosteal elevation and subperiosteal new bone formation at 2 years of age, **(B).** (From Chamberlain DS, Whitaker J, Silverman FN: Idiopathic osteoarthropathy and cranial defects in children (familial idiopathic osteoarthropathy). *A.J.R.* 93:408, 1965. Used by permission.)

REFERENCES

Chamberlain DS, Whitaker J, Silverman FN: Idiopathic osteoarthropathy and cranial defects in children (familial idiopathic osteoarthropathy). *A.J.R.* 93:408, 1965.
Currarino G, et al.: Familial idiopathic osteoarthropathy. *A.J.R.* 85:633, 1961.
Diren HB, et al.: Primary hypertrophic osteoarthropathy. *Pediatr. Radiol.* 16:231, 1986.
Reginato AJ, et al.: Familial idiopathic hypertrophic osteoarthropathy and cranial suture defects in children. *Skeletal Radiol.* 8:105, 1982.

OSTEOLYSIS CLASSIFICATION

1. Phalangeal: Several forms.
2. Carpal and tarsal: (a) Francois and others (autosomal recessive); (b) with nephropathy (autosomal dominant).
3. Miscellaneous: (a) Hajdu-Cheney form (autosomal dominant); (b) Winchester form (autosomal recessive): (c) Torg form (autosomal recessive); (d) other forms.

OSTEOLYSIS (FAMILIAL EXPANSILE)

Synonyms: Familial expansile osteolysis; Osterberg syndrome.

Mode of Inheritance: Autosomal dominant, with the disease affecting at least 5 generations of a family, involving a total of 40 of the 90 members of the family evaluated (only a single family has been reported).

Clinical Manifestations: (a) *bone pain* (limbs only) with onset varied from the teenage years to middle age, some lesions painless; (b) pathological fracture; (c) *deafness* with onset often before 10 years of age: middle-ear type (ossicular involvement) followed by inner-ear involvement (conductive hearing loss in younger patients, mixed conductive and sensorineural deafness in older patients); (d) progressive tooth mobility, spontaneous tooth fracture, pulpitis; (e) high serum alkaline phosphatase levels, normal serum calcium and phosphorus values.

Radiologic Manifestations: (a) bone changes before any localized lesions: slight modeling abnormality of the long bones, distorted trabecular pattern (tightly meshed appearance); (b) *focal expanding bone lesions*: rounded area of the loss of trabeculae (metaphyseal, diaphyseal), with a gradual and progressive increase in size and endosteal scalloping and tunneling of the cortex, involvement of the whole bone, in some cases leaving a very fine cortical shell, longitudinal collapse of the bone in some patients; lesions rare in the girdles and axial skeleton; (c) bone scintigraphy: greater uptake of the isotope in the tibias as compared with the femora, focal increase in uptake at the site of the radiographic abnormalities; (d) *extensive resorption of dental roots*.

Differential Diagnosis: Paget disease; fibrous dysplasia; osteitis fibrosa cystica (Fig SY−O−8).

REFERENCE

Osterberg PH, et al.: Familial expansile osteolysis. A new dysplasia. *J. Bone Joint Surg. [Br.]* 70:255, 1988.

OSTEOLYSIS (GORHAM)

Synonyms: Gorham syndrome; Gorham-Stout syndrome; disappearing-bone disease; phantom bone.

Pathology: Nonmalignant proliferation of thin-walled vessels within the disappearing bones; bone replaced by fibrous tissue, no regeneration of the vanished bone; no healing at the fracture sites; increased numbers of osteoclasts.

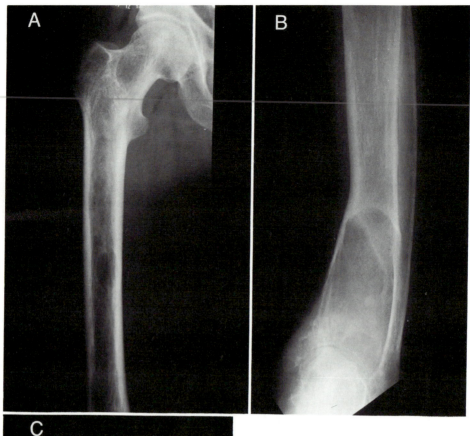

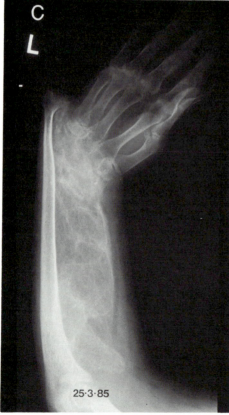

FIG SY−O−8.
Osteolysis (familial expansile osteolysis): examples of focal disease in the early stage **(A)**, intermediate stage **(B)** and late stage **(C)**. (From Wallace RGH: *A Study of a Familial Bone Dysplasia* (thesis). The Queen's University of Belfast, 1987; Osterberg PH, Wallace RGH, Adams DA, et al.: Familial expansile osteolysis. A new dysplasia. *J. Bone Joint Surg. [Br.]* 70:255, 1988. Used by permission.)

Clinical Manifestations: Onset usually in childhood or young adult life: (a) *progressive deformity without systemic findings, with or without overlying skin or soft-tissue angiomas;* (b) *pain;* (c) *increased focal skin temperature (thermography);* (d) *chylous or serosanguineous pleural effusion;* (e) spinal cord transection, paraplegia; (f) death may result from thoracic cage involvement; partial remission may occur.

Radiologic Manifestations: (a) *patchy osteoporosis in the early stage; progressive, extensive, partial, or total unicentric bone resorption (one or more bones may be involved);* (b) tapering of the end of the bone involved; (c) may cross the joint; (d) no evidence of reossification; (e) pathological fracture; (f) ^{99m}Tc pyrophosphate scan: decreased isotope uptake in affected areas, rarely increased uptake.

Differential Diagnosis: Angiomatosis.

REFERENCES

Abraham J, et al.: Massive osteolysis in an infant. *A.J.R.* 135:1084, 1980.

Cannon SR: Massive osteolysis. A review of seven cases. *J. Bone Joint Surg. [Br.]* 68:24, 1986.

Choma ND, et al.: Gorham's syndrome: A case report and review of the literature. *Am. J. Med.* 83:1151, 1987.

Feigl D: Gorham's disease of the clavicle with bilateral pleural effusions. Eight years later. *Chest* 92:189, 1987.

Gorham LW, et al.: Disappearing bones: A rare form of massive osteolysis: Report of two cases, one with autopsy findings. *Am. J. Med.* 17:674, 1954.

Gorham LW, Stout AP: Massive osteolysis (acute spontaneous absorption of bone, phantom bone, disappearing bone): Its relation to hemangiomatosis. *J. Bone Joint Surg. [Am.]* 37:985, 1955.

Hejgaard N, et al.: Massive Gorham osteolysis of the right hemipelvis complicated by chylothorax: Report of a case in a 9-year-old boy successfully treated by pleurodesis. *J. Pediatr. Orthop.* 7:96, 1987.

Joseph J, et al.: Disappearing bone disease: A case report and review of the literature. *J. Pediatr. Orthop.* 7:584, 1987.

Kolář J, et al.: Langfristige Teilremission des Gorhamschen Syndroms. *Fortschr. Rontgenstr.* 134:214, 1981.

Mathias K, et al.: Gorham-Stout-Syndrom der Mandibula. *Radiologe* 26:440, 1986.

Pastakia B, et al.: Seventeen year follow-up and autopsy findings in a case of massive osteolysis. *Skeletal Radiol.* 16:291, 1987.

OSTEOLYSIS WITH NEPHROPATHY

Synonym: Multicenteric osteolysis with nephropathy.

Mode of Inheritance: Sporadic; autosomal dominant.

Clinical Manifestations: Onset of symptoms in early childhood: (a) multifocal *progressive deformities;* (b) shortening of the extremities; (c) *chronic progressive nephropathy*

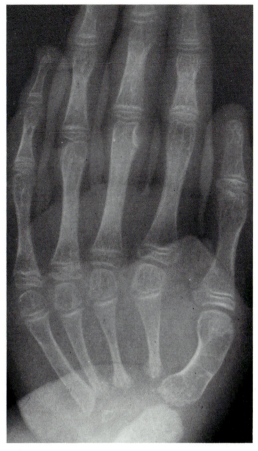

FIG SY–O–9.
Osteolysis with nephropathy: progressive symmetrical osteolysis involving the wrists, elbows, and feet in association with renal failure and hypertension. Resorption of the carpal bones and distal portion of the ulna with prominent shortening and tapering of the second to fourth metacarpals was present at age 14. (From Macpherson RI, Walker RD, Kowall MH: Essential osteolysis with nephropathy. *J. Can. Assoc. Radiol.* 24:98, 1973. Used by permission.)

with azotemia, hypertension, and finally death in adult life; (d) micrognathia, high-arched palate.

Radiologic Manifestations: (a) *progressive disappearance of bones, in particular carpals and tarsals;* partial resorption of adjacent tubular bones ("sucked candy" appearance of the tubular bones); (b) shortening and bowing of tubular bones; (c) flattening—loss of normal curvature and osteoporosis of carpal and tarsal bones prior to the development of osteolysis.

Differential Diagnosis: Juvenile rheumatoid arthritis; Winchester syndrome; etc. (Fig SY–O–9).

REFERENCES

Bèbe M: Acro-ostéolyse essentielle, anomalies squelettiques congénitales et néphropathie chronique avec insuffisance rénale (Maladie de Julien Marie et M. Dérot). *Ann. Pediatr. (Paris)* 21:537, 1974.

Bennett WM, et al.: Nephropathy of idiopathic multicentric osteolysis. *Nephron* 25:134, 1980.
Carnevale A, et al.: Idiopathic multicentric osteolysis with facial anomalies and nephropathy. *Am. J. Med. Genet.* 26:877, 1987.
Erickson CM, et al.: Carpal-tarsal osteolysis. *J. Pediatr.* 93:779, 1978.
Hardegger F, et al.: The syndrome of idiopathic osteolysis. Classification, review, and case report. *J. Bone Joint Surg. [Br.]* 67:89, 1985.
Lemaitre L, et al.: Carpal and tarsal osteolysis. *Pediatr. Radiol.* 13:219, 1983.
Macpherson RI, et al.: Essential osteolysis with nephropathy. *J. Can. Assoc. Radiol.* 24:98, 1973.
Marie J, et al.: Acro-ostéolyse essentielle compliquée d'insuffisance rénale d'évolution fatale. *Presse Med.* 71:249, 1963.
Marie J, et al.: Polydystrophies squelettiques avec ostéolyse progressive, *Arch. Fr. Pediatr.* 8:752, 1951.
Pai GS, et al.: Idiopathic multicenteric osteolysis: Report of two new cases and a review of the literature. *Am. J. Med. Genet.* 29:929, 1988.
Tuncbilek E, et al.: Carpal-tarsal osteolysis. *Pediatr. Radiol.* 15:255, 1985.
Tyler T, et al.: Idiopathic multicenteric osteolysis. *A.J.R.* 126:23, 1976.
Vichi GF, et al.: Case report 401. Idiopathic carpal/tarsal osteolysis (ICTO) associated with nephropathy. *Skeletal Radiol.* 15:665, 1986.

OSTEOLYSIS WITHOUT NEPHROPATHY

Synonym: Hereditary multicentric osteolysis.

Mode of Inheritance: Autosomal dominant or X-linked dominant; less commonly reported as recessive.

Clinical Manifestations: Onset of symptoms in early childhood: (a) arthritic complaints; (b) swelling of joints and soft-tissue thickening followed by a period of progressive deformity; collapse in the wrists, ankles, etc.

Radiologic Manifestations: (a) demineralization in the early stage; (b) collapse, sclerosis, and bone resorption (carpals, tarsals, elbows, shoulders), etc.

Note: Short stature, mental retardation, severe distal osteolysis with a characteristic appearance (maxillary hypoplasia, relative exophthalmos) and an autosomal recessive transmission has been reported as a subtype of essential osteolysis (Petit et al.).

REFERENCES

Amin PH, et al.: Essential osteolysis of carpal and tarsal bones. *Br. J. Radiol.* 51:539, 1978.
Beals RK, et al.: Carpal and tarsal osteolysis: A case report and a review of the literature. *J. Bone Joint Surg. [Am.]* 57:681, 1975.
Fryns JP, et al.: Carpal and tarsal osteolysis. *Ann. Genet. (Paris)* 23:123, 1980.
Hemingway AP, et al.: Familial vanishing limbs: Four generations of idiopathic multicentric osteolysis. *Clin. Radiol.* 34:585, 1983.
Petit P, et al.: Distal osteolysis, short stature, mental retardation, and characteristic facial appearance: Delineation of an autosomal recessive subtype of essential osteolysis. *Am. J. Med. Genet.* 25:537, 1986.
Sauvegrain J, et al.: Ostéolyse multicentrique a transmission récessive. Quatre cas dans une nouvelle famille. *Ann. Radiol. (Paris)* 24:638, 1981.
Tookman AG, et al.: Idiopathic multicentric osteolysis with acroosteolysis. A case report. *J. Bone Joint Surg. [Br.]* 67:86, 1985.
Torg J, et al.: Hereditary multicentric osteolysis with recessive transmission: New syndrome. *J. Pediatr.* 75:243, 1969.
Tyler T, et al.: Idiopathic multicentric osteolysis. *A.J.R.* 126:23, 1976.

OSTEOMA CUTIS, FAMILIAL

Synonym: Familial ectopic ossification.

Mode of Inheritance: Dominant trait.

Clinical Manifestations: (a) *subcutaneous areas of thickening* at various sites, subcutaneous mobile lumps; (b) normal values for serum calcium, phosphorus, and alkaline phosphatase.

Radiologic Manifestations: *Ectopic bone masses;* in one case strands and sheets of bone extending along muscle planes out into soft tissues from the pelvis and limb bone in a lower limb (unique case reported by Gardner et al.).

Differential Diagnosis: Surgical scar; chronic venous insufficiency; pseudohypoparathyroidism; scleroderma; dermatomyositis; etc.

REFERENCES

Fawcett HA, et al.: Hereditary osteoma cutis. *J. R. Soc. Med.* 76:697, 1983.
Gardner RJM, et al.: Familial ectopic ossification. *J. Med. Genet.* 25:113, 1988.
Peterson WC, et al.: Primary osteoma of the skin. *Arch. Dermatol.* 87:626, 1963.

OSTEOPOROSIS (IDIOPATHIC JUVENILE)

Synonym: Juvenile osteoporosis.

Mode of Inheritance: Not definitely known, autosomal recessive has been suggested.

Frequency: Rare.

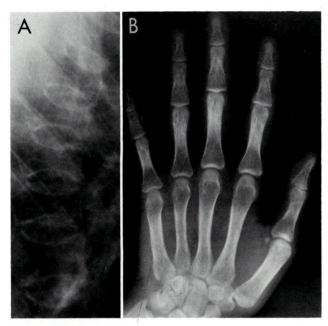

FIG SY–O–10.
Osteoporosis (idiopathic juvenile) in a 15-year-old female with severe hip pain of a 2-month duration and loss of 2 to 3 inches in height over the preceding 18 months. **A,** vertebral bodies markedly osteoporotic and endplates concave. **B,** bones of the hand demineralized, cortices thinned. (From Gooding CA, Ball JH: Idiopathic juvenile osteoporosis. *Radiology* 93:1349, 1969. Used by permission.)

Clinical Manifestations: *Onset at 3 to 12 years of age;* (a) abnormal gait; (b) *pain in the feet, spine, or elsewhere;* (c) small stature; (d) usually a negative calcium balance; (e) low plasma calcitriol (1,25-dihydroxycholecalciferol) and normal serum calcifediol (25-hydroxycholecalciferol) levels; (f) spontaneous resolution of the osteoporosis following puberty.

Radiologic Manifestations: (a) *abrupt development of osteoporosis,* becoming progressively more severe for a time and then becoming stabilized; (b) vertebral collapse; (c) *fractures* of long bones; (d) skeletal maturation retardation (Fig SY–O–10).

REFERENCES

Gooding CA, Ball JH: Idiopathic juvenile osteoporosis. *Radiology* 93:1349, 1969.

Houang MTV, et al.: Idiopathic juvenile osteoporosis. *Skeletal Radiol.* 3:17, 1978.

Lachmann D, et al.: A care-report of idiopathic juvenile osteoporosis with particular reference to 47-calcium absorption. *Eur. J. Pediatr.* 125:265, 1977.

Marder HK, et al.: Calciterol deficiency in juvenile osteoporosis. *Am. J. Dis. Child.* 136:914, 1982.

Schippers JC: A case of spontaneous general osteoporosis in girl 10 years old. *Monatschr. Kindergeneesk.* 8:109, 1938.

Smith R: Idiopathic juvenile osteoporosis. *Am. J. Dis. Child.* 133:889, 1979.

Smith R: Idiopathic osteoporosis in the young. *J. Bone Joint Surg. [Br.]* 62:417, 1980.

Stöver B, et al.: Idiopathische juvenile Osteoporose. *Fortschr. Rontgenstr.* 121:435, 1974.

Teotia M, et al.: Idiopathic juvenile osteoporosis. *Am. J. Dis. Child.* 133:894, 1979.

Towbin R, et al.: Generalized osteoporosis with multiple fractures in an adolescent. *Invest. Radiol.* 16:171, 1981.

OSTEOPOROSIS OF THE HIP (TRANSIENT)

Synonym: Transient osteoporosis of the hip.

Frequency: Uncommon in adults; extremely rare in children.

Clinical Manifestations: (a) *hip pain* of one to several months' duration, referred to the knee in some cases; (b) joint fluid may be increased in quantity, laboratory studies compatible with sterile synovitis; (c) synovial biopsy findings may be normal or show mild chronic inflammatory changes; (d) occasional elevation of the erythrocyte sedimentation rate.

Radiologic Manifestations: (a) *generalized demineralization of the femoral head,* with a lesser degree of demineralization of the acetabulum and femoral neck, gradual improvement and *recovery in 2 to 6 months,* no joint narrowing; (b) computed tomography: osteoporosis, joint effusion; (c) bone scintigraphy: increased uptake with positive findings before plain radiographic detection of the disease; (d) magnetic resonance imaging (MRI): decreased signal intensity of bone marrow in the femur on T_1-weighted image, increased signal intensity on T_2-weighted images, joint effusion, regression of MR images within 6 to 10 months (associated with clinical improvement).

REFERENCES

Arnstein AR: Regional osteoporosis. *Orthop. Clin. North Am.* 3:585, 1972.

Beaulieu JG, et al.: Transient osteoporosis of the hip in pregnancy: Review of the literature and a case report. *Clin. Orthop.* 115:165, 1976.

Bloem JL: Transient osteoporosis of the hip: MR imaging. *Radiology* 167:753, 1988.

Dihlmann VW, et al.: Diagnostic algorithms for transitory osteoporosis of the hip using computed tomography. *A.J.R.* 141:625, 1983.

Kaplan SS, et al.: Transient osteoporosis of the hip. A case report and review of the literature. *J. Bone Joint Surg. [Am.]* 67:490, 1985.

Nicol RO, et al.: Transient osteopaenia of the hip in children. *J. Pediatr. Orthop.* 4:590, 1984.

Shifrin LZ, et al.: Idiopathic transient osteoporosis of the hip. *J. Bone Joint Surg. [Br.]* 69:769, 1987.

Wilson AJ, et al.: Transient osteoporosis: Transient bone marrow edema. *Radiology* 167:757, 1988.

OTODENTAL DYSPLASIA

Mode of Inheritance: Autosomal dominant.

Frequency: Very rare.

Clinical and Radiologic Manifestations: (a) abnormal crown morphology of the teeth (large and bulbous crowns), obliteration of the normal relationship between cusps and grooves, absence of premolars in some cases; (b) denticles and taurodontism; (c) progressive sensorineural hearing loss.

REFERENCES

Cook RA, et al.: Otodental dysplasia: A five year study. *Ear Hear.* 2:90, 1981.
Levin LS, et al.: Otodental dysplasia: A "new" ectodermal dysplasia. *Clin. Genet.* 8:136, 1975.

OTO-ONYCHO-PERONEAL SYNDROME

Mode of Inheritance: Possibly autosomal recessive.

Frequency: Two male siblings.

Clinical Manifestations: (a) low-set and rotated large ears, unfolded helix, prominent anthelix, hypoplastic lobules; (b) partial aplasia of the nails; (c) other reported abnormalities: immobility of several interphalangeal joints, dolichocephaly, flaring of the temporal region.

Radiologic Manifestations: Aplasia of the fibulas in one sibling and proximal hypoplasia of the fibulas in the other sibling.

REFERENCES

Pfeiffer RA: The oto-onycho-peroneal syndrome. A probably new genetic entity. *Eur. J. Pediatr.* 138:317, 1982.

OTO-PALATO-DIGITAL SYNDROME, TYPE 1

Synonyms: Taybi syndrome; OPD-1 syndrome.

Mode of Inheritance: X-linked with lesser expression in females.

Frequency: Rare; according to Wiedemann et al., including the cases presented in their textbook, 69 cases in males and 34 in females were known up to 1981. Some of these cases may have represented OPD-2 syndrome.

Clinical Manifestations: (a) *short stature (most);* (b) *characteristic craniofacial features:* frontal bossing, prominent occiput, prominent supraorbital ridges, flat face, broad nasal root, antimongoloid slant of the palpebral fissures, microstomia; (c) *cleft palate;* (d) *conductive deafness;* (e) *short, broad*

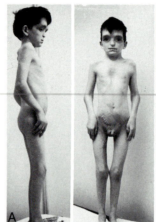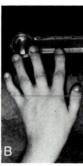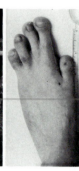

FIG SY—O—11.
Oto-palato-digital syndrome, type 1. **A,** 9-year-old patient with short stature, characteristic craniofacial features (frontal bossing, prominent occiput, prominent supraorbital ridges, flat face, broad nasal root, and microstomia). Note the elbow flexion. **B,** short broad thumbs and great toes and broad terminal phalanges of the other digits. (From Taybi H: Generalized skeletal dysplasia with multiple anomalies. A note on Pyle's disease. *A.J.R.* 88:450, 1962. Used by permission.)

thumbs and great toes and broad terminal phalanges of the other digits; (f) *limited elbow motion;* (g) *syndactyly of the toes;* (h) *nail dystrophy.*

Radiologic Manifestations: (a) *thick and dense base of the skull, prominence of the supraorbital ridges, steep clivus, poor pneumatization of the frontal and sphenoid sinuses,* delayed closure of the anterior fontanelle, small mandible; (b) *poor development of the mastoids, dense middle-ear ossicles;* (c) posterior defect of the neural arch of the vertebrae; (d) dislocation of the radial heads; (e) flat acetabulum, coxa valga; (f) mild lateral bowing of femora; (g) *carpal anomalies:* transverse capitate, comma-shaped trapezoid, carpal fusions, supernumerary carpal bones; (h) *tarsal anomalies:* fusion, anomalous fifth metatarsal, extra calcaneal ossification center; (i) *short thumbs and great toes,* large cone-shaped epiphysis of the distal phalanx of the thumbs and great toes; (j) partial anodontia, impacted teeth; (k) *other reported abnormalities:* bowing of the long bones, widened lower thoracic and lumbosacral spinal canal, small pedicles, hip and elbow subluxation, etc. (Figs SY—O—11 and SY—O—12).

REFERENCES

Buran DJ, et al.: The otopalatodigital syndrome. *Arch. Otolaryngol.* 85:394, 1967.
Dudding BA, et al.: The oto-palato-digital syndrome: A new symptom-complex consisting of deafness, dwarfism, cleft palate, characteristic facies, and a generalized bone dysplasia. *Am. J. Dis. Child.* 113:214, 1967.

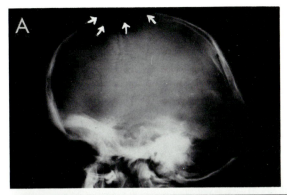

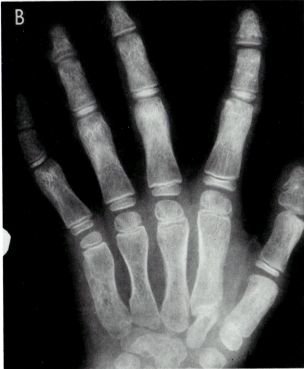

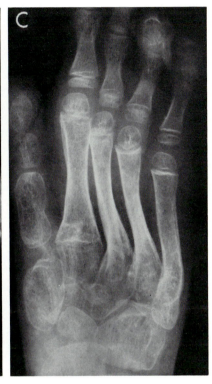

FIG SY–O–12.
Oto-palato-digital syndrome, type 1, in a 9-year-old boy with a small trunk and extremities in comparison with a prominent skull, hypertelorism, receding eyes, microstomia, and semiflexed elbows. **A,** roentgenogram of the skull shows dense bone, in particular at the base, a widely open anterior fontanelle *(arrows)*, deep upper occipital region, heavy supraorbital ridge, steep clivus, lack of pneumatization of the frontal and sphenoid sinuses, and sclerotic changes in the mastoid regions. **B,** malformed carpal bones, abnormal tubulation of metacarpals and phalanges, and a large and cone-shaped epiphysis of the thumb. **C,** tarsal and metatarsal bones abnormally formed; note the shortness of the first metatarsal and phalanges of the great toe. (From Taybi H: Generalized skeletal dysplasia with multiple anomalies. *A.J.R.* 88:450, 1962. Used by permission.)

Gall JC Jr, et al.: Oto-palato-digital syndrome: Comparison of clinical and radiographic manifestations in males and females. *Am. J. Hum. Genet.* 24:24, 1972.

Gorlin RJ: Oto-palato-digital syndrome. *Am. J. Dis. Child.* 114:215, 1967.

Langer LO: The roentgenographic features of the oto-palato-digital (OPD) syndrome. *A.J.R.* 100:63, 1967.

Pazzaglia UE, et al.: Oto-palato-digital syndrome in four generations of a large family. *Clin. Genet.* 30:338, 1986.

Plenier V, et al.: Le syndrome otopalato-digital. *Rev. Stomatol. Chir. Maxillofac.* 84:322, 1983.

Poznanski AK, et al.: The hand in the oto-palato-digital syndrome. *Ann. Radiol. (Paris)* 16:203, 1973.

Rosenbaum S, et al.: The oto-palato-digital syndrome. *Rev. Brasil. Genet.* 9:341, 1986.

Salinus CF, et al.: Variable expression in otopalatodigital syndrome: *Birth Defects* 15:329, 1979.

Spranger J: Pattern recognition in bone dysplasias. *Prog. Clin. Biol. Res.* 200:315, 1985.

Szabó L, et al.: Das Oto-palato-digitale Syndrom (Taybi). *Z. Orthop.* 115:75, 1977.

Taybi H: Generalized skeletal dysplasia with multiple anomalies. *A.J.R.* 88:450, 1962.

Wiedemann H-R, Grosse K-R, Dibbern H: *An Atlas of Characteristic Syndromes. A Visual Aid to Diagnosis.* Chicago, Year Book Medical Publishers Inc, 1985, pp. 16–17.

OVARIAN HYPERSTIMULATION SYNDROME

Clinical Manifestations: Onset of symptoms usually 5 to 7 days after ovulation; mild to severe manifestations: (a) mild form: lower abdominal discomfort, no significant weight gain, *enlarged ovaries (less than 5 cm in average diameter)*; (b) severe form: *ovarian enlargement more than 10 cm in average diameter, hemoconcentration, hypotension, oliguria, electrolyte imbalance;* (c) other reported abnormalities: adult respiratory distress syndrome, occurrence of the syndrome after follicular aspiration, occurrence of the syndrome in preterm infants (estradiol-producing ovarian cysts).

Radiologic Manifestations: (a) *enlarged ovaries mainly due to the presence of multiple thin-walled cysts,* often located in the periphery; (b) *ascites, pleural effusion;* (c) complication: ovarian rupture or torsion.

REFERENCES

McArdle CR, et al.: Ovarian hyperstimulation syndrome. *A.J.R.* 135:835, 1980.

Ritchie WGM: Sonographic evaluation of normal and induced ovulation. *Radiology* 161:1, 1986.
Sedin G, et al.: Ovarian hyperstimulation syndrome in preterm infants. *Pediatr. Res.* 19:548, 1985.
Van Der Merwe JP, et al.: Severe ovarian hyperstimulation after follicular aspiration. *S. Afr. Med. J.* 73:426, 1988.
Zosmer A, et al.: Adult respiratory distress syndrome complicating ovarian hyperstimulation syndrome. *Fertil. Steril.* 47:524, 1987.

OVARIAN VEIN SYNDROME

Clinical and Radiologic Manifestations: *Obstruction of the distal part of the ureter by the ovarian vein;* symptoms often in parous women and exceptionally in children or nulliparous women; (a) *abdominal pain,* abdominal colic, pain in the sacral area and thighs; (b) nausea, vomiting; (c) pyelonephritis, obstructive nephropathy; (d) *ovarian vein (unilateral, occasionally bilateral) dilatation.*

REFERENCES

De Schepper A, et al.: Computed tomographic diagnosis of dilated ovarian veins in a case of "ovarian vein syndrome". *Eur. J. Radiol.* 3:324, 1983.
Hubmer G: The ovarian vein syndrome. *Eur. Urol.* 4:263, 1978.

PACHYDERMOPERIOSTOSIS

Synonyms: Touraine-Solente-Golé syndrome; idiopathic hypertrophic osteoarthropathy; primary hypertrophic osteoarthropathy.

Mode of Inheritance: Autosomal dominant with marked variability in expressivity; 85% reported cases in males.

Clinical Manifestations: Onset of symptoms around puberty: (a) *coarsening of facial features (thickening and folding of the skin);* (b) *spadelike enlargement of the hands and feet;* (c) *digital clubbing;* (d) cylindrical thickening of the legs and forearms; (e) *furrowing and oiliness of the skin;* (f) excessive sweating; (g) *cutis verticis gyrata* (bulldog scalp); (h) joint effusion.

Radiologic Manifestations: (a) *early stage: symmetrical excessive subperiosteal new bone formation of the distal segment of the long bones and metacarpals, metatarsals, and proximal phalanges;* (b) *advanced stage:* (1) *all bones with the exception of the skull may be involved, with marked subperiosteal bone formation;* (2) *ossification of the ligaments and tendons;* (3) *joint effusion;* (4) *joint ankylosis;* (5) acroosteolysis; (6) scintigraphic findings: diffuse uptake along the cortical margins of the long bones (parallel tract or double-stripe sign).

Differential Diagnosis: Secondary hypertrophic osteoarthropathy.

Notes: (a) the clinical manifestations of the syndrome may be complete (pachydermia, periostitis, cutis verticis gyrata) or incomplete (absence of pachydermia and cutis verticis gyrata); (b) the syndrome usually progresses slowly for about 10 years and is followed by a quiescent period (Fig SY−P−1).

REFERENCES

deVries N, et al.: Case report 399: Pachydermoperiostosis (primary hypertrophic osteoarthropathy). *Skeletal Radiol.* 15:658, 1986.

Fournier AM, et al.: Pachydermopériostose. *J. Radiol. Electrol.* 54:417, 1973.

Friedreich N: Hyperostose des gesammten Skelettes. *Virchows Arch. [A]* 43:83, 1868 (quoted by Rimoin DL).

Guyer PB, et al.: Pachydermoperiostosis with acroosteolysis. *J. Bone Joint Surg. [Br.]* 60:219, 1978.

Hedayati H, et al.: Acrolysis in pachydermoperiostosis. *Arch. Intern. Med.* 140:1087, 1980.

Herbert DA, et al.: Idiopathic hypertrophic osteoarthropathy (pachydermoperiostosis). *West. J. Med.* 134:354, 1981.

Joseph B, et al.: Acro-osteolysis associated with hypertrophic pulmonary osteoarthropathy and pachydermoperiostosis. *Radiology* 154:343, 1985.

Kozlowski K, et al.: Idiopathic hypertrophic osteoarthropathy (report of a further case with brief literature review). *Australas. Radiol.* 27:291, 1983.

Mottahedeh P, et al.: Touraine-Solente-Golé syndrom (Pachydermopériostose) *Acta Madica Iranica* 22:10, 1980.

Rimoin DL: Pachydermoperiostosis (idiopathic clubbing and periostosis): Genetic and physiologic considerations. *N. Engl. J. Med.* 272:923, 1965.

Sirinavin C, et al.: Digital clubbing, hyperhidrosis, acroosteolysis and osteoporosis. A case resembling pachydermoperiostosis. *Clin. Genet.* 22:83, 1982.

Touraine A, Solente G, Golé L: Un syndrome ostéodermopathique: La pachydermie plicaturée avec pachypériostose des extrémités. *Presse Med.* 43:1820, 1935.

PAGET-SCHROETTER SYNDROME

Synonym: Effort-induced thrombosis.

Pathology: *Primary venous obstruction of an upper extremity in the axillary region.*

Clinical Manifestations: (a) rapid or gradual onset of pain, redness, tenderness, *increased venous pressure in an upper limb;* (b) *cordlike masses in the axilla;* (c) marked venous collateral circulation of the arm and shoulder (infrared photography).

Radiologic Manifestations: *Site of venous obstruction and collateral circulation* demonstrable by venography.

REFERENCES

Brüster H, et al.: Diagnose und Therapiekontrolle des Paget-von Schroetter-Syndroms. *Radiologe* 20:141, 1980.

Hughes ESR: Venous obstruction in upper extremity (Paget-Schroetter's syndrome): Review of 320 cases. *Int. Abstr. Surg.* 88:89, 1949.

Paget J: *Clinical Lectures and Essays.* London, Longmans, Green & Co., 1875.

Parienty J-R, et al.: Syndrome de Paget-von Schrötter. *Ann. Radiol. (Paris)* 8:331, 1965.

Sanghavi ST, et al.: Paget-Schroetter syndrome. *J. Postgrad. Med.* 29:175, 1983.

Schrötter L: Erkrankungen der Gefässe, in Nothnagel CWH (ed.): *Handbuch der Pathologie und Therapie.* Wein, Holder, 1884.

Smith-Behn J, et al.: Primary thrombosis of the axillary/subclavian vein. *South Med. J.* 79:1176, 1986.

Steinberg I: Angiographic features of primary venous ob-

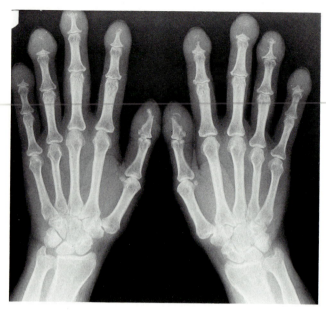

FIG SY–P–1.
Pachydermoperiostosis with acro-osteolysis in a 42-year-old woman with pronounced clubbing of her fingers. (From Guyer PB, Bruton FJ, Wren NWG: Pachydermoperiostosis with acro-osteolysis. *J. Bone Joint Surg. [Br.]* 60:219, 1978. Used by permission.)

struction of upper extremity: Paget–von Schrötter syndrome. *A.J.R.* 98:388, 1966.
Zigun JR, et al.: "Effort" thrombosis (Paget-Schroetter's syndrome) secondary to martial arts training. *Am. J. Sports Med.* 16:189, 1988.

PALLISTER-HALL SYNDROME

Synonym: Hypothalamic hamartoblastoma-hypopituitarism, imperforate anus–postaxial polydactyly

Frequency: Rare.

Clinical and Radiologic Manifestations: (a) congenital hypothalamic hamartoblastoma; (b) hypopituitarism; (c) imperforate anus; (d) postaxial polydactyly; (e) neonatally lethal malformation syndrome; (f) other reported abnormalities: unusual facies, laryngeal cleft, abnormal lung lobulation, renal agenesis and/or renal dysplasia, short fourth metacarpals, nail dysplasia, multiple buccal frenula, microcephalus, congenital heart disease, hypoadrenalism, intrauterine growth retardation.

Note: It has been suggested that the Pallister-Hall syndrome and severe Smith-Lemli-Opitz syndrome are the same.

REFERENCES

Clarren SK, et al.: Congenital hypothalamic hamartoblastoma, hypopituitarism, imperforate anus, and postaxial polydactyly—a new syndrome? II. Neuropathological considerations. *Am. J. Med. Genet.* 7:75, 1980.
Donnai D, et al: Smith-Lemli-Opitz syndrome: Do they include the Pallister-Hall syndrome (letter)? *Am. J. Med. Genet.* 28:741, 1987.
Haas JE, et al.: Hypothalamic hamartoblastoma, hypoendocrinism, and hypomelia: A new syndrome? *Lab. Invest.* 42:172, 1980.
Hall JG, Pallister PD, et al.: Congenital hypothalamic hamartoblastoma, hypopituitarism, imperforate anus, and postaxial polydactyly—A new syndrome? I: Clinical, causal, and pathologic considerations. *Am. J. Med. Genet.* 7:47, 1980.
Huff DS, et al.: Pallister-Hall syndrome (letter). *N. Engl. J. Med.* 306:430, 1982.

PALLISTER-KILLIAN SYNDROME

Synonyms: Isochromosome 12p mosaicism; Pallister mosaic aneuploidy; Pallister/Teschler-Nicola/Killian syndrome.

Frequency: Rare.

Clinical Manifestations: (a) *craniofacial features:* "coarse" face, prominent forehead, sparse scalp hair, sparse eyebrows, hypertelorism, epicanthal folds, flat bridge of the nose, macrostomia, macroglossia, abnormal ears, highly arched palate; (b) *hypotonia* in newborns; (c) *isochromosome 12p mosaicism* (isochromosome usually absent in cultured lymphocytes but present in fibroblasts); (d) other reported abnormalities: large size at birth, accessory nipples, prognathism in adulthood, pigmentary dysplasia of the skin, bitemporal alopecia, umbilical hernia, lymphedema, optic hypoplasia, cataracts, etc.

Radiologic Manifestations: (a) limbs: *distal digital hypoplasia, shortness of the long bones;* (b) other reported abnormalities: urogenital sinus anomaly, ventricular system dilatation (computed tomography), skeletal maturation retardation, imperforate anus, etc.

REFERENCES

Kawashima H: Skeletal anomalies in a patient with the Pallister/Teschler-Nicola/Killian syndrome. *Am. J. Med. Genet.* 27:285, 1987.
Killian W, et al.: Case report 102: Abnormal hair, craniofacial dysmorphism, and severe mental retardation—a new syndrome? *J. Clin. Dysmorphol.* 1:6, 1983.
Lin AE, et al.: Case of Pallister-Killian syndrome with imperforate anus. (letter) *Am. J. Med. Genet.* 31:705, 1988.
Reynolds JF, et al.: Isochromosome 12p mosaicism (Pallister mosaic aneuploidy or Pallister-Killian syndrome): Report of 11 cases. *Am. J. Med. Genet.* 27:257, 1987.
Teschler-Nicola M, Killian W: Case report 72: Mental retardation, unusual facial appearance, abnormal hair. *Syndrome Ident.* 7:6, 1981.
Wenger SL, et al.: Risk effect of maternal age in Pallister i(12p) syndrome. *Clin. Genet.* 34:181, 1988.

PANCOAST SYNDROME

Pathology: Destructive lesion of the thoracic inlet (neoplastic, traumatic, inflammatory, etc.) with involvement of the brachial and sympathetic plexus of nerves.

Clinical Manifestations: (a) *pain* in the shoulder region with radiation into the axilla, toward the scapula, and along the ulnar aspect of the arm; (b) *muscular atrophy* and weakness of the muscles of the hand; (c) *Horner syndrome;* (d) compression of blood vessels causing edema; (e) hoarseness.

Radiologic Manifestations: (a) apical thoracic density in the form of a cap or a mass; (b) bone destruction (ribs, vertebrae); (c) indentation of the esophagus by a mass; (d) percutaneous needle biopsy under fluoroscopy guidance.

REFERENCES

Hare ES: Tumor involving certain nerves. *London Med. Gazette* 23:16, 1838.

O'Connell RS, et al.: Superior sulcus tumor: Radiographic diagnosis and workup. *A.J.R.* 140:25, 1983.

Omenn GS: Pancoast syndrome due to metastatic carcinoma from the uterine cervix. *Chest* 60:268, 1971.

Pancoast HK: Superior pulmonary sulcus tumor: Tumor characterized by pain, Horner's syndrome, destruction of bone, and atrophy of hand muscles. *J.A.M.A.* 99:1391, 1932.

Simpson FG, et al.: Pancoast's syndrome associated with invasive aspergillosis. *Thorax* 41:156, 1986.

Stathatos C, et al.: Pancoast's syndrome due to hydatid cysts of the thoracic outlet. *J. Thorac. Surg.* 58:764, 1969.

PANCREATIC DISEASE, SUBCUTANEOUS FAT NECROSIS, AND POLYSEROSITIS

Clinical and Radiologic Manifestations: (a) *pancreatic disease:* acute or chronic pancreatitis, traumatic pancreatitis, pancreatic carcinoma; (b) *polyserositis:* pleural effusion, pericardial effusion, ascites, arthritis; (c) *subcutaneous fat necrosis;* (d) eosinophilia; (e) possible contribution of immune-mediated injury.

REFERENCE

Potts DE, et al.: Syndrome of pancreatic disease, subcutaneous fat necrosis and polyserositis. *Am. J. Med.* 58:417, 1975.

PANCREATITIS, HEREDITARY

Synonym: Hereditary pancreatitis.

Mode of Inheritance: Autosomal dominant.

Clinical Manifestations: (a) *recurrent acute epidoses of abdominal pain beginning in infancy or childhood;* (b) failure to thrive; (c) *elevated serum amylase level;* (d) other reported abnormalities: malabsorption.

Radiologic Manifestations: (a) *pancreatic calcification;* (b) *pancreatic enlargement, edema, ductal dilatation, pseudocyst;* (c) other reported abnormalities: ascites, pleural effusion, pseudocyst of the mediastinum, portal vein thrombosis, splenic vein thrombosis, etc.

Differential Diagnosis: Nonhereditary pancreatitis; idiopathic fibrosing pancreatitis.

REFERENCES

Atkinson GO, et al.: Idiopathic fibrosing pancreatitis: A cause of obstructive jaundice in childhood. *Pediatr. Radiol.* 18:28, 1988.

Confort MW, et al.: Pedigree of a family with hereditary chronic relapsing pancreatitis. *Gastroenterology* 21:54, 1952.

Ghishan FK, et al.: Chronic relapsing pancreatitis in childhood. *J. Pediatr.* 102:514, 1983.

Ginies JL, et al.: Faux kyste mediastinal au cours d'une pancréatite hereditaire. *Arch. Fr. Pediatr.* 43:709, 1986.

McElroy R, et al.: Hereditary pancreatitis in a kinship associated with portal vein thrombosis. *Am. J. Med.* 52:228, 1972.

Weizman Z, et al.: Acute pancreatitis in childhood. *J. Pediatr.* 113:24, 1988.

PAPILLON-LEFÈVRE SYNDROME

Synonyms: Hyperkeratosis palmoplantaris and periodontoclasia; hyperkeratosis palmoplantaris with periodontosis; maladie de Meleda.

Mode of inheritance: Autosomal recessive.

Frequency: Over 160 published cases (Pareek et al).

Clinical Manifestations: Onset of symptoms in infancy: (a) hyperkeratosis of the palm, sole, ankle, elbow, and knee, with centripetal extension of the keratoses to the limbs and trunk; (b) periodontopathy, gingival swelling and erythema, loosening of the teeth, deep periodontal pockets of infection, loss of teeth; (c) abnormally thin cementum, extensive destruction of the periodontal ligament, severe inflammation of the soft tissues (microscopic examination).

Radiologic Manifestations: (a) dural and choroidal calcifications; (b) *marked destruction of supporting alveolar bone with teeth soon becoming mobile and prematurely lost* (deciduous and permanent teeth); (c) atrophy of the alveolar process following a period of bone destruction; (d) almost completely edentulous by the age of 17 years; (e) other reported associated findings: skeletal maturation retardation, osteoporosis.

REFERENCES

Gorlin RJ, et al.: The syndrome of palmar-plantar hyperkeratosis and premature peridontal destruction of the teeth: A clinical and genetic analysis of the Papillon-Lefèvre syndrome. *J. Pediatr.* 65:895, 1964.
Nazzaro V, et al.: Papillon-Lefevre syndrome. Ultrastructural study and successful treatment with acitretin. *Arch. Dermatol.* 124:533, 1988.
Papillon MM, Lefèvre P: Deux cas de keratodermie palmaire et plantaire symétrique familiale (maladie de Meleda) chez le frère et la soeur: Coexistence dans les deux cas d'altérations dentaires graves. *Bull. Soc. Fr. Dermatol. Syph.* 31:82, 1924.
Pareek SS, et al.: Papillon-Lefevre syndrome. A report of six cases in one family. *Int. J. Dermatol.* 25:638, 1986.
Vrahopoulos TP, et al.: Ultrastructure of the periodontal lesion in a case of Papillon-Lefevre syndrome (PLS). *J. Clin. Periodontol.* 15:17, 1988.

PARIETAL "FORAMINA"–CLAVICULAR HYPOPLASIA

Mode of Inheritance: Autosomal dominant.

Frequency: Very rare.

Clinical Manifestations: (a) macrocephaly, high forehead, occipital hair tuft; (b) hypertelorism, short nasal septum, microtia, atretic ear canal.

Radiologic Manifestations: (a) congenital parietal defects; (b) distal hypoplasia of the clavicles (Fig SY–P–2).

REFERENCES

Eckstein HB, et al.: Congenital parietal "foramina" associated with faulty ossification of the clavicles. *Br. J. Radiol.* 36:220, 1963.
Golabi M, et al.: Parietal foramina clavicular hypoplasia. An autosomal dominant syndrome. *Am. J. Dis. Child.* 138:596, 1984.

PARINAUD SYNDROME

Clinical Manifestations: Diplopia, ptosis, or separation of the eyelids; paralysis of conjugate upward movement of the eye without paralysis of convergence; retraction; nystagmus; wide pupils; papilledema.

Radiologic Manifestations: Intracranial lesions: neoplasms, inflammations, hemorrhage, small vascular lesions, hydrocephalus, etc.

REFERENCES

Hamer J, et al.: Parinaud's syndrome in non-tumorous hydrocephalic intracranial hypertension. *Neuropaediatrie* 7:217, 1976.
Martin X, et al.: Ophthalmia nodosa and the oculoglandular syndrome of Parinaud. *Br. J. Ophthalmol.* 70:536, 1986.
Parinaud H: *Le Strabisme et Son Traitement.* Paris, G. Doin & Co., 1899.
Pierrot-Deseilligny CH, et al: Parinaud's syndrome. Electrooculographic and anatomical analyses of six vascular cases with deductions about vertical gaze organization in the premotor structures. *Brain* 105:667, 1982.
Slavin ML: Gaze palsy associated with viral syndrome. *Am. J. Ophthalmol.* 100:468, 1985.

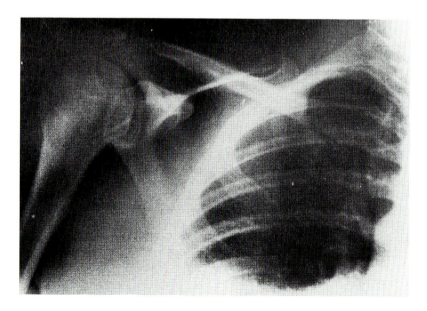

FIG SY–P–2.
Parietal foramina–clavicular hypoplasia in a 33-year-old male. Hypoplasia of the lateral segment of the clavicle is present. (From Golabi M, Carey J, Hall BD: Parietal foramina clavicular hypoplasia. *Am. J. Dis. Child.* 138:596, 1984. Used by permission.)

PATELLA APLASIA, COXA VARA, TARSAL SYNOSTOSIS

Mode of Inheritance: Reported in a mother and her two children.

Clinical and Radiologic Manifestations: (a) bilateral hip dysplasia, coxa vara, hypoplasia of the descending ramus of the pubic bone; (b) patella aplasia; (c) moderate femoral hypoplasia; (d) talocalcaneal synostosis, absence of one metatarsal and oligodactyly.

REFERENCE

Goeminne L, et al.: Congenital coxa vara, patella aplasia and tarsal synostosis. A new inherited syndrome. *Acta Genet. Med. Gemellol. (Roma)* 19:534, 1970.

PATELLA HYPOPLASIA

Clinical and Radiologic Manifestations: (a) pes planus, bilateral brachydactyly of the fourth toes, unilateral tarsal fusion (talo-navicular); (b) hypoplasia and subluxation of the patellae; (c) absence of ischial tuberosities; (d) gracile fibulas; (e) "winging" of scapulae, mild thoracic scoliosis and lumbar lordosis.

REFERENCE

Sandhaus YS, et al.: A new patella syndrome. *Clin. Genet.* 31:143, 1987.

PATTERSON SYNDROME

Synonym: Pseudoleprechaunism.

Clinical Manifestations: (a) normal birth weight; bodily disproportion noted at birth with large hands, feet, nose, and ears; (b) cutis laxa present from birth; (c) generalized bronzed hyperpigmentation present from birth; (d) hirsutism; (e) mental retardation; (f) epilepsy; (g) kyphoscoliosis; (h) deformities of the extremities with swelling in joint regions related to bone deformities; (i) endocrine disorders: hyperadrenocorticism, cushinoid features, diabetes mellitus; premature adrenarche with elevated dehydroepiandrosterone and androstenedione levels; (j) survival beyond infancy.

Radiologic Manifestations: (a) thickening of the cranial vault and base of the skull, thickening and deformity of facial bones; (b) deformed vertebral bodies with irregular and dense endplates, platyspondyly of the cervical vertebrae, hypoplasia of the odontoid process, anterior displacement of the atlas, ovoid configuration of the thoracic and lumbar vertebrae; (c) marked deformity of ribs, clavicles, and scapulae; (d) pro-

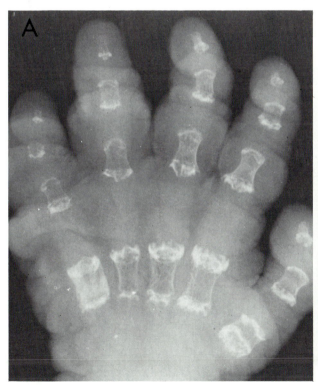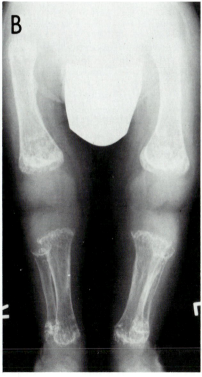

FIG SY—P—3.
Patterson syndrome in a 7-year-old male with "dysendocrinism" present from birth. **A** and **B,** marked cutis gyrata of the hand, very marked delay in skeletal maturation, poor enchondral bone for- mation, irregular metaphyseal ossification, and sclerotic metaphyseal changes. (From Patterson JH: Presentation of a patient with leprechaunism. *Birth Defects* 5(4):117, 1969. Used by permission.)

gressive deformity and failure of ossification of the pubic bones, ischia, triradiate cartilages, and margins of the sacroiliac joints; flattening and irregularity of the acetabular roofs; (e) shortness and deformity of the tubular bones with poor enchondral bone formation, irregular metaphyseal ossification, and sclerotic metaphyseal changes; (f) severe skeletal maturation retardation (Fig SY–P–3).

Note: The Patterson syndrome should be differentiated from leprechaunism or Donohue syndrome (intrauterine disproportionate dwarfism, failure to thrive, coarse and grotesque facies, large hands and feet, endocrine disorders, large phallus, breast hypertrophy, hirsutism, progressive marasmus, severe skeletal maturation retardation, death in infancy).

REFERENCES

Cantani A, et al.: Un syndrome polydysmorphique rare: Le lepréchaunisme. Revue des quarante-neuf cas publiés dans la littérature. *Ann. Genet.* 30:221, 1987.

David TJ, et al.: The Patterson syndrome, leprechaunism, and pseudoleprechaunism. *J. Med. Genet.* 18:294, 1981.

Donahue WL: Clinicopathologic conference at the Hospital for Sick Children: Dysendocrinism. *J. Pediatr.* 32:739, 1948.

Fürste HO, et al.: Leprechaunismus (Donohue-Syndrom). Klinische und pathologisch-anatomische Befunde. *Helv. Paediatr. Acta* 39:95, 1984.

Patterson JH: Presentation of a patient with leprechaunism. *Birth Defects* 5(4):117, 1969.

Szilagyi PG, et al.: Pancreatic exocrine aplasia, clinical features of leprechaunism, and abnormal gonadotropin regulation. *Pediatr. Pathol.* 7:51, 1987.

PELVIC DYSPLASIA–ARTHROGRYPOTIC LOWER LIMBS

Mode of Inheritance: Autosomal recessive has been suggested (two sisters).

Clinical and Radiologic Manifestations: (a) arthrogrypotic changes in the lower limbs; (b) pelvic dysplasia: markedly widened triradiate cartilage, irregular and notched acetabula, marked hypoplasia of the ilia, notched iliac wings, delayed ossification of the capital femoral ossification centers.

Differential Diagnosis: Scapuloiliac dysostosis (pelvis-shoulder dysplasia.

REFERENCE

Ray S, et al.: Pelvic dysplasia associated with arthrogrypotic changes in the lower extremities. A new syndrome. *Clin. Orthop.* 207:99, 1986.

PENA-SHOKEIR SYNDROME

Synonyms: Pena-Shokeir syndrome, type I; fetal akinesia deformation sequence.

Mode of Inheritance: Sporadic; autosomal recessive; genetic heterogeneity; intrafamilial heterogeneity.

Frequency: Approximately 60 published cases to 1986 (Hall).

Clinical Manifestations and Pathology: (a) *intrauterine growth retardation;* (b) *facial dysmorphism: low-set and malformed ears, hypertelorism, epicanthal folds, small mandible, depressed nasal tip;* (c) limb anomalies: small or prominent joints, fixed joints in flexion or extension position, lack of normal growth, clubfoot, camptodactyly; (e) short umbilical cord, polyhydramnios; (f) other reported abnormalities: pterygia, short neck, central nervous system (brain dysgenesis including hydrocephalus, microgyria, oligogyria, hypoplastic optic nerves, cortical ectopia of the cerebellum, cerebellar hypoplasia, absent septum pellucidum, cavum septum pellucidum, hydranencephaly, absent olfactory nerves, spinal cord dysgenesis), craniofacial (short palpebral fissures, ptosis, cleft palate, cleft lip, long philtrum, choanal atresia), limb (postaxial polydactyly, duplicated thumb, proximal radioulnar synostosis, dislocated radial head, syndactyly/oligodactyly), cardiovascular (cyanotic and noncyanotic heart defects, coarctation of the aorta, etc), laryngeal stenosis, genitourinary (undescended testes, hypospadias, urachal anomalies, duplicated vagina and uterus), endocrine (thyroid hypoplasia, adrenal hypoplasia), alimentary system (imperforate anus, ectopic anus), skin (pigmented nevi, hypertrichosis); (g) perinatal death, some surviving infancy.

Radiologic Manifestations: (a) prenatal ultrasonography: hydramnios, hydrops/edema, scalp edema, micrognathia/retrognathia, restricted limb movement, decreased/absent fetal breathing, small narrow chest, absent stomach echo, arthrogryposis, rocker-bottom/clubfoot, fixed flexion of the knees, fixed extension of the knees, fixed flexion of the elbows, flexion deformities of the wrists and ankles, depressed nasal tip, deformed ears, camptodactyly, shortness of the long bones, kyphosis of the thoracic spine, cryptorchidism, reduced muscle bulk; (b) postnatal: (1) limbs: thin, gracile, sticklike or cylindrical long bones, talipes equinovarus, camptodactyly, subluxation at the interphalangeal joints of the fingers, dislocations (hips, knees, etc.), fracture; (2) thin ribs, small thorax, pulmonary hypoplasia; (3) other reported abnormalities: scoliosis, vertebral segmentation anomalies, extra ribs, various urinary system anomalies, renal hamartomas, renal cysts, intestinal malrotation, etc.

Differential Diagnosis: Arthrogryposis multiplex congenita; cerebro-oculo-facio-skeletal syndrome (Pena-Shokeir II syndrome); Neu-Laxova syndrome; lethal multiple pterygium syndrome (Fig SY–P–4).

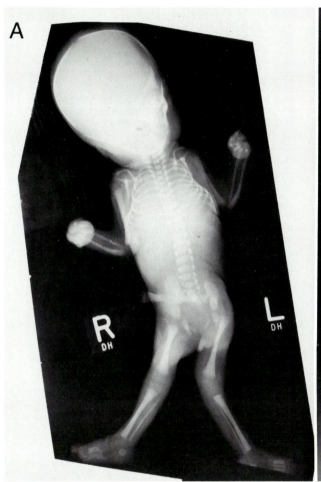

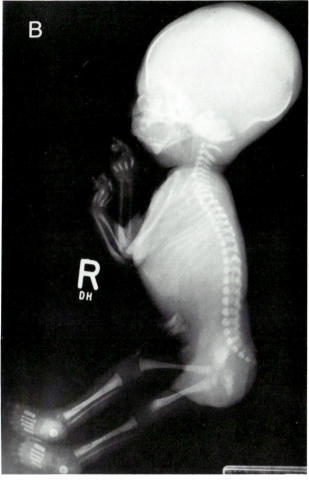

FIG SY–P–4.
Pena-Shokeir syndrome: anteroposterior **(A)** and lateral **(B)** views of a stillborn female infant with micrognathia, gracile bones, and fixed deformities of many joints. (From Houston CS, Shokeir MHK: Separating Pena-Shokeir I syndrome from the "arthrogryposis basket". *J. Can. Assoc. Radiol.* 32:215, 1981. Used by permission.)

REFERENCES

Agapitos M, et al: Arthrogryposis multiplex congenita, Pena-Shokeir phenotype, with gastroschisis and agenesis of the leg. *Pediatr. Pathol.* 8:409, 1988.

Hageman G, et al.: The heterogeneity of the Pena-Shokeir syndrome. *Neuropediatrics* 18:45, 1987.

Hall JG: Invited editorial comment: Analysis of Pena Shokeir phenotype. *Am. J. Med. Genet.* 25:99, 1986.

Houston CS, et al.: Separating Pena-Shokeir I syndrome from the "arthrogryposis basket". *J. Can. Assoc. Radiol.* 32:215, 1981.

Ohlsson A, et al.: Prenatal sonographic diagnosis of Pena-Shokeir syndrome type I, or fetal akinesia deformation sequence. *Am. J. Med. Genet.* 29:59, 1988.

Pena SD, Shokeir MHK: Syndrome of camptodactyly, multiple ankyloses facial anomalies, and pulmonary hypoplasia: A lethal condition. *J. Pediatr.* 85:373, 1974.

PENDRED SYNDROME

Mode of Inheritance: Autosomal recessive.

Frequency: 1 to 8:100,000 adults, equal in both sexes; 6% to 10% of the patients with congenital deafness (Früs et al.).

Clinical Manifestations: (a) *congenital perceptive hearing loss*; (b) *goiter (euthyroid or hypothyroid)*; (c) *pathological perchlorate test findings*; (d) other reported abnormalities: *thyroid carcinoma*.

Radiologic Manifestations: (a) *goiter*; (b) Mondini defect (malformation of the cochlea: partial aplasia resulting in 1 to 1½ coils instead of the normal 2½ to 2¾ coils, with the middle and apical coils sharing a common cloaca).

Note: Please refer to Deaf mutism-goiter-euthyroidism syndrome.

REFERENCES

Bergstrom L: Pendred's syndrome with atypical features. *Ann. Otol. Rhinol. Laryngol.* 89:135, 1980.

Das VK: Pendred's syndrome with episodic vertigo, tinnitus and vomiting and normal bithermal caloric responses. *J. Laryngol. Otol.* 101:721, 1987.
Fraser GR: Association of congenital deafness with goiter (Pendred's syndrome): A study of 207 families. *Ann. Hum. Genet.* 28:201, 1965.
Friis J, et al.: Thyroid function in patients with Pendred's syndrome. *J. Endocrinol. Invest.* 11:97, 1988.
Illum P: Thyroid carcinoma in Pendred's syndrome. *J. Laryngol. Otol.* 92:435, 1978.
Johnsen T, et al.: Pendred's syndrome. Acoustic, vestibular and radiological findings in 17 unrelated patients. *J. Laryngol. Otol.* 101:1187, 1987.
Medeiros-Neto GA, et al.: Thyroidal iodoproteins in Pendred's syndrome. *J. Clin. Endocrinol.* 28:1205, 1968.
Pendred V: Deaf-mustism and goiter. *Lancet* 2:532, 1896.
van Wouwe JP, et al.: A patient with dup(10p)del(8q) and Pendred syndrome. *Am. J. Med. Genet.* 24:211, 1986.

PERICARDITIS-ARTHRITIS-CAMPTODACTYLY

Synonyms: Camptodactyly-arthropathy-pericarditis syndrome; CAP syndrome; PAC syndrome.

Mode of Inheritance: Five of seven siblings in one family; also a report of a sporadic case.

Clinical and Radiologic Manifestations: Onset of symptoms in childhood: (a) constrictive pericarditis; (b) arthritis, primarily affecting the large joints; (c) camptodactyly, bilateral and symmetrical, secondary to flexion of the flexor tendons at the proximal interphalangeal joint level.

Differential Diagnosis: Juvenile rheumatoid arthritis; systemic lupus erythematosus; mulibrey nanism.

REFERENCES

Goldman H, et al.: Familial pericarditis, arthritis, and camptodactyly. *N. Engl. J. Med.* 310:127, 1984.
Laxer RM, et al.: The camptodactyly-arthropathy-pericarditis syndrome: Case report and literature review. *Arthritis Rheum.* 29:439, 1986.
Martinez-Lavin M, et al.: Familial syndrome of pericarditis, arthritis, and camptodactyly. *N. Engl. J. Med.* 309:224, 1983.

PERLMAN SYNDROME

Mode of Inheritance: Appears to be autosomal recessive.

Frequency: Nine published cases (Greenberg et al.).

Clinical and Radiologic Manifestations: (a) facial features: round fullness, hypotonic with open mouth, long upper lip inverted V-shaped upper lip, micrognathia, serrated upper alveolar edge, darwinian tubercle of the ears, upsweep of the anterior scalp hairline; (b) fetal gigantism; (c) Wilms tumor; (d) renal dysplasia; (e) hyperplasia of the endocrine pancreas; (f) mental retardation; (g) other reported abnormalities: diaphragmatic hernia, cardiovascular defect, hypospadias, polysplenia.

REFERENCES

Greenberg F, et al.: Expanding the spectrum of the Perlman syndrome. *Am. J. Med. Genet.* 29:773, 1988.
Neri G, et al.: The Perlman syndrome: Familial renal dysplasia with Wilms tumor, fetal gigantism and multiple congenital anomalies. *Am. J. Med.* 19:195, 1984.
Perlman M: Perlman syndrome: Familial renal dysplasia with Wilms tumor, fetal gigantism, and multiple congenital anomalies (letter). *Am. J. Med. Genet.* 25:793, 1986.
Perlman M, et al.: Renal hamartomas and nephroblastomatosis with fetal gigantism: A familial syndrome. *J. Pediatr.* 83:414, 1973.
Perlman M, et al.: Syndrome of fetal gigantism, renal hamartomas and nephroblastomatosis with Wilms' tumour. *Cancer* 35:1212, 1975.

PERSISTENT MÜLLERIAN DUCT SYNDROME

Mode of Inheritance: Autosomal recessive.

Clinical and Radiologic Manifestations: An intersex disorder (pseudohermaphroditism): (a) male with unilateral or bilateral cryptorchidism; (b) normal external male genitalia; (c) inguinal hernia; (d) female genital organs (uterus and fallopian tubes) located in the inguinal canal; (e) malignancies.

Differential Diagnosis: Mixed gonad dysgenesis (ambiguous genitalia, unilateral testis and a streak gonad on the contralateral side, persistent müllerian duct structures, usually a chromosome mosaicism of XO/XY).

REFERENCES

Beheshti M, et al.: Familial persistent müllerian duct syndrome. *J. Urol.* 131:968, 1984.
Kazim E: Intra-abdominal seminomas in persistent müllerian duct syndrome. *Urology* 26:290, 1985.
Mouli K, et al.: Persistent müllerian duct syndrome in a man with transverse testicular ectopia. *J. Urol.* 139:373, 1988.
Nilson O: Hernia uteri inguinalis beim Manne. *Acta Chir. Scand.* 83:231, 1939.
Snow BW, et al.: Testicular tumor in patient with persistent müllerian duct syndrome. *Urology* 26:495, 1985.

PERSISTING MESONEPHRIC DUCT SYNDROME

Clinical and Radiologic Manifestations: The triad: (a) persistence of the mesonephric duct, genitourinary anomalies; (b) rectal anomalies: imperforate anus, anal stenosis, H-type urethroanal fistula, anteriorly displaced rectum; (c) anomalies of renal ascent or morphology: pelvic kidney, hydronephrosis, multicystic kidney, crossed renal ectopia, retroiliac artery ureter, unilateral absence of kidney.

REFERENCE

Vordermark JS II: The persisting mesonephric duct syndrome: The description of a new syndrome. *J. Urol.* 130:958, 1983.

PEUTZ-JEGHERS SYNDROME

Mode of Inheritance: Autosomal dominant; familial incidence in about 50%.

Frequency: Uncommon.

Clinical Manifestations: (a) *brown or black pigmentations* of the lips, buccal mucosa, face, palms, and soles; (b) hamartomatous polyps causing recurrent abdominal pain, alimentary tract bleeding, and anemia; (c) intussusception resulting from a polyp, rectal prolapse; (d) malignant degeneration of the polyps rare; (e) increased incidence of ovarian cysts and tumors (5%) (sex cord tumor); (f) high risk of development of neoplasms (18 times greater than is expected in the general population): gastrointestinal carcinomas, nongastrointestinal carcinomas, multiple myeloma, testicular neoplasms; (g) other reported abnormalities: extragastrointestinal polyps (urinary tract, bronchus, nose), enteritis cystica profunda, etc.

Radiologic Manifestations: (a) *alimentary tract polyposis,* intussusception; (b) extragastrointestinal polyps (rare): urinary tract, bronchus, and nose (Figs SY–P–5 and SY–P–6).

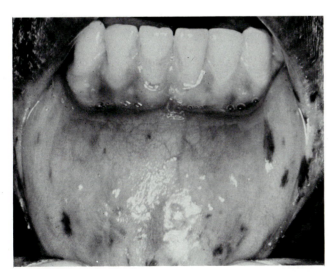

FIG SY–P–5.
Peutz-Jeghers syndrome in a 21-year-old male. Melanotic macules are present on the mucosal surface of the lower lip. (From Godard JE, Dodds WJ, Phillips JC, et al.: Peutz-Jeghers syndrome: Clinical and roentgenographic features. *A.J.R.* 113:316, 1971. Used by permission.)

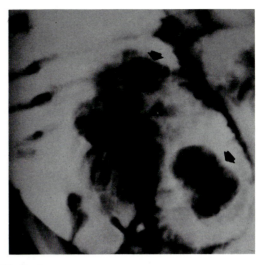

FIG SY–P–6.
Peutz-Jeghers syndrome in a 14-year-old male. Two large polyps are present in the terminal ileum *(arrows).* An ileocolic intussusception was seen to form and reduce during fluoroscopy. (From Godard JE, Dodds WJ, Phillips JC, et al.: Peutz-Jeghers syndrome: Clinical and roentgenographic features. *A.J.R.* 113:316, 1971. Used by permission.)

REFERENCES

Anderson NJ, et al.: Peutz-Jeghers syndrome with cervical adenocarcinoma and enteritis cystica profunda. *West J. Med.* 141:242, 1984.

Giardiello FM, et al.: Increased risk of cancer in the Peutz-Jeghers syndrome. *N. Engl. J. Med.* 316:1511, 1987.

Godard JE, et al.: Peutz-Jeghers syndrome: Clinical and roentgenographic features. *A.J.R.* 113:316, 1971.

Gürses N, et al.: Peutz-Jeghers syndrome: A clinical study of a large family in two generations. *Z. Kinderchir.* 41:364, 1986.

Hutchinson J: Pigmentation of lips and mouth. *Arch. Surg.* 7:290, 1896.

Jeghers H, et al.: Generalized intestinal polyposis and melanin spots of the oral mucosa, lips, and digits: A syndrome of diagnostic significance. *N. Engl. J. Med.* 241:993, 1949.

Linos DA, et al.: Does Peutz-Jeghers syndrome predispose to gastrointestinal malignancy? A later look. *Arch. Surg.* 116:1182, 1981.

Peutz JLA: Over een zeer merkwaardige, gecombinerde familiare polyposis van de slijmvliezen van den tractus intestinalis met die van de neuskeelholte en gepaard met eigenaardige pigmentaties van huiden slijmvliezen. *Ned. Mschr. Geneeskd.* 10:134, 1921.

Ryo UY, et al.: Extensive metastases in Peutz-Jeghers syndrome. *J.A.M.A.* 239:2268, 1978.

Sommerhaug RG, et al.: Peutz-Jeghers syndrome and ureteral polyposis. *J.A.M.A.* 211:120, 1970.

Tovar JA, et al.: Peutz-Jeghers syndrome in children: Report of two cases and review of the literature. *J. Pediatr. Surg.* 18:1, 1983.

Walecki JK, et al.: Ultrasound contribution to diagnosis of Peutz-Jeghers syndrome. *Pediatr. Radiol.* 14:62, 1984.

Weber FP: Patches of deep pigmentation of oral mucous membrane not connected with Addison's disease. *Q. J. Med.* 12:404, 1919.

Wilson DM, et al.: Testicular tumors with Peutz-Jeghers syndrome. *Cancer* 57:2238, 1986.

PHALANGEAL MICROGEODIC SYNDROME OF INFANCY

Frequency: Approximately 40 published cases, mostly from Japan (Meller et al.).

Clinical Manifestations: Onset of symptoms at about 18 months to 2 years of age: (a) *swelling, redness, heat, and minimal pain in the fingers;* (b) spontaneous *regression* of clinical manifestations within a few months; (c) unknown cause.

Radiologic Manifestations: *Small lacunae in the middle and distal phalanges* of affected fingers, mild widening of involved phalanges.

Notes: (a) about 75% of reported cases have been from Japan, with symptoms developing in winter; (b) the mean age of onset of symptoms of the Japanese cases was 6½ years, which is older than originally reported by Maroteaux (18 months to 2 years) (Fig SY–P–7).

REFERENCES

Kaibara N, et al.: Phalangeal microgeodic syndrome in childhood: Report of seven cases and review of the literature. *Eur. J. Pediatr.* 136:41, 1981.

MacCarthy J, et al.: Phalangeal microgeodic syndrome of infancy. *Arch. Dis. Child.* 51:473, 1976.

Maroteaux P: Cinq observations d'une affection microgéodique des phalanges du nourrisson d'étiologie inconnue. *Ann. Radiol. (Paris)* 13:229, 1970.

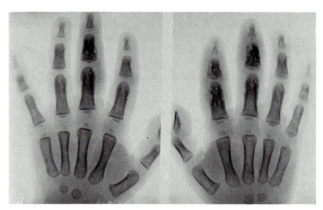

FIG SY–P–7.
Phalangeal microgeodic syndrome of infancy in a 2-year-old male. Small lacunae are seen in the phalanges. (From Maroteaux P: Cinq observations d'une affection microgéodique des phalanges du nourrisson d'étiologie inconnue. *Ann. Radiol. (Paris)* 13:229, 1970. Used by permission.)

Meller Y, et al.: Phalangeal microgeodic syndrome in childhood. *Acta Orthop. Scand.* 53:553, 1982.

Sugiura Y, et al.: Bone changes of unknown etiology affecting phalanges of fingers in children: Report of eight cases. *Pediatr. Radiol.* 4:243, 1976.

PHILLIPS-GRIFFITHS SYNDROME

Mode of Inheritance: Report of a brother and sister.

Clinical and Radiologic Manifestations: (a) bilateral macular coloboma; (b) cleft palate; (c) digital anomalies.

REFERENCE

Phillips CI, Griffiths DL: Macular coloboma and skeletal abnormalities. *Br. J. Ophthalmol.* 53:346, 1969.

PICK DISEASE

Mode of Inheritance: Autosomal dominant.

Pathology: (a) symmetrical lobar or circumscribed atrophy (frontal lobes more than temporal lobes, parietal and occipital lobes rarely affected); (b) Pick cells and Pick inclusion bodies.

Clinical Manifestation: Dementia.

Radiologic Manifestations: Loss of tissue (localized and symmetrical, often lobar) associated with an increased volume of the frontal interhemispheric space, the sylvian fissure, and the frontal horns.

REFERENCES

Groen JJ, et al.: Computed tomography in Pick's disease: Findings in a family affected in three consecutive generations. *J. Comput. Assist. Tomogr.* 6:907, 1982.

Groen JJ, et al.: Hereditary Pick's disease: Second reexamination of a large family and discussion of other hereditary cases, with particular reference to electroencephalography and computerized tomography. *Brain* 105:443, 1982.

Munoz-Garcia D, et al.: Classic and generalized variants of Pick's disease: A clinicopathological, ultrastructural, and immunocytochemical comparative study. *Ann. Neurol.* 16:467, 1984.

Pick A: Ueber die Benziehungen der senilen Hirnatrophie zur Aphasie. *Prager Med. Wochenschr.* 17:165, 1892.

PICKWICKIAN SYNDROME

Clinical Manifestations: (a) *marked obesity;* (b) *somnolence;* (c) narrow oropharynx (computed tomography), *cardiorespiratory insufficiency with decreased alveolar ventilation;* (d) intermittent cyanosis; (e) periodic respiration, decreased hypoxic ventilatory drive, sleep apnea, arrhythmias, serious elevation of both pulmonary and systemic pressures;

(f) secondary polycythemia; (g) myoclonic twitching; (h) right ventricular hypertrophy; (i) right ventricular failure (in an advanced stage).

Radiologic Manifestations: (a) cardiomegaly; (b) normal or prominent pulmonary vasculature.

REFERENCES

Dickens C: *The Posthumous Papers of the Pickwick Club.* London, Chapman & Hall, 1837.

Özsoylu S, et al.: Pickwickian syndrome related to central nervous system leukemia. *Am. J. Dis. Child.* 140:503, 1986.

Phillipson EA: Pickwickian, obesity-hypoventilation, or fee-fi-fo-fum syndrome. *Am. Rev. Respir. Dis.* 121:781, 1980.

Rapoport DM, et al.: Hypercapnia in the obstructive sleep apnea syndrome. A reevaluation of the "pickwickian syndrome". *Chest* 89:627, 1986.

Simpser MD, et al.: Sleep apnea in a child with the pickwickian syndrome. *Pediatrics* 60:290, 1977.

Stark VP, et al.: Diagnostik der obstruktiven Schlafapnoe (Pickwickian Syndrome). Wertigkeit der Computertomographie. *Fortschr. Rontgenstr.* 140:46, 1984.

Zwillich CW, et al.: Decreased hypoxic ventilatory drive in the obesity-hypoventilation syndrome. *Am. J. Med.* 59:343, 1975.

PLEONOSTEOSIS

Synonym: Léri syndrome.

Mode of Inheritance: Autosomal dominant with good penetrance and variable expression.

Frequency: Rare.

Clinical Manifestations: (a) shortness of stature; (b) mongoloid facies; (c) short and spadelike hands; (d) broad thumbs in the valgus position; (e) genu recurvatum; (f) flexion contractures of the digits of the hands and feet; (g) cubitus valgus; (h) limitation of motion of the joints; (i) carpal tunnel syndrome, Morton metatarsalgia.

Radiologic Manifestations: (a) increase in width of the bones, in particular those of the hands, feet, and vertebrae; (b) bizarre enlargement of the posterior neural arches of the cervical vertebrae (Rukavina et al.), a relative decrease in the anteroposterior diameter of the vertebral bodies of L_2 and L_3; (c) flexion contractures of the digits of the hands and feet; (d) other reported abnormalities: skeletal maturation retardation, ischemic necrosis of the femoral heads, spinal cord compression.

REFERENCES

Friedman M, et al.: Léri's pleonosteosis. *Br. J. Radiol.* 54:517, 1981.

Hilton RC, et al.: Léri's pleonosteosis. *Q. J. Med.* 49:419, 1980.

Léri A: Dystrophie osseuse generalisée congénitale et héréditaire: La pleonostéose familiale. *Presse Med.* 30:13, 1922.

Metcalfe RA, et al.: Spinal cord compression in Léri's pleonosteosis. *Br. J. Radiol.* 58:117, 1985.

Rukavina JG, et al.: Léri's pleonosteosis: A study of a family with a review of the literature. *J. Bone Joint Surg. [Am.]* 41:397, 1959.

Shaw DG: Léri's pleonosteosis. *Br. J. Radiol.* 54:819, 1981.

Watson-Jones R: Léri's pleonosteosis, carpal tunnel compression of the median nerves and Morton's metatarsalgia. *J. Bone Joint Surg. [Br.]* 31:560, 1949.

PLUMMER-VINSON SYNDROME

Synonym: Paterson-Brown-Kelly syndrome.

Clinical Manifestations: Most patients are middle-aged women: (a) glossitis; mucosal changes in the mouth, pharynx, and proximal segment of the esophagus *(webs, bands, mucosal folds)* causing dysphagia; (b) *simple hypochromic anemia;* (c) achlorhydria; (d) other reported abnormalities: spoon-shaped fingernails, splenomegaly, association with Kartagener syndrome, postcricoid carcinoma.

Radiologic Manifestations: (a) web in the hypopharynx or cervical esophagus; (b) spasm in the pharynx or esophagus.

REFERENCES

Beitman RG, et al.: Oral manifestations of gastrointestinal disease. *Dig. Dis. Sci.* 26:741, 1981.

Kelly AB: Spasm at the entrance to the oesophagus. *J. Laryngol. Otol.* 34:285, 1919.

Miller G: Patterson-Kelly, Plummer-Vinson syndrome (letter). *Dig. Dis. Sci.* 25:813, 1980.

Nicoli F, et al.: Radiologic and endoscopic diagnosis in Plummer-Vinson syndrome. *Rays* 11:51, 1986.

Paterson DR: A clinical type of dysphagia. *J. Laryngol. Otol.* 34:289, 1919.

Plummer HS: Diffuse dilatation of the esophagus without anatomic stenosis (cardiospasm): A report of ninety-one cases. *J.A.M.A.* 58:2013, 1912.

Todd NW Jr, et al.: A patient with Kartagener and Paterson-Brown-Kelly syndromes. *J.A.M.A.* 234:1248, 1975.

Vinson PP: Hysterical dysphagia. *Minn. Med.* 5:107, 1922.

POEMS SYNDROME

Synonyms: Takatsuki syndrome; PEP syndrome; Crow-Fukase syndrome.

Definition: *P*lasma cell dyscrasia-polyneuropathy-*O*rganomegaly, *E*ndocrinopathy, *M* protein, and *S*kin changes.

Clinical Manifestations: (a) *polyneuropathy:* peripheral neuropathy, papilledema, increased cerebrospinal fluid pro-

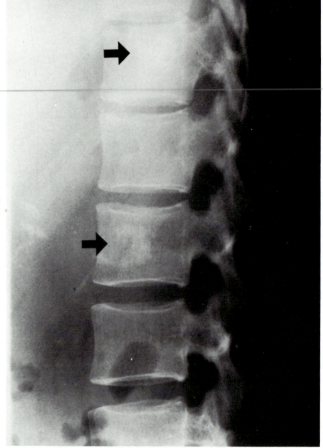

FIG SY−P−8.
POEMS syndrome. A lateral roentgenogram of the lumber spine in a
37-year-old female shows patchy sclerosis in the L_1 and L_3 vertebral
bodies *(arrows).* (From Tanaka O, Ohsawa T: The POEMS syndrome:
Report of three cases with radiographic abnormalities. *Radiologe*
24:472, 1984. Used by permission.)

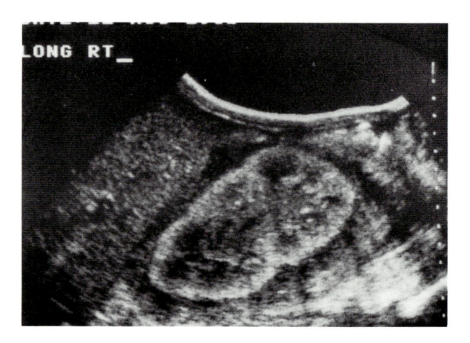

FIG SY−P−9.
POEMS syndrome in a 44-year-old man. A sagittal ultrasonogram
shows renal enlargement with the length measuring over 13 cm.
Note the increased echogenicity of the renal cortex. (From Arenson AM, et al.: Renal ultrasound in POEMS syndrome. *J. Clin. Ultrasound* 13:208, 1985. Used by permission.)

tein concentration; (b) *organomegaly* (hepatomegaly, splenomegaly, renomegaly), lymphadenopathy; (c) *endocrinopathy:* gynecomastia, impotence, amenorrhea, glucose intolerance, adrenal insufficiency, hypothyroidism; (d) *M protein:* IgA, IgG, marrow plasma cells, IgG κ monoclonal gammopathy; (e) *skin changes:* hyperpigmentation, thickening, hirsutism, hyperhidrosis; (f) other reported abnormalities: peripheral edema, ascites, pleural effusion, fever, finger clubbing, white fingernails, malabsorption, verrucous angiomas, association with giant lymph node hyperplasia (Castleman disease), infiltrative orbitopathy, optic disk edema, intracranial hypertension, thyroid nodule with evidence of thyroiditis (biopsy), microangiopathic glomerulopathy, association with myeloma (the disease may be a variant of myeloma), presentation as systemic sclerosis, etc.

Radiologic Manifestations: (a) single or multiple sclerotic ringlike lytic or mixed sclerotic and lytic bone lesions (most common in the spine, pelvis, and ribs; also reported in the skull and long bones), "ivory vertebra," coarse bony trabeculae, cortical thickening, diffuse calvarial thickening; (b) enlarged, prominent, echogenic kidneys; (c) infiltrative orbitopathy: diffuse swelling of the posterior orbital contents (pattern similar to orbital pseudotumors).

Note: Polyneuropathy may be absent (Figs SY–P–8 and SY–P–9).

REFERENCES

Arenson AM, et al.: Renal ultrasound in POEMS syndrome. *J. Clin. Ultrasound* 13:208, 1985.

Bitter MA, et al.: Giant lymph node hyperplasia with osteoblastic bone lesions and the POEMS (Takatsuki's) syndrome. *Cancer* 56:188, 1985.

Bourdette DN, et al.: Infiltrative orbitopathy, optic disc edema, and POEMS. *Neurology* 34:532, 1984.

Fam AG, et al.: POEMS syndrome: Study of a patient with proteinuria, microangiopathic glomerulopathy, and renal enlargement. *Arthritis Rheum.* 29:233, 1986.

Morrow JS, et al.: POEMS syndrome: Studies in a patient with an IgG-κ M protein but no polyneuropathy. *Arch. Intern. Med.* 142:1231, 1982.

Nakanishi T, et al.: The Crow-Fukase syndrome: A study of 102 cases in Japan. *Neurology* 34:712, 1984.

Resnick D, et al.: Plasma-cell dyscrasia with polyneuropathy, organomegaly, endocrinopathy, M-protein, and skin changes: The POEMS syndrome. *Radiology* 140:17, 1981.

Tanaka O, et al.: The POEMS syndrome: Report of three cases with radiographic abnormalities. *Radiologe* 24:472, 1984.

Viard J-P, et al.: POEMS syndrome presenting as systemic sclerosis. Clinical and pathologic study of a case with microangiopathic glomerular lesions. *Am. J. Med.* 84:524, 1988.

POLAND SYNDROME

Synonym: Poland anomaly.

Frequency: 1:30,000 live births; over 400 published cases to 1984 (Gausewitz et al.).

Clinical Manifestations: (a) *partial or complete absence of pectoralis muscles* (often the sternocostal head of the pectoralis major); (b) *anomalies of the ipsilateral upper limb;*

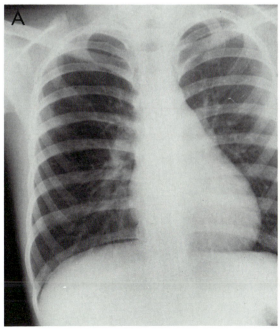
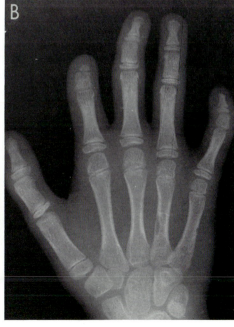

FIG SY–P–10.
Poland syndrome in a 10-year-old female. **A,** hyperlucency of the right side of the chest resulting from hypoplasia of the pectoralis muscles. **B,** hypoplasia and dysplasia of the phalanges of the right hand. (Courtesy of Children's Hospital of San Francisco.)

type 1, five digits present (normal or hypoplastic); type 2, absent central digits, functional border digits; type 3, no functional digits, more severe absence deformities than in type 2; type 4, absent thumb, radial ray defects; abnormalities of the muscles and tendons of the hand and forearm; (c) posterior shoulder girdle abnormalities; (d) other reported anomalies: hypoplasia of the breast and nipple, supernumerary nipple, leukemia, B-cell lymphoma, morning glory syndrome, dextrocardia, Möbius syndrome, undescended testes, facial paralysis, cleft lip, cutaneous problems, body asymmetry.

Radiologic Manifestations: (a) *syndactyly*, polydactyly, hypoplasia of the arm and hand, absence of metacarpals and phalanges; (b) *relative hyperlucency of the ipsilateral hemithorax;* (c) absence of a normal axillary fold on the affected side, deficient or absent pectoral muscle; (d) other reported anomalies: rib deformities, lung herniation, plagiocephaly, congenital hip dislocation, renal anomalies (agenesis, hypoplasia), elevated scapula, scoliosis, vertebral anomalies, sternal anomalies, hypoplastic scapula, absent infraspinatus, absent serratus anterior, etc.

Notes: (a) a nongenetic malformation syndrome, more than one member of a family reported in two second cousins; (b) subclavian artery supply disruption in the early embryonic life has been suggested as an etiologic factor; (c) Poland-Möbius syndrome refers to patients with the features of both syndromes (Fig SY—P—10).

REFERENCES

Beals RK, et al.: Congenital absence of pectoral muscles: A review of twenty-five patients. *Clin. Orthop.* 119:166, 1976.

Bosch-Banyeras JM, et al.: Poland-Möbius syndrome associated with dextrocardia. *J. Med. Genet.* 21:70, 1984.

Bouwes Bavinck JN, et al.: Subclavian artery supply disruption sequence: Hypothesis of a vascular etiology for Poland, Klippel-Feil, and Möbius anomalies. *Am. J. Med. Genet.* 23:903, 1986.

David TJ: Familial Poland anomaly. *J. Med. Genet.* 19:293, 1982.

Demos TC, et al.: Computed tomography of partial unilateral agenesis of the pectoralis muscles. *J. Comput. Assist. Tomogr.* 9:558, 1985.

Esquembre C, et al.: Poland syndrome and leukaemia. *Eur. J. Pediatr.* 146:444, 1987.

Fontaine G, et al.: Le syndrome de Poland-Möbius. A propos de 2 observations. *Arch. Fr. Pediatr.* 41:351, 1984.

Gausewitz SH, et al: Severe limb deficiency in Poland's syndrome. *Clin. Orthop.* 185:9, 1984.

Hanka SS, et al.: Dextrocardia associated with Poland's syndrome. *J. Pediatr.* 86:312, 1975.

Hegde HR, et al.: Posterior shoulder girdle abnormalities with absence of pectoralis major muscle. *Am. J. Med. Genet.* 13:285, 1982.

Hershatter BW, et al.: Poland's syndrome and lymphoma. *Am. J. Dis. Child.* 137:1211, 1983.

Ireland DCR, et al.: Poland's syndrome: A review of forty-three cases. *J. Bone Joint Surg. [Am.]* 58:52, 1976.

Parker DL, et al.: Poland-Möbius syndrome. *J. Med. Genet.* 18:317, 1981.

Pišteljić DT, et al.: Poland syndrome associated with 'morning glory' syndrome (coloboma of the optic disc). *J. Med. Genet.* 23:364, 1986.

Poland A: Deficiency of the pectoralis muscles. *Guys Hosp. Rep.* 6:191, 1841.

Ravitch M: Poland's syndrome—A study of an eponym. *Plast. Reconstr. Surg.* 59:508, 1977.

Risseeuw GA, et al: Poland's syndrome: Including ultrasonography of the pectoralis muscle as a new diagnostic modality. *J. Belge Radiol.* 68:231, 1985.

Senrui H, et al.: Anatomical findings in the hands of patients with Poland's syndrome. Report of four cases. *J. Bone Joint Surg. [Am.]* 64:1079, 1982.

POLYCYSTIC KIDNEY DISEASE (PKD)
Classification:

1. Recessive PKD (infantile PKD).
2. Dominant PKD (adult PKD).
3. Polycystic kidney disease in tuberous sclerosis.
4. Glomerulocystic kidney disease (cystic dilatation of the Bowman space and the first portion of the proximal convuluted tubules.
5. Medullary-type polycystic kidney disease, autosomal dominant.
6. Familial medullary polycystic kidney associated with congenital blindness, cataract, etc.

Genetic Notes: (a) two genetic markers closely linked to adult polycystic kidney disease on chromosome 16 are the α-globin cluster at a recombination frequency of approximately 5% and phosphoglycolate phosphatase; (b) prenatal diagnosis of dominant PKD by means of a linked DNA probe derived from the α-globin region; (c) most sporadic cases of polycystic kidney disease probably represent the recessive form of the disease; (d) the incidence of dominant PKD is about 1 in 1,000.

Clinical Notes: (a) recessive PKD is manifested in infancy (including neonatal lethal) or childhood, the dominant PKD may be manifested during infancy (including neonatal) or childhood, a family history and evaluation of other members of the family is very important for classification in the questionable cases; (b) PKD may be associated with hepatic fibrosis (hepatic fibrosis—renal cystic disease), cystic liver disease, cystic disease of other organs, and Caroli syndrome.

Radiologic Notes: (a) prenatal diagnosis of recessive PKD (RPKD): oligohydramnios, enlarged fetal abdominal circumference, renomegaly, increased renal echogenicity, cysts; (b) prenatal diagnosis of autosomal dominant PKD (DPKD) is possible (renal enlargement, increased renal echogenicity, cyst); (c) radiological features of DPKD in children: "macroscopic" renal cysts (rarely lacking on ultrasound or computed tomography [CT], even distribution of contrast material in the renal cortex and medulla [CT], absence of tu-

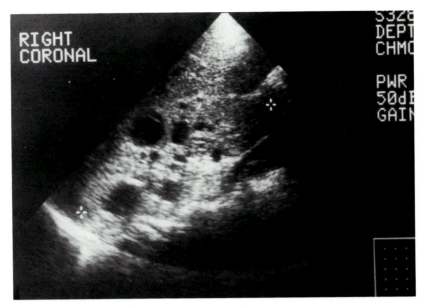

FIG SY—P—11.
Polycystic kidney disease (adult) in a 15-year-old male with a history of hematuria.
(Courtesy of Peter E. Kane, M.D., Children's Hospital Medical Center, Oakland, Calif.)

bular enlargement on excretory urography, normal liver echogenicity (echogenicity of the kidneys equal or less than that of the liver), may develop a liver cyst in adulthood; (d) radiological features of RPKD in children: streaky pattern of enlarged collecting tubules on excretory urography, echogenicity of the kidney higher than that of the liver, persistence of contrast material in the renal cortex longer than normal (CT), lacelike medullary renal cysts, absence of "macroscopic" renal cysts, obscure renal contour on ultrasonographic examination, liver texture suggesting periportal fibrosis; (e) multiple liver cysts common in DPKD in adults but not detectable in infants and children with this type of PKD; (f) single or multiple high-density (56 to 98 Hounsfield units) renal cysts on nonenhanced CT studies in adult polycystic kidney disease (DPKD), hepatic fibrosis and portal hypertension in RPKD is progressive with a changing pattern over a period of several years; (g) associated abnormalities with DPKD: cerebral aneurysm(s), cerebral hemorrhage, polycystic liver disease with an incidence ranging from 15% to 75% (it has been suggested that adult polycystic liver disease is an entity of its own and presents independently of adult polycystic kidney disease), perinephric hemorrhage (originating from an underlying hemorrhagic cyst), cholangiocellular carcinoma, persistent primitive trigeminal artery, cavum septi pellucidi and cerebral aneurysm in association with DPKD in a patient (Figs SY—P—11 and SY—P—12).

REFERENCES

Böhm N, et al.: Multiple acyl-CoA dehydrogenation deficiency (glutaric aciduria type II), congenital polycystic kidneys, and symmetric warty dysplasia of the cerebral cortex in two newborn brothers. II. Morphology and pathogenesis. *Eur. J. Pediatr.* 139:60, 1982.

Cole BR, et al.: Polycystic kidney disease in the first year of life. *J. Pediatr.* 111:693, 1987.

Fairley KF, et al.: Familial visual defects associated with polycystic kidney and medullary sponge kidney. *Br. Med. J.* 1:1060, 1963.

Fitch SJ, et al.: Ultrasonographic features of glomerulocystic disease in infancy: Similarity of infantile polycystic kidney disease. *Pediatr. Radiol.* 16:400, 1986.

Goldman SH, et al: Hereditary occurrence of cystic disease of renal medulla. *N. Engl. J. Med.* 274:984, 1966.

Harris R: Adult polycystic kidney disease. *J. Med. Genet.* 24:449, 1987.

Hossack KF, et al.: Echocardiographic findings in autosomal dominant polycystic kidney disease. *N. Engl. J. Med.* 319:907, 1988.

Kääriäinen H: Polycystic kidney disease in children: A genetic and epidemiological study of 82 Finnish patients. *J. Med. Genet.* 24:474, 1987.

Kääriäinen H, et al.: Dominant and recessive polycystic kidney disease in children: Classification by intravenous pyelography, ultrasound, and computed tomography. *Pediatr. Radiol.* 18:45, 1988.

Karhunen PJ, et al.: Adult polycystic liver and kidney diseases are separate entities. *Clin. Genet.* 30:29, 1986.

Kimberling WJ, et al.: Linkage heterogeneity of autosomal dominant polycystic kidney disease. *N. Engl. J. Med.* 319:913, 1988.

Landais P, et al.: Cholangiocellular carcinoma in polycystic kidney and liver disease. *Arch. Intern. Med.* 144:2274, 1984.

Lazarou LP, et al.: Adult polycystic kidney disease and linked RFLPs at the globin locus: A genetic study in the South Wales population. *J. Med. Genet.* 24:466, 1987.

Levine E, et al.: Liver cysts in autosomal-dominant polycystic kidney disease: Clinical and computed tomographic study. *A.J.R.* 145:229, 1985.

Levine E, et al.: Perinephric hemorrhage in autosomal domi-

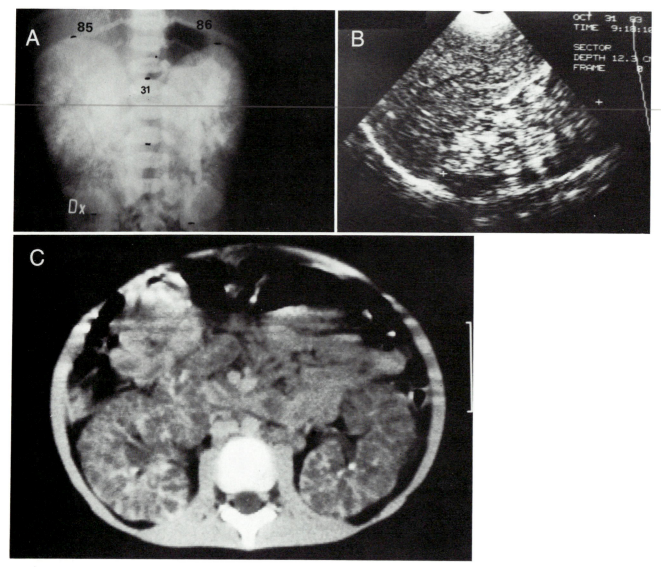

FIG SY–P–12.
Polycystic kidney disease (recessive). **A,** newborn. Excretory urography shows gross renal enlargement and accumulation of contrast medium in dilated tubules. **B,** 7-year-old patient with increased renal echogenicity that exceeds that of the liver, an obscure renal contour, and no detectable cysts. **C,** 7-year-old patient. CT shows lacelike medullary cysts and accentuation of contrast medium in the cortex. (From Kääriäinen H, Jääskeläinen J, Kivisaari L, et al.: Dominant and recessive polycystic kidney disease in children: Classification by intravenous pyelography, ultrasound and computed tomography. *Pediatr. Radiol.* 18:45, 1988. Used by permission.)

nant polycystic kidney disease: CT and MR findings. *J. Comput. Assist. Tomogr.* 11:108, 1987.

Luthy DA, et al.: Infantile polycystic kidney disease: Observations from attempts at prenatal diagnosis. *Am. J. Med. Genet.* 20:505, 1985.

Matsumura M, et al.: Persistent primitive trigeminal artery, cavum septi pellucidi, and associated cerebral aneurysm in a patient with polycystic kidney disease: Case report. *Neurosurgery* 16:395, 1985.

Melson GL, et al.: The spectrum of sonographic findings in infantile polycystic kidney disease with urographic and clinical correlations. *J. Clin. Ultrasound* 13:113, 1985.

Meziane MA, et al.: Computed tomography of high density renal cysts in adult polycystic kidney disease. *J. Comput. Assist. Tomogr.* 10:767, 1986.

Pierson M, et al.: Une curieuse association malformative congénitale et familiale atteignant l'oeil et le rein. *J. Genet. Hum.* 12:184, 1963.

Premkumar A, et al.: The emergence of hepatic fibrosis and portal hypertension in infants and children with autosomal recessive polycystic kidney disease. Initial and follow-up sonographic and radiographic findings. *Pediatr. Radiol.* 18:123, 1988.

Pretorius DH, et al.: Diagnosis of autosomal dominant polycystic kidney disease in utero and in the young infant. *J. Ultrasound Med.* 6:249, 1987.

Reeders ST, et al.: Prenatal diagnosis of autosomal dominant polycystic kidney disease with a DNA probe. *Lancet* 2:6, 1986.

Reeders ST, et al.: Two genetic markers closely linked to adult polycystic kidney disease on chromosome 16. *Br. Med. J.* 292:851, 1986.

Taitz LS, et al.: Screening for polycystic kidney disease: Importance of clinical presentation in the newborn. *Arch. Dis. Child.* 62:45, 1987.

Wakabayashi T, et al.: Polycystic kidney disease and intracranial aneurysms: Early angiographic diagnosis and early operation of the unruptured aneurysm. *J. Neurosurg.* 58:488, 1983.

Whelton A, et al.: Renal medullary cystic disease: A family study. *Birth Defects* 10(4):154, 1974.

Zerres K, et al.: Cystic kidneys. Genetics, pathologic anatomy, clinical picture, and prenatal diagnosis. *Hum. Genet.* 68:104, 1984.

POLYDACTYLY, SYNDACTYLY, AND OLIGODACTYLY, APLASIA OR HYPOPLASIA OF FIBULA, HYPOPLASIA OF PELVIS AND BOWING OF FEMORA

Mode of Inheritance: Autosomal recessive presumed (a family of Turkish-Arabian descent).

Clinical and Radiologic Manifestations: Hypoplasia of pelvis, congenital dislocation of hip, severe bowing of femur, aplasia or hypoplasia of fibula, absence or coalescence of tarsal bones, absence of various metatarsals, hypoplasia and aplasia of toes, clinodactyly, hypoplasia of fingers and fingernails, postaxial polydactyly.

Differential Diagnosis: Femur-fibula-ulna syndrome.

REFERENCES

Fuhrmann W, et al.: Poly-, syn- and oligodactyly, aplasia or hypoplasia of fibula, hypoplasia of pelvis and bowing of femora in three sibs—a new autosomal recessive syndrome. *Eur. J. Pediatr.* 133:123, 1980.

Fuhrmann W, et al.: A new autosomal recessive skeletal dyslplasia syndrome—prenatal diagnosis and histopathology, in, Papadatos CJ, Bartsocas CS (eds): *Skeletal Dysplasias.* New York, Alan R. Liss, 1982, pp 519–524.

POLYPOSIS SYNDROMES

1. Familial juvenile-type polyposis coli: autosomal dominant transmission.

2. Familial polyposis of the entire gastrointestinal tract: often juvenile type.

3. Familial gastric polyposis.

4. Generalized juvenile polyposis with pulmonary arteriovenous malformation (a mother and her daughter).

5. Familial polyposis of the colon (familial adenomatosis coli): autosomal dominant transmission with about one third sporadic, very high risk (approaching 100%) of colon carcinoma, extracolonic-associated abnormalities rare (duodenal polyps; gastric polyps; multiple endocrine neoplasia [MEN], type 2b; brain tumor; papillary and follicular thyroid tumors; carcinoid in the stomach; adrenal adenoma; adrenal carcinoma; adenocarcinoma of the gallbladder; malignancies in the periampullar region; congenital hypertrophy of the retinal pigment epithelium; childhood hepatoblastoma with a family history of polyposis coli; occult radiopaque jaw lesions, which are good predictors of polyp development in kindreds with adenomatous polyposis and jaw lesions; desmoid tumors).

6. Peutz-Jeghers syndrome.

7. Gardner syndrome.

8. Intestinal polyposis with exostoses (a family report).

9. Cronkhite-Canada syndrome.

10. Cowden syndrome.

11. Turcot syndrome.

12. Ruvalcaba-Myhre-Smith syndrome.

REFERENCES

Baker RH, et al.: Hyperpigmented lesions of the retinal pigment epithelium in adenomatous polyposis. *Am. J. Med. Genet.* 31:427, 1988.

Bartram CI, et al.: Colonic polyp patterns in familial polyposis. *A.J.R.* 142:305, 1984.

Bombi JA, et al.: Polyposis coli associated with adenocarcinoma of the gallbladder. Report of a case. *Cancer* 53:2561, 1984.

Bussey HJR: *Familial Polyposis Coli.* Baltimore, Johns Hopkins University Press, 1975.

Cox KL, et al.: Hereditary generalized juvenile polyposis associated with pulmonary arteriovenous malformation. *Gastroenterology* 78:1566, 1980.

dos Santos JG, et al.: Familial gastric polyposis: A new entity. *J. Genet. Hum.* 28:293, 1980.

Fuchs GA: Multiple kartilaginaere Exostosen bei Kolon- und Magen-polypose: Millelungen einer neuen vom Gardner-syndrom abweichenden erblichen Kombinationserkrankung. *Dtsch. Med. Wochenschr.* 100:2316, 1975.

Jones IT, et al.: Desmoid tumors in familial polyposis coli. *Ann. Surg.* 204:94, 1986.

Keating MA, et al.: Hamartoma of the bladder in a 4-year-old girl with hamartomatous polyps of the gastrointestinal tract. *J. Urol.* 138:366, 1987.

Kingston JE, et al.: Association between hepatoblastoma and polyposis coli. *Arch. Dis. Child.* 58:959, 1983.

Lynch HT, et al.: Congenital hypertrophy of retinal pigment epithelium in non-Gardner's polyposis kindreds. *Lancet* 2:333, 1987.

Maeda M, et al.: Radiological features of familial polyposis coli: Grouping by polyp profusion. *Br. J. Radiol.* 57:217, 1984.

Offerhaus GJA, et al.: Occult radiopaque jaw lesions in familial adenomatous polyposis coli and hereditary non-polyposis colorectal cancer. *Gastroenterology* 93:490, 1987.

Perkins JT, et al.: Adenomatous polyposis coli and multiple

endocrine neoplasia type 2b. A pathogenetic relationship. *Cancer* 55:375, 1985.

Smith HJ, et al.: Umbilicated adenomas in familial polyposis coli: Radiologic and histologic correlation (case report). *A.J.R.* 147:61, 1986.

Stevenson JK, et al.: Unfamiliar aspects of familial polyposis coli. *Am. J. Surg.* 152:81, 1986.

Yonemoto RH, et al.: Familial polyposis of the entire gastrointestinal tract. *Arch. Surg.* 99:427, 1969.

POLYSPLENIA SYNDROME

Mode of Inheritance: Autosomal recessive has been suggested in some familial cases; X-linked recessive also has been documented.

Frequency: 146 autopsy-proved cases reviewed by Peoples et al.; underreported.

Pathology: (a) levoisomerism (two lobes in each lung, bilateral hyparterial bronchi); (b) *congenital heart disease* (high incidence of atrial septal defect, anomalous pulmonary veins, bilateral superior vena cava, and azygos continuation of the inferior vena cava), preduodenal portal vein, morphological left ventricular outflow obstruction, duplication of the inferior vena cava; (c) hepatic symmetry, extrahepatic biliary atresia, absent gallbladder; (d) other reported abnormalities: a case with camptomelia, cervical lymphocele, polycystic dysplasia, short gut and polysplenia, Hodgkin disease, dynein arm defect, gastrointestinal duplication, etc.

Clinical Manifestations: Congenital heart disease.

Radiologic Manifestations: (a) various imaging modalities (ultrasound, computed tomography; scintigraphy, standard radiography) showing the thoracic and abdominal anomalies enumerated under Pathology; (b) *arteriographic demonstration* of a common celiac-mesenteric artery and *multiple spleens;* (c) other reported abnormalities: esophageal atresia, tracheoesophageal atresia, malrotation of the bowel, vertebral anomalies, renal anomalies (agenesis, cyst, etc.), ovarian cyst, spontaneous splenic infarction, dextrocardia.

Notes: (a) not all patients with polysplenia have congenital heart disease; (b) Some variants of polysplenia syndrome are (1) externally bilobed lungs with a normal bronchial branch pattern, congenital heart disease, intestinal malrotation, short pancreas; (2) pulmonary isomerism of the right lung type, congenital heart disease, pulmonary and systemic venous abnormalities, malrotation of the intestine with multiple spleens; (3) asplenia in one sibling and polysplenia in another sibling has been reported in some families (Fig SY–P–13).

REFERENCES

Abramson SJ, et al.: Biliary atresia and noncardiac polyspenic syndrome: US and surgical considerations. *Radiology* 163:377, 1987.

Arnold GL, et al.: Probable autosomal recessive inheritance of polysplenia, situs inversus and cardiac defects in an Amish family. *Am. J. Med. Genet.* 16:35, 1983.

Boyer B, et al.: Polysplénie avec duplication de la veine cave inférieure. *J. Radiol.* 68:285, 1987.

Cumming WA, et al.: Campomelia, cervical lymphocele, polycystic dysplasia, short gut, polysplenia. *Am. J. Med. Genet.* 25:783, 1986.

Curran JG, et al.: Hodgkin's disease in a patient with polysplenia. *Br. J. Radiol.* 60:929, 1987.

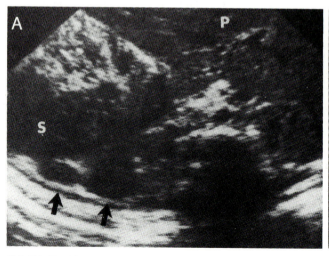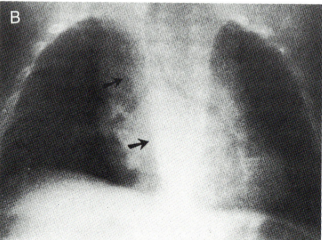

FIG SY–P–13.

Polysplenia syndrome. **A,** a transverse sonogram of the upper portion of the abdomen reveals a right-sided stomach *(S),* a preduodenal portal vein *(P),* and multiple spleens *(arrows).* **B,** a high-kilovoltage magnification chest radiograph shows bilateral hyparterial bronchi, a dilated azygos vein *(upper arrow),* and azygous continuation of the inferior vena cava *(lower arrow).* (From Abramson SJ, Berdon WE, Altman RP, et al.: Biliary atresia and noncardiac polysplenic syndrome: US and surgical considerations. *Radiology* 163:377, 1987. Used by permission.)

de la Monte SM, et al.: Sisters with polysplenia. *Am. J. Med. Genet.* 21:171, 1985.

Landing BH: Five syndromes (malformation complexes) of pulmonary symmetry, congenital heart disease, and multiple spleens. *Pediatr. Pathol.* 2:125, 1984.

Mathias RS, et al.: X-linked laterality sequence: Situs inversus, complex cardiac defects, splenic defects. *Am. J. Med. Genet.* 28:111, 1987.

Opitz JM: Editorial comment on the paper by de la Monte and Hutchins on familial polyasplenia. *Am. J. Med. Genet.* 21:175, 1985.

Paddock RJ, et al.: Polysplenia syndrome: Spectrum of gastrointestinal congenital anomalies. *J. Pediatr. Surg.* 17:563, 1982.

Peoples WM, et al.: Polysplenia: A review of 146 cases. *Pediatr. Cardiol.* 4:129, 1983.

Roguin N, et al.: Angiography of azygos continuation of inferior vena cava in situs ambiguus with left isomerism (polysplenia syndrome) *Pediatr. Radiol.* 14:109, 1984.

Shadle CA, et al.: Spontaneous splenic infarction in polysplenia syndrome. *J. Comput. Assist. Tomogr.* 6:177, 1982.

Shen-Schwarz S, et al.: Meckel syndrome with polysplenia: Case report and review of the literature. *Am. J. Med. Genet.* 31:349, 1988.

Sullivan RF, et al.: A case of biliary atresia and polysplenia. Evaluation by hepatobiliary scintigraphy. *Clin. Nucl. Med.* 12:55, 1987.

Tonkin ILD, et al.: Visceroatrial situs abnormalities: Sonographic and computed tomographic appearance. *A.J.R.* 138:509, 1982.

Vossen PG, et al.: Computed tomography of the polysplenia syndrome in the adult. *Gastrointest. Radiol.* 12:209, 1987.

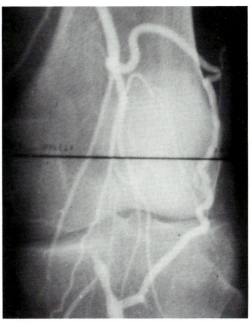

FIG SY–P–14.
Popliteal artery entrapment syndrome in a 39-year-old male with a clinical history of pain of several months duration in his left calf that was precipitated by walking. The left popliteal space shows medial displacement of the left popliteal artery. Note the large collateral artery. (From Turner GR, Gosney WG, Ellingson W, et al.: Popliteal artery entrapment syndrome. *J.A.M.A.* 208:692, 1969. Used by permission.)

POPLITEAL ARTERY ENTRAPMENT SYNDROME

Pathology: (a) occlusion of the popliteal artery often caused by an anomalous course of the artery in relation to the medial head of the gastrocnemius; (b) variants: mild deviation of the artery's course behind the tibial head with combined entrapment of the popliteal vein and artery, entrapment caused by fascial slips impinging on a normally located popliteal artery.

Clinical Manifestations: (a) *unilateral intermittent claudication (foot, calf muscles) usually in young male adults;* (b) *numbness, tingling, or coolness of the foot relieved by leg position changes;* (c) *ischemic symptoms after vigorous exercises;* (d) *absent or decreased ankle pulses, diminished resting ankle/brachial pressure index.*

Radiologic Manifestations: (a) *arteriographic demonstration of segmental occlusion and medial displacement of the popliteal artery,* stress runoff technique (active plantar flexing against a foot board) may be necessary to show the obstruction; (b) thrombotic occlusion of the calf arteries as a complication; (c) Doppler study (circulatory abnormalities) (Fig SY–P–14).

REFERENCES

Gaines VD, et al.: Popliteal entrapment syndrome. *Cardiovasc. Intervent. Radiol.* 8:156, 1985.

Goebel VN, et al.: CT-Aspekt der häufigsten Variante des Entrapmentsyndroms der Arteria poplitea. *Fortschr. Röntgenstr.* 142:698, 1985.

Greenwood LH, et al.: Popliteal artery entrapment: Importance of the stress runoff for diagnosis. *Cardiovasc. Intervent. Radiol.* 9:93, 1986.

Jeffery PC, et al.: Popliteal artery entrapment syndrome. A report of 2 cases. *S. Afr. Med. J.* 67:692, 1985.

Klooster NJJ, et al.: Popliteal artery entrapment syndrome. *Fortschr. Röntgenstr.* 148:624, 1988.

Metges PJ, et al.: L'artère poplitée piégée. *J. Radiol.* 62:331, 1981.

Stuart TPA: Note on a variation in the course of the popliteal artery. *J. Anat. Physiol.* 13:162, 1879.

Turner GR, et al.: Popliteal artery entrapment syndrome. *J.A.M.A.* 208:692, 1969.

PORENCEPHALY (FAMILIAL)

Synonym: Familial porencephaly.

Mode of Inheritance: Consistent with an autosomal dominant trait, with variable expression and reduced penetrance.

Clinical and Radiologic Manifestations: Presumed to be of prenatal origin: (a) hemiplegia; (b) seizures; (c) cerebral ventricular dilatation, most prominent in the frontal horn region; irregular outline of the lateral ventricular wall; porencephalia; (d) absence of a history of known etiology (infection, vascular disruption, trauma, severe maternal hypoxia, central nervous system hemorrhage).

REFERENCES

Berg RA, et al.: Familial porencephaly. *Arch. Neurol.* 40:567, 1983.
Haar L, et al.: Hereditary nonprogressive athetotic hemiplegia: A new syndrome. *Neurology* 27:849, 1977.
Zonana J, et al.: Familial porencephaly and congenital hemiplegia. *J. Pediatr.* 109:671, 1986.

POSTAXIAL ACROFACIAL DYSOSTOSIS SYNDROME

Synonym: Miller syndrome.

Frequency: 12 cases (Donnai et al., Meinecke et al., Fryns et al.).

Clinical and Radiologic Manifestations: (a) malar hypoplasia, lower lid ectropion, micrognathia, cleft palate, cleft

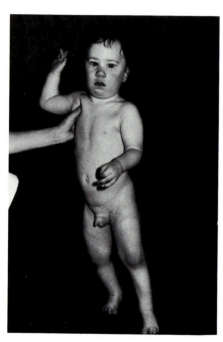

FIG SY–P–15.
Postaxial acrofacial dysostosis: Hypotelorism (interpupillary distance: 3rd percentile), upward slant of a short palpebral fissure, malar hypoplasia, marked retrognathia, and absence of the fifth rays. (From Meinecke P, Wiedemann H-R: Robin sequence and oligodactyly in mother and son—Probably a further example of postaxial acrofacial dysostosis syndrome. *Am. J. Med. Genet.* 27:953, 1987. Used by permission.)

lip, cup-shaped ears, hypotelorism, upward slant of short palpebral fissures; (b) absence of the fifth digit, aplasia or hypoplasia of the fifth ray of the hand (unilateral or bilateral), shortened forearm, ulnar hypoplasia, short radius, proximally inserted thumbs; (c) absent fifth toes, absent third and fourth toes in some (Fig SY–P–15).

REFERENCES

Donnai D, et al.: Postaxial acrofacial dysostosis (Miller) syndrome. *J. Med. Genet.* 24:422, 1987.
Fryns JP, et al.: Acrofacial dysostosis with postaxial limb deficiency. *Am. J. Med. Genet.* 29:205, 1988.
Meinecke P, et al.: Robin sequence and oligodactyly in mother and son—Probably a further example of the postaxial acrofacial dysostosis syndrome. *Am. J. Med. Genet.* 27:953, 1987.
Miller M, Fineman R, Smith DW: Postaxial acrofacial dysostosis syndrome. *J. Pediatr.* 95:970, 1979.

POSTCARDIOTOMY SYNDROME

Synonym: Postpericardiotomy syndrome.

Clinical Manifestations: Onset of symptoms weeks or months after a surgical procedure (closed or open heart surgery): (a) *chest pain*; (b) *fever*; (c) muscle and joint pain; (d) cough; (e) *pericardial friction rubs*; (f) dyspnea; (g) elevated leukocyte count and erythrocyte sedimentation rate; (h) relief of symptoms with salicylates or corticosteroids; (i) high titer of heart reactive antibody; (j) postpericardiotomy syndrome as a cause of intracardiac pericardial baffle obstruction.

Radiologic Manifestations: (a) *pericardial effusion* (serous or serosanguineous); (b) pleural effusion; (c) basilar pulmonary infiltrates; (d) absence of frank congestive heart failure; (e) cardiac tamponade (rare).

REFERENCES

Engle MA, et al.: The postpericardiotomy syndrome and antiheart antibodies. *Circulation* 49:401, 1974.
Kaminsky ME, et al.: Postpericardiotomy syndrome. *A.J.R.* 138:503, 1982.
Kaye D, et al.: Probable postcardiotomy syndrome following implantation of a transvenous pacemaker: Report of the first case. *Am. Heart J.* 90:627, 1975.
King TE, et al.: Cardiac tamponade complicating the postpericardiotomy syndrome. *Chest* 83:500, 1983.
Kron IL, et al.: Late cardiac tamponade in children. A lethal complication. *Ann. Surg.* 199:173, 1984.
Luken JA, et al.: Post-pericardiotomy syndrome as a cause of intracardiac pericardial baffle obstruction. *Pediatr. Cardiol.* 7:58, 1986.
Soloff LA, et al.: Reactivation of rheumatic fever following mitral commissurotomy. *Circulation* 8:481, 1953.
Stelzner TJ, et al.: The pleuropulmonary manifestations of the postcardiac injury syndrome. *Chest* 84:383, 1983.

POSTCHOLECYSTECTOMY SYNDROME

Clinical Manifestations: *Recurrence of symptoms* present prior to cholecystectomy (abdominal pain, nausea, vomiting, etc.).

Radiologic Manifestations: (a) *detection of abnormalities undiagnosed prior to cholecystectomy* (by ultrasonography, scintigraphy, fine-needle cholangiography, and endoscopic retrograde cholepancreatography techniques): retained stones, ampulary stenosis (stenosis of the sphincter of Oddi, papilla of Vater stenosis, or papillary stenosis), juxtapapillary diverticula, benign stricture, cancer of the bile duct, pancreatic disease, dysfunction of the sphincter; (b) *diagnosis of conditions not related to the biliary system undetected prior to surgery.*

REFERENCES

Ayre-Smith G: Fine needle cholangiography in postcholecystectomy patients. *A.J.R.* 130:697, 1978.
Dreiling DA: The postcholecystectomy syndrome. *Am. J. Dig. Dis.* 7:603, 1962.
Gregg JA, et al.: Postcholecystectomy syndrome and its association with ampullary stenosis. *Am. J. Surg.* 139:374, 1980.
Tulassay Z, et al.: Endoscopy in postcholecystectomy syndrome. *Lancet* 2:800, 1980.
Zeman RK, et al.: Postcholecystectomy syndrome: Evaluation using biliary scintigraphy and endoscopic retrograde cholangiopancreatography. *Radiology* 156:787, 1985.

POSTCOARCTECTOMY SYNDROME

Synonym: Syndrome of "mesenteric arteritis."

Etiology: Related to postoperative paradoxical hypertension; the precise physiological reason not fully known.

Pathology: (a) hemorrhagic areas in the bowel wall; (b) arterial and venous thrombosis; (c) necrosis and ulceration of the bowel, perforation; (d) inflammatory cellular infiltrate of the bowel wall.

Clinical Manifestations: Onset of symptoms usually after the second postoperative day: (a) abdominal pain, tenderness, distension, ileus, vomiting, melena; (b) fever; (c) hypertension; (d) leukocytosis.

Radiologic Manifestations: (a) adynamic ileus with dilated bowel loops seen on plain film; (b) contrast study demonstrating *edema of the bowel with thickening of mucosal folds*; (c) stenosis of the bowel at the site of scarring as a late sequela; (d) vasoconstriction: beading, segmental constriction, dilatation, and stretching; delayed distal progression of the contrast medium (Fig SY–P–16).

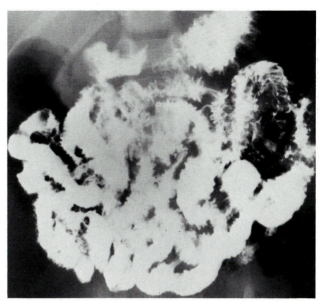

FIG SY–P–16.
Postcoarctectomy syndrome in a 4-year-old male who developed vomiting, abdominal pain distention, and a rise in blood pressure on the second day following resection of coarctation of the aorta. A contrast study of the bowel 5 days following a surgical procedure shows thickening of the mucosal folds. (Courtesy of Dr. Robert S. Arkoff, San Francisco.)

REFERENCES

Depoix-Joseph J-P, et al.: Les complications digestives de la cure chirurgicale de la coarctation de l'aorte. *Arch. Fr. Pediatr.* 36:347, 1979.
Ho ECK, et al.: The syndrome of "mesenteric arteritis" following surgical repair of aortic coarctation: Report of nine cases and review of the literature. *Pediatrics* 49:40, 1972.
Kawauchi M, et al.: Angiographic demonstration of mesenteric arterial changes in postcoarctectomy syndrome. *Surgery* 98:602, 1985.
Mays ET, et al.: Postcoarctectomy syndrome. *Arch. Surg.* 91:58, 1965.
Pomar JL, et al.: Mesenteric arteritis complicating surgical repair of coarctation of the aorta. Angiographic findings and management. *Chest* 82:509, 1982.
Sealy WC: Indications for surgical treatment of coarctation of the aorta. *Surg. Gynecol. Obstet.* 97:301, 1953.

POSTGASTRECTOMY "SYNDROMES"

1. Dumping syndrome.
2. Malabsorption syndrome.
3. Alkaline gastritis (reflux gastritis).
4. Anemia.
5. Bone disease (osteomalacia, osteoporosis).
6. Afferent loop syndrome.
7. Postvagotomy-functional syndrome.
8. Neurological complications (hypoglycemia, vitamin B_{12} deficiency).

9. Cancer of the gastric remnant.
10. Bezoar.
11. Jejunogastric intussusception.
12. Weight loss.

REFERENCES

Meshkinpour H, et al.: Reflux gastritis syndrome. *Dig. Dis.* 5:146, 1987.
Cooperman AM: Postgastrectomy syndromes. *Surg. Annu.* 13:139, 1981.

POSTMYOCARDIAL INFARCTION SYNDROME

Synonym: Dressler syndrome.

Clinical Manifestations: Onset usually after a *latency period* of 1 to several weeks following myocardial infarction: (a) *chest pain;* (b) *fever;* (c) *polyserositis* (pericardium, pleura); (d) increased erythrocyte sedimentation rate; (e) leukocytosis; (f) tendency to recurrence; (g) heart-specific antibodies; (h) ST-segment changes diagnostic of pericarditis (rare).

Radiologic Manifestations: (a) *enlargement of the cardiopericardial shadow;* (b) *pleural effusion* (in some); (c) *pulmonary infiltrates* (in some); (d) widening of the upper portion of the mediastinum (one third of cases); (e) echocardiogram of pericardial effusion.

REFERENCES

Dressler W: A post-myocardial infarction syndrome. *J.A.M.A.* 160:379, 1956.
Krainin FM, et al.: Infarction-associated pericarditis. Rarity of diagnostic electrocardiogram. *N. Engl. J. Med.* 311:1211, 1984.
Levin EJ, et al.: Dressler syndrome (postmyocardial infarction syndrome). *Radiology* 87:731, 1966.
Lichstein E, et al.: Current incidence of postmyocardial infarction (Dressler's) syndrome. *Am. J. Cardiol.* 50:1269, 1982.
Williams RKT, et al.: Postcoronary pain and the postmyocardial infarction syndrome. *Br. Heart J.* 51:327, 1984.

POTTER SEQUENCE

Synonyms: Potter syndrome; oligohydramnios tetrad (facial features, limb malformations, pulmonary hypoplasia, and classically, renal agenesis); Potter facies; renofacial dysplasia; renal nonfunction syndrome; renal nonfunction sequence.

Mode of Inheritance: Risk of recurrence of about 6%; autosomal recessive, autosomal dominant (unilateral renal anomaly in a parent), and X-linked recessive patterns of inheritance have been suggested.

Frequency: About 0.25% of live-born babies (Helin et al.).

Pathology: (a) renal agenesis, hypoplasia or cystic dysplastic kidneys, obstructive uropathy, etc; (b) bilateral pulmonary hypoplasia; (c) brain dysgenesis: small brain, defects in neural migration, cerebellar heterotopia, abnormal hippocampi, abnormal lamination of the cerebral cortex.

Clinical Manifestations: (a) Potter facies: flattened facies, widely spaced eyes, low-set large and floppy ears, micrognathia, a prominent fold that arises at the inner canthus and extends downward and laterally below the eyes; (b) excessively lax skin in some; (c) limb-positioning defects (rocker-bottom feet, etc.); (d) fetal growth deficiency; (e) other reported abnormalities: spadelike hand, hyperextensible knee joints, absent abdominal musculature, imperforate anus, chromosomal abnormalities (trisomy 7, balanced translocation, deletion of chromosome 15, ring chromosome 4 mosaicism, etc.), Holzgreve-Wagner-Rehder syndrome (Potter sequence with persistent buccopharyngeal membrane type II, postaxial polydactyly, cleft palate, cardiac anomalies, intesti-

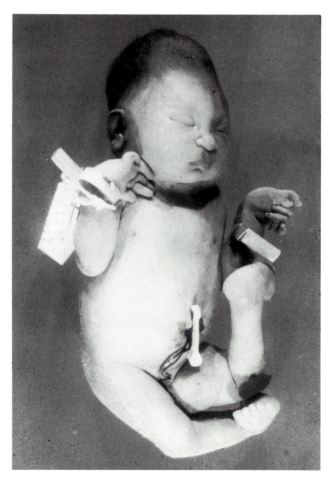

FIG SY—P—17.
Infant with the Potter sequence and chromosome abnormality 46,XX6q+. Note the joint contractures and abnormal thumbs. (From Curry CJR, Jensen K, Holland J, et al.: The Potter sequence: A clinical analysis of 80 cases. *Am. J. Med. Genet.* 19:679, 1984. Used by permission.)

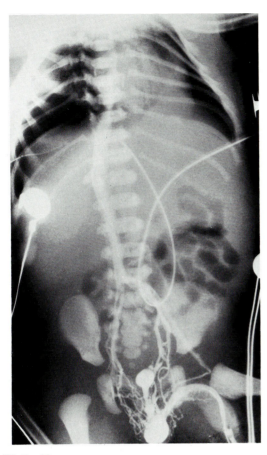

FIG SY–P–18.
Potter sequence in a newborn in whom respiratory distress and pneumothorax developed after birth. A cystourethrogram shows opacification of the very small bladder and extensive venous opacification with drainage into the inferior vena cava. Note also the right pneumothorax and bell-shaped thorax with slanting ribs. Autopsy revealed an absence of kidneys and ureters. (Courtesy of Dr. Peter E. Kane, Department of Radiology, Children's Hospital Medical Center, Oakland, Calif.)

nal nonfixation, intrauterine growth retardation), etc.; (f) stillborn or death soon after birth.

Radiologic Manifestations: (a) prenatal diagnosis (ultrasonography): severe oligohydramnios, renal agenesis or dysplasia, limb deformities, fetal growth retardation; (b) *pneumothorax, pneumomediastinum, decreased thoracic volume, bell-shaped thorax, poorly expanded and "structureless" lung (pulmonary hypoplasia)*; (c) ultrasonogram: absent kidneys, cystic kidneys, large adrenal glands mimicking the presence of kidneys; (d) *cystogram: small bladder, reflux of contrast material into unused ureters, extension of contrast material into the prostatic bed, intravasation of contrast material into the pelvic vein and drainage into the inferior vena cava;* (e) clubfoot.

Notes: (a) ultrasonographic screening for parents and siblings of infants born with agenesis or dysgenesis of both kidneys or with agenesis of one kidney and dysgenesis of the other kidney has been recommended (Roodhooft et al.); (b) prenatal ultrasonographic screening of subsequent pregnancy strongly recommended; (c) a combination of pneumomediastinum/pneumothorax and a bell-shaped chest contour should suggest the possibility of renal dysgenesis in the infants with an incomplete clinical picture of Potter syndrome (Figs SY–P–17 and SY–P–18).

REFERENCES

Clark RD: del(15)(q22q24) syndrome with Potter sequence (letter). *Am. J. Med. Genet.* 19:703, 1984.

Côté GB: Potter's syndrome and chromosomal anomalies. *Hum. Genet.* 58:220, 1981.

Curry CJR, et al.: The Potter sequence: A clinical analysis of 80 cases. *Am. J. Med. Genet.* 19:679, 1984.

Fryns JP, et al.: Ring chromosome 4 mosaicism and Potter sequence. *Ann. Genet. (Paris)* 31:120, 1988.

Grunnet ML, et al.: Brain abnormalities in infants with Potter syndrome (oligohydramnios tetrad). *Neurology* 31:1571, 1981.

Helin I, et al.: Prenatal diagnosis of Potter's syndrome by ultrasound. *Acta Paediatr. Scand.* 72:939, 1983.

Holzgreve W, et al.: Bilateral renal agenesis with Potter phenotype, cleft palate, anomalies of the cardiovascular system, skeletal anomalies including hexadactyly and bifid metacarpal. A new syndrome? *Am. J. Med. Genet.* 18:177, 1984.

Legius E, et al.: Holzgreve-Wagner-Rehder syndrome: Potter sequence associated with persistent buccopharyngeal membrane. A second observation. *Am. J. Med. Genet.* 31:269, 1988.

Leonidas JC, et al.: Radiographic chest contour and pulmonary air leaks in oligohydramnios-related pulmonary hypoplasia (Potter's syndrome). *Invest. Radiol.* 17:6, 1982.

Pflueger SMV, et al.: Trisomy 7 and Potter syndrome. *Clin. Genet.* 25:543, 1984.

Potter EL: Facial characteristics of infants with bilateral renal agenesis. *Am. J. Obstet. Gynecol.* 51:885, 1946.

Roodhooft AM, et al.: Familial nature of congenital absence and severe dysgenesis of both kidneys. *N. Engl. J. Med.* 310:1341, 1984.

Schmidt W, et al.: Genetics, pathoanatomy and prenatal diagnosis of Potter I syndrome and other urogenital tract diseases. *Clin. Genet.* 22:105, 1982.

Wolf EL, et al.: Diagnosis of oligohydramnios-related pulmonary hypoplasia (Potter syndrome): Value of portable voiding cystourethrography in newborns with respiratory distress. *Radiology* 125:769, 1977.

PRADER-WILLI SYNDROME

Synonyms: Prader-Labhart-Willi syndrome; H₃O syndrome.

Mode of Inheritance: Very low recurrence risk in siblings.

Frequency: About 1:10,000 births; over 500 published cases (Butler et al., 1986).

Clinical Manifestations: (a) short stature; (b) *obesity;* (c) *neonatal hypotonia;* (d) strabismus, misrouting of retinal-ganglion fibers at the optic chiasm in association with abnormal evoked potentials indistinguishable from those recorded in human albinos; (e) narrow anterior bifrontal diameter; (f) *hypogonadism* (small penis, undescended testes, low plasma gonadotropin levels); sexual maturation normal, retarded, or advanced; (g) *small hands and feet;* (h) *mental retardation;* (i) *diabetes mellitus or abnormal glucose tolerance test results;* (j) obesity-hypoventilation syndrome, disturbances of sleep-wakefulness patterns, excessive daytime sleepiness, etc.; (k) chromosomal aberrations: chromosome 15 abnormalities in about half of the patients with the syndrome (interstitial deletion of the proximal long arm of chromosome 15, duplication in the proximal half of 15q, terminal deletion of the distal part of Xq.

Radiologic Manifestations: No characteristic findings, reported abnormalities: (a) *acromicria;* (b) retarded skeletal maturation; (c) skull changes such as microcrania, increased sutural serration, wormian bones, short mandible with increased mandibular angle, small sella turcica area in the lateral projection, absent frontal sinuses, slight ventricular dilatation; (d) dental caries; (e) scoliosis; (f) coxa valga; (g) asymmetry of the length of the limbs; (h) varying degrees of syndactyly, misplaced thumb; (i) hip dislocation; (j) osteoporosis; (k) distinguishable metacarpophalangeal pattern profile in those with interstitial deletion of the long arm of chromosome 15 and those without this chromosomal abnormality; (1) other reported abnormalities: premature coronary artery atherosclerosis, hypopigmentation (cutaneous and ocular), abnormal dermatoglyphic features (displacement of the axial triradius away from the normal proximal position, an excess of whorls primarily on the thumbs, radial termination of the palmar A mainline, and a lack of arches on the big toe), leukemia.

Note: The patients with chromosome deletion have been reported to have lighter hair, eye, and skin color, greater sum sensitivity, and higher intelligence scores than do the patients with normal chromosomes.

REFERENCES

Bray GA, et al.: The Prader-Willi syndrome: A study of 40 patients and a review of the literature. *Medicine (Baltimore)* 62:59, 1983.

Butler MG, et al.: Clinical and cytogenetic survey of 39 individuals with Prader-Labhart-Willi syndrome. *Am. J. Med. Genet.* 23:793, 1986.

Butler MG, et al.: Metacarpophalangeal pattern profile analysis in Prader-Willi syndrome. A follow-up report on 38 cases. *Clin. Genet.* 28:27, 1985.

Cassidy SB: Prader-Willi syndrome. *Curr. Probl. Pediatr.* 14:5, 1984.

Creel DJ, et al.: Abnormalities of the central visual pathways in Prader-Willi syndrome associated with hypopigmentation. *N. Engl. J. Med.* 314:1606, 1986.

deFrance HF, et al.: Duplication in chromosome 15q in a boy with the Prader-Willi syndrome; further cytogenetic confusion. *Clin. Genet.* 26:379, 1984.

Hall BD: Leukaemia and the Prader-Willi syndrome. *Lancet* 1:46, 1986.

Ishikawa T, et al.: Prader-Willi syndrome in two siblings: One with normal karyotype, one with a terminal deletion of distal Xq. *Clin. Genet.* 32:295, 1987.

Lamb AS, et al.: Premature coronary artery atherosclerosis in a patient with Prader-Willi syndrome. *Am. J. Med. Genet.* 28:873, 1987.

Laurance BM, et al.: Prader-Willi syndrome after age 15 years. *Arch. Dis. Child.* 56:181, 1981.

Ledbetter DH, et al.: Chromosome 15 abnormalities and the Prader-Willi syndrome: A follow-up report of 40 cases. *Am. J. Hum. Genet.* 34:278, 1982.

Pearson KD, et al.: Roentgenographic manifestations of the Prader-Willi syndrome. *Radiology* 100:369, 1971.

Prader A, Labhart A, and Willi H: Ein Syndrom von Adipositas, Kleinwuchs, Kryptorchismus und Oligophrenie nach myatonieartigem Zustand im Neugeborenenalter. *Schweiz. Med. Wochenschr.* 86:1260, 1956.

Reed T, et al.: Dermatoglyphic features in Prader-Willi syndrome with respect to chromosomal findings. *Clin. Genet.* 25:341, 1984.

Uehling D: Cryptorchidism in the Prader-Willi syndrome. *J. Urol.* 124:103, 1980.

Vela-Bueno A, et al.: Sleep in the Prader-Willi syndrome. Clinical and polygraphic findings. *Arch. Neurol.* 41:294, 1984.

Wiesner GL, et al.: Hypopigmentation in the Prader-Willi syndrome. *Am. J. Hum. Genet.* 40:431, 1987.

PROGERIA

Synonym: Hutchinson-Gilford syndrome.

Mode of Inheritance: Rare familial cases in siblings and monozygotic twins; autosomal recessive in some cases.

Frequency: 1:8 million births (Gamble).

Clinical Manifestations: Onset of symptoms in the second year of life: (a) *typical facies* (old man appearance in childhood), frontal and parietal bossing, poor midface development, hypoplastic mandible, thin and beaked nose, delayed dentition, crowded teeth; (b) *dwarfism;* (c) *"horse-riding" stance;* (d) *alopecia;* (e) brown pigmented areas on the trunk, *skin atrophy,* hypoplasia of the nails, prominent subcutaneous veins; (f) joint deformity, muscular atrophy, pointed end of short distal phalanges; (g) high and squeaky voice; (h) atheromatosis, systemic hypertension, myocardial infarction, congestive heart failure, premature death (in the early teens); (i) insulin resistance, increased secretion of fibronectin and collagen; (j) scleroderma.

Radiologic Manifestations: (a) *hypoplastic facial bones, in particular the mandible; bitemporal bossing; thin cranial vault;* sutural bones; strips of unossified membrane of the cranial vault; delay in closure of cranial sutures and fontanelles;

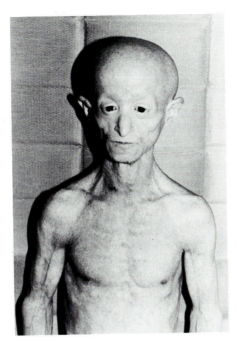

FIG SY–P–19.
Progeria syndrome (Hutchinson-Gilford) in a 45-year-old man. Note the alopecia, craniofacial disproportion, prominent eyes, sculptured nose, and micrognathia. (From Ogihara T, Hata T, Tanaka K, et al.: Hutchinson-Gilford progeria syndrome in a 45-year-old man. *Am. J. Med.* 81:135, 1986. Used by permission.)

(b) *slender long bones, coxa valga;* (c) *pointed distal phalanges, progressive acro-osteolysis of the terminal phalanges;* (d) *short and thin clavicles, progressive thinning and resorption of the distal portions of the clavicles and ribs, thin ribs;* (e) *pathological fractures;* (f) *bone age usually normal;* (g) *osteoporosis;* (h) *infantile vertebrae;* (i) *delayed eruption of*

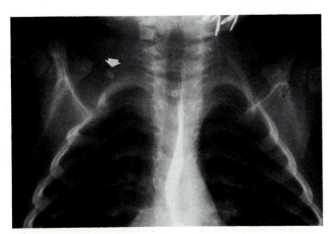

FIG SY–P–20.
Progeria: partial resorption of the first four ribs on each side. The left clavicle has been completely resorbed, and only a small remnant of the right clavicle persists *(arrow).* (From Ozonoff MB, Clemett AR: Progressive osteolysis in progeria. *A.J.R.* 100:75, 1967. Used by permission.)

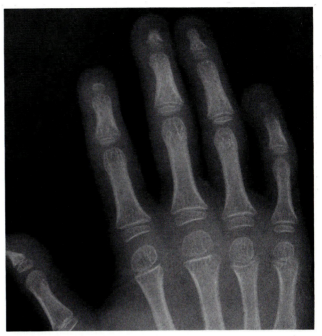

FIG SY–P–21.
Progeria: resorption of the ungual tuft with preservation of soft tissues. (From Margolin FR, Steinbach HL: Progeria: Hutchinson-Gilford syndrome. *A.J.R.* 103:173, 1968. Used by permission.)

teeth, overcrowded teeth; (j) other reported abnormalities: carotid artery aneurysm, progressive hip dislocation, etc.

Differential Diagnosis: Acrogeria; Werner syndrome; Cockayne syndrome (Figs SY–P–19 to SY–P–21).

REFERENCES

Darlington GJ, et al.: Sister chromatid exchange frequencies in progeria and Werner syndrome patients. *Am. J. Hum. Genet.* 33:762, 1981.

de Martinville B, et al.: Progeria de Gilford-Hutchinson à début néonatal chez des jumeaux monozygotes. *Arch. Fr. Pediatr.* 37:679, 1980.

Dyck JD, et al.: Management of coronary artery disease in Hutchinson-Gilford syndrome. *J. Pediatr.* 111:407, 1987.

Franklyn PP: Progeria in siblings. *Clin. Radiol.* 27:327, 1976.

Gabr M, et al.: Progeria: A pathologic study. *J. Pediatr.* 57:70, 1960.

Gamble JG: Hip disease in Hutchinson-Gilford progeria syndrome. *J. Pediatr. Orthop.* 4:585, 1984.

Gilford H: Progeria: A form of senilism. *Practitioner* 73:188, 1904.

Green LN: Progeria with carotid artery aneurysms: Report of a case. *Arch. Neurol.* 38:659, 1981.

Hutchinson J: Case of congenital absence of hair with atrophic condition of the skin and its appendages. *Lancet* 1:923, 1886.

Maciel AT: Evidence for autosomal recessive inheritance of progeria (Hutchinson-Gilford). *Am. J. Med. Genet.* 31:483, 1988.

Macleod W: Progeria. *Br. J. Radiol.* 39:224, 1966.

Maquart FX, et al.: Increased secretion of fibronectin and collagen by progeria (Hutchinson-Gilford) fibroblasts. *Eur. J. Pediatr.* 147:442, 1988.

Margolin FR, Steinbach HL: Progeria: Hutchinson-Gilford syndrome. *A.J.R.* 103:173, 1968.

Moen C: Orthopaedic aspects of progeria. *J. Bone Joint Surg. [Am.]* 64:542, 1982.

Ogihara T, et al.: Hutchinson-Gilford progeria syndrome in a 45-year-old man. *Am. J. Med.* 81:135, 1986.

Ozonoff MB, Clemett AR: Progressive osteolysis in progeria. *A.J.R.* 100:75, 1967.

Rosenbloom AL, et al.: Progeria: Insulin resistance and hyperglycemia. *J. Pediatr.* 102:400, 1983.

PROGRESSIVE FAMILIAL ENCEPHALOPATHY–BASAL GANGLIA CALCIFICATION

Clinical and Radiologic Manifestations: (a) encephalopathy in infancy; (b) microcephaly; (c) chronic cerebrospinal fluid pleocytosis; (d) basal ganglia calcification.

REFERENCES

Aicardi J, et al.: A progressive familial encephalopathy in infancy with calcifications of the basal ganglia and chronic cerebrospinal fluid lymphocytosis. *Ann. Neurol.* 15:49, 1984.

Mehta L, et al.: Familial calcification of the basal ganglia with cerebrospinal fluid pleocytosis. *J. Med. Genet.* 23:157, 1986.

PROSTAGLANDIN-INDUCED PERIOSTITIS

Etiology: Long-term (several weeks to several months) prostaglandin (E_1 and E_2) infusion.

Clinical Manifestations: (a) *swelling and tenderness of the limb(s)*; (b) other reported abnormalities: widening of cranial sutures, digital swelling.

Radiologic Manifestations: *Laminar symmetrical subperiosteal bone formation, particularly in the diaphyseal areas of the long bones,* also noted in the rib and scapulum; remodeling in the follow-up.

Differential Diagnosis: Caffey disease; vitamin and mineral deficiencies; leukemia; metastatic disease; physiological subperiosteal bone formation of infancy; etc.

Notes: (a) other complications of prostaglandin E infusions are hyperthermia, hypotension, skin flushing, edema, diarrhea, apnea, bradycardia, slight elevation of the alkaline phosphatase concentration; (b) the bone manifestations are probably dose related.

REFERENCES

Høst A, et al.: Reversibility of cortical hyperostosis following long-term prostaglandin E_1 therapy in infants with ductus-dependent congenital heart disease. *Pediatr. Radiol.* 18:149, 1988.

Ringel RE, et al.: Prostaglandin-induced periostitis: A complication of long-term PGE_1 infusion in an infant with congenital heart disease. *Radiology* 42:657, 1982.

Sharp C, et al.: Digital swelling following long-term administration of prostaglandin E_1 in an infant. *Clin. Pediatr. (Phila)* 26:302, 1987.

Ueda K, et al.: Cortical hyperostosis following long-term administration of prostaglandin E_1 in infants with cyanotic congenital heart disease. *J. Pediatr.* 97:834, 1980.

PROTEUS SYNDROME

Pathology: A congenital hamartomatous disorder with neurocutaneous manifestations (tissues of mesodermal and

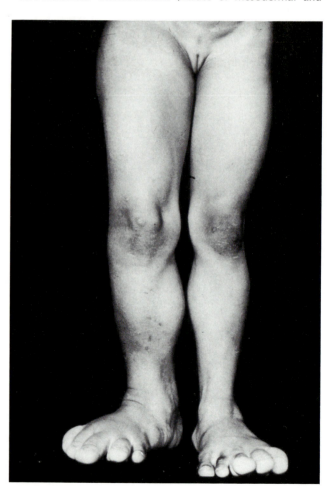

FIG SY–P–22.
Proteus syndrome. A hyperpigmented right leg, a right leg larger than the left, and bilateral macrodactyly are present. (From Clark RD, Donnai D, Rogers J, et al.: Proteus syndrome: An expanded phenotype. *Am. J. Med. Genet.* 27:99, 1987. Used by permission.)

ectodermal origin): (a) thickening of the palms and soles, hyperkeratosis and increased collagen, fine cytoplasmic projections of basal cells into the dermoepidermal junction; (b) "tumors": lipomas (subcutaneous, abdominal), hemangiomas, lymphangiomas, hamartomas.

Frequency: More than 50 published cases (Viljoen et al., 1988).

Clinical Manifestations: (a) craniofacial: *macrocephaly*, broad depressed nasal bridge and/or beaked nose, asymmetry, frontal bossing, skull protuberances (frontotemporal, parieto-occipital, external auditory canals, the alveolar ridges,

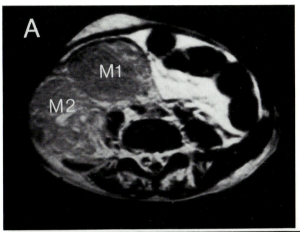

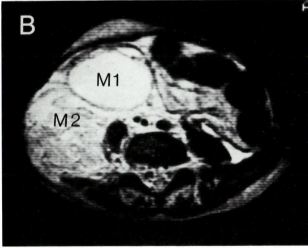

FIG SY−P−23.
Proteus syndrome. **A,** magnetic resonance imaging (TR/TE 2000/27). A T_2 image of the lower portion of the abdomen shows low-intensity signals from masses M1 and M2. **B,** greater T_2 weighting (TR/TE 2000/70) shows the signal intensity increased in M1, which suggests a predominantly fluid nature. M2 gave a lower signal because it contains more solid material. Biopsy confirmed this to be lymphangiomatous and fibrofatty tissue. (From Cremin BJ, Viljoen DL, Wynchank S, et al.: The Proteus syndrome: The magnetic resonance and radiological features. *Pediatr. Radiol.* 17:486, 1987. Used by permission.)

etc.); (b) *partial gigantism* of the hands and/or feet, usually asymmetrical involvement, hemihypertrophy; (c) *skin lesions: epidermal nevi, hyperkeratosis, thickening of the skin and subcutaneous tissue of the palms and soles (gyriform), nodular hypertrophy (subcutaneous masses), lipomas, vascular anomalies, depigmentation, pigmented lesions;* (d) *limb asymmetry (segmental, total);* (e) eye abnormalities: strabismus, epibulbar tumor, enlarged eye, myopia, anisocoria, heterochromia irides, unilateral microphthalmos, cataract, retinal detachment, chorioretinitis, nystagmus, ptosis; (f) other reported abnormalities: height increase, shortness, seizure disorder, mental retardation, muscle atrophy, scoliosis, kyphosis, pectus excavatum, elbow ankylosis, angulation defects of the knees, elongation of the neck and trunk, increased abdominal girth (subcutaneous fat), dilated subcutaneous veins, malformed ears, highly arched palate, peg-shaped teeth, macro-orchidism, penile hypertrophy.

Radiologic Manifestations: (a) *macrocrania, exostoses, cranial hyperostosis,* wide subdural space, dilated ventricles, cerebral atrophy; (b) *limbs: overgrowth of adipose tissues and bones, in particular the hands and feet; macrodactyly;* etc.; (c) very high or wide irregularly shaped vertebrae, intervertebral disk dystrophy, megaspondylodysplasia, long neck and/or trunk, kyphoscoliosis; (d) abnormal ribs and scapulae (hypertrophy, etc.); (e) intra-abdominal masses (lipoma, lymphangioma).

Differential Diagnosis: Klippel-Trenaunay-Weber syndrome; neurofibromatosis; Riley-Smith syndrome; Maffucci syndrome; Bannayan syndrome; Zonana syndrome (macrocephaly with multiple lipomas and hemangiomas); encephalocraniocutaneous lipomatosis.

Note: The syndrome is named after the Greek god Proteus ("the polymorphous"), who could change his shape at will (Figs SY−P−22 and SY−P−23).

REFERENCES

Azouz EM, et al.: Radiologic findings in the Proteus syndrome. *Pediatr. Radiol.* 17:481, 1987.

Burgio GR, et al.: Further and new details on the Proteus syndrome. *Eur. J. Pediatr.* 143:71, 1984.

Clark RD, et al.: Proteus syndrome: An expanded phenotype. *Am. J. Med. Genet.* 27:99, 1987.

Costa T, et al.: Proteus syndrome: Report of two cases with pelvic lipomatosis. *Pediatrics* 76:984, 1985.

Cremin BJ, et al.: The Proteus syndrome: The magnetic resonance and radiological features. *Pediatr. Radiol.* 17:486, 1987.

Gorlin RJ: Proteus syndrome. *J. Clin. Dysmorphol.* 2:8, 1984.

Mücke J, et al.: Variability in the Proteus syndrome: Report of an affected child with progressive lipomatosis. *Eur. J. Pediatr.* 143:320, 1985.

Viljoen DL, et al.: Cutaneous manifestations of the Proteus syndrome. *Pediatr. Dermatol.* 5:14, 1988.

Viljoen DL, et al.: Proteus syndrome in Southern Africa: Natural history and clinical manifestations in six individuals. *Am. J. Med. Genet.* 27:87, 1987.

Viljoen DL, et al.: Proteus syndrome in South Africa: Natural history and clinical manifestations in 10 individuals. Presented at the Birth Defect Meeting, Baltimore, 1988.

Wiedemann H-R: Encephalocraniocutaneous lipomatosis and Proteus syndrome (letter). *Am. J. Med. Genet.* 25:403, 1986.

Wiedemann H-R, et al.: The proteus syndrome. Partial gigantism of the hands and/or feet, nevi, hemihypertrophy, subcutaneous tumors, macrocephaly or other skull anomalies and possible accelerated growth and visceral affections. *Eur. J. Pediatr.* 140:5, 1983.

PRUNE-BELLY SYNDROME

Synonyms: Eagle-Barrett syndrome; prune-belly sequence.

Mode of Inheritance: Most reported cases in males (95%); rare occurrence in siblings.

Frequency: Approximately 450 cases reported in the world literature (Greskovich et al.); about 1:40,000 live births.

Pathology (not included under clinical or radiological manifestations): (a) alimentary system (30% of cases): malrotation (most common anomaly), mesenteric anomalies, obstruction (atresia, stenosis), volvulus, imperforate anus, intussusception, cloaca, Meckel diverticulum, duplication, biliary malformation, gastroschisis; (b) respiratory system: lung hypoplasia, cystic adematoid malformation of the lung; (c) malformations of a bulbous or pendulous urethra and/or corporeal bodies of the penis: dilatation of the bulbous urethra, fusiform megalourethra, dorsal chordee, penile torsion; (d) other reported abnormalities: absent limb, giant fetal abdominal cyst, anencephaly, retroperitoneal germ cell tumor, cystic dysplasia of the adrenal glands, etc.

Clinical Manifestations: (a) *partial or complete absence of abdominal musculature;* (b) *dysplasia of the urinary tract;* (c) skeletal abnormalities: talipes equinovarus (in about 40% of the patients), limb deformities, etc.; (d) association with other syndromes: Potter, Turner, EEC, Beckwith-Wiedemann, chromosome anomalies (Down, trisomy 18, etc.), Hirschsprung; (e) genital anomalies: *undescended testes,* aplasia of the external genitalia, megalourethra; (f) congenital heart disease; (g) other reported abnormalities: pectus carinatum, microcephaly, splenic torsion, pulmonary artery stenosis associated with mental retardation and hearing defects.

Radiologic Manifestations: (a) *flabby abdomen;* (b) gaseous distension of the bowel; (c) flared iliac wings, wide interpubic distance; (d) dysplastic kidneys, pyelocaliectasis, dilated and tortuous ureters, large bladder with an irregular contour, patent urachus, tapering of the base of the bladder extending to the posterior urethra, prostatic maldevelopment,

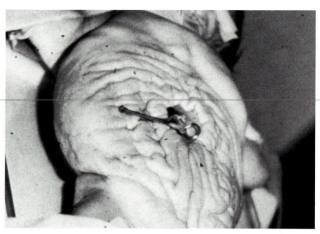

FIG SY–P–24.
Prune-belly syndrome and an open urachus in a neonate.

megalourethra, dilated utricle, bladder wall calcification, renal calcification, urethral stenosis, urethral valve; (e) pulmonary hypoplasia, lobar atelectasis, pneumonias; (f) musculoskeletal abnormalities: meningomyelocele, scoliosis, torticollis, pectus carinatum, pectus excavatum, arthrogryposis, clubfoot, valgus foot, lower limb hemimelia, toe syndactyly, hip dysplasia, metatarsus varus, polydactyly, flaring of costal margins; (g) intrauterine ultrasonography: laxity of the abdominal wall, urinary system anomalies, ascites (may be transient), fetal hydrops, limb anomalies, oligohydramnios or polyhydramnios.

Notes: (a) affected females usually have milder urologic abnormalities; (b) the pathogenesis of prune-belly syndrome is controversial: stretching of the abdominal wall due to a dilated urinary system, in particular, megalocystis as the etiologic factor rather than a primary abdominal wall muscular anomaly; prostatic hypoplasia associated with a functional urethral obstruction; etc.

Differential Diagnosis: Posterior urethral valve (Figs SY–P–24 and SY–P–25).

REFERENCES

Aaronson IA: Posterior urethral valve masquerading as the prune belly syndrome. *Br. J. Urol.* 55:508, 1983.

Adeyokunnu AA, et al.: Prune belly syndrome in two siblings and a first cousin. *Am. J. Dis. Child.* 136:23, 1982.

Alford BA, et al.: Pulmonary complications associated with the prune-belly syndrome. *Radiology* 129:401, 1978.

Aliabadi H, et al.: Splenic torsion and the prune belly syndrome. *Pediatr. Surg. Int.* 2:369, 1987.

Amacker EA, et al.: An association of prune belly anomaly with trisomy 21. *Am. J. Med. Genet.* 23:919, 1986.

Beckmann H, et al.: Prune belly sequence associated with trisomy 13 (letter). *Am. J. Med. Genet.* 19:603, 1984.

Berdon WE, et al.: The radiologic and pathologic spectrum of the prune belly syndrome. *Radiol. Clin. North Am.* 15:83, 1977.

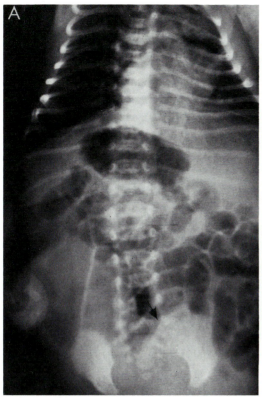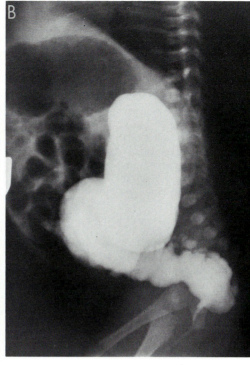

FIG SY–P–25.
Prune-belly syndrome in a 3-day-old male with a deficiency of abdominal musculature and bilateral cryptorchidism. **A,** pneumomediastinum, flabby abdomen with bulging flanks, bowel distension, calcification of the lower portion of the abdomen in the wall of the urachus *(arrow),* and flared iliac wings. **B,** voiding cystourethrogram: markedly dilated ureters, deformed bladder, abnormal bladder outlet, and a relatively narrow urethra.

Burton BK, et al.: Prune belly syndrome: Observations supporting the hypothesis of abdominal overdistention. *Am. J. Med. Genet.* 17:669, 1984.

Cawthern TH, et al.: Prune belly syndrome associated with Hirschsprung's disease. *Am. J. Dis. Child.* 133:652, 1979.

Christopher CR, et al.: Ultrasonic diagnosis of prune-belly syndrome. *Obstet. Gynecol.* 59:391, 1982.

Eagle JF, Barrett GS: Congenital deficiency of abdominal musculature with associated genitourinary abnormalities. *Pediatrics* 6:721, 1950.

Frydman M, et al.: Chromosome abnormalities in infants with prune belly anomaly: Associated with trisomy 18. *Am. J. Med. Genet.* 15:145, 1983.

Gaboardi F, et al.: Prune-belly syndrome: Report of three siblings. *Helv. Paediatr. Acta* 37:283, 1982.

Garris J, et al.: The ultrasound spectrum of prune-belly syndrome. *J. Clin. Ultrasound* 8:117, 1980.

Greskovich FJ III, et al.: The prune belly syndrome: A review of its etiology, defects, treatment and prognosis. *J. Urol.* 140:707, 1988.

Hodes ME, et al.: Prune belly syndrome in an anencephalic male. *Am. J. Med. Genet.* 14:37, 1983.

Holzgreve W: Prenatal diagnosis of persistent common cloaca with prune belly and anencephaly in the second trimester. *Am. J. Med. Genet.* 20:729, 1985.

Honoré LH: Benign cystic dysplasia of the adrenal glands in a case of prune belly syndrome. *J. Pediatr.* 123:562, 1980.

Ivarsson S, et al.: Coexisting ectrodactyly-ectodermal dysplasia-clefting (EEC) and prune belly syndromes. Report of a case. *Acta Radiol.* 23:287, 1982.

Jaffe R, et al.: Giant fetal abdominal cyst. Ultrasonic diagnosis and management. *J. Ultrasound Med.* 6:45, 1987.

Kirks DR, Taybi H: Prune belly syndrome. An unusual cause of neonatal abdominal calcification. *A.J.R.* 123:778, 1975.

Knight JA, et al.: Association of the Beckwith-Wiedemann and prune belly syndromes. *Clin. Pediatr. (Phila.)* 19:485, 1980.

Kroovand RL, et al.: Urethral and genital malformations in prune belly syndrome. *J. Urol.* 127:94, 1981.

Kuruvilla AC, et al.: Congenital cystic adenomatoid malformation of the lung associated with prune belly syndrome. *J. Pediatr. Surg.* 23:370, 1987.

Lee SM: Prune-belly syndrome in a 54-year old man. *J.A.M.A.* 237:2216, 1977.

Lockhart JL, et al.: Siblings with prune belly syndrome and associated pulmonary stenosis, mental retardation, and deafness. *Urology* 14:140, 1979.

Lubinsky M, et al.: The association of "prune belly" with Turner's syndrome. *Radiology* 134:1171, 1980.

Lubinsky M, et al.: Transient fetal hydrops and "prune belly" in one identical female twin. *N. Engl. J. Med.* 308:256, 1983.

Meizner I, et al.: Prenatal ultrasonic diagnosis of the

extreme form of prune belly syndrome. *J. Clin. Ultrasound* 13:581, 1985.

Moerman P, et al.: Pathogenesis of the prune-belly syndrome: A functional urethral obstruction caused by prostatic hypoplasia. *Pediatrics* 73:470, 1984.

Orvis BR, et al.: Testicular histology in fetuses with prune belly syndrome and posterior urethral valves. *J. Urol.* 139:335, 1988.

Parker RW: Case of an infant in whom some of the abdominal muscles were absent. *Trans. Clin. Soc. London* 28:201, 1895.

Pramanik AK, et al.: Prune belly syndrome associated with Potter (renal nonfunction) syndrome. *Am. J. Dis. Child.* 131:672, 1977.

Reinig JW, et al.: CT evaluation of the prune belly syndrome. *J. Comput. Tomogr.* 5:548, 1981.

Ringert RH, et al.: Congenital megalourethra associated with prune belly syndrome. *Z. Kinderchir.* 23:414, 1978.

Sayre R, et al.: Prune belly syndrome and retroperitoneal germ cell tumor. *Am. J. Med.* 81:895, 1986.

Silverman FN, et al.: Congenital absence of the abdominal muscles associated with malformation of the genitourinary and alimentary tracts: Report of cases and review of literature. *Am. J. Dis. Child.* 80:91, 1950.

Teramoto R, et al.: Splenic torsion with prune belly syndrome. *J. Pediatr.* 98:91, 1981.

Tuch BA, et al.: Prune-belly syndrome: A report of twelve cases and review of the literature. *J. Bone Joint Surg. [Am.]* 60:109, 1978.

Walker J, et al.: Prune belly syndrome associated with exomphalos and anorectal agenesis. *J. Pediatr. Surg.* 22:215, 1987.

Weber ML, et al.: Prune belly syndrome associated with congenital cystic adenomatoid malformation of the lung. *Am. J. Dis. Child.* 132:316, 1978.

Willert C, et al.: Association of prune belly syndrome and gastroschisis. *Am. J. Dis. Child.* 132:526, 1978.

PSEUDARTHROSIS OF THE CLAVICLE (FAMILIAL)

Mode of Inheritance: Male-to-male transmission in three generations.

Clinical and Radiologic Manifestations: Almost always occurs on the right side, bilateral in 10% of the cases: (a) "bump" in the midportion of the clavicle; (b) hypermobility at the site of the pseudarthrosis; (c) defect in the midportion of the clavicle without callus formation or other manifestation of a healing fracture.

Differential Diagnosis: Cleidocranial dysostosis; post-traumatic pseudarthrosis.

REFERENCE

Gibson DA, et al.: Congenital pseudoarthrosis of the clavicle. *J. Bone Joint Surg. [Br.]* 52:629, 1970.

PSEUDOTUMOR CEREBRI SYNDROME

Synonym: Benign intracranial hypertension.

Definition and Diagnostic Criteria: (a) *increased intracranial pressure in the absence of an intracranial mass;* (b) *normal cerebrospinal fluid (CSF) composition;* (c) *papilledema;* (d) *normal or small ventricles.*

Clinical Manifestations: (a) headaches, dizziness, nausea, blurring, obscurations, scotomas, diplopia, tinnitus, parethesias, alteration of consciousness; (b) papilledema, sixth-nerve palsy, visual field defect, enlarged blind spots, decreased or permanent loss of visual acuity, horizontal nystagmus; (c) normal CSF chemistry and cytology; (d) other reported abnormalities: visual loss (10% to 26% of patients), facial diplegia, facial pain, significant delayed pattern reversal of visual evoked potentials.

Association With: (a) dural sinus thrombosis; (b) inflammatory diseases of the paranasal sinuses, mastoids, middle ears, or respiratory tract; (c) endocrine disturbances (hypoparathyroidism, corticosteroid therapy, menarche, corticosteroid withdrawal, Addison disease, Cushing syndrome, adrenal adenoma, hypothyroidism, therapy for juvenile hypothyroidism); (d) galactosemia; (e) allergy; (f) vitamin A intoxication; tetracycline; indomethacin; diphtheria, tetanus, and pertussis immunization; ketoprofen in Bartter syndrome; nalidixic acid; lithium carbonate; (g) gastroenteritis; (h) head trauma; (i) maple syrup urine disease; (j) severe respiratory distress in cystic fibrosis (raised venous pressure due to in-

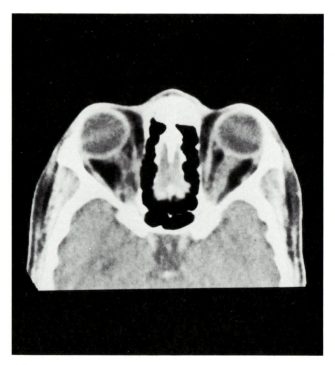

FIG SY–P–26.
Pseudotumor cerebri: papilledema in both eyes. An axial transverse computed tomographic scan of the orbits shows the grossly thickened optic nerves resulting from chronic papilledema. (From O'Reilly GV, Hammerschlag SB, Bergland, RM, et al.: Pseudotumor cerebri: Computed tomography of resolving papilledema. *J. Comput. Assist. Tomogr.* 7:364, 1983. Used by permission.)

creased intrathoracic pressure); (k) vitamin D—deficiency rickets; (l) insecticide/herbicide exposure; (m) systemic lupus erythematosus; (n) familial (associated with obesity); (o) empty sella syndrome; (p) others: Lyme disease, Guillain-Barré syndrome, rapid weight gain during treatment of children with malnutrition, obstructive nephropathy, empty sella syndrome, etc.

Radiologic Manifestations: (a) widening of sutures, demineralization of the dorsum sella, deepening of the pituitary fossa; (b) lateral ventricle smaller than normal (in some), narrow basal cisterns, thickened optic nerves associated with papilledema; (c) magnetic resonance imaging: increased signals in the periventricular white matter suggesting diffuse low-level edema (Fig SY—P—26).

REFERENCES

Ahlskog JE, et al.: Pseudotumor cerebri. *Ann. Intern. Med.* 97:249, 1982.

Bouygues D, et al.: Hypertension intracrânienne benigne du nourrisson et de l'enfant. *Ann. Pediatr. (Paris)* 27:286, 1980.

Britton C, et al.: Pseudotumor cerebri, empty sella syndrome, and adrenal adenoma. *Neurology* 30:292, 1980.

Carlow TJ, et al.: Controversies in diagnosis and management of pseudotumor cerebri (letter). *Arch. Neurol.* 44:128, 1987.

DeJong AR, et al.: Pseudotumor cerebri and nutritional rickets. *Eur. J. Pediatr.* 143:219, 1985.

Digre KB, et al.: Pseudotumor cerebri in men. *Arch. Neurol.* 45:866, 1988.

Donaldson JO, et al.: Pseudotumor cerebri in an obese woman with Turner syndrome. *Neurology* 31:758, 1981.

Dunsker SB, et al.: Pseudotumor cerebri associated with idiopathic cryofibrinogenemia: Report of a case. *Arch. Neurol.* 23:120, 1970.

Hart RG, et al.: Pseudotumor cerebri and facial pain. *Arch. Neurol.* 39:440, 1982.

Jacob J, et al.: Increased intracranial pressure after diphtheria, tetanus and pertussis immunization. *Am. J. Dis. Child.* 133:217, 1979.

Jenkyn LR: Insecticide/herbicide exposure, aplastic anaemia and pseudotumour cerebri. *Lancet* 2:368, 1979.

Kiwak KJ, et al.: Benign intracranial hypertension and facial diplegia. *Arch. Neurol.* 41:787, 1984.

Konomi H, et al.: Indomethacin causing pseudotumor cerebri in Bartter's syndrome. *N. Engl. J. Med.* 298:855, 1978.

Larizza D, et al.: Ketoprofen causing pseudotumor cerebri in Bartter's syndrome. *N. Engl. J. Med.* 300:796, 1979.

Lessell S, et al.: Permanent visual impairment in childhood pseudotumor cerebri. *Arch. Neurol.* 43:801, 1986.

Litman N, et al.: Galactokinase deficiency presenting as pseudotumor cerebri. *J. Pediatr.* 86:410, 1975.

McVie R: Abnormal TSH regulation, pseudotumor cerebri, and empty sella after replacement therapy in juvenile hypothyroidism. *J. Pediatr.* 105:768, 1984.

Mor F, et al.: Evidence on computed tomography of pseudotumour cerebri in hypoparathyroidism. *Br. J. Radiol.* 61:158, 1988.

Moser FG, et al.: MR imaging of pseudotumor cerebri. *A.J.R.* 150:903, 1988.

Noetzel MJ, et al.: Pseudotumor cerebri associated with obstructive nephropathy. *Pediatr. Neurol.* 2:238, 1986.

Nonne M: Der Pseudotumor cerebri. *Neue Dtsch. Chir.* 10:107, 1914.

O'Reilly GV, et al.: Pseudotumor cerebri: Computed tomography of resolving papilledema. *J. Comput. Assist. Tomogr.* 7:364, 1983.

Powers JM, et al.: Pseudotumor cerebri due to partial obstruction of the sigmoid sinus by a cholesteatoma. *Arch. Neurol.* 43:519, 1986.

Press OW, et al.: Pseudotumor cerebri and hypothyroidism. *Arch. Intern. Med.* 143:167, 1983.

Quincke H: Ueber Meningitis serosa und verwandte Zustände. *Dtsch. Z. Nervenheilkd.* 9:149, 1896—1897.

Rao KG: Pseudotumor cerebri associated with nalidixic acid. *Urology* 4:204, 1974.

Raucher HS, et al.: Pseudotumor cerebri and Lyme disease: A new association. *J. Pediatr.* 107:931, 1985.

Repka MX, et al.: Pseudotumor cerebri. *Am. J. Ophthalmol.* 98:741, 1984.

Roach ES, et al.: Increased intracranial pressure following treatment of cystic fibrosis. *Pediatrics* 66:622, 1980.

Ropper AH, et al.: Mechanism of pseudotumor in Guillain-Barré syndrome. *Arch. Neurol.* 41:259, 1984.

Rush JA: Pseudotumor cerebri. Clinical profile and visual outcome in 63 patients. *Mayo Clin. Proc.* 55:541, 1980.

Saul RF, et al.: Pseudotumor cerebri secondary to lithium carbonate. *J.A.M.A.* 253:2869, 1985.

Saxena VK, et al.: Pseudotumor cerebri: A complication of parenteral hyperalimentation. *J.A.M.A.* 235:2124, 1976.

Sørensen PS, et al.: Endocrine studies in patients with pseudotumor cerebri. Estrogen levels in blood and cerebrospinal fluid. *Arch. Neurol.* 43:902, 1986.

Sørensen PS, et al.: Visual evoked potentials in pseudotumor cerebri. *Arch. Neurol.* 42:150, 1985.

Spector RH, et al.: Pseudotumor cerebri caused by a synthetic vitamin A preparation. *Neurology* 34:1509, 1984.

Traviesa DC, et al.: Familial benign intracranial hypertension. *J. Neurol. Neurosurg. Psychiatry* 39:420, 1976.

Van Dop C, et al.: Pseudotumor cerebri associated with initiation of levothyroxine therapy for juvenile hypothyroidism. *N. Engl. J. Med.* 308:1076, 1983.

Vogel R, et al.: Increased intracranial pressure in galactosemia. *Clin. Pediatr. (Phila.)* 15:386, 1976.

Wall M, et al.: Visual loss in pseudotumor cerebri. Incidence and defects related to visual field strategy. *Arch. Neurol.* 44:170, 1987.

PSEUDOXANTHOMA ELASTICUM

Synonyms: Grönblad-Strandberg syndrome; Grönblad-Strandberg-Touraine syndrome; Darier syndrome.

Mode of Inheritance: Heterogeneity; autosomal recessive; autosomal dominant.

Frequency: Estimated at between 1:70,000 and 1:160,000 adults (Belli et al.).

Pathology: (a) degeneration in collagenous-elastic tissue, fragmentation and clumping of elastic tissues in the deep dermis; (b) narrowed arterial lumen due to medial thickening, invasion of the media by irregular and anarchic elastic fibers, fragmentation of the elastic laminae, calcific deposition; (c) endocardial thickening; (d) mucosal lesions.

Clinical Manifestations: (a) *xanthoma-like skin lesions* of flexural folds: yellowish, grouped papules and plaques; redundant skin fold formation; (b) diminished vision, *angioid streaks of the retina* (cracks in a membrane beneath the retina); (c) cardiovascular manifestations: premature atherosclerosis, intermittent claudication, diminished peripheral pulses, angina pectoris, abdominal pain, systemic hypertension, restrictive cardiomyopathy, mitral valve prolapse, etc.; (d) hemorrhage: gastrointestinal tract, retina, kidneys, bladder, uterus, nose, joints, subarachnoid space; (e) other reported abnormalities: association with polyposis coli, abnormal phosphorus and vitamin D metabolism, abnormal placenta (small cotyledon and more numerous than normal, etc.), intrauterine growth retardation of the infant born to a mother with the disease.

Radiologic Manifestations: (a) *vascular, dermal, and periarticular calcifications;* (b) ischemic resorption of the terminal phalanges; (c) *vascular abnormalities:* aortic dilatation, occlusion of the peripheral arteries with marked collateral circulation, arteriosclerotic plaques and occlusion of the major vessels in young adults, arteriovenous fistulas, tortuosity of arteries, carotid rete mirabile, irregularity of the walls of brachiocephalic vessels; (d) restrictive cardiomyopathy; (e) myocardial infarction; (f) fibro-osseous metaplasia of the long bones, dysplasia of the vertebrae; (g) fine punctate opacities in the lung.

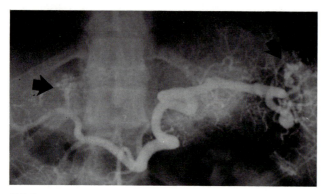

FIG SY—P—27.
Pseudoxanthoma elasticum in a 36-year-old female who had had an episode of hematemesis and a clinical diagnosis of pseudoxanthoma elasticum. Abdominal angiography showed an area of marked tortuosity and irregular narrowing distal to the origin of the superior mesenteric artery. Angiomatous malformations are shown *(arrows)* in the spleen and liver in this selective celiac arteriogram. (From Bardsley JL, Koehler PR: Pseudoxanthoma elasticum: Angiographic manifestations in abdominal vessels. *Radiology* 93:559, 1969. Used by permission.)

Notes: (a) Grönblad-Strandberg syndrome represents the combination of retinal angioid streaks and pseudoxanthoma elasticum; (b) classification (Pope, 1974b, 1975): (1) autosomal recessive, type I: moderate vascular and retinal involvement, "peau d'orange" flexural skin lesions; (2) autosomal recessive, type II: skin lesions, no systemic involvement, very rare; (3) autosomal dominant, type I: severe retinal and cardiovascular degeneration, cutaneous lesions; (4) autosomal dominant, type II: mild retinal and cardiovascular manifestations, macular skin changes, blue sclerae, hyperextensible joints, high-arched palate, myopia (Fig SY—P—27).

REFERENCES

Bardsley JL, Koehler PR: Pseudoxanthoma elasticum: Angiographic manifestations in abdominal vessels. *Radiology* 93:559, 1969.

Belli A, et al.: Visceral angiographic findings in pseudoxanthoma elasticum. *Br. J. Radiol.* 61:368, 1988.

Darier J: Pseudoxanthoma elasticum. *Monatsschr. Prakt. Dermatol.* 23:609, 1896.

di Matteo J, et al.: Les manifesations cardiovasculaires de l'élastorrhexie systématisée (syndrome de Grönblad-Strandberg-Touraine). *Ann. Med. Interne (Paris)* 134:470, 1983.

Elejalde R, et al.: Manifestations of pseudoxanthoma elasticum during pregnancy: A case report and review of the literature. *Am. J. Med. Genet.* 18:755, 1984.

Grönblad E: Angioid streaks: Pseudoxanthoma elasticum, Vorläufige Mitteilung. *Acta Ophthalmol.* 7:329, 1929.

Irani C, et al.: Pseudoxanthome élastique avec insuffisance aortique et hypertension artérielle chez un enfant de douze ans. *Arch. Fr. Pediatr.* 41:337, 1984.

James AE Jr, et al.: Roentgen findings in pseudoxanthoma elasticum (PXE). *A.J.R.* 106:642, 1969.

Lebwohl M, et al.: Diagnosis of pseudoxanthoma elasticum by scar biopsy in patients without characteristic skin lesions. *N. Engl. J. Med.* 317:347, 1987.

Lebwohl MG, et al.: Pseudoxanthoma elasticum and mitral-valve prolapse. *N. Engl. J. Med.* 307:228, 1982.

Mallette LE, et al.: Heritable syndrome of pseudoxanthoma elasticum with abnormal phosphorus and vitamin D metabolism. *Am. J. Med.* 83:1157, 1987.

Mamtora H, et al.: Pulmonary opacities in pseudoxanthoma elasticum: Report of two cases. *Br. J. Radiol.* 54:65, 1981.

Navarro-Lopez F, et al.: Restrictive cardiomyopathy in pseudoxanthoma elasticum. *Chest* 78:113, 1980.

O'Holleran M, et al.: Pseudoxanthoma elasticum and polyposis coli. *Arch. Surg.* 116:476, 1981.

Pope FM: Autosomal dominant pseudoxanthoma elasticum. *J. Med. Genet.* 11:152, 1974a.

Pope FM: Historical evidence for the genetic heterogeneity of pseudoxanthoma elasticum. *Br. J. Dermatol.* 92:493, 1975.

Pope FM: Two types of autosomal recessive pseudoxanthoma elasticum. *Arch. Dermatol.* 110:209, 1974b.

Prick JJG, et al.: Radiodiagnostic signs in pseudoxanthoma elasticum generalisatum (dysgenesis elastofibrillaris mineralisans). *Clin. Radiol.* 28:549, 1977.

Renie WA, et al.: Pseudoxanthoma elasticum: High calcium intake in early life correlates with severity. *Am. J. Med. Genet.* 19:235, 1984.

Rios-Montenegro EN, et al.: Pseudoxanthoma elasticum: Association with bilateral carotid rete mirabile and unilateral carotid-cavernous sinus fistula. *Arch. Neurol.* 26:151, 1972.

Schachnar L, et al.: Pseudoxanthoma elasticum with severe cardiovascular disease in a child. *Am. J. Dis. Child.* 127:571, 1974.

Strandberg J: Pseudoxanthoma elasticum. *Z. Haut. Geschwulsporsch. Krankh.* 31:689, 1929.

Touraine A: L'elastorrhexie systematisée. *Bull. Soc. Fr. Dermatol. Syph.* 47:255, 1940.

Viljoen DL, et al.: Heterogeneity of pseudoxanthoma elasticum: Delineation of a new form? *Clin. Genet.* 32:100, 1987.

PTERYGIUM SYNDROMES

Neck Pterygium (Webbed Neck)

Association With: (a) chromosomal syndromes: trisomy 21, trisomy 13, Turner syndrome, etc.; (b) Noonan syndrome; (c) Nielson syndrome: short stature, cleft palate, camptodactyly, vertebral fusion; (d) Golden-Lakim syndrome: dolichocephaly, small mandible, pointed facies, bifid uvula, pectus excavatum, kyphoscoliosis, flexion deformity of the knees without webbing, pes cavus, clubfoot, etc.; (e) LEOPARD syndrome; (f) fetal alcohol syndrome; (g) multiple pterygium syndrome; (h) pterygium colli medianum and midline cervical cleft.

Pterygium Syndromes and Syndromes with Limb Pterygia

Classification—Genetic (Hall et al., 1982): (a) autosomal dominant forms: popliteal pterygium syndrome, antecubital pterygium syndrome, multiple pterygium-ptosis-skeletal abnormalities syndrome; (b) autosomal recessive forms: multiple pterygium syndrome, lethal multiple pterygium syndrome, lethal pterygium syndrome with facial cleft (Bartsocas-Papas), popliteal pterygium with ectodermal dysplasia.

Description:

(A) POPLITEAL PTERYGIUM SYNDROME: (a) autosomal dominant inheritance with variable expressivity and incomplete penetrance, autosomal recessive transmission has also been suggested; (b) *lower lip pits, cleft lip/palate*, micrognathia, ankyloblepharon filiforme, syngnathia; (c) *popliteal web in severe cases extending from the hip to the heel, intercrural pterygium*; (d) *genitourinary anomalies*: cryptorchidism, ambiguous genitalia, absent or cleft scrotum, hypoplasia or aplasia of the labia majora; (e) *skeletal anomalies*: syndactyly of the hands and feet, hypoplasia or aplasia of the digits, toenail dysplasia, fusion of the interphalangeal joints, valgus or varus deformities of the feet, talipes equinovarus, hypoplasia of the tibia, bipartate or absent patella, low acetabular angle, scoliosis, lordosis, rib anomalies; (f) other reported abnormalities: growth retardation, mental retardation, hernia, etc.

(B) ANTECUBITAL PTERYGIUM SYNDROME: (a) autosomal dominant inheritance with some reduction in penetrance; (b) *web extending across the cubital fossa*; (c) *skeletal anomalies*: sub-

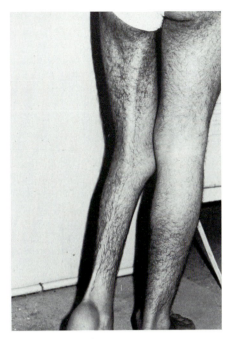

FIG SY–P–28.
Popliteal pterygium in a 15-year-old patient. Note the ischiocalcaneal cord, flexion contracture of the knee, and hypotrophy of the left leg. (From Herold HZ, Shmueli G, Baruchin AM: Popliteal pterygium syndrome. *Clin. Orthop.* 209:194, 1986. Used by permission.)

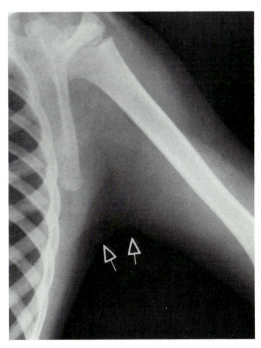

FIG SY–P–29.
Multiple pterygium syndromes in a 3½-year old female with low-set ears; a broad-tipped and deformed nose; pterygium of the neck, both axillae, and the right popliteal region (a 15-degree flexion contracture); and cleft palate (repaired). A webbed axilla is seen on this roentgenogram *(arrows)*.

luxation of the radial head, maldevelopment of the radio-ulnar joint, aplasia of the trochlea of the humerus; (d) *cleft palate.*

(C) MULTIPLE PTERYGIUM-PTOSIS-SKELETAL ABNORMALITIES SYNDROME (FRIAS): Autosomal dominant: (a) multiple pterygia; (b) ptosis of the eyelids, antimongoloid slanting of the palpebral fissures; (c) skeletal anomalies: vertebral anomalies, scoliosis, pelvic dysplasia, camptodactyly, fusion of the tarsal bones.

(D) MULTIPLE PTERYGIUM SYNDROME (ESCOBAR SYNDROME): (a) autosomal recessive mode of inheritance; (b) *webbing of variable severity and distribution (neck, axilla, elbow, intercrural, knee, digits;* (c) *short stature;* (d) *orofacial anomalies:* epicanthal folds or hypertelorism, long philtrum, antimongoloid palpebral fissures, low-set ears, micrognathia, eyelid ptosis, cleft palate, down-turned corners of the mouth; (e) *musculoskeletal abnormalities:* multiple flexion contractures, rib anomalies, vertebral anomalies, scoliosis, lordosis, congenital hip dislocation, flexion deformity of the fingers, soft-tissue syndactyly of the fingers, rocker-bottom feet, talipes equinovarus; (f) *genital anomalies:* cryptorchidism, hypoplasia or absent labia majora; (g) other reported abnormalities: hypoplastic nipples, umbilical hernia, inguinal hernia, low posterior hairline, muscular hypoplasia, mental retardation, etc.

(E) LETHAL MULTIPLE PTERYGIUM SYNDROME: (a) antimongoloid slant of the eyes, hypertelosism, cleft palate and lips, low-set ears; (b) cutaneous syndactyly of the fingers; (c) pterygium (neck, axilla, chin, antecubital, knee); (d) genital abnormalities; (e) various skeletal anomalies (limbs, trunk); (f) hydrops fetalis; (g) cystic hygroma; (h) hydranencephaly.

(F) LETHAL PTERYGIUM SYNDROME WITH FACIAL CLEFT (BARTSOCAS-PAPAS SYNDROME): (a) low birth weight; (b) microcephaly, ankyloblepharon, corneal ulceration, filiform band between the jaws, cleft palate and lips, hypoplastic nose, apparently low-set ears; (c) lanugo hair; (d) absent thumb/finger syndactyly, equinovarus/syndactyly of the toes; (e) bilateral popliteal pterygium; (f) hypoplastic nails; (g) genital abnormalities; (h) synostosis of the hands and feet.

Miscellaneous

(A) Progressive form of multiple pterygium syndrome in association with nemalin myopathy (Papadia et al., 1987); (B) multiple pterygia, camptodactyly, facial anomalies, cystic hygroma, hypoplastic lungs and heart, skeletal anomalies (Chen et al.); (C) multiple pterygium syndrome complicated by malignant hyperthermia (Robinson et al.) (Figs SY—P—28 to SY—P—30; Table SY—P—1).

REFERENCES

Addison A, et al.: Flexion contractures of the knee associated with popliteal webbing. *J. Pediatr. Orthop.* 3:376, 1983.

Bixler D, et al.: Popliteal pterygium syndrome in monozygous twins. *Birth Defects* 10:167, 1974.

Chen H, et al.: Syndrome of multiple pterygia, camptodactyly, facial anomalies, hypoplastic lungs and heart, cystic hygroma, and skeletal anomalies: Delineation of a new entity and review of lethal forms of multiple pterygium syndrome. *Am. J. Med. Genet.* 17:809, 1984.

Escobar V, et al.: Multiple pterygium syndrome. *Am. J. Dis. Child.* 132:609, 1978.

Escobar V, et al.: The popliteal pterygium syndrome. A phenotypic and genetic analysis. *J. Med. Genet.* 15:35, 1978.

Frohlich GS, et al.: Popliteal pterygium syndrome: Report of a family. *J. Pediatr.* 90:91, 1977.

Froster-Iskenius UG, et al.: An unusual bendlike web in an infant with lethal multiple pterygium syndrome. *Am. J. Med. Genet.* 30:763, 1988.

Fryns JP, et al.: Cystic hygroma and multiple pterygium syndrome. *Ann. Genet. (Paris)* 27:252, 1984.

Fryns JP, et al.: Multiple pterygium syndrome type Escobar in two brothers. Follow-up data from childhood to adulthood. *Eur. J. Pediatr.* 147:550, 1988.

Godbersen S, et al.: Pterygium colli medianum and midline cervical cleft: Midline anomalies in the sense of a developmental field defect. *Am. J. Med. Genet.* 27:719, 1987.

Golden RL, Lakim H: The form fruste in Marfan's syndrome. *N. Engl. J. Med.* 260:797, 1959.

Hall JG, et al.: Limb pterygium syndromes: A review and report of eleven patients. *Am. J. Med. Genet.* 12:377, 1982.

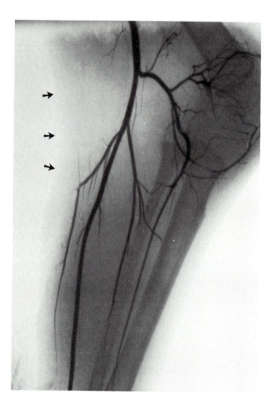

FIG SY—P—30.
Popliteal pterygium syndrome in a boy with popliteal webbing, webbing of the eyelids, intraoral webbing, lower lip pits, a bilateral cleft lip and palate, syndactyly of several pairs of toes, dysplasia of the toenails, and a cleft scrotum. The father was affected by the same syndrome. Arteriography of the lower limb demonstrates an abnormally dorsal position of the popliteal artery. Note the popliteal pterygium *(arrows).* (Courtesy of Dr. Corning Benton, Cincinnati.)

TABLE SY—P—1.

Distinguishing Features of Multiple and Popliteal Pterygium Syndromes*

	Multiple Pterygium Syndrome	Popliteal Pterygium Syndrome
Clinical features	Popliteal webs Neck webs Elbow webs Axillary webs Vertebral abnormalities Spindling or clawing of fingers Genital and palate anomalies may occur but less frequently than in popliteal pterygium syndrome Normal intelligence	Popliteal webs Cleft palate/cleft lip Lower lip congenital sinuses Genital anomalies Syndactyly of toes Toenail anomalies Normal intelligence
Genetics	Autosomal recessive	Autosomal dominant with incomplete penetrance and variable expressivity
Differential diagnosis	Syndromes Turner Noonan LEOPARD	Isolated cleft palate or cleft lip Van der Waude syndrome

*From Addison A, Webb PJ: Flexion contractures of the knee associated with popliteal webbing. *J. Pediatr. Orthop.* 3:376, 1983. Used by permission.

Hall JG: The lethal multiple pterygium syndromes (editorial). *Am. J. Med. Genet.* 17:803, 1984.

Herold HZ, et al.: Popliteal pterygium syndrome. *Clin. Orthop.* 209:194, 1986.

Martin NJ, et al.: Lethal multiple pterygium syndrome: Three consecutive cases in one family. *Am. J. Med. Genet.* 24:295, 1986.

Mbakop A, et al.: Lethal multiple pterygium syndrome: Report of a new case with hydranencephaly. *Am. J. Med. Genet.* 25:575, 1986.

McKeown CME, et al.: An autosomal dominant multiple pterygium syndrome. *J. Med. Genet.* 25:96, 1988.

Nielson H: Dystrophia brevicollis congenita. *Hospitalstidende* 77:403, 1934.

Papadia F, et al.: Nosological difference between the Bartsocas-Papas syndrome and lethal multiple pterygium syndrome (letter). *Am. J. Med. Genet.* 29:699, 1988.

Papadia F, et al.: Progressive form of multiple pterygium syndrome in association with nemalin-myopathy: Report of a female followed for twelve years. *Am. J. Med. Genet.* 26:73, 1987.

Papadia F, et al.: The Bartsocas-Papas syndrome: Autosomal recessive form of popliteal pterygium syndrome in a male infant. *Am. J. Med. Genet.* 17:841, 1984.

Pashayan H: Bilateral aniridia, multiple webs and severe mental retardation in a 47, XXY/48, XXXXY mosaic. *Clin. Genet.* 4:126, 1973.

Ramer JC, et al.: Multiple pterygium syndrome. An overview. *Am. J. Dis. Child.* 142:794, 1988.

Robinson LK, et al.: Multiple pterygium syndrome: A case complicated by malignant hyperthermia. *Clin. Genet.* 32:5, 1987.

Shun-Shin M: Congenital web formation. *J. Bone Joint Surg. [Br.]* 36:268, 1954.

Stoll C, et al.: Familial pterygium syndrome. *Clin. Genet.* 18:317, 1980.

Temtamy S, McKusick VA: Pterygium syndromes. *Birth Defects* 14:469, 1978.

Thompson EM, et al.: Multiple pterygium syndrome: Evolution of the phenotype. *J. Med. Genet.* 24:733, 1987.

Tolmie JL, et al.: A lethal multiple pterygium syndrome with apparent X-linked recessive inheritance. *Am. J. Med. Genet.* 27:913, 1987.

Trèlat U: Sur une vice conformation très râre de la lèvre inférieure. *J. Med. Chir. Prat.* 40:442, 1869.

Tuerk D, et al.: The surgical treatment of congenital webbing (pterygium of the popliteal area). *Plast. Reconstr. Surg.* 56:339, 1975.

Wallis CE, et al.: Autosomal dominant antecubital pterygium: Syndromic status substantiated. *Clin. Genet.* 34:64, 1988.

PULMONARY ALVEOLAR MICROLITHIASIS

Mode of Inheritance: Autosomal recessive; about half of reported cases are familial.

Clinical Manifestations: The age range is from newborn to 80 years: (a) *cough, dyspnea,* chest aches; (b) pulmonary function tests: *restrictive dysfunction, hypoxia;* (c) transbronchial biopsy: *laminated concretions (microliths).*

Radiologic Manifestations: (a) *very fine diffuse sandlike micronodulation involving both lungs,* the lower two thirds of lungs more involved; (b) computed tomography (CT): diffuse pulmonary infiltrative pattern with CT density of *calcification;*

(c) scintigraphy: *intense uptake of the tracer (*^{99m}*Tc diphosphonate) in the lungs.*

Differential Diagnosis: Metastatic and dystrophic pulmonary calcification of various etiologic origin.

REFERENCES

Balikian JP, et al.: Pulmonary alveolar microlithiasis: Report of five cases with special reference to roentgen manifestations. *A.J.R.* 103:508, 1968.

Caffrey PR, et al.: Pulmonary alveolar microlithiasis occurring in premature twins. *J. Pediatr.* 66:758, 1965.

Cale WF, et al.: Transbronchial biopsy of pulmonary alveolar microlithiasis. *Arch. Intern. Med.* 143:358, 1983.

Friedreich N: Corpora amylacea in den Lungen. *Virchows Arch [A]* 9:613, 1856.

Harbitz F: Extensive calcification of the lungs as a distinct disease. *Arch. Intern. Med.* 21:139, 1918.

Prakash UBS, et al.: Pulmonary alveolar microlithiasis. A review including ultrastructural and pulmonary function studies. *Mayo Clin. Proc.* 58:290, 1983.

PULMONARY VALVE DYSPLASIA SYNDROME

Mode of Inheritance: Possible genetic recessive factors.

Clinical Manifestations: (a) clinical and laboratory findings similar to those of pulmonary valvular stenosis but without a pulmonary ejection click; (b) *unusual facies (hypertelorism, epicanthal folds, low-set ears);* (c) *small stature;* (d) *mental retardation.*

Radiologic Manifestations: (a) right ventricular obstruction *with thickening and immobility of pulmonary valve leaflets without "doming"*; (b) *absence of annular hypoplasia;* (c) presence of *three distinct valve cusps* without commissural fusion.

REFERENCES

Koretzky ED, et al.: Congenital pulmonary stenosis resulting from dysplasia of valve. *Circulation* 40:43, 1969.

Linde LM, et al.: Pulmonary valvular dysplasia: A cardiofacial syndrome. *Br. Heart J.* 35:301, 1973.

QUADRILATERAL SPACE SYNDROME

Etiology: Compression of the posterior humeral circumflex artery (PHCA) and axillary nerve in the quadrilateral space.

Clinical Manifestations: Usual occurrence in young adults: *Intermittent paresthesia in the upper limb during forward flexion, abduction, or both; aggravation of the symptoms with external rotation of the humerus.*

Radiologic Manifestation: *Obstruction of the PHCA with the arm in abduction and external rotation.*

REFERENCES

Cormier PJ, et al.: Quadrilateral space syndrome: A rare cause of shoulder pain. *Radiology* 167:797, 1988.

Cahill BR, Palmer RE: Quadrilateral space syndrome. *J. Hand Surg.* 8:65, 1983.

R

RADIAL HYPOPLASIA–TRIPHALANGEAL THUMBS–HYPOSPADIAS–MAXILLARY DIASTEMA

Mode of Inheritance: Autosomal dominant.

Clinical and Radiologic Manifestations: (a) bilateral, symmetrical, fingerlike, nonopposable triphalangeal thumbs; (b) shortened forearms and hypoplastic radii, radial deviation of the hands; (c) hypospadias in the affected males; (d) anterior maxillary diastema.

Differential Diagnosis: Aase syndrome; Holt-Oram syndrome; Nager syndrome of acrofacial dysostosis; TAR syndrome; Fanconi anemia.

REFERENCE

Schmitt E, et al.: An autosomal dominant syndrome of radial hypoplasia, triphalangeal thumbs, hypospadias, and maxillary diastema. *Am. J. Med. Genet.* 13:63, 1982.

RADIAL RAY APLASIA–RENAL ANOMALIES

Mode of Inheritance: Autosomal dominant most likely.

Clinical and Radiologic Manifestations: (a) bilateral absence of the radius and thumb; (b) renal anomalies: solitary kidney, crossed fused ectopy; (c) short stature, external ear malformation, high frequency of chromosome breaks in lymphocytes (son).

Differential Diagnosis: (radial ray aplasia or hypoplasia): Holt-Oram; IVIC; Fanconi anemia; TAR; familial ray defect in association with renal disease (possible autosomal recessive [Siegler et al.]).

REFERENCES

Siegler RL, et al.: Upper limb anomalies and renal disease. *Clin. Genet.* 17:117, 1980.
Sofar S, et al.: Radial ray aplasia and renal anomalies in father and son: A new syndrome. *Am. J. Med. Genet.* 14:151, 1983.

RADIAL RAY HYPOPLASIA SYNDROME

Mode of Inheritance: Autosomal dominant.

Clinical and Radiologic Manifestations: (a) radial ray hypoplasia of variable severity ranging from a totally absent radius, first metacarpal, and phalangeal bones to hypoplastic carpal and metacarpal bones and a triphalangeal thumb; (b) choanal stenosis; (c) esotropia.

REFERENCE

Goldblatt J, et al.: New autosomal dominant radial ray hypoplasia syndrome. *Am. J. Med. Genet.* 28:647, 1987.

RADIO-DIGITO-FACIAL DYSPLASIA

Mode of Inheritance: Probably autosomal recessive.

Clinical and Radiologic Manifestations: (a) severe prenatal onset of dwarfism; (b) bilateral radial hypoplasia, malformation of the thumbs (hypoplasia, proximally placed), clinodactyly of the fifth fingers; (c) minor facial dysmorphism: fish mouth, mild micrognathia, slightly receding forehead, anteverted external nares; (d) psychomotor retardation.

REFERENCE

Similä S, et al.: Radio-digito-facial dysplasia associated with dwarfism. *Helv. Paediatr. Acta* 38:81, 1983.

RAEDER SYNDROME

Synonym: Raeder paratrigeminal syndrome.

Etiology: A lesion near the ascending sympathetic chain in the neck distal to the superior cervical ganglion; the lesions include trauma, tumor, infections, embolization of the gasserian ganglion, perivasculitis brought on by exertion, lesions of the internal carotid artery in the region of the ascending sympathetic chain (inflammation, hemorrhage, dissection, pseudoaneurysm), syphilitic aortitis.

Clinical Manifestations: (a) *unilateral ptosis of the eye and miosis of the pupil, conjunctival injection and tearing;* (b) *headaches;* (c) *ipsilateral facial sweating preserved.*

Radiologic Manifestations: Demonstration of the etiologic factors: sinusitis, vascular abnormalities, tumor, etc.

REFERENCES

Brandel JP, et al.: Syndrome de Raeder dû a une dissection carotidienne. *Presse Med.* 16:541, 1987.

Healy JF, et al.: Raeder syndrome associated with lesions of the internal carotid artery. *Radiology* 141:101, 1981.

Mokri B: Raeder's paratrigeminal syndrome. Original concept and subsequent deviations. *Arch. Neurol.* 39:395, 1982.

RAMON SYNDROME

Mode of Inheritance: Consanguineous parents.

Frequency: Fewer than ten published cases (Pina-Neto et al.).

Clinical Manifestations: (a) *cherubism;* (b) *gingival fibromatosis;* (c) *epilepsy;* (d) *mental deficiency;* (e) other reported abnormalities: stunted growth, hypertrichosis, rheumatoid arthritis (in one family).

Radiologic Manifestations: *Fibrous dysplasia of the jaw* ("soap bubble," multilocular, with bone distension and thinning of the cortex of the maxilla and mandible).

REFERENCES

Pina-Neto JM, et al.: Cherubism, gingival fibromatosis, epilepsy, and mental deficiency (Ramon syndrome) with juvenile rheumatoid arthritis. *Am. J. Med. Genet.* 25:433, 1986.

Ramon Y, et al.: Gingival fibromatosis combined with cherubism. *Oral Surg.* 24:436, 1967.

RAYNAUD SYNDROME

Synonym: Raynaud disease.

Clinical Manifestations: Occurrence primarily in young adults without known associated disease: (a) *symptoms developing with exposure to cold or in association with emotional upset;* (b) *symmetrical involvement of hands;* (c) *usually absence of gangrene, but if present, limited to the skin of the fingertips;* (d) *normal pulse;* (e) *absence of recognition of the underlying disorder as a cause of the symptom complex;* (f) *recurrence of symptoms for at least 2 years without detection of the underlying cause;* (g) frequent digital telangiectases, digital edema and elevated levels of immunoglobulins in the patients being anticentromere antibody–positive.

Radiologic Manifestations: (a) *absence of filling of the distal parts of the digital arteries;* (b) *diminished caliber of digital arteries.*

Note: Raynaud phenomenon (vasomotor disorder manifested by pallor and cyanosis of the distal parts of the extremities) occurs in association with various diseases: chronic renal insufficiency, hepatitis, malignant neoplasms, scleroderma, disseminated lupus erythematosus, etc.

REFERENCES

Allen EV: The peripheral arteries in Raynaud's disease: An arteriographic study of living subjects. *Proc. Mayo Clin.* 12:187, 1937.

Allen EV, Brown GE: Raynaud's disease. A clinical study of 147 cases. *J.A.M.A.* 99:1472, 1932.

Balas P, et al.: Raynaud's phenomenon: Primary or secondary causes. *Arch. Surg.* 114:1174, 1979.

Porter JM, et al.: The clinical significance of Raynaud's syndrome. *Surgery* 80:756, 1976.

Raynaud AGM: *De L'asphyxie Locale et de la Gangrène Symétrique des Extremités* (thesis). Paris, 1862.

Samani D, et al.: Orthopaedic complications of Raynaud syndrome. *J. Bone Joint Surg. [Am.]* 69:1093, 1987.

Sarkozi J, et al.: Significance of anticentromere antibody in idiopathic Raynaud's syndrome. *Am. J. Med.* 83:893, 1987.

Sayre JW: Raynaud's disease presenting in a 5-month-old-male infant. *Pediatrics* 52:412, 1973.

von Wagner H-H, et al.: Der differentialdiagnostische Stellenwert des Handarteriogramms beim primären und sekundären Raynaud-Syndrom. *Fortschr. Rontgenstr.* 142:10, 1985.

Wegelius U: Angiography of the hand. *Acta Radiol.* 315(suppl.):91, 1972.

RECTAL ULCER SYNDROME

Synonym: Solitary rectal ulcer syndrome.

Clinical Manifestations: (a) rectal bleeding; (b) long history of defecation disorders; (c) *benign mucosal lesion in the distal anterior wall of the rectum.*

Radiologic Manifestations: (a) granularity of the rectal mucosa, thickened rectal folds, rectal stricture; (b) defecography: *intussusception of the rectal wall, rectocele, rectal prolapse, failure of relaxation of the puborectalis that prevents passage of a bolus, abnormal perineal descent* (Fig SY–R–1).

REFERENCES

Goei R, et al.: Solitary rectal ulcer syndrome: Findings at barium enema study and defecography. *Radiology* 168:303, 1988.

Goei R, et al.: The solitary rectal ulcer syndrome: Diagnosis with defecography. *A.J.R.* 149:933, 1987.

Madigan MR, et al.: Solitary ulcer of the rectum. *Gut* 10:871, 1969.

Rutter KR, et al.: The solitary ulcer syndrome of the rectum. *Clin. Gastroenterol.* 4:505, 1975.

RED-EYED SHUNT SYNDROME

Etiology: Carotid-cavernous fistula.

Clinical Manifestations: (a) red eye, proptosis, dilated episcleral vessels, increased intraocular pressure, pain, diplo-

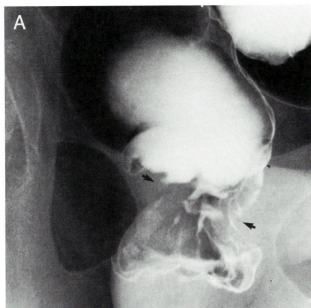

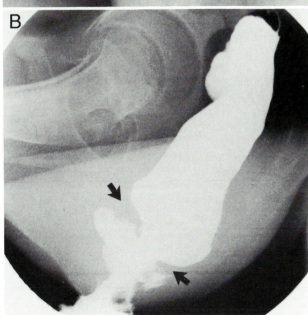

FIG SY—R—1.
Rectal ulcer syndrome in a 19-year-old man with a history of frequent defecation, straining, a sense of incomplete evacuation, and rectal bleeding. **A,** an anteroposterior radiograph shows circular narrowing of the distal portion of the rectum *(arrows).* **B,** during straining, defecography shows infoldings on the anterior and posterior rectal wall that form an intussusception *(arrows).* (From Goei R, Baeten C, Janevski B, et al.: The solitary rectal ulcer syndrome: Diagnosis with defecography. *A.J.R.* 149:933, 1987. Used by permission.)

pia, exophthalmos, limited eye motion; (b) noise in the head, bruit.

Radiologic Manifestations: (a) dilated superior ophthalmic vein (ultrasonography); (b) carotid-cavernous fistula.

REFERENCE

Phelps CD, et al.: The diagnosis and prognosis of atypical carotid-cavernous fistula (red-eyed shunt syndrome). *Am. J. Ophthalmol.* 93:423, 1982.

REFLEX SYMPATHETIC DYSTROPHY SYNDROME

Synonyms: Causalgia; Sudeck atrophy; alogoneurodystrophy (reflex sympathetic dystrophy after minor trauma); reflex dystrophy; reflex neurovascular dystrophy.

Etiologies and Associated Conditions: (a) trauma: fracture, sprain, laceration, contusion, crush injury, electrical or thermal burn, spinal cord injury, etc.; (b) postoperative: hip or knee surgery, ganglion excision, Dupuytren contracture repair, carpal tunnel decompression; (c) neurological disorders: head trauma, cerebrovascular accident, spinal cord disorders, myelography, peripheral nerve injury, peripheral nerve entrapment; (d) intrathoracic diseases: myocardial infarction (shoulder-hand syndrome), thoracic or cardiac surgery, infection; (e) other: cervical osteoarthritis, herpes zoster, neoplasm, metabolic bone disease, drugs, idiopathic (about 25% of cases), etc.

Clinical Manifestations: (a) pain, tenderness, hyperesthesia; (b) swelling with or without pitting edema; (c) dystrophic changes: atrophy, nail dystrophy, hypertrichosis, hyperhidrosis; (d) vasomotor changes: erythema, cyanosis, Raynaud phenomenon; (e) decreased hand/finger movement.

Radiologic Manifestations: Radiographic manifestations not evident for 1 to 2 months from the onset of symptoms: (a) *patchy osteopenia in the involved area,* best demonstrated by fine-detail radiography; (b) metaphyseal, subperiosteal, and subarticular radiolucent bands (bone resorption), subchondral bone erosion, juxta-articular erosions; (c) *decreased or increased uptake or radionuclide in the affected site (decreased or increased blood flow);* (d) variants of osteoporosis: radial type involving only one or two rays of the hand or foot; zonal type with an area of demineralization confined initially to a small segment of bone (femoral head, femoral condyle, etc.); (e) thermography: hypothermia in the majority of cases, hyperthermia in others.

Differential Diagnosis: Rheumatoid arthritis; tenosynovitis; sprain; malingering; etc.

Notes: (a) plain roentgenograms and bone scan results may be normal in the early stage of the disease; (b) the prognosis is usually better in children as compared with adults; (c)

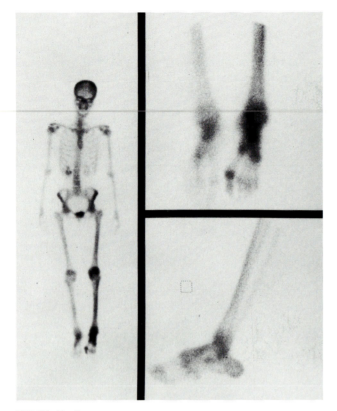

FIG SY–R–2.
Reflex sympathetic dystrophy in a 31-year-old woman who had severe left ankle pain for approximately 7 weeks after a twisting injury. A hyperemic response of reflex sympathetic dystrophy in the left lower extremity and involvement proximally to the left hemipelvis is present (2-hour whole-body image and spot views after the administration of 15 mCi of ^{99m}Tc methylene diphosphonate). Radiographs demonstrated severe bone demineralization in the left foot, tibia, and fibula. (From Heck LL: Recognition of atypical reflex sympathetic dystrophy. *Clin. Nucl. Med.* 12:925, 1987. Used by permission.)

three-phase radionuclide bone scanning is recommended; (d) chronic facial pain may represent a manifestation of reflex sympathetic dystrophy of the face. (e) 135 cases in the pediatric age group reported (Doury et al.) (Fig SY–R–2).

REFERENCES

Doury P, et al.: L'algodystrophie de l'enfant. *Ann. Pediatr. (Paris)* 35:469, 1988.
Genant HK, et al.: The reflex sympathetic dystrophic syndrome. *Radiology* 117:21, 1975.
Griffiths HJ, et al.: Juxta-articular erosions in reflex sympathetic dystrophy. *Acta Radiol.* 29:183, 1988.
Heck LL: Recognition of atypical reflex sympathetic dystrophy. *Clin. Nucl. Med.* 12:925, 1987.
Helms CA, et al.: Segmental reflex sympathetic dystrophy syndrome. *Radiology* 135:67, 1980.
Holder LE, et al.: Reflex sympathetic dystrophy in the hands: Clinical and scintigraphic criteria. *Radiology* 152:517, 1984.
Jaeger B, et al.: Reflex sympathetic dystrophy of the face. Report of two cases and a review of the literature. *Arch. Neurol.* 43:693, 1986.
Katz MM, et al.: Reflex sympathetic dystrophy affecting the knee. *J. Bone Joint Surg. [Br.]* 69:797, 1987.
Labenne M, et al.: L'algodystrophie, une affection peu connue chez l'enfant. Revue générale à propos de quatre cas. *Ann. Pediatr. (Paris)* 34:603, 1987.
Laxer RM, et al.: Technetium 99m–methylene diphosphonate bone scans in children with reflex neurovascular dystrophy. *J. Pediatr.* 106:437, 1985.
Lemahieu R-A, et al.: Reflex sympathetic dystrophy: An underreported syndrome in children? *Eur. J. Pediatr.* 147:47, 1988.
Lightman HI, et al.: Thermography in childhood reflex sympathetic dystrophy. *J. Pediatr.* 111:551, 1987.
Schwartzman RJ, et al.: Reflex sympathetic dystrophy. A review. *Arch. Neurol.* 44:555, 1987.
Smith DL, et al.: Reflex sympathetic dystrophy syndrome. Diagnosis and management. *West. J. Med.* 147:342, 1987.
Sudeck P: Ueber die akute entzündliche Knochenatrophie. *Arch. Klin. Chir. (Berlin)* 62:147, 1900.

REIFENSTEIN SYNDROME

Synonym: Hereditary familial hypogonadism.

Mode of Inheritance: Consistent with X-linked recessive inheritance.

Frequency: Rare.

Clinical Manifestations: (a) *hypospadias;* (b) *postpubertal testicular atrophy;* (c) *azoospermia and infertility;* (d) *weak or absent virilization;* (e) *gynecomastia;* (f) high excretion of follicle-stimulating hormone, normal level of 17-ketosteroids; (g) testicular biopsy: Leydig cell hyperplasia, atrophic seminiferous tubules, and interstitial fibrosis; spermatogenesis in some.

Radiologic Manifestations: (a) hypospadias; (b) prostatic utricle (in some).

REFERENCES

Bowen P, et al.: Hereditary male pseudohermaphroditism with hypogonadism, hypospadias and gynecomastia: Reifenstein's syndrome. *Ann. Intern. Med.* 62:252, 1965.
Flatau E, et al.: Response to LH-RH and HCG in two brothers with Reifenstein syndrome. *Helv. Paediatr. Acta* 30:377, 1975.
Jones LW, et al.: Reifenstein's syndrome: Hereditary familial hypogonadism with hypospadias and gynecomastia. *J. Urol.* 104:608, 1970.
Reifenstein EC Jr: Hereditary familial hypogonadism. *Proc. Am. Fed. Clin. Res.* 3:86, 1947.
Schweikert HU, et al.: Clinical and endocrinological characterization of two subjects with Reifenstein syndrome associated with qualitative abnormalities of the androgen receptor. *Horm. Res.* 25:72, 1987.

Wieacker P, et al.: Linkage analysis with RFLPs in families with androgen resistance syndromes: Evidence for close linkage between the androgen receptor locus and the DXS1 segment. *Hum. Genet.* 76:248, 1987.

REITER SYNDROME

Clinical Manifestations: (a) *urethritis;* (b) *arthritis;* (c) *conjunctivitis, iritis;* (d) *mucocutaneous lesions* (balanitis, keratodermia, buccal ulcerations, erythema, etc.); (e) diarrhea; (f) myocarditis, pericarditis, cardiac conduction abnormalities; (g) neuritis; (h) association with HLA-B27 antigen; (i) other reported manifestations: recurrent peritonitis, co-occurrence with acquired immunodeficiency, arthritis presumably caused by *Chlamydia* in Reiter syndrome.

Radiologic Manifestations: (a) *bone erosion and joint effusion* (heels, toes, and sacroiliac joints in particular), massive synovial hypertrophy; (b) *arthritis mutilans* of the feet; (c) tendonitis with *periostitis* of or adjacent to sites of tendon insertions (plantar surface of the calcaneus, the major site); (d) aortic insufficiency in some (late in the course of the disease) resulting from dilatation of the aortic valve ring, distal aortitis (aortic narrowing); (e) lateral vertebral hyperostosis with bridging around the cartilaginous disk, cervical spine involvement rare (anterior atlantoaxial dislocation, craniovertebral lesions typical for rheumatoid arthritis, spondylitis typical for ankylosing spondylitis, anterior ossification); (f) radionuclide imaging: increased focal uptake of ^{99m}Tc pyrophosphate.

REFERENCES

Calabro JJ, et al.: Reiter's syndrome in siblings. *J.A.M.A.* 238:2494, 1977.

Fiessinger N, Leroy E: Contribution à l'étude d'une épidémie de dysenterie dans la Somme (juillet-octobre 1916). *Bull. Mem. Soc. Med. Hop. (Paris)* 40:2030, 1916.

Finder JG, et al.: Massive synovial hypertrophy in Reiter's syndrome. A case report. *J. Bone Joint Surg. [Am.]* 65:555, 1983.

Ishikawa H, et al.: Arthritis presumably caused by *Chlamydia* in Reiter syndrome. Case report with electron microscopic studies. *J. Bone Joint Surg. [Am.]* 68:777, 1986.

Keat A: Reiter's syndrome and reactive arthritis in perspective. *N. Engl. J. Med.* 309:1606, 1983.

Khalkhali I, et al.: Bone imaging of the heel in Reiter's syndrome. *A.J.R.* 132:110, 1979.

Latchaw RE, et al.: Reiter disease with atlantoaxial subluxation. *Radiology* 126:303, 1978.

Martel W, et al.: Radiologic features of Reiter disease. *Radiology* 132:1, 1979.

Moisanen A, et al.: Cervical spine involvements in Reiter's syndrome. *Fortschr. Rontgenstr.* 141:84, 1984.

Morgan SH, et al.: Distal aortitis complicating Reiter's syndrome. *Br. Heart J.* 52:115, 1984.

Paulus HE, et al.: Aortic insufficiency in five patients with Reiter's syndrome. *Am. J. Med.* 53:464, 1972.

Reiter H: Ueber eine bisher unerkannte Spirochäteninfektion (Spirochätosis arthritica). *Dtsch. Med. Wochenschr.* 42:1535, 1916.

Resnick D, et al.: Calcaneal abnormalities in articular disorders. *Radiology* 125:355, 1977.

Rosenberg AM, et al.: Reiter's disease in children. *Am. J. Dis. Child.* 133:394, 1979.

Ruppert GB, et al.: Cardiac conduction abnormalities in Reiter's syndrome. *Am. J. Med.* 73:335, 1982.

Stadalnick RC, et al.: Sesamoid periostitis in the thumb in Reiter's syndrome. *J. Bone Joint. Surg. [Am.]* 57:279, 1975.

Sundaram M, et al.: Paravertebral ossification in psoriasis and Reiter's disease. *Br. J. Radiol.* 48:628, 1975.

Waelsch L: Üeber chronische, nicht gonorrhoische Urethritis. *Arch. Dermatol. Syph. (Berlin)* 123:1089, 1916.

Weisman LF, et al.: Reiter's syndrome and recurrent peritonitis after appendectomy. *Surgery* 101:508, 1987.

Winchester R, et al.: The co-occurrence of Reiter's syndrome and acquired immunodeficiency. *Ann. Intern. Med.* 106:19, 1987.

RELAPSING POLYCHONDRITIS

Synonyms: Polychondritis; polychondropathy.

Frequency: Over 400 published cases (Michet et al.).

Pathology: Segmental necrotizing glomerulonephritis; arteritis; vascular sclerosis; laminated subintimal fibroplasia; loss of basophilic staining of the cartilage; destruction of cartilage and replacement of cartilage by fibrous tissue.

Clinical Manifestations: (a) fever, anorexia, weight loss; (b) *auricular chondritis,* painful erythematous swelling of the external ear, cauliflower ear deformity, conductive deafness, neurosensory deafness due to inner ear involvement; (c) *arthralgia and arthritis* of large or small joints, tendinitis; (d) *chest pain due to costochondritis, hoarseness, cough, dyspnea, laryngeal and tracheal tenderness,* aphonia and airway obstruction due to edema, collapse of the trachea and cricoid rings, pulmonary function test abnormalities reflecting the upper airway obstruction; (e) *nasal chondritis,* swelling and tenderness, saddle nose deformity; (f) episcleritis, conjunctivitis, iritis, exophthalmos; (g) cardiovascular manifestations: myocarditis, dilatation of the cardiac valvular ring, aortic insufficiency; (h) cutaneous lesions; (i) antibodies to type II collagen; (j) nephropathy; (k) nervous system complications: confusion, disorientation, nystagmus, facial weakness, cerebral vasculitis.

Radiologic Manifestations: (a) *calcification of the external ear cartilage,* collapse of the cartilage of the nose; (b) *arthritis,* usually polyarthritis, with small and large joints involved; joint space narrowing; cartilage destruction; osseous erosions; "arthritis mutilans"; osteopenia; "periostitis" of the bones adjacent to involved joints; (c) cardiomegaly; aortic ring dilatation; aortic, mitral, and tricuspid insufficiency; aortic aneurysm; (d) severe chronic lung disease resulting from dissolution of the cartilaginous structure of air passages, deformity of the tracheobronchial tree, enlargement and irregularity of the cartilages of the larynx and tracheal rings,

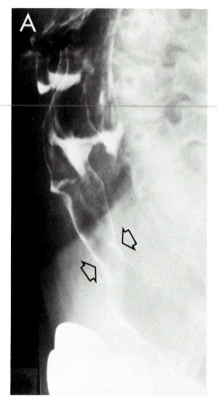

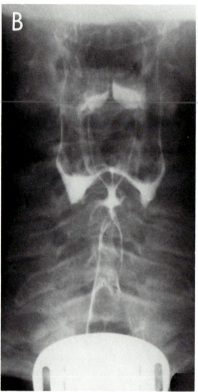

FIG SY–R–3.

A and **B,** relapsing polychondritis in a 35-year-old woman. A contrast laryngogram shows a short stenotic segment of the trachea *(arrows).* (From Kilman WJ: Narrowing of the airway in relapsing polychondritis. *Radiology* 126:373, 1978. Used by permission.)

edema, fibrosis, calcification; (e) ureteral obstruction due to association with retroperitoneal fibrosis.

Note: In the MAGIC (mouth and genital ulcers with inflamed cartilage) syndrome coexistence of the clinical features of relapsing polychondritis and Behçet syndrome have been reported (Figs SY–R–3 and SY–R–4).

REFERENCES

Blau EB: Relapsing polychondritis and retroperitoneal fibrosis in an 8-year old boy. *Am. J. Dis. Child.* 130:1149, 1976.

Braunstein EM, et al.: Radiological aspects of the arthropathy of relapsing polychondritis. *Clin. Radiol.* 30:441, 1979.

Casselman JW, et al.: Polychondritis affecting the laryngeal cartilages: CT findings. *A.J.R.* 150:355, 1988.

Chang-Miller A, et al.: Renal involvement in relapsing polychondritis. *Medicine (Baltimore)* 66:202, 1987.

Cipriano PR, et al.: Multiple aortic aneurysms in relapsing polychondritis. *Am. J. Cardiol.* 37:1097, 1976.

Firestein GS, et al.: Mouth and genital ulcers with inflamed cartilage: MAGIC syndrome. Five patients with features of relapsing polychondritis and Behçet's disease. *Am. J. Med.* 79:65, 1985.

Foidart JM, et al.: Antibodies to type II collagen in relapsing polychondritis. *N. Engl. J. Med.* 299:1203, 1978.

Gagnerie F, et al.: Exophtalmie au cours de la polychondrite atrophiante. Deux observations. *Presse Med.* 16:968, 1987.

Im JG, et al.: CT manifestations of tracheobronchial involvement in relapsing polychondritis. *J. Comput. Assist. Tomogr.* 12:792, 1988.

Jaksch-Wartenhorst R: Polychondropathia. *Wien Arch. Intern. Med.* 6:93, 1923.

Kilman WJ: Narrowing of the airway in relapsing polychondritis. *Radiology* 126:373, 1978.

Mendelson DS, et al.: Relapsing polychondritis studied by computed tomography. *Radiology* 157:489, 1985.

Michet CJ, et al.: Relapsing polychondritis. Survival and predictive role of early disease manifestations. *Ann. Intern. Med.* 104:74, 1986.

Mohsenifar Z, et al.: Pulmonary function in patients with relapsing polychondritis. *Chest* 81:711, 1982.

Rogers PH, et al.: Relapsing polychondritis with insulin resistance and antibodies to cartilage. *Am. J. Med.* 55:243, 1973.

Stewart SS, et al.: Cerebral vasculitis in relapsing polychondritis. *Neurology* 38:150, 1988.

Sundaram MBM, et al.: Nervous system complications of relapsing polychondritis. *Neurology* 33:513, 1983.

Treves R, et al.: Surdité totale au cours d'une polychondrite chronique atrophiante. *Nouv. Presse Med.* 8:1605, 1979.

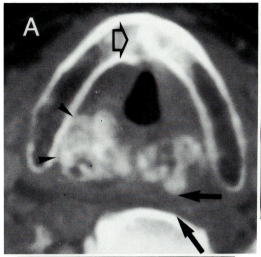

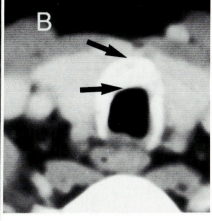

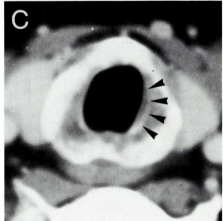

FIG SY–R–4.
Relapsing polychondritis. **A,** a computed tomographic (CT) scan at the level of the vocal cords shows both arytenoid cartilages being enlarged and irregular. The right arytenoid cartilage obliterates the space between the thyroid and arytenoid cartilages and makes contact with the thyroid cartilage *(arrowheads).* Arytenoid cartilages nearly touch in the midline. The left arytenoid cartilage compresses on the hypopharynx *(black arrows).* The anterior portion of the thyroid cartilage is also thickened *(open arrow),* and the vocal cords are swollen. **B,** a CT scan at the level of the first tracheal ring shows thickening of the tracheal ring, especially the anterior part *(black arrows).* There is no significant narrowing of the airway lumen at this level. **C,** a CT scan shows circumferential thickening of the cricoid cartilage and edema of the mucosa *(arrowheads).* (From Casselman JW, Lehmahieu SF, Peene P, et al.: Polychondritis affecting the laryngeal cartilage: CT findings. *A.J.R.* 150:355, 1988. Used by permission.)

RENAL, GENITAL, AND EAR ANOMALIES

Frequency: Three families (King et al.).

Clinical Manifestations: (a) *vaginal atresia;* (b) *abnormal pinna, low-set ears, stenosis of the external auditory canal, mild deafness;* (c) other reported abnormalities: lacrimal duct obstruction, myopia, beaked nose, micrognathia, maxillary hypoplasia, crowded teeth, atrial septal defect, abnormal dermatoglyphics, hypoplastic areolae, umbilical hernia, hydrocephalus, anteriorly placed stenotic rectum, etc.

Radiologic Manifestations: (a) *renal anomalies:* agenesis, dysgenesis; (b) *middle ear:* malformed ossicles; (c) *skeletal anomalies:* clinodactyly, short fourth metacarpals, congenital separation of the pubic symphysis, spina bifida occulta.

REFERENCES

King LA, et al.: Syndrome of genital, renal, and middle ear anomalies: A third family and report of a pregnancy. *Obstet. Gynecol.* 69:491, 1987.

Turner G: A second family with renal, vaginal, and middle ear anomalies. *J. Pediatr.* 76:641, 1970.

Winter JD, et al.: A familial syndrome of renal, genital, and middle ear anomalies. *J. Pediatr.* 72:88, 1968.

RENAL-HEPATIC-PANCREATIC DYSPLASIA

Clinical, Pathological, and Radiologic Manifestations: (a) renal malformations: cystic dysplasia, abnormally differentiated ducts, deficient nephron differentiation, renal insufficiency; (b) hepatic malformations: enlarged portal areas containing numerous elongated biliary "profiles," perilobular fibrosis, cholestasis, intrahepatic ductal dilatation, chronic jaundice; (c) pancreatic anomalies: fibrosis, cysts, diminution of parenchymal tissue, insulin-dependent diabetes mellitus; (c) death: neonatal or in the first year of life.

REFERENCES

Bernstein J, et al.: Renal-hepatic-pancreatic dysplasia: A syndrome reconsidered. *Am. J. Med. Genet.* 26:391, 1987.
Ivemark BI, et al.: Familial dysplasia of kidneys, liver and pancreas. A probably genetically determined syndrome. *Acta Paediatr. Scand.* 48:1, 1959.

RENDU-OSLER-WEBER SYNDROME

Synonyms: Hereditary hemorrhagic telangiectasia; Osler-Weber-Rendu disease; Osler disease.

Mode of Inheritance: Autosomal dominant.

Frequency: Uncommon.

Pathology: (a) *skin telangiectases;* (b) *mucous membrane: telangiectases, arteriovenous malformations;* (c) *pulmonary arteriovenous fistulas (in about 50% of patients);* (d) *central nervous system: telangiectases, arteriovenous malformations, aneurysms;* (e) *hepatic fibrotic arteriovenous malformations, systemic arteriovenous shunts, hepatic artery–portal vein shunts, intrahepatic portosystem shunts;* (f) *retinal telangiectases.*

Clinical Manifestations: (a) *skin telangiectasis;* (b) *epistaxis,* hematuria, upper and lower alimentary tract hemorrhage (endoscopic demonstration), hemoptysis, hemothorax, intracranial hemorrhage, intraocular hemorrhage; (c) *symptoms related to pulmonary arteriovenous fistulas:* dyspnea, cyanosis, clubbing, extracardiac murmur, hypoxemia, polycythemia, secondary cerebral ischemia, paradoxical cerebral embolism, brain abscess; (d) seizures, motor/sensory deficit; (e) hepatomegaly, hepatic bruit; (f) high output failure due to hyperdynamic circulation; (g) portal hypertension, portosystemic encephalopathy due to intrahepatic portosystemic shunts.

Radiologic Manifestations: (a) angiographic demonstration of *angiodysplasias:* aneurysms, arteriovenous communications, conglomerate masses of angiectasia, capillary angiodysplasic lesions, phlebectasia, angiomas; (b) liver imaging: dilated hepatic artery, multiple arteriovenous malformations, abnormal echogenicity of the liver.

Notes: (a) a pair of identical twins with hereditary hemorrhagic telangiectasia concordant with cerebrovascular arteriovenous malformations has been reported; (b) among the etiologic factors in young persons with stroke, hereditary hemorrhagic telangiectasia should be considered and its manifestations sought (Figs SY–R–5 and SY–R–6).

REFERENCES

Babington BG: Hereditary epistaxis. *Lancet* 2:362, 1865.
Cloogman HM, et al.: Hereditary hemorrhagic telangiectasia: Sonographic findings in the liver. *Radiology* 150:521, 1984.
Cynamon HA, et al.: Multiple telangiectases of the colon in childhood. *J. Pediatr.* 112:928, 1988.
Daly JJ, et al.: The liver in hereditary hemorrhagic telangiectasia (Osler-Weber-Rendu disease). *Am. J. Med.* 60:723, 1976.
Danchin N, et al.: Osler-Weber-Rendu disease with multiple intrahepatic arteriovenous fistulas. *Am. Heart J.* 105:856, 1983.
Halpern M, et al.: Hereditary hemorrhagic telangiectasia: An angiographic study of abdominal visceral angiodysplasias associated with gastrointestinal hemorrhage. *Radiology* 90:1143, 1968.
Legg JW: A case of haemophilia complicated with multiple naevi. *Lancet* 2:856, 1876.
Lesser BA, et al.: Identical twins with hereditary hemorrhagic telangiectasia. Concordant for cerebrovascular arteriovenous malformations. *Am. J. Med.* 81:931, 1986.
McCue CM, et al.: Pulmonary arteriovenous malformations related to Rendu-Osler-Weber syndrome. *Am. J. Med. Genet.* 19:19, 1984.
Mirra JM, et al.: Skeletal hemangiomatosis in association with hereditary hemorrhagic telangiectasia. *J. Bone Joint Surg. [Am.]* 55:850, 1973.
Osler W: On a family form of recurring epistaxis, associated with multiple telangiectasis of skin and mucous membranes. *Bull. Johns Hopkins Hosp.* 12:333, 1901.
Peery WH: Clinical spectrum of hereditary hemorrhagic telangiectasia (Osler-Weber-Rendu disease). *Am. J. Med.* 82:989, 1987.
Pillon B, et al.: Aspects angiographiques et possibilités de l'angiographie thérapeutique dans les localisations digestives de la maladie de Rendu-Osler. *Ann. Radiol. (Paris)* 24:551, 1981.
Radtke WE, et al.: Misdiagnosis of atrial septal defect in patients with hereditary telangiectasia (Osler-Weber-Rendu disease) and hepatic arteriovenous fistulas. *Am. Heart J.* 95:235, 1978.
Rendu M: Epistaxis repétées chez un sujet porteur de petits angiomes cutanés et muqueux. *Bull. Mem. Soc. Med. Hop. (Paris)* 13:731, 1896.
Weber FP: Multiple hereditary developmental angiomata (telangiectases) of the skin and mucous membranes associated with recurring hemorrhages. *Lancet* 2:160, 1907.

RESPIRATORY DISTRESS SYNDROME

Synonyms: RDS; hyaline membrane disease.

Pathophysiology: Pulmonary immaturity: surfactant deficiency; highly compliant chest wall, pulmonary overperfusion (left-to-right shunting through the ductus arteriosus).

Clinical Manifestations: Symptoms developing soon after birth: tachypnea, grunting, cyanosis in room air, chest retraction, abdominal protrusion.

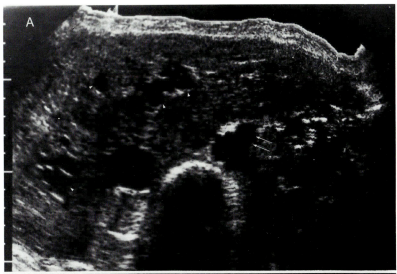

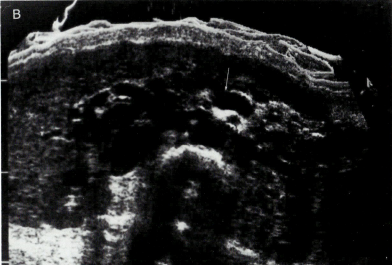

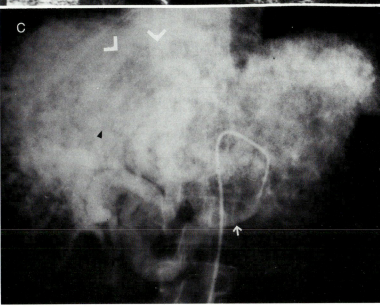

FIG SY−R−5.
Rendu-Osler-Weber syndrome. **A,** a transverse scan of the upper portion of the abdomen shows a prominent celiac axis originating from the aorta *(arrows)*. Multiple arteriovenous malformations are present in the liver *(arrowheads)*. **B,** a transverse scan through the porta hepatis with multiple prominent vascular structures mimicks dilated biliary ducts. An enlarged common hepatic artery is present *(arrow)* along with an incidental right renal cyst *(arrowhead)*. **C,** arterial phase of a hepatic arteriogram. An enlarged hepatic artery *(arrow)*, numerous arteriovenous malformations *(arrowhead)*, and early draining hepatic veins *(V)* are confirmed. (From Cloogman HM, DiCapo RD: Hereditary hemorrhagic telangiectasis: Sonographic findings in the liver. *Radiology* 150:521, 1984. Used by permission.)

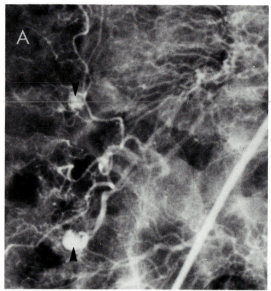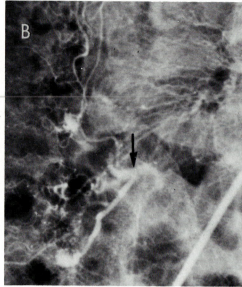

FIG SY−R−6.
Rendu-Osler-Weber syndrome: angiectatic arteriovenous dysplasia. **A,** arterial phase *(arrowheads);* arterial angiectatic masses. **B,** early opacification of dense draining veins *(arrow).* (From Halpern M, Turner AF, Citron BP, : Hereditary hemorrhagic telangiectasia:

An angiographic study of abdominal visceral angiodysplasias associated with gastrointestinal hemorrhage. *Radiology* 90:1143, 1968. Used by permission.)

Radiologic Manifestations: (a) *fine reticulogranular pattern of the lung;* (b) *air bronchogram caused by peribronchial atelectasis, alveolar opacification;* (c) findings may be minimal to severe (total lung opacification), generalized or localized in distribution, symmetrical or asymmetrical.

REFERENCES

Ablow RC, et al.: Localized roentgenographic pattern of hyaline membrane disease. *A.J.R.* 112:23, 1971.
Bertrand J-M, et al.: The long-term pulmonary sequelae of prematurity: The role of familial airway hyperreactivity and the respiratory distress syndrome. *N. Engl. J. Med.* 312:742, 1985.
Giedion A, et al.: Acute pulmonary x-ray changes in hyaline membrane disease treated with artificial ventilation and positive end-expiratory pressure (PEEP). *Pediatr. Radiol.* 1:145, 1973.
Isdale JM, et al.: The value of radiography in the initial grading of the idiopathic respiratory distress syndrome. *S. Afr. Med. J.* 56:707, 1979.
Singleton EB: Respiratory distress syndrome, in Kaufmann HJ (ed.): *Progress in Pediatric Radiology* Basel, S. Karger AG, 1967, vol. 1, p. 109.
Stark AR, et al.: Respiratory distress syndrome. *Pediatr. Clin. North Am.* 33:533, 1986.
Tchou CS, et al.: Asymmetric distribution of the roentgen pattern in hyaline membrane disease. *J. Can. Assoc. Radiol.* 23:85, 1972.
Tudor L, et al.: The value of radiology in the idiopathic respiratory distress syndrome: A radiological and pathological correlation study. *Clin. Radiol.* 27:65, 1976.

RETT SYNDROME

Mode of Inheritance: Rare familial cases: maternal cousins, half-sisters with the same mother, in one of dizygotic twins, monozygotic twins; occurring only in girls.

Pathology: Brain biopsy: white matter disease, many neurons and oligodendroglia containing membrane-bound electron-dense inclusions with a distinct lamellar and granular substructure.

Clinical Manifestations: (a) *normal prenatal and perinatal period; normal psychomotor development through the first 6 months of life;* (b) *normal head size at birth, deceleration of head growth;* (c) *deterioration of higher brain function:* loss of purposeful hand skills, severely impaired expressive and receptive language, apparent mental retardation; (d) other reported abnormalities: autism, seizures, breathing dysfunction, spasticity, choreoathetosis, lactic acidemia, growth retardation, scoliosis, renovascular hypertension; (e) electroencephalography: *slowing and disorganization of background activity while awake, multifocal epileptiform discharges, intermittent high-amplitude discharges during sleep.*

Radiologic Manifestations: (a) cerebral atrophy in some cases; (b) abnormal positron-emission tomographic scan results of the brain (decreased metabolic activity in some areas).

REFERENCES

Al-Mateen M, et al.: Rett syndrome. A commonly overlooked progressive encephalopathy in girls. *Am. J. Dis. Child.* 140:761, 1986.

Keret D, et al.: Scoliosis in Rett syndrome. *J. Pediatr. Orthop.* 8:138, 1988.

Moeschler JB, et al.: Rett syndrome: Natural history and management. *Pediatrics* 82:1, 1988.

Naidu S, et al.: Rett syndrome: Positron emission tomography metabolic-clinical correlates (abstract). *Ann. Neurol.* 24:305, 1988.

Oldfors A, et al.: Rett syndrome: Spinal cord neuropathology. *Pediatr. Neurol.* 4:172, 1988.

Papadimitriou JM, et al.: Rett syndrome: Abnormal membrane-bound lamellated inclusions in neurons and oligodendroglia. *Am. J. Med. Genet.* 29:365, 1988.

Partington MW: Rett syndrome in monozygotic twins. *Am. J. Med. Genet.* 29:633, 1988.

The Rett syndrome diagnostic criteria work group: Diagnostic criteria for Rett syndrome. *Ann. Neurol.* 23:425, 1988.

Trauner DA, et al.: Electroencephalographic abnormalities in Rett syndrome. *Pediatr. Neurol.* 3:331, 1987.

Uhari M, et al.: Renovascular hypertension in a child with Rett's syndrome. *Acta Paediatr. Scand.* 76:372, 1987.

REYE SYNDROME

Clinical Manifestations: (a) *history of recent viral infection or "upper respiratory tract infection"*; (b) *vomiting*; (c) *encephalopathy*: marked cerebral edema, delirium, seizures, hyperpnea, irregular deep respiration, decerebrate posturing, increased intracranial pressure, normocellular and sterile cerebrospinal fluid (CSF), normal CSF protein levels, coma; (d) *hepatomegaly, acute liver failure, abnormal liver function test results;* (e) hematologic and metabolic abnormalities: increased leukocyte count, ammonia, serum aminotransferases, prothrombine time, creatine phosphokinase, serum short- and medium-chain fatty acids, aminoacids (lysine, glutamine, alanine, α-amino-*N*-butyrate), lactic acid, uric acid, blood urea nitrogen, amylase, CSF glutamine and catecholamine; decreased serum and CSF glucose levels and serum C1 and C1s complement activity; respiratory alkalosis; metabolic acidosis; (f) acute renal failure; (g) acute pancreatitis; (h) fatty degeneration of the liver and other viscera; (i) central retinal vein occlusion.

Radiologic Manifestations: (a) *cerebral edema* presenting as a low density in deep white matter with subcortical sparing, effacement of sulci and compression of the ventricles; (b) *brain atrophy*, predominantly in the frontal lobe in the chronic phase; (c) *fatty liver*.

Differential Diagnosis: Inborn errors of metabolism with "Reye syndrome–like" presentation (Green et al.).

Notes: (a) the cause of Reye syndrome is uncertain; the role of viral infection, aspirin, and genetic predisposition is not definitely known; (b) in grade 1 Reye syndrome, there is milder neurological involvement; the presenting manifestations may be vomiting and liver dysfunction; (c) liver biopsy has been considered to be necessary for an accurate diagnosis and exclusion of other causes of acute encephalopathy.

REFERENCES

Atkins JN, et al.: Reye's syndrome in the adult patient. *Am. J. Med.* 67:672, 1979.

Baliga R, et al.: Acute renal failure in Reye's syndrome. *Am. J. Dis. Child.* 133:1009, 1979.

Chu AB, et al.: Reye's syndrome. Salicylate metabolism, viral antibody levels, and other factors in surviving patients and unaffected family members. *Am. J. Dis. Child.* 140:1009, 1986.

Daniels SR, et al.: Scientific uncertainties in the studies of salicylate use and Reye's syndrome. *J.A.M.A.* 249:1311, 1983.

Edwards KM, et al.: Reye's syndrome associated with adenovirus infections in infants. *Am. J. Dis. Child.* 139:343, 1985.

Ellis GH, et al.: Pancreatitis and Reye's syndrome. *Am. J. Dis. Child.* 133:1014, 1979.

Faraj BA, et al.: Hypercatecholaminemia in Reye's syndrome. *Pediatrics* 73:481, 1984.

Green CL, et al.: Inborn errors of metabolism and Reye syndrome: Differential diagnosis. *J. Pediatr.* 113:156, 1988.

Heubi JE, et al.: Grade I Reye's syndrome—Outcome and predictors of progression to deeper coma grades. *N. Engl. J. Med.* 311:1539, 1984.

Kimura A, et al.: Necessity of liver biopsy for accurate diagnosis of Reye's syndrome. *J. Pediatr. Gastroenterol. Nutr.* 6:153, 1987.

Lichtenstein PK, et al.: Grade I Reye's syndrome. A frequent cause of vomiting and liver dysfunction after varicella and upper-respiratory-tract infection. *N. Engl. J. Med.* 309:133, 1983.

Meythaler JM, et al.: Reye's syndrome in adults. Diagnostic considerations. *Arch. Intern. Med.* 147:61, 1987.

Pollack JD: *Reye's syndrome, Proceedings.* New York, Grune & Stratton, 1975.

Reye RDK, et al.: Encephalopathy and fatty degeneration of the viscera: A disease entity in childhood. *Lancet* 2:749, 1963.

Ruskin JA, et al.: CT findings in adult Reye syndrome. *A.J.N.R.* 6:446, 1985.

Shimizu M, et al.: Ultrasonically undetectable fatty liver in acute fatty liver of pregnancy and Reye's syndrome. *J. Clin. Ultrasound* 13:679, 1985.

Smith P, et al.: Central retinal vein occlusion in Reye's syndrome. *Arch. Ophthalmol.* 98:1256, 1980.

Trauner DA: Reye's syndrome. *West. J. Med.* 141:206, 1984.

Volk DM: Reye's syndrome. An update for the practicing physician. *Clin. Pediatr. (Phila.)* 20:505, 1981.

RICHTER SYNDROME

Definition: Development of histiocytic lymphoma with generalized manifestations in a patient with chronic lymphocytic leukemia.

Frequency: Occurrence in 3% to 10% of patients with chronic lymphocytic leukemia (Cohen et al.).

Clinical Manifestations: Abrupt onset of symptoms: (a) fever, increasing lymphadenopathy, weight loss, abdominal pain; (b) progression of hepatosplenomegaly; (c) fulminant illness, death usually in 2 to 6 months.

Radiologic Manifestations: (a) marked lymphadenopathy; (b) hepatosplenomegaly, focal low-density (computed tomography) lesions within the liver; (c) lytic bone lesions.

REFERENCES

Cohen LM, et al.: CT manifestations of Richter syndrome. *J. Comput. Assist. Tomogr.* 11:1007, 1987.
Heslop HE, et al.: Sustained complete remission in Richter's syndrome. *Cancer* 59:1036, 1987.
Olson M, et al.: CT characteristics of a hyperdense renal mass due to Richter syndrome. *J. Comput. Assist. Tomogr.* 12:669, 1988.
Suster S, et al.: A reappraisal of Richter's syndrome. Development of two phenotypically distinctive cell lines in a case of chronic lymphocytic leukemia. *Cancer* 59:1412, 1987.
Trump DL, et al.: Richter's syndrome: Diffuse histiocytic lymphoma in patients with chronic lymphocytic leukemia. A report of five cases and review of the literature. *Am. J. Med.* 68:539, 1980.

RIEGER SYNDROME

Synonym: Iris-dental dysplasia syndrome.

Mode of Inheritance: Autosomal dominant with almost complete penetrance and variability in expression.

Frequency: Rare.

Clinical Manifestations: (a) facial features: underdeveloped maxilla, relative prognathism, protruding lower lip, broad and flat nasal root, mild telecanthus with or without hypertelorism; (b) eye *abnormalities: aniridia or hypoplastic iris,* bands of iris stroma, iris coloboma, glaucoma, ectopic pupil, anterior polar cataracts, optic atrophy, microcornea or megalocornea, deep anterior chamber, strabismus, pseudohypertelorism; (c) other reported abnormalities: myotonic dystrophy, muscular dystrophy, growth hormone deficiency; (d) periumbilical skin projection (75% of cases), exomphalos; (e) chromosomal abnormalities: interstitial deletion 4q, partial monosomy 21q22.2, partial deletion of the short arm of chromosome 10, etc.

Radiologic Manifestations: (a) *tooth abnormalities:* hypodontia, microdontia, peg- or conical-shaped teeth, malocclusion; (b) dysgnathia: hypoplasia of the maxilla, relative prominence of the mandible; (c) associated reported abnormalities: arachnodactyly, polydactyly, scoliosis, kyphosis, cardiac malformations, hydrocephalus, syringomyelia, imper-

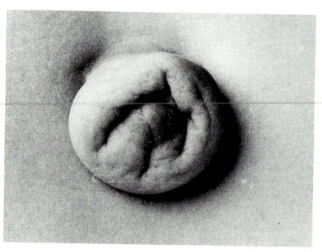

FIG SY−R−7.
Rieger syndrome: umbilicus of a child with a characteristic projection of the periumbilical skin. (From Reddihough DS, Rogers JG, Keith CG: Rieger syndrome with exomphalos. *Aust. Pediatr. J.* 18:130, 1982. Used by permission.)

forate anus, umbilical hernia, hip dislocation, brachydactyly, clinodactyly, partial absence of the facial bones, empty sella, peripheral pulmonary hypoplasia, Meckel diverticulum, etc. (Fig SY−R−7).

REFERENCES

Feingold M, et al.: Rieger's syndrome. *Pediatrics* 44:564, 1969.
Hervé J, et al.: Monosomie partielle du bras court d'un chromosome 10, associée a un syndrome de Rieger et a un deficit immunitaire partiel, type di George. *Ann. Pediatr. (Paris)* 31:77, 1984.
Judisch GF, et al.: Rieger's syndrome—A case report with a 15-year follow-up. *Arch. Ophthalmol.* 97:2120, 1979.
Langdon JD, Rieger's syndrome. *Oral Surg.* 30:788, 1970.
Ligutić I, et al.: Interstitial deletion 4q and Rieger syndrome. *Clin. Genet.* 20:323, 1981.
Nielsen F, et al.: A case of partial monosomy 21q22.2 associated with Rieger's syndrome. *J. Med. Genet.* 21:218, 1984.
Reddihough DS, et al.: Rieger syndrome with exomphalos. *Aust. Paediatr. J.* 18:130, 1982.
Rieger H: Beiträge zur Kenntnis seltener Missbildungen der Iris.; über Hypoplasie des Irisvorderblattes mit Verlagerung und Entrundung der Pupille. *Arch. F. Ophthalmol.* 133:602, 1935.
Sadeghi-Nejad A, et al.: Autosomal dominant transmission of isolated growth hormone deficiency in iris-dental dysplasia (Rieger's syndrome). *J. Pediatr.* 85:644, 1974.
Wolpert SM: Empty sella and Rieger's anomaly. *N. Engl. J. Med.* 304:1177, 1981.

RIGHT MIDDLE LOBE SYNDROME

Pathology: (a) bronchial obstruction; (b) chronic inflammation, pneumonia, bronchiectasis.

Clinical Manifestations: (a) cough, wheezing, recurrent pneumonia; (b) bronchial narrowing may be detectable on endoscopy.

Radiologic Manifestations: (a) *total or partial atelectasis of the right middle lobe;* (b) bronchography may or may not reveal the presence of bronchial narrowing.

REFERENCES

Culiner MM: The right middle lobe syndrome: Non-obstructive complex. *Dis. Chest* 50:57, 1966.

Early GL, et al.: Right middle lobe syndrome due to an endobronchial angiofibroma. *Arch. Intern. Med.* 143:560, 1983.

Graham EA, et al.: "Middle lobe syndrome." *Postgrad. Med.* 4:29, 1948.

Khoury MB, et al.: CT of obstructive lobar collapse. *Invest. Radiol.* 20:708, 1985.

Lindskog GE, et al.: Middle lobe syndrome. *N. Engl. J. Med.* 253:489, 1955.

Rosenbloom SA, et al.: Peripheral middle lobe syndrome. *Radiology* 149:17, 1983.

Saterfiel JL, et al.: Computed tomography of combined right upper and middle lobe collapse. *J. Comput. Assist. Tomogr.* 12:383, 1988.

RIGID SPINE SYNDROME

Frequency: Rare.

Clinical Manifestations: (a) restricted spinal flexion, overextended spine, fibrous shortening of the extensor muscles; (b) reduced muscle size; (c) loss of adipose tissue; (d) myopathic pattern on electromyographic examination; (e) elevated serum creatine phosphokinase level; (f) muscle biopsy: variation in fiber size; (g) other reported abnormalities: joint contractures, scoliosis, restrictive respiratory insufficiency with reduced vital capacity, fatal cardiomyopathy (hypertrophy of the interventricular septum and posterior left ventricular wall).

Radiologic Manifestations: Progressive limitation of flexion and extension of the cervical spine, wide separation of the laminae of C_1 and C_2 with the cervical spine in a neutral position ("alligator sign"—referring to the shape of the alligator's open mouth).

Differential Diagnosis: Congenital muscular dystrophies, Emery-Dreifuss myopathy; myosclerosis.

Note: It has been suggested that this syndrome may be an X-linked disorder and possibly related to Emery-Dreifuss muscular dystrophy (Wettstein et al.).

REFERENCES

Dubowitz V: Rigid spine syndrome: A muscle syndrome in search of a name. *Proc. R. Soc. Med.* 66:219, 1973.

Echenne B, et al.: Congenital muscular dystrophy and rigid spine syndrome. *Neuropediatrics* 14:97, 1983.

Emery AE, et al.: Unusual type of benign X-linked muscular dystrophy. *J. Neurol. Neurosurg. Psychiatry* 29:338, 1966.

Giannini S, et al.: Surgical correction of cervical hyperextension in rigid spine syndrome. *Neuropediatrics* 19:105, 1988.

Serratrice G, et al.: Le syndrome de la colonne vertébrale rigide et ses frontières nosologiques. Deux observations. *Presse Med.* 13:1129, 1984.

Tariieu M, et al.: Syndrome de la colonne raide. Aspect d'hypotrophie et prédominance des fibres musculaires de type 1. *Arch. Fr. Pediatr.* 43:115, 1986.

Wettstein A, et al.: Rigid spine-syndrom. *Verh. Dtsch. Ges. Neurol.* 2:812, 1983.

RILEY-DAY SYNDROME

Synonym: Familial dysautonomia.

Mode of Inheritance: Autosomal recessive; most cases in Ashkenazi Jews.

Frequency: 27/100,000 in Israel 1977 to 1981 (Maayan, et al.).

Clinical Manifestations: (a) *dysautonomia* manifested by (1) fever; (2) skin blotching; (3) excessive sweating; (4) cool extremities; (5) reduced pain and taste sensation; (6) hypolacrimation; (7) corneal hypoesthesia and corneal ulceration; (8) episodic vomiting; (9) episodic hypertension and postural hypotension; (10) difficulty in swallowing, regurgitation, structural abnormalities of the myenteric (Auerbach) plexus demonstrated by a flat-mount preparation of the esophagus and stomach; (11) diminished gag reflex; (b) *motor incoordination;* (c) *emotional lability;* (d) absence of fungiform papillae of the tongue; (e) recurrent pneumonia, pulmonary function abnormalities (reduced diffusion, lung restriction, resting hypoxemia, arterial oxygen desaturation with exercise, marked irregularity of the breathing pattern during sleep, etc.); (f) obstetric problems (Axelrod et al.): meconium staining (36%), breech presentation (31%), variable decelerations (29%), premature rupture of membranes (29%), fetal bradycardia (15%), Apgar score $\leq$7 (5 minutes) (13%), cesarean section (19%), low vacuum extraction (6%); (g) neonatal problems: poor or no suck reflex (62%), hypotonia (32%), hypothermia (26%), aspiration (20%), lethargy (14%), respiratory distress (14%), pneumothorax (12%), difficulty initiating respirations (10%), necrotizing enterocolitis (4%), hyperthermia (2%), arrhythmia (2%), apnea (2%); (h) histamine test very important in suspected neonatal cases; (i) other reported abnormalities: short stature, mental retardation, loss of the histamine flare response, myocardial infarction, subarachnoid hemorrhage, uremia, unexplained sudden death, bilateral lack of induced vestibular response to the caloric test, recurrent osteomyelitis, drooling of saliva, loss of deep tendon reflexes, ataxia, convulsions, breath-holding spells, frequency of urination, symmetrical degeneration of the fasciculus interfascicularis in the dorsal aspect of the spinal tract and sparsity of myelinated fibers in the dorsal roots, associated with congenital megacolon and sural nerve axonal degeneration in a non-Jewish girl, etc.

Radiologic Manifestations: (a) *swallowing difficulty*: incoordination in deglutition and closure of the larynx resulting in tracheal aspiration, delayed relaxation of the cricopharyngeus; (b) *incoordination between the esophageal peristaltic wave and the lower esophageal sphincter*, dilatation and atonicity of the esophagus, poor emptying of the esophagus in the horizontal position; (c) small-bowel distension, megacolon; (d) retarded skeletal maturation; (e) recurrent pneumonia; (f) other reported abnormalities: kyphoscoliosis, increased incidence of fractures and aseptic necrosis, neuropathic knee joint, hip dislocation, pes cavus, microcephaly, hydrocephalus, craniofacial disproportion (small face), congenital heart disease, irregular pulmonary aeration, interstitial fibrosis, peribronchial thickening, atelectasis.

REFERENCES

Ariel I: Structural abnormalities of the myenteric (Auerbach's) plexus in familial dysautonomia (Riley-Day syndrome) as demonstrated by flat-mount preparation of the esophagus and stomach. *Pediatr. Pathol.* 4:89, 1985.

Axelrod FB, et al.: Neonatal recognition of familial dysautonomia. *J. Pediatr.* 110:946, 1987.

Axelrod FB, et al.: Progressive sensory loss in familial dysautonomia. *Pediatrics* 67:517, 1981.

Azizi E, et al.: Congenital megacolon associated with familial dysautonomia. *Eur. J. Pediatr.* 142:68, 1984.

Clayson D, et al.: Personality development and familial dysautonomia. *Pediatrics* 65:269, 1980.

Fishbein D, et al.: Pulmonary manifestations of familial dysautonomia in an adult. *Am. J. Med.* 80:709, 1986.

Grünebaum M: Radiological manifestations in familial dysautonomia. *Am. J. Dis. Child.* 128:176, 1974.

Grünebaum M: The "chest-abdomen sign" in familial dysautonomia. *Br. J. Radiol.* 48:23, 1975.

Guzzetta F, et al.: Familial dysautonomia in a non-Jewish girl, with histological evidence of progression in the sural nerve. *Dev. Med. Child. Neurol.* 28:62, 1986.

Gyepes MT, et al.: Familial dysautonomia: The mechanism of aspiration. *Radiology* 91:471, 1968.

Kaplan M, et al.: Diagnosis of familial dysautonomia in the neonatal period. *Acta Paediatr. Scand.* 74:131, 1985.

Kirkpatrick RH, et al.: Roentgenographic findings in familial dysautonomia. *Radiology* 68:654, 1957.

Klebanoff MA, et al.: Familial dysautonomia associated with recurrent osteomyelitis in a non-Jewish girl. *J. Pediatr.* 96:75, 1980.

Maayan CH, et al.: Incidence of familial dysautonomia in Israel 1977–1981. *Clin. Genet.* 32:106, 1987.

Mitnick JS, et al.: Aseptic necrosis in familial dysautonomia. *Radiology* 142:89, 1982.

Reshef R, et al.: Myocardial infarction associated with the Riley-Day syndrome. *Am. Heart J.* 94:486, 1977.

Riley CM, Day RL, et al.: Central autonomic dysfunction with defective lacrimation: Report of five cases. *Pediatrics* 3:468, 1949.

Siggers DC, et al.: Vestibular dysfunction in familial dysautonomia (The Riley-Day syndrome). *Arch. Dis. Child.* 50:890, 1975.

Yoslow W, et al.: Orthopedic defects in familial dysautonomia: A review of sixty-five cases. *J. Bone Joint Surg. [Am.]* 53:1541, 1971.

Ziegler MG: Deficient sympathetic nervous response in familial dysautonomia. *N. Engl. J. Med.* 294:630, 1976.

RILEY-SMITH SYNDROME

Synonym: Macrocephaly-pseudopapilledema-hemangiomata syndrome.

Mode of Inheritance: Probably autosomal dominant.

Clinical Manifestations: (a) *macrocephaly* (present at birth); (b) *pseudopapilledema*; (c) *multiple hemangiomas*; (d) normal vision and intelligence; (e) recurrent respiratory infections with chronic lung manifestations.

Radiologic Manifestations: (a) *macrocrania*; (b) increased thickness of the cranial bones; (c) *normal pneumoencephalogram* (performed in one patient).

Note: Since this syndrome, Bannayan syndrome, and Ruvalcaba-Myhre-Smith (Ruvalcaba-Myhre) syndrome share several important features, the name of "macrocephaly, hamartomas and papilledema syndrome" has been proposed to include all the above as a single entity (Dvir et al.).

REFERENCES

Dvir M, et al.: Heredofamilial syndrome of mesodermal hamartomas, macrocephaly, and pseudopapilledema. *Pediatrics* 81:287, 1988.

Riley HD Jr, Smith WR: Macrocephaly, pseudopapilledema and multiple hemangiomata: A previously undescribed heredofamilial syndrome. *Pediatrics* 26:293, 1960.

ROBERTS SYNDROME

Synonyms: Appelt-Gerken-Lenz syndrome; cleft lip/palate and tetraphocomelia; tetraphocomelia–cleft palate syndrome; SC–phocomelia syndrome; pseudothalidomide syndrome.

Mode of Inheritance: Autosomal recessive.

Frequency: Rare.

Clinical and Radiologic Manifestations: (a) *low birth weight*; (b) *facial dysmorphism*: ocular hypertelorism, hypoplastic nasal alae, bilateral cleft lip/palate and protrusion of the intermaxillary portion of the upper jaw, abnormal pinnae, micrognathia; (c) exophthalmos, cataracts, corneal opacity, colobomas of the eyelids; (d) *limb anomalies*: phocomelia, oligodactyly, flexion contractions; (e) *genital anomalies*: prominence of the phallus, cryptorchidism, enlarged clitoris, enlarged labia minora, cleft labia minora, septate vagina, hypospadias; (f) other reported abnormalities: psychomotor re-

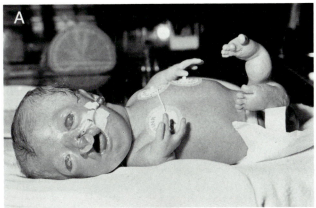

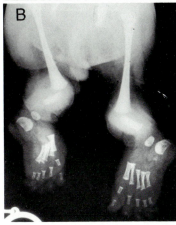

FIG SY—R—8.
Roberts syndrome in a newborn. Note the corneal opacity, bilateral cleft lip and maxilla, and reduction anomalies of the limbs **(A and B).** (From Römke C, Foster-Iskenius U, Heyne K, et al.: Roberts syndrome and SC phocomelia. A single genetic entity. *Clin. Genet.* 31:170, 1987. Used by permission.)

tardation; clinodactyly; clubfoot; thrombocytopenia; contracture in the knee joints; renal anomalies; persistent branchial arches; congenital heart disease; abnormally straight, often rodlike chromosomes, some with a railroad track appearance; nail hypoplasia; dermatoglyphic abnormalities; nuchal cystic hygroma; frontal encephalocele; hydrocephalus; facial hemangioma; fine, thin, silver-blond hair, etc.

Differential Diagnosis: TAR syndrome; thalidomide syndrome (Fig SY—R—8).

REFERENCES

Fryns JP, et al.: The Roberts tetraphocomelia syndrome: Identical limb defects in two siblings. *Ann. Genet.* 30:243, 1987.

Graham JM Jr, et al.: Nuchal cystic hygroma in a fetus with presumed Roberts syndrome (letter). *Am. J. Med. Genet.* 15:163, 1983.

Herrmann J, et al.: The SC phocomelia and the Roberts syndrome: Nosologic aspects. *Eur. J. Pediatr.* 125:117, 1977.

Louie E, et al.: Roberts' syndrome. II. Aberrant Y chromosome behavior. *Clin. Genet.* 19:71, 1981.

Parry DM, et al.: SC phocomelia syndrome, premature centromere separation, and congenital cranial nerve paralysis in two sisters, one with malignant melanoma. *Am. J. Med. Genet.* 24:653, 1986.

Roberts JB: A child with double cleft of lip and palate, protrusion of the intermaxillary portion of the upper jaw and imperfect development of the bones of the four extremities. *Ann. Surg.* 70:252, 1919.

Römke C, et al.: Roberts syndrome and SC phocomelia. A single genetic entity. *Clin. Genet.* 31:170, 1987.

Zergollern L, et al.: Four siblings with Robert's syndrome. *Clin. Genet.* 21:1, 1982.

ROBIN SEQUENCE

Synonyms: Robin syndrome; Pierre Robin syndrome; Pierre Robin complex; Robin anomaly.

Mode of Inheritance: No known genetic pattern. Familial cases have been reported.

Clinical Manifestations: (a) *micrognathia*; (b) *cleft palate* (U shaped); (c) *glossoptosis*; (d) association with various syndromes: Stickler, chromosomal abnormalities, Möbius, Joubert, X-linked hydrocephalus, Treacher Collins, deLange, Marden-Walker, arthrogryposis, cerebro-costo-mandibular, Nager, femoral hypoplasia, Beckwith-Wiedemann, velocardiofacial, Stevenson, CHARGE, fetal alcohol, hydantoin, trimethadione, amniotic band, campomelic dysplasia, diastrophic dysplasia, spondyloepiphyseal dysplasia congenita, Andre, congenital myotonic dystrophy, etc.; (e) other reported associated abnormalities: mental retardation (in 20%), various limb anomalies (amelia, congenital amputations, syndactyly, clubfoot, hyperphalangia-clinodactyly of the index finger), cor pulmonale, oligodactyly in a mother and son, congenital heart disease (ventricular septal defect, atrial septal defect, patent ductus arteriosus, etc.), upper airway obstruction, cardiopulmonary manifestations (cor pulmonale, cardiomegaly, pulmonary edema, cyanosis), sleep disturbances, apnea, etc.

Radiologic Manifestations: (a) *hypoplasia of the mandible;* (b) *cleft palate;* (c) *upper airway obstruction;* (d) other reported associated abnormalities: congenital heart disease, pulmonary hypertension with cardiomegaly and pulmonary edema, various anomalies of the upper and lower limbs, combined occipitoatlantoaxial hypermobility with anterior and posterior arch defects of the atlas.

Note: About 30% of patients with so-called Robin syndrome develop the full clinical picture of the Stickler syndrome.

REFERENCES

Andre M, et al.: Abnormal facies, cleft palate, and generalized dysostosis: A lethal X-linked syndrome. *J. Pediatr.* 98:747, 1981.

Carey JC, et al.: The Robin sequence as a consequence of malformation, dysplasia, and neuromuscular syndromes. *J. Pediatr.* 101:858, 1982.

Dykes EH, et al.: Pierre Robin syndrome and pulmonary hypertension. *J. Pediatr. Surg.* 20:49, 1985.

Gamble JG, et al.: Combined occipitoatlantoaxial hypermobility with anterior and posterior arch defects of the atlas in Pierre-Robin syndrome. *J. Pediatr. Orthop.* 5:475, 1985.

Hanson JW, et al.: U-shaped palatal defect in the Robin anomalad: Developmental and clinical relevance. *J. Pediatr.* 87:30, 1975.

Johnson GM, et al.: Cor pulmonale in severe Pierre Robin syndrome. *Pediatrics* 65:152, 1980.

Meinecke P, et al.: Robin sequence and oligodactyly in mother and son—Probably a further example of the postaxial acrofacial dysostosis syndrome. *Am. J. Med. Genet.* 27:953, 1987.

Pearl W: Congenital heart disease in the Pierre Robin syndrome. *Pediatr. Cardiol.* 2:307, 1982.

Pratt AE: The Pierre Robin syndrome. *Br. J. Radiol.* 39:390, 1966.

Randall P, et al.: Pierre Robin and the syndrome that bears his name. *Cleft Palate J.* 2:237, 1965.

Robin P: La chute de la base de la langue: Considerée comme une nouvelle cause de gêne dans la respiration naso-pharyngienne. *Bull. Acad. Natl. Med. (Paris)* 89:37, 1923.

Robinow M, et al.: Robin sequence and oligodactyly in a mother and son. *Am. J. Med. Genet.* 25:293, 1986.

Shah CV, et al.: Cardiac malformations with facial clefts with observation on the Pierre Robin syndrome. *Am. J. Dis. Child.* 119:238, 1970.

Sheffield LJ, et al.: A genetic follow-up study of 64 patients with the Pierre Robin complex. *Am. J. Med. Genet.* 28:25, 1987.

Silengo MC, et al.: Pierre Robin syndrome with hyperphalangism-clinodactylysm of the index finger: A possible new palato-digital syndrome. *Pediatr. Radiol.* 6:178, 1977.

Singh RP, et al.: Pierre Robin syndrome in siblings. *Am. J. Dis. Child.* 120:560, 1970.

Spier S, et al.: Sleep in Pierre Robin syndrome. *Chest* 90:711, 1986.

Stevenson RE, et al.: A digito-palatal syndrome with associated anomalies of the heart, face and skeleton. *J. Med. Genet.* 17:238, 1980.

ROMBERG SYNDROME

Synonyms: Hemifacial atrophy; Parry-Romberg syndrome; progressive hemifacial atrophy.

Mode of Inheritance: No definite genetic predisposition; few familial cases have been reported.

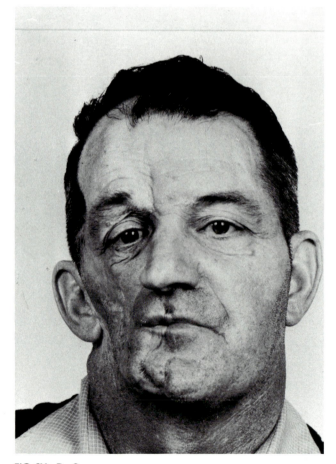

FIG SY–R–9.
Romberg syndrome: hemifacial atrophy in a 58-year-old man with clinical manifestations dating back to early childhood. (From Asher SW, Berg BO: Progressive hemifacial atrophy. Report of three cases, including one observed over 43 years and computed tomographic findings. *Arch. Neurol.* 39:44, 1982. Used by permission.)

Frequency: Rare.

Clinical Manifestations: Progressive disease with an onset in childhood or early adult life: (a) *wasting of soft tissues on one side of the face* with sharp vertical delineation between normal and abnormal sides (coup de sabre); (b) alopecia, poliosis, focal pigmentary changes of the skin; (c) *neurological disorders:* trigeminal neuralgia; ataxia; Horner syndrome; migraine; epilepsy, especially jacksonian motor and sensory types; abnormal electroencephalographic findings; (d) *ocular complications:* enophthalmos, rarely exophthalmos, eyelid atrophy, blepharoptosis, blepharophimosis, loss of cilia, pupillary abnormalities, extraocular muscle weakness, iridocyclitis, refractive changes; (e) other reported abnormalities: involvement of the ear, larynx, esophagus, diaphragm, and kidney; ipsilateral or contralateral involvement of the trunk and extremities; Ewing sarcoma; association with localized scleroderma on the trunk and limb (possibly "scleroderma en coup de sabre" and Romberg syndrome representing manifestations of the same entity); presence of antinuclear antibodies in serum; hemiplegic migraine; etc.

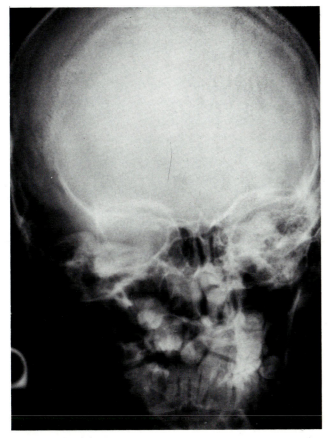

FIG SY–R–10.
Romberg syndrome in a 13-year-old female with a history of progressive right hemiatrophy and brown pigmentation in the right infraorbital region. The symptoms began at 5 years of age. Bone atrophy with right hemifacial distribution is present.

Radiologic Manifestations: (a) *bone atrophy corresponding to sites of soft-tissue atrophy* (shorter body and ramus of the mandible and a delay in development of the angle, etc.); (b) delay in eruption of teeth on the involved side; (c) other reported abnormalities: porencephalia, intracranial calcification (occipital lobe), nonenhancing area of increased density in the parietal lobe, hyperdense areas in the brain (computed tomography) (Figs SY–R–9 and SY–R–10).

REFERENCES

Asher SW, et al.: Progressive hemifacial atrophy. Report of three cases, including one observed over 43 years, and computed tomographic findings. *Arch. Neurol.* 39:44, 1982.

Lewkonia RM, et al.: Progressive hemifacial atrophy (Parry-Romberg syndrome). Report with review of genetics and nosology. *Am. J. Med. Genet.* 14:385, 1983.

Muchnick RS, et al.: Ocular manifestations and treatment of hemifacial atrophy. *Am. J. Ophthalmol.* 88:889, 1979.

Paradise JE, et al.: Progressive facial hemiatrophy. Report of a case associated with Ewing's sarcoma. *Am. J. Dis. Child.* 134:1065, 1980.

Parry CH: Collections from the unpublished medical writings of the late Caleb H. Parry (London, Underwoods, 1825) (quoted from Rogers BO), p. 478.

Rogers BO: Progressive facial hemiatrophy: Romberg's disease; a review of 772 cases. Proceedings of the Third International Conference on Plastic Surgery. *Excerpta Med. Int. Cong. Series* 66:681, 1963.

Romberg MH: *Klininische Ergebnisse.* Berlin, Forstner, 1846 (quoted from Rogers BO), p. 75.

Sagild JC, et al.: Hemiplegic migraine and progressive hemifacial atrophy. *Ann. Neurol.* 17:620, 1985.

Schwartz RA, et al.: Myopathy associated with sclerodermal facial hemiatrophy. *Arch. Neurol.* 38:592, 1981.

Tirosh E, et al.: Hemifacial atrophy (Romberg's syndrome). *Am. J. Dis. Child.* 134:884, 1980.

ROSSELLI-GULIENETTI SYNDROME

Clinical and Radiologic Manifestations: (a) ectodermal dysplasia: anhidrosis, hypotrichosis, microdontia, nail dysplasia; (b) deformity of the fingers and toes; (c) cleft lip and palate; (d) mental retardation.

REFERENCES

Bowen P, et al.: Ectodermal dysplasia, mental retardation, cleft lip/palate and other anomalies in three sibs. *Clin. Genet.* 9:35, 1976.

Rosselli D, Guienetti R: Ectodermal dysplasia. *Br. J. Plast. Surg.* 14:190, 1961.

ROTATOR CUFF IMPINGEMENT SYNDROME

Synonym: Shoulder impingement syndrome.

Pathophysiological Mechanism: Entrapment of the soft-tissue structures under the coracoacromial arc.

Pathology: Rotator cuff tendonitis; fibrosis; rupture.

Clinical Manifestations: *Pain during abduction and external rotation of the arm.*

Radiologic Manifestations: (a) *subacromial proliferation of bone, spurring of the interior aspect of the acromioclavicular joint, degenerative changes in the humeral tuberosities;* (b) arthrogram: *tear;* (c) magnetic resonance imaging: *increased signal intensity in the tendinous portion of the rotator cuff* (due to degeneration and inflammation).

REFERENCES

Beltran J, et al.: Rotator cuff lesions of the shoulder: Evaluation by direct sagittal CT arthrography. *Radiology* 160:161, 1986.

Cone RO III, et al.: Shoulder impingement syndrome: Radiographic evaluation. *Radiology* 150:29, 1984.

Hardy DC, et al.: The shoulder impingement syndrome: Prevalence of radiographic findings and correlation with response to therapy. *A.J.R.* 147:557, 1986.

Kieft GJ, et al.: Rotator cuff impingement syndrome: MR imaging. *Radiology* 166:211, 1988.

Seeger LL, et al.: Shoulder impingement syndrome: MR findings in 53 shoulders. *A.J.R.* 150:343, 1988.

ROTHMUND-THOMSON SYNDROME

Synonym: Poikiloderma congenita.

Mode of Inheritance: Autosomal recessive; possible genetic heterogeneity.

Frequency: Rare.

Clinical Manifestations: Onset of symptoms in infancy: (a) *erythema progressing to atrophy; depigmentation, hyperpigmentation, scaling, and telangiectasia of the skin;* a peculiar marmoration skin pattern; (b) *partial or total alopecia,* missing or sparse eyebrows and eyelashes; (c) *defective nails;* (d) *hypogonadism;* (e) *cataract;* (f) *short distal portions of the limbs;* (g) dwarfism (in about 50% of cases); (h) mental deficiency; (i) saddle nose; (j) defective teeth: microdontia, delayed eruption, supernumerary teeth, missing teeth, multiple crown malformations; (k) sensitivity to light; (l) other reported abnormalities: soft-tissue contracture, anemia, osteogenic sarcoma, growth hormone deficiency, small hands, arterial hypertension, glaucoma.

Radiologic Manifestations: Nonspecific findings: (a) osteoporosis; (b) osteosclerosis; (c) short and broad phalanges, metacarpals, and metatarsals; absent thumb; (d) mild epiphyseal dysostosis and metaphyseal sclerosis in some long bones, radial hypoplasia or agenesis, knee subluxation; (e)

phalangeal tuft resorption; (f) flattened and elongated vertebral bodies; (g) cystic bone changes; (h) soft-tissue calcification, decreased subcutaneous tissues; (i) microdontia and occasionally anodontia.

REFERENCES

Dechenne Ch, et al.: Un cas de maladie de Rothmund-Thomson avec hypertension. *Ann. Pediatr. (Paris)* 29:665, 1982.

Hall JG, et al.: Rothmund-Thomson syndrome with severe dwarfism. *Am. J. Dis. Child.* 134:165, 1980.

Kassner EG, et al.: Rothmund-Thomson syndrome (poikiloderma congenitale) associated with mental retardation, growth disturbance, and skeletal features. *Skeletal Radiol.* 2:99, 1977.

Kaufmann S, et al.: Growth hormone deficiency in the Rothmund-Thomson syndrome. *Am. J. Med. Genet.* 23:861, 1986.

Kozlowski K, et al.: Osteosarcoma in a boy with Rothmund-Thomson syndrome. *Pediatr. Radiol.* 10:42, 1980.

Maurer RM, et al.: Rothmund's syndrome: A cause of resorption of phalangeal tufts and dystrophic calcification. *Radiology* 89:706, 1967.

Nathanson M, et al.: Syndrome de Rothmund-Thomson avec glaucome. Etude endocrinienne. *Ann. Pediatr. (Paris)* 30:520, 1983.

Plantin P, et al.: Poïkilodermie de Rothmund-Thomson. A propos due suivi sur vingt ans d'un cas déjà présenté dans la petite enfance. *Ann. Pediatr. (Paris)* 34:635, 1987.

Rothmund A: Ueber Cataracten in Verbindung mit einer eigentümlichen Hautdegeneration. *Graefes Arch. Ophthalmol.* 14:159, 1868.

Sfar Z, et al.: Le syndrome de Rothmund-Thomson. A propos de quatre cas. *Ann. Pediatr. (Paris)* 35:501, 1988.

Starr DG, et al.: Non-dermatological complications and genetic aspects of the Rothmund-Thomson syndrome. *Clin. Genet.* 27:102, 1985.

Thomson MS: An hitherto undescribed familial disease. *Br. J. Dermatol.* 35:455, 1923.

RUBINSTEIN-TAYBI SYNDROME

Mode of Inheritance: Unknown; familial occurrence in nontwin siblings and in twins (concordant and discordant); recurrence in siblings with parental consanguinity; suggested risk of occurrence in siblings: about 1%.

Frequency: Estimated to be 1:300,000; 1 case per 300 institutionalized subjects; approximatley 600 published cases; more than 120 publications related to the syndrome (Berry, Wood and Rubinstein).

Clinical Manifestations: (a) *characteristic facies* (small head; beaked or straight nose; nasal septum extending below the alae; apparent hypertelorism; antimongoloid slant of the palpebral fissures; high-arched palate; abnormalities in position, rotation, size, or shape of the ears; mild retrognathia); (b) *broad thumb,* especially the distal phalanx (described as spatulate, short, stubby, flat, wide, or clubbed); angulated thumb (hitchhiker thumb, hammerhead thumb, viper-type proximal phalanx) in about one third of the cases; broad fingers, especially the distal phalanges; clinodactyly of the fourth and fifth fingers; polydactyly of the little finger; (c) *broad and large great toe,* angular deformity (medial or lateral) of the great toe, clinodactyly of the fourth toes; (d) *mental, motor, social, and language retardation;* (e) short stature; (f) incomplete or delayed descent of the testes in males; (g) other reported abnormalities: electroencephalographic abnormalities, refractive errors, excess dermal ridge patterning in the thenar and first interdigital areas of the palm, nevus flammeus, anterior scalp hair upsweep (moderate to severe), peculiar grimacing smile, overlapping toes, heavy or high-arched eyebrows, epicanthi, long eyelashes, nasolacrimal duct obstruction, constricted palate resembling a curved Chinese roof, dental abnormalities (talon cusps, crowding of teeth, double rows of teeth), eye abnormalities (strabismus, cataracts, glaucoma, colobomas, refractive errors), flattening of the fingernails, hypoplasia of the toenails, skin manifestations (paronychia, tendency to keloids, hypertrichosis, seborrheic dermatitis, unusual dermatoglyphics), joint laxity, brisk reflexes, awkward gait, flatfeet, slight hip and knee flexion, malignancy (leukemia, nasopharyngeal rhabdomyosarcoma).

Radiologic Manifestations: (a) *short and wide terminal phalanx of the thumbs* (broadness mainly localized to the distal phalanx and involving both soft tissues and bone), a hole or distal notch in the distal phalanx that suggests an attempt at duplication, no true duplication (Wood and Rubinstein), "delta deformity" of the proximal phalanx of the thumbs that causes angulation in about 40% of the cases (Wood and Rubinstein), *short, wide, and tufted terminal phalanges of the finger (in the majority);* (b) short and wide terminal phalanx of the great toes, duplication in the proximal and distal phalanges of the great toes, "kissing delta phalanx" of the great toes in association with duplication (fused epiphyses), hallux valgus; (c) flaring of the ilia (small iliac index); (d) skeletal maturation retardation; (e) other reported abnormalities: large foramen magnum, congenital heart defects (in 25% of cases, patent ductus arteriosus and ventricular septal defect are the most common anomalies), gastroesophageal reflux, urinary tract anomalies, various skeletal anomalies (prominent forehead, large anterior fontanelle, parietal foramina, vertebral anomalies, sternal anomalies, dislocation of the patellae, syndactyly, polydactyly, clinodactyly of the fifth finger), absence of the corpus callosum.

Differential Diagnosis: (a) hitchhiker thumb: Apert syndrome, diastrophic dysplasia, Pfeiffer syndrome, chromosome 13 trisomy; (2) facial appearance: Seckel syndrome, Hallermann-Streiff syndrome, Treacher Collins syndrome, a dominantly inherited syndrome with some features similar to Rubinstein-Taybi syndrome (Cotsirilos et al.).

Note: Over 500 individuals with the syndrome were the subject of a review by Dr. Jack Rubinstein at the Ninth Annual David W. Smith Workshop on Malformations and Morphogenesis, August 7, 1988, Oakland, California; most of the

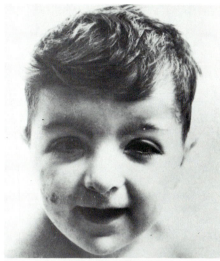

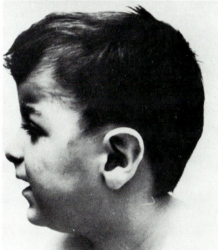

FIG SY—R—11.
Rubinstein-Taybi syndrome in a 3-year-old male with mental retardation and an unusual facial appearance. (From Rubinstein JH, Taybi H: Broad thumbs and toes and facial abnormalities. A possible mental retardation syndrome. *Am. J. Dis. Child.* 105:88, 1963. Used by permission.)

information had been reported in the article by Wood and Rubinstein; the historical aspect of the original description of the syndrome was also presented at this meeting by Drs. Rubinstein and Taybi (Figs SY—R—11 and SY—R—12).

REFERENCES

Allanson JE: The changing face: Rubinstein-Taybi syndrome (abstract). Presented at the 9th Annual David W. Smith Workshop on Malformations and Morphogenesis, Oakland, Calif. August 3–7, 1988.

Baker MA: Dental and oral manifestations of Rubinstein-Taybi syndrome: Report of case. *A.S.D.C. J. Dent. Child.* 54:369, 1987.

Baraitser M, et al.: The Rubinstein-Taybi syndrome: Occur-

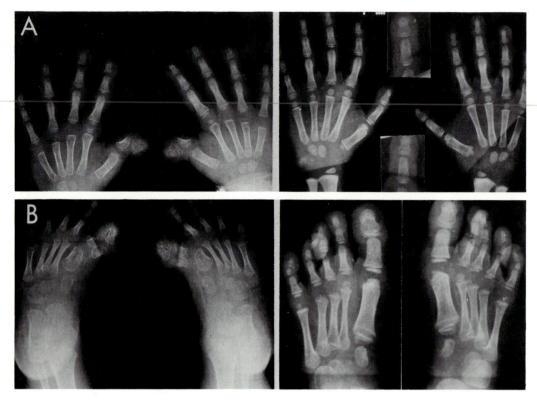

FIG SY−R−12.

Rubinstein-Taybi syndrome. **A,** hands of two patients: *left,* trapezoid deformity of the proximal phalanges of the thumbs, incurving of the thumb and wide distal phalanges of all digits; *right,* broad distal phalanges of all digits. **B,** feet of the same patients: *left,* medial incurving of the toes, trapezoid deformity of the first metatarsals and duplication of the phalanges of the toes; *right,* broad great toes. (From Taybi H, Rubinstein JH: Broad thumbs and toes and unusual facial features: A probable mental retardation syndrome. *A.J.R.* 93:362, 1965. Used by permission.)

rence in two sets of identical twins. *Clin. Genet.* 23:318, 1983.

Berry AC: Rubinstein-Taybi syndrome. *J. Med. Genet.* 24:562, 1987.

Bonassi E, et al.: Aspetti rieducativi nella sindrome di Rubinstein-Taybi. Illustrazione di 4 casi clinici. *Minerva Pediatr.* 27:218, 1975.

Borzani M, et al.: La sindrome di Rubinstein-Taybi. Descrizione di tre nuovi casi con particolare riguardo agli aspetti radiologici. *Minerva Pediatr.* 32:547, 1980.

Buchinger G, et al.: Rubinstein-Taybi-Syndrom bei wahrscheinlich einigen Zwillingen und drei weiteren Kindern Gleichzeitige Korrecktur einer Fehldiagnose. *Klin. Paediatr.* 185:296, 1973.

Char F: Rubinstein-Taybi syndrome in blacks. Followup from infancy to late childhood (abstract). Presented at the 9th Annual David W. Smith Workshop on Malformations and Morphogenesis, Oakland, Calif., August 3–7, 1988.

Cotsirilos P, et al.: Dominant inheritance of a syndrome similar to Rubinstein-Taybi. *Am. J. Med. Genet.* 26:85, 1987.

Gardner DG, et al.: Talon cusps: A dental anomaly in the Rubinstein-Taybi syndrome. *Oral. Surg.* 47:519, 1979.

Grunow JE: Gastroesophageal reflux in Rubinstein-Taybi syndrome. *J. Pediatr. Gastroenterol. Nutr.* 1:273, 1982.

Halamek LP, et al.: Rubinstein-Taybi syndrome in two siblings of a first cousin marriage (abstract). Presented at the 9th Annual David W. Smith Workshop on Malformations and Morphogenesis, Oakland, Calif., August 3–7, 1988.

Hall BD: Keloids in Rubinstein-Taybi syndrome (abstract). Presented at the 9th Annual David W. Smith Workshop on Malformations and Morphogenesis, Oakland, Calif., August 3–7, 1988.

Hennekam RCM, et al.: Rubinstein-Taybi syndrome in the Netherlands (abstract). Presented at the 9th Annual David W. Smith Workshop on Malformations and Morphogenesis, Oakland, Calif., August 3–7, 1988.

Jonas DM, et al.: Rubinstein-Taybi syndrome and acute leukemia. *J. Pediatr.* 92:851, 1978.

Kajii T: Monozygotic twins discordant for Rubinstein-Taybi syndrome. *J. Med. Genet.* 18:312, 1981.

Kinirons MJ: Oral aspects of Rubinstein-Taybi syndrome. *Br. Dent. J.* 154:46, 1983.

Matsoukas J: Fatherhood of the so-called Rubinstein-Taybi syndrome. *Am. J. Dis. Child.* 126:860, 1973 (refer to Pouce bot arqué en forte abduction-extension et autres symptomes concomitants. *Rev. Chir. Orthop.* 43:142, 1957.).

Neuhold VA, et al.: Taybi-Rubinstein syndrom: Der Stellenwert des Röntgenbilder. *Fortschr. Röntgentr.* 150:49, 1989.

Robson MJ, et al.: Cervical spondylolisthesis and other skeletal abnormalities in Rubinstein-Taybi syndrome. *J. Bone Joint Surg. [Br.]* 62:297, 1980.

Rubinstein JH: Broad thumbs—hallux syndrome, in *The Proceedings of the 13th International Congress of Pediatrics.* Vienna, Austria, 1971, pp. 471–476.

Rubinstein JH, Taybi H: Broad thumbs and toes and facial abnormalities: A possible mental retardation syndrome. *Am. J. Dis. Child.* 105:588, 1963.

Selmanowitz VJ, et al.: Rubinstein-Taybi syndrome. Cutaneous manifestations and colossal keloids. *Arch. Dermatol.* 117:504, 1981.

Smith DW, et al.: Scalp hair patterning as a clue to early fetal brain development. *J. Pediatr.* 83:374, 1973.

Sobel RA, et al.: Rubinstein-Taybi syndrome and nasopharyngeal rhabdomyosarcoma. *J. Pediatr.* 99:1000, 1981.

Stevens CA, et al.: Rubinstein-Taybi syndrome—a natural history study (abstract). Presented at the 9th Annual David W. Smith Workshop on Malformations and Morphogenesis, Oakland, Calif., August 3–7, 1988.

Taybi H: Broad thumbs and great toes, facial abnormalities, and mental retardation syndrome, Symposium 10: The Rubinstein-Taybi syndrome, in Richards BW (ed.): *Proceedings, The First Congress of the International Association for the Scientific Study of Mental Deficiency.* Montpellier, France, 1967, pp. 596–599.

Taybi H, Rubinstein JH: Broad thumbs and toes and unusual facial features: A probable mental retardation syndrome. *A.J.R.* 93:362, 1965.

Wood VE, Rubinstein JH: Surgical treatment of the thumb in the Rubinstein-Taybi syndrome. *J. Hand Surg. [Br.]* 12:166, 1987.

RÜDIGER SYNDROME

Mode of Inheritance: Possibly autosomal recessive.

Frequency: Single family reported by Rüdiger et al.

Clinical and Radiologic Manifestations: (a) coarse facial features, flat nasal bridge, stubby nose, protuberant upper lip; (b) thickened palms and soles with an abnormal dermatoglyphic pattern, short digits, palmar flexion contracture, hypoplastic fingernails; (c) hydronephrosis due to ureteral stenosis, bicornuate uterus; (d) inguinal hernia; (e) low-pitched hoarse voice; (f) failure to develop motor control, bifid uvula, etc.

REFERENCE

Rüdiger RA, et al.: Severe developmental failure with coarse facial features, distal limb hypoplasia, thickened palmar creases, bifid uvula, and ureteral stenosis: A previously unidentified familial disorder with lethal outcome. *J. Pediatr.* 79:977, 1971.

RUTHERFURD SYNDROME

Mode of Inheritance: Autosomal dominant with high degree of penetrance.

Clinical Manifestations: (a) *corneal dystrophy;* (b) *hypertrophy of the gums;* (c) *failure of tooth eruption,* dentigerous cyst; (d) mental retardation, aggressive behavior.

Radiologic Manifestations: (a) deciduous teeth unerupted; (b) resorption of unerupted teeth.

REFERENCES

Houston IB, et al.: Rutherfurd's syndrome: A familial oculo-dental disorder. *Acta Paediatr. Scand.* 55:233, 1966.

Rutherfurd ME: Three generations of inherited dental defects. *Br. Med. J.* 2:9, 1931.

RUTLEDGE LETHAL MULTIPLE CONGENITAL ANOMALY SYNDROME

Mode of Inheritance: Autosomal recessive.

Clinical and Radiologic Manifestations: (a) micrognathia, V-shaped upper lip, microglossia, thick alveolar ridges, highly arched palate, closed fontanelles, inclusion cysts of the tongue, apparently low-set ears, webbed neck; (b) joint contracture, mesomelic dwarfism, clubfeet, four-finger creases, digital anomalies; (c) other abnormalities: am-

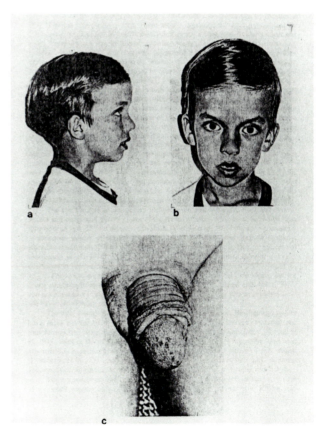

FIG SY–R–13.
Ruvalcaba-Myhre-Smith syndrome in a 7½-year-old patient with macrocephaly, hamartomatous intestinal polyps, and café au lait spots on the penis. (From DiLiberti JH, Weleher RG, Budden S: Ruvalcaba-Myhre-Smith syndrome: A case with probable autosomal-dominant inheritance and additional manifestations. *Am. J. Med. Genet.* 15:491, 1983. Used by permission.)

biguous genitalia, widely spaced nipples, oligopapillary renal hypoplasia, congenital heart defects, cerebellar hypoplasia, pulmonary hypoplasia, etc.

REFERENCE

Rutledge JC, et al.: A "new" lethal multiple congenital anomaly syndrome: Joint contractures, cerebellar hypoplasia, renal hypoplasia, urogenital anomalies, tongue cysts, shortness of limbs, eye abnormalities, defects of the heart, gallbladder agenesis, and ear malformations. *Am. J. Med. Genet.* 19:255, 1984.

RUVALCABA-MYHRE-SMITH SYNDROME

Mode of Inheritance: Probably autosomal dominant.

Clinical Manifestations: (a) *pigmented macules on the penis;* (b) *macrocephaly;* (c) *hamartomatous intestinal polyposis;* (d) other reported abnormalities: delayed psychomotor development in childhood, prominent Schwalbe lines, prominent corneal nerves, lipid storage myopathy (increased numbers of neural lipid droplets, the type 2 fibers consistently smaller than expected; abnormal electromyographic findings).

Radiologic Manifestations: *Gastrointestinal polyposis* (diffuse).

Differential Diagnosis: Gardner syndrome; familial colonic polyposis; juvenile polyposis; Peutz-Jeghers syndrome, Cronkhite-Canada syndrome (Fig SY−R−13).

REFERENCES

DiLiberti JH, et al.: A new lipid storage myopathy observed in individuals with Ruvalcaba-Myhre-Smith syndrome. *Am. J. Med. Genet.* 18:163, 1984.

DiLiberti JH, et al.: Ruvalcaba-Myhre-Smith syndrome: A case with probable autosomal-dominant inheritance and additional manifestations. *Am. J. Med. Genet.* 15:491, 1983.

Foster MA, et al.: Ruvalcaba-Myhre-Smith syndrome: A new consideration in the differential diagnosis of intestinal polyposis. *Gastrointest. Radiol.* 11:349, 1986.

Gretzula JC, et al.: Ruvalcaba-Myhre-Smith syndrome. *Pediatr. Dermatol.* 5:28, 1988.

Halal F: Cerebral gigantism, intestinal polyposis, and pigmentary spotting of the genitalia (letter). *Am. J. Med. Genet.* 15:161, 1983.

Ruvalcaba RHA, Myhre S, Smith DW: Sotos syndrome with intestinal polyposis and pigmentary changes of the genitalia. *Clin. Genet.* 18:413, 1980.

SANDIFER SYNDROME

Frequency: Over 30 published cases (Keren et al., Nanayakkara et al.).

Clinical Manifestations: *Abnormal movement or positioning of the head, neck, and upper part of trunk during or after eating*, i.e., sudden extension, continual movement from side to side, and flexion of the upper portion of the trunk and neck.

Radiologic Manifestations: With the clinically described contortions, the gastroesophageal junction rises, and the upper portion of the stomach enters the thoracic cavity *(hiatal hernia)*.

Differential Diagnosis: Tics; seizures.

Notes: (a) torticollis has been reported in association with gastroesophageal reflux without a hiatal hernia; (b) a penetrating impacted star-shaped foreign body in the esophagus has been reported with the "Sandifer movements"; (c) two of the original cases reported by Kinsbourne were the cases of the neurologist Paul Sandifer whose name is associated with the syndrome.

REFERENCES

Hadari A, et al.: Sandifer's syndrome—A rare complication of hiatal hernia. *Z. Kinderchir.* 39:202, 1984.
Keren G, et al.: Sandifer's syndrome following reverse gastric tube operation (Gavriliu's operation). *J. Pediatr. Surg.* 18:632, 1983.
Kinsbourne M: Hiatus hernia with contortions of the neck. *Lancet* 1:1058, 1964.
Nanayakkara CS, et al.: Sandifer syndrome: An overlooked diagnosis? *Dev. Med. Neurol.* 27:816, 1985.
Ramenofsky ML, et al.: Gastroesophageal reflux and torticollis. *J. Bone Joint Surg. [Am.]* 60:1140, 1978.
Smallpiece CJ, et al.: Sandifer's syndrome: A new cause. *Thorax* 37:634, 1982.
Sutcliffe J: Torsion spasms and abnormal postures in children with hiatus hernia: Sandifer's syndrome, in Kaufmann HJ (ed.): *Progress in Pediatric Radiology.* Basel, Karger, 1969, vol. 2, p. 190.

SARCOIDOSIS

Clinical Manifestations: (a) *general symptoms:* fever, weight loss, dyspnea, productive or nonproductive cough, chest pain, wheezing; (b) extrathoracic manifestations: skin, eyes, central nervous system, kidney, testicles, salivary glands, nose, paranasal sinuses, larynx, liver with or without obstructive jaundice, peripheral lymphadenopathy, abdominal pain, nausea, vomiting, skeletal pain, muscular pain, arthralgia, arthritis; (c) laboratory findings: low-grade anemia; hypercalcemia; hypercalciuria; high levels of serum alkaline phosphatase and cholesterol; elevated serum globulin levels, particularly the γ fraction, elevation of the serum angiotensin-converting enzyme level, chronic thrombocytopenia; (d) immunologic changes: depression of delayed-type hypersensitivity, hyperactive circulating antibody response, Kveim-Siltzback test phenomenon; (e) arrhythmias, conduction disturbances, cardiomyopathy.

Radiologic Manifestations: (a) cardiorespiratory: laryngeal obstruction (laryngeal infiltration, epiglottic and subglottic polypoid masses, tracheal stenosis), eggshell calcification in the hilar and mediastinal lymph nodes, pulmonary artery narrowing, computed tomographic (CT) demonstration of increased lung density, granulomatous nodules, tracheal compression, bullae, pulmonary infiltrates, fibrosis and end-stage lung disease, chylothorax, pleural thickening, fibrothorax, pleural effusion, mediastinal emphysema, pneumothorax, hilar haze, cystic bronchial dilatation, thick wall cavities, atelectasis, cardiomegaly, cardiac failure, pericardial effusion, cardiomyopathy, left ventricular aneurysm; (b) *skeletal system:* oval or spheroid *lytic lesion of the phalanges*, "lace work" type of destructive lesions of the phalanges, lytic lesion and subperiosteal new bone formation of the long bones, radiolucent calvarial defects, scattered radiodense lesions, arthritis; (c) *urinary tract:* enlargement of the kidneys due to sarcoid granulomas, poor concentration of contrast medium on excretory urography, ureteral obstruction; (d) nodular lymphoid hyperplasia of the small intestine, antral and pyloric stiffening and narrowing, gastric and duodenal ulcers, abnormal mucosal pattern, saccules; (e) central nervous system (cerebral hemispheres, cerebellar and mesencephalic structures, cranial nerves, particularly II and VII, and pituitary gland most common sites; brain stem and spinal cord less common sites): (1) meningeal lesions causing nodular granulomatous masses, adhesive meningitis causing obstructive hydrocephalus, communicating hydrocephalus with sarcoid arachnoiditis; (2) intraparenchymal lesions; CT demonstration of a contrast-enhanced mass or masses; hypodense white matter lesions (CT), great variability on magnetic resonance imaging (isointense or hypointense relative to the cerebral cortex on T_1- and T_2-weighted images or hyperintense on T_2-weighted images); (f) *salivary glands:* ectasia, spreading apart of the ducts in the early phase, displacement of the ducts due to swelling in the later phase, and finally destruction of the duct system; (g) radioisotope scanning: (1) ^{99m}Tc pyrophosphate or pyrodiphosphate compounds: uptake in the involved regions:

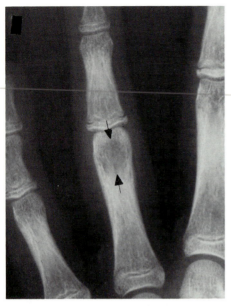

FIG SY–S–1.
Sarcoidosis in a 15-year-old female with an oval lytic lesion of the proximal phalanx of the fourth digit *(arrows).*

bones, lacrimal glands, salivary glands, paranasal sinuses, mediastinum, lung, inguinal areas; (2) ^{67}Ga citrate: uptake in pulmonary and extrapulmonary foci; (h) orbital sarcoidosis: lacrimal glands, optic nerve and its sheath, ocular bulb, anterior uveitis, choroid with subretinal fluid collection; (i) other reported abnormalities: association with liver cirrhosis, splenomegaly, protein-losing enteropathy; granulomatous biliary tract obstruction, association with tumoral calcinosis, abdominal adenopathy, pancreatic involvement, hepatomegaly, splenomegaly, heterogeneous enhancement of the spleen with hypodense areas within the spleen, female pelvic visceral involvement (Fig SY–S–1).

REFERENCES

Battesti JP, et al.: Pulmonary sarcoidosis with an alveolar radiographic pattern. *Thorax* 37:448, 1982.

Bekerman C, et al.: The role of gallium-67 in the clinical evaluation of sarcoidosis. *Semin. Roentgenol.* 20:400, 1985.

Berkmen YM: Radiologic aspects of intrathoracic sarcoidosis. *Semin. Roentgenol.* 20:356, 1985.

Besnier E: Lupus pernio de la face, synovites fongueuses (scrofulotuberculeuses) symétriques des extrémités supérieures. *Ann. Dermatol. Syph. (Paris)* 10:333, 1889.

Bloom R, et al.: Granulomatous biliary tract obstruction due to sarcoidosis. *Am. Rev. Respir. Dis.* 117:783, 1978.

Boeck C: Multiple benign sarcoid of the skin. *J. Cutan. Genitourin. Dis.* 17:543, 1889.

Campo RV, et al.: Choroidal granuloma in sarcoidosis. *Am. J. Ophthalmol.* 97:419, 1984.

Chiang R, et al.: Empty sella turcica in intracranial sarcoidosis. Pituitary insufficiency, primary polydipsia, and changing neuroradiologic findings. *Arch. Neurol.* 41:662, 1984.

Chiles C, et al.: Radiographic manifestations of cardiac sarcoid. *A.J.R.* 145:711, 1985.

Dalley RW, et al.: Computed tomography of calvarial and petrous bone sarcoidosis. *J. Comput. Assist. Tomogr.* 11:884, 1987.

Davis SD, et al.: Nodular lymphoid hyperplasia of the small intestine and sarcoidosis. *Arch. Intern. Med.* 126:668, 1970.

Deutch SJ, et al.: Abdominal lymphadenopathy in sarcoidosis. *J. Ultrasound Med.* 6:237, 1987.

Dubois PJ, et al.: Computed tomography of sarcoidosis of the optic nerve. *Neuroradiology* 24:179, 1983.

Duszlak EJ Jr, et al.: Pelvic sarcoidosis. *J. Comput. Assist. Tomogr.* 6:1032, 1982.

Field SK, et al.: Sarcoidosis presenting as chronic thrombocytopenia. *West. J. Med.* 146:481, 1987.

Finke R, et al.: Sarcoidosis and immunocytoma. *Am. J. Med.* 80:939, 1986.

Forman MB, et al.: Radionuclide imaging in myocardial sarcoidosis. Demonstration of myocardial uptake of technetium pyrophosphate 99m and gallium. *Chest* 83:578, 1983.

Friedman HZ, et al.: Sarcoidosis of the pancreas. *Arch. Intern. Med.* 143:2182, 1983.

Gilman MJ, et al.: CT attenuation values of lung density in sarcoidosis. *J. Comput. Assist. Tomogr.* 7:407, 1983.

Godin E, et al.: Acro-ostéosclerose au cours de la maladie de Besnier-Boeck-Schaumann. *J. Radiol. Electrol.* 58:115, 1977.

Grossman H, et al.: Radiographic features of sarcoidosis in pediatric patients. *Semin. Roentgenol.* 20:393, 1985.

Guilford WB, et al.: Sarcoidosis presenting as a rib fracture. *A.J.R.* 139:608, 1982.

Haas GP, et al.: Testicular sarcoidosis: Case report and review of the literature. *J. Urol.* 135:1254, 1986.

Hayes WS, et al.: MR and CT evaluation of intracranial sarcoidosis. *A.J.R.* 149:1043, 1987.

Hitchon PW, et al.: Sarcoidosis presenting as an intramedullary spinal cord mass. *Neurosurgery* 15:86, 1984.

Iko BO, et al.: Multifocal defects and spenomegaly in sarcoidosis: A new scintigraphic pattern. *J. Natl. Med. Assoc.* 74:739, 1982.

Iko BO, et al.: Sarcoidosis of the parotid gland. *Br. J. Radiol.* 59:547, 1986.

Johnson DG, et al.: Ga-67 uptake in the lung in sarcoidosis. *Radiology* 150:551, 1984.

Kelly RB, et al.: MR demonstration of spinal cord sarcoidosis: Report of a case. *A.J.N.R.* 9:197, 1988.

Ketonen L, et al.: Hypodense white matter lesions in computed tomography of neurosarcoidosis. *J. Comput. Assist. Tomogr.* 10:181, 1986.

Leeds NE, et al.: Neurosarcoidosis of the brain and meninges. *Semin. Roentgenol.* 20:387, 1985.

Le Verger JC, et al.: Sarcoïdose et hypertension portale. *J. Gastroenterol. Clin. Biol.* 1:661, 1977.

Maddrey WC: Sarcoidosis and primary biliary cirrhosis. Associated disorders? *N. Engl. J. Med.* 308:588, 1983.

Mathieu D, et al.: Computed tomography of splenic sarcoidosis. *J. Comput. Assist. Tomogr.* 10:679, 1986.

Meranze S, et al.: Retroperitoneal manifestations of sarcoidosis on computed tomography. *J. Comput. Assist. Tomogr.* 9:50, 1985.

Merten DF, et al.: Pulmonary sarcoidosis in childhood. *A.J.R.* 135:673, 1980.

Miller A: The vanishing lung syndrome associated with pulmonary sarcoidosis. *Br. J. Dis. Chest* 75:209, 1981.

Mirfakhraee M, et al.: Virchow-Robin space: A path of spread in neurosarcoidosis. *Radiology* 158:715, 1986.

Naveau B: Manifestations articulaires de la sarcoïdose. *Ann. Med. Interne (Paris)* 135:105, 1984.

Oven TJ, et al.: Lytic lesion of the sternum. Rare manifestation of sarcoidosis. *Am. J. Med.* 80:285, 1986.

Pattishall EN, et al.: Childhood sarcoidosis. *J. Pediatr.* 108:169, 1986.

Popović OS, et al.: Sarcoidosis and protein losing enteropathy. *Gastroenterology* 78:119, 1980.

Rabinowitz JG, et al.: The usual unusual manifestations of sarcoidosis and the "hilar haze"—A new diagnostic aid. *A.J.R.* 120:821, 1974.

Rockoff SD, et al.: Unusual manifestations of thoracic sarcoidosis. *A.J.R.* 144:513, 1985.

Rudzki C, et al.: Chronic intrahepatic cholestasis of sarcoidosis. *Am. J. Med.* 59:373, 1975.

Sacher M, et al.: Computed tomography of bilateral lacrimal gland sarcoidosis. *J. Comput. Assist. Tomogr.* 8:213, 1984.

Saraux H: Manifestations oculaires de la sarcoïdose. *Ann. Med. Interne (Paris)* 135:109, 1984.

Sartosis DJ, et al.: Musculoskeletal manifestations of sarcoidosis. *Semin. Roentgenol.* 20:376, 1985.

Schaumann J: Etude sur le lupus pernio et ses rapports avec le sarcoïdes et la tuberculose. *Ann. Dermatol. Syph.* 5:357, 1917.

Schoenfeld RH, et al.: Unilateral ureteral obstruction secondary to sarcoidosis. *Urology* 25:57, 1985.

Sharma OP: Hypercalcemia in sarcoidosis. The puzzle finally solved. *Arch. Intern. Med.* 145:626, 1985.

Sharma OP: Sarcoidosis: Clinical, laboratory, and immunologic aspects. *Semin. Roentgenol.* 20:340, 1985.

Signorini E, et al.: Rare multiple orbital localizations of sarcoidosis. *Neuroradiology* 26:145, 1984.

Solomon A, et al.: Computed tomography in pulmonary sarcoidosis. *J. Comput. Assist. Tomogr.* 3:754, 1979.

Som PM, et al.: Parotid gland sarcoidosis and the CT sialogram. *J. Comput. Assist. Tomogr.* 5:674, 1981.

Som PM, et al.: Sarcoidosis of the optic nerve. *J. Comput. Assist. Tomogr.* 6:614, 1982.

Visco JJ, et al.: Sarcoidosis of the larynx. *Radiology* 131:636, 1979.

Wolpe FM, et al.: Tumoral calcinosis associated with sarcoidosis and positive bone and gallium imaging. *Clin. Nucl. Med.* 12:529, 1987.

SCAPULOILIAC DYSOSTOSIS (KOSENOW-SINIOS)

Synonym: Pelvis-shoulder dysplasia.

Mode of Inheritance: Probably autosomal dominant; possible new mutation.

Frequency: Four published cases (Blane et al.).

Clinical Manifestations: Varied, not consistent: microphthalmos, ectopic pupils, coloboma of the retina, corneal opacification, malformed and low-set ears, narrow external auditory canal, ocular hypertelorism, coloboma of the eyelids, absent lacrimal puncta, micrognathia, waddling gait.

Radiologic Manifestations: (a) *extreme hypoplasia of the scapula and ilium;* (b) *hypoplasia of the clavicle;* (c) lordosis of lumbosacral spine, rounded appearance of the lumbar vertebral bodies in infancy; (d) faulty development of ribs, overconstriction of the shaft of the femora and tibias; (e) other reported abnormalities: cranium bifidum, micrognathia, radioulnar synostosis, synostosis of the distal portions of the clavicles to the scapulae, clinodactyly of the fingers, simple partial syndactyly.

Note: A sister and brother with some features of this dystosis (scapular and iliac hypoplasia) in addition to congenital dwarfism and rhizomelia have been reported from North Africa (Cousin et al.) (Fig SY−S−2).

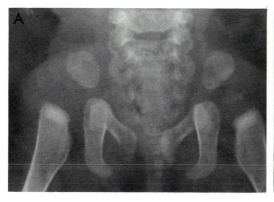
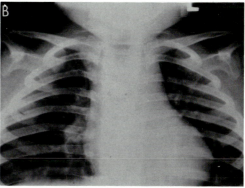

FIG SY−S−2.
Scapuloiliac dysostosis. **A,** extreme hypoplasia of the ilium in a 5-month-old girl. **B,** bilateral cervical ribs, straight clavicles, and scapular dysplasia in the same patient at 20 months of age. (From Kosenow W, Niederle J, Sinios A: Becken-Schulter dysplasia. *Fortschr. Rontgenstr.* 113:39, 1970. Used by permission.)

REFERENCES

Blane CE, et al.: Scapuloiliac dysostosis. *Br. J. Radiol.*
    57:526, 1984.
Cousin J, et al.: Dysplasie pelvi-scapulaire familiale avec
    anomalies épiphysaires, nanisme et dysmorphies: Un nou-
    veau syndrome?. *Arch. Fr. Pediatr.* 39:173, 1982.
Kosenow W, Niederle J, Sinios A: Becken-Schulter
    Dysplasie. *Fortschr. Rontgenstr.* 113:39, 1970.
Thomas PS, et al.: Pelvis-shoulder dysplasia. *Pediatr. Radiol.*
    5:219, 1977.

SCHILDER DISEASE

Pathology: A diffuse demyelinating disease with the lesions often in the centrum semiovale and occipital lobes; focal necrotic foci with cavitation; etc.

Clinical Manifestations: Slowly progressive or episodic
course: (a) pyramidal tract signs, blindness, deafness, extraocular muscle paralysis, nystagmus, dysarthria; (b) psychiatric disturbances, mental retardation.

Radiologic Manifestations: (a) computed tomography:
decreased density in the periventricular white matter, ventricular dilatation; (b) magnetic resonance imaging: course of demyelination from the periventricular white matter distally (increased signal intensity on T_2-weighted images.

Note: The neurological manifestation of adrenoleukodystrophy has been referred to as Schilder disease.

REFERENCES

Cobb SR, et al.: Wallerian degeneration in a patient with
    Schilder disease: MR imaging demonstration. *Radiology*
    162:521, 1987.
Konkol RJ, et al.: Schilder's disease: Additional aspects and
    a therapeutic option. *Neuropediatrics.* 18:149, 1987.
Poser CM, et al.: Schilder's myelinoclastic diffuse sclerosis.
    Pediatrics 77:107, 1986.
Schilder P: Zur Kenntnis der sogenannten diffusen Sklerose.
    Z. Ges. Neurol. Psychol. 10:1, 1912.

SCHINZEL-GIEDION SYNDROME

Mode of Inheritance: Autosomal recessive.

Frequency: Rare.

Clinical Manifestations: (a) severe midface hypoplasia,
choanal stenosis; (b) congenital heart defect; (c) clubfeet; (d)
hypertrichosis, hypoplasia of the dermal ridges; (e) other abnormalities: failure to thrive, epilepsy, profound motor and
intellectual retardation, postaxial hexadactyly, mesomelic
brachymelia, narrow fingernails, etc.

Radiologic Manifestations: (a) short and sclerotic base of
the skull, steep base of the skull, wide supraoccipital "syn-

chondrosis," multiple wormian bones, orbital hypertelorism,
wide cranial sutures and fontanelles; (b) increased density of
long tubular bones and vertebrae, hypoplastic or aplastic pubic bones, moderate mesomelic brachymelia, short first
metacarpals, hypoplasia of the distal phalanges in the hands
and feet; (c) congenital hydronephrosis and hydroureter.

REFERENCES

Kelley RI, et al.: Congenital hydronephrosis, skeletal dyspla-
    sia, and severe developmental retardation: The Schinzel-
    Giedion syndrome. *J. Pediatr.* 100:943, 1982.
Schinzel A: A syndrome of midface retraction, multiple ra-
    diological anomalies, renal malformations and hyper-
    trichosis. *Hum. Genet.* 62:382, 1982.
Schinzel A, Giedion A: A syndrome of severe midface re-
    traction, multiple skull anomalies, clubfeet, and cardiac
    and renal malformations in sibs. *Am. J. Med. Genet.*
    1:361, 1978.

SCHWARZ-LÉLEK SYNDROME

Mode of Inheritance: No known genetic pattern.

Clinical Manifestations: Normal at birth; onset in childhood: (a) *enlargement of the head, marked frontal bossing;*
(b) *thick mandible;* (c) *genu recurvatum.*

Radiologic Manifestations: (a) *marked hyperostosis and
sclerosis of the skull,* in particular, in the frontal and occipital
regions; obliteration of the paranasal sinuses; (b) *bowing of
humeri and femora;* (c) *widening of long bones* similar to that
in Pyle disease.

REFERENCES

Gorlin RJ, et al.: Genetic craniotubular bone dysplasias and
    hyperostoses: A critical analysis. *Birth Defects* 5(4):79,
    1969.
Lélek I: Camurati-Engelmannshe Erkrankung. *Fortschr. Ront-
    genstr.* 94:702, 1961.
Schwarz E: Craniometaphyseal dysplasia. *A.J.R.* 84:461,
    1960.

SCHWARTZ-JAMPEL SYNDROME

Synonyms: Chondrodystrophic myotonia; osteochondro-
muscular dystrophy.

Mode of Inheritance: Autosomal recessive, variable expressivity.

Frequency: Uncommon.

Clinical Manifestations: Progressive disease with an onset of symptoms in infancy: (a) *masklike facies, blepharophimosis, microstomia, recessed chin, full cheeks;* (b) *short stature, stiff posture, short neck, short trunk,* pectus carinatum,

kyphosis or kyphoscoliosis; (c) *prolonged myotonic responses,* firm hypertrophic muscles, muscular weakness and wasting; (d) *large-joint stiffness and contracture;* (e) high-pitched voice; (f) immunologic abnormalities (humoral and cellular); (g) manifestations in neonates: short stature, contractures, myotonia (electromyographic, clinical), muscle hypertrophy, muscle rigidity, choking, respiratory difficulty, apnea, abnormal facies (blepharophimosis, microstomia, etc); (h) compression myelopathy.

Radiologic Manifestations: (a) triangular deformity of the pelvis, flared iliac wings; (b) *hip disorders:* coxa vara or coxa valga, delay in appearance of femoral head ossification, fragmentation of the femoral head, flat femoral head, slipped capital femoral epiphysis; (c) slender diaphysis of the long bones; (d) scoliosis, kyphoscoliosis, flattening of the vertebral bodies, basilar invagination; (e) pectus carinatum; (f) increased bone density in neonates; (g) ultrasound: increased echogenicity of muscle; computed tomography: increased muscle bulk with normal attenuation (Fig SY−S−3).

REFERENCES

Aberfeld DC, et al.: Myotonia, dwarfism, diffuse bone disease, and unusual ocular and facial abnormalities (a new syndrome). *Brain* 88:313, 1965.

Calzolari C, et al.: Schwartz-Jampel syndrome with singular skeletal alterations. *Riv. Ital. Pediatr.* 8:265, 1982.

Edwards WC, et al.: Chondrodystrophic myotonia (Schwartz-Jampel syndrome): Report of a new case and follow-up of patients initially reported in 1969. *Am. J. Med. Genet.* 13:51, 1982.

Farrell SA, et al.: Neonatal manifestations of Schwartz-Jampel syndrome. *Am. J. Med. Genet.* 27:799, 1987.

Ferrannini E, et al.: Schwartz-Jampel syndrome with autosomal-dominant inheritance. *Eur. Neurol.* 21:137, 1982.

Horan F, et al.: Orthopaedic aspects of the Schwartz syndrome. *J. Bone Joint Surg. [Am.]* 57:542, 1975.

Pavone L, et al.: Immunologic abnormalities in Schwartz-Jampel syndrome. *J. Pediatr.* 98:512, 1981.

Schwartz O, Jampel RS: Congenital blepharophimosis associated with a unique generalized myopathy. *Arch. Ophthalmol.* 68:52, 1962.

Seay AR, et al.: Malignant hyperpyrexia in a patient with Schwartz-Jampel syndrome. *J. Pediatr.* 93:83, 1983.

Smith DL, et al.: Compressive myelopathy in the Schwartz-Jampel syndrome. *Ann. Neurol.* 9:497, 1981.

Stewart SR, et al.: Immunologic profile of the Schwartz-Jampel (osteo-chondro-muscular dystrophy) syndrome. *J. Pediatr.* 96:958, 1980.

SCIMITAR SYNDROME

Synonyms: Pulmonary venolobar syndrome; venolobar syndrome; Halarz syndrome.

Mode of Inheritance: Some familial cases have been reported (autosomal dominant).

Pathology: (a) hypoplasia of the right lung and right pulmonary artery; (b) dextroposition of the heart; (c) anomalous systemic vessels to an abnormal segment originating totally or in part from the thoracic aorta, abdominal aorta, or even the celiac axis; (d) anomalous venous drainage of part or all of

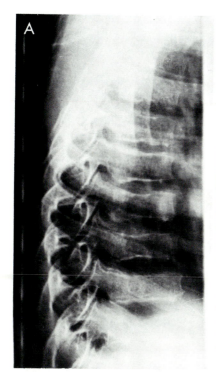
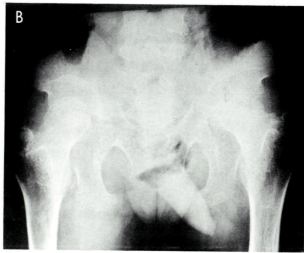

FIG SY−S−3.
Schwartz-Jampel syndrome. **A,** platyspondyly. **B,** pelvic dysplasia, coxa vara, flattening of the capital femoral epiphysis. (From Horan F, Beighton P: Orthopedic aspects of Schwartz syndrome. *J. Bone Joint Surg. [Am.]* 57:542, 1974. Used by permission.)

the right lung usually into the inferior vena cava, portal vein, hepatic vein, or rarely the lower right atrium; (e) anomalies of the diaphragm on the affected side (accessory diaphragm, hernia, cyst); (f) extrapleural soft tissues replacing missing lobe(s); (g) associated congenital heart defects (atrial septal defect, coarctation of the aorta, ventricular septal defect, patent ductus arteriosus, tetralogy of Fallot, etc.).

Clinical Manifestations: May be asymptomatic or symptomatic: (a) recurrent respiratory infection; (b) decrease in breath sounds on the right side of the chest; (c) small right hemithorax.

Radiologic Manifestations: (a) *shift of the heart and mediastinum to the right*; (b) unsharp right cardiac border (due to a strong rotation of the heart into the right hemithorax) and right hemidiaphragm; (c) *scimitar-shaped vein located in the right supradiaphragmatic region and draining into the inferior vena cava* (partial or total anomalous drainage), other forms of anomalous venous drainage: "double-scimitar" venous drainage into the inferior vena cava, simultaneous venous return from the right lung to both the inferior vena cava and the left atrium or scimitar-type vein draining into the left atrium without connection to the inferior vena cava, association with a crossover lung segment, left-sided scimitar syndrome (anomalous left pulmonary venous drainage to the inferior vena cava and through the pericardiophrenic vein to the innominate vein); (d) computed tomography (CT): hyparterial relationship of the right bronchus to the pulmonary artery, the course and drainage site of the scimitar vein, mediastinal shift, unusual fissures, abnormal bronchial tree, and pulmo-

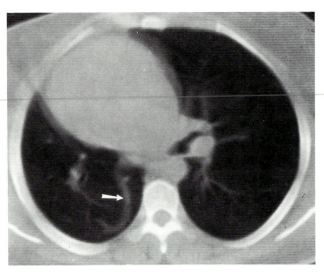

FIG SY–S–5.
Scimitar syndrome. A CT scan at the level of the left lower bronchus shows a strong mediastinal shift to the right, abnormal lucency of the right lung, and disordered vascularity. The large scimitar vein *(arrow)* curving posteriorly is connected to the hilum (probably to the left atrium) at this level and on the lower section was shown to be connected to the inferior vena cava. (From Godwin JD, Traver RD: Scimitar syndrome: Four new cases examined with CT. *Radiology* 159:15, 1986. Used by permission.)

nary lobation; (e) bronchiectasis of the right lung (Figs SY–S–4 and SY–S–5).

REFERENCES

Bennet J, et al.: Le syndrome de Halasz. *Ann. Radiol. (Paris)* 18:271, 1975.

Blaysat G, et al.: Le syndrome du cimeterre du nourrisson. Physiopathologie et déductions thérapeutiques dans 12 cas. *Arch. Fr. Pediatr.* 44:245, 1987.

Clements BS, et al.: The crossover lung segment: Congenital malformation associated with a variant of scimitar syndrome. *Thorax* 42:417, 1987.

Cooper G: Case of malformation of the thoracic viscera: Consisting of imperfect development of right lung, and transposition of the heart. *Lond. Med. Gaz.* 18:600, 1836.

Dische MR, et al.: Horseshoe lung associated with a variant of the "scimitar" syndrome. *Br. Heart J.* 36:617, 1974.

Felson B: Scimitar syndrome: Four new cases examined with CT (letter). *Radiology* 162:581, 1987.

Gikonyo DK, et al.: Scimitar syndrome in neonates: Report of four cases and review of the literature. *Pediatr. Cardiol.* 6:193, 1986.

Godwin JD, et al.: Scimitar syndrome: Four new cases examined with CT. *Radiology* 159:15, 1986.

Halasz N, et al.: Bronchial and arterial anomalies with drainage of the right lung into the inferior vena cava. *Circulation* 14:826, 1956.

Haworth SG, et al.: Pulmonary hypertension in scimitar syndrome in infancy. *Br. Heart J.* 50:182, 1983.

Mardini MK, et al.: Anomalous left pulmonary venous drainage to the inferior vena cava and through the pericardio-

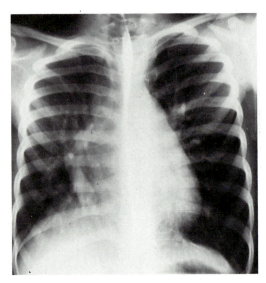

FIG SY–S–4.
Scimitar syndrome in a 5-year-old female. Note the slightly smaller right hemithorax as compared with the left, the minimal shift of the heart to the right, the indistinct right cardiac border, and the scimitar-shape anomalous vein. (From Gwinn JL, Barnes GR Jr: Radiological case of the month. *Am. J. Dis. Child.* 114:585, 1967. Used by permission.)

phrenic vein to the innominate vein: Left-sided scimitar syndrome. *Am. Heart J.* 101:860, 1981.

Morgan JR, et al.: Syndrome of hypoplasia of the right lung and dextroposition of the heart: "Scimitar sign" with normal pulmonary venous drainage. *Circulation* 43:27, 1971.

Osborn AG, et al.: Unusual venous drainage patterns in the scimitar syndrome. *Radiology* 113:601, 1974.

Partridge JB, et al.: Scimitar et cetera—the dysmorphic right lung. *Clin. Radiol.* 39:11, 1988.

Pearl W: Scimitar variant. *Pediatr. Cardiol.* 8:139, 1987.

Platia EV, et al.: Scimitar syndrome with peripheral left pulmonary artery branch stenoses. *Am. Heart J.* 107:594, 1984.

Tomsick TA, et al.: The congenital pulmonary venolobar syndrome in three successive generations. *J. Can. Assoc. Radiol.* 27:196, 1976.

SCLERODERMA

Synonyms: Progressive systemic sclerosis; systemic scleroderma; acrosclerosis syndromes.

Clinical Manifestations: Chronic or subacute course involving *several systems:* (a) *skin edema, induration, and finally atrophy;* (b) gangrene of the extremities; (c) joint pain; (d) *Raynaud phenomenon* (in about 60%), microangiopathy evaluated by dynamic fluorescence videomicroscopy; (e) dysphagia, nausea and vomiting, constipation, or diarrhea, abdominal distension, intestinal pseudo-obstruction, secondary malabsorption (abnormal intraluminal bacterial flora), fecalith formation associated with constipation, acute abdominal manifestation (obstruction, bowel perforation, peritonitis, bowel infarction, hemorrhage due to telangiectasia); (f) pericardial disease (acute process with chest pain, dyspnea, fever and a precardial friction rub or a chronic picture of pericardial effusion), myocardial fibrosis (diffuse and patchy distribution, abnormalities of myocardial perfusion), disorders of cardiac rhythm and conduction; (g) diminished ventilatory function of the lung (interstitial fibrosis with distortion of smaller airways and bronchiolectasis, arterial abnormalities), pulmonary hypertension, etc; (h) other reported abnormalities: pulmonary hypertension, cor pulmonale, malabsorption syndrome, scleroderma renal crisis, association with hypothyroidism or hyperthyroidism, impotence, etc.

Radiologic Manifestations: (a) *extremities:* (1) *absorption of the distal phalanges,* absorption of carpal bones and the distal portions of the radius and ulna (rare); (2) periarticular soft-tissue swelling, *joint destruction;* (3) *soft-tissue calcification;* (4) generalized osteoporosis; (5) carpal synostosis; (6) periosteal new bone formation of the long bones; (7) thickening of the skin (ultrasonographic measurement of the finger: 3.3 ± 0.7 mm as compared with normal control subjects of 2.5 ± 0.2 mm); (b) *alimentary tract:* (1) *wide and atonic esophagus* with decreased peristalsis, stricture, Barrett esophagus; (2) *atonic dilated stomach;* (3) gastroesophageal reflux; (4) *dilatation and sacculation of the small bowel* with decreased motility and peristaltic activity, prolonged transit time, increased fluid, diverticula, packed valvulae; (5) *areas*

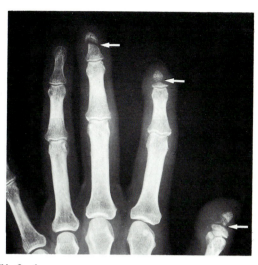

FIG SY–S–6.
Scleroderma: osseous resorption *(arrows)* as transverse bands across the shafts of the distal phalanges. (From Bassett LW, Block KLN, Furst DE, et al.: Skeletal findings in progressive systemic sclerosis (scleroderma). *A.J.R.* 136:1121, 1981. Used by permission.)

of sacculation and narrowing of the colon and thickened longitudinal folds in the narrowed segment, increased fluid, postevacuation residua, increased length, lack of haustrations, megacolon; (c) *chest:* (1) rib erosion; (2) *cardiomegaly;* (3) small *cystic areas in the lung;* (4) *diffuse lung fibrosis,* in particular, in the lower lobes; (5) pericardial effusion; (d) *teeth:* widening of the periodontal membrane; (e) other reported abnormalities: resorption of ribs and the medial ends of the clavicles, ankylosis of the interphalangeal joints, intra-articular calcification associated with bone erosion, dilatation of the pulmonary artery and main branches in patients with pulmonary arterial hypertension, diffuse spotty lucencies on the nephrogram phase of renal arteriography, corrugated mucosal pattern of the esophagus, atypical wide-mouthed esophageal diverticula, etc.

Notes: Tuft resorption and soft-tissue calcification in the fingers are more common in child scleroderma; small-bowel involvement, hand contractures, and erosive arthropathy are less frequent in child as compared with adult scleroderma (Fig SY–S–6).

REFERENCES

Agha FP, et al.: Barrett's esophagus complicating scleroderma. *Gastrointest. Radiol.* 10:325, 1985.

Åkesson A, et al.: Ultrasound examination of skin thickness in patients with progressive systemic sclerosis (scleroderma). *Acta. Radiol.* 27:91, 1986.

Bassett LW, et al.: Skeletal findings in progressive systemic sclerosis (scleroderma). *A.J.R.* 136:1121, 1981.

Bollinger A, et al.: Microangiopathy of progressive systemic sclerosis. Evaluation by dynamic fluorescence videomicroscopy. *Arch. Intern. Med.* 146:1541, 1986.

Brower AC, et al.: Unusual articular changes of the hand in scleroderma. *Skeletal Radiol.* 4:119, 1979.

Campbell WL, et al.: Specificity and sensitivity of esophageal motor abnormality in systemic sclerosis (scleroderma) and related diseases: A cineradiography study. *Gastrointest. Radiol.* 11:218, 1986.

Drane WE, et al.: Progressive systemic sclerosis: Radionuclide esophageal scintigraphy and manometry. *Radiology* 160:73, 1986.

Elke M, et al.: Histologische Befunde an umschriebenen arrodierten Rippen bei Lungenfibrose im Verlaufe von Sklerodermie. *Arch. Klin. Med.* 212:73, 1966.

Horowitz AL, et al.: The "hide-bound" small bowel of scleroderma: Characteristic mucosal fold pattern. *A.J.R.* 119:332, 1973.

Nicholson D, et al.: Progressive systemic sclerosis and Graves' disease. *Arch. Intern. Med.* 146:2350, 1986.

Nowlin NS, et al.: Impotence in scleroderma. *Ann. Intern. Med.* 104:794, 1986.

Owens GR, et al.: Cardiopulmonary manifestations of systemic sclerosis. *Chest* 91:118, 1987.

Resnick D, et al.: Selective involvement of the first carpometacarpal joint in scleroderma. *A.J.R.* 131:283, 1978.

Rohrmann CA, et al.: Radiologic and histologic differentiation of neuromuscular disorders of the gastrointestinal tract: Visceral myopathies, visceral neuropathies, and progressive systemic sclerosis. *A.J.R.* 143:933, 1981.

Shamberger RC, et al.: Progressive systemic sclerosis resulting in megacolon. *J.A.M.A.* 250:1063, 1983.

Shanks MJ, et al.: Radiographic findings of scleroderma in childhood. *A.J.R.* 141:657, 1983.

Singsen BH: Scleroderma in childhood. *Pediatr. Clin. North Am.* 33:1119, 1986.

Steigerwald JC, et al.: Bone resorption of the ribs and pulmonary function in progressive systemic sclerosis. *Chest* 68:838, 1975.

Texier L, et al.: Aspects cutaneo-muqueux des sclérodermies. *Ann. Med. Interne. (Paris)* 135:580, 1984.

Traub YM, et al.: Hypertension and renal failure (scleroderma renal crisis) in progressive systemic sclerosis. Review of a 25-year experience with 68 cases. *Medicine (Baltimore)* 62:335, 1983.

Ungerer RG, et al.: Prevalence and clinical correlates of pulmonary arterial hypertension in progressive systemic sclerosis. *Am. J. Med.* 75:65, 1983.

von Reinbold WD, et al.: Benignes Pneumoperitoneum bei progressiver Systemsklerose. *Fortschr. Rontgenstr.* 144:115, 1986.

Winograd J, et al.: The spotted nephrogram of renal scleroderma. *A.J.R.* 126:734, 1976.

SEA-BLUE HISTIOCYTE SYNDROME

Clinical Manifestations: (a) *abnormal cells (histiocytes) containing large blue cytoplasmic granules in the bone marrow, skin, lung, gastrointestinal tract, nervous system, spleen*; (b) *splenomegaly, hepatomegaly, progressive hepatic cirrhosis, lymphadenopathies*; (c) *periodic hemorrhagic diathesis associated with thrombocytopenia*; (d) other reported abnormalities: retinal involvement, nervous system involvement, association with cholesterol ester storage disease, etc.

Radiologic Manifestations: (a) pulmonary nodular densities, hilar adenopathy; (b) *hepatosplenomegaly.*

REFERENCES

Ashwal S, et al.: A new form of sea-blue histiocytosis associated with progressive anterior horn cell and axon degeneration. *Ann. Neurol.* 16:184, 1984.

Besley GTN, et al.: Cholesterol ester storage disease in an adult presenting with sea-blue histiocytosis. *Clin. Genet.* 26:195, 1984.

Jones B, et al.: Sea-blue histiocyte disease in siblings. *Lancet* 2:73, 1970.

Sawitsky A, et al.: An unidentified reticuloendothelial cell in bone marrow and spleen: Report of two cases with histochemical studies. *Blood* 9:977, 1954.

Zina AM, et al.: Sea-blue histiocyte syndrome with cutaneous involvement. Case report with ultrastructural findings. *Dermatologica* 174:39, 1987.

SEAT BELT SYNDROME

Clinical Manifestations: Trauma in persons wearing lap seat belts who are involved in high-speed collisions that results from acute flexion over the seat belt; contusion of the anterior abdominal wall usually present.

Radiologic Manifestations: (a) *"Chance fracture" of the vertebrae* (flexion fractures of the lumbar spine consisting of horizontal splitting of the vertebral body and posterior arch that is accompanied by separation of the posterior elements), simple compression fractures of the lumbar vertebrae, *various degrees of disruption of the posterior elements,* fracture and subluxation of the upper thoracic vertebrae; (b) abdominal visceral injuries: liver, spleen, pancreas, kidneys, bladder, pregnant uterus, bowel, mesentery, omentum; (c) vascular injuries (chest and abdomen); (d) heart contusion; (e) disruption of the abdominal wall musculature.

REFERENCES

Chance GQ: Note on type of flexion fracture of the spine. *Br. J. Radiol.* 21:452, 1948.

Dehner JR: Seat belt injuries of the spine and abdomen. *A.J.R.* 111:833, 1971.

Hampson S, et al.: Fractures of the upper thoracic spine—and addition to the "seat-belt" syndrome. *Br. J. Radiol.* 57:1033, 1984.

Taylor GA, et al.: Lap-belt injuries of the lumbar spine in children: A pitfall in CT diagnosis. *A.J.R.* 150:1355, 1988.

Wagner AC: Disruption of abdominal wall musculature: Unusual feature of seat belt syndrome. *A.J.R.* 133:753, 1979.

Woelfel GF, et al.: Severe thoracic and abdominal injuries associated with lap-harness seatbelts. *J. Trauma* 24:166, 1984.

SECKEL SYNDROME

Synonyms: Bird-headed dwarfism; Virchow-Seckel dwarfism.

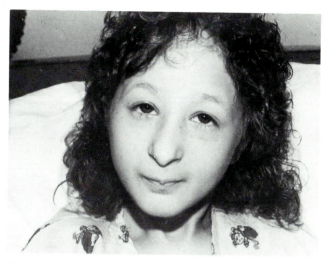

FIG SY–S–7.
Seckel syndrome in a 12-year-old girl. (From Butler MG, Hall BD, Maclean RN, et al.: Do some patients with Seckel syndrome have hematological problems and/or chromosome breakage? *Am. J. Med. Genet.* 27:645, 1987. Used by permission.)

Mode of Inheritance: Probably autosomal recessive.

Frequency: Uncommon.

Clinical Manifestations: (a) *low birth weight, dwarfism;* (b) *mental retardation;* (c) *bird-headed appearance* (microcephaly, beaklike protrusion of the nose, hypoplasia of the cheek bones, prominent eyes, ocular hypertelorism, micrognathia; (d) other reported abnormalities: low-set ears, lobeless ears, high-arched or cleft palate, cryptorchidism, various urogenital anomalies, flexion contracture of the elbows, hypoplastic anemia, pancytopenia, chromosomal instability.

Radiologic Manifestations: (a) *microcrania, ocular hypertelorism, hypoplasia of the maxillae and mandible;* (b) hand and wrist: ivory epiphyses, cone-shaped epiphyses in the proximal phalanges, disharmoic skeletal maturation (carpals, phalanges), alteration in tubular bone length, small carpal bones, angular carpal bone configuration, normal or increased cortical thickness of the metacarpals, incurving of the distal phalanges, clubbing of fingers, hypoplastic thumb; (c) other reported abnormalities: premature closure of cranial sutures, missing or atrophic teeth, kyphoscoliosis, sternal anomalies, absence of patellae, absence of tibiofibular joints, short fibulas, dislocations (hip, knee, elbow), rhizomelic shortening of the humeri and femora (Fig SY–S–7).

REFERENCES

Amici G, et al.: Sindrome di Seckel. *Minerva Pediatr.* 29:2077, 1977.
Bass HN, et al.: Seckel syndrome with disproportional dwarfism. *Birth Defects* 12(6):139, 1976.
Butler MG, et al.: Do some patients with Seckel syndrome have hematological problems and/or chromosome breakage? *Am. J. Med. Genet.* 27:645, 1987.
Cervenka J, et al.: Seckel's dwarfism: Analysis of chromosome breakage and sister chromatid exchanges. *Am. J. Dis. Child.* 133:555, 1979.
Lilleyman JS: Constitutional hypoplastic anemia associated with familial "bird-headed" dwarfism (Seckel syndrome). *Am. J. Pediatr. Hematol. Oncol.* 6:207, 1984.
Majewski F, et al.: Studies of microcephalic primordial dwarfism 1: Approach to a delineation of the Seckel syndrome. *Am. J. Med. Genet.* 12:7, 1982.
Poznanski AK, et al.: Radiological findings in the hand in Seckel syndrome (bird-headed dwarfism). *Pediatr. Radiol.* 13:19, 1983.
Seckel HPG: *Bird-headed Dwarfs: Studies in Developmental Anthropology Including Human Proportions.* Springfield, Ill., Charles C. Thomas Publisher, 1960.
Toudic L, et al.: Nanism intra-uterin majeur avec dysmorphies et encéphalopathie profond du type nanisme à tête d'oiseau (Virchow-Seckel). *Ann. Pediatr. (Paris)* 24:653, 1977.

SENIOR SYNDROME

Clinical Manifestations: (a) *short stature at birth;* (b) *minute toenails* (one or more small toes bilaterally); (c) other reported abnormalities: mild intellectual impairment, broad nose, wide mouth, incurving of the fifth fingers.

Radiologic Manifestations: Short middle phalanges of the fifth fingers, fusion of the middle and distal phalanges of the fifth toes.

REFERENCES

Mace JW, et al.: Short stature and onychodysplasia: Report of a case resembling Senior syndrome. *Am. J. Dis. Child.* 125:114, 1973.
Senior B: Impaired growth and onychodysplasia: Short children with tiny toenails. *Am. J. Dis. Child.* 122:7, 1971.

SÉZARY SYNDROME

Clinical and Radiologic Manifestations: (a) erythroderma, intractable itching; (b) Sézary cells (abnormal lymphocytes) in the skin and peripheral blood; (c) lymphadenopathy; (d) other reported abnormalities: hyperpigmentation, loss of hair, loss or thickening of the nails, hyperkeratosis of the palms and soles, visceral involvement, oral mucosal lesions (enlarged tongue, tenderness, etc.), IgE hyperimmunoglobulinemia and storage histiocytosis, etc.

Note: Sézary syndrome is an epidermotropic variant of cutaneous T-cell lymphoma.

REFERENCES

Kuhn BS, et al.: Intraoral manifestations of Sézary's syndrome: Report of a case. *J. Oral Maxillofac Surg.* 46:303, 1988.

Miyayama H, et al.: Massive IgE-hyperimmunoglobulinemia and storage histiocytosis in Sézary syndrome. A postmortem study. *Cancer* 53:1869, 1984.

Paradinas FJ, et al.: Visceral lesions in an unusual case of Sézary's syndrome. *Cancer* 33:1068, 1974.

Sausville EA, et al.: Histopathologic staging at initial diagnosis of mycosis fungoides and the Sézary syndrome. Definition of three distinctive prognostic groups. *Ann. Intern. Med.* 109:372, 1988.

Sézary A: Nouvelle réticulose cutanée: La réticulose maligne leucémique à histomonocytes monstrueux et à forme d'erythrodermie oedémateuse et pigmentée. *Ann. Dermatol. Syph.* 9:5, 1944.

Willemze R: Recent developments in the early diagnosis of mycosis fungoides and Sézary's syndrome. *Eur. J. Cancer Clin. Oncol.* 23:1581, 1987.

SHAH-WAARDENBURG SYNDROME

Synonyms: Waardenburg-Shah syndrome; Hirschsprung disease with pigmentary anomaly.

Mode of Inheritance: Autosomal recessive.

Frequency: Rare.

Clinical and Radiologic Manifestations: (a) white forelock; (b) isochromia iridis; (c) long-segment Hirschsprung disease.

REFERENCES

Ambani LM: Waardenburg and Hirschsprung syndromes. *J. Pediatr.* 102:802, 1983.

Farndon PA, et al.: Waardenburg's syndrome associated with total aganglionosis. *Arch. Dis. Child.* 58:932, 1983.

Shah KN, et al.: White forelock, pigmentary disorder of irides, and long segment Hirschsprung's disease, possible variant of Waardenburg's syndrome. *J. Pediatr.* 99:432, 1981.

SHAPIRO SYNDROME

Clinical Manifestations: (a) *spontaneous relapsing hypothermia*; (b) *episodic hyperhidrosis*; (c) abnormal electroencephalographic findings; (d) other reported abnormalities: seizures, primary organic polydipsia, insufficient antidiuretic hormone secretion, pituitary dwarfism, precocious puberty, behavioral disturbances during attack.

Radiologic Manifestations: *Agenesis of the corpus callosum.*

REFERENCES

Dutan G, et al.: Syndrome de Shapiro. *Pediatrie* 30:117, 1975.

Guihard J, et al.: Hypothermie spontané récidivante avec agénésie du corps calleux: Syndrome de Shapiro (nouvelle observation). *Ann. Pediatr. (Paris)* 18:645, 1971.

LeWitt PA, et al.: Episodic hyperhidrosis, hypothermia, and agenesis of corpus callosum. *Neurology* 33:1122, 1983.

Shapiro WR, et al.: Spontaneous recurrent hypothermia accompanying agenesis of corpus callosum. *Brain* 92:423, 1969.

SHEEHAN SYNDROME

Pathology: *Necrosis of the pituitary during the postpartum period*, secondary atrophy: thyroid, adrenal cortex, ovaries.

Clinical Manifestations: *Acute postpartum shock followed by asthenia, failure of lactation, amenorrhea or menstrual irregularity, pallor, anorexia, brachycardia, hypotension, weight loss, cachexia, clinical manifestations of hypothyroidism, adrenal insufficiency, and gonadal insufficiency.*

Radiologic Manifestations: (a) *small sella turcica* reported in 10 of 14 patients several years after the onset of symptoms; (b) "empty sella," hypodensity (computed tomography) in the area of the hypophysis with preservation of the pituitary stalk.

REFERENCES

Fleckman AM, et al.: Empty sella of normal size in Sheehan's syndrome. *Am. J. Med.* 75:585, 1983.

Hazard J, et al.: Aspect actuel du syndrome de Sheehan. Vingt observations. *Ann. Med. Interne (Paris)* 136:21, 1985.

Meador CK, et al.: The sella turcica in postmortem pituitary necrosis (Sheehan's syndrome). *Ann. Intern. Med.* 65:259, 1966.

Reye von: Die ersten klinischen Symptom bei Schwund des Hypophysenvorderlappens (Simmondssche Krankheit) und ihre erfolgreiche Behandlung. *Dtsch. Med. Wochenschr.* 54:696, 1928.

Sheehan HL: Post-partum necrosis of the anterior pituitary. *J. Pathol. Bacteriol.* 45:189, 1937.

Sheehan HL: Simmonds's disease due to postpartum necrosis of the anterior pituitary. *Q. J. Med.* 8:277, 1939.

Simmonds M: Ueber Hypophysisschwund mit tödlichem Ausgang. *Dtsch. Med. Wochenschr.* 40:322, 1914.

Tolis G, et al.: Sheehan's syndrome: In vivo diagnosis with the use of computerized axial tomography and pituitary provocative testing. *Fertil. Steril.* 41:146, 1984.

SHONE SYNDROME

Clinical and Radiologic Manifestations: (a) "parachute mitral valve"; (b) supravalvular ring of the left atrium; (c) subaortic stenosis; (d) coarctation of the aorta.

REFERENCE

Shone JD, et al.: The developmental complex of "parachute mitral valve," supravalvular ring of left atrium, subaortic stenosis, and coarctation of aorta. *Am. J. Cardiol.* 11:714, 1963.

SHORT-BOWEL SYNDROME

Etiology: (a) congenital; (b) acquired (postsurgical), in particular, in cases with an absence of the distal portion of the ileum and ileocecal valve or resection of more than two thirds of the small bowel.

Clinical Manifestations: *Diarrhea, steatorrhea, dehydration, malnutrition, failure to thrive, vomiting, gastric hypersecretion,* metabolic acidosis due to D-lactic acidosis related to abnormal intestinal bacterial flora, oxaluria.

Pathology: *Adaptation changes in the bowel wall* (increased diameter of the intestine; increase in villus height; increase in crypt depth; hyperplasia-increased cell proliferation and migration rate; increased rate of DNA synthesis and total DNA, RNA, and protein concentrations; increase in water, electrolyte, and nutrient transport per centimeter of small intestine; increase in mucosal enzymes per centimeter of small intestine; changes in tissue metabolism accompanied by regeneration and growth).

Radiologic Manifestations: *increased diameter of the small intestine, thickening and hypertrophy of the bowel wall.*

Note: A syndrome with autosomal recessive inheritance and a congenitally short small bowel in association with malrotation, functional intestinal obstruction, and in a high percentage of cases, hypertrophic pyloric stenosis has been reported (Royer et al. and others).

REFERENCES

Grosfeld JL, et al.: Short bowel syndrome in infancy and childhood. Analysis of survival in 60 patients. *Surgery* 151:41, 1986.

Hermier M, et al.: D'un nouveau cas de grêle court congénital avec malrotation intestinale. *Arch. Fr. Pediatr.* 33:251, 1976.

Kemperdick H, et al.: Small bowel aplasia combined with duodenal atresia and malrotation of the colon (short bowel syndrome). *Z. Kinderchir.* 17:217, 1975.

Kerner JA Jr, et al.: The medical and surgical management of infants with the short bowel syndrome. *J. Perinatol.* 5:13, 1984.

Lin C-H, et al.: Nutritional assessment of children with short-bowel syndrome receiving home parenteral nutrition. *Am. J. Dis. Child.* 141:1093, 1987.

Royer P, et al.: Le syndrome familial de grêle court avec malrotation intestinal et sténose hypertrophique du pylore chez le nourrisson. *Arch. Fr. Pediatr.* 31:223, 1974.

Sansaricq C, et al.: Familial congenital short small bowel with associated defects. *Clin. Pediatr. (Phila.)* 23:453, 1983.

Schoorel EP, et al.: D-lactic acidosis in a boy with short bowel syndrome. *Arch. Dis. Child.* 55:810, 1980.

Scully JM, et al.: Serum gastrin concentration in infants with short gut syndrome. *J. Pediatr. Surg.* 11:315, 1976.

Shawis RN, et al.: Functional intestinal obstruction associated with malrotation and short small-bowel. *J. Pediatr. Surg.* 19:172, 1984.

Sheldon GF: Role of parenteral nutrition in patients with short bowel syndrome. *Am. J. Med.* 67:1021, 1979.

Wilmore DW: Factors correlating with successful outcome following extensive intestinal resection in the newborn infant. *J. Pediatr.* 80:88, 1972.

SHPRINTZEN-GOLDBERG SYNDROME

Clinical and Radiologic Manifestations: Reported in two unrelated children: (a) craniosynostosis; (b) exophthalmos; (c) maxillary and mandibular hypoplasia; (d) soft-tissue hypertrophy of the palatal shelves; (e) low-set, pliable auricles; (f) arachnodactyly; (g) abdominal hernias; (h) obstructive apnea; (i) mental retardation, development delay; (j) joint contractures.

REFERENCE

Shprintzen RJ, Goldberg RB: A recurrent pattern syndrome of craniosynostosis associated with arachnodactyly and abdominal hernias. *J. Craniofac. Genet. Dev. Biol.* 2:65, 1982.

SHY-DRAGER SYNDROME

Synonym: Progressive autonomic nervous system failure (PAF).

Mode of Inheritance: Possibly autosomal dominant.

Pathology: Symmetrical degeneration in the intermediolateral columns, hypothalmus, caudate nuclei, Onuf nucleus of the sacral cord.

Clinical Manifestations: (a) *orthostatic hypotension* without acceleration of the pulse; (b) *urinary and fecal incontinence,* abnormal urodynamic study results (detrusor areflexia, detrusor hyperreflexia, lower neuron lesion involving periurethral striated muscle); (c) *erectile impotence;* (d) *anhidrosis;* (e) other reported abnormalities: paralysis of the laryngeal abductor muscles, association with pheochromocytoma, iris atrophy, external ocular palsies, rigidity, tremor, fasciculations, myasthenia, anterior horn cell neuropathy.

Radiologic Manifestations: (a) magnetic resonance imaging: a decrease in signal intensity of the putamina, particularly along their lateral and posterior portions (T_2-weighted sequences and T_1-weighted spin-echo sequences); (b) open vesical neck at rest.

REFERENCES

Chadenas D, et al.: Pheochromocytome associé a un syndrome de dysautonomie de Shy et Drager. *Presse Med.* 16:965, 1987.

Drayer BP, et al.: Parkinson plus syndrome: Diagnosis using high field MR imaging of brain iron. *Radiology* 159:493, 1986.

Gilmartin JJ, et al.: Upper airway obstruction complicating the Shy-Drager syndrome. *Thorax* 39:313, 1984.

Kachi T, et al.: Effect of L-threo-3,4-dihydroxyphenylserine on muscle sympathetic nerve activities in Shy-Drager syndrome. *Neurology* 38:1091, 1988.

Lewis P: Familial orthostatic hypotension. *Brain* 87:719, 1964.

Pastakia B, et al.: Multiple system atrophy (Shy-Drager syndrome): MR imaging. *Radiology* 159:499, 1986.

Salinas JM, et al.: Urological evaluation in the Shy-Drager syndrome. *J. Urol.* 135:741, 1986.

Shy GM, Drager GA: A neurologic syndrome associated with orthostatic hypotension: A clinical-pathologic study. *Arch. Neurol.* 2:511, 1960.

Wheeler JS, et al.: Voiding dysfunction in Shy-Drager syndrome. *J. Urol.* 134:362, 1985.

SILVER-RUSSELL SYNDROME

Synonyms: Silver syndrome; Russell-Silver syndrome.

Mode of Inheritance: Autosomal dominant and X-linked transmissions have been suggested in some families.

Frequency: Uncommon.

Clinical Manifestations: (a) *low birth weight* at full term; (b) *short stature;* (c) facial or limb asymmetry in some cases; (d) *pseudohydrocephalic appearance,* frontal bossing, *small triangular face,* small mandible; (e) downturned corners of the mouth ("shark mouth"); (f) short and/or incurved fifth fingers; (g) mental retardation; (h) endocrine abnormalities: abnormal pattern of sexual development (increased serum or urinary gonadotropin levels in the prepubertal age, precocious sexual development, premature mucosal esterogenation, sexual ambiguity), growth hormone deficiency, corticotropin deficiency, panhypopituitarism; (i) other reported abnormalities: cryptorchidism, clitoromegaly, chromosome abnormalities (trisomy 18 mosaicism, deletion of the short arm of chromosome 18), syndactyly, poor muscular development, mental retardation, urinary tract infections, large anterior fontanelle, hypoglycemia, café au lait spots, syndactyly of the feet, disproportionately short arms, difficult pregnancy, blue sclerae in infancy, 47,XXY karyotype.

Radiologic Manifestations: (a) *hand: clinodactyly; fifth, middle, or distal phalangeal hypoplasia;* syndactyly; Kirner deformity; ivory epiphysis; second metacarpal pseudoepiphysis; (b) *asymmetry;* (c) *skeletal maturation retardation,* difference in skeletal maturation of the two sides; (d) other re-

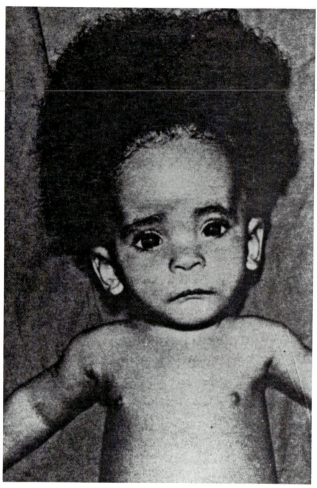

FIG SY–S–8.
Silver-Russell syndrome: broad prominent forehead, relative smallness of the lower portion of the face, pointed chin, downturned edges of the mouth, and thin vermilion border of the lips. (From Patton MA: Russell-Silver syndrome. *J. Med. Genet.* 25:557, 1988. Used by permission.)

ported abnormalities: elbow dislocation, hip dislocation, irregularities of the end plates of the vertebrae, hypoplasia of the sacrum and coccyx, renal anomalies (horseshoe kidney, etc.).

Differential Diagnosis: Chromosomal abnormalities (18p-, 18 trisomy/normal mosaicism, triploid/normal mosaicism, etc); mulibrey nanism; Noonan syndrome.

Notes: The extreme clinical diversity and the nonspecificity of the diagnostic criteria for the "syndrome" are responsible for the inclusion of heterogeneous conditions with overlapping clinical features under the title of Silver-Russell syndrome; there has been a question as to whether the syndromes described by Silver and Russell represent a single condition or two separate ones (Figs SY–S–8 and SY–S–9).

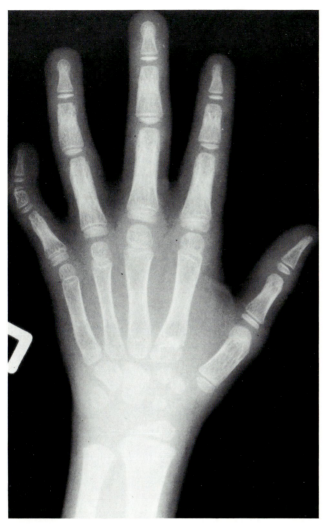

FIG SY–S–9.
Silver-Russell syndrome: hand and wrist radiograph of an 8-year-old boy with ivory epiphyses of the distal phalanges. No 2 to 4 digits, clinodactyly with a short fifth middle phalanx, pseudoepiphysis of the second metacarpal, and delayed bone age are present. (From Herman TE, Crawford JD, Cleveland RH, et al.: Hand radiographs in Russell-Silver syndrome. *Pediatrics* 79:743, 1987. Used by permission.)

REFERENCES

Arai Y, et al.: Horseshoe kidney in Russell-Silver syndrome. *Urology* 31:321, 1988.

Cassidy SB, et al.: Russell-Silver syndrome and hypopituitarism. Patient report and literature review. *Am. J. Dis. Child.* 140:155, 1986.

Davies PSW, et al.: Adolescent growth and pubertal progression in the Silver-Russell syndrome. *Arch. Dis. Child.* 63:130, 1988.

Escobar V, et al.: Phenotypic and genetic analysis of the Silver-Russell syndrome. *Clin. Genet.* 13:278, 1978.

Fjord M, et al.: Deletion short arm 18 and Silver-Russell syndrome. *Acta Paediatr. Scand.* 67:101, 1978.

Gardner LI: The lessons of Polyploidy. Relation to congenital asymmetry and the Russell-Silver syndrome. *Am. J. Dis. Child.* 136:292, 1982.

Gareis FJ, et al.: The Russell-Silver syndrome without asymmetry. *J. Pediatr.* 79:775, 1971.

Hansen KK, et al.: Silver-Russell syndrome with unusual findings. *Pediatrics* 79:125, 1987.

Haslam RHA, et al.: Renal abnormalities in the Russell-Silver syndrome. *Pediatrics* 51:216, 1973.

Herman TE, et al.: Hand radiographs in Russell-Silver syndrome. *Pediatrics* 79:743, 1987.

LeGoffe J-Y, et al.: Puberté précoce et syndrome de Silver: Une association inhabituelle. *Arch. Fr. Pediatr.* 34:899, 1977.

Marks LJ: The Silver-Russell syndrome. A case with sexual ambiguity and a review of the literature. *Am. J. Dis. Child.* 131:447, 1977.

Moseley JE, et al.: The Silver syndrome: Congenital asymmetry, short stature and variations in sexual development; roentgen features. *A.J.R.* 97:74, 1966.

Nishi Y, et al.: Silver-Russell syndrome and growth hormone deficiency. *Acta Paediatr. Scand.* 71:1035, 1982.

Partington MW: X-linked Russell-Silver syndrome (abstract). *Proc. Greenwood Genet. Center* 4:139, 1985.

Partington MW: X-linked short stature with skin pigmentation: Evidence for heterogeneity of the Russell-Silver syndrome. *Clin. Genet.* 29:151, 1986.

Russell A: Syndrome of "intra-uterine" dwarfism recognizable at birth with craniofacial dysostosis, disproportionately short arms and other anomalies (5 examples). *Proc. R. Soc. Med.* 47:1040, 1954.

Saal HM, et al.: Reevaluation of Russell-Silver syndrome. *J. Pediatr.* 107:733, 1985.

Silver HK, et al.: Syndrome of congenital hemihypertrophy, shortness of stature and elevated urinary gonadotropins. *Pediatrics* 12:368, 1953.

Specht EE, et al.: Orthopaedic considerations of Silver's syndrome. *J. Bone Joint Surg. [Am.]* 55:1502, 1973.

Szalay GC: Russell-Silver dwarfism (letter). *J. Pediatr.* 108:1037, 1986.

Willems PJ, et al.: Activation of fatty acid oxidation in the Silver-Russell syndrome and the Brachmann-deLange syndrome. *Am. J. Med. Genet.* 30:865, 1988.

SIMPSON-GOLABI-BEHMEL SYNDROME

Synonyms: Golabi-Rosen syndrome; gigantism-dysplasia syndrome.

Mode of Inheritance: X-linked recessive with partial expression in some of the carriers.

Frequency: Very rare.

Clinical and Radiologic Manifestations: (a) *prenatal and postnatal overgrowth;* (b) *mental retardation;* (c) *"coarse" facial appearance, short and broad upturned nose, large mouth, submucous cleft/cleft palate, hypertelorism, grooved lower lip/tongue/gingiva;* (d) *other reported abnormalities: hepato-splenomegaly, bowel obstruction, Meckel diverticulum, large/cystic kidneys, undescended testes, inguinal hernia, coccygeal skin tag, sacral anomalies and a tail bone, hy-*

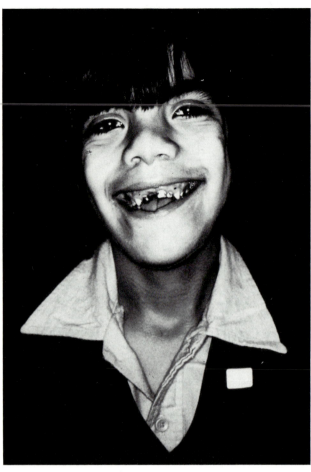

FIG SY–S–10.
Simpson-Golabi-Behmel syndrome in a 7-year-old boy with a coarse facial appearance, a short broad nose with an upturned ridged nasal tip, a large mouth, hypertelorism, and downslanted palpebral fissures. (From Golabi M, Rosen L: A new X-linked mental retardation-overgrowth syndrome. *Am. J. Med. Genet.* 17:345, 1984. Used by permission.)

poplasia of the distal phalanges, syndactyly of the second and third fingers and toes, tibial clinodactyly of the second toes, ulnar clinodactyly of the second fingers, postaxial polydactyly, supernumerary nipples (Fig SY–S–10).

REFERENCES

Golabi M, Rosen L: A new X-linked mental retardation-overgrowth syndrome. *Am. J. Med. Genet.* 17:345, 1984.
Kajii T, et al.: The Golabi-Rosen syndrome (letter). *Am. J. Med. Genet.* 19:819, 1984.
Neri G, et al.: Simpson-Golabi-Behmel syndrome: An X-linked encephalo-tropho-schisis syndrome. *Am. J. Med. Genet.* 30:287, 1988.
Opitz JM: The Golabi-Rosen syndrome—Report of a second family. *Am. J. Med. Genet.* 17:359, 1984.
Opitz JM, et al.: Simpson-Golabi-Behmel syndrome: Follow-up of the Michigan family. *Am. J. Med. Genet.* 30:301, 1988.

SINGLETON-MERTEN SYNDROME

Mode of Inheritance: No known genetic factor.

Frequency: Extremely rare.

Clinical Manifestations: Onset of symptoms in childhood: (a) history of *fever of unknown origin in early infancy, muscular weakness, poor development*; (b) *abnormal dentition*; (c) normal serum calcium, phosphorus, and alkaline phosphatase levels; (d) other reported abnormalities: chronic psoriasiform skin lesions, glaucoma, photosensitivity, hypertension, heart block, foot deformities.

Radiologic Manifestations: (a) skeletal demineralization; (b) *expanded shafts of metacarpals and phalanges with widened medullary cavities*; (c) *cardiomegaly*; (d) *intramural calcification of the proximal segment of the aorta* with extension into the descending aorta; aortic and mitral valve calcification; (e) other reported abnormalities: shallow acetabular fossa, subluxation of the femoral head, coxa valga, soft-tissue calcification between the radius and ulna, hypoplastic distal radial epiphysis, constriction of the proximal part of the shaft of the radius, acro-osteolysis, equinovarus foot deformity (Fig SY–S–11).

REFERENCES

Gay BB, et al.: A syndrome of widened medullary cavities of bone, aortic calcification, abnormal dentition, and muscular weakness (the Singleton-Merten syndrome). *Radiology* 118:389, 1976.
Singleton EB, Merten DF: An unusual syndrome of widened medullary cavities of the metacarpals and phalanges, aortic calcification and abnormal dentition. *Pediatr. Radiol.* 1:2, 1973.

SJÖGREN SYNDROME

Synonyms: Sicca syndrome; Gougerot-Sjögren syndrome; Gougerot-Houwer-Sjögren syndrome; Gougerot-Mikulicz-Sjögren syndrome.

Definition and Classification: An autoimmune exocrinopathy with production of multiple antibodies, lymphocytic infiltration of glandular and extraglandular organs, and polyclonal B-cell proliferation: (a) primary; (b) secondary: rheumatoid arthritis, systemic lupus erythematosus, etc.

Clinical Manifestations: Onset of symptoms usually in middle age (women in particular): (a) *xerostomia*; (b) *pharyngolaryngitis sicca*; (c) *rhinitis sicca*; (d) *keratoconjunctivitis*; (e) *painless swelling of the parotid glands*; (f) *polyarthritis* (in 50% to 60%); (g) rapid destruction of the teeth; (h) dry skin and vagina; (i) chronic bronchitis, recurrent pneumonitis, interstitial lymphocytic pneumonia, restrictive ventilatory impairment, interstitial fibrosis, small-airway disease, desiccation of the upper respiratory tract, large-airway obstruction, pleuritic pain; (j) central nervous system disease (in approxi-

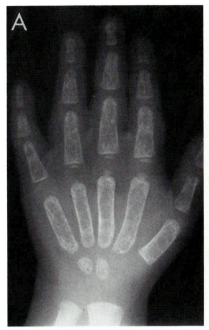

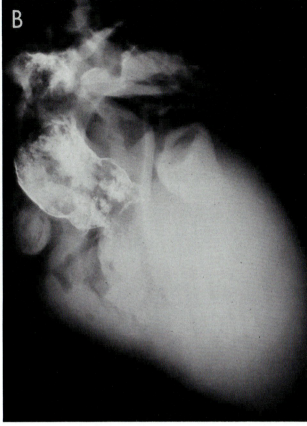

FIG SY–S–11.
Singleton-Merten syndrome in a 2-year-old child with a clinical history of increasing fatigability and intermittent fever. **A,** diffuse osteoporosis was found in a bone survey. Note the thinned cortices and hyperlucent expansion of the medullary space. **B,** gross cardiomegaly, extensive calcification of the aorta involving the aortic root and ascending aorta, and pulmonary edema were present at 4 years of age. A radiogram of a postmortem specimen shows aortic calcification including calcification of the aortic valve. (From Singleton EB, Merten DF: An unusual syndrome of widened medullary cavities of the metacarpals and phalanges, aortic calcification and abnormal dentition. *Pediatr. Radiol.* 1:2, 1973. Used by permission.)

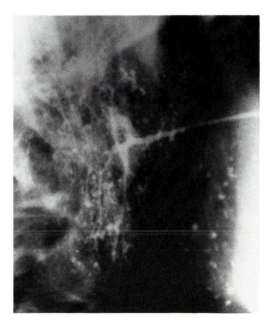

FIG SY–S–12.
Sjögren syndrome. A parotid sialogram shows peripheral cylindric and punctate sialectases. (From Gonzalez L, Mackenzie AH, Tarar RA: Parotid sialography in Sjögren's syndrome. *Radiology* 97:91, 1970. Used by permission.)

mately 20% of patients with primary Sjögren syndrome): the clinical picture resembling multiple sclerosis, aseptic meningoencephalitis, vasculitic neuropathy, psychiatric abnormalities (affective disturbances, etc.), hemiparesis, transient aphasia; (k) other reported abnormalities: renal tubular acidosis (in 20%), lymphoproliferative neoplasms, sclerosing cholangitis in association with pancreatitis, hypothyroidism, acrosclerosis associated with telangiectasis and myxedema, inclusion body myositis, retroperitoneal fibrosis, association with HLA-DR3, autoimmune hemolytic anemia in sisters, adherence of lipstick to the teeth, association with the CREST syndrome, increased HLA-B8 in primary sicca syndrome, infrequent familial occurrence, Raynaud phenomenon, etc.

Radiologic Manifestations: (a) *sialectasia* (punctate, globular, cavitary, and destructive types), atrophy of the salivary ducts, enlarged hetergeneously echogenic salivary glands, bilateral cystic lesions; (b) *various chest findings:* reticular-nodular infiltrate, patchy infiltrate, hilar lymph node enlargement, bronchiectasis; (c) lymphographic abnormalities (enlarged nodes with a foamy reticular pattern); (d) destructive juxta-articular changes; (e) nephrocalcinosis; (f) renal rickets; (g) mucosal atrophy of the esophagus, achalasia of the cardia, gastric hypersecretion; (h) nonenhancing (computed tomographic) lucencies in the brain in patients with clinical manifestations in the central nervous system; the lesions best detected by magnetic resonance imaging (predominantly within the subcortical and periventricular white matter); (i) other reported abnormalities: enlarged mediastinal nodes, distended gallbladder, etc. (Fig SY–S–12).

REFERENCES

Albert J, et al.: Association d'un syndrome de Gougerot-Sjögren et d'un syndrome C.R.S.T. avec calcifications intraarticulaires et lésions ostéolytiques inhabituelles. *J. Radiol.* 63:757, 1982.

Alexander EL, et al.: Magnetic resonance imaging of cerebral lesions in patients with the Sjögren syndrome. *Ann. Intern. Med.* 108:815, 1988.

Alexander EL, et al.: Neurologic complications of primary Sjögren's syndrome. *Medicine (Baltimore)* 61:247, 1982.

Alexander EL, et al.: Primary Sjögren's syndrome with central nervous system disease mimicking multiple sclerosis. *Ann. Intern. Med.* 104:323, 1986.

Allard PH, et al.: Pneumonie interstitielle lymphocytaire au cours d'un syndrome de Gougerot-Sjögren avec slérodermie. *Ann. Med. Interne (Paris)* 135:431, 1984.

Andonopoulos AP, et al.: CT evaluation of mediastinal lymph nodes in primary Sjögren syndrome. *J. Comput. Assist. Tomogr.* 12:199, 1988.

Arrago JP, et al.: Syndrome de Gougerot-Sjögren. Etude fonctionnelle des glandes salivaires par la scintigraphie. *Presse Med.* 13:209, 1984.

Balafrej M, et al.: Acrosclérose, syndrome de Gougerot-Sjögren myxoedème et anticorps anti-centromère. *Ann. Med. Interne (Paris)* 138:185, 1987.

Boling EP, et al.: Primary Sjögren's syndrome and autoimmune hemolytic anemia in sisters. A family study. *Am. J. Med.* 74:1066, 1983.

Bradus RJ, et al.: Parotid gland: US findings in Sjögren syndrome. Work in progress. *Radiology* 169:749, 1988.

Chisholm DM, et al.: Hydrostatic sialography as an index of salivary gland disease in Sjögren's syndrome. *Acta Radiol.* 11:577, 1971.

Deprettere AJ, et al.: Diagnosis of Sjögren's syndrome in children. *Am. J. Dis. Child.* 142:1185, 1988.

Gentric A, et al.: Fibrose rétropéritonéale idiopathique et syndrome de Gougerot-Sjögren. *Presse Med.* 16:1702, 1987.

Gonzalez L, et al.: Parotid sialography in Sjögren's syndrome. *Radiology* 97:91, 1970.

Gougerot H: Insuffisance progressive et atrophie des glandes salivaires et muqueuses de la bouche, des conjonctives (et parfois des muqueuses nasale, laryngée, vulvaire). "Secheresse" de la bouche, des conjunctives, etc. *Bull. Soc. Fr. Derm. Syph.* 32:376, 1925.

Gutmann L, et al.: Inclusion body myositis and Sjögren's syndrome. *Arch. Neurol.* 42:1021, 1985.

Hradský M, et al.: Oesophageal abnormalities in Sjögren's syndrome. *Scand. J. Gastroenterol.* 2:200, 1967.

Koivukangas T, et al.: Sjögren's syndrome and achalasia of the cardia in two siblings. *Pediatrics* 51:943, 1973.

Lichtenfeld JL, et al.: Familial Sjögren's syndrome with associated primary salivary gland lymphoma. *Am. J. Med.* 60:286, 1976.

Malinow KL, et al.: Neuropsychiatric dysfunction in primary Sjögren's syndrome. *Ann. Intern. Med.* 103:344, 1985.

Molina R, et al.: Primary Sjögren's syndrome in men. Clinical, serologic, and immunogenetic features. *Am. J. Med.* 80:23, 1986.

Moutsopoulos HM, et al.: Genetic differences between primary and secondary sicca syndrome. *N. Engl. J. Med.* 301:761, 1979.

Reveille JD, et al.: Primary Sjögren's syndrome and other autoimmune diseases in families. *Ann. Intern. Med.* 101:748, 1984.

Ruiz-Arguelles GJ: The "lipstick-on-teeth" sign in Sjögren's syndrome. *N. Engl. J. Med.* 315:1030, 1986.

Silbiger ML, et al.: Sjögren's syndrome: Its roentgenographic features. *A.J.R.* 100:554, 1967.

Sjögren H: Zur Kenntnis der Keratoconjunctivitis sicca. *Acta Ophthalmol. Copenh* (suppl. 2):1–151, 1933.

Tanaka K et al.: Sjögren's syndrome with abnormal manifestations of the gallbladder and central nervous system. *J. Pediatr. Gastroenterol. Nutr.* 4:148, 1985.

Vermylen C, et al.: Sjögren's syndrome in a child. *Eur. J. Pediatr.* 144:266, 1985.

Versapuech JM, et al.: Cholangite sclérosante, pancréatite chronique et syndrome de Sjögren. *Ann. Med. Interne. (Paris)* 137:147, 1986.

Wemeau JL, et al.: Hypothyroïdie et syndrome de Gougerot-Sjögren. *Ann. Med. Interne. (Paris)* 134:288, 1983.

Whittingham S, et al.: Serological diagnosis of primary Sjögren's syndrome by means of human recombinant La (SS-B) as nuclear antigen. *Lancet* 1:1, 1987.

SJÖGREN-LARSSON SYNDROME

Mode of Inheritance: Autosomal recessive, variable expressivity.

Frequency: Approximately 200 published cases (Gomori et al.).

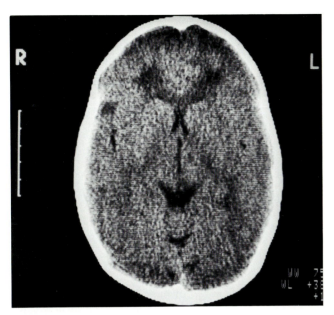

FIG SY—S—13.

Sjögren-Larsson syndrome: Noncontrast enhanced CT showing white matter hypodensity. Note the lucencies located particularly around the frontal horns and the central part of the lateral ventricles and in the supraventricular region of the centrum semi ovale and, in a lesser degree, extending to the occipital region. (From Mulder LJMM, et al.: Cranial CT in the Sjögren-Larsson syndrome. *Neuroradiology* 29:560, 1987. Used by permission.)

Clinical Manifestations: A neurocutaneous syndrome: (a) *congenital ichthyosis;* (b) *pyramidal tract spasticity;* (c) *mental retardation,* speech defects; (d) *short stature;* (e) prenatal diagnosis: skin biopsy (hyperkeratosis); (f) other reported abnormalities: chorioretinal pigmentary and degenerative changes, congenital cerebral spastic diplegia, diminished sweating except the face and dorsum of the hands, defective sweating, hypertelorism, dermatoglyphic anomalies, dental dysplasia.

Radiologic Manifestations: (a) computed tomography (CT): hypodensity in the supratentorial white matter, diffuse cortical hypertrophy, internal hydrocephalus; (b) short metacarpals and metatarsals, basilar impression, epiphyseal-metaphyseal dysplasia, foot deformities and flexion contractures, hypertelorism, widening of the symphysis pubis, hypoplasia of the femoral heads, retarded skeletal maturation, dental hypoplasia, kyphosis (Fig SY—S—13).

REFERENCES

Avigan J, et al.: Sjögren-Larsson syndrome: Δ^5- and Δ^6-fatty acid desaturases in skin fibroblasts. *Neurology* 35:401, 1985.

Gedde-Dahl T Jr, et al.: Autosomal recessive ichthyosis in Norway. II. Sjögren-Larsson—like ichthyosis without CNS or eye involvement. *Clin. Genet.* 25:242, 1984.

Gomori JM, et al.: Computed tomography in Sjögren-Larsson syndrome. *Neuroradiology* 29:557, 1987.

Gustavson KH, et al.: Dermatoglyphic patterns in the Sjögren-Larsson syndrome. *Clin. Genet.* 17:120, 1980.

Holmgren G., et al.: Urinary amino acids and organic acids in the Sjögren-Larsson syndrome. *Clin. Genet.* 20:64, 1981.

Kousseff BG, et al.: Prenatal diagnosis of Sjögren-Larsson syndrome. *J. Pediatr.* 101:998, 1982.

Mulder LJMM, et al.: Cranial CT in the Sjögren-Larsson syndrome. *Neuroradiology* 29:560, 1987.

Ozonoff MB, et al.: Sjögren-Larsson syndrome with epiphyseal-metaphyseal dysplasia. *A.J.R.* 118:187, 1973.

Probst FP, et al.: Cranial CT in the Sjögren-Larsson syndrome. *Neuroradiology* 21:101, 1981.

Selmanowitz VJ, et al.: The Sjögren-Larsson syndrome. *Am. J. Med.* 42:412, 1967.

Sjögren T, Larsson T: Oligophrenia in combination with congenital ichthyosis and spastic disorders. *Acta Psychiatr. Scand.* 32(suppl. 113):1, 1957.

Sten J, et al.: Sjögren-Larsson syndrome in Sweden. A clinical, genetic and epidemiological study. *Clin. Genet.* 19:233, 1981.

SLEEP APNEA SYNDROME

Nosology (Association of Sleep Disorder Centers): (a) sleep apnea: pauses in nocturnal breathing lasting 10 seconds or longer; (b) sleep apnea syndrome: multiple obstructive or mixed apneas with repetitive episodes of inordinately loud snoring and excessive daytime sleepiness.

Clinical Manifestations: (a) disturbed sleep, snoring, excessive daytime somnolence; (b) obesity; (c) cardiopulmonary abnormalities: arterial hypertension, nocturnal cardiac arrhythmias, cor pulmonale; (d) nocturnal polysomnographic recording: obstructive apneic episodes.

Radiologic Manifestations: (a) airway obstruction (somnofluoroscopy): type 1, obstruction at the level of the soft palate only; type 2, obstruction occurs initially at the level of the soft palate followed by closure of the more distal part of the airway; type 3, obstruction initially occurs distal to the soft palate; airway at the soft-palate level may close or remain open; (b) computed tomography: measurement of tongue size in order to evaluate its predictive value for the result of corrective surgery (uvulopalatopharyngoplasty); (c) pulmonary edema.

REFERENCES

Association of Sleep Disorder Centers: Diagnostic classification of sleep and arousal disorders. 1st ed. *Sleep* 2:1, 1979.

Berry DTR, et al.: Sleep apnea syndrome. A critical review of the apnea index as a diagnostic criterion. *Chest* 86:529, 1984.

Chaudhary BA, et al.: Pulmonary edema as a presenting feature of sleep apnea syndrome. *Chest* 82:122, 1982.

Guilleminault C, et al.: Women and the obstructive sleep apnea syndrome. *Chest* 93:104, 1988.

Hegstrom T, et al.: Obstructive sleep apnea syndrome: Preoperative radiologic evaluation. *A.J.R.* 150:67, 1988.

Hultcrantz E, et al.: Sleep apnea in children without hypertrophy of the tonsils. *Clin. Pediatr. (Phila.)* 27:350, 1988.

Katsantonis GP, et al.: Somnofluoroscopy: Its role in the selection of candidates for uvulopalatopharyngoplasty. *Otolaryngol Head Neck Surg* 94:56, 1986.

Larsson SG, et al.: Computed tomography of the oropharynx in obstructive sleep apnea. *Acta Radiol.* 29:401, 1988.

SMALL LEFT COLON SYNDROME

Clinical Manifestations: (a) *symptoms of intestinal obstruction within the first 2 days of life;* (b) high incidence of an association with maternal diabetes; (c) other associated conditions: hypoglycemic cardiomyopathy, persistent fetal circulation, meconium plug, maternal ingestion of psychotropic drugs, association with neonatal intussusception, association with cystic fibrosis, occurrence in twins.

Radiologic Manifestations: (a) *intestinal distension;* (b) *significant narrowing of the colon extending from the splenic flexure to the anus;* (c) intestinal perforation (small bowel, colon); (d) association with meconium plug syndrome; (e) increased subcutaneous fat thickness in infants of diabetic or gestational diabetic mothers (Fig SY–S–14).

Differential Diagnosis: Hirschsprung disease.

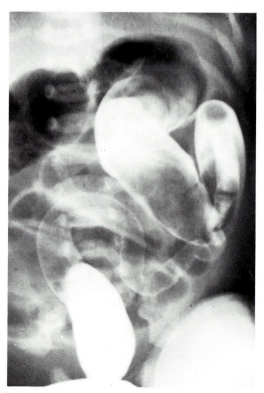

FIG SY–S–14.
Small left colon syndrome in a male newborn with clinical symptoms of intestinal obstruction. Narrowing of the sigmoid and descending colon is present. The meconium plug is outlined by contrast material.

REFERENCES

Berdon WE, et al.: Neonatal small left colon syndrome: Its relationship to aganglionosis and meconium plug syndrome. *Radiology* 125:457, 1977.

Cohen MD, et al.: Neonatal small left colon syndrome in twins. *Gastrointest. Radiol.* 7:283, 1982.

Davis WS, et al.: Neonatal small left colon syndrome. *A.J.R.* 120:322, 1974.

Davis WS, et al.: Neonatal small left colon syndrome: Occurrence in asymptomatic infants of diabetic mothers. *Am. J. Dis. Child.* 129:1024, 1975.

Ellerbroek C, et al.: Neonatal small left colon in an infant with cystic fibrosis. *Pediatr. Radiol.* 16:162, 1986.

Falterman CG, et al.: Small left colon syndrome associated with maternal ingestion of psychotropic drugs. *J. Pediatr.* 97:308, 1980.

Fotter R: Das "neonatal small left colon syndrome." *Fortschr. Rontgenstr.* 134:324, 1981.

Hall SL, et al.: Neonatal intussusception associated with neonatal small left colon syndrome. *Clin. Pediatr. (Phila.)* 26:191, 1987.

Kuhns LR, et al.: Fat thickness in the neonatal small left colon syndrome. *A.J.R.* 126:538, 1976.

Nixon GW, et al.: Intestinal perforation as a complication of the neonatal small left colon syndrome. *A.J.R.* 125:75, 1975.

Rangecroft L: Neonatal small left colon syndrome. *Arch. Dis. Child.* 54:635, 1979.

SMITH-LEMLI-OPITZ SYNDROME

Synonym: RSH syndrome.

Mode of Inheritance: Autosomal recessive.

Frequency: Estimated to be 1:40,000 births; male-to-female ratio of 3:1 (Joseph et al.).

Clinical Manifestations: Symptoms present at birth: (a) *low birth weight, failure to thrive;* (b) *hypotonia at birth,* progressive spasticity in childhood; (c) moderate to severe *mental retardation;* (d) *typical facies:* microcephaly, blepharoptosis, inner epicanthal folds, strabismus, short nose with a broad bridge, anteverted nostrils, broad maxillary anterior alveolar ridge, micrognathia, slanted auricles or low-set ears; (e) short neck; (f) short and narrow shoulders; (g) *urogenital anomalies:* hypospadias, cryptorchidism, cleft scrotum; pseudohermaphroditism, micropenis, microurethra, hypoplastic scrotum, 46,XY with female external genitalia; (h) ocular abnormalities: absence of lacrimal punctae, posterior synechiae, cataracts, ptosis, epicanthal folds, choroidal hemangioma, pale disks, neuronal atrophy; (i) other reported abnormalities: cleft palate, sacral dimple, abnormal electroencephalographic and electrocardiographic findings, acrocyanosis of the hands and feet, hypoplasia of the thymus, irritability, typical shrill screaming, frequent vomiting and regurgitation, abnormal dermatoglyphics, Hirschsprung disease.

Radiologic Manifestations: (a) *microcephaly;* scaphocephaly; micrognathia; mild to moderate hydrocephalus in-

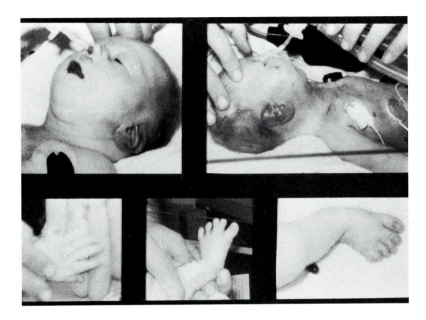

FIG SY—S—15.
Smith-Lemli-Opitz syndrome in a patient shortly after birth. Note the micrognathia, large low-set ears *(upper row)*, postaxial polydactyly of the left hand *(bottom left)*, bilateral syndactyly between the second and third toes, and postaxial polydactyly of the right foot. (From Bialer MG, Penchaszadeh VB, Kahn E, et al.: Female external genitalia and müllerian duct derivatives in a 46,XY infant with the Smith-Lemli-Opitz syndrome. *Am. J. Med. Genet.* 28:723, 1987. Used by permission.)

volving one or more ventricles; hypoplasia of the frontal lobes, the corpus callosum, the cerebellum, and the brain stem; irregular frontal gyri; pachygyria; (b) *soft-tissue syndactyly of the second and third toes;* (c) swallowing mechanism dysfunction in early infancy, gastroesophageal regurgitation and recurrent pneumonia; (d) urinary tract anomalies: ureteropelvic junction obstruction, vesicoureteral reflux, hydronephrosis, collecting system duplication, positional renal abnormalities, renal cystic dysplasia, renal agenesis, etc.; (e) other reported abnormalities: congenital heart disease; pyloric stenosis; polydactyly; brachydactyly; hypoplasia of the thumbs, which are low-set on the hands; clubfoot; stippled epiphyses.

Differential Diagnosis: Pallister-Hall syndrome; Meckel syndrome.

Note: Smith-Lemli-Opitz syndrome, type II features: *male pseudohermaphroditism, postaxial hexadactyly, congenital heart disease, cleft palate,* Hirschsprung disease, unilobated lungs, large adrenals, pancreatic islet cell hyperplasia, *early lethality* (Fig SY—S—15).

REFERENCES

Akl KF, et al.: The Smith-Lemli-Opitz syndrome. *Clin. Pediatr. (Phila.)* 16:665, 1977.

Bialer MG, et al.: Female external genitalia and müllerian duct derivatives in a 46,XY infant with the Smith-Lemli-Opitz syndrome. *Am. J. Med. Genet.* 28:723, 1987.

Cruveiller J, et al.: Nanisme de Smith-Lemli-Opitz. A propos de quatre observations. Revue de litérature. *Ann. Pediatr. (Paris)* 24:843, 1977.

Curry CJR, et al.: Smith-Lemli-Opitz syndrome—Type II: Multiple congenital anomalies with male pseudohermaphroditism and frequent early lethality. *Am. J. Med. Genet.* 26:45, 1987.

Donnai D, et al.: Smith-Lemli-Opitz syndromes: Do they include the Pallister-Hall syndrome (letter)? *Am. J. Med. Genet.* 28:741, 1987.

Fine RN, et al.: Smith-Lemli-Opitz syndrome: Radiologic and postmortem findings. *Am. J. Dis. Child.* 115:483, 1968.

Joseph DB, et al.: Genitourinary abnormalities associated with the Smith-Lemli-Opitz syndrome. *J. Urol.* 137:719, 1987.

Kim EH, et al.: Smith-Lemli-Opitz syndrome associated with Hirschsprung disease, 46,XY female karyotype, and total anomalous pulmonary venous drainage. *J. Pediatr.* 106:861, 1985.

Kretzer FL, et al.: Ocular manifestations of the Smith-Lemli-Opitz syndrome. *Arch. Ophthalmol.* 99:2000, 1981.

Lowry RB: Variability in the Smith-Lemli-Opitz syndrome: Overlap with the Meckel syndrome (editorial). *Am. J. Med. Genet.* 14:429, 1983.

Marion RW, et al.: Computed tomography of the brain in the Smith-Lemli-Opitz syndrome. *J. Child. Neurol.* 2:198, 1987.

Nevo S, et al.: Smith-Lemli-Opitz syndrome in an inbred family. *Am. J. Dis. Child.* 124:431, 1972.

Opitz JM, et al.: Smith-Lemli-Opitz (RSH) syndrome bibliography. *Am. J. Med. Genet.* 28:745, 1987.

Penchaszadeh VB: The nosology of the Smith-Lemli-Opitz syndrome (editorial). *Am. J. Med. Genet.* 28:719, 1987.

Retbi JM, et al.: Syndrome de Smith-Lemli-Opitz et pseudo-hermaphrodisme masculin. *Ann. Pediatr. (Paris)* 28:55, 1981.

Smith DW, Lemli L, Opitz JM: A newly recognized syndrome of multiple congenital anomalies. *J. Pediatr.* 64:210, 1964.

SNAPPING HIP SYNDROME

Synonym: Snapping tendon syndrome.

Etiology: Abnormalities of the fascia lata, gluteus maximus muscle, or ileopsoas tendon (snapping of the iliopsoas tendon over the iliopectineal eminence, etc.).

Clinical Manifestations: Pain and an audible snapping of the hip with motion.

Radiologic Manifestations: (a) computed tomography: inflamed iliopsoas bursa; (b) a negative defect impression of the ligament on the contrast-filled bursa is seen during hip motion at fluoroscopy; (c) tendinography and evaluation of the snapping with hip motion (fluoroscopic observation).

REFERENCES

Binnie JF: Snapping hip. *Ann. Surg.* 58:59, 1913.
Schaberg JE, et al.: The snapping hip syndrome. *Am. J. Sports Med.* 12:361, 1984.
Staple TW, et al.: Snapping tendon syndrome: Hip tenography with fluoroscopic monitoring. *Radiology* 166:873, 1988.

SNEDDON SYNDROME

Clinical Manifestations: (a) *skin lesion: livedo reticularis;* (b) *ischemic cerebrovascular disease;* (c) lupus anticoagulant and anticardiolipin antibodies (in the absence of systemic lupus erythematosus).

Radiologic Manifestations: Occluded or normal vessels; atypical moyamoya.

REFERENCES

Levine SR, et al.: Sneddon's syndrome: An antiphospholipid antibody syndrome? *Neurology* 38:798, 1988.
Robollo M, et al.: Livedo reticularis and cerebrovascular lesions (Sneddon's syndrome: Clinical, radiologic and pathologic features in eight cases. *Brain* 106:965, 1983.
Rumpl E, et al.: Cerebrovascular lesions in livedo reticularis (Sneddon syndrome): A progressive cerebrovascular disorder? *J. Neurol.* 231:324, 1985.
Sneddon JB: Cerebral-vascular lesions in livedo reticularis. *Br. J. Dermatol.* 77:180, 1965.

SORSBY SYNDROME

Mode of Inheritance: Autosomal dominant.

Frequency: 11 members of a single family (Thompson et al.).

Clinical and Radiologic Manifestations: (a) bilateral macular colobomas, horizontal pendular nystagmus, visual loss; (b) hand and foot anomalies: shortening of the middle and terminal phalanges of the second to fifth digits, absent or hypoplastic nails, broad or bifid thumbs and halluces, syndactyly, absence of the distal phalanges (in some); (c) other reported abnormalities: unilateral absence of a kidney, duplication of the uterus and vagina.

REFERENCES

Thompson EM, et al.: Sorsby syndrome: A report on further generations of the original family. *J. Med. Genet.* 25:313, 1988.
Sorsby A: Congenital coloboma of the macula, together with an account of the familial occurrence of bilateral macular coloboma in association with apical dystrophy of the hands and feet. *Br. J. Ophthalmol.* 19:65, 1935.

SOTOS SYNDROME

Synonym: Cerebral gigantism.

Mode of Inheritance: Sporadic; autosomal dominant and autosomal recessive modes of inheritance have been suggested in some families; male-to-male transmission also reported.

Frequency: More than 200 published cases (Kaneko et al.).

Clinical Manifestations: (a) *acromegalic appearance;* (b) *characteristic facial features* (large head, prominent forehead and supraorbital ridges, antimongoloid slant of the eyes, ocular hypertelorism, prominent jaw, high-arched palate); (c) *very rapid growth in height and weight* (above the 90th percentile); (d) mental retardation; (e) absence of precocious sexual development; (f) *large hands and feet;* (g) *poor motor coordination;* (h) other reported abnormalities: premature eruption of teeth, feeding difficulties in infancy, autonomic failure with persistent fever, thyrotoxicosis, Kocher-Debré-Sémélaigne syndrome, Wilms tumor, hepatoma, pigmented nevus, osteochondroma, cavernous hemangioma, glucose intolerance, low somatomedin levels, increased urinary excretion of 17-ketosteroids and 17-hydroxysteroids, early sexual development, retinal degeneration, congenital heart defects, thin and brittle nails, etc.

Radiologic Manifestations: (a) *large dolichocephalic skull,* ocular hypertelorism, high-rising orbital roofs, normal-size sella turcica; (b) *advanced skeletal maturation;* (c) *disproportionately large hands and feet,* abnormal metacarpophalangeal pattern profile (a major peak in the proximal phalangeal area and a smaller peak in the metacarpal area,

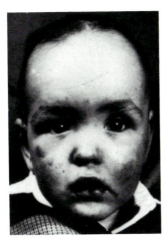

FIG SY—S—16.
Sotos syndrome in a 2.75-year-old boy with a birth weight of 4 kg and a birth length of 56 cm. (From Wit JM, Beemer FA, Barth PG, et al.: Cerebral gigantism (Sotos syndrome). Compiled data of 22 cases. Analysis of clinical features, growth and plasma somatomedin. *Eur. J. Pediatr.* 144:131, 1985. Used by permission.)

with the distal hand bones being relatively short; heterogeneity in the profile); (d) other reported abnormalities: dilated cerebral ventricles, cavum septum pellucidum, cavum velum interpositum, posteriorly inclined dorsum sella turcica, presence of an anterior fontanelle bone, vertebra plana, interver-

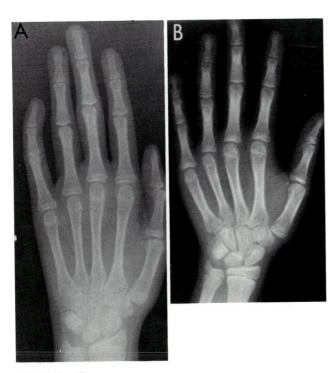

FIG SY—S—17.
Sotos syndrome in a 12½-year-old mentally retarded female who is large for her age. Note the large size of her hand. **A,** compared with that of another patient of same age. **B,** skeletal maturation is 13 years, 9 months when compared with the standards.

tebral disk herniation, kyphosis or kyphoscoliosis, syndactyly, unequal leg length, absent corpus callosum, hydronephrosis, functional megacolon.

Differential Diagnosis: Cerebral gigantism of hypothalamic origin.

Note: Due to the clinical picture of Sotos syndrome in patients with fragile X chromosome, a search for this chromosomal abnormality has been recommended in all cases of cerebral gigantism (Figs SY—S—16 and SY—S—17).

REFERENCES

Adam KAR, et al.: Cerebral gigantism with hydronephrosis: A case report. *Clin. Genet.* 29:178, 1986.

Bale AE, et al.: Familial Sotos syndrome (cerebral gigantism): Craniofacial and psychological characteristics. *Am. J. Med. Genet.* 20:613, 1985.

Beemer FA, et al.: Cerebral gigantism (Sotos syndrome) in two patients with fra (X) chromosomes. *Am. J. Med. Genet.* 23:221, 1986.

Butler MG, et al.: Metacarpophalangeal pattern profile analysis in Sotos syndrome: A follow-up report on 34 subjects. *Am. J. Med. Genet.* 29:143, 1988.

Evans PR: Sotos' syndrome (cerebral gigantism) with peripheral dysostosis. *Arch. Dis. Child.* 46:199, 1971.

Halal F: Male to male transmission of cerebral gigantism. *Am. J. Med. Genet.* 12:411, 1982.

Kaneko H, et al.: Congenital heart defects in Sotos sequence. *Am. J. Med. Genet.* 26:569, 1987.

Lecornu M, et al.: Gigantisme cérébral chez des jumeaux. *Arch. Fr. Pediatr.* 33:277, 1976.

Livieri C, et al.: Retinal degeneration in Sotos' syndrome. *Helv. Paediat. Acta* 37:93, 1982.

Maldonado V, et al.: Cerebral gigantism associated with Wilms' tumor. *Am. J. Dis. Child.* 138:486, 1984.

Ranke MB, et al.: Cerebral gigantism of hypothalamic origin. *Eur. J. Pediatr.* 140:109, 1983.

Sotos JF, et al.: Cerebral gigantism. *Am. J. Dis. Child.* 131:625, 1977.

Sotos JF, et al.: Cerebral gigantism in childhood: A syndrome of excessively rapid growth with acromegalic features and a nonprogressive neurologic disorder. *N. Engl. J. Med.* 271:109, 1964.

Sugarman GI, et al.: A case of cerebral gigantism and hepatocarcinoma. *Am. J. Dis. Child.* 131:631, 1977.

Whitaker MD, et al.: The hypothalamus and pituitary in cerebral gigantism. A clinicopathologic and immunocytochemical study. *Am. J. Dis. Child.* 139:679, 1985.

Winship IM: Sotos syndrome—autosomal dominant inheritance substantiated. *Clin. Genet.* 28:243, 1985.

Wilson TA, et al.: Cerebral gigantism and thyrotoxicosis. *J. Pediatr.* 96:685, 1980.

Wit JM, et al.: Cerebral gigantism (Sotos syndrome). Compiled data of 22 cases. Analysis of clinical features, growth and plasma somatomedin. *Eur. J. Pediatr.* 144:131, 1985.

SPLENIC FLEXURE SYNDROME

Synonyms: Acute flexura lienalis syndrome; Payr syndrome.

Clinical Manifestations: (a) left upper abdominal pain; (b) tenderness over the left upper portion of the abdomen; (c) abdominal distension in some.

Radiologic Manifestations: (a) *localized gaseous distension of the splenic flexure of the colon* with contrast studies demonstrating interposition of the splenic flexure of the colon between the diaphragm, stomach, and spleen.

Note: The existence of the syndrome is questionable.

REFERENCES

Kozlowski K: Acute flexura lienalis syndrome. *Am. J. Dis. Child.* 122:239, 1971.
Machella TE, et al.: Observations on the splenic flexure syndrome. *Ann. Intern. Med.* 37:543, 1952.
Oppermann HC, et al.: Das Flexura-lienalis-Syndrom in Kindesalter. *Z. Kinderchir.* 22:33, 1977.

Payr E: Ueber eine eigentümliche, durch abnorm starke Klickunge und Adhäsionen bedinge gucartige Stenose der Flexura lienalis und hepatice coli. *Verh. Dtsch. Keng. Inn. Med.* 27:276, 1910.

SPLENOGONADAL FUSION/LIMB DEFORMITY

Classification and Pathology: (a) types: (1) continuous splenogonadal fusion: spleen connected to the left gonad by a cord of splenic or fibrous tissue or by bandlike masses of splenic tissue; (2) accessory splenic tissue attached to the gonad; (b) other associated anomalies: limb defects, abnormal fissures of the lungs, hypoplastic lungs, congenital cardiovascular defects, left diaphragmatic hernia, partial situs inversus, Meckel diverticulum, bilobed spleen, hepatolienal fusion, abnormal fissuring of the spleen, accessory spleen, anal malformations, adrenogonadal fusion, hypoplasia of the adrenals, hypospadias, double uterus, abnormal fissures of the liver, microgastria, etc.

Frequency: Approximately 90 published cases (Tank et al.).

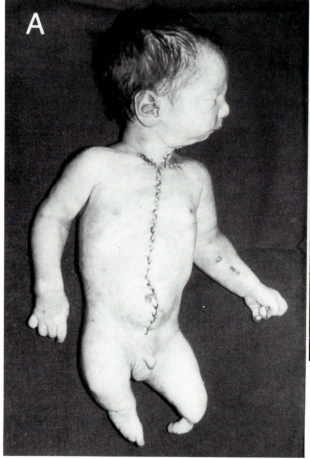

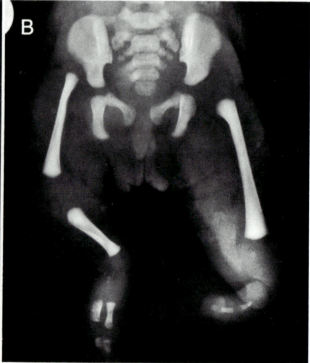

FIG SY–S–18.
Splenogonadal fusion syndrome. **A,** postmortem photograph of an infant with peromelia of the lower limbs and micrognathia. **B,** roentgenogram of the lower limbs. The right femur is shorter than the left one is, and an absent left tibia and fibula, short right tibia and absent right fibula, and feet deformity are present. At postmortem examination fusion of a splenic mass and the left testicle ventral to the left kidney was found. (From Gouw ASH, Elema JD, Bink-Boelkens TE, et al.: The spectrum of splenogonadal fusion. Case report and review of 84 reported cases. *Eur. J. Pediatr.* 144:316, 1985. Used by permission.)

Clinical Manifestations: (a) *limb malformation* (amelia, peromelia, phocomelia, ectromelia, hemimelia, clubfoot); (b) *inguinal hernia, cryptorchidism, scrotal "mass," pain in the scrotal region;* (c) other reported abnormalities: micrognathia, asymmetrical skull, Möbius syndrome, etc.

Radiologic Manifestations: (a) ^{99m}Tc sulfur colloid imaging for *ectopic splenic tissue localization;* (b) *limb anomalies;* (c) hip dislocation.

Note: In one third of the patients with splenogonadal fusion (usually the continuous type) other congenital defects are present (Fig SY—S—18).

REFERENCES

Gouw ASH, et al.: The spectrum of splenogonadal fusion. Case report and review of 84 reported cases. *Eur. J. Pediatr.* 144:316, 1985.

Hines JR, Eggum PR: Spleno-gonadal fusion causing bowel obstruction. *Arch. Surg.* 83:887, 1961.

Kufaas T, et al.: Splenogonadal fusion. *Z. Kinderchir.* 38:232, 1983.

Mandell GA, et al.: A case of microgastria in association with splenic-gonadal fusion. *Pediatr. Radiol.* 13:95, 1983.

Markiewicz C, et al.: Fusion spléno-gonadique. A propos de 3 observations. *Chir. Pediatr.* 27:216, 1986.

Mhiri MN, et al.: Douleur scrotale gauche révélatrice d'une rate accessoire en ectopie paragonadique. *Arch. Fr. Pediatr.* 45:123, 1988.

Pauli RM, et al.: Limb deficiency and splenogonadal fusion. *Am. J. Med. Genet.* 13:81, 1982.

Tank ES, et al.: Splenic gonadal fusion. *J. Urol.* 139:798, 1988.

SPLIT-HAND AND SPLIT-FOOT DEFORMITIES

Synonyms: Lobster-claw deformity; ectrodactyly.

Definition: Defect in development of the central rays of the extremities; in the monodactylous type, the fifth digit is usually present.

Types: (a) isolated malformation; (b) part of a syndrome.

Syndromes (Temtamy and McKusick)

1. Split hand with orofacial malformations: (a) EEC syndrome (Ectrodactyly, Ectodermal dysplasia, Cleft lip/palate); (b) split hand/split foot with mandibulofacial dysostosis.
2. Split hand with perceptive deafness.
3. Split hand with congenital nystagmus, fundal changes, and cataract (Karsch-Neugebauer syndrome).
4. Anonychia with ectrodactyly.
5. Acrorenal syndrome (Dieker-Opitz syndrome, Curran syndrome).
6. Aplasia of the tibia with split-hand and -foot deformity (autosomal dominant in most families).
7. X-chromosomally inherited split-hand and split-foot anomaly.

REFERENCES

Ahmad M, et al.: X-chromosomally inherited split-hand/split-foot anomaly in a Pakistani kindred. *Hum. Genet.* 75:169, 1987.

Bujdoso G, et al.: Monodactylous splithand-splitfoot. A malformation occurring in three distinct genetic types. *Eur. J. Pediatr.* 133:207, 1980.

David TS: The differential diagnosis of the cleft hand and cleft foot malformations. *Hand* 6:58, 1974.

Dieker H, Opitz JM: Associated acral and renal malformations. *Birth Defects* 5(3):68, 1969.

Lees DH, et al.: Anonychia with ectrodactyly: Clinical and linkage data. *Ann. Hum. Genet.* 22:69, 1957.

Leiter E, et al.: Genitourinary tract anomalies in lobster claw syndrome. *J. Urol.* 115:339, 1975.

Maisels DD: Lobster claw deformities of the hand. *Hand* 2:79, 1970.

Majewski F, et al.: Aplasia of tibia with split-hand/split-foot deformity. Report of six families with 35 cases and considerations about variability and penetrance. *Hum. Genet.* 70:136, 1985.

Neugebauer H: Spalthand-und-fuss mit familiärer Besonderheit. *Z. Orthop.* 95:500, 1962.

Patterson TJS, et al.: Cranio-facial dysostosis and malformations of the feet. *J. Med. Genet.* 1:112, 1964.

Pilarski RT, et al.: Karsch-Neugebauer syndrome: Split foot/split hand and congenital nystagmus. *Clin. Genet.* 27:97, 1985.

Rüdiger RA, et al.: Association of ectrodactyly, ectodermal dysplasia, cleft lip-palate: The EEC syndrome. *Am. J. Dis. Child.* 120:160, 1970.

Salmon MA, et al.: The nasolacrimal duct and split hand/split foot syndrome. *Dev. Med. Child Neurol.* 19:418, 1977.

Temtamy S, McKusick VA: Split hands as a part of syndromes. *Birth Defects* 14(3):157, 1978.

Viljoen DL, et al.: The split-hand and split-foot anomaly in a Central African Negro population. *Am. J. Med. Genet.* 19:545, 1984.

Wildervanck LS: Perceptive deafness associated with split hand and foot. A new syndrome? *Acta Genet.* 13:161, 1963.

SPLIT NOTOCHORD SYNDROME

Synonym: Combined anterior and posterior spina bifida.

Frequency: 11 cases of split notochord with a dorsal enteric fistula. and 12 cases of splitting of the spine (Pathak et al. and others).

Pathology: (a) *vertebral anomalies: anterior and posterior spina bifida;* (b) *neural anomalies:* split notochord, meningomyelocele, meningocele, developmental anomalies of the hindbrain and cervical spinal cord; (c) *visceral anomalies:*

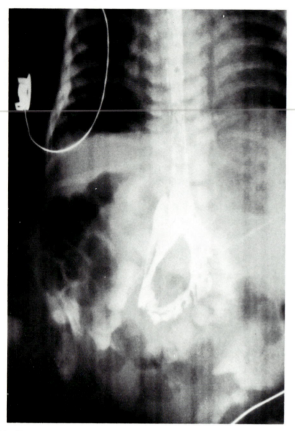

FIG SY–S–19.
Split notochord syndrome in a newborn with exstrophy of the bladder and lumbar abnormalities with meconium draining through the dorsal fistula in the lumbar region. Myelography demonstrates total lumbar rachischisis.

mediastinal cysts of foregut origin (neuroenteric cysts); enteric duplication; diaphragmatic hernia; imperforate anus; dorsal enteric fistula (passage of bowel through the spinal cleft); partial agenesis of the colon; malrotation of the bowel; common mesentery; malformed kidney; bicornuate uterus; enteric fistula opening into the rectum, sigmoid, closed colonic loop, or lower part of the small intestine.

Clinical Manifestations: (a) external deformities related to the anomalies listed under Pathology (spina bifida cystica, enteric fistula, etc.); (b) neurological deficit associated with spinal cord anomalies.

Radiologic Manifestations: (a) spina bifida (anterior and posterior); (b) spinal cord and nerve defects, split cord; (c) intestinal anomalies including intestinal herniation through the dorsal cleft; (d) genitourinary anomalies; (e) neuroenteric cyst (Fig SY–S–19).

REFERENCES

Bentley JFR, et al.: Developmental posterior enteric remnants and spinal malformations. *Arch. Dis. Child.* 35:76, 1960.

Crowe JE, et al.: Radiological case of the month: Split notochord syndrome. *Am. J. Dis. Child.* 132:814, 1978.
Faris JC, et al.: The split notochord syndrome. *J. Pediatr. Surg.* 10:467, 1975.
Gupta DK, et al.: Split notochord syndrome presenting with meningomyelocoele and dorsal enteric fistula. *J. Pediatr. Surg.* 22:382, 1987.
Kheradpir MH, et al.: Dorsal herniation of the gut with posterior opening of the terminal colon: A rare manifestation of the split notochord syndrome. *Z. Kinderchir.* 38:186, 1983.
Pathak VB, et al.: Double split of notochord with massive prolapse of the gut. *J. Pediatr. Surg.* 23:1039, 1988.

SPONDYLOCOSTAL DYSOSTOSIS

Synonyms: Spondylocostal dysplasia; costovertebral dysplasia; hereditary costovertebral dysplasia.

Mode of Inheritance: Autosomal dominant; autosomal recessive; occurrence in identical twins.

Frequency: Uncommon.

Clinical Manifestations: (a) *dwarfism with a short trunk and neck, limited rotatory movement of the spine, normal limbs,* increase in the anteroposterior diameter of the chest; (b) nerve root compression; (c) usually normal life expectancy.

Radiologic Manifestations: (a) *vertebral anomalies:* "block" vertebrae, hemivertebrae, "butterfly" vertebrae, sagittal clefts; (b) *rib anomalies:* hypoplasia, fusion, reduced number; (c) normal skull and limb bones; (d) urinary system anomalies; (e) congenital heart defects.

Differential Diagnosis: Spondylothoracic dysostosis (Jarcho-Levin syndrome); COVESDEM (costovertebral segmentation defect with mesomelia) syndrome.

Notes: The distribution of vertebral anomalies does not seem to be helpful in the differential diagnosis of spondylothoracic dysostosis and spondylocostal dysostosis; The dysostosis and deformities are generally more severe in spondylothoracic dysostosis (Jarcho-Levin syndrome) (Fig SY–S–20).

REFERENCES

Aymé S, et al.: Spondylocostal/spondylothoracic dysostosis: The clinical basis for prognosticating and genetic counseling. *Am. J. Med. Genet.* 24:599, 1986.
Beighton P, et al.: Spondylocostal dysostosis in South African sisters. *Clin. Genet.* 19:23, 1981.
Casamassima AC, et al.: Spondylocostal dysostosis associated with anal and urogenital anomalies in a Mennonite sibship. *Am. J. Med. Genet.* 8:117, 1981.
Delgoffe C, et al.: Dysostoses spondylocostales et cardiopathies congénitales. *Ann. Pediatr. (Paris)* 29:135, 1982.
Devos EA, et al.: Spondylocostal dysostosis and urinary tract

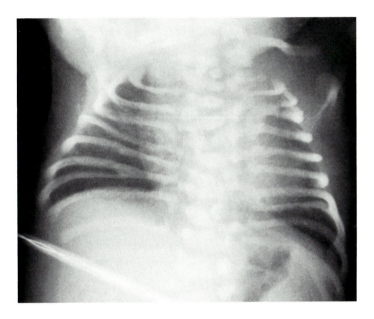

FIG SY—S—20.
Spondylocostal dysostosis, dominant type, in a newborn female with truncal dwarfism, a prominent occiput, and normal limbs. Block vertebrae, hemivertebrae, butterfly vertebrae, and rib anomalies (dysplasia, fusion, and abnormal position) are present. Vertebral anomalies were also noted in the cervical and lum- bosacral segments. The father (of Puerto Rican origin) had similar rib and vertebral anomalies in the cervical, thoracic, and lum- bosacral regions. The cranium and limbs of the father appeared normal. (Courtesy of Dr. Robert E. Sharkey, Hayward, Calif.)

anomaly: Definition and review of an entity. *Eur. J. Pediatr.* 128:7, 1978.

Fogarty EE, et al.: Spondylocostal dysplasia in identical twins. *J. Pediatr. Orthop.* 5:720, 1985.

Kozlowski K: Spondylo-costal dysplasia. A further report— review of 14 cases. *Fortschr. Rontgenstr.* 140:204, 1984.

Kozlowski K, et al.: Spondylo-costal dysplasia—Severe and moderate types (report of 8 cases). *Australas. Radiol.* 25:81, 1981.

Rimoin DL, et al.: Spondylocostal dysplasia: A dominantly inherited form of short-trunked dwarfism. *Am. J. Med.* 45:948, 1968.

Roberts AP, et al.: Spondylothoracic and spondylocostal dy- sostosis. Hereditary forms of spinal deformity. *J. Bone Joint Surg. [Br.]* 70:123, 1988.

Silengo MC, et al.: Recessive spondylocostal dysostosis: Two new cases. *Clin. Genet.* 13:289, 1978.

Wadia RS, et al.: Recessively inherited costovertebral seg- mentation defect with mesomelia and peculiar facies (COVESDEM syndrome). A new genetic entity? *J. Med. Genet.* 15:123, 1978.

Zeller CH, et al.: Dysostose spondylocostale avec polydac- tylie. *J. Radiol.* 63:355, 1982.

STAGNANT SMALL-BOWEL SYNDROME

Synonyms: Small-intestinal stasis syndrome; stagnant loop syndrome.

Etiology: Small-bowel stenosis or stricture; gastrocolic fistula; ileocolic fistula; small-bowel diverticula; Crohn dis- ease; blind loop (segment of the small intestine completely bypassed); blind pouch (side-to-side anastomosis associated with persistence of the residual afferent and efferent ends of the intestine).

Pathology: Hypertrophy of the bowel wall, edema, in- flammation, and ulceration.

Clinical Manifestations: (a) *weight loss, growth retarda- tion, malnutrition;* (b) *abdominal cramp, abdominal disten- sion;* (c) *malabsorption;* (d) *macrocytic anemia;* (e) *multiple vitamin deficiencies;* (f) abnormal jejunal bile acid concen- tration due to abnormal bacterial flora; (g) other reported ab- normalities: bleeding, arthritis-dermititis syndrome, spinocer- ebellar degeneration in the blind loop syndrome with vitamin E malabsorption.

Radiologic Manifestations: (a) spherical, tubular, or club-shaped gas-containing structures on plain films of the abdomen; (b) pseudotumor if filled with fluid or food debris, *demonstration of distended bowel by a contrast study of the bowel.*

REFERENCES

Botsford TW, et al.: Blind pouch syndrome. A complication of side to side intestinal anastomosis. *Am. J. Surg.* 113:486, 1967.

Brin MF, et al.: Blind loop syndrome, vitamin E malabsorp- tion, and spinocerebellar degeneration. *Neurology* 35:338, 1985.

Camúñez F, et al.: Percutaneous duodenostomy in blind loop syndrome. *A.J.R.* 150:1199, 1988.

Hurtubise M, et al.: Stenose de l'intestin grêle: Syndrome de l'anse stagnante associé et malabsorption. *J. Can. Assoc. Radiol.* 25:227, 1974.

Klinkhoff AV, et al.: Postgastrectomy blind loop syndrome and the arthritis-dermatitis syndrome. *Arthritis Rheum.* 28:214, 1985.

Maglinte DDT: "Blind pouch" syndrome: A cause of gastrointestinal bleeding. *Radiology* 132:314, 1979.

Northfield TC, et al.: Value of small intestinal bile acid analysis in the diagnosis of the stagnant loop syndrome. *Gut* 14:341, 1973.

Salonen IS, et al.: Intestinal blind pouch- and blind loop-syndrome in children operated previously for congenital duodenal obstruction. *Ann. Chir. Gynaecol. Fenn.* 65:38, 1976.

Sternowsky HJ, et al.: Severe iron deficiency anemia from intestinal blood loss in connatal blind loop syndrome. *Z. Kinderchir.* 17:29, 1975.

STEAL SYNDROMES (VASCULAR)

1. Subclavian.
2. Aortoiliac.
3. Coronary.
4. Celiac.
5. Spinal.
6. Renal-splanchnic.
7. Mesenteric.
8. Pulmonary artery–subclavian (congenital).
9. Thyrocervical.
10. Pulmonary (coronary artery to bronchial artery to pulmonary artery branch).
11. External carotid (vertebral to external carotid artery, due to proximal external carotid artery occlusion).
12. Reno-celiac (through the inferior phrenic and suprarenal arteries).
13. Pulmonary (pulmonary arteriovenous fistula).
14. Vertebral artery (aberrant vertebral artery originating from the descending aorta, distal to aortic coarctation).
15. Vascular steal associated with a vein of Galen aneurysm that affects the ophthalmic artery and branches of the middle and anterior cerebral arteries.
16. Pelvic steal (external iliac, causing impotence).

REFERENCES

Bates ER, et al.: Coronary artery steal: Demonstration by digital coronary radiography. *Radiology* 154:61, 1985.

Fried R, et al.: Congenital pulmonary arteriovenous fistula producing pulmonary arterial steal syndrome. *Pediatr. Cardiol.* 2:313, 1982.

Fujii S, et al.: Coronary steal in Takayasu's aortitis. *Am. Heart J.* 109:596, 1985.

Goldwasser B, et al.: Impotence due to the pelvic steal syndrome: Treatment by iliac transluminal angioplasty. *J. Urol.* 133:860, 1985.

Grossman RI, et al.: Vascular steal associated with vein of Galen aneurysm. *Neuroradiology* 26:381, 1984.

Hesse SJ, et al.: True and false external carotid steals. *Clin. Radiol.* 24:303, 1974.

Homan RW, et al.: Quantification of intracerebral steal in patients with arteriovenous malformation. *Arch. Neurol.* 43:779, 1986.

Kinkhabwala M, et al.: "Intersplanchnic steal syndrome": Another cause for reversible distal colon ischemia. *Br. J. Radiol.* 47:729, 1974.

Kusske JA, et al.: Embolization and reduction of the "steal" syndrome in cerebral arteriovenous malformations. *J. Neurosurg.* 40:313, 1974.

Pirker E: Der nutritive Effekt der "Klassischen" Steal-Syndrom. *Fortschr. Rontgenstr.* 131:461, 1979.

Rosenbusch G, et al.: Reno-zöliakales Steal-Phänomen: Aa. phreniacae inferiores et suprarenales als Kollateralen fur den Truncus coeliacus. *Fortschr. Rontgenstr.* 122:218, 1975.

Spindola-Franco H, et al.: Pulmonary steal syndrome: An unusual case of coronary-bronchial pulmonary artery communication. *Radiology* 126:25, 1978.

Stoesslein F, et al.: Aberrant vertebral artery originating from the descending aorta: A new congenital steal syndrome in coarctation. *Eur. J. Radiol.* 2:157, 1982.

STEELE-RICHARDSON-OLSZEWSKI SYNDROME

Clinical and Radiologic Manifestations: (a) supranuclear ophthalmoplegia, pseudobulbar palsy, dystonia, axial rigidity, dementia ("subcortical dementia"); (b) cerebellar and pyramidal signs and symptoms minor or absent; (c) positron-emission tomography: a global decrease in blood flow and oxygen utilization, more marked in the frontal region.

REFERENCES

Leenders KL, et al.: Steele-Richardson-Olszewski syndrome. Brain energy metabolism, blood flow and fluorodopa uptake measured by positron emission tomography. *Brain* 111:615, 1988.

Richardson JC, Steele J, Olszewski J: Supranuclear ophthalmoplegia, pseudobulbar palsy, nuchal dystonia and dementia: A clinical report on eight cases of 'heterogenous system degeneration.' *Trans. Am. Neurol. Assoc.* 88:25, 1963.

Steele JC, Richardson JC, Olszewski J: Progressive supranuclear palsy: A heterogeneous degeneration involving the brainstem, basal ganglia and cerebellum with vertical gaze and pseudobulbar palsy, nuchal dystonia and dementia. *Arch. Neurol.* 10:333, 1964.

STERNAL-CARDIAC MALFORMATIONS ASSOCIATION

Clinical Manifestations: (a) *sternal deformity:* pectus carinatum, anterior sternal defect, etc.; (b) *congenital heart disease:* patent ductus arteriosus, ventricular septal defect, atrial septal defect, tetralogy of Fallot, transposition of the great arteries, etc.; (c) other reported abnormalities: micrognathia, clubfeet, hemifacial microsomia, microphthalmos, tracheo-esophageal fistula, congenital laryngeal stridor, dolichocephalic skull, etc.

Radiologic Manifestations: *Various sternal anomalies:* premature sternal fusion including chondromanubrial deformity (marked posterior angulation), delayed ossification of the mesosternum, multiple manubrial ossification centers, sternal defects (including Cantrell syndrome), etc.

Note: (a) the premature obliteration of the sternal sutures in association with pectus carinatum has been referred to Currarino-Silverman syndrome; (b) the incidence of congenital heart disease in the patients with sternal anomalies has been reported to be 18% (Lees et al.).

REFERENCES

Currarino G, Silverman FN: Premature obliteration of the sternal sutures and pigeon-breast deformity. *Radiology* 70:532, 1958.

Kim OH, et al.: Delayed sternal ossification in infants with congenital heart disease. *Pediatr. Radiol.* 10:219, 1981.

Lees RF, et al.: Sternal anomalies and congenital heart disease. *A.J.R.* 124:423, 1975.

Shamberger RC, et al.: Surgical correction of chondromanubrial deformity (Currarino-Silverman syndrome). *J. Pediatr. Surg.* 23:319, 1988.

Steiner RM, et al.: Absent mesosternum in congenital heart disease. *A.J.R.* 127:923, 1976.

STERNAL MALFORMATION/VASCULAR DYSPLASIA ASSOCIATION

Clinical and Radiologic Manifestations: (a) sternal (complete or partial, including the cleft to the xiphoid); (b) hemangiomas, telangiectasis (face, scalp, neck, trunk, upper respiratory tract, abdominal); (c) other reported abnormalities: skin changes over the sternal defect, absent pericardium, cleft lip, micrognathia.

REFERENCES

Hersh JH, et al.: Sternal malformation/vascular dysplasia association. *Am. J. Med. Genet.* 21:177, 1985.

Kaplan LC, et al.: Anterior midline defects: Association with ectopia cordis or vascular dysplasia defines two distinct entities (letter). *Am. J. Med. Genet.* 21:203, 1985.

STERNO-COSTO-CLAVICULAR HYPEROSTOSIS

Synonyms: Hyperostosis (multiple); Köhler disease; acquired hyperostosis syndrome.

Frequency: Approximately 40 published cases (Toloune et al.).

Clinical Manifestations: (a) *pain in the upper part of the chest and shoulder, limitation of motion, exacerbation and remission;* (b) intermittent pustular, exfoliative dermatitis of the palms and soles; (c) moderate elevation of the sedimentation rate and C-reactive protein concentration, elevated serum globulin levels (α_1 and α_2), polyclonal gammapathy, mildly elevated serum alkaline phosphatase concentration; (d) biopsy: nonsuppurative acute and chronic inflammation of bones, muscles, and entheses; ligamentous fibrosis; ligamentous ossification; lymphocytes, plasma cells, and polymorphonuclear leukocytes within the wall of small vessels; (e) frequent occurrence in Japanese patients.

Radiologic Manifestations: (a) *hyperostosis and cortical thickening,* (clavicles, sternum, upper ribs, etc.), sclerotic changes in the sacroiliac joint region; (b) *increased uptake on skeletal scintigraphy;* (c) other reported abnormalities: pleural effusion, pulmonary infiltrates.

REFERENCES

Aberle DR, et al.: Sternocostoclavicular hyperostosis affecting the sternum, medial ends of the clavicles and upper segments of the anterior ribs (case report 407). *Skeletal Radiol.* 16:70, 1987.

Beraneck L, et al.: Hyperostose multiple avec sacro-iliite unilaterale. Une nouvelle spondyloarthropathie. *Presse Méd.* 13:2001, 1984.

Bjorkstein B, et al.: Chronic recurrent multifocal osteomyelitis and pustulosis palmoplantaris. *J. Pediatr.* 93:227, 1978.

Dihlmann VW, et al.: Das akquierte Hyperostose-Syndrom (AHS). Synthese aus 13 eigenen Beobachtungen von sternokostoklavikulärer. Hyperostose und über 300 Fällen aus der Literatur—Teil 1. *Fortschr. Rontgenstr.* 149:386, 1988.

Köhler H, et al.: Sternocostoclavicular hyperostosis: Painful swelling of the sternum, clavicles, and upper ribs. *Ann. Intern. Med.* 87:192, 1977.

Resnick D: Sternocostoclavicular hyperostosis. *A.J.R.* 135:1278, 1980.

Sartoris DJ, et al.: Sternocostoclavicular hyperostosis: A review and report of 11 cases. *Radiology* 159:125, 1986.

Toloune F, et al.: Hyperostose sterno-costo-claviculaire (maladie de Köhler). une nouvelle observation. *J. Radiol.* 69:419, 1988.

STEVENS-JOHNSON SYNDROME

Etiology: Various agents have been implicated: infections, drugs, collagen diseases, contactants, foods, visceral malignancies, radiation therapy.

Clinical Manifestations: (a) *systemic symptoms;* (b) *erythema multiforme;* (c) *vesicular lesions of the mucous membranes (stomatitis, urethritis, conjunctivitis);* (d) other reported abnormalities: esophageal stricture, ulcerative colitis, ulcerative proctitis, nephritis, nephrotic syndrome, uremia, pericarditis, pericardial effusion, atrial arrhythmias, blind-

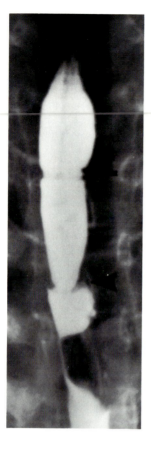

FIG SY−S−21.
Stevens-Johnson syndrome. An esophagogram shows a short (3 mm) segment of mild (1.4 cm) narrowing *(arrow)* and a web with marked compromise (4 mm) of the lumen *(arrowhead)*. (From Peters ME, Gourley G, Mann FA: Esophageal stricture and web secondary to Stevens-Johnson syndrome. *Pediatr. Radiol.* 13:290, 1982. Used by permission.)

ness, anonychia, oral mucosal scarring, familial occurrence (rare), chronic obliterative bronchitis, dysphagia.

Radiologic Manifestations: (a) patchy atypical pneumonia, pneumothorax, pneumomediastinum, subcutaneous emphysema; (b) cardiomegaly (pericardial effusion); (c) calcification of the bladder wall; (d) esophageal stricture, obliteration of the piriform sinus (Fig SY−S−21).

REFERENCES

Edwards C, et al.: Mycoplasma pneumonia, Stevens-Johnson syndrome, and chronic obliterative bronchitis. *Thorax* 38:867, 1983.
Fischer PR, et al.: Familial occurrence of Stevens-Johnson syndrome. *A. J. Dis. Child.* 137:914, 1983.
Ginsburg CM: Stevens-Johnson syndrome in children. *Pediatr. Infect. Dis.* 1:155, 1982.
Hansen RC: Blindness, anonychia, and oral mucosal scarring as sequelae of the Stevens-Johnson syndrome. *Pediatr. Dermatol.* 1:298, 1984.
Hernborg A: Stevens-Johnson syndrome after mass prophy-
laxis with sulfadoxine for cholera in Mozambique. *Lancet* 2:1072, 1985.
Hessl JM, et al.: Stevens-Johnson syndrome with vesical calcification: A case report. *J. Urol.* 107:662, 1972.
Howell CG, et al.: Esophageal stricture secondary to Stevens-Johnson syndrome. *J. Pediatr. Surg.* 22:994, 1987.
Kalb RE, et al.: Stevens-Johnson syndrome due to mycoplasma pneumoniae in an adult. *Am. J. Med.* 79:541, 1985.
Peters ME, et al.: Esophageal stricture and web secondary to Stevens-Johnson syndrome. *Pediatr. Radiol.* 13:290, 1983.
Stevens AM, Johnson FC: A new eruptive fever associated with stomatitis and ophthalmia: Report of two cases in children. *Am. J. Dis. Child.* 24:526, 1922.
Virant FS, et al.: Multiple pulmonary complications in a patient with Stevens-Johnson syndrome. *Clin. Pediatr. (Phila.)* 23:412, 1984.
Yetiv JZ, et al.: Etiologic factors of the Stevens-Johnson syndrome. *South. Med. J.* 73:599, 1980.

STEWART-BERGSTROM SYNDROME

Mode of Inheritance: Autosomal dominant (one family).

Clinical and Radiologic Manifestations: (a) *arthrogryposis-like deformity of distal parts of the extremities* (contracture, limitation of movement); (b) *sensorineural deafness*.

REFERENCE

Stewart JM, Bergstrom L: Familial hand abnormalities and sensorineural deafness: A new syndrome. *J. Pediatr.* 78:102, 1971.

STEWART-TREVES SYNDROME

Definition: Lymphangiosarcoma developing in lymphedematous extremities following radical mastectomy.

REFERENCES

Miettinen M, et al.: Postmastectomy angiosarcoma (Stewart-Treves syndrome). Light-microscopic, immunohistological, and ultrastructural characteristics of two cases. *Am. J. Surg. Pathol.* 7:329, 1983.
Noguchi M, et al.: Stewart-Treves syndrome. A report of two cases with a review of Japanese literature. *Jpn. J. Surg.* 17:407, 1987.
Stewart F-W, Treves N: Lymphangiosarcoma after postmastectomy lymphedema: Report of 6 cases in elephantiasis chirurgica. *Cancer* 1:64, 1948.
Tomita K, et al.: Lymphangiosarcoma in postmastectomy lymphedema (Stewart-Treves syndrome): Ultrastructural and immunohistologic characteristics *J. Surg. Oncol.* 38:275, 1988.

STICKLER SYNDROME

Synonyms: Arthro-ophthalmopathy; Wagner-Stickler syndrome.

Mode of Inheritance: Autosomal dominant; phenotype variability in families.

Clinical Manifestations: (a) severe *progressive myopia* to minus 18 D, retinal detachment, glaucoma, amblyopia; (b) depressed nasal bridge, maxillary hypoplasia, long philtrum; (c) progressive sensorineural hearing loss; (d) *cleft palate;* (e) *enlarged wrist, knee, and ankle joints at birth;* hypermobility of the joints; limitation of mobility of the joints in some cases; joint pain; dislocated patella; marfanoid body build; (f) Robin syndrome in a newborn in association with hypotonicity and hyperextensibility of the joints; (g) other reported abnormalities: malocclusion and dental maleruption, supernumerary digits, short fourth metacarpal, mental retardation, lenticular opacities, increased urinary hydroxyproline excretion, mitral valve prolapse (in about 45%).

Radiologic Manifestations: (a) narrowness of the diaphyses of long bones, thin cortices, normal width of the metaphyses, *irregularity in ossification, flattening and underdevelopment of some epiphyses,* coxa valga, wide femoral neck, subluxation of the femoral head, protrusio acetabuli, hypoplasia of the iliac wings; (b) *irregularity of the end plates of the vertebrae,* Scheuermann-like changes, thoracic kyphosis, anterior wedging of the vertebral bodies, scoliosis.

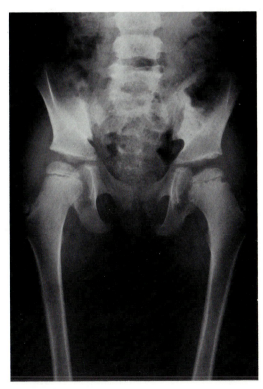

FIG SY−S−22.
Stickler syndrome in an 8-year-old female with hypoplasia of the iliac wing, narrow sciatic notches, flattening and irregularity of the femoral epiphyses, a wide femoral neck, and coxa valga. (From Spranger JW: Arthro-ophthalmopathia hereditaria. *Ann. Radiol. (Paris)* 11:359, 1968 Used by permission.)

Differential Diagnosis: Marshall syndrome: some have suggested that the Marshall and Stickler syndromes represent the same entity and have recommended that the term Marshall-Stickler syndrome be used; this recommendation has been rejected by others.

Note: About 30% of patients with the so-called Robin syndrome develop the full clinical picture of the Stickler syndrome (Fig SY−S−22).

REFERENCES

Aymé S, et al.: The Marshall and Stickler syndromes: Objective rejection of lumping. *J. Med. Genet.* 21:34, 1984.

Beals RK: Hereditary arthro-ophthalmopathy (The Stickler syndrome). *Clin. Orthop.* 125:32, 1977.

Blair NJ, et al.: Hereditary progressive arthroophthalmopathy of Stickler. *Am. J. Ophthalmol.* 88:876, 1979.

Kozlowski K, et al.: Stickler syndrome. *Pediatr. Radiol.* 3:230, 1975.

Liberfarb RM, et al.: The Wagner-Stickler syndrome: A study of 22 families. *J. Pediatr.* 99:394, 1981.

Spranger JW: Arthro-ophthalmopathia hereditaria. *Ann. Radiol. (Paris)* 11:359, 1968.

Stickler GB, et al.: Hereditary progressive arthroophthalmopathy. *Mayo Clin. Proc.* 40:433, 1965.

Stickler GB, et al.: Hereditary progressive arthroophthalmopathy II. Additional observations on vertebral abnormalities, a hearing defect, and a report of a similar case. *Mayo Clin. Proc.* 42:495, 1967.

Taillard F, et al.: Syndrome de Marshall ou syndrome de Stickler? Discussion a propos d'une famille. *Ann. Pediatr. (Paris)* 34:279, 1987.

Wagner H: Ein bisher unbekanntes Erbleiden des Auges (Degeneratio hyaloideo-retinalis hereditaria), beobachtet im Kanton Zurich. *Klin. Monatsbl. Augenheilkd.* 100:840, 1938.

STIFF-MAN SYNDROME

Synonym: Moersch-Woltmann syndrome.

Frequency: Rare.

Clinical Manifestations: (a) *progressive symmetrical muscle rigidity,* in particular, those of the back (extensors) and abdominal wall; (b) *painful muscle spasms* with profuse sweating and tachycardia that are precipitated by stimuli or movements; (c) increased tendon reflexes (occasionally); (d) *movement in block* (tin soldier); (e) *electromyography:* continuous motor unit activity with superimposed bursts (at rest or with activity) that are abolished by nerve block, curare, general anesthesia, sleep, and benzodiazepines; (f) other reported abnormalities: sudden death, increased immuno−gamma globulin G and acute-phase protein levels in the spinal fluid.

Radiologic Manifestations: (a) fractures resulting from muscular spasm; (b) hypertrophic arthropathy of the spinal column; (c) computed tomography: cerebral atrophic changes.

Note: Clinical and electrophysiological features similar to this syndrome have been reported in association with encephalomyelitis.

REFERENCES

Daras M, et al.: "Stiff-man syndrome" in an adolescent. *Pediatrics* 67:725, 1981.

Drake ME: Stiff-man syndrome and dementia. *Am. J. Med.* 74:1085, 1983.

Goetz CG, et al.: On the mechanism of sudden death in Moersch-Woltman syndrome. *Neurology* 33:930, 1983.

Maida E, et al.: Stiff-man syndrome with abnormalities in CSF and computerized tomography findings. *Arch. Neurol.* 37:182, 1980.

Masson C, et al.: Amnésie, syndrome de l'homme raide. Manifestations révélatrices d'une encéphalomyélite paranéoplasique. *Ann. Med. Interne (Paris)* 138:502, 1987.

Moersch FP, Woltmann HW: Progressive fluctuating muscular rigidity and spasm ("stiff-man" syndrome): Report of a case and some observations in 13 other cases. *Proc. Staff Meet. Mayo Clin.* 31:421, 1956.

Moore WT, et al.: Familial dwarfism and "stiff joints": Report of a kindred. *Arch. Intern. Med.* 115:398, 1965.

Olafson RA, et al.: "Stiff-man" syndrome: A review of the literature: Report of three additional cases and discussion of pathophysiology and therapy. *Proc. Staff Meet. Mayo Clin.* 39:131, 1964.

STRAIGHT BACK SYNDROME

Synonym: Sternospinal cardiac compression.

Clinical Manifestations: (a) dyspnea (rare); (b) *ejection systolic murmur at the base of the heart or a late systolic murmur;* (c) right axis deviation, an rSr' pattern in lead V_1; (d) pressure gradient between the right and main pulmonary arteries; (e) pectus excavatum; (f) other reported abnormalities: mitral valve prolapse, bicuspid aortic valve.

Radiologic Manifestations: (a) *straight dorsal spine;* (b) *narrow anteroposterior diameter of the thoracic cage;* (c) *heart flattened* and displaced to the left; (d) prominent pulmonary artery segment, prominent right hilus and pulmonary vasculature in the right lower lung field; (e) pulmonary venous obstruction and dilatation (very rare).

REFERENCES

Ansari A: The "straight back" syndrome: Current perspective more often associated with valvular heart disease than pseudoheart disease: A prospective clinical, electrocardiographic, roentgenographic, and echocardiographic study of 50 patients. *Clin. Cardiol.* 8:290, 1985.

Kumar UN, et al.: Abnormal pulmonary vasculature in an asymptomatic man. *Chest* 70:527, 1976.

Matsuo S, et al.: Straight back syndrome. *Am. Heart J.* 86:828, 1973.

Rawlings MS: The "straight back" syndrome: A new cause of pseudoheart disease. *Am. J. Cardiol.* 5:333, 1960.

Twigg HL, et al.: Straight back syndrome: Radiographic manifestations. *Radiology* 88:274, 1967.

STURGE-WEBER SYNDROME

Synonym: Encephalotrigeminal angiomatosis.

Mode of Inheritance: No definite evidence of heredity, almost always sporadic in occurrence.

Frequency: Uncommon.

Pathology: (a) angiomatous skin lesions; (b) venous angiomas (leptomeninges, choroid plexus in association with enlargement of the choroid plexus), cerebrovascular thromboses; (c) calcium deposition around blood vessels.

Clinical Manifestations: (a) *angiomatous lesions (port-wine nevi) of the face* in a trigeminal facial distribution, gingiva and alveolar ridges; (b) choroidal angioma of the eye with secondary buphthalmos and glaucoma; (c) *contralateral hemiplegia,* homonymous hemianopia, (d) *seizures;* (e) *mental retardation;* (f) decreased regional cerebral blood flow in the areas of the lesions (xenon 133 inhalation technique); (g) other reported abnormalities: external ear deformity, coarctation of the aorta, coloboma of the iris, cortical blindness, Klippel-Trenaunay syndrome.

Radiologic Manifestations: (a) *skull asymmetry* with a smaller hemicranium on the involved side, enlarged vascular channels of the skull, enlarged frontal sinus (rare), occasionally ipsilateral enlargement of a hemicranium; (b) *double-contour "gyriform" patterns of intracranial calcification* in the subcortical region, primarily in the parietal and occipital regions; (c) brain scan: widened cap of radioactivity over the affected cerebral convexity, identical radioactivity in hemispheres in studies performed 1–3 hours following the injection of isotope material; (d) *dilatation of the lateral ventricle on the affected side* and widening of the subarachnoid space resulting from brain atrophy; (e) angiography: arterial occlusion (rare), *capillary or venous angiomatous stains, various venous abnormalities* (nonfilling of the superior sagittal sinus; tortuosity; segmental ectasia; bizarre course of the cerebral veins and absence, deformity, and caliber irregularities of the deep veins); (f) computed tomography: cerebral calcification (unilateral or bilateral), contrast enhancement of leptomeningeal angiomatosis, ipsilateral cortical atrophy, enlargement of the ipsilateral ventricle, decreased (very rarely increased) volume of the ipsilateral hemicranium, enlarged subarachnoid space in cases with an enlarged ipsilateral hemicranium; enlargement and increased enhancement of the choroid plexus on the same side as the facial and intracranial lesions; (g) magnetic resonance imaging: accelerated myelination in the abnormal cerebral hemisphere; (h) other reported abnormalities: megalencephaly and hydrocephalus due to impaired cerebral venous return, development of abnormal drainage channels via the periorbital veins in association with an absence of the deep cerebral veins, atypical in-

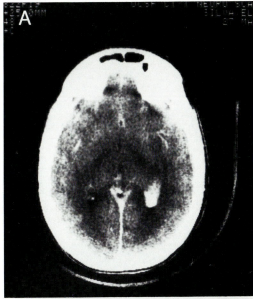

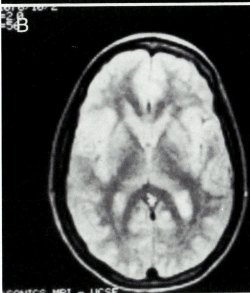

FIG SY—S—23.

Sturge-Weber syndrome: angiomatous malformations of the choroid plexus. **A,** contrast computed tomography shows increased enhancement of the glomus of the choroid plexus on the left (the side of the facial port-wine stain). **B,** a magnetic resonance scan using a T_2-weighted spin-echo technique (TR, 2000; TE, 56 ms) shows increased intensity in the same location. (From Stimac GK, Soloman MA, Newton TH: CT and MR of angiomatous malformations of the choroid plexus in patients with Sturge-Weber disease. *A.J.N.R.* 7:623, 1986. Used by permission.)

tracranial calcifications (bilateral in about 15% of the cases); calcifications contralateral to the bulk of the facial nevus; isolated frontal lobe calcification; intracranial calcification and abnormalities of the superficial cortical veins with pathological features of Sturge-Weber syndrome without facial angioma; (j) glaucoma and calcified choroidal angioma (Fig SY—S—23).

REFERENCES

Alonso A, et al.: Intracranial calcification in a neonate with the Sturge-Weber syndrome and additional problems. *Pediatr. Radiol.* 8:39, 1979.

Ambrosetto P, et al.: Sturge-Weber syndrome without port-wine facial nevus. Report of 2 cases studied by CT. *Child. Brain* 10:387, 1983.

Chaudary RR, et al.: Sturge-Weber syndrome with extensive intracranial calcifications contralateral to the bulk of the facial nevus, normal intelligence, and absent seizure disorder. *A.J.N.R.* 8:736, 1987.

Deutsch J, et al.: Kombination von Sturge-Weber und Klippel-Trenaunay syndrom. *Klin. Paediatr.* 188:464, 1976.

Di Trapani G, et al.: Light microscopy and ultrastructural studies of Sturge-Weber disease. *Child. Brain* 9:23, 1982.

Dulac O, et al.: Maladie de Sturge-Weber. Intérêt de l'analyse topgraphique de l'angiome cutané pour le diagnostic d'angiome pial associé. *Arch. Fr. Pediatr.* 39:155, 1982.

Enjolras O, et al.: Facial port-wine stains and Sturge-Weber syndrome. *Pediatrics* 76:48, 1985.

Fishman MA, et al.: Megalencephaly due to impaired cerebral venous return in a Sturge-Weber variant syndrome. *J. Child Neurol.* 1:115, 1986.

Garcia JC, et al.: Recurrent thrombotic deterioration in the Sturge-Weber syndrome. *Child. Brain* 8:427, 1981.

Hatfield M, et al.: Isolated frontal lobe calcification in Sturge-Weber syndrome. *A.J.N.R.* 9:203, 1988.

Jacoby CG, et al.: Accelerated myelination in early Sturge-Weber syndrome. Demonstrated by MR imaging. *J. Comput. Assist. Tomogr.* 11:226, 1987.

Kuhl DE, et al.: The brain scan in Sturge-Weber syndrome. *Radiology* 103:621, 1972.

Probst FP: Vascular morphology and angiographic flow pattern in Sturge-Weber angiomatosis: Facts, thoughts and suggestions. *Neuroradiology* 20:73, 1980.

Riela AR, et al.: Regional cerebral blood flow characteristics of the Sturge-Weber syndrome. *Pediatr. Neurol.* 1:85, 1985.

Stimac GK, et al.: CT and MR of angiomatous malformations of the choroid plexus in patients with Sturge-Weber disease. *A.J.N.R.* 7:623, 1986.

Sturge WA: A case of partial epilepsy apparently due to a lesion of one of the vasomotor centers of the brain. *Trans. Clin. Soc. (London)* 12:162, 1879; also *Br. Med. J.* 1:704, 1879.

Taly AB, et al.: Sturge-Weber-Dimitri disease without facial nevus. *Neurology* 37:1063, 1987.

Weber FP: Right-sided hemi-hypotrophy resulting from right-sided congenital spastic hemiplegia, with a morbid condition of the left side of the brain, revealed by radiograms. *J. Neurol. Psychopathol.* 3:134, 1922.

SUBAORTIC STENOSIS—SHORT STATURE

Synonym: Onat syndrome.

Mode of Inheritance: Reported in a family in which the parents were second cousins.

Clinical and Radiologic Manifestations: (a) short stature, hoarseness, obstructive lung disease, upturned nose, inguinal hernia; (b) discrete subaortic stenosis.

REFERENCE

Onat A, et al.: Discrete subaortic stenosis as part of a short stature syndrome. *Hum. Genet.* 65:331, 1984.

SUBCLAVIAN STEAL SYNDROME

Pathophysiology: Circulation to an arm via the vertebral artery in a patient with subclavian or innominate artery obstruction proximal to the origin of the vertebral artery with ischemia of the brain and/or arm as a result.

Etiology: Arteriosclerosis; thrombosis; tumor; Takayasu syndrome; congenital anomaly (hypoplasia, atresia, or isolation of the subclavian artery with a right or cervical aortic arch; vascular rings; coarctation of the aorta with obliteration of the subclavian artery orifice); extravascular obstruction due to a fibrous band and surgically corrected congenital anomalies; granulation tissue secondary to cannulation of an artery; trauma; surgical procedure (Blalock-Taussig procedure); subclavian artery aneurysm; etc.;

Clinical Manifestations: (a) *pain and numbness of the arm and hand, claudication;* (b) *dizziness, light-headedness, syncopal episodes, headache, vertigo,* visual defect, coldness, fatigue during activity, aphasia, hearing loss, etc; (c) absent radial pulse, a difference in brachial artery pressure greater than 20 mm Hg, supraclavicular bruit; (d) congenital subclavian steal usually asymptomatic in childhood.

Radiologic Manifestations: (a) angiographic demonstration of *arterial obstruction to an arm and reverse direction of flow of contrast medium from the vertebral artery to the arm,* increased or decreased jugular vein opacity as compared with the opposite side; (b) Doppler ultrasound: delay in pulse-wave propagation in an artery relative to the opposite side.

REFERENCES

Arevalo F, et al.: Bilateral subclavian steal syndrome. *A.J.R.* 127:668, 1976.

Aveback P: Unusual cause of subclavian-steal syndrome. *N. Engl. J. Med.* 295:1262, 1976.

Baker RA, et al.: Segmental intervertebral anastomosis in subclavian steal. *Br. J. Radiol.* 48:101, 1975.

Berguer R, et al.: Noninvasive diagnosis of reversal of vertebral artery blood flow. *N. Engl. J. Med.* 302:1349, 1980.

Bloch S, et al.: The subclavian steal syndrome. *Clin. Radiol.* 27:483, 1976.

Brill CB, et al.: Isolation of the right subclavian artery with subclavian steal in a child with Klippel-Feil anomaly: An example of the subclavian artery supply disruption sequence. *Am. J. Med. Genet.* 26:933, 1987.

Contorni L: The true story of the "subclavian steal syndrome" or "Harrison and Smyth's syndrome." *J. Cardiovasc. Surg.* 14:408, 1973.

Erbstein RA, et al.: Subclavian artery steal syndrome: Treatment by percutaneous transluminal angioplasty. *A.J.R.* 151:291, 1988.

Garcia OL, et al.: Congenital bilateral subclavian steal. *Am. J. Cardiol.* 44:101, 1979.

Kotval PS, et al.: Doppler diagnosis of intermittent subclavian steal during systole caused by axillary-axillary bypass graft. *J. Ultrasound Med.* 7:593, 1988.

McCormick TL, et al.: Subclavian steal syndrome: Is venous-phase angiography meaningful? *Radiology* 138:93, 1981.

Midglez FM, et al.: Subclavian steal syndrome in the pediatric age group. *Ann. Thorac. Surg.* 24:252, 1977.

Motarjeme A, et al.: Percutaneous transluminal angioplasty for treatment of subclavian steal. *Radiology* 155:611, 1985.

Nalbantgil I, et al.: Venous-phase angiography in subclavian-steal syndrome. *Radiology* 128:411, 1978.

Otto R, et al.: Subclavian aneurysm producing the subclavian steal syndrome. *Cardiovasc. Intervent. Radiol.* 9:90, 1986.

Perraudin ML, et al.: Syndrome de vol sous-clavier congénital avec arc aortique droit. *Ann. Pediatr. (Paris)* 28:45, 1981.

Reivich M, et al.: Reversal of blood flow through the vertebral artery and its effect on cerebral circulation. *N. Engl. J. Med.* 265:878, 1961.

Rowe DM, et al.: Right subclavian steal associated with aberrant right subclavian artery. *A.J.N.R.* 9:604, 1988.

Takahashi M, et al.: Congenital subclavian steal associated with an unusual type of right aortic arch. *Cardiovasc. Intervent. Radiol.* 4:136, 1981.

SUPERIOR MESENTERIC ARTERY SYNDROME

Synonyms: Arteriomesenteric duodenal compression; Wilkie syndrome.

Definition: Compression of the third portion of the duodenum secondary to an increase in acuteness of the aortosuperior mesenteric artery angle.

Etiology: Congenital rapid weight loss; rapid growth without weight gain; hyperextension of the vertebral column (body brace, cast); duodenal hypotonia.

Clinical Manifestations: *Postprandial epigastric fullness, nausea, vomiting,* abdominal cramps, weight loss, *slender habitus.*

Radiologic Manifestations: (a) *dilatation of the duodenum proximal to a vertical linear extrinsic pressure defect of third portion of the duodenum;* marked "to-and-fro" peristaltic waves proximal to the obstruction; gastric dilatation (in some, relief of the obstruction in the prone position; (b) *narrow aortomesenteric angle* (10 to 12 degrees as compared with the normal of 45 to 65 degrees) and a *decrease in the aortomesenteric distance* (2 to 3 mm as compared with the normal of 7 to 20 mm).

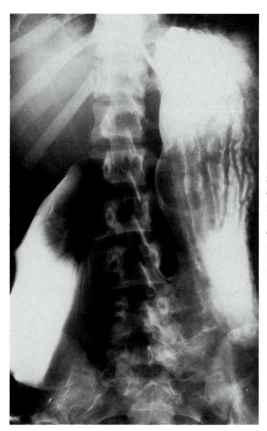

FIG SY–S–24.
Superior mesenteric artery syndrome in a 16-year-old female who had been in good health until a "boil" developed on her right nasolabial fold followed by pneumonia and meningitis. At admission to Children's Hospital of San Francisco 19 days after the onset of the disease, she was in a cachectic state with abdominal distension and massive gastric fluid retention. Marked dilatation of the proximal segment of the duodenum with a sharp distal cutoff is seen. Conservative management failed, and finally duodenojejunostomy was performed. (Courtesy of Dr. Robert S. Arkoff, San Francisco.)

Differential Diagnosis: Extrinsic "masses" (hematoma, neoplasm, aneurysm, mesenteric arteriovenous fistula, etc.) (Fig SY–S–24).

REFERENCES

Altman DH, et al.: Superior mesenteric artery syndrome in children. *A.J.R.* 118:104, 1973.

Amy BW, et al.: Superior mesenteric artery syndrome associated with scoliosis treated by a modified Ladd procedure. *J. Pediatr. Orthop.* 5:361, 1985.

Burrington JD: Superior mesenteric artery syndrome in children. *Am. J. Dis. Child.* 130:1367, 1976.

Burrington JD, et al.: Obstruction of duodenum by superior mesenteric artery: Does it exist in children? *J. Pediatr. Surg.* 9:733, 1974.

Gottrand F, et al.: Le syndrome de la pince mésentérique (cas radiologique du mois). *Arch. Fr. Pediatr.* 43:811, 1986.

Hines JR, et al.: Superior mesenteric artery syndrome. Diagnostic criteria and therapeutic approaches. *Am. J. Surg.* 148:630, 1984.

Lescher TJ, et al.: Superior mesenteric artery syndrome in thermally injured patients. *J. Trauma* 19:567, 1979.

Ptasznik J, et al.: Obstruction of the third portion of the duodenum. *Australas. Radiol.* 30:19, 1986.

Reed JK, et al.: Traumatic mesenteric arteriovenous fistula presenting as the superior mesenteric artery syndrome. *Arch. Surg.* 121:1209, 1986.

Shandling B: The so-called superior mesenteric artery syndrome. *Am. J. Dis. Child.* 130:1371, 1976.

Von Rokitansky C: *Lehrbuch der pathologischen anatomie,* Vienna, Braumüller & Seidel, 1855–1861, p. 187, quoted by Shandling.

Wilkie DPD: Chronic duodenal ileus. *Br. Med. J.* 2:793, 1921.

SUPERIOR VENA CAVA SYNDROME

Etiology: (a) mediastinitis; (b) mediastinal tumors; (c) vascular (aneurysms, fistula, vasculitis, thrombosis, long-term peritoneovenous shunt, transvenous pacemaker implantation), after the Mustard procedure, central venous catheter sequela (Broviac or Hickman catheters); (d) pneumomediastinum, pneumothorax; (e) mediastinal hematoma; (f) other reported causes: Behçet syndrome, silicosis, sarcoidosis, etc.

Clinical Manifestations: (a) headache, vertigo, somnolence, syncope, convulsions; (b) hoarseness, respiratory distress; (c) epistaxis; (d) cyanosis and edema of the face, neck, shoulder, and arms; (e) *engorgement and tortuosity of veins of the neck, thorax, and arms;* (f) vascular congestion of the eyes and nasal mucosa.

Radiologic Manifestations: (a) irregular *widening of the mediastinum,* tortuous density parallel to the spine (azygos and hemiazygos), dilated left superior intercostal vein, rib

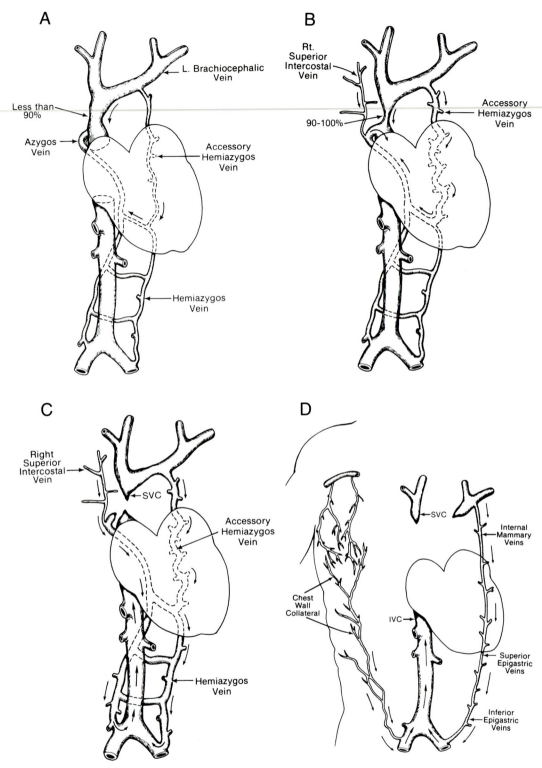

FIG SY–S–25.

Diagrams of the superior vena cava syndrome. **A,** type I: partial obstruction (up to 90% stenosis) of the SVC with patency of the azygos–right atrial pathway. **B,** type II: near complete to complete obstruction (90% to 100%) of the SVC with patency and antegrade flow in the azygos–right atrial pathways. **C,** type III: near complete to complete obstruction (90% to 100%) of the SVC with reversal of the azygos blood flow. **D,** type IV: complete obstruction of the SVC and one or more of the major caval tributaries including the azygos systems (*IVC* = inferior vena cava). (From Stanford W, Doty DB: The role of venography and surgery in the management of patients with superior vena cava obstruction. *Ann. Thorac. Surg.* 41:158, 1986. Used by permission.)

notching (rare); (b) hydrothorax, hydropericardium; (c) *venographic demonstration of the site of obstruction and collaterals* (between the innominate tributaries and azygos tributaries, between the superior vena cava [SVC] and inferior vena caval systems along the posterior and anterior portions of the trunk, collaterals between the arm and thorax, between the anterior and posterior veins and collaterals across the midline); (d) radionuclide venography; (e) computed tomography: SVC obstruction (demonstration of the etiologic factor), increased size and greater numbers of chest wall collaterals; (f) ultrasonography: absence of normal respiratory rhythmicity and response to a sudden sniff maneuver (venous collapse in a rapid, transient manner secondary to the sudden decrease in intrathoracic pressure); (g) communicating hydrocephalus secondary to SVC obstruction (Fig SY–S–25).

REFERENCES

Bankoff MS, et al.: Bronchogenic cyst causing superior vena cava obstruction: CT appearance. *J. Comput. Assist. Tomogr.* 9:951, 1985.

Bechtold RE, et al.: Superior vena caval obstruction: Detection using CT. *Radiology* 157:485, 1985.

Bertrand M, et al.: Iatrogenic superior vena cava syndrome. A new entity. *Cancer* 54:376, 1984.

Carter MM, et al.: The "aortic nipple" as a sign of impending superior vena caval syndrome. *Chest* 87:775, 1985.

Conte FA, et al.: Superior vena cava syndrome and bilateral subclavian vein thrombosis. CT and radionuclide venography correlation. *Clin. Nucl. Med.* 11:698, 1986.

Crowley DC, et al.: Superior vena cava obstruction: Complication of pulmonary artery ectasia in levo-transposition of the great arteries. *Cardiovasc. Intervent. Radiol.* 4:27, 1981.

Curci MR, et al.: Bilateral chylothorax in a newborn. *J. Pediatr. Surg.* 15:663, 1980.

Danilowicz D, et al.: Superior vena caval syndrome after Mustard repair: Surgical decompression using a saphenous vein homograft. *Am. Heart J.* 101:862, 1981.

Drane WE, et al.: Obstruction of the superior vena cava or its major tributaries demonstrated by Bolus-injection excretory urography. *Radiology* 144:499, 1982.

Eckhauser FE, et al.: Superior vena cava obstruction associated with long-term peritoneovenous shunting. *Ann. Surg.* 190:758, 1979.

Good JT, et al.: Superior vena cava syndrome as a cause of pleural effusion. *Am. Rev. Respir. Dis.* 125:246, 1982.

Gooding GAW, et al.: Obstruction of the superior vena cava or subclavian veins: Sonographic diagnosis. *Radiology* 159:663, 1986.

Hershey CO, et al.: Transient superior vena cava syndrome due to propylthiouracil therapy in intrathoracic goiter. *Chest* 79:356, 1981.

Issa PY, et al.: Superior vena cava syndrome in childhood: Report of ten cases and review of the literature. *Pediatrics* 71:337, 1983.

Markowitz RI, et al.: Communicating hydrocephalus secondary to superior caval obstruction. Occurrence after Mustard's operation for transposition of the great arteries. *Am. J. Dis. Child.* 138:638, 1984.

Matherne GP, et al.: Cine computed tomography for diagnosis of superior vena cava obstruction following the Mustard operation. *Pediatr. Radiol.* 17:246, 1987.

Mendelson DS, et al.: Computed tomography of mediastinal collaterals in SVC syndrome. *J. Comput. Assist. Tomogr.* 12:884, 1988.

Or I, et al.: Pacemaker implantation in a patient with a Behçet's disease. Associated with superior vena cava obstruction. *Cardiovasc. Intervent. Radiol.* 9:13, 1986.

Phillips PL, et al.: Syphilitic aortic aneurysm presenting with the superior vena cava syndrome. *Am. J. Med.* 71:171, 1981.

Sculier JP, et al.: Superior vena caval obstruction syndrome in small cell lung cancer. *Cancer* 57:847, 1986.

Serdarevic M, et al.: Das Vena Cava superior-Syndrom-Klinik, Ätiologie und casuistische Beiträge. *Radiologe* 24:286, 1984.

Stanford W, et al.: Superior vena cava obstruction: A venographic classification. *A.J.R.* 148:259, 1987.

Stanford W, et al.: The role of venography and surgery in the management of patients with superior vena cava obstruction. *Ann. Thorac. Surg.* 41:158, 1986.

Weiss KS, et al.: Radiation-induced leiomyosarcoma of the great vessels presenting as superior vena cava syndrome. *Cancer* 60:1238, 1987.

SWEET SYNDROME

Clinical Manifestations: (a) *fever;* (b) *raised painful plaques on the extremities, face, and neck;* (c) dense dermal cellular infiltrate with neutrophils; (d) polymorphonuclear leukocytosis; (e) association with malignancies (hematologic, in particular, acute myelogenous leukemia), myeloproliferative disorders, lymphoproliferative disorders, myelodysplastic syndrome.

Radiologic Manifestations: Pulmonary infiltrates (case report).

REFERENCES

Cohen PR, et al.: Sweet's syndrome and malignancy. *Am. J. Med.* 82:1220, 1987.

Grigsby PW, et al.: Sweet's syndrome in association with solid tumors. *Am. J. Med.* 82:1084, 1987.

Lazarus AA, et al.: Pulmonary involvement in Sweet's syndrome (acute febrile neutrophilic dermatosis). Preleukemic and leukemic phases of acute myelogenous leukemia. *Chest* 90:922, 1986.

Sweet RD: An acute febrile neutrophilic dermatosis. *Br. J. Dermatol.* 76:349, 1964.

SWYER-JAMES SYNDROME

Synonyms: Unilateral hyperlucent lung syndrome; Macleod syndrome; Swyer-James-Macleod syndrome.

Etiology: (a) sequela of various lung insults: bronchiolitis, bronchiolitis obliterans, measles, *Mycoplasma pneumoniae,* pertussis, adenovirus pneumonia, foreign-body aspiration, hydrocarbon pneumonia, radiotherapy; (b) idiopathic.

Clinical Manifestations: (a) history of recurrent pulmonary infection in childhood; (b) usually asymptomatic in adult life; however, the subject may have a cough, chronic and repeated pulmonary infections, decreased exercise tolerance, hemoptysis, and arterial blood desaturation.

Radiologic Manifestations: (a) unilateral small, hyperlucent lung (or lobe); (b) *poor air exchange* and change of lung density between inspiration and expiration; (c) *diminished* pulmonary vasculature, small hilar shadow of the involved side; (d) bronchographic demonstration of *dilatation of the bronchi and lack of alveolization of the contrast medium* (pruned-tree appearance), hyperdistensible bronchial diameter shown by functional bronchography (inflation under 50 cm H_2O pressure); (e) angiographic demonstration of *diminished size and number of pulmonary vessels in the portion of the involved lung;* (f) radioimaging: decreased perfusion and ventilation seen on an isotope scan of the lung, may reveal

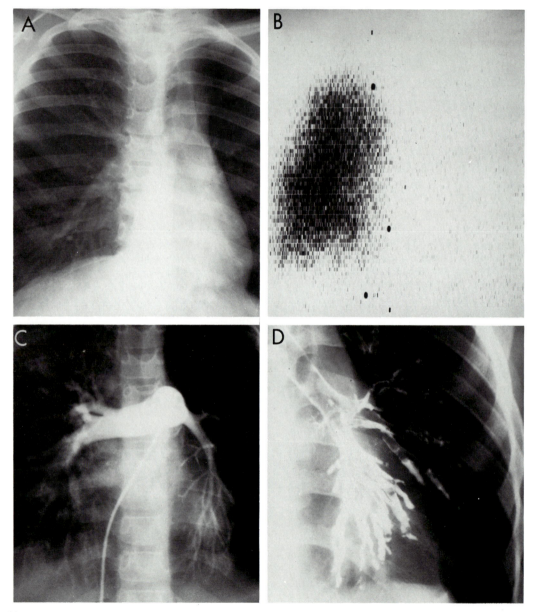

FIG SY–S–26.
Swyer-James syndrome in a 7-year-old male with a history of multiple episodes of pneumonitis from the age of 1 year. The patient was asymptomatic at time of this examination. **A,** the left lung is small and hyperlucent. **B,** a complete absence of perfusion of the left lung is noted on a lung scan. **C,** the left main pulmonary artery is small, and there is a lack of terminal arterial and capillary filling. **D,** bronchiectatic changes in left lower lobe and lingula and lesser changes in the remainder of the left lung. (From Kogutt MS, Swischuk LE, Goldblum R: Swyer-James syndrome (unilateral hyperlucent lung) in children. *Am. J. Dis. Child.* 125:614, 1973. Used by permission.)

otherwise unsuspected bilateral involvement; (g) other reported abnormalities: unilateral pulmonary edema (Swyer-James syndrome protecting the affected lung from pulmonary edema).

Differential Diagnosis: Bronchial obstruction; congenital hypoplastic pulmonary artery; unilateral external muscular anomalies; etc. (Fig SY–S–26).

REFERENCES

Daniel TL, et al.: Swyer-James syndrome—unilateral hyperlucent lung syndrome. A case report and review. *Clin. Pediatr. (Phila.)* 23:393, 1984.

Giedion A, et al.: Normal and abnormal variations of bronchial diameter in functional bronchography. *Ann. Radiol. (Paris)* 27:265, 1984.

Hekali P, et al.: Chronic unilateral hyperlucent lung. A consecutive series of 40 patients. *Fortschr. Rontgenstr.* 136:41, 1982.

Kogutt MS, Swischuk LE, Goldblum R: Swyer-James syndrome (unilateral hyperlucent lung) in children. *Am. J. Dis. Child.* 125:614, 1973.

Macleod WM: Abnormal transradiancy of one lung. *Thorax* 9:147, 1954.

Macpherson RI, et al.: Unilateral hyperlucent lung: A complication of viral pneumonia. *J. Can. Assoc. Radiol.* 20:225, 1969.

O'Dell CW Jr, et al.: Ventilation-perfusion lung impinges in the Swyer-James syndrome. *Radiology* 121:423, 1976.

Peters ME, et al.: Swyer-James-Macleod syndrome: A case with a baseline normal chest radiograph. *Pediatr. Radiol.* 12:211, 1982.

Stokes D, et al.: Unilateral hyperlucent lung (Swyer-James syndrome) after severe *Mycoplasma pneumoniae* infection. *Am. Rev. Respir. Dis.* 117:145, 1978.

Swyer PR, James GCW: A case of unilateral pulmonary emphysema. *Thorax* 8:133, 1953.

Vanker EA: Asymmetrical pulmonary oedema due to Swyer-James syndrome. *Br. J. Radiol.* 60:1126, 1987.

SYNDROME OF INAPPROPRIATE SECRETION OF ANTIDIURETIC HORMONE

Synonyms: Inappropriate secretion of antidiuretic syndrome; SIADH.

Etiology: Ectopic production of antidiuretic hormone induced by nonosmotic stimuli: (a) neoplasia at various sites, in particular, bronchogenic carcinoma; (b) infections in various organs; (c) central nervous diseases including trauma, infection, vascular occlusion, neoplasm, vasculitis, multiple sclerosis, cerebral atrophy, hypoplastic corpus callosum, surgery; (d) drugs; (e) others: acute asthma, acute bronchitis, chronic obstructive pulmonary disease, pneumothorax, cystic fibrosis, psychosis, following spinal fusion, etc.

Types: (a) transient and self-limited; (b) chronic and persistent.

Clinical Manifestations: (a) normovolemic or near-normovolemic hyponatremia in a patient with unrestricted water intake; (b) inappropriately high urine osmolarity; (c) high urinary excretion of sodium; (d) normal renal function; (e) correction of the hyponatremia by fluid restriction.

Radiologic Manifestations: Those of the etiologic factors.

REFERENCES

Bartter FC, et al.: The syndrome of inappropriate secretion of antidiuretic hormone. *Am. J. Med.* 42:790, 1967.

Bell GR, et al.: The syndrome of inappropriate antidiuretic-hormone secretion following spinal fusion. *J. Bone Joint Surg. [Am.]* 68:720, 1986.

Benfield GFA, et al.: Status asthmaticus and the syndrome of inappropriate secretion of antidiuretic hormone. *Thorax* 37:147, 1982.

Braden G, et al.: Syndrome of inappropriate antidiuresis in Waldenström's macroglobulinemia. *Am. J. Med.* 80:1242, 1986.

Chemtob S, et al.: Syndrome of inappropriate secretion of antidiuretic hormone in enteroviral meningitis. *Am. J. Dis. Child.* 139:292, 1985.

Dall BE, et al.: Syndrome of inappropriate anti-diuretic hormone secretion complicating metrizamide myelography. *J. Bone Joint Surg. [Am.]* 70:142, 1988.

Goldstein CS, et al.: Idiopathic syndrome of inappropriate antidiuretic hormone secretion possibly related to advanced age. *Ann. Intern. Med.* 99:185, 1983.

Greenbaum-Lefkoe B, et al.: Syndrome of inappropriate antidiuretic hormone secretion. A complication of high-dose intravenous melphalan. *Cancer* 55:44, 1985.

Kramer DS, et al.: Acute psychosis, polydipsia, and inappropriate secretion of antidiuretic hormone. *Am. J. Med.* 75:712, 1983.

Littlewood TJ, et al.: Syndrome of inappropriate antidiuretic hormone secretion due to treatment of lung cancer with cisplatin. *Thorax* 39:636, 1984.

Ravikumar TS, et al.: The syndrome of inappropriate ADH secretion secondary to vinblastine-bleomycin therapy. *J. Surg. Oncol.* 24:242, 1983.

Sklar C, et al.: Chronic syndrome of inappropriate secretion of antidiuretic hormone in childhood. *Am. J. Dis. Child.* 139:733, 1985.

Stagg MP, et al.: Chronic lymphocytic leukemic meningitis as a cause of the syndrome of inappropriate secretion of antidiuretic hormone. *Cancer* 60:191, 1987.

SYNDROME X

Clinical and Radiologic Manifestations: (a) angina on effort; (b) positive exercise test findings; (c) no demonstrable coronary stenosis (angiography) or coronary vasospasm; (d) echocardiographically silent myocardial ischemia during dipyridamole echocardiography test; (e) no other explanation for the symptoms (hypertension, valve disease, cardiomyopathy).

Note: These patients are considered to have functional rather than anatomic ischemia.

REFERENCES

Favaro L, et al.: Sex differences in exercise induced left ventricular dysfunction in patients with syndrome X. *Br. Heart J.* 57:232, 1987.

Kemp HG: Left ventricular function in patients with the anginal syndrome and normal coronary arteriograms. *Am. J. Cardiol.* 32:375, 1973.

Picano E, et al.: Usefulness of a high-dose dipyridamole-chocardiography test for diagnosis of syndrome X. *Am. J. Cardiol.* 60:508, 1987.

Turiel M, et al.: Pain threshold and tolerance in women with syndrome X and women with stable angina pectoris. *Am. J. Cardiol.* 60:503, 1987.

T

TABATZNIK SYNDROME

Mode of Inheritance: Autosomal dominant.

Clinical Manifestations: (a) cardiac arrhythmias; (b) sloping shoulders, hypoplastic deltoid muscles, short arm.

Radiologic Manifestations: Upper limb deformities: flaring of lower end of humerus, flaring and obliquity of distal end of radius, absent styloid process of ulna, shortening and hypoplasia of fourth and fifth metacarpals, brachytelephalangy.

REFERENCE

Temtamy S, McKusick VA: Heart-hand syndrome II (Tabatznik syndrome). *Birth Defects* 14(3):241, 1978.

TAKAYASU ARTERITIS

Synonyms: Aortitis syndrome; middle aortic syndrome; aortic arch syndrome; pulseless disease; aortoarteritis; etc.

Clinical Manifestations: Two clinical stages: early systemic, followed by an occlusive phase. (a) asthenia, weight loss, fever; (b) dyspnea, palpitations, angina pectoris, myocardial infarction, hemoptysis, intermittent claudication; (c) pulse deficit, vascular bruit, heart failure, mitral insufficiency, aortic insufficiency, pericardial rub, elevated blood pressure; (d) headache, syncope, seizures, visual disturbances, amblyopia, retinopathy, hemiplegia, paraplegia, abnormal fundi; (e) abdominal pain, diarrhea, vomiting; (f) other reported abnormalities: association with tuberculosis, arthralgia, peripheral gangrene, annuloaortic ectasia associated with Hashimoto disease, close association with two B-cell alloantigens; (g) occurrence of familial cases.

Radiologic Manifestations: Multiple and diffuse arterial involvement: (a) *partial or total systemic arterial obstruction,* single or multiple sites, particularly the aorta and major branches (carotids at their origin and subclavian arteries where they pass over the ribs, renal and visceral branches); (b) the pulmonary artery and its branches may also be involved; (c) *extensive collateral circulation,* bronchial-pulmonary artery communication, coronary-bronchial artery communication (coronary steal); (d) other reported abnormalities: pleural effusion, rib notching, hilar adenopathy, pulmonary hypertension associated with a prominent pulmonary artery, decreased pulmonary vascularity, widening of the ascending aorta, irregularity of aortic contour, saccular or fusiform aneurysm, heart failure, aortic wall thickening, aortic wall calcification, aortic pseudoanurysm, abnormal cerebral metabolic parameters shown by positron-emission tomography (Fig SY–T–1).

REFERENCES

Amparo EG, et al.: Magnetic resonance imaging of aortic disease: Preliminary results. *A.J.R.* 143:1203, 1984.

Dubourg O, et al.: Aortite de Takayasu. Exploration de l'aorte et de ses branches par angiographie numérisée et echographie bidimensionnelle. *Presse Med.* 14:23, 1985.

Fujii S, et al.: Coronary steal in Takayasu's aortitis. *Am. Heart J.* 109:596, 1985.

Grollman JH Jr, Hanafee W: The roentgen diagnosis of Takayasu's arteritis. *Radiology* 83:387, 1964.

Haas A, et al.: Takayasu's arteritis presenting as pulmonary hypertension. *Am. J. Dis. Child.* 140:372, 1986.

Hardoff R, et al.: Radionuclide demonstration of systemic arterial supply to the lung in Takayasu's arteritis. *Clin. Nucl. Med.* 12:479, 1987.

Hayashi K, et al.: Initial pulmonary artery involvement in Takayasu arterites. *Radiology* 159:401, 1986.

Hayashi K, et al.: Takayasu's arteritis: Decrease in aortic wall thickening following steroid therapy, documented by CT. *Br. J. Radiol.* 59:281, 1986.

Ishikawa K: Natural history and classification of occlusive thromboartopathy (Takayasu's disease). *Circulation* 57:27, 1978.

Kawai T, et al.: Pleural effusion associated with aortitis syndrome. *Chest* 68:826, 1975.

Kohrman MH, et al.: Takayasu arteritis: A treatable cause of stroke in infancy. *Pediatr. Neurol.* 2:154, 1986.

Lewis VD, et al.: The midaortic syndrome: Diagnosis and treatment. *Radiology* 167:111, 1988.

Liu YQ: Radiology of aortoarteritis. *Radiol. Clin. North Am.* 23:671, 1985.

Masuzawa T, et al.: Pulseless disease associated with multiple intracranial aneurysms. *Neuroradiology* 28:17, 1986.

Miller DL, et al.: Vascular imaging with MRI: Inadequacy in Takayasu's arteritis. Compared with angiography. *A.J.R.* 146:949, 1986.

Numano F, et al.: Takayasu's disease in twin sisters: Possible genetic factors. *Circulation* 58:173, 1978.

Pantell RH, et al.: Takayasu's arteritis: The relationship with tuberculosis. *Pediatrics* 67:84, 1981.

Peterson IM, et al.: Aortic pseudoaneurysm complicating Takayasu disease: CT appearance. *J. Comput. Assist. Tomogr.* 10:676, 1986.

Shimokawa H, et al.: Annuloaortic ectasia in a case of Takayasu's arteritis associated with Hashimoto's disease. *Br. Heart J.* 49:94, 1983.

Takayasu M: Case with peculiar changes in retinal vessels. *Acta Soc. Ophthalmol. Jpn.* 12:554, 1908.

Théron J, et al.: Takayasu's arteritis of the aortic arch: Endo-

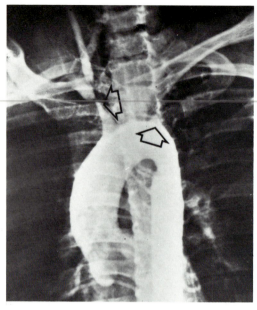

FIG SY–T–1.
Takayasu arteritis in a 19-year-old female with right-sided weakness and aphasia. An aortic arch study demonstrates occlusion of the left subclavian and left common carotid arteries and partial obstruction of the innominate artery. The arch is slightly narrowed in its distal portion. *Arrows* point to vessels with a flame-shaped configuration characteristic of the disease. (From Grollman JH Jr, Hanafee W: The roentgen diagnosis of Takayasu's arteritis. *Radiology* 83:387, 1964. Used by permission.)

vascular treatment and correlation with positron emission tomography. *A.J.N.R.* 8:621, 1987.

Volkman DJ, et al.: Association between Takayasu's arteritis and a B-cell alloantigen in North Americans. *N. Engl. J. Med.* 306:464, 1982.

Yamato M, et al.: Takayasu arteritis: Radiographic and angiographic findings in 59 patients. *Radiology* 161:329, 1986.

TAR SYNDROME

Synonym: Thrombocytopenia-absent radius syndrome.

Mode of Inheritance: Pattern consistent with autosomal recessive; great intrafamilial and interfamilial variability (skeletal, hematologic, gastrointestinal, and cardiac abnormalities); consanguinity in a family.

Frequency: 40 published cases (1969) plus 60 cases in the English language literature published after 1969 (Hedberg et al.).

Clinical Manifestations: (a) *congenital deformity of the forearm and hand* (often bilateral) with the hand at right angles to the forearm, thumb always present, hypoplasia of muscles and soft tissues in the arms and shoulder; (b) hemorrhagic tendencies caused by *thrombocytopenia,* with onset at birth or shortly thereafter; decrease in the number and sever-

ity of the thrombocytopenic episodes in most cases; (c) *myeloid leukemoid reactions* and eosinophilia; (d) *hypercellular bone marrow and congenital absence or marked reduction of megakaryocytes* without a reduction in other elements of the bone marrow; (e) congenital heart defects; (tetralogy of Fallot, atrial septal defect and ventricular septal defect, etc.) in 22% of the reported cases; (f) other reported abnormalities: short stature, other skeletal anomalies, facial dysmorphism, trisomy 18, cutaneous hemangioma, cleft palate, dorsal pedal edema (lasting 3 to 18 months), hyperhidrosis, vomiting and diarrhea, gastrointestinal bleeding, mental retardation (secondary to intracranial hemorrhage), milk allergy, lactose intolerance, redundant nuchal skin folds, hypogammaglobulinemia, tetraphocomelia, lower-limb abnormalities (stiff or subluxing knees, etc.), ptosis, hypertelorism, dysseborrheic dermatitis leading to bleeding in the skin, glaucoma (related to intraocular bleeding).

Radiologic Manifestations: (a) bilateral absent radii with or without other upper-limb anomalies: short and malformed ulna, absent ulna, abnormal humerus, absent humerus in 5% to 10% of cases with digits arising from the shoulder, hypoplastic digits, hypoplastic or fused phalanges, carpal bone hypoplasia or fusion, hypoplastic or absent middle phalanx of the fifth digit; (b) shoulder anomalies: absent or hypoplastic glenoid fossa, acromium, scapula, or clavicle; lateral clavic-

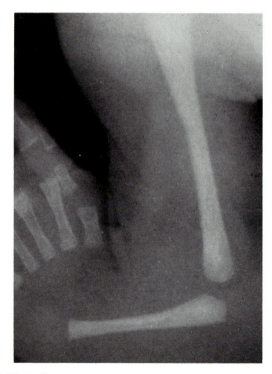

FIG SY–T–2.
TAR syndrome in a newborn female with deformed upper limbs, ecchymosis, rectal bleeding, and a very low platelet count. Bone marrow aspiration revealed almost no megakaryocytes. The radius is absent on the right side. A total absence of ossification of the radius and ulna was noted on the left side.

TABLE SY–T–1.

Comparison of TAR, Fanconi Anemia, Holt-Oram Syndrome, and SC Phocomelia/Roberts Syndrome*

Syndrome	Hematologic	Skeletal	Other	Genetic	Prognosis
TAR	Thrombocytopenia prominent Other cell lines normal Onset of thrombocytopenia usually in infancy	Bilateral absence of radii Thumbs always present Intercalary involvement Lower extremities involved less than the upper	Cardiac anomalies common	Normal chromosomes Possibly autosomal recessive (see the text)	Excellent if survival past the first year
Fanconi anemia	Thrombocytopenia may presage eventual aplastic anemia Onset of aplastic anemia rarely in the first year usually between the ages of 5–10 yr	Absent thumbs Terminal skeletal defects	Renal anomalies Hyperpigmentation	Abnormal breaks, gaps, and rearrangements Autosomal recessive	Poor without transplantation High risk of malignancy
Holt-Oram	Normal hematologically	Characteristic thumb defects Terminal upper extremity defects	Cardiac defects common	Normal chromosomes Autosomal dominant	Good, depending on cardiac anomaly
Roberts/SC phocomelia	Clinically significant thrombocytopenia not reported	Tetraphocomelia Cleft lip and palate Thumbs sometimes present	Numerous dysmorphic features Multiple malformations	Subtle centromeric puffing noted in some cases Autosomal recessive	Failure to thrive

*From Hedberg VA, Lipton JM: Thrombocytopenia with absent radii. A review of 100 cases. *Am. J. Pediatr. Hematol. Oncol.* 10:51, 1988. Used by permission.

ular hook; (c) lower-limb anomalies: hip dislocation, phocomelia, coxa valga, genu varum, subluxed knee, hypoplastic or absent patella, patellar dislocation, femoral and tibial torsion, abnormal tibiofibular joint, clubfoot, abnormal toe placement; (d) other reported abnormalities: minor vertebral anomaly, minor rib anomaly, hypoplasia of the mandible and maxilla, pancreatic cyst, uterine anomalies, Meckel diverticulum, unilateral absent kidney, esophageal anomalies, etc.

Differential Diagnosis: Fanconi anemia; Holt-Oram syndrome; Roberts/SC phocomelia.

Note: TAR is derived from Thrombocytopenia–Absent Radius syndrome (Fig SY–T–2; Table SY–T–1).

REFERENCES

Adeyokunnu AA: Radial aplasia and amegakaryocytic thrombocytopenia (TAR syndrome) among Nigerian children. *Am. J. Dis. Child.* 138:346, 1984.

Anyane-Yeboa K, et al.: Tetraphocomelia in the syndrome of thrombocytopenia with absent radii (TAR syndrome). *Am. J. Med. Genet.* 20:571, 1985.

Bernhard WG, et al.: Congenital leukemia. *Blood* 6:990, 1951.

Greenwald HM, et al.: Congenital essential thrombocytopenia. *Am. J. Dis. Child.* 38:1245, 1929.

Gross H, et al.: Kongenitale hypoplastische Thrombopenie mit Radiusaplasie: Ein Syndrom multipler Abartungen. *Neue Oesterr. Z. Kinderheilkd.* 1:574, 1956.

Hall JG: Thrombocytopenia and absent radius (TAR) syndrome. *J. Med. Genet.* 24:79, 1987.

Hall JG, et al.: Thrombocytopenia with absent radius. *Medicine (Baltimore)* 18:411, 1969.

Hedberg VA, et al.: Thrombocytopenia with absent radii. A review of 100 cases. *Am. J. Pediatr. Hematol. Oncol.* 10:51, 1988.

Le Marec B, et al.: Genetic counselling in a case of TAR syndrome where the father presented malformations of the feet. *Clin. Genet.* 34:104, 1988.

Schnur RE, et al.: Thrombocytopenia with absent radius in a boy and his uncle. *Am. J. Med. Genet.* 28:117, 1987.

Schoenecker PL, et al.: Dysplasia of the knee associated with the syndrome of thrombocytopenia and absent radius. *J. Bone Joint Surg. [Am.]* 66:421, 1984.

Teufel M, et al.: Consanguinity in a Turkish family with thrombocytopenia with absent radii (TAR) syndrome. *Hum. Genet.* 64:94, 1983.

Thévenieau D, et al.: Anomalies du membre supérieur, thrombopénie et thrombopathie. A propos de trois observations. *Arch. Fr. Pediatr.* 35:631, 1978.

TETHERED CORD SYNDROME

Synonyms: Tethered filum terminale; filum terminale syndrome; tethered conus syndrome.

Pathology: Low-placed conus as a single malformation or associated with a local neuroectodermal anomaly (lipoma, epidermoid or dermoid, cord duplication or cord dysgenesis, diastematomyelia, adhesions).

Clinical Manifestations: Initial symptoms often in childhood: (a) *weakness, painful or numb lower limbs, spastic gait, muscle atrophy, neurogenic bladder, bladder dysfunction* (flaccid bladder, uninhibited bladder, mixed bladder dysfunction), *scoliosis, foot deformities;* (b) *external evidence of spinal dysrhaphia:* hypertrichosis, dermoids, subcutaneous lipomas, sinus tracts.

Radiologic Manifestations: (a) *single or multiple vertebral bifid arches, wide interpediculate distances, kyphoscoliosis,* increased lumbar lordotic curve; (b) *wide dural sac, low filum terminale,* abnormal position and angle of the nerve roots, *cord splitting, tethering bands, tethering masses (dermoid, lipomatous tissue,* etc.).

Note: Primary tethered cord includes the anomalies referred to under Pathology and excludes anomalies associated with overt meningomyelocele and tethering of the cord secondary to myelomeningocele repair.

REFERENCES

Chaseling RW, et al.: Meningoceles and the tethered cord syndrome. *Child. Nerv. Syst.* 1:105, 1985.
Fitz CR, et al.: The tethered conus. *A.J.R.* 125:515, 1975.
Hellstrom WJG, et al.: Urological aspects of the tethered cord syndrome. *J. Urol.* 135:317, 1986.
Holtzman RNN, et al.: *The Tethered Spinal Cord.* New York, Thieme-Stratton Inc., 1985.
Pang D, et al.: Tethered cord syndrome in adults. *J. Neurosurg.* 57:32, 1982.
Raghavendra BN, et al.: The tethered spinal cord: Diagnosis by high-resolution real-time ultrasound. *Radiology* 149:123, 1983.
Sarwar M, et al.: Primary tethered cord syndrome: A new hypothesis of its origin. *A.J.N.R.* 5:235, 1984.
Simon RH, et al.: Tethered spinal cord in adult siblings. *Neurosurgery* 8:241, 1981.
Wortsman J, et al.: Spinal meningeal AVM supplied from the internal iliac artery associated with tethered cord syndrome in an adult: Case report. *J. Can. Assoc. Radiol.* 34:323, 1983.

THALIDOMIDE EMBRYOPATHY

Etiology: Maternal ingestion of thalidomide (α-phthalimidoglutarimide) early in pregnancy.

Clinical Manifestations: (a) *various limb anomalies;* (b) other reported malformations: broad nasal bridge, microphthalmos, ear deformities, teeth defects, cardiac anomalies, renal and intestinal malformations, cerebral defects, absent appendix, hypertrophic pyloric stenosis, etc.

Radiologic Manifestations: *Limb anomalies: preaxial reduction in size or number of skeletal elements:* amelia, proximal phocomelia, radial forearm anomalies, digits usually present, hip dislocation.

REFERENCES

Lenz W, et al.: Die Thalidomid-Embryopathie. *Dtsch. Med. Wochenschr.* 87:1232, 1962.
Lenz W: Das Thalidomid-Syndrom. *Fortschr. Med.* 81:148, 1963.
McBride WG: Thalidomide and congenital abnormalities. *Lancet* 2:1358, 1961.
Schäfer KH, et al: Infantile hypertrophic pyloric stenosis after prenatal exposure to thalidomide. *Eur. J. Pediatr.* 146:63, 1987.
Smithells RW: Thalidomide, absent appendix, and sweating. *Lancet* 1:1042, 1978.
Taussig HB: A study of German outbreak of phocomelia: The thalidomide syndrome. *J.A.M.A.* 180:1106, 1962.
Wiedemann H-R, et al.: Zur Frage der derzeitigen Haufung von Gliedmassen-Fehlbildungen. *Med. Monatsschr.* 12:816, 1961.

THE 3-M SYNDROME

Synonym: The Three M syndrome.

Mode of Inheritance: Autosomal recessive.

Frequency: Rare.

Clinical Manifestations: (a) *low birth weight, proportionate dwarfism;* (b) *frontal bossing,* hatched-shaped craniofacial configuration, *large head for height, triangular-shaped face, flattened malar region, prominent ears, short nose with upturned nares, prominent mouth or full lips, long philtrum, small pointed chin;* (c) other reported abnormalities: dysplastic/prominent ears, hyperlordosis, short fifth fingers, short and broad neck, prominent trapezius muscles, short thorax, pectus carinatum or excavatum, transverse grooves of the anterior portion of the chest wall, winged scapulae, abnormal teeth, hyperextensible joints, diastasis recti.

Radiologic Manifestations: (a) *slender tubular bones,* slender ribs; (b) short fifth digits, prominent heels, pes planus, decreased extension of the elbows, congenital hip dislocation, flaring iliac wings, shortened anteroposterior diameter of the lumbar vertebral bodies, irregularity of end plates, spina bifida occulta, small pelvis, short femoral necks; (c) osteoporotic appearance; (d) delayed bone age.

Note: M is the first letter of the last name of three of the authors of the original article (see the references) (Fig SY−T−3).

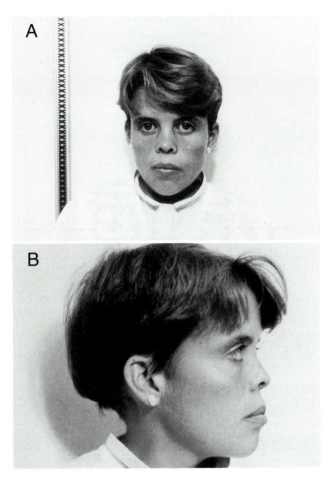

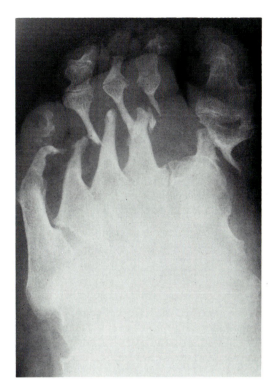

FIG SY–T–3.

The 3-M syndrome in a 29-year-old female. Note the frontal boss-ing, flattened malar regions, upturned nares, long philtrum, and full lips. (From Hennekam RCM, Bijlsma JB, Spranger J: Further de-lineation of the 3-M syndrome with review of the literature. *Am. J. Med. Genet.* 28:195, 1987. Used by permission.)

REFERENCES

Cantú J-M, et al.: 3-M slender-boned nanism. *Am. J. Dis. Child.* 135:905, 1981.

Hennekam RCM, et al.: Further delineation of the 3-M syn-drome with review of the literature. *Am. J. Med. Genet.* 28:195, 1987.

Miller JD, McKusick VA, Malvaux P, et al.: The 3-M syn-drome: A heritable low birthweight dwarfism. *Birth De-fects* 11:39, 1975.

Spranger J, et al.: A new familial intrauterine growth retarda-tion syndrome: The "3-M syndrome." *Eur. J. Pediatr.* 123:115, 1976.

Van Goethem H, et al.: The 3-M syndrome. *Helv. Paediat. Acta* 42:159, 1987.

THEVENARD SYNDROME

Synonym: Acrodystrophic neuropathy.

FIG SY–T–4.

Thevenard syndrome in a 36-year-old female with peripheral sen-sory impairment and painless perforating ulcers on the soles. Shown are extensive bone destruction of the metatarsopha-langeal and a loss of the metatarsal heads and base of the pha-langes. (From Banna M, Foster JB: Roentgenologic features of acrodystrophic neuropathy. *A.J.R.* 115:186, 1972. Used by permis-sion.)

Mode of Inheritance: Autosomal dominant; sporadic cases are common.

Clinical Manifestations: Onset of symptoms often at pu-berty: (a) *peripheral sensory impairment*; (b) *trophic changes and ulcer with the sole of the foot as the primary site*; (c) ele-*phant foot*; (d) vasomotor disturbance; (e) hypertrichosis.

Radiologic Manifestations: Lesions often limited to the lower extremities: (a) *acro-osteolysis*; (b) *destruction of meta-tarsophalangeal joints*; (c) Charcot arthropathy of the lower limbs with effusion; (d) hemarthrosis; (e) osteoporosis; (f) pathological fractures; (g) dislocation (Fig SY–T–4).

REFERENCES

Banna M, Foster JB: Roentgenologic features of acrodystro-phic neuropathy. *A.J.R.* 115:186, 1972.

Thevenard A: L'acropathie ulcéro-mutilante familiale. *Rev. Neurol.* 74:193, 1942.

THICKENED CORTICAL BONES AND CONGENITAL NEUTROPENIA

Mode of Inheritance: Three sisters have been reported with this combination.

Frequency: Single report (Boechat et al.).

Clinical and Radiologic Manifestations: (a) congenital neutropenia; (b) recurrent infections; (c) thickening of the ribs and cortical thickening of the tubular bones.

Differential Diagnosis: Shwachman syndrome, cartilage-hair hypoplasia, Fanconi pancytopenia, Chédiak-Higashi syndrome (Fig SY–T–5).

REFERENCE

Boechat MI, et al.: Thickened cortical bones in congenital neutropenia. *Pediatr. Radiol.* 17:124, 1987.

THIEMANN DISEASE

Synonym: Familial osteoarthropathy of the fingers.

Mode of Inheritance: Autosomal dominant.

Clinical Manifestations: Onset of symptoms usually before 25 years of age: (a) swelling of the interphalangeal joints of the fingers; (b) normal laboratory test results.

Radiologic Manifestations: (a) abnormalities of the epiphyses of the middle and proximal phalanges: flattening, fragmentation, increased radiographic opacity (dense epiphysis, ivory epiphysis), broadening; (b) late changes: osteoarthritis, sometimes simulating Heberden and Bouchard nodes.

REFERENCES

Allison AC, et al.: Familial osteoarthropathy of the fingers. *J. Bone Joint Surg. [Br.]* 40:538, 1958.
Giedion A: Acrodysplasias: Peripheral dysostosis, acrodysostosis and Thiemann's disease. *Clin. Orthop.* 114:107, 1976.
Thiemann H: Juvenile epiphysenstörungen. *Fortschr. Rontgenstr.* 14:79, 1909.
Trippel JG: Eine Sippe mit Thiemannscher Erkrankung. *Helv. Med. Acta* 17:59, 1950.
van der Laan JG, et al.: Ivory and dense epiphyses of the hand: Thiemann disease in three sisters. *Skeletal Radiol.* 15:117, 1986.

THORACIC OUTLET SYNDROME

Synonym: Neurovascular compression syndrome.

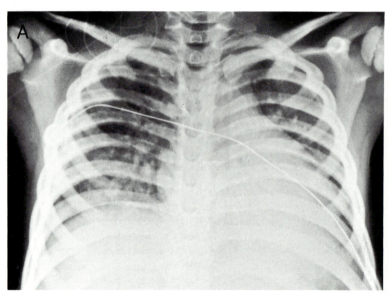
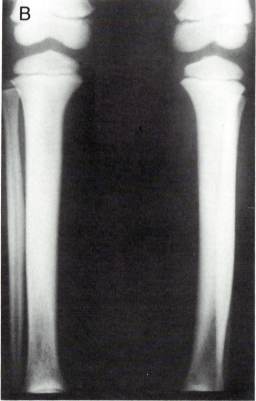

FIG SY–T–5.
Thickened cortical bones in congenital neutropenia. **A,** a chest radiograph shows thickening of the ribs. **B,** cortical thickening involving diaphysis of both tibias and fibulas. (From Boechat MI, Gormley LS, O'Laughlin BJ: Thickened cortical bones in congenital neutropenia. *Pediatr. Radiol.* 17:124, 1987. Used by permission.)

Etiology: Congenital fibrous or muscular band anomalies; hypertrophy of the pectoralis minor or scalenus anticus muscles; cervical rib; anomalies of the first thoracic rib; costoclavicular compression; hyperabduction compression; anomalous clavicle; fracture of the clavicle; retrosternal dislocation of the clavicle; subacromial dislocation of the humeral head; enlargement of the transverse process of C_7; clavicular deformities (tumor, callus); spinal curvature in association with rib abnormalities; poor posture resulting in narrowing of the space between the first rib and clavicle; soft-tissue injuries; the syndrome of sternocostoclavicular hyperostosis; "the droopy shoulder syndrome."

Clinical Manifestations: (a) *pain* (chest wall, shoulder, arm, hand); (b) *numbness*; tetany of the hand; (c) *skin color changes*; (d) *claudications*; (e) *bruit* in the supraclavicular or infraclavicular fossae, diminished pulse and lower blood pressure on the affected side; (f) *wasting* of hand muscles, weakness and wasting in the forearm; (g) functional abnormalities shown by sensory and motor conduction studies, quantitative electromyography, and somatosensory evoked potentials.

Radiologic Manifestations: (a) arteriographic demonstration of the site and severity of *arterial obstruction (usually the second portion of the subclavian artery), venous obstruction* (in some); (b) radioisotope demonstration of flow reduction; (c) abnormal arterial flow detectable by using Doppler technique (decreased or discontinuation of flow during postural tests); (d) osteoporosis of the phalanges (in patients with emboli); (e) *bone abnormalities:* abnormal cervical transverse process, rudimentary rib, abnormalities of the first thoracic

vertebra and corresponding ribs, clavicular deformities, previous thoracoplasty.

Differential Diagnosis: Angina pectoris (Fig SY–T–6).

REFERENCES

Capistrant TD: Thoracic outlet syndrome in whiplash injury. *Ann. Surg.* 185:175, 1977.

Desoutter P, et al.: Syndrome vasculaire de la traversée thoracobrachiale par cal fracturaire hypertrophique de la clavicule. *J. Radiol.* 62:401, 1981.

Fields WS, et al.: Thoracic outlet syndrome: Review and reference to stroke in a major league pitcher. *A.J.R.* 146:809, 1986.

Gangabar DM, et al.: Retrosternal dislocation of the clavicle producing thoracic outlet syndrome. *J. Trauma* 18:369, 1978.

Godfrey NF, et al.: Thoracic outlet syndrome mimicking angina pectoris with elevated creatine phosphokinase values. *Chest* 83:461, 1983.

Huffman JD: Electrodiagnostic techniques for and conservative treatment of thoracic outlet syndrome. *Clin. Orthop.* 207:21, 1986.

Jerrett SA, et al.: Thoracic outlet syndrome. Electrophysiologic reappraisal. *Arch. Neurol.* 41:960, 1984.

Jirik FR, et al.: Clavicular hyperostosis with enthesopathy, hypergammaglobulinemia, and thoracic outlet syndrome. *Ann. Intern. Med.* 97:48, 1982.

Lagerquist LG, et al.: Thoracic outlet syndrome with tetany of the hands. *Am. J. Med.* 59:281, 1975.

Roos DB: Congenital anomalies associated with thoracic outlet syndrome: Anatomy, symptoms, diagnosis, and treatment. *Am. J. Surg.* 132:771, 1976.

Roos DB: Thoracic outlet syndromes: Update 1987. *Am. J. Surg.* 154:568, 1987.

Smith T, et al.: Diagnosis of thoracic outlet syndrome. Value of sensory and motor conduction studies and quantitative electromyography. *Arch. Neurol.* 44:1161, 1987.

Swift TR, et al.: The droopy shoulder syndrome. *Neurology* 34:212, 1984.

Tomsick TA, et al.: Thoracic outlet syndrome associated with rib fusion and cervicothoracic scoliosis. *J. Can. Assoc. Radiol.* 25:211, 1974.

Vin F, et al.: Syndrome de la traversée thoraco-brachiale. Valeur des explorations artérielles non vulnérantes. *Presse Med.* 15:1709, 1986.

Walker OM, et al.: Coexistent ipsilateral subclavian steal and thoracic outlet compression syndromes. *J. Thorac. Cardiovasc. Surg.* 69:874, 1974.

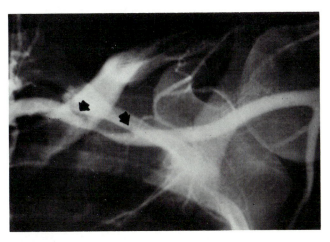

FIG SY–T–6.
Thoracic outlet syndrome in a 20-year-old male with numbness and tingling of both upper extremities. Note the ridgelike compression of the subclavian artery resulting from effacement of the vessel against the first rib and reflecting the inherent tightness of the costoclavicular space. (From Lang EK: Arteriographic diagnosis of thoracic outlet syndromes. *Med. Times* 97:195, 1969. Used by permission.)

THORACIC-PELVIC DYSOSTOSIS

Mode of Inheritance: Reported in a mother and her son.

Clinical and Radiologic Manifestations: (a) small chest and protuberant abdomen in the infant, mild respiratory distress in the postnatal period; (b) shortness of ribs; (c) small ilium, pelvic inlet, and sciatic notches.

REFERENCE

Bankier A, et al.: Thoracic-pelvic dysostosis: A 'new' autosomal dominant form. *J. Med. Genet.* 20:276, 1983.

TIBIAL HEMIMELIA

Classification: (a) autosomal dominant: (1) tibial hemimelia-foot polydactyly-triphalangeal thumbs syndrome (Werner syndrome); (2) tibial hemimelia diplopodia syndrome; (3) tibial hemimelia–split hand/foot syndrome; (4) tibial hemimelia-micromelia-trigonobrachycephaly syndrome; (5) others; (b) autosomal recessive suggested in some cases.

REFERENCES

Emami-Ahiri Z, et al.: Bilateral absence of the tibia in three sibs. *Birth Defects* 10(5):197, 1974.
Richieri-Costa A: Tibial hemimelia–cleft lip/palate in a Brazilian child born to consanguineous parents. *Am. J. Med. Genet.* 28:325, 1987.
Richieri-Costa A, et al.: Tibial hemimelia: Report on 37 new cases, clinical and genetic considerations. *Am. J. Med. Genet.* 27:867, 1987.

TIETZE SYNDROME

Synonyms: Costosternal syndrome; parasternal chondrodynia; costochondritis.

Clinical Manifestations: (a) subacute or acute onset of *painful nonsuppurative tumefaction* at the costal cartilage; (b)

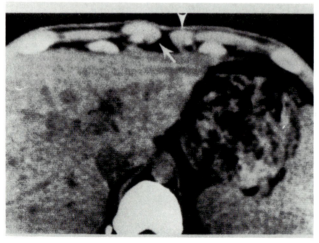

FIG SY–T–7.
Tietze syndrome in a 19-year-old male patient with painful tender swelling of the right seventh costochondral junction for 1 month. Bulbous enlargement *(arrow)* of the right seventh costal cartilage as compared with the opposite normal cartilage *(arrowhead)* is evident. (From Edelstein G, Levitt RG, Slaker DP: Computed tomography of Tietz syndrome. *J. Comput. Assist. Tomogr.* 8:20, 1984. Used by permission.)

self-limiting and of unknown etiology; (c) commonly involves the second right or left costal cartilages.

Radiologic Manifestations: (a) *soft-tissue swelling* in the tangential view; (b) computed tomography: enlargement of the costal cartilage, ventral angulation of the involved costal cartilage, calcification within the cartilaginous mass, compression of the pectoralis muscle anteriorly and the pleura and lung parenchyma posteriorly (Fig SY–T–7).

REFERENCES

Edelstein G, et al.: Computed tomography of Tietze syndrome. *J. Comput. Assist. Tomogr.* 8:20, 1984.
Hamburg C, et al.: Reliability of computed tomography in the initial diagnosis and follow-up. Evaluation of Tietze's syndrome: Case report with review of the literature. *Comput. Tomogr.* 11:83, 1987.
Jurik AG, et al.: Radiographic findings in patients with clinical Tietze syndrome. *Skeletal Radiol.* 16:517, 1987.
Kessel I, et al.: Tietze's syndrome in childhood. *Acta Paediatr. Scand.* 56:557, 1967.
Szántó VD: Verbreiterung des retrosternalen Weichteilschattens beim Tietze-Syndrom. *Fortschr. Rontgenstr.* 139:456, 1983.
Tietze A: Ueber eine eigenartige Häufung von Fällen mit Dystrophie der Rippenknorpel. *Berl. Klin. Wochenschr.* 58:829, 1921.
Wiedemann H-R: Tietze-Syndrom (Chondroosteopathia costalis tuberosa) im frühen Kindesalter. *Helv. Paediatr. Acta* 27:25, 1972.

TOLOSA-HUNT SYNDROME

Synonyms: Painful ophthalmoplegia; superior orbital fissuritis.

Clinical Manifestations: (a) *recurrent or steady retro-orbital pain of various intensity and duration, spontaneous remissions;* (b) *ophthalmoplegia;* third, fourth, and sixth nerves; first division of the fifth cranial nerve; periarterial sympathetic fibers; and the optic nerve; (c) *nonspecific inflammation (granulomatous) in the cavernous sinus or superior orbital fissure or at both sites;* (d) pain is steroid responsive.

Radiologic Manifestations: (a) *orbital venography: occlusion of the superior ophthalmic vein, collateral venous flow, poor opacification or obliteration of the cavernous sinus;* (b) carotid arteriography: narrowing of the cavernous segment of the internal carotid artery, arterial stationary wave phenomenon; (c) computed tomography: cavernous sinus inflammation.

Differential Diagnosis: Orbital apex pseudotumor (suggested to be considered part of the spectrum of the Tolosa-Hunt syndrome); tumors presenting with manifestations of cavernous sinus syndrome; aneurysm (Fig SY–T–8).

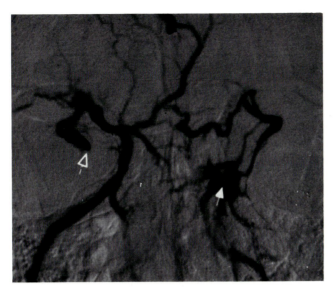

FIG SY–T–8.
Tolosa-Hunt syndrome: transfrontal orbital venogram in a 43-year-old man with symptoms of pain behind the right eye; diplopia and drooping of the right upper lid show a complete occlusion of the right superior ophthalmic vein *(open arrow)*. The carotid artery *(closed arrow)* is identified as a filling defect in the normal left cavernous sinus. There is no filling of the right cavernous sinus. (From Sondheimer FK, Knapp J: Angiographic finding in the Tolosa-Hunt syndrome: Painful ophthalmoplegia. *Radiology* 106:105, 1973. Used by permission.)

REFERENCES

Campbell RJ, et al.: Painful ophthalmoplegia (Tolosa-Hunt variant): Autopsy findings in a patient with necrotizing intracavernous carotid vasculitis and inflammatory disease of the orbit. *Mayo Clin. Proc.* 62:520, 1987.
Coppeto JR, et al.: Tolosa-Hunt syndrome with proptosis mimicked by giant aneurysm of posterior cerebral artery. *Arch. Neurol.* 38:54, 1981.
Hannerz J, et al.: Orbital phlebography in patients with Tolosa-Hunt's syndrome in comparison with normal subjects. *Acta Radiol.* 25:457, 1984.
Hunt WE: Tolosa-Hunt syndrome: One cause of painful ophthalmoplegia. *J. Neurosurg.* 44:544, 1976.
Hunt WE, et al.: Painful ophthalmoplegia: Its relation to indolent inflammation of the cavernous sinus. *Neurology* 11:56, 1961.
Kwan ESK, et al.: Tolosa-Hunt syndrome revisited: Not necessarily a diagnosis of exclusion. *A.J.R.* 150:413, 1988.
Rapin F, et al.: Ophtalmoplégie douloureuse de Tolosa-Hunt. *Arch. Fr. Pediatr.* 44:299, 1987.
Sondheimer FK, Knapp J: Angiographic finding in the Tolosa-Hunt syndrome: Painful ophthalmoplegia. *Radiology* 106:105, 1973.
Spector RH, et al.: The "sinister" Tolosa-Hunt syndrome. *Neurology* 36:198, 1986.
Tolosa E: Periarteritic lesion of carotid siphon with clinical features of carotid infraclinoidal aneurysm. *J. Neurol. Neurosurg. Psychiatry* 17:300, 1954.

TORRE SYNDROME

Synonym: Muir-Torre syndrome.

Clinical and Radiologic Manifestations: (a) multiple sebaceous adenomas of the skin; (b) internal carcinoma: endometrial, gastrointestinal.

REFERENCES

Banse-Kupin L, et al: Torre's syndrome: Report of two cases and review of the literature. *J. Am. Acad. Dermatol.* 10:803, 1984.
Bitran J, et al.: Multiple sebaceous gland tumors and internal carcinoma: Torre's syndrome. *Cancer* 33:835, 1974.
Grignon DJ, et al.: Transitional cell carcinoma in the Muir-Torre syndrome. *J. Urol.* 138:406, 1987.
Torre D: Multiple sebaceous gland tumors. *Arch. Dermatol.* 98:549, 1968.

TOWNES-BROCKS SYNDROME

Synonym: Anus-hand-ear syndrome.

Mode of Inheritance: Autosomal dominant; intrafamilial variability.

Frequency: 40 cases in seven families (De Vries–Van Der Weerd, et al.).

Clinical and Radiologic Manifestations: (a) *imperforate anus*; (b) *triphalangeal thumbs*; (c) *lop ears*; (d) *sensorineural deafness*; (e) other reported abnormalities: pes planus, supernumerary thumb, clinodactyly of the fifth toes, fusion of the metatarsals, supernumerary thumbs, hypoplastic thumb, congenital heart disease, etc.

REFERENCES

Alysworth AS: The Townes-Brocks syndrome: A member of the anus-hand-ear family of syndromes (abstract). *Am. J. Hum. Genet.* 37:43, 1985.
De Vries–Van Der Weerd M-ACS, et al.: A new family with Townes-Brocks syndrome. *Clin. Genet.* 34:195, 1988.
Monteiro de Pina-Neto J: Phenotypic variability in Townes-Brocks syndrome. *Am. J. Med. Genet.* 18:147, 1984.
Reid IS, Turner G: Familial anal abnormality. *J. Pediatr.* 88:992, 1976.
Townes PL, Brocks ER: Hereditary syndrome of imperforate anus and hand, foot and ear anomalies. *J. Pediatr.* 81:321, 1972.

TOXIC SHOCK SYNDROME

Etiology: Association with infection by *Staphylococcus aureus* and some other organisms: vaginal tampons, sinusitis, postoperative, nasal packing, ureterolithotomy, bacterial croup, etc.

Clinical Manifestations: (a) intense myalgia; (b) high fever; (c) skin rash and desquamation; (d) vomiting and diarrhea; (e) abnormal renal and liver function test findings; sterile pyuria; immature granulocytic leukocytosis; low platelet count; coagulation abnormalities; hypocalcemia; low serum albumin and total protein concentrations; elevation of blood urea nitrogen, alanine transaminase, bilirubin, and creatine kinase levels; (f) hypotension, syncope; (g) disorientation, alteration in consciousness without focal neurological signs when fever or hypotension are absent.

Radiologic Manifestations: (a) ultrasonography of the liver: increased brightness of portal vein wall echoes, diminished echogenicity of the liver parenchyma; (b) adult respiratory distress syndrome, pulmonary edema, cardiac failure.

REFERENCES

Barbour SD, et al.: Toxic-shock syndrome associated with nasal packing: Analogy to tampon-associated illness. *Pediatrics* 73:163, 1984.
Chenaud M, et al.: Bacterial croup and toxic shock syndrome. *Eur. J. Pediatr.* 145:306, 1986.
Dunn SR, et al.: Toxic shock syndrome following ureterolithotomy. *J. Urol.* 128:1305, 1982.
Griffith JA, et al.: Toxic shock syndrome and sinusitis—A hidden site of infection. *West J. Med.* 148:580, 1988.
Gysler M: Toxic shock syndrome—A synopsis. *Pediatr. Clin. North Am.* 28:431, 1981.
Lieberman JM, et al.: Toxic shock syndrome: Sonographic appearance of the liver. *A.J.R.* 137:606, 1981.
Morrison VA, et al.: Postoperative toxic shock syndrome. *Arch. Surg.* 118:791, 1983.
Tofte RW, et al.: Clinical and laboratory manifestations of toxic shock syndrome. *Ann. Intern. Med.* 96:843, 1982.
Wiesenthal AM, et al.: Toxic shock syndrome in children aged 10 years or less. *Pediatrics* 74:112, 1984.

TREACHER COLLINS SYNDROME

Synonyms: Mandibulofacial dysostosis; Franceschetti-Klein syndrome; Franceschetti-Zwahlen-Klein syndrome; Berry–Treacher Collins syndrome; first-arch syndrome; Treacher Collins–Franceschetti syndrome.

Mode of Inheritance: Autosomal dominant.

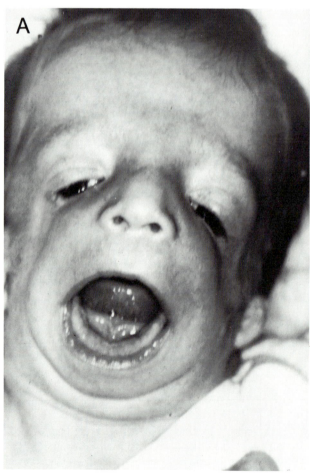

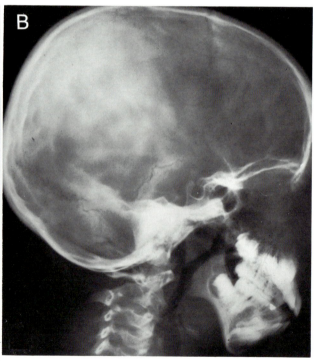

FIG SY–T–9.
Treacher Collins syndrome. **A,** typical facial features. **B,** Lateral film of the skull. Note the characteristic bowing of the lower border of the mandible. This peculiar downward curve of the horizontal portion of the ramus of the mandible is pathognomonic of this syndrome. Note the hypoplastic acellular mastoids with absent external auditory canals. Note the constriction of the air-outlined pharynx, particularly at the level of the oropharynx.

(From Mafee MF, Shild JA, Kumar A, et al.: Radiographic features of the ear-related developmental anomalies in patients with mandibulofacial dysostosis. *Int. J. Pediatr. Otorhinolaryngol.* 7:229, 1984. Used by permission.)

Frequency: Uncommon.

Clinical Manifestations: (a) *hypoplasia of the face with sunken cheek bones, malformed ear* (hypoplastic auricle and stenosis or atresia of the external meatus), macrostomia, high-arched palate, blind fistulas between the auricle and the corner of the mouth, extra rudimentary ear tags, obliteration of the nasal frontal angle; (b) *antimongoloid slant of the palpebral fissure; coloboma in the outer portion of the lower lid* and, in some cases, the upper lid; partial or total absence of the lower eyelashes; (c) conductive deafness; (d) dental anomalies, malocclusion of the teeth; (e) projection of scalp hair onto the lateral aspect of the cheek; (f) other reported abnormalities: microphthalmos, choanal atresia, absence of the parotid gland, congenital heart disease, malformation of limbs, cryptorchidism, mental retardation, trisomy 11q ter by t(11;22) translocation.

Radiologic Manifestations: (a) *hypoplasia of the malar bones,* agenesis of the malar bones, obtuse angle of the mandible, concave curvature of the horizontal ramus of the mandible, malocclusion, absence of palatine bones, cleft palate, *hypogenesis or agenesis of the mandible;* (b) *underdeveloped paranasal sinuses and mastoids,* absence of ossicles of the middle ear, deficient cochlea and vestibular apparatus; (c) hypoplasia or absence of the external auditory canal; hypoplasia or absence of the tympanic cavity; closed middle-ear cavity by a thick osseous atretic plate; absence or dysplastic and rudimentary ossicles; presence of a single large conglomerate incudomalleal mass attached to the atretic

plate, epitympanum, or both; hypoplasia or absence of the mastoid; inner-ear abnormalities rare (deficient cochlea and vestibular apparatus); closed oval window; abnormal course of the facial nerve canal; (d) vertebral anomalies (in some); (e) pharyngeal hypoplasia, narrowing of the anteroposterior diameter of the pharynx; (f) midtrimester sonographic diagnosis (micrognathia and microtia) (Fig SY–T–9 and SY–T–10).

REFERENCES

Berry GA: Note on congenital defect (coloboma) of lower lid, Report 12, pt 3. *Royal London Ophthalmologic Hospital.* January 1889, pp. 225–357.

Chabrolle JP, et al.: Un syndrome de dysostose mandibulo-faciale associé a une anomalie chromosomique. *Ann. Pediatr. (Paris)* 34:641, 1987.

Crane JP, et al.: Midtrimester sonographic diagnosis of mandibulofacial dysostosis. *Am. J. Med. Genet.* 25:251, 1986.

Franceschetti A: Un syndrome nouveau: La dysostose mandibulo-faciale. *Bull. Schweiz. Akad. Med. Wiss.* 1:60, 1944.

Franceschetti A, Klein D: The mandibulo-facial dysostosis: A new hereditary syndrome. *Acta Ophthalmol. (Copenh.)* 27:143, 1949.

Lowry RB, et al.: Mandibulofacial dysostosis in Hutterite sibs: A possible recessive trait. *Am. J. Med. Genet.* 22:501, 1985.

Mafee MF, et al.: Radiographic features of the ear-related developmental anomalies in patients with mandibulofacial dysostosis. *Int. J. Pediatr. Otorhinolaryngol.* 7:229, 1984.

Shprintzen RJ, et al.: Pharyngeal hypoplasia in Treacher Collins syndrome. *Arch. Otolaryngol.* 105:127, 1979.

Sulik KK, et al.: Mandibulofacial dysostosis (Treacher Collins Syndrome): A new proposal for its pathogenesis. *Am. J. Med. Genet.* 27:359, 1987.

Treacher Collins E: Case with symmetrical congenital notches in the outer part of each lower lid and defective development of malar bones. *Trans. Ophthalmol. Soc. U.K.* 20:190, 1900.

TRICHO-DENTO-OSSEOUS SYNDROME

Mode of Inheritance: Autosomal dominant.

Frequency: Rare.

Clinical Manifestations: (a) dark, *very curly scalp hair* that straightens by the second decade of life; (b) pitted dysplastic enamel, discoloration, eruption defects, etc.; (c) *nail defects:* thinness of the nails, splitting of superficial layers of the nails.

Radiologic Manifestations: (a) *sclerosis of the base of the skull and mastoids,* short mandibular rami, obtuse mandibular angle; (b) *mild to moderate hyperostosis of the cortex of the tubular bones, sclerosis of the provisional zone of calcification;* (c) *dental defects:* hypoplasia of the enamel, delayed formation and eruption of teeth, early loss of teeth, discol-

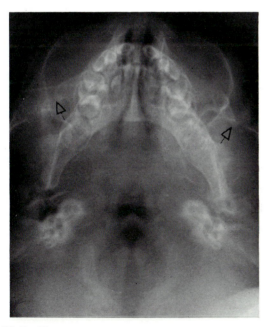

FIG SY–T–10.
Treacher Collins syndrome in a newborn female infant with the typical facial appearance of the syndrome and micrognathia. Hypoplasia of the malar bones is shown in this basilar view of the skull *(arrows).* (Courtesy of The Children's Hospital of San Francisco.)

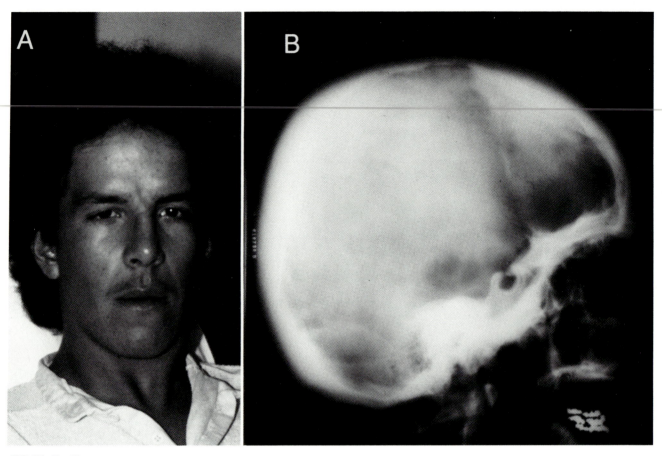

FIG SY—T—11.
Tricho-dento-osseous syndrome. **A,** fuzzy hair. **B,** increased density at the base of the skull. (From Quattromani F, Shapiro SD, Young RS, et al.: Clinical heterogeneity in the tricho-dento-osseous syndrome. *Hum. Genet.* 64:116, 1983. Used by permission.)

ored teeth, hypocalcification, enlarged pulp chambers, taurodontism of the molars, dental abscess.

Note: Variant of the syndrome (Quattromani et al.): hair and teeth morphology similar to that described above in association with skeletal dysplasia consisting of sclerosis and thickening of the calvarium with long bones that show subtle undertubulation but no sclerosis (Fig SY—T—11).

REFERENCES

Crawford JL: Concomitant taurodontism and amelogenesis imperfecta in the American Caucasian. *J. Dent. Child.* 37:171, 1970.

Leisti J, et al.: A new type of autosomal dominant trich-dento-osseous syndrome (abstract). *Birth Defects* 11:58, 1978.

Lichtenstein J, et al.: The tricho-dento-osseous (TDO) syndrome. *Am. J. Hum. Genet.* 24:569, 1972.

Quattromani F, et al.: Clinical heterogeneity in the tricho-dento-osseous syndrome. *Hum. Genet.* 64:116, 1983.

Robinson GC, et al.: Hereditary enamel hypoplasia: Its association with characteristic hair structure. *Pediatrics* 37:498, 1966.

Shapiro SD, et al.: Tricho-dento-osseous syndrome: Heterogeneity or clinical variability. *Am. J. Med. Genet.* 16:225, 1983.

TRICHO-ODONTO-ONYCHIAL DYSPLASIA

Mode of Inheritance: Probably autosomal recessive.

Frequency: Four siblings.

Clinical and Radiologic Manifestations: (a) severe hypotrichosis, dystrophic nails; (b) hypoplasia of the enamel leading to secondary adontia; (c) bone deficiency of the frontoparietal region; (d) other anomalies: supernumerary nipples, nevus pigmentosus, etc.

REFERENCE

Pinheiro M, et al.: Trichodontoonychial dysplasia—A new mesoectodermal dysplasia. *Am. J. Med. Genet.* 15:67, 1983.

TRICHORRHEXIS NODOSA SYNDROME

Synonyms: Pollitt syndrome; trichothiodystrophy—neurocutaneous syndrome; trichothiodystrophy syndrome of Pollitt.

Mode of Inheritance: Autosomal recessive has been suggested.

Frequency: 51 cases (Chapman), 25 of 51 from one Amish community in northern Indiana.

Clinical Manifestations: (a) *low birth weight, mental and physical retardation;* (b) *brittle hair, sulfur deficient (cystine deficient), nail dysplasia;* (c) other reported abnormalities: ichthyosis, collodeon membrane, cryptorchidism, decreased fertility, cataracts (small and punctate), photosensitivity, frequent infections (pneumonia, otitis, mastoiditis, sinusitis, pyelonephritis), etc.

Radiologic Manifestations: (a) axial osteosclerosis; (b) peripheral osteopenia; (c) retarded skeletal maturation; (d) kyphosis.

REFERENCES

Chapman S: The trichothiodystrophy syndrome of Pollitt. *Pediatr. Radiol.* 18:154, 1988.
Jackson CE, et al.: Brittle hair with short stature, intellectual impairment and decreased fertility: An autosomal recessive syndrome in an Amish kindred. *Pediatrics* 54:201, 1974.
Pollitt RJ, et al.: Sibs with mental and physical retardation and trichorrhexis nodosa with abnormal amino acid composition of the hair. *Arch. Dis. Child.* 43:211, 1968.

TRIGONOCEPHALY, FAMILIAL

Mode of Inheritance: Autosomal dominant.

Clinical and Radiologic Manifestations: (a) trigonocephaly, premature fusion of the metopic suture; (b) other abnormalities: mild synophrys, hypotelorism, unilateral preauricular ear tag, omphalocele, hemivertebra, minor malformations of the fingers and toes; (c) normal intelligence.

Differential Diagnosis: Opitz trigony syndrome (C syndrome); chromosomal aberration syndromes; holoprosencephaly; familial trigonocephaly-short stature-developmental delay (Say-Meyer); sporadic trigonocephaly.

REFERENCES

Frydman M, et al.: Trigonocephaly: A new familial syndrome. *Am. J. Med. Genet.* 18:55, 1984.
Hunter AGW, et al.: Trigonocephaly and associated minor anomalies in mother and son. *J. Med. Genet.* 13:77, 1976.
Say B, Meyer J: Familial trigonocephaly associated with short stature and developmental delay. *Am. J. Dis. Child.* 135:711, 1981.

TRIPLOIDY

Frequency: 1% of all conceptions; live birth in only 1 in every 10,000 of these pregnancies (Jacobs et al.).

Clinical and Radiologic Manifestations:
(A) PRENATAL: (a) fetal growth retardation; (b) body asymmetry (relatively large head), hydrocephalus; (c) oligohydramnios; (d) abnormally large and/or hydropic placenta; (e) genetic amniocentesis: 69 chromosomes.
(B) POSTNATAL: (a) low birth weight; (b) hypotonia; (c) facial asymmetry, cleft lip/palate, low-set ears, colobomas, microphthalmos, hypertelorism; (d) syndactyly, clubfoot, simian creases, etc.; (e) multiple congenital anomalies involving every organ system: central nervous system (hydrocephalus, absent corpus callosum, meningomyelocele, holoprosencephaly, Arnold-Chiari malformation, etc.), congenital heart defects, genitourinary anomalies, etc.

REFERENCES

Benacerraf, BR: Intrauterine growth retardation in the first trimester associated with triploidy. *J. Ultrasound Med.* 7:153, 1988.
Bendon RW, et al.: Prenatal detection of triploidy. *J. Pediatr.* 112:149, 1988.
Crane JP, et al.: Antenatal ultrasound findings in fetal triploidy syndrome. *J. Ultrasound Med.* 4:519, 1985.
Edwards MT, et al.: Prenatal sonographic diagnosis of triploidy. *J. Ultrasound Med.* 5:279, 1986.
Jacobs PA, et al.: Human triploidy: Relationship between parental origin of the additional complement and development of partial hydatidiform mole. *Ann. Hum. Genet.* 46:223, 1982.
Rubinstein JB, et al.: Placental changes in fetal triploidy syndrome. *J. Ultrasound Med.* 5:545, 1986.

TROELL-JUNET SYNDROME

Clinical and Radiologic Manifestations: Predilection for women: (a) *acromegaly;* (b) *toxic goiter* (usually nodular); (c) *diabetes mellitus;* (d) *hyperostosis of the vault of the skull.*

REFERENCES

Junet R: Une forme rare d'hyperthyréose: L'hyperostose de la voûte crânienne des acromégaliques hyperthyroïdiens (syndrome de Troell-Junet). *Helv. Med. Acta* 22:167, 1955.
Junet RM: *Histopathologie du Squelette Acromegalique et Ses Modifications Sous L'influence de L'hyperthyroidisme* (thesis 1681). Geneva, 1938.
Moore S: The Troell-Junet syndrome. *Acta Radiol.* 39:485, 1953.
Troell A: "Syndroma morgagni" hos patienter med samtidig akromegali och tyreotoxikos. *Sven. Lak.* 35:763, 1938.

TROUSSEAU SYNDROME

Clinical and Radiological Manifestations: (a) recurrent migratory thrombophlebitis and arterial thrombosis; (b) neoplastic disease.

REFERENCES

Bell WR, et al.: Trousseau's syndrome. Devastating coagulopathy in the absence of heparin. *Am. J. Med.* 79:423, 1985.
Dey HM, et al.: Radiogallium hot spleen in Trousseau's syndrome with splenic vein occlusion. *Clin. Nucl. Med.* 9:640, 1986.
Trousseau A: *Phlegmasia Alba Dolens. Clinique Medicale de Hotel-Dieu de Paris.* London, New Sydenham Society, 1868, vol. 3, p. 695.

TUBEROUS SCLEROSIS

Synonym: Bourneville-Pringle syndrome.

Mode of Inheritance: Autosomal dominant with variable expressivity and pleiotropism; fresh mutation; evidence presented in support of an assignment of the gene for tuberous sclerosis to the distal portion of the long arm of chromosome 9.

Frequency: Between 1:10,000 and 1:150,000 births (Martin et al.).

Clinical Manifestations: (a) skin lesions: *fibrous-angiomatous lesions* (adenoma sebaceum), "shagreen patches,"

café au lait spots, forehead plaque, ash leaf—shaped depigmented macules, leathery skin in the lower part of the trunk, subungual fibroma; (b) *neurological manifestations:* seizures, spasms in infancy, mental deficiency, developmental deficiency, increased intracranial pressure, psychiatric disorder; (c) *cardiovascular abnormalities:* hypertension, aneurysms, cardiac rhabdomyoma, Wolff-Parkinson-White, extra systoles, conduction blocks, tachycardias, sinus bradycardia, renal vascular hypertension, etc; (d) *renal manifestations:* renal enlargement (cysts, hamartoma, carcinoma), renal failure, renal and perirenal hemorrhage (may cause death), hematuria; (e) *respiratory system:* cor pulmonale, pneumothorax, chylothorax; (f) *retinal phakoma;* (g) other reported associated abnormalities: hydrops fetalis, gynecomastia, sexual precocity, tumors (hamartoma, renal cell carcinoma, benign teratoma, lymphangioma, eosinophilic adenoma and acromegalic gigantism, sacrococcygeal chordoma), acanthosis nigricans, hepatic angiomyolipoma and a para-aortic lymph node containing foci of angiomyolipoma (associated with renal angiomyolipoma), pitted enamel hypoplasia, isosexual precocity, hypothalamic endocrine disorders, etc.

Radiologic Manifestations: (a) central nervous system: (1) computed tomography (CT): calcification, subependymal nodules, parenchymal hamartomas (cortical tubers) with less attenuation than in the surrounding brain tissue, hypendense lesions (rare), tubers not usually enhanced by contrast material; (2) magnetic resonance imaging (MRI): subependymal nodules of intermediate signal intensity; parenchymal hamartomas with long T_1 and T_2 relaxation characteristics; MRI superior to CT, particularly for cortical tubers, cystic lesions

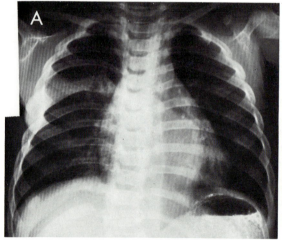
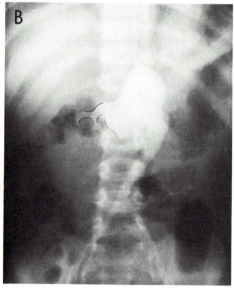

FIG SY—T—12.
Tuberous sclerosis in a child 6 months of age. Chest radiography shows large sclerotic right 5th, 10th, and 11th ribs. A mediastinal mass is seen in the retrocardiac region and represents a fusiform aneurysm of the distal third of the dorsal aorta, which was resected and successfully replaced by a homograft. **B,** an aorto-gram at 2½ years of age demonstrates an aneurysm of the abdominal aorta below a previous hemograft and obstruction of the left renal artery. (From Dutton RV, Singleton EB: Tuberous sclerosis: A case report with aortic aneurysm and unusual rib changes. *Pediatr. Radiol.* 3:184, 1975. Used by permission.)

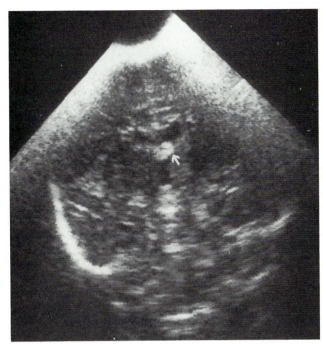

FIG SY–T–13.
Tuberous sclerosis. An ultrasonogram in an infant through the bodies of the lateral ventricle demonstrates an echogenic subependymal nodule *(arrow)* along the floor of the left lateral ventricle, adjacent to the foramen of Monro. (From Legge M, Sauerbrei E, Macdonald A: Intracranial tuberous sclerosis in infancy. *Radiology* 153:667, 1984. Used by permission.)

and heterotopic clusters; high-signal lesions in the cerebellum; (3) ultrasonography: densely echogenic periventricular nodules; (4) hypometabolic cortical lesions demonstrated by positron-emission tomography; (5) miscellaneous: hydrocephalus due to obstruction, neoplasm (giant-cell astrocytomas or higher-grade gliomas), arterial ectasia, and occlusion; (b) *cardiovascular system:* cardiac rhabdomyoma or hamartoma, arterial aneurysm, coaractation of the abdominal aorta

and renal artery stenosis, cardiogenic emboli, cardiac failure; (c) *respiratory system:* interstitial reticular infiltrates that may progress to honeycomb lung, cor pulmonale, pulmonary cyst, pulmonary lymphangioma, chylothorax, spontaneous pneumothorax; (d) *urinary system:* single or multiple renal masses: (1) angiomyolipomas (ultrasonographic demonstration of a cluster of internal echoes at both low and high gain, plain film and CT demonstration of intrarenal fat density,

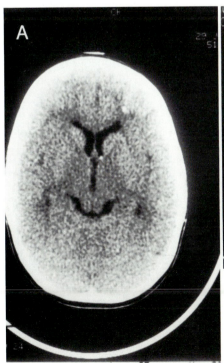

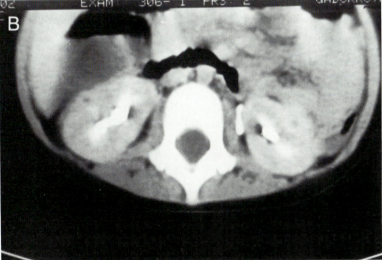

FIG SY–T–14.
Tuberous sclerosis in a 2-year-old boy with a history of recurrent seizures. **A,** calcification in the left frontal lobe and paraventricular calcification. **B,** CT of the upper portion of the abdomen shows multiple small renal cysts. (Courtesy of Peter E. Kane, M.D., Children's Hospital Medical Center, Oakland, Calif.)

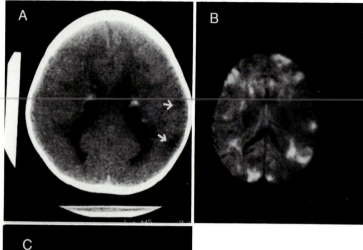

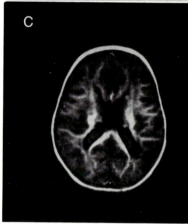

FIG SY–T–15.
Tuberous sclerosis: cerebral abnormalities. **A,** unenhanced transaxial CT image shows multiple calcified subependymal nodules. The parenchymal hamartomatous lesions are hypoattenuated *(arrows).* **B,** SE 2000/84 (TR ms/TE ms) transaxial MR image shows multiple parenchymal foci of increased signal intensity. **C,** IR 2000/28/369 (TR ms/TE ms/TI ms) transaxial MR image shows periventricular nodules of intermediate signal intensity and parenchymal hamartomas of decreased signal intensity. (From Altman NR, Purser RK, Post MJD: Tuberous sclerosis: Characteristics at CT and MR imaging. *Radiology* 167:527, 1988. Used by permission.)

stretching of the calyces on excretory urography, angiographic demonstration of hypervascularity and irregular outpouchings from interlobular and interlobar arteries); (2) renal cysts similar to adult polycystic disease; (3) renal cell carcinoma, Wilms tumor; (4) intratumoral and perirenal hemorrhage; (5) berry aneurysms of intrarenal arteries, spontaneous intraperitoneal rupture of a kidney; (e) *skeletal system:* patchy localized sclerotic densities in the skull, vertebrae, pelvis, and long bones; cystlike defects in the phalanges, metatarsals, and metacarpals; localized periosteal thickening along the shaft of the tubular bones; rib expansion and sclerosis; exostosis and enostosis of the tubular bones; thinning of the occipital bone in association with a cortical tuber adjacent to the thinned bone (case report); clivus chordoma (case report) (Figs SY–T–12 through SY–T–16).

REFERENCES

Alkalay AL, et al.: Spontaneous regression of cardiac rhabdomyoma in tuberous sclerosis. *Clin. Pediatr. (Phila.)* 26:532, 1987.

Altman NR, et al.: Tuberous sclerosis: Characteristics at CT and MR imaging. *Radiology* 167:527, 1988.

Avni EF, et al.: L'atteinte rénale dans la sclérose tubéreuse de Bourneville. *Ann. Radiol. (Paris)* 27:207, 1984.

Blumenkopf B, et al.: Tuberous sclerosis and multiple intracranial aneurysms. *Neurosurgery* 17:797, 1985.

Couture A, et al.: Diagnostic neonatal par ultrasons d'une sclérose tubéreuse de Bourneville a forme cardiaque et cérébrale (cas radiologique du mois). *Arch. Fr. Pediatr.* 43:345, 1986.

de Tinguy du Pouet M, et al.: Troubles endocriniens hypothalamiques révélateurs d'une sclérose tubéreuse de Bourneville. *Presse Med.* 14:599, 1985.

Dutton RV, et al.: Tuberous sclerosis: A case report with aortic aneurysm and unusual rib changes. *Pediatr. Radiol.* 3:184, 1975.

Earthman WJ, et al.: Angiomyolipomas in tuberous sclerosis: Subselective embolotherapy with alcohol, with long-term follow-up study. *Radiology* 160:437, 1986.

Fleury P, et al.: The incidence of hepatic hamartomas in tuberous sclerosis. Evaluation by ultrasonography. *Fortschr. Rontgenstr.* 146:694, 1987.

Flynn PM, et al.: Coarctation of the aorta and renal artery stenosis in tuberous sclerosis. *Pediatr. Radiol.* 14:337, 1984.

Fryer AE, et al.: Evidence that the gene for tuberous sclerosis is on chromosome 9. *Lancet* 1:659, 1987.

Fryer AE, et al.: Forehead plaque: A presenting skin sign in tuberous sclerosis. *Arch. Dis. Child.* 62:292, 1987.

Gibbs JL: The heart and tuberous sclerosis. An echocardiographic and electrocardiographic study. *Br. Heart J.* 54:596, 1985.

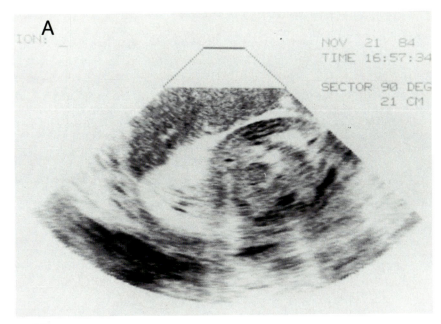

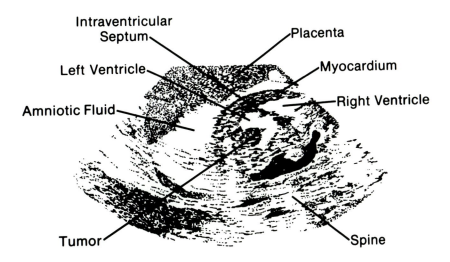

FIG SY−T−16.
Tuberous sclerosis: intracardiac tumor (rhabdomyoma). In utero ultrasonography shows polyhydramnios and a tumor arising from the lateral wall of the left ventricle immediately below the mitral valve. (From Stanford W, Abu-Yousef M, Smith W: Intracardiac tumor (rhabdomyoma) diagnosed by in utero ultrasound: A case report. *J. Clin. Ultrasound* 15:337, 1987. Used by permission.)

Grether P, et al.: Wilms' tumor in an infant with tuberous sclerosis. *Ann. Genet. (Paris)* 30:183, 1987.

Hoffman WH, et al.: Acromegalic gigantism and tuberous sclerosis. *J. Pediatr.* 93:478, 1978.

Hunt A, et al.: Psychiatric disorder among children with tuberous sclerosis. *Dev. Med. Child. Neurol.* 29:190, 1987.

Jayakar PB, et al.: Tuberous sclerosis and Wolff-Parkinson-White syndrome. *J. Pediatr.* 108:259, 1986.

Kandt RS, et al.: Tuberous sclerosis with cardiogenic cerebral embolism: Magnetic resonance imaging. *Neurology* 35:1223, 1985.

Kingsley DPE, et al.: Tuberous sclerosis: A clinicoradiological evaluation of 110 cases with particular reference to atypical presentation. *Neuroradiology* 28:38, 1986.

Legge M, et al.: Intracranial tuberous sclerosis in infancy. *Radiology* 153:667, 1984.

Luna CM, et al.: Pulmonary lymphangiomyomatosis associated with tuberous sclerosis. *Chest* 88:473, 1985.

Lygidakis NA, et al.: Pitted enamel hypoplasia in tuberous sclerosis patients and first-degree relatives. *Clin. Genet.* 32:216, 1987.

Mandia SE, et al.: Spontaneous intraperitoneal rupture of a kidney in a patient with tuberous sclerosis. *J. Urol.* 136:83, 1986.

Martin N, et al.: MRI evaluation of tuberous sclerosis. *Neuroradiology* 29:437, 1987.

Medley BE, et al.: Tuberous sclerosis. *Semin. Roentgenol.* 11:35, 1976.

Mitnick JS, et al.: Cystic renal disease in tuberous sclerosis. *Radiology* 147:85, 1983.

Ng SH, et al.: Tuberous sclerosis with aortic aneurysm and rib changes: CT demonstration. *J. Comput. Assist. Tomogr.* 12:666, 1988.

Oppenheimer EY, et al.: The late appearance of hypopigmented maculae in tuberous sclerosis. *Am. J. Dis. Child.* 139:408, 1985.

Östör AG, et al.: Tuberous sclerosis initially seen as hydrops fetalis. *Arch. Pathol. Lab. Med.* 102:34, 1978.

Pinto-Lord MC, et al.: Hyperdense cerebral lesion in childhood tuberous sclerosis: Computed tomographic demonstration and neuropathologic analysis. *Pediatr. Neurol.* 2:245, 1986.

Pringle JJ: A case of congenital adenoma sebaceum. *Br. J. Dermatol.* 2:1, 1890.

Raghavendra BN, et al.: Small angiomyolipoma of the kidney: Sonographic-CT evaluation. *A.J.R.* 141:575, 1983.

Roach ES, et al.: Magnetic resonance imaging in tuberous sclerosis. *Arch. Neurol.* 44:301, 1987.

Root AW, et al.: Gonadotrop-independent isosexual precocity in a boy with tuberous sclerosis: Effect of ketoconazole. *J. Pediatr.* 109:1012, 1986.

Scappaticci S, et al.: Chromosome abnormalities in tuberous sclerosis. *Hum. Genet.* 79:151, 1988.

Schroeder BA, et al.: Clivus chordoma in a child with tuberous sclerosis: CT and MR demonstration. *J. Comput. Assist. Tomogr.* 11:195, 1987.

Scotti LN, et al.: The value of CT in genetic counseling in tuberous sclerosis. *Pediatr. Radiol.* 9:1, 1980.

Stanford W, et al.: Intracardiac tumor (rhabdomyoma) diagnosed by in utero ultrasound: A case report. *J. Clin. Ultrasound* 15:337, 1987.

Stillwell TJ, et al.: Renal lesions in tuberous sclerosis. *J. Urol.* 138:477, 1987.

Szelies B, et al.: Hypometabolic cortical lesions in tuberous sclerosis with epilepsy: Demonstration by positron emission tomography. *J. Comput. Assist. Tomogr.* 7:946, 1983.

Terada T, et al.: Tuberous sclerosis with an atypical radiological skull change: Case report. *Neurosurgery* 16:804, 1985.

Weinblatt ME, et al.: Renal cell carcinoma in patients with tuberous sclerosis. *Pediatrics* 80:898, 1987.

TUMORAL CALCINOSIS

Synonyms: Calcinosis, tumoral; hyperphosphatemic tumoral calcinosis; tumoral calcinosis; diaphysitis and hyperphosphatemia.

Mode of Inheritance: Autosomal recessive in most cases; autosomal dominant with variable clinical expressivity in one family (Lyles et al.); more commonly reported in blacks.

Frequency: Rare.

Clinical Manifestations: Onset of symptoms in the first or second decade of life: (a) *painless, hard, large, or small mass or masses over the extensor surface of joints*; (b) limitation of joint motions, inhibition of normal muscular function in association with large calcific masses; (c) progressive increase in the size of masses; (d) hyperphosphatemia with an elevated tubular maximum for phosphate in relation to the glomerular filtration rate, elevated 1,25-dihydroxyvitamin D levels, normocalcemia, normal renal function; (e) sinus formation associated with a whitish, chalky discharge to the skin (amorphic Ca apatite); (f) other reported abnormalities: elevated sedimentation rate, erythematous rash and involvement of the mucous membranes (gingivitis, perlèche, hoarseness) preceding the development of calcified nodules, acrocyanosis, palmoplantar hyperhidrosis, hyperglobulinemia.

Radiologic Manifestations: (a) *dense round or oval-shaped calcium deposits in the juxta-articular regions* that measure from a few millimeters to several centimeters in diameter; may have a multinodular appearance; hip, elbow, shoulder, ankle, wrist, and foot the most common sites; sedimentation of calcified material within fluid-filled cysts; (b) "diaphysitis" (subperiosteal new bone formation); (c) vascular calcification, calcinosis cutis.

Differential Diagnosis: Calcinosis universalis and circumscripta, vitamin D intoxication, milk-alkali syndrome, chronic renal disease, hypoparathyroidism, pseudohypoparathyroidism, dermatomyositis, sarcoidosis, primary hyperparathyroidism.

Note: Due to overlapping reactive diaphyseal new bone formation in association with hyperphosphatemic tumoral

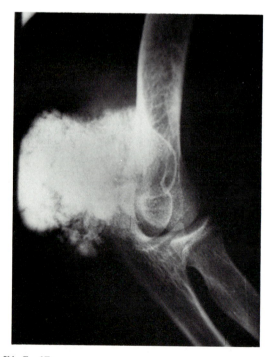

FIG SY–T–17.
Tumoral calcinosis in a 15-year-old male with two masses, one in the left elbow and one in the right buttock. Multilocular calcifications with no attachment to elbow joint are present. Radiolucent septa are shown in the calcified mass. (From Yaghmai I, Mirbod P: Tumoral calcinosis. *A.J.R.* 111:573, 1971. Used by permission.)

calcinosis in three children and the syndrome of hyperostosis and hyperphosphatemia, the possibility of the two conditions representing manifestations of a hereditary disorder of calcium and phosphorus metabolism has been suggested (Clarke et al.) (Fig SY–T–17).

REFERENCES

Clarke E, et al.: Tumoral calcinosis, diaphysitis, and hyperphosphatemia. *Radiology* 151:643, 1984.
Croock AD, et al.: Tumoral calcinosis presenting as adhesive capsulitis: Case report and literature. *Arthritis Rheum.* 30:455, 1987.
Durat MH: Tumeurs multiples et singulaires des bourses sereuses. *Bull. Mem. Soc. Anat. (Paris)* 74:725, 1899.
Giard A: Sur la calcification tibernale. *C.R. Soc. Biol.* 10:1015, 1898.
Gordon LF, et al.: Computed tomography in soft tissue calcification layering. *J. Comput. Assist. Tomogr.* 8:71, 1984.
Heydemann JS, et al.: Tumoral calcinosis in a child. *J. Pediatr. Orthop.* 8:474, 1988.
Inclán A, et al.: Tumoral calcinosis. *J.A.M.A.* 121:490, 1945.
Lyles K, et al.: Genetic transmission of tumoral calcinosis, autosomal dominant with variable clinical expressivity. *J. Clin. Endocrinol. Metab.* 60:1093, 1985.
Manaster BJ, et al.: Tumoral calcinosis: Serial images to monitor successful dietary therapy. *Skeletal Radiol.* 8:123, 1982.
Metzker A, et al.: Tumoral calcinosis revisited—common and uncommon features. Report of ten cases and review. *Eur. J. Pediatr.* 147:128, 1988.
Steinherz R, et al.: Elevated serum calcitriol concentrations do not fall in response to hyperphosphatemia in familial tumoral calcinosis. *Am. J. Dis. Child.* 139:816, 1985.
Teissir LJ: *Du Diabete Phosphatique,* (thesis). Paris, 1877; cited in Davis H, Moe PJ: *Pediatrics* 24:780, 1959.
Yaghmai I, Mirbod P.: Tumoral calcinosis. *A.J.R.* 111:573, 1971.

TUOMAALA SYNDROME

Mode of Inheritance: Probably autosomal recessive.

Frequency: No new references (1968 to 1988).

Clinical and Radiologic Manifestations: (a) maxillary hypoplasia, relative prognathism; (b) ocular anomalies: antimongoloid slanting of the eyes, distichiasis, strabismus, nystagmus, lenticular opacities, foveal hypoplasia, myopia; (c) skin dyspigmentation; (d) congenital edentia; (e) brachydactyly.

REFERENCE

Tuomaala P, Haapanen E: Three siblings with similar anomalies in the eyes, bones and skin. *Acta Ophthalmol.* 46:365, 1968.

TURCOT SYNDROME

Synonym: Glioma-polyposis syndrome.

Mode of Inheritance: Autosomal recessive considered most likely; autosomal dominant with variable expressivity also has been suggested.

Frequency: Over 20 published cases (Chowdhary et al., Lewis et al.).

Clinical and Radiologic Manifestations: *Familial polyposis of the colon* in association with a *malignant tumor of the central nervous system* (glioblastoma and/or medulloblastoma).

Notes: (a) occurrence of central nervous system malignancy has been reported in some members of the families with Gardner syndrome or familial polyposis; (b) it has been proposed that Turcot syndrome patients be divided into type I (only siblings affected) and type II (two or more generations with colonic polyposis); in addition nonfamilial cases also have been reported.

REFERENCES

Baughman FA Jr, et al.: The glioma-polyposis syndrome. *N. Engl. J. Med.* 281:1345, 1969.
Chowdhary UM, et al.: Turcot syndrome (glioma polyposis). Case report. *J. Neurosurg.* 63:804, 1985.
Everson RB, et al.: Familial glioblastoma with hepatic focal nodular hyperplasia. *Cancer* 38:310, 1976.
Lewis JH, et al.: Turcot's syndrome. Evidence for autosomal dominant inheritance. *Cancer* 51:524, 1983.
McKusick VA: Genetic factors in intestinal polyposis. *J.A.M.A.* 182:271, 1962.
Radin DR, et al.: Turcot syndrome: A case with spinal cord and colonic neoplasms. *A.J.R.* 142:475, 1984.
Todd DW, et al.: A family affected with intestinal polyposis and gliomas. *Ann. Neurol.* 9:390, 1981.
Turcot J, et al.: Malignant tumors of the central nervous system associated with familial polyposis of the colon: Report of two cases. *Dis. Colon Rectum* 2:465, 1959.

TWIN-TO-TWIN TRANSFUSION SYNDROME

Synonyms: Fetal transfusion syndrome; fetofetal transfusion syndrome.

Clinical Manifestations: (a) one of the twins sharing placental circulation is *anemic,* and the other is *plethoric;* caused by twin-to-twin vascular anastomosis and an imbalanced placental circulation favoring one twin; (b) *disparity of body size, recipient twin being larger;* (c) polyhydramnios; (d) donor twin with blueberry muffin–like macules and papules associated with cutaneous erythropoiesis; (e) perinatal death in a high percentage of cases.

Radiological Manifestations: (a) *cardiomegaly* and radiographic manifestation of *cardiac failure in the anemic twin;*

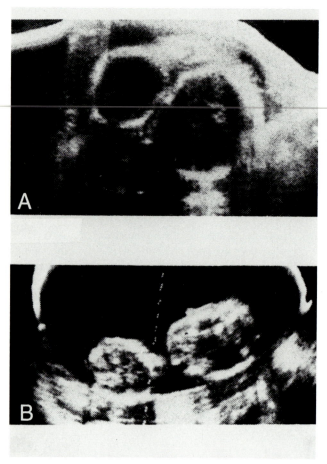

FIG SY–T–18.
Twin-to-twin transfusion syndrome: Ultrasonography at 28 weeks of gestation. A cross section of the heads **(A)** and a cross section of the abdomen **(B)** shows disparity in size of the twins. (From Brennan JN, Diwan RV, Rosen MG, et al.: Fetofetal transfusion syndrome: Prenatal ultrasonographic diagnosis. *Radiology* 143:535, 1982. Used by permission.)

(b) *cardiomegaly in the plethoric twin;* increased pulmonary vasculature; (c) fetal ultrasonography: significant difference in the size of fetuses of the same sex; disparity in size between the amniotic sacs (polyhydramnios in the recipient's sac and oligoamnios in the donor's sac); disparity between the size or number of the vessels in the umbilical cords; a single placenta with areas of disparity in echogenicity; hydrops in either fetus; enlarged heart, kidneys, and muscular mass of the recipient fetus; difference in the urinary bladder size (full bladder in the recipient fetus and empty bladder in the donor fetus); abnormal peak systolic velocity-to-end diastolic velocity ratio (Doppler ultrasound) (Fig SY–T–18).

REFERENCES

Ashley WE, et al.: Twin-to-twin transfusion: Cause of increased pulmonary vasculature in the newborn. *A.J.R.* 137:617, 1981.

Brennan JN, et al.: Fetofetal transfusion syndrome: Prenatal ultrasonographic diagnosis. *Radiology* 143:535, 1982.

Elejalde BR, et al.: Diagnosis of twin to twin transfusion syndrome at 18 weeks of gestation. *J. Clin. Ultrasound* 11:442, 1983.

Klingberg WG, et al.: Placental parabiotic circulation of single-ovum human twins. *Am. J. Dis. Child.* 90:519, 1955.

Portal P: *The Compleat Practice of Men and Women Midwives.* London, Clark, 1705; cited by Elejalde et al.

Pretorius DH, et al.: Doppler ultrasound of twin transfusion syndrome. *J. Ultrasound Med.* 7:117, 1988.

Schwartz JL, et al.: Twin transfusion syndrome causing cutaneous erythropoiesis. *Pediatrics* 74:527, 1984.

ULNA AND FIBULA DUPLICATION (HEREDITARY)

Mode of Inheritance: A father and his daughter affected.

Clinical and Radiologic Manifestations: (a) "peculiar facies," nasal clefts; (b) ulnar and fibular dimelia, absent radius and tibia; (c) other abnormalities: polydactyly, syndactyly, carpal fusion, duplication of the calcaneus and cuboid, four cuneiforms, etc.

REFERENCES

Sandrow RE, et al.: Hereditary ulnar and fibular dimelia with peculiar facies. A case report. *J. Bone Joint Surg.* [Am.] 52:367, 1970.

ULNAR-MAMMARY SYNDROME

Synonyms: Schinzel syndrome; ulnar-mammary syndrome, type Pallister.

Mode of Inheritance: Autosomal dominant with full penetrance and highly variable expression.

Frequency: 12 published cases (Schinzel).

Clinical Manifestations: (a) *ulnar finger and fibular toe ray defects*; (b) *delayed growth and onset of puberty*; (c) *obesity*; (d) *hypogenitalism and diminished sexual activity*; (e) *hypoplasia of the nipples and apocrine glands, diminished ability to perspire*; (f) other reported abnormalities: pyloric stenosis, anal atresia, anal stenosis, subglottic stenosis, imperforate hymen, inguinal hernia, sparse axillary hair, no body odor.

Radiological Manifestations: (a) *limb anomalies*: short, crooked, and stiff terminal phalanges of the fifth fingers; absence of the fifth finger ray, absence of the fourth and fifth finger rays, absence of the third to the fifth finger rays; hypoplastic or absent ulna; postaxial polydactyly of the hand; hypoplastic humerus, scapula, clavicle, and pectoralis major muscle; short, stiff, and crooked terminal phalanges of toes 4 and 5; (b) hypodontia; (c) renal malformations (Fig SY–U–1).

REFERENCES

Gilly E: Absence complète des mammales chez une femme mère. Atrophie du membre superieur droit. *Courrier Med.* 32:27, 1882.
Hecht JT, et al.: The Schinzel syndrome in a mother and daughter. *Clin. Genet.* 25:63, 1984.
Pallister PD, et al.: Studies of malformation syndromes in man. XXXXII: A pleiotropic dominant mutation affecting skeletal, sexual and apocrine-mammary development. *Birth Defects* 12:247, 1976.
Schinzel A: Ulnar-mammary syndrome. *J. Med. Genet.* 24:778, 1987.
Schinzel A, et al: The ulnar-mammary syndrome: An autosomal dominant pleiotropic gene. *Clin. Genet.* 32:160, 1987.

URETHRAL SYNDROME IN WOMEN

Etiology: Acute, subacute, or chronic nonspecific inflammation of the proximal part of the urethra, paraurethral ducts and glands, and bladder neck.

Clinical Manifestations: (a) dysuria; (b) edematous and hyperemic external urethral orifice; narrowing of the urethral lumen; inflammatory changes of the trigone, bladder neck, and urethra; (c) high incidence of pyelonephritis.

Radiologic Manifestations: (a) indentation at the base of the bladder, edematous pedunculated or sessile polyps most often located in the anterior aspect of the bladder neck; (b) periurethral calcification.

Note: The Subcommittee of the Research Council Bacteriuria Committee has recommended that the term *urethral syndrome* not be used because it causes confusion.

REFERENCES

Jackson EA: Urethral syndrome in women. *Radiology* 119:287, 1976.
Brumfitt W, et al.: Urethral syndrome or dysuria/frequency syndrome: A terminological and microbiological dilemma. *Lancet* 1:1066, 1982.
Report by member of the Medical Research Council Bacteriuria Committee: Recommended terminology of urinary tract infection. *Br. Med. J.* 2:717, 1979.

UROFACIAL SYNDROME

Synonym: Ochoa syndrome.

Mode of Inheritance: Autosomal recessive.

Clinical Manifestations: (a) *"inverse" facial expression when laughing*; (b) diurnal and/or nocturnal enuresis, recurrent urinary tract infections; (c) hypertension associated with urinary system disease; (d) *cystometric studies: hypertonic,*

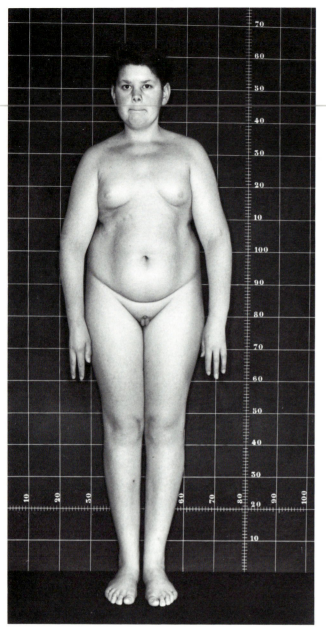

FIG SY—U—1.
Ulnar-mammary syndrome in a 19-year, 5-month-old male patient. Note the pseudogynecomastia, obesity, hypoplastic, underpigmented nipples, small genitalia, and ulnar ray defects. A micropenis, beginning pubic growth, and a hypoplastic and empty scrotum are present. (From Schinzel A, et al.: The ulnar-mammary syndrome: An autosomal dominant pleiotropic gene. *Clin. Genet.* 32:160, 1987. Used by permission.)

hyperreflexic type of bladder with uninhibited contractions of the detrusor muscle in most patients; (e) *constipation* in about two thirds of the cases.

Radiological Manifestations: (a) vesicoureteral reflux (unilateral or bilateral), trabeculated bladder; spastic posterior urethra at the level of the external sphincter in most patients, significant residual urine after voiding; (b) clubbing of the calices, hydronephrosis, scarring, small kidney size (manifestations of chronic pyelonephritis) (Fig SY—U—2).

REFERENCES

Elejalde R: Genetic and diagnostic considerations in three families with abnormalities of facial expression and congenital urinary obstruction: "The Ochoa syndrome." *Am. J. Med. Genet.* 3:97, 1979.
Hinman F Jr: Nonneurogenic neurogenic bladder (the Hinman syndrome)—15 years later. *J. Urol.* 136:769, 1986.
Ochoa B, Gorlin RJ: Urofacial (Ochoa) syndrome. *Am. J. Med. Genet.* 27:661, 1987.

UROGENITAL ADYSPLASIA (HEREDITARY)

Mode of Inheritance: Autosomal dominant with incomplete penetrance and variable expression.

Clinical and Radiologic Manifestations: (a) *unilateral or bilateral renal agenesis (or severe dysplasia);* (b) Potter sequence in infants with bilateral renal agenesis/dysplasia; (c) *genital anomalies;* (d) extragenitourinary anomalies (less frequent than in sporadic cases); (e) ultrasound study of the kidneys of parents, siblings, and other relatives recommended (unilateral or bilateral renal agenesis).

REFERENCES

Al Saadi AA, et al.: A family study of renal dysplasia. *Am. J. Med. Genet.* 19:669, 1984.
Biedel CW, et al.: Müllerian anomalies and renal agenesis: Autosomal dominant urogenital adysplasia. *J. Pediatr.* 104:861, 1984.
McPherson E, et al.: Dominantly inherited renal adysplasia. *Am. J. Med. Genet.* 26:863, 1987.

USHER SYNDROME

Mode of Inheritance: Autosomal recessive, 100% penetrance.

Frequency: Estimated to be 3:100,000; between 3% and 6% in the congenitally deaf population (Karjalainen et al.).

Clinical Manifestations: (a) *congenital hearing loss;* (b) *night blindness, retinitis pigmentosa* (RP); (c) mental disturbance; vestibular dysfunction.

Radiological Manifestations: Computed tomography: abnormal hindbrain circulation (focal areas of both delayed and diminished circulation of the cerebellar hemisphere); cerebellar atrophy.

Notes: Classification into four groups: type 1, profound congenital hearing loss and onset of RP before puberty; type

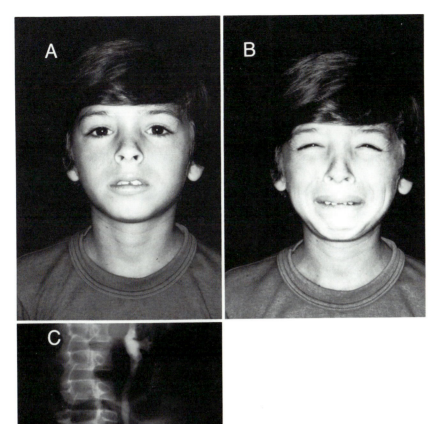

FIG SY–U–2.
Urofacial syndrome. **A,** normal facial expression. **B,** inverted facial expression when laughing. **C,** voiding cystourethrography shows a trabeculated bladder with left vesicoureteral reflux and "spasmodic" constriction of the posterior urethra. (From Ochoa B, Gorlin RJ: Urofacial (Ochoa) syndrome. *Am. J. Med. Genet.* 27:661, 1987. Used by permission.)

2, moderate to severe hearing loss from birth and RP appearing at puberty; type 3, progressive hearing loss and RP apparent at puberty; type 4, sex-linked inheritance.

REFERENCES

Davenport SLH, et al.: Usher's syndrome in four hard-of-hearing siblings. *Pediatrics* 62:578, 1978.

Grøndahl J: Estimation of prognosis and prevalence of retinitis pigmentosa and Usher syndrome in Norway. *Clin. Genet.* 31:255, 1987.

Karjalainen S, et al.: An unusual otological manifestation of Usher's syndrome in four siblings. *Clin. Genet.* 24:273, 1983.

Kumar A, et al.: Vestibular and auditory function in Usher's syndrome. *Ann. Otol. Rhinol. Laryngol.* 93:600, 1984.

Usher CH: Bowman's lecture: On a few hereditary eye affections. *Trans. Ophthalmol. Soc. U.K.* 55:164, 1935.

Von Graefe A: Exceptionelles Verhalten des Gesichtsfeldes bei Pigmententartung der Netzhaut. *Graefes Arch. Klin. Exp. Ophthalmol.* 4:250, 1958.

VAQUEZ-OSLER SYNDROME

Clinical Manifestations: (a) *hematopoietic proliferation;* (b) *erythrocytosis;* (c) *increase in blood viscosity;* (d) *cyanosis;* (e) nervous system manifestations (vertigo, headache); (f) visual disturbances (blurred vision, scotoma, diplopia); (g) cardiovascular manifestations (intermittent claudication, angina pectoris, venous thrombosis, thrombophlebitis; (h) hemorrhage at different sites; (i) gastrointestinal symptoms; (j) plethora; (k) *splenomegaly;* (l) hepatomegaly (in some).

Radiologic Manifestations: (a) *pulmonary vascular distension;* (b) cardiomegaly (in 25% of cases); (c) pulmonary infarction; (d) vascular thrombosis; (e) gout; (f) urinary tract calculi.

REFERENCES

Berbis P, et al.: Severe erosive lichen planus and polycythemia vera in an adolescent. *Dermatologica* 174:244, 1987.

Fiandra O, et al.: Circulation pulmonaire dans la polyglobulie vraie: Etude angiocardiographique. *Ann. Radiol. (Paris)* 4:537, 1961.

Gemelli A, et al.: Study of left ventricular function using systolic time intervals in a group of patients with polycythemia vera (Vaquez-Osler disease). *Minerva Med.* 75:2667, 1984.

Osler W: Chronic cyanosis with polycythaemia and enlarged spleen: A new clinical entity. *Am. J. Med. Sci.* 126:187, 1903.

Pitman RG, et al.: The radiological appearances of the chest in polycythemia vera. *Clin. Radiol.* 12:276, 1961.

Vaquez HM: Sur une form spéciale de cyanose s'accompagnant d'hyperglobulie excessive et persistante. *C.R. Soc. Biol. (Paris)* 44:384, 1892.

VASCULAR SYNDROMES

Description: See Table SY–V–1.

REFERENCES

Avasthey P, et al.: Primary pulmonary hypertension, cerebrovascular malformation, and lymphoedema feet in a family. *Br. Heart J.* 30:769, 1968.

Beers CV, et al.: Tumors and short toe—a dihybrid pedigree. A family history showing the inheritance of hemangioma and metatarsus atavicus. *J. Hered.* 33:366, 1942.

Bicknell JM, et al.: Familial cavernous angiomas. *Arch. Neurol.* 35:746, 1978.

Burke EC, et al.: Disseminated hemangiomatosis. *Am. J. Dis. Child.* 108:418, 1964.

Bussone G, et al.: Divry-Van Bogaert syndrome. Clinical and ultrastructural findings. *Arch. Neurol.* 41:560, 1984.

Dobyns WB, et al.: Familial cavernous malformations of the central nervous system and retina. *Ann. Neurol.* 21:578, 1987.

Gluszcz A, et al.: Familial syndrome of general dysplasia of the connective tissue and of the vascular system associated with angioblastoma of the spinal canal. *Pol. Med. J.* 2:924, 1963.

Hayman LA, et al.: Familial cavernous angiomas: Natural history and genetic study over 5-year period. *Am. J. Med. Genet.* 11:147, 1982.

Kaplan P, et al.: A spinal arteriovenous malformation with hereditary cutaneous hemangiomas. *Am. J. Dis. Child.* 130:1329, 1976.

Kikuchi K, et al.: Wyburn-Mason syndrome: Report of a rare case with computed tomographic and angiographic evaluations. *Comput. Tomogr.* 12:111, 1988.

Leiber B: Angeborene supraumbilikale Mittelbauchrhaphe (SMBR) and kavernose Gesichtschamangiomatose—ein neues Syndrom? *Monatsschr. Kinderheilkd.* 130:84, 1982.

Leipner VN, et al: Röntgenbefunde bei einer angiomatösen Dysplasie (Typ Weber). *Fortschr. Rontgenstr.* 142:571, 1985.

Michels VV, et al.: Familial cavernous angiomas of the central nervous system and retina (abstract). *Am. J. Hum. Genet.* 37:69, 1985.

Pasyk KA, et al.: Familial vascular malformations. Report of 25 members of one family. *Clin. Genet.* 26:221, 1984.

Picard L, et al.: Angiomatose myelencéphalo-occipitale: Form postérieure du syndrome de Bonnet-Dechaume et Blanc. *Ann. Radiol. (Paris)* 16:499, 1973.

Wyburn-Mason R: Arterio-venous aneurysm of midbrain and retina, facial naevi and mental changes. *Brain* 66:163, 1943.

Zaremba J, et al.: Hereditary neurocutaneous angioma: A new genetic entity? *J. Med. Genet.* 16:443, 1979.

VATER ASSOCIATION

Synonyms: VACTEL; VACTERL; VACTER.

Definition: Association of some or all of the following anomalies:

V: Vertebral anomalies, Vascular anomalies.
A: Anal anomalies, Auricular defects.
C: Cardiovascular anomalies.
T: Tracheoesophageal fistula.
E: Esophageal atresia, Esophageal ring.
R: Renal anomalies, Radial defects, Rib anomalies.
L: Limb anomalies.

TABLE SY—V—1.

Vascular "Syndromes"

Name	Description
Sturge-Weber	Nevus flammeus and cerebral angiomatosis
von Hippel–Lindau	Angiomatosis of the retina and cerebellum
Wyburn-Mason	Arteriovenous aneurysm of the retina and midbrain
Blue rubber bleb nevus	Cavernous lesions of the skin and gastrointestinal tract
Louis-Barr	Ataxia, telangiectasia
Rendu-Osler-Weber	Hereditary hemorrhagic telangiectasia
Fabry	Angiokeratoma corporis diffusum
Riley-Smith	Angiomatosis of the skin, macrocephaly, and pseudopapilledema
Klippel-Trenauney-Weber	Nevus vasculosus and tissue hypertrophy
Maffucci	Dyschondroplasia and angiomas
Burke et al.	Angiomatosis of the skin and CNS
Kasabach-Merritt	Hemangiomas associated with thrombocytopenia
Bannayan	Macrocephaly and multiple hamartomas, hemangiomas
Dirvy–van Bogaert	Corticomeningeal angiomatosis, telangiectatic "marbled skin"; autosomal recessive
Familial cerebral arteriovenous malformations	CNS complications (hemorrhage, seizures, etc.)
Familial vascular malformations (Pasyk et al.)	Most with cavernous hemangiomas, some with arteriovenous malformations and capillary hemangiomas (not involving the CNS)
Familial cavernous malformations of the CNS (Bicknell et al., Hayman et al.)	CNS complication (hemorrhage, seizure, etc.
Hemangiomatosis—cerebellar angioblasma (Gluszcz et al.)	Cutaneous hemangiomatosis, acrocyanosis, hyperflexibility of the joints, phimosis; reported in 4 sibs
Hereditary neurocutaneous angioma	Skin hemangioma and multiple dilated thin-walled cerebral vessels; reported in 3 generations
Lymphedema and cerebral arteriovenous anomaly (Avasthey et al.)	Lymphedema of the feet and cerebral arteriovenous malformation; reported in a mother and sons

Frequency: Estimated to be about 1:3,500 (Corcorman et al.).

Etiology: A defective mesodermal development during embryogenesis before the 35th day of gestation due most likely to various causes; genetic factors probably not involved; recurrence within a sibship reported; exposure to progesterones and estrogens has been suggested as an etiologic factor.

Clinical and Radiologic Manifestations: (a) vertebral anomalies: aplasia, dysplasia, hypoplasia, scoliosis; (b) vascular anomalies (cardiovascular anomalies): ventricular septal defect, patent ductus arteriosus, tetralogy of Fallot, single ventricle, transposition of the great arteries, etc.; (c) anorectal malformations: anal atresia most common; (d) tracheoesophageal fistula; (e) renal anomalies: aplasia, dysplasia, cysts, hydronephrosis, ectopia, persistent urachus, vesicoureteral reflux, ureteropelvic junction obstruction, etc.; (f) radial dysplasia, hypoplasia of the thumb, triphalangeal thumb, radial polydactyly, radial aplasia, etc.; (g) other reported skeletal abnormalities: rib anomalies; sternal anomalies; Sprengel deformity; hypoplasia of the humerus; radioulnar synostosis; midline anomalies of the hand; absence of the pubis, femur, tibia, fibula, and two rays of the foot; clinodactyly; syndactyly; hypoplastic middle phalanx of the fifth digit; malposition of the digits; etc.; (h) other reported abnormalities: genital and gonadal anomalies, single umbilical artery, inguinal hernia, small intestinal defects, choanal atresia, cleft lip and/or palate, central nervous system anomalies (hydrocephalus, absent corpus callosum, etc.), tracheal agenesis, etc.; (i) postnatal growth deficiency (Fig SY—V—1).

REFERENCES

Aleksic S, et al.: Neural defects in Say-Gerald (VATER) syndrome. *Child's Brain* 11:255, 1984.

Auchterlonie IA, et al.: Recurrence of the VATER association within a sibship. *Clin. Genet.* 21:122, 1982.

Barnes JC, et al.: The VATER Association. *Radiology* 126:445, 1978.

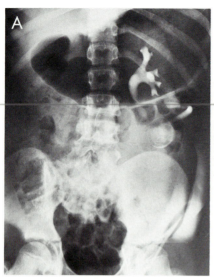
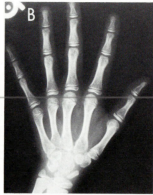
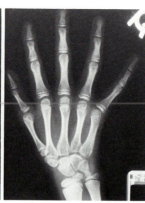

FIG SY–V–1.
VATER association. The patient was treated in the neonatal period for a tracheoesophageal fistula and anal atresia. Bilateral hydronephrosis was diagnosed in the first month of life. Right nephroureterectomy was performed at 2 years of age. **A,** an excretory urogram at the age of 12 years shows cutaneous ureterostomy on the left side. Note the partial absence of the sacrum. **B,** radiograms of the hands at 12 years of age show a relative smallness of the right thumb and the first and second metacarpals. The right hand is smaller than the left. (From Taybi H: Urinary tract manifestations of multisystem diseases in children, in Margulis AR, Gooding CA (eds): *Diagnostic Radiology.* San Francisco, University of California, 1979, p. 141.

Barry JE, et al.: The VATER Association: One end of a spectrum of anomalies. *Am. J. Dis. Child.* 128:769, 1974.
Baumann W, et al.: VATER-oder VACTERL-Syndrom. *Klin. Paediatr.* 188:328, 1976.
Briard ML, et al.: Association VACTERL et hydrocéphalie: Une nouvelle entité familiale. *Ann. Genet. (Paris)* 27:220, 1984.
Claiborne AK, et al.: Prenatal and postnatal sonographic delineation of gastrointestinal abnormalities in a case of the VATER syndrome. *J. Ultrasound Med.* 5:45, 1986.
Corcornan et al.: *Lancet* 2:981, 1975.
Czeizel A, et al.: An aetiological study of the VACTERL-association. *Eur. J. Pediatr.* 144:331, 1985.
Dewar CR, et al.: Tracheoesophageal fistula and associated malformations. *West. J. Med.* 128:370, 1978.
Fernbach SK, et al.: The expanded spectrum of limb anomalies in the VATER association. *Pediatr. Radiol.* 18:215, 1988.
Heyman MB, et al.: Esophageal muscular ring and the VACTERL association: A case report. *Pediatrics* 67:683, 1981.
Khoury MJ, et al.: A population study of the VACTERL association: Evidence for its etiologic heterogeneity. *Pediatrics* 71:815, 1983.
Knowles S, et al.: Pulmonary agenesis as part of the VACTERL sequence. *Arch. Dis. Child.* 63:723, 1988
Lawhon SM, et al.: Orthopaedic aspects of the VATER association. *J. Bone J. Surg. [Am.]* 68:424, 1986.
Mapstone CL, et al.: Analysis of growth in the VATER association. *Am. J. Dis. Child.* 140:386, 1986.
Milstein JM, et al.: Tracheal agenesis in infants with VATER association. *Am. J. Dis. Child.* 139:77, 1985.
Quan L, et al.: The VATER association: Vertebral defects and atresia, tracheoesophageal fistula with esophageal atresia, radial dysplasia. *Birth Defects* 8:75, 1972.
Reinberg Y, et al.: Wilms tumor and the VATER association. *J. Urol.* 140:787, 1988.

Say B, Gerald PS: A new polydactyly, imperforate anus, vertebral anomalies syndrome. *Lancet* 2:688, 1968.
Smith DW: The VATER Association. *Am. J. Dis. Child.* 128:767, 1974.
Touloukian RJ, et al.: High proximal pouch esophageal atresia with vertebral, rib, and sternal anomalies: An additional component to the VATER association. *J. Pediatr. Surg.* 23:76, 1988.
Uehling DT, et al.: Urologic implications of the VATER association. *J. Urol.* 129:352, 1983.
Weaver DD, et al.: The VATER association. *Am. J. Dis. Child.* 140:225, 1986.

VELO-CARDIO-FACIAL SYNDROME

Synonym: Shprintzen syndrome.

Mode of Inheritance: Probably autosomal dominant.

Frequency: Uncommon.

Clinical and Radiological Manifestations: (a) *facial dysmorphism:* prominent nose with a broad, often squared root, narrow alar base, malar flatness, vertical maxillary excess, retrusion of the chin, malocclusion, narrow palpebral fissures, occasionally malformed auricles; (b) *cleft palate or occult submucous cleft;* (c) *cardiac malformations:* ventricular septal defect with or without a right-sided aortic arch, etc.; (d) *learning disability,* mental retardation; (e) other reported abnormalities: microcephaly, small stature, slender hands and digits, inguinal hernia, Robin malformation sequence, platybasia, ophthalmologic abnormalities (tortuous retinal vessels, small optic disks, embryotoxon, cataracts, coloboma, unilateral microphthalmos), facial asymmetry,

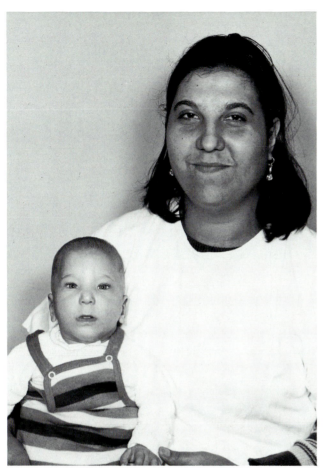

FIG SY—V—2.
Velocardiofacial syndrome in a mother and daughter with a long face, narrow and receding forehead, hypertelorism, upslanting palpebral fissures, prominent nasal bridge, long nose with hypoplastic alae, short upper lip, small mandible, and normal ears. (From Meinecke P, Beemer FA, Schinzel A, et al.: The velo-cardio-facial (Shprintzen) syndrome. Clinical variability in eight patients. *Eur. J. Pediatr.* 145:539, 1986. Used by permission.)

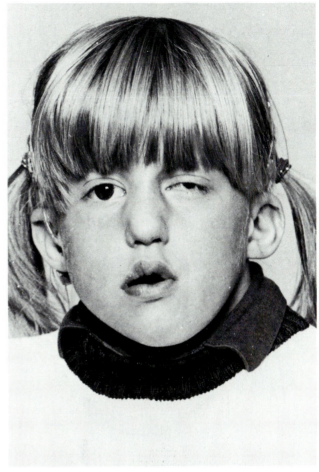

FIG SY—V—3.
Velocardiofacial syndrome. Note the asymmetrical face (smaller on the left), left microphthalmos, left facial paresis, small anomalous ears, and short neck. (From Beemer FA, de Nef JJEM, Delleman JW, et al.: *Am. J. Med. Genet.* 24:541, 1986. Used by permission.)

unilateral facial paresis, short neck, possibly holoprosencephaly, sensorineural hearing loss, pharyngeal hypotonia.

Differential Diagnosis: CHARGE association (Figs SY—V—2 and SY—V—3).

REFERENCES

Beemer FA, et al.: Additional eye findings in a girl with the velo-cardio-facial syndrome (letter). *Am. J. Med. Genet.* 24:541, 1986.

Meinecke P, et al.: The velo-cardio-facial (Shprintzen) syndrome. Clinical variability in eight patients. *Eur. J. Pediatr.* 145:539, 1986.

Shprintzen RJ: Reply from Dr. Shprintzen. *Am. J. Med. Genet.* 28:753, 1987.

Shprintzen RJ, et al.: The expanded velo-cardio-facial syndrome (VCF): Additional features of the most common clefting syndrome (abstract). *Am. J. Hum. Genet.* 37:77, 1985.

Shprintzen RJ, et al.: The velo-cardio-facial syndrome: A clinical and genetic analysis. *Pediatrics* 67:167, 1981.

Strong WB: Familial syndrome of right-sided aortic arch, mental deficiency, and facial dysmorphism. *J. Pediatr.* 73:882, 1968.

Wraith JE, et al.: Velo-cardio-facial syndrome presenting as holoprosencephaly. *Clin. Genet.* 27:408, 1985.

Young D, et al.: Cardiac malformations in the velo-cardio-facial syndrome. *Am. J. Cardiol.* 46:643, 1980.

VESICOURETERAL REFLUX (FAMILIAL)

Mode of Inheritance: Genetic transmission probably polygenic; X-linked reported; familial incidence of 8% to 32%; 45% incidence in asymptomatic siblings in one report (Van den Abbeele et al.).

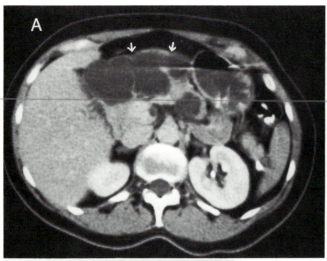
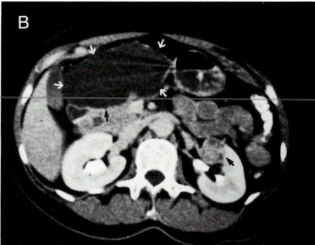

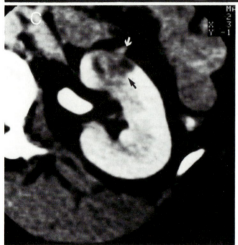

FIG SY–V–4.
von Hippel–Lindau syndrome: multiple simple pancreatic cysts and left renal carcinoma. **A,** body of the pancreas replaced by multiple cysts *(arrows)*. **B,** large cysts *(arrows)* involve the pancreatic head; a 2.5-cm solid mass *(lower right arrow)* arises in the left kidney (attenuation value after contrast, 88 H). **C,** left renal cell carcinoma *(black arrow)* shows early extension *(white arrow)* into perinephric fat. (From Levine E, Collins DL, Horton WA, et al.: CT screening of the abdomen in von Hippel–Lindau disease. *A.J.R.* 139:505, 1982. Used by permission.)

Clinical and Radiologic Manifestations: (a) symptomatic (urinary tract infection, etc.) or asymptomatic sibling(s); (b) radionuclide cystography ideal for screening of sibling(s) (low gonadal radiation).

REFERENCES

Middleton GW, et al.: Sex-linked familial reflux. *J. Urol.* 114:36, 1975.
Noe HN: The relationship of sibling reflux to index patient dysfunctional voiding. *J. Urol.* 140:119, 1988.
Van den Abbeele AD, et al.: Vesicoureteral reflux in asymptomatic siblings of patients with know reflux: Radionuclide cystography. *Pediatrics* 79:147, 1987.

VON HIPPEL–LINDAU SYNDROME

Synonym: Hippel-Lindau syndrome.

Mode of Inheritance: Autosomal dominant transmission with variable penetrance and delayed expression; reported in identical twins.

Frequency: Uncommon.

Pathology: (a) *retina: hemangioblastoma;* (b) *central nervous system: hemangioblastoma* (cerebrum, cerebellum, medulla oblongata, spinal cord), syringomyelia, meningioma, arteriovenous malformation of the cervical spinal cord; (c) genitourinary system: kidney (hemangioblastoma, hypernephroma, adenoma, cyst), bladder (hemangioblastoma), epididymis (cyst, clear-cell papillary cystadenoma of epididymis presenting as infertility, hypernephroid tumor); (d) pancreas: hemangioblastoma, cyst, cystadenoma; (e) liver: angioma, cyst, adenoma; (f) spleen: angioma; (g) adrenal gland: pheochromocytoma, cyst; (h) lung: cyst; (i) bone: cyst, hemangioma; (j) skin and mucosa: nevus, café au lait spots, etc.; (k) other reported lesions: omental cyst, mesenteric cyst, paraganglioma.

Clinical Manifestations: Onset of symptoms often in the third to fifth decades of life: (a) *visual:* hemorrhage, retinal detachment, glaucoma, uveitis, etc.; (b) *neurological:* related to cerebral, cerebellar, and spinal cord lesions; (c) polycythemia; (d) hypertension.

Radiological Manifestations: (a) *masses* at various sites demonstrable by different radiological techniques: ultrasonography, computed tomography (CT), magnetic resonance imaging, angiography; (b) brain scintigraphy: various intracranial lesions; (c) calcification: orbit, brain.

Notes: Recommended screening program (Green et al.): (1) annual ophthalmologic examination for members at risk and every 6 months for the individuals with any manifestation of the disease; (2) annual measurement of blood pressure and urinary catecholamine level; (3) annual neurological examination of those at risk; (4) brain imaging in the teens as a baseline study and annually in patients with any other signs of the disease; (5) baseline CT scanning of abdomen in the mid-20s; (6) annual ultrasonography of the abdomen (Fig SY−V−4).

REFERENCES

Coulam CM, et al.: Hippel-Lindau syndrome. *Semin. Roentgenol.* 11:61, 1976.

Fill WL, et al.: The radiographic manifestations of von Hipple-Lindau disease. *Radiology* 133:289, 1979.

Go RCP, et al.: Segregation and linkage analyses of von Hippel Lindau disease among 220 descendants from one kindred. *Am. J. Hum. Genet.* 26:131, 1984.

Green JS, et al.: Von Hippel−Lindau disease in a Newfoundland kindred. *Can. Med. Assoc. J.* 134:133, 1986.

Hippel E, von: Vorstellung eines Patienten mit einem sehr ungewöhnlichen Aderhautleiden: Bericht ü d. 24. *Versammlung Ophthalmol. Ges.* 269, 1895.

Hubschmann OR, et al.: Von Hippel−Lindau disease with multiple manifestations: Diagnosis and management. *Neurosurgery* 8:92, 1981.

Huson SM, et al.: Cerebellar haemangioblastoma and von Hippel−Lindau disease. *Brain* 109:1297, 1986.

Jennings AM, et al.: Von Hippel−Lindau disease in a large British family: Clinicopathological features and recommendations for screening and follow-up. *Q. J. Med.* 66:233, 1988.

Levine E, et al.: CT screening of the abdomen in von Hippel−Lindau disease. *A.J.R.* 139:505, 1982.

Lindau A: Studien über Kleinhirnzysten. *Acta Pathol. Microbiol. Scand.* Suppl. 1:1, 1926.

Loughlin KR, et al.: Urological management of patients with von Hippel−Lindau disease. *J. Urol.* 136:789, 1985.

Malek RS, et al.: Renal cell carcinoma in von Hippel−Lindau syndrome. *Am. J. Med.* 82:236, 1987.

Sato Y, et al.: Hippel-Lindau disease: MR imaging. *Radiology* 166:241, 1988.

Seitz ML, et al.: Von Hippel−Lindau disease in an adolescent. *Pediatrics* 79:632, 1987.

Wesolowski DP, et al.: Hippel-Lindau syndrome in identical twins. *Br. J. Radiol.* 54:982, 1981.

Witten FR, et al.: Bilateral clear cell papillary cystadenoma of the epididymides presenting as infertility: An early manifestation of Von Hippel−Lindau's syndrome. *J. Urol.* 133:1062, 1985.

W SYNDROME

Synonym: Pallister W syndrome.

Mode of Inheritance: Consistent with X-linked trait (reported in two brothers).

Clinical Manifestations: (a) prematurity, mental retardation, seizures, slight spasticity, tremor; (b) craniofacial abnormalities (frontal prominence, anterior cowlick, hypertelorism, antimongoloid slanting of the palpebral fissures, alternating internal strabismus, flat and broad bridge and tip of the nose, incomplete medial oral cleft, markedly short and high mandible.

Radiologic Manifestations: Cubitus valgus, subluxation at the proximal radio-ulnar joints, short ulnae, lateral bowing of radii, camptodactyly, clinodactyly.

REFERENCE

Pallister PD, et al.: The W Syndrome. *Birth Defects* 10(7):51, 1974.

WAARDENBURG SYNDROME

Mode of Inheritance: Autosomal dominant; penetrance of the gene as measured by dystopia canthorum (in type 1) has been estimated to be 83%.

Frequency: Estimated to be 1:42,000 (Senrui et al.).

Clinical Manifestations: (a) *type 1 with dystopia canthorum (most cases)*, type 2 without dystopia canthorum; (b) *pigmentary disorders of the eyes:* heterochromia of the iris, pigmentary disorders of the fundus, etc.; (c) *hypertelorism,* broad and high nasal root; (d) *hyperplasia of the medial segment of the eyebrows, confluent eyebrows:* (e) *congenital partial or total sensorineural deafness;* (f) *partial albinism* (poliosis, white forelock), premature graying of hair, vitiligo; (g) other reported abnormalities: ptosis, thin nose with flaring alae nasae, prominent ears, Cupid's bow configuration of the lips, dacrocystitis, lack of a frontonasal angle, prominent mandible, cleft or high-arched palate, seizures (associated with a wide subarachnoid space), anal atresia, tracheoesophageal fistula with esophageal atresia, congenital clasped thumb in three generations of one family.

Radiologic Manifestations: Tomography of the middle and inner ears: absence of an oval window, thickened wall of the labyrinth, dysplasia of the semicircular canal.

Differential Diagnosis: Klein-Waardenburg syndrome; Waardenburg-Shah syndrome (Shah-Waardenburg syndrome, Hirschsprung disease with pigmentary anomaly): familial white forelock and white eyebrows and eyelashes, isochromia iridis, long-segment Hirschsprung disease, parental consanguinity in some families (Fig SY–W–1).

REFERENCES

Arias S: Genetic heterogeneity in the Waardenburg syndrome. *Birth Defects* 7(4):87, 1971.

Currie ABM, et al.: Associated developmental abnormalities of the anterior end of the neural crest: Hirschsprung's disease—Waardenburg's syndrome. *J. Pediatr. Surg.* 21:248, 1986.

Delleman JW, et al.: Ophthalmological findings in 34 patients with Waardenburg syndrome. *J. Pediatr. Ophthalmol. Strabismus* 15:341, 1978.

Klein D: Albinisme partiel (leucisme) avec surdi-mutite, blepharophimosis et dysplasie myo-osteo-articulaire. *Helv. Paediatr. Acta* 5:38, 1950.

Mallory SB, et al.: Waardenburg's syndrome with Hirschsprung's disease: A neural crest defect. *Pediatr. Dermatol.* 3:119, 1986.

Meire F, et al.: Waardenburg syndrome, Hirschsprung megacolon, and Marcus Gunn ptosis. *Am. J. Med. Genet.* 27:683, 1987.

Nemansky J, et al.: Tomographic findings of the inner ears of 24 patients with Waardenburg's syndrome. *A.J.R.* 124:250, 1975.

Nutman J, et al.: Anal atresia and the Klein-Waardenburg syndrome. *J. Med. Genet.* 18:239, 1981.

Nutman J, et al.: Possible Waardenburg syndrome with gastrointestinal anomalies. *J. Med. Genet.* 23:175, 1986.

Preus M, et al.: Waardenburg syndrome—penetrance of major signs. *Am. J. Med. Genet.* 15:383, 1983.

Sanyas P, et al: Un syndrome de Waardenburg associé a une crise épileptique géneralisée. Étude tomodensitométrique cérébrale. *Ann. Pediatr. (Paris)* 29:142, 1982.

Schweitzer VG, et al.: Waardenburg's syndrome: A case report with CT scanning and cochleovestibular evaluation. *Int. J. Pediatr. Otorhinolaryngol.* 7:311, 1984.

Senrui H, et al.: Congenital clasped thumb combined with Waardenburg syndrome in three generations of one family: An undescribed congenital anomalies complex. *J. Pediatr. Orthop.* 4:472, 1984.

Shah KN, et al.: White forelock, pigmentary disorder of irides, and long segment Hirschsprung disease: Possible variant of Waardenburg syndrome. *J. Pediatr.* 99:432, 1981.

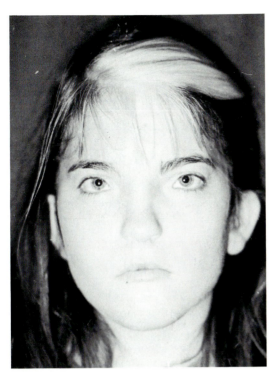

FIG SY–W–1.
Waardenburg syndrome in an 18-year-old female with the characteristic facial feature. Note the white forelock. (From Goodman RM, Oelsner G, Berkenstadt M, et al.: Absence of a vagina and right sided adnexa uteri in the Waardenburg syndrome: A possible clue to the embryological defect. *J. Med. Genet.* 25:355, 1988. Used by permission.)

Van der Hoeve J: Abnome Länge der Tränenröhrohen mit Amyloblepharon. *Klin. Monatsbl. Augenheilkd.* 56:232, 1916; cited by Currie.
Waardenburg PJ: A new syndrome combining development anomalies of the eyelids, eyebrows and nose root with pigmentary defects of iris and head hair and with congenital deafness. *Am. J. Hum. Genet.* 3:195, 1951.

WAARDENBURG ANOPHTHALMIA SYNDROME

Synonyms: Anophthalmos-syndactyly; anophthalmos–limb anomalies; anophthalmia, type Waardenburg.

Mode of Inheritance: Consistent with autosomal recessive; parental consanguity.

Clinical and Radiologic Manifestations: (a) *anophthalmia* (unilateral, bilateral), small orbit(s); (b) *limb anomalies* (distal): syndactyly of the fingers, absent fused metacarpals, camptodactyly, syndactyly of the toes, oligodactyly of the toes; (c) other reported abnormalities: clubfoot, mental retardation.

REFERENCES

Richieri-Costa A, et al.: Autosomal recessive anophthalmia with multiple congenital abnormalities—type Waardenburg. *Am. J. Med. Genet.* 14:607, 1983.
Traboulsi EI, et al.: Waardenburg's recessive anophthalmia syndrome. *Ophthalmic Paediatr. Genet.* 4:13, 1984.
Waardenburg PJ: Autosomally-recessive anophthalmia with malformations of the hands and feet, in Waardenburg PJ, et al. (eds.): *Genetics and Ophthalmology.* Assen, Royal Van Gorcum, 1961, vol. 1, p. 773.

WALDENSTRÖM MACROGLOBULINEMIA

Synonym: Waldenström syndrome.

Clinical Manifestations: A well-differentiated B-cell lymphoplasmacytic neoplasm: (a) common presentations: weakness, fatigue, anemia, bleeding, lymphadenopathy, hepatosplenomegaly; (b) uncommon presentations: pulmonary disease, Raynaud phenomenon, renal disease, hyperviscosity syndrome, peripheral neuropathy, central nervous system manifestations (stroke, focal or multifocal brain syndromes); (c) hyperglobulinemia, increased macroglobulin levels, presence in the blood of a monoclonal IgM paraprotein that is made by a clone of transformed immature B lymphocytes, elevated sedimentation rate; (d) other reported abnormalities: association with Guillain-Barré syndrome, hypercalcemia, syndrome of inappropriate antidiuresis, chronic liver disease, renal amyloidosis, myelopathy due to meningeal involvement.

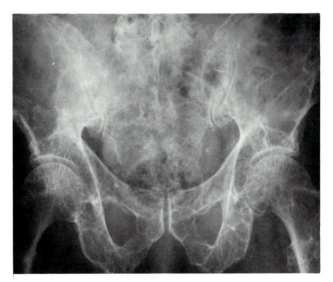

FIG SY–W–2.
Waldenström syndrome in a 65-year-old male with a 2-year history of anemia, increased incidence of infection, and pain in the bones of the back, ribs, and right leg. Extensive osteolysis and expansion throughout the pelvis are present. (From Vermess M, Pearson KD, Einstein AB, et al.: Osseous manifestations of Waldenström's macroglobulinemia. *Radiology* 102:497, 1972. Used by permission.)

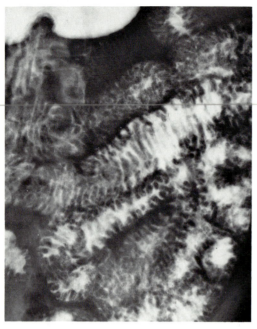

FIG SY–W–3.
Waldenström syndrome in a 55-year-old female with steatorrhea, a total serum protein level of 6.2, and an albumin content of 3.2 gm/100 ml. A contrast study demonstrates the wide caliber of the small bowel and uniformly thickened mucosal folds. (From Khilnani MT, Keller RJ, Cuttner J: Macroglobulinemia and steatorrhea: Roentgen and pathologic findings in the intestinal tract. *Radiol. Clin. North Am.* 7:43, 1969. Used by permission.)

Radiologic Manifestations: (a) the proteinaceous material causing obstruction and dilatation of the intestinal lymphatics and the lacteals in the tips of the villi: thickening of the bowel wall and mucosal folds, dilatation, "sandlike" fine granular pattern due to micronodules, chronic obstruction, higher than normal incidence of neoplasms; (b) *bones*: demineralization, punched-out osteolytic lesions, cystlike lesions, expansile lesions, compression of the vertebral bodies; (c) *reticuloendothelial system*: hepatosplenomegaly; lymphadenopathy (enlarged reticular appearance on lymphangiography); abnormal liver, spleen, and bone marrow isotope scans findings; (d) *chest*: pleural and pericardial effusion, heart failure, extramedullary hematopoiesis, recurrent pneumonia, chronic pulmonary infiltrate, pulmonary edema, pseudotumors in the lung that may cavitate; (e) *central nervous system*: subarachnoid or subdural hemorrhage, focal hemorrhage; (f) *urinary system*: poor renal function.

Differential Diagnosis: Chronic lymphocytic leukemia; lymphocytic lymphoma; multiple myeloma; osteolytic metastases; diseases with diffuse osteopenia (mastocytosis, acute hyperthyroidism, hyperparathyroidism with "brown tumors", osteomalacia) (Figs SY–W–2 and SY–W–3).

REFERENCES

Blattner WA, et al.: Waldenström's macroglobulinemia and autoimmune disease in a family. *Ann. Intern. Med.* 93:830, 1980.
Braden GL, et al.: Syndrome of inappropriate antidiuresis in Waldenström's macroglobulinemia. *Am. J. Med.* 80:1242, 1986.
Casassus Ph, et al.: Hypercalcemie compliquant une maladie de Waldenström: Revelation d'un syndrome de Richter. *Ann. Med. Interne (Paris)* 134:130, 1983.
Chelazzi G, et al.: Aspects radiologiques des manifestations thoraciques de la macroglobulinémi de Waldenström. *Ann. Radiol. (Paris)* 18:721, 1975.
Dellagi K, et al: Neuropathie périphérique de la macroglobulinemie de Waldenström. *Presse Med.* 13:1199, 1984.
Jensen DM, et al.: Chronic liver disease manifesting as Waldenström's macroglobulinemia. *Arch. Intern. Med.* 142:2318, 1982.
Khilnani MT, et al.: Macroglobulinemia and steatorrhea: Roentgen and pathologic findings in the intestinal tract. *Radiol. Clin. North Am.* 7:43, 1969.
Kobayashi H, et al.: Two cases of pulmonary Waldenström's macroglobulinemia. *Chest* 88:297, 1985.
Meyer C, et al.: Amylose rénale révélant une macroglobulinémie de Waldenström. *Presse Med.* 13:2020, 1984.
Neiman HL, et al.: Pulmonary and pleural manifestations of Waldenström's macroglobulinemia. *Radiology* 107:301, 1973.
Renner RR, et al.: Roentgenologic manifestations of primary macroglobulinemia (Waldenström). *A.J.R.* 113:499, 1971.
Ries CA: Waldenström's macroglobulinemia (Medical Staff Conference) *West J. Med.* 148:320, 1988.
Sundaram M, et al.: Case Report 215. *Skeletal Radiol.* 9:132, 1982.
Taillan B, et al.: Association maladie de Waldenström-syndrome de Guillain-Barré. *Presse Med.* 14:844, 1985.
Vermess M, et al.: Osseous manifestations of Waldenström's macroglobulinemia. *Radiology* 102:497, 1972.
Waldenström J: Incipient myelomatosis or "essential" hyperglobulinemia with fibrinogenopenia: A new syndrome? *Acta Med. Scand.* 117:216, 1944.
Woimant F, et al.: Myélopathie révelatrice d'une macroglobulinémie. *Ann. Med. Interne (Paris)* 136:121, 1985.

WALKER-WARBURG SYNDROME

Synonyms: Hydrocephalus-agyria-retinal dysplasia syndrome; HARD (±E) syndrome; Warburg syndrome; Chemke syndrome; Pagon syndrome; cerebro-ocular dysgenesis.

Frequency: Approximately 40 published cases.

Clinical and Radiologic Manifestations: (a) *hydrocephalus* (H), *agyria* (A), *retinal dysplasia* (RD), with or without *encephalocele* (±E); (b) other reported abnormalities: cerebellar dysplasia, agenesis of the corpus callosum, lack of cortical laminar structure, hypoplastic white matter, Dandy-Walker anomaly, Arnold-Chiari malformation, stenosis of the aqueduct of Sylvius, etc.

REFERENCES

Aymé S, et al.: HARD (±E) syndrome: Report of a sixth family with support for autosomal-recessive inheritance. *Am. J. Med. Genet.* 14:759, 1983.

Burton BK, et al.: Walker-Warburg syndrome with cleft lip and cleft palate in two sibs. *Am. J. Med. Genet.* 27:537, 1987.

Chemke J, et al.: A familial syndrome of central nervous system and ocular malformations. *Clin. Genet.* 7:1, 1975.

Crowe C, et al.: The prenatal diagnosis of Warburg syndrome (abstract). *Am. J. Hum. Genet.* 37:214, 1985.

Dobyns WB, et al.: Syndromes with lissencephaly. II: Walker-Warburg and cerebro-oculo-muscular syndromes and a new syndrome with type II lissencephaly. *Am. J. Med. Genet.* 22:157, 1985.

Farrell SA, et al.: Prenatal diagnosis of retinal detachment in Walker-Warburg syndrome. *Am. J. Med. Genet.* 28:619, 1987.

Pagon RA, et al.: Hydrocephalus, agyria, retinal dysplasia, encephalocele (HARD ± E) syndrome: An autosomal recessive condition. *Birth Defects* 14(6B):233, 1978.

Walker AE: Lissencephaly. *Arch. Neurol. Psychiatry* 48:13, 1942.

Warburg M: Aetiological heterogeneity and morphological similarity in congenital retinal nonattachment and falciform folds. *Trans. Ophthalmol. Soc. U.K.* 9:272, 1979.

WALLENBERG SYNDROME

Synonym: Lateral medullary syndrome.

Etiology: Occlusion of the vertebral artery or its branches.

Clinical and Radiologic Manifestations: (a) vertigo, nausea, vomiting; (b) dysarthria, dysphagia, nystagmus, ipsilateral Horner syndrome, ipsilateral vocal cord paralysis, ipsilateral facial pain sensation impairment, contralateral pain perception below the face; (c) magnetic resonance imaging (MRI): medullary infarction.

Notes: (a) MRI is more sensitive in detecting the medullary infarction; (b) demyelinating diseases may present as Wallenberg syndrome.

REFERENCES

Houi K, et al.: Wallenberg's syndrome on MRI. *Neuroradiology* 29:117, 1987.

Ross MA, et al.: Magnetic resonance imaging in Wallenberg's lateral medullary syndrome. *Stroke* 17:542, 1986.

Smith DB, et al.: Demyelinating disease presenting as Wallenberg's syndrome. Report of a patient. *Stroke* 12:877, 1981.

Wallenberg A: Acute Bulbaraffection (Embolie der Art. cerebellar post. inf. sinister?). *Arch. Psychiatrie* 24:509, 1895.

WARFARIN EMBRYOPATHY

Synonyms: Cumarin embryopathy; coumadin embryopathy; fetal warfarin syndrome.

Etiology: Maternal ingestion of vitamin K antagonist anticoagulant in the first trimester of pregnancy.

Clinical Manifestations: (a) *craniofacial dysmorphism*: frontal bossing, underdeveloped nasal cartilages, small and upturned nose, choanal stenosis, hypertelorism, poorly developed hypoplastic ears, large tongue; (b) blindness, optic atrophy, cataract, microphthalmos, prominent eyes, small

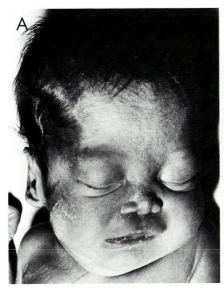
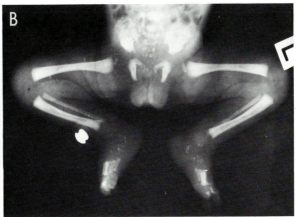

FIG SY—W—4.
Warfarin embryopathy in a newborn female with facial dysmorphism (collapsed nasal bridge) **(A)** and stippled calcification in the feet, hips, and sacrum **(B)**. (From Whitfield MF: Chondrodysplasia punctata after warfarin in early pregnancy. Case report and summary of the literature. *Arch. Dis. Child.* 55:139, 1980. Used by permission.)

eyelids; (c) *short neck;* (d) *low birth weight, short limbs, brachydactyly,* hypoplastic nails; (e) *respiratory difficulties;* (f) mental retardation; (g) other reported abnormalities: hydrocephalus, occipital meningocele, deafness, seizures, hypotonia, large clitoris, congenital heart disease, asplenia syndrome.

Radiological Manifestations: (a) *stippled calcification* (tubular bones, vertebrae, calcanei, ribs, pelvis, nose), tracheal cartilage calcification; (b) *short and broad hands, short distal phalanges, short long bones;* (c) *skull anomalies:* prominent occiput, extra fontanelles, frontal bossing; (d) radiodense skeleton (Fig SY—W—4).

REFERENCES

Cox DR, et al.: Asplenia syndrome after fetal exposure to warfarin. *Lancet* 2:1134, 1977.

Guillot M, et al.: Embryo-foetopathie coumarinique et maladie des epiphyses ponctuées. *Arch. Fr. Pediatr.* 36:63, 1979.

Hall JG: Maternal and fetal sequelae of anticoagulation during pregnancy. *Am. J. Med.* 68:122, 1980.

Johnson JF: Coumadin-induced chondrodysplasia punctata with increased skeletal density. *Skeletal Radiol.* 3:244, 1979.

Pawlow VI, et al.: Kumarin-embryopathie. *Z. Klin. Med.* 440:885, 1985.

Struwe FE, et al.: Coumarin-embryopathie. *Radiologe* 24:68, 1984.

Tamburrini O, et al.: Chondrodysplasia punctata after warfarin. Case report with 18-month follow-up. *Pediatr. Radiol.* 17:323, 1987.

Whitefield MF: Chondrodysplasia punctata after warfarin in early pregnancy. Case report and summary of the literature. *Arch. Dis. Child.* 55:139, 1980.

WATERHOUSE-FRIDERICHSEN SYNDROME

Clinical and Radiologic Manifestations: (a) fulminant bacterial sepsis, in particular, meningococcal septicemia; (b) disseminated intravascular coagulation (DIC); (c) shock; (d) bilateral adrenal hemorrhage (echo-free, mixed, or echogenic ultrasonographic picture).

Notes: (a) adrenocortical insufficiency is potentially reversible; (b) DIC in meningicoccemia may result in severe metaphyseal-epiphyseal changes (irregular ball-and-socket deformities).

REFERENCES

Friderichsen C: Nebennieren-apoplexie bei kleinen Kinderh. *Jahrb. Kinderh.* 87:109, 1918.

Lanman JT: Adrenal steroids in meningococcemia. *J. Pediatr.* 46:724, 1955.

Patriquin HB, et al.: Late sequelae of infantile meningococcemia in growing bones of children. *Radiology* 141:77, 1981.

Sarnaik AP, et al.: Ultrasound diagnosis of adrenal hemorrhage in meningococcemia. *Pediatr. Radiol.* 18:427, 1988.

Waterhouse R: A case of suprarenal apoplexy. *Lancet* 1:577, 1911.

WEAVER SYNDROME

Synonym: Weaver-Smith syndrome.

Frequency: Eight males and two females (Thompson et al.).

Clinical Manifestations: (a) *craniofacial features: broad forehead, flat occiput, large ears, ocular hypertelorism, prominent or long philtrum, relative micrognathia* associated with difficulty in swallowing; (b) *prenatal and postnatal growth excess;* (c) limb abnormalities: prominent fingerpads, camptodactyly, clinodactyly, broad thumbs, thin and deep-set nails, limited elbow or knee extension, foot deformities (clubfoot, calcaneovalgus, metatarsus adductus, pes cavus); (d) neurological manifestations: hypertonia, hypotonia, development delay, hoarse low-pitched voice; (e) other reported abnormalities: excess loose skin, umbilical hernia, diastasis recti, inguinal hernia, inverted nipples, etc.; (f) female-to-male ratio: 1:4.

Radiologic Manifestations: (a) *accelerated osseous maturation;* (b) small iliac wings, coxa valga, wide femoral necks, widened proximal femoral heads, widened distal portions of the femora and ulnae, unilateral distally dislocated ulna.

Differential Diagnosis: Marshall-Smith syndrome; Beckwith-Wiedemann syndrome; Sotos syndrome (Fig SY—W—5).

REFERENCES

Amir N, et al: Weaver-Smith syndrome. A case study with long-term follow-up. *Am. J. Dis. Child.* 138:1113, 1984.

Ardinger HH, et al.: Further delineation of Weaver syndrome. *J. Pediatr.* 108:228, 1986.

Farrell SA, et al.: Weaver syndrome with pes cavus. *Am. J. Med. Genet.* 21:737, 1985.

Fitch N: Update on the Marshall-Smith-Weaver controversy (letter). *Am. J. Med. Genet.* 20:559, 1985.

Roussounis SH, et al.: Siblings with Weaver syndrome. *J. Pediatr.* 102:595, 1983.

Thompson EM, et al.: A girl with the Weaver syndrome. *J. Med. Genet.* 24:232, 1987.

Weaver DD, Graham CB, Thomas IT, Smith DW: A new overgrowth syndrome with accelerated skeletal maturation, unusual facies, and camptodactyly. *J. Pediatr.* 84:547, 1974.

WEBER-CHRISTIAN SYNDROME

Synonyms: Weber-Christian panniculitis; Weber-Christian disease; Pfeifer-Weber-Christian syndrome.

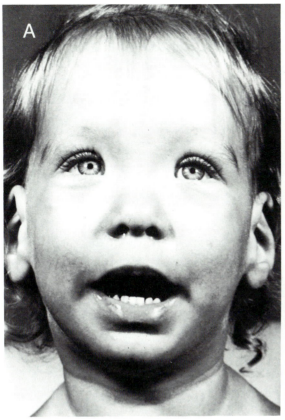 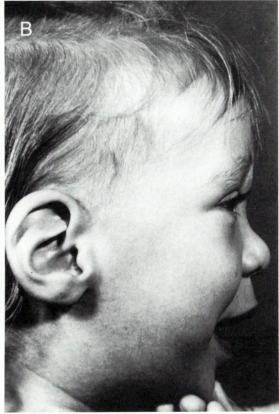

FIG SY–W–5.
A and **B,** Weaver syndrome. Note the broad forehead, hypertelorism, flat nasal bridge, long philtrum, large ears, and micrognathia. (From Ardinger HH, Hanson JW, Harrod MJE, et al.: Further delineation of Weaver syndrome. *J. Pediatr.* 108:228, 1986. Used by permission.)

Pathology: Nonsuppurative nodular panniculitis: infiltration of fatty tissues by inflammatory cells leading to fat necrosis and fibrosis; sites: subcutaneous fat; visceral, omental, and mesenteric fat; pericardiac fat; pancreas; kidney; adrenal glands; etc.

Clinical Manifestations: Most patients are middle-aged women: (a) *tenderness and skin redness followed by skin pigmentation and finally atrophy*, nodules, fever, arthritis/arthralgias, myalgia; (b) pulmonary, cardiac, or alimentary tract manifestations (rare); recurrent pneumonia; abdominal symptoms related to mesenteric panniculitis; liver cirrhosis; (c) hepatosplenomegaly (in some); (d) elevated erythrocyte sedimentation rate, anemia, leukopenia, hypocomplementemia, circulating 7S Igm or immune complexes (at the times of active symptoms); (e) association with other disorders: diabetes mellitus, pancreatitis, tuberculosis, autoimmune and collagen vascular diseases, malignant neoplasms, nephrotic syndrome, erythema nodosum, acute myelogenous leukemia, rheumatoid arthritis, systemic lupus erythematosus, sarcoid, immune complex glomerulonephritis, α_1-antitrypsin deficiency (two members of a family), chronic active hepatitis.

Radiologic Manifestations: Nonspecific findings: (a) *calcification of nodules;* (b) myocardosis with myocardial decompensation, coronary occlusion resulting from pericardial fibrosis; (c) pancreatitis, bone lesion related to pancreatitis (demineralization, destructive lesions in the hands and feet in association with periosteal reaction, pathological fracture); (d) granulomatous pneumonitis; (e) ileus caused by inflammatory changes of the bowel wall or mesentery; (f) other reported abnormalities: liver cirrhosis, retroperitoneal fibrosis, sterile splenic abscess, xanthogranoloma of the dura and leptomeninges (nonsuppurative inflammatory condition), sclerosing panniculitis of the mesentery (Fig SY–W–6).

REFERENCES

Bernstein JR: Nonsuppurative nodular panniculitis (Weber-Christian disease). An unusual cause of mammary calcifications. *J.A.M.A.* 238:1942, 1977.
Christian HA: Relapsing febrile nodular nonsuppurative panniculitis. *Arch. Intern. Med.* 42:338, 1928.
Clark P, et al.: Genetic study of a family with two members with Weber-Christian disease (panniculitis) and alpha 1 antitrypsin deficiency. *Am. J. Med. Genet.* 13:57, 1982.
Dupont AG, et al.: Weber-Christian panniculitis with membranous glomerulonephritis. *Am. J. Med.* 75:527, 1983.
Edge J, et al.: Weber-Christian panniculitis and chronic active hepatitis. *Eur. J. Pediatr.* 145:227, 1986.

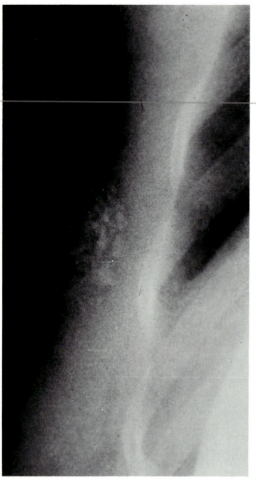

FIG SY−W−6.
Weber-Christian syndrome: calcified area in the left mammary of a 22-year-old female. (From Leonhardt T: A case of Weber-Christian disease; roentgenographically demonstrable mammary calcifications. *Am. J. Med.* 44:140, 1968. Used by permission.)

Gilchrist TC, et al.: A unique case of atrophy of the fatty layer of the skin preceded by the ingestion of the fat by large phagocytic cells, macrophages. *Johns Hopkins Hosp. Bull* 27:291, 1916.

Legmann P, et al.: Syndrome de Weber-Christian et affections pancreatiques. A propos d'un cas avec revue de la littérature. *J. Radiol.* 67:625, 1986.

Lemley DE, et al.: Sterile splenic abscesses in systemic Weber-Christian disease. Unique source of abdominal pain. *Am. J. Med.* 83:567, 1987.

Leonhardt T: A case of Weber-Christian disease with roentgenographically demonstrable mammary calcifications. *Am. J. Med.* 44:140, 1968.

Panush RS, et al.: Weber-Christian disease. Analysis of 15 cases and review of the literature. *Medicine (Baltimore)* 64:181, 1985.

Pfeifer V: Ueber einen Fall von herdweiser Atrophie des subkutanen Fettgewebes. *Dtsch. Arch. Klin. Med.* 50:438, 1892.

Pick P, et al.: Xanthrogranuloma of the dura in systemic Weber-Christian disease. *Neurology* 33:1067, 1983.

Sorensen RU, et al.: Ten-year course of early-onset Weber-Christian syndrome with recurrent pneumonia: A suggestion for pathogenesis. *Pediatrics* 78:115, 1986.

Srivastava RN, et al.: Weber-Christian disease with nephrotic syndrome. *Am. J. Dis. Child.* 127:420, 1974.

Stack J, et al.: Imaging of a case of sclerosing panniculitis. *Br. J. Radiol.* 59:1119, 1986.

Vassall JH II: Weber-Christian panniculitis with immune complex glomerulonephritis. *J. Natl. Med. Assoc.* 77:237, 1985.

Weber FP: A case of relapsing nonsuppurative nodular panniculitis showing phagocytosis of subcutaneous fat-cells by macrophages. *Br. J. Dermatol.* 37:301, 1925.

Zheutlin N, et al.: X-Ray sign in Weber-Christian disease. *J.A.M.A.* 189:580, 1964.

WEGENER GRANULOMATOSIS

Synonym: Lethal granulomatosis.

Pathology: *Angiitis, focal necrosis, and a granulomatous reaction beginning in the respiratory tract; progressive involvement of other tissues, including the development of focal necrotizing glomerulonephritis.*

Clinical Manifestations: May occur at any age, most common between the third and fifth decade of life; infrequent in children: (a) malaise, weight loss, fever, night sweats, vertigo; (b) *rhinorrhea, crust formation,* and obstruction of nasal passages; *dysosmia; ozena;* otitis media; mastoiditis; (c) dyspnea, *hemoptysis,* hoarseness, stridor; (d) ocular manifestations: nasolacrimal duct obstruction, optic nerve involvement, ocular muscle involvement, conjunctivitis, episcleritis, corneoscleral ulceration, uveitis, scleritis, vasculitis of the retina and optic nerve, orbital cellulitis, proptosis, retinal hemorrhage; (e) purpura, telangiectasia; (f) *albuminuria, hematuria, casts in the urine,* uremia; (g) anemia, leukocytosis, eosinophilia; (h) other reported abnormalities: cardiac involvement (coronary arteritis, pericarditis, arrhythmias), breast involvement (may be present before the development of typical clinical manifestations of the disease), gangrene of the feet.

Radiologic Manifestations: (a) initial osteoporosis of midline facial structures; (b) *tumorlike soft-tissue encroachment on the nasal passages and sinuses* and reactive bone changes (sclerosis), computed tomographic demonstration of orbital mass(es), bone and sinus destruction, trabecular bone formation within the sinuses, optic nerve involvement, compression of the optic nerve, retinal venous congestion and edema of the optic disk in association with a retrobulbar mass, flattening of the posterior aspect of the globe, extraocular muscle thickening, often bilateral orbital lesions, mastoiditis, invasion of cavernous sinus; (c) airway obstruction: subglottic mass, mass between the trachea and esophagus, tracheal stenosis, bronchial narrowing; (d) *granulomatous lung changes: solitary or multiple irregular nodular densities, cavitation of nodules,* patchy infiltrates, miliary lesions, reduced lung volume and diffusing capacity, atelectasis associated with endotracheal lesions, pleural thickening and effusion, spontaneous pneumothorax, pulmonary edema, bronchiectasis; (e) pericarditis, pericardial effusion; (f) urinary system: necrotizing urethritis, prostatic involvement, ureteral obstruction due to vasculitis, angiographic abnormalities (panarteritis nodosa, intrarenal arterial aneurysms, lumen variations and occlusions), spontaneous perinephritic hematoma; (g) other reported abnormalities: breast involvement mimicking carcinoma (mammography), cerebral vasculitis, cerebral edema, intracerebral hemorrhage.

REFERENCES

Allen DC, et al.: Pathology of the heart and the cardiac conduction system in Wegener's granulomatosis. *Br. Heart J.* 52:674, 1984.

Bennett RW, et al.: Wegener's granulomatosis presenting as vertigo. *West J. Med.* 146:359, 1987.

Bullen CL, et al.: Ocular complications of Wegener's granulomatosis. *Ophthalmology* 90:279, 1983.

Cohen MI, et al.: Tracheal and bronchial stenosis associated with mediastinal adenopathy in Wegener granulomatosis: CT findings. *J. Comput. Assist. Tomogr.* 8:327, 1984.

Deininger HK: Wegener granulomatosis of the breast. *Radiology* 154:59, 1985.

Farrelly CA: Wegener's granulomatosis: A radiological review of the pulmonary manifestations at initial presentation and during relapse. *Clin. Radiol.* 33:545, 1982.

Fowler M, et al.: Wegener granulomatosis. Unusual cause of necrotizing urethritis. *Urology* 14:66, 1979.

Goldberg AL, et al.: Wegener granulomatosis invading the cavernous sinus: A CT demonstration. *J. Comput. Assist. Tomogr.* 7:701, 1983.

Göthlin J, et al.: Renal and hepatic angiography in the late phase of Wegener's granulomatosis (WG). *Fortschr. Rontgenstr.* 136:338, 1982.

Hall SL, et al.: Wegener granulomatosis in pediatric patients. *J. Pediatr.* 106:739, 1985.

Hearne CB, et al.: Survival after intracerebral hemorrhage in Wegener's granulomatosis. *West. J. Med.* 137:431, 1982.

Jaspan T, et al.: Spontaneous pneumothorax in Wegener's granulomatosis. *Thorax* 37:774, 1982.

Kedziora JA, et al.: Limited form of Wegener's granulomatosis in ulcerative colitis. *A.J.R.* 125:127, 1975.

Lampman JH, et al.: Subglottic stenosis in Wegener's granulomatosis. *Chest* 79:230, 1981.

Maguire R, et al.: Unusual radiographic features of Wegener's granulomatosis. *A.J.R.* 130:233, 1978.

Monahan DW, et al.: Retinal hemorrhages as a disease parameter in Wegener's granulomatosis. *J. Natl. Med. Assoc.* 76:518, 1984.

Neumann G, et al.: Wegener's granulomatosis in childhood. Review of the literature and case report. *Pediatr. Radiol.* 14:267, 1984.

Paling MR, et al.: Paranasal sinus obliteration in Wegener granulomatosis. *Radiology* 144:539, 1982.

Phillips RW, et al.: Wegener's granulomatosis and gangrene in the feet. *Ann. Intern. Med.* 99:571, 1983.

Rouffiat J, et al.: Les lésions pulmonaires de la maladie de Wegener. *Ann. Radiol. (Paris)* 28:43, 1985.

Schiavone WA, et al.: Unusual cardiac complications of Wegener's granulomatosis. *Chest* 88:745, 1985.

Stein MG, et al.: Computed tomography of diffuse tracheal stenosis in Wegener granulomatosis. *J. Comput. Assist. Tomogr.* 10:868, 1986.

Stillwell TJ, et al.: Prostatic involvement in Wegener's granulomatosis. *J. Urol.* 138:1251, 1987.

Wechsler RJ, et al.: Chest radiograph in lymphomatoid granulomatosis: Comparison with Wegener granulomatosis. *A.J.R.* 142:79, 1984.

Wegener F: Ueber generalisierte, septische Gegasserkrankungen. *Verh. Dtsch. Ges. Pathol.* 29:202, 1936.

Yamashita Y, et al.: Cerebral vasculitis secondary to Wegener's granulomatosis: Computed tomography and angiographic findings. *J. Comput. Tomogr.* 10:115, 1986.

WEILL-MARCHESANI SYNDROME

Synonyms: Marchesani syndrome; spherophakia-brachymorphia syndrome; congenital mesodermal dysmorphodystrophy.

Mode of Inheritance: Genetic heterogeneity: most cases autosomal recessive, some autosomal dominant.

Frequency: Approximately 70 published cases to 1983 (Bebe).

Clinical Manifestations: (a) short stature with *disproportionate shortening of the limbs, in particular, distally;* (b) *spherophakia, microphakia, myopia,* ectopia lentis, glaucoma; (c) craniofacial features: pug nose, depressed nasal bridge, broad head, mild maxillary hypoplasia, narrow palate; (d) cardiovascular defects; (e) other reported abnormalities: malformed and malaligned teeth, hypertrophy of the limb muscles.

Radiological Manifestations: (a) *brachycephaly* or *scaphocephalic skull,* shallow orbits, hypotelorism, small maxillae and zygomatic arches; (b) *short metacarpals, metatarsals, and phalanges;* (c) skeletal maturation retardation; (d) other reported abnormalities: short and wide diaphyses, thin cortices, mild epiphyseal deformities, slight anterior rounded appearance of the vertebrae, narrow spinal canal, thinness of disk spaces, widened ribs, thickening of the skull vault.

REFERENCES

Bebe M: Les syndrome de Weill-Marchesani. A propos d'une observation. *Ann. Pediatr. (Paris)* 30:673, 1983.

Ferrier S, et al.: Le syndrome de Marchesani (sphérophakie-brachymorphie). *Helv. Paediatr. Acta* 35:185, 1980.

Gorlin RJ: Spherophakia-brachymorphia syndrome (Weill-Marchesani). *Semin. Roentgenol.* 8:236, 1973.

Marchesani O: Brachydactylie und angeborene Kugellinse als Systemarkrankung. *Klin. Monatsbl. Augenheilkd.* 103:392, 1939.

Weill G: Ectopie des cristallins et malformations générales. *Ann. D'ocul.* 169:21, 1932.

Young ID, et al.: Weill-Marchesani syndrome in mother and son. *Clin. Genet.* 30:475, 1986.

WEISMANN-NETTER SYNDROME

Synonyms: Weismann-Netter and Stuhl syndrome; tibio-peroneal diaphyseal toxopachyostosis.

Mode of Inheritance: Sporadic and familial cases (siblings, mother, and children, involvement over three generations through the female line); autosomal or X-linked dominant a good possibility.

Frequency: 40 published cases (Robinow et al).

Clinical Manifestations: (a) *dwarfism;* (b) *"saber shin"* deformity of the legs, usually bilateral, occasionally unilateral; (c) other reported abnormalities: anemia, goiter, mild mental retardation (20% of cases).

Radiological Manifestations: (a) *anterior bowing of the tibia and fibula with thickening of the posterior cortices* and distortion of the bony trabeculae in the midshafts; (b) other reported abnormalities: bowing of long bones (radius, ulna, femur), thickening of the cortex of tubular bones, small pelvis with "squaring" of the iliac wings, kyphoscoliosis, dural calcification, exaggerated trabeculation of the carpals and epiphyses of the metacarpals and phalanges, thinness of the posterior aspect of the ribs and exaggerated downward angulation.

Bone Biopsy: Normal bone.

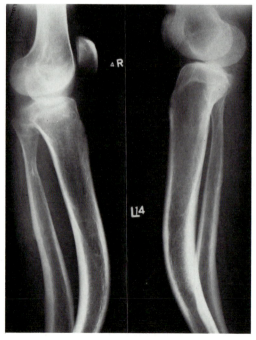

FIG SY–W–7.
Weismann-Netter syndrome in a 93-year-old male with anterior bowing of both legs and anterior bowing of the tibia and fibula with posterior cortical thickening. (From Alavi SM, Keats TE: Toxopachyostéose diaphysaire tibiopéronière (Weismann-Netter syndrome). *A.J.R.* 118:314, 1973. Used by permission.)

Differential Diagnosis: Syphilis; healed rickets; prenatal bowing; fibrous dysplasia; etc. (Fig SY–W–7).

REFERENCES

Alavi SM, Keats TE: Toxopachyostéose diaphysaire tibio-péronière (Weismann-Netter syndrome). *A.J.R.* 118:314, 1973.

Amendola MA, et al.: Weismann-Netter-Stuhl syndrome: Toxopachyostéose diaphysaire tibiopéronière. *A.J.R.* 135:1211, 1980.

Azimi F, et al.: Weismann-Netter-Stuhl syndrome (toxopachyostéose diaphysaire tibiopéronière). *Br. J. Radiol.* 47:618, 1977.

Hiller HG, et al.: Weismann-Netter syndrome (toxopachyostéose diaphysaire tibio-péronière). *Australas. Radiol.* 20:174, 1976.

Robinow M, et al.: The Weismann-Netter syndrome. *Am. J. Med. Genet.* 29:573, 1988.

Roca M, et al.: Le syndrome de Weismann-Netter-Stuhl. A propos de deux nouveaux cas. *Ann. Radiol. (Paris)* 30:401, 1987.

Weismann-Netter R, Stuhl L: D'une ostéopathie congenitale eventuellement familiale surtout definie par l'incurvation antero-postérieure et l'épaississement des deux os de la jambe (toxopachyostéose diaphysaire tibio-péronière). *Presse Med.* 62:1618, 1954.

WERDNIG-HOFFMANN DISEASE

Synonyms: Muscular atrophy (infantile); spinal muscular atrophy I; amyotonia congenita; Oppenheim disease.

Mode of Inheritance: Autosomal recessive.

Frequency: Uncommon.

Pathology: Degeneration of anterior horn cells of the spinal cord.

Clinical Manifestations: Onset before birth (30%) or soon after birth: (a) generalized *hypotonia,* expressionless face (facial muscle involvement); (b) *weakness;* (c) *diminished reflexes;* (d) recurrent pneumonia; (e) diaphragmatic paralysis causing respiratory failure in infancy, chest asymmetries; (f) median age of death: 7 months.

Radiologic Manifestations: (a) muscular atrophy and *replacement of muscle fibers by intramuscular fat;* (b) overtubulation of long bones; osteoporosis; birth fracture; congenital hip dislocation; flexion deformities, especially of the hands; (c) bell-shaped thoracic cage, plastic bowing of the ribs, diaphragmatic paralysis; (d) pharyngeal-laryngeal functional deficit, recurrent lung collapse and pneumonia.

Differential Diagnosis: Osteogenesis imperfeta (osteopenia, fractures).

REFERENCES

Burke SW, et al.: Birth fractures in spinal muscular atrophy. *J. Pediatr. Orthop.* 6:34, 1986.

Caro PA, et al.: Plastic bowing of ribs in children. *Skeletal Radiol.* 17:255, 1988.

Gay BB, et al.: Roentgenologic evaluation of disorders of muscle. *Semin. Roentgenol.* 8:25, 1973.

Grünebaum M, et al.: The pharyngo-laryngeal deficit in the acute form of infantile spinal muscular atrophy (Werdnig-Hoffmann disease). *Pediatr. Radiol.* 11:67, 1981.

Hoffmann J: Weitere Beiträge zur Lehre von der progressiven neurotischen Muskeldystrophie. *Dtsch. Z. Nervenheilkd.* 1:95, 1891.

Kuzubars S, et al.: Preservation of the phrenic motoneurons in Werdnig-Hoffmann disease. *Ann. Neurol.* 9:506, 1981.

McWilliam RC, et al.: Diaphragmatic paralysis due to spinal muscular atrophy. An unrecognised cause of respiratory failure in infancy? *Arch. Dis. Child.* 60:145, 1985.

Werdnig G: Zwei frühinfantile hereditäre Fälle von progressiver Muskelatrophie unter dem Bilde der dystrophie, aber auf neurotischer. *Grundlage. Arch. Psychiatr.* 22:437, 1891.

Gebhart E, et al.: Spontaneous and induced chromosomal instability in Werner syndrome. *Hum. Genet.* 80:135, 1988.

Goto M, et al.: Family analysis of Werner's syndrome: A survey of 42 Japanese families with a review of the literature. *Clin. Genet.* 19:8, 1981.

Jacobson HG, et al.: Werner's syndrome: A clinical-roentgen entity. *Radiology* 74:373, 1961.

Ohno T, et al.: Life span elongation of Werner's syndrome fibroblasts by co-culture with origin-defective SV-40 DNA transformed cells. *Hum. Genet.* 68:209, 1984.

Rosen RS, et al.: Werner's syndrome. *Br. J. Radiol.* 43:193, 1970.

Saeki H, et al.: Bladder carcinoma with Werner syndrome. *Urology* 30:494, 1987.

Salk D: Werner's syndrome: A review of recent research with an analysis of connective tissue metabolism, growth control of cultured cells, and chromosomal aberrations. *Hum. Genet.* 62:1, 1982.

Tri TB, et al.: Congestive cardiomyopathy in Werner's syndrome. *Lancet* 1:1052, 1978.

Werner CWO: *Ueber Katarakt in Verbindung mit Sklerodermie* (doctoral dissertation). Kiel, West Germany, 1904.

WERNER SYNDROME

Synonyms: Progeria adultorum; adult progeria.

Mode of Inheritance: Autosomal recessive.

Frequency: Rare.

Clinical Manifestations: (a) *premature aging* with an onset after adolescence (premature grayness, alopecia, loss of pubic and axillary hair, atrophy of muscle and subcutaneous tissues); (b) *cataract*; (c) scleromatous skin changes; (d) abnormal *high-pitched voice*; (e) *short stature* with a relatively large trunk and spindly extremities; (f) *impotence and sterility*; (g) atherosclerosis; (h) organic brain syndrome; (i) coexistence of malignant tumors (in 10%); (j) adult-type diabetes; (k) somatic chromosome aberrations (chromosome instability) in multiple tissues in vivo and in vitro.

Radiologic Manifestations: (a) soft-tissue atrophy; (b) *osteoporosis*; (c) *atherosclerosis with calcification;* (d) soft-tissue calcification (in particular, ligamentous about the knees); (e) osteoarthritis of the peripheral joints; (f) spondylosis deformans; (g) neurotrophic bone changes; (h) coronary artery disease, congestive heart failure, cardiomyopathy.

REFERENCES

Cerimele D, et al.: High prevalence of Werner's syndrome in Sardinia. Description of six patients and estimate of the gene frequency. *Hum. Genet.* 62:25, 1982.

Darlington GJ, et al.: Sister chromatid exchange frequencies in progeria and Werner syndrome patients. *Am. J. Hum. Genet.* 33:762, 1981.

WERNICKE-KORSAKOFF SYNDROME

Clinical Manifestations: Most common occurrence in chronic alcoholics; an inborn disorder in metabolism (presumably autosomal recessive) with clinical manifestations presented only when the diet is deficient in thiamine: (a) confusion, loss of memory, seizures, etc.; (b) ataxia; (c) ophthalmoplegia.

Radiologic Manifestations: Symmetrical, low-density thalmic lesions (computed tomography).

REFERENCES

Blass JP, et al.: Abnormality of a thiamine-requiring enzyme in patients with Wernicke-Korsakoff syndrome. *N. Engl. J. Med.* 297:1367, 1977.

Blass JP, et al.: Genetic factors in Wernicke-Korsakoff syndrome. *Alcoholism Clin. Exp. Res.* 3:126, 1979.

Leigh D, et al.: Wernicke-Korsakoff syndrome in monozygotic twins: A biochemical peculiarity. *Br. J. Psychiatry* 139:156, 1981.

McDowell JR, et al.: Computed tomographic findings in Wernicke-Korsakoff syndrome. *Arch. Neurol.* 41:454, 1984.

Nixon PK, et al.: An erythrocyte transketolase isoenzyme pattern associated with Wernicke-Korsakoff syndrome. *Eur. J. Clin. Invest.* 14:278, 1984.

WET LUNG SYNDROME

Synonym: Transient tachypnea of the newborn.

Probable Pathophysiology: Delay in removal of alveolar fluid.

Clinical Manifestations: (a) *tachypnea beginning at birth or shortly after birth* and lasting 2 to 5 days; (b) retraction; (c) grunting respiration; (d) mild cyanosis (in some); (e) echocardiography: increased left ventricular pre-ejection period-to-ejection time ratio in the classic (mild) form; increased left ventricular pre-ejection period-to-ejection time ratio and right ventricular pre-ejection-to-ejection time ratio in the severe form, generalized myocardial failure, pulmonary hypertension, and right-to-left shunting.

Radiologic Manifestations: (a) borderline heart size or minimal cardiomegaly; (b) *prominent vascular markings;* (c) *widened interlobar fissures,* minimal fluid in costophrenic angles; (d) Kerley lines (rare); (e) *resolution of above findings within a few hours to 5 days.*

Differential Diagnosis: Group B streptococcal sepsis; polycythemia; pulmonary lymphangiectasis; congenital cardiovascular diseases with obstructive pulmonary venous return.

Notes: (a) low neonatal serum protein levels may be associated with the wet lung syndrome; (b) transient worsening of pulmonary parenchymal opacities and appearance of pleural effusion may occasionally present as an atypical picture of the syndrome.

REFERENCES

Avery ME, et al.: Transient tachypnea of newborn: Possible delayed resorption of fluid at birth. *Am. J. Dis. Child.* 111:380, 1966.
Bloom BT, et al.: Wet lung syndrome. *Am. J. Dis. Child.* 140:969, 1986.
Glasier CM, et al.: Progressive chest radiographic changes in wet lung disease. *Am. J. Perinatol.* 2:198, 1985.
Halliday HL, et al.: Transient tachypnoea of the newborn: Two distinct clinical entities? *Arch. Dis. Child.* 56:322, 1981.
Kuhn JP, et al.: Roentgen findings in transient tachypnea of the newborn. *Radiology* 92:751, 1969.
Rawlings JS, et al: Radiological case of the month. *Am. J. Dis. Child.* 139:1233, 1985.
Wesenberg RL, et al.: Radiological findings in wet-lung disease. *Radiology* 98:69, 1971.

WEYERS ACRODENTAL DYSOSTOSIS

Synonym: Acrofacial dysostosis.

Mode of Inheritance: Autosomal dominant.

Frequency: Very rare.

Clinical and Radiologic Manifestations: (a) *postaxial polydactyly of the hands and feet;* (b) *dental anomalies* (shape, number, implantation of the upper and lower incisors); (c) mandibular cleft; (d) other reported abnormalities: radial clinodactyly and hypoplasia of the nails of the fifth fingers, partial syndactyly of the second and third toes.

REFERENCES

Curry CJ, et al.: Polydactyly, conical teeth, nail dysplasia, and short limbs: A new autosomal dominant malformation syndrome. *Birth Defects* 15(5B):253, 1979.
Roubicek M, et al.: Syndrome of polydactyly, conical teeth and nail dysplasia (letter). *Am. J. Med. Genet.* 20:205, 1985.
Roubicek M, et al.: Weyers acrodental dysostosis in a family. *Clin. Genet.* 26:587, 1984.
Shapiro SD, et al.: Curry-Hall syndrome. *Am. J. Med. Genet.* 17:579, 1984.
Weyers H: Hexadactylie, Unterkieferspalt und Oligodontie, ein neuer Syndromenkomplex (Dysostosis acro-facialis). *Ann. Paediatr. (Basel)* 181:45, 1953.
Weyers H: Uber eine korrelierte Missbildung der Kiefer—und Extremittätenakren (Dysostosis acro-facialis). *Fortschr. Rontgenstr.* 77:562, 1952.

WEYERS SYNDROME OF DEFICIENCY OF ULNAR AND FIBULAR RAYS

Frequency: Extremely rare.

Clinical and Radiologic Manifestations: (a) *deficiency of the ulnar and fibular rays;* (b) other reported abnormalities: antecubital pterygia, reduced sternal segments, renal anomalies, cleft lip/palate, hypoplasia of the maxilla, dental deformities.

REFERENCES

Elejalde BR, et al.: Prenatal diagnosis of Weyers syndrome (deficient ulnar and fibular rays with bilateral hydronephrosis). *Am. J. Med. Genet.* 21:439, 1985.
Weyers H: Das Oligodactylie Syndrom des Menschen und seine Parallelmutation bei der Hausmaus. *Ann. Paediatr. (Basel)* 189:351, 1957.

WIEDEMANN-RAUTENSTRAUCH SYNDROME

Synonyms: Progeroid syndrome, neonatal; neonatal progeroid syndrome.

Mode of Inheritance: Autosomal recessive.

Frequency: Six published cases (Rudin et al.).

Clinical Manifestations: (a) *smallness for age, growth deficiency;* (b) craniofacial features: *progeroid face,* hydrocephaloid skull, widely open sutures, persistently open fontanelle, prominent scalp veins, sparse scalp hair, low-set ears, hypoplasia of the facial bones, beaked-shaped nose, natal teeth; (c) *large hands and feet with long fingers and toes;* (d) *generalized paucity of subcutaneous fat, prominence of muscles*

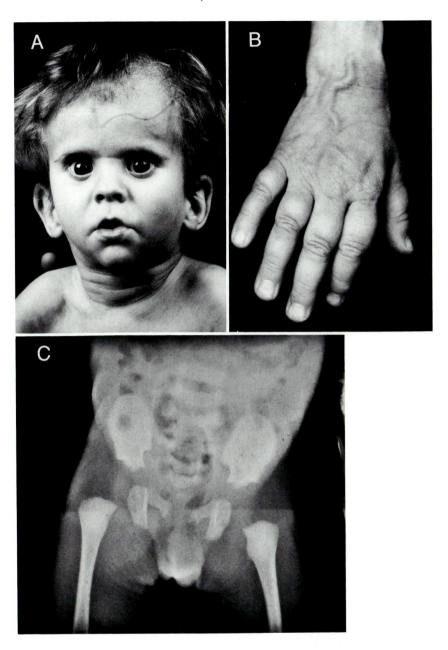

FIG SY—W—8.
Wiedemann-Rautenstrauch syndrome. **A,** progeroid facial features of a male at 20 months of age. **B,** paradoxical cushions of subcutaneous fat between the finger joints; prominent, enlarged veins. **C,** radiograph of the pelvis at birth: hypoplastic os ilium with a trident configuration of the acetabula. (From Rudin C, Thommen L, Fliegel C, et al.: The neonatal pseudo-hydrocephalic progeroid syndrome (Wiedemann-Rautenstrauch). Report of a new patient and review of the literature. *Eur. J. Pediatr.* 147:433, 1988. Used by permission.)

and veins, paradoxical fat accumulation during infancy (buttocks, flanks, anogenital area); (e) demyelination of the central nervous system with lesions characteristic of pure sudanophilic leukodystrophy (a case report, Martin et al.).

   Radiologic Manifestations: *Large neurocranium; wide cranial sutures; abnormally small, dense, unerupted teeth; small ilium in a neonate with a "trident configuration" of the acetabula* (Fig SY—W—8).

REFERENCES

Devos EA, et al.: The Wiedemann-Rautenstrauch or neonatal progeroid syndrome. *Eur. J. Pediatr.* 136:245, 1981.
Martin JJ, et al.: The Wiedemann-Rautenstrauch or neonatal progeroid syndrome. Neuropathological study of a case. *Neuropediatrics* 15:43, 1984.
Rautenstrauch T, et al.: Progeria: A cell culture study and clinical report of familial incidence. *Eur. J. Pediatr.* 124:101, 1977.

Rudin C, et al.: The neonatal pseudo-hydrocephalic progeroid syndrome (Wiedemann-Rautenstrauch). Report of a
new patient and review of the literature. *Eur. J. Pediatr.*
147:433, 1988.
Wiedemann HR: An unidentified neonatal progeroid syndrome: Follow-up report. *Eur. J. Pediatr.* 130:65, 1979.

WILDERVANCK SYNDROME

Synonym: Cervico-oculo-acoustic syndrome.

Mode of Inheritance: Unknown; almost exclusively affects females.

Frequency: Uncommon.

Clinical Manifestations: (a) *congenital perceptive deafness;* (b) *retraction of the bulb* in one or both eyes, *Duane
syndrome* (narrowing of the palpebral fissure(s) on adduction), *abducens paralysis;* (c) other reported abnormalities: facial hypoplasia, facial and cranial asymmetry, preauricular
appendages, subconjunctival lipoma, defective teeth, Klippel-Feil deformity, subluxation of the lens, facial paralysis,
cervical encephalocele.

Radiological Manifestations: (a) *fused cervical vertebrae,*
fused upper thoracic vertebrae, occipitocervical fusion, occipital vertebrae, spina bifida occulta; (b) constricted internal
auditory meatus, underdevelopment of the bony labyrinth
(cochlea and vestibular apparatus), often an absence of semi-

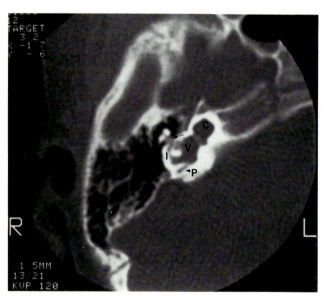

FIG SY–W–9.
Wildervanck syndrome. axial computed tomography of the right
temporal bone shows a cystic cochlea *(c)*, a dilated vestibule *(v)*,
and posterior *(p)* and lateral *(l)* semicircular canals. Notice the abnormally thick stapes crura *(arrow)*. (From Schild JA, Mafee MF,
Miller MF: Wildervanck syndrome—The external appearance and
radiologic findings. *Int. J. Pediatr. Otorhinolaryngol.* 7:305, 1984.
Used by permission.)

circular canals, Mondini deformity, stapes anomaly, etc. (Fig
SY–W–9).

REFERENCES

Cremers CWRJ, et al.: Hearing loss in the cervico-oculo-
acoustic (Wildervanck) syndrome. *Arch. Otolaryngol.*
110:54, 1984.
Giroud M, et al.: Les anomalies radiologiques dans le syndrome de Wildervanck. *J. Radiol.* 64:131, 1983.
Schild JA, et al.: Wildervanck syndrome—The external appearance and radiologic findings. *Int. J. Pediatr. Otorhinolaryngol.* 7:305, 1984.
Strisciuglio P, et al.: Wildervanck's syndrome with bilateral
subluxation of lens and facial paralysis. *J. Med. Genet.*
20:72, 1983.
Wildervanck LS: Een geval van aandoening van Klippel-Feil
gecombinurd met abducens paralyse, retractio bulbi en
doofstomheid. *Ned. Tijdschr. Geneeskd.* 96:2752, 1952.
Wildervanck LS: Een cervico-oculo-acousticus syndroom.
Ned. Tijdschr. Geneeskd. 104:2600, 1960.
Wildervanck LS, et al.: Radiological examination of the inner ear of deaf-mute presenting the cervico-
oculo-acusticus syndrome. *Acta Otolaryngol.* 61:445,
1966.

WILLIAMS SYNDROME

Synonyms: Idiopathic hypercalcemia-supravalvular aortic stenosis syndrome; elfin facies syndrome; Williams-
Beuren syndrome.

Mode of Inheritance: Autosomal dominant for supravalvular aortic stenosis; Williams syndrome described in
monozygotic twins and second cousins; supravalvular aortic
stenosis and Williams syndrome have been considered the
ends of a spectrum for an autosomal dominant gene defect of
variable penetrance and expression.

Frequency: Gene frequency at least 1:10,000 (Burn).

Clinical Manifestations: (a) *facial dysmorphism:* broad
forehead, medial eyebrow flare, depressed nasal bridge, anteverted and small nose, full and heavy cheeks, long philtrum, pointed chin, widely opened mouth, pouting lips, ocular hypotelorism, prominent ears, periorbital fullness, strabismus, blue eyes with a stellate pattern of the iris, malocclusion
of the teeth; (b) *growth deficiency;* (c) mild to moderate *mental retardation;* overly affectionate, trusting, and outgoing personality; gross and fine motor deficiencies; delayed language
development; talkative; good articulation skills; hypersensi-
tive to sound; (d) impaired calcitonin secretion, persistently
elevated 1,25-dihydroxyvitamin D levels (case report), hypercalcemia in infancy possibly caused by an abnormality in the
regulation of circulating 25-hydroxyvitamin D; (e) *cardiovascular diseases,* systemic hypertension secondary to peripheral
vascular anomalies; (f) dental anomalies: late eruption, microdontia, small roots, invagination of the incisors, malocclusion, pathological folding of the buccal mucosa; (g) other re-

REFERENCES

Böttiger LE, et al.: Wissler's syndrome. *Acta Med. Scand.* 174:415, 1963.

Campanacci D: Sindrome di Wissler-Fanconi in adulti. *G. Clin. Med.* 52:475, 1971.

Fanconi G: Ueber einen Fall von Subsepsis allergica Wissler. *Helv. Paediatr. Acta* 1:532, 1946.

Ström J: Wissler's syndrome. *Acta Paediatr. Scand.* 54:91, 1965.

Wissler H: Ueber eine besondere Form sepsisähnlicher Krankheiten (Subsepsis hyperergica). *Monatsschr. Kinderheilkd.* 94:1, 1943.

WOLFF-PARKINSON-WHITE SYNDROME

Clinical and Radiologic Manifestations: (a) *abnormal electrocardiographic pattern: short PR interval, widened QRS complex, initial delta wave;* (b) association with cardiac and noncardiac diseases: Ebstein anomaly of the tricuspid valve, idiopathic hypertrophic subaortic stenosis, congenitally corrected transposition of the great arteries, congenital hydrops, episodic appearance of supraventricular tachycardia, hand and foot anomalies; (c) abnormal echographic pattern of left ventricular posterior wall and interventricular septum motions.

REFERENCES

Angel J, et al.: Idiopathic hypertrophic subaortic stenosis and Wolff-Parkinson-White syndrome. *Chest* 68:248, 1975.

Hishida H, et al.: Echocardiographic patterns of ventricular contraction in the Wolff-Parkinson-White syndrome. *Circulation* 54:567, 1976.

Lauener P-A, et al.: Congenital hydrops and WPW syndrome. *Pediatr. Cardiol.* 6:113, 1985.

Nakajima K, et al.: Congenitally corrected transposition of the great arteries associated with the pre-excitation syndrome. *Clin. Nucl. Med.* 11:564, 1986.

Niarchos AP, et al.: Association of Wolff-Parkinson-White syndrome with congenital abnormalities of hands and feet. *Br. Heart J.* 36:409, 1974.

Robinson K, et al.: Wolff-Parkinson-White syndrome: Atrial fibrillation as the presenting arrhythmia. *Br. Heart J.* 59:578, 1988.

Wolff L, Parkinson J, White PD: Bundle-branch block with short P−R interval in healthy young people prone to paroxysmal tachycardia. *Am. Heart J.* 5:685, 1930.

WRINKLY SKIN SYNDROME

Mode of Inheritance: Autosomal recessive most likely; consanguinity.

Clinical and Radiological Manifestations: (a) *wrinkly skin of the dorsum of the hands and feet, increased palmar and plantar creases, prominent vein pattern, skin hypoelasticity, dry skin;* (b) small for gestational age, failure to thrive, developmental delay, hypotonia; (c) *microcephaly,* brachycephaly, midface hypoplasia; (d) *decreased muscle mass, winged scapulae;* (e) congenital hip "dysplasia," joint hyperextensibility; (f) mental retardation; (g) other reported abnormalities: kyphosis, lordosis, scoliosis, myopia, chorioretinitis, transverse wrinkling of the abdomen, atrial septal aneurysm.

Differential Diagnosis: Cutis laxa; geoderma osteodysplastica; pseudoxanthoma elasticum.

Note: The reported cases have been from the Middle East (Jewish and Arab) (Fig SY−W−13).

REFERENCES

Casamassima AC, et al.: Wrinkly skin syndrome: Phenotype and additional manifestations. *Am. J. Med. Genet.* 27:885, 1987

Gazit ERM, et al.: The wrinkly skin syndrome: A new heritable disorder of connective tissue. *Clin. Genet.* 4:186, 1973.

Karrar ZA, et al.: The wrinkly skin syndrome: A report of two siblings from Saudi Arabia. *Clin. Genet.* 23:308, 1983.

YELLOW NAIL SYNDROME

Synonym: Yellow nails-bronchiectasis-lymphedema syndrome.

Frequency: Over 60 published cases (Coche et al.).

Clinical Manifestations: Onset of symptoms in adult life, onset in childhood rare: (a) *thickened, smooth, and discolored (yellow or green) nails with transverse ridging and excessive curvature; onycholysis;* (b) *primary lymphedema* (edema of the ankles and, occasionally, of the upper extremities, face, and thorax); (c) chronic cough; (d) propensity to malignancy; (e) other reported abnormalities: incomplete form of the syndrome; association with malignancies, immunologic disorders (hypogammaglobulinemia, IgM deficiency, IgA deficiency), thyroid disorders (thyrotoxicosis, thyroid deficiency, etc.), rheumatoid arthritis, tuberculosis.

Radiological Manifestations: (a) recurrent pleural effusion, pericardial effusion, chylothorax; (b) *bronchiectasis;* (c) sinusitis; (d) *hypoplasia of the lymphatic system.*

Note: The typical components of the triad of yellow discoloration of the nails, lymphedema, and chronic respiratory tract disease may not be present, or they may appear at different intervals (months to years) (Fig SY−Y−1).

REFERENCES

Angelillo VA, et al.: Yellow nail syndrome with reduced glucose level in pleural fluid. *Chest* 75:83, 1979.

Beer DJ, et al.: Pleural effusion associated with primary lymphadema: A perspective on the yellow nail syndrome. *Am. Rev. Respir. Dis.* 117:595, 1978.

Coche G, et al.: Le syndrome des ongles jaunes. A propos d'un cas. Revue de ses principales manifestations radiologiques. *J. Radiol.* 67:435, 1986.

Levillain Cl, et al.: Syndrome des ongles jaunes. Revue de la littérature à propos de deux cas associés a un cancer. *Ann. Med. Interne (Paris)* 135:440, 1984.

Magid M, et al.: The yellow nail syndrome in an 8-year-old girl. *Pediatr. Dermatol.* 4:90, 1987.

Samman PD, et al.: The "yellow nail" syndrome. *Br. J. Dermatol.* 76:153, 1964.

Thomas PS, et al.: Yellow nail syndrome and bronchial carcinoma. *Chest* 92:191, 1987.

Valmary J, et al.: Une cause rare de chylothorax: Le syndrome des ongles jaunes. *Presse Med.* 15:1640, 1986.

Wakasa M, et al.: Yellow nail syndrome associated with chronic pericardial effusion. *Chest* 92:366, 1987.

YOUNG SYNDROME

Synonyms: Sinusitis-infertility syndrome; Barry-Perkins-Young syndrome.

Mode of Inheritance: Possibly autosomal recessive.

Clinical Manifestations: (a) azoospermia owing to bilateral epididymal obstruction; (b) chronic and recurrent upper and lower respiratory infections.

Radiological Manifestations: (a) sinusitis; (b) bronchitis, bronchiectasis.

Differential Diagnosis: Cystic fibrosis; ciliary dyskinesia (immotile-cilia syndrome).

REFERENCES

Handelsman DJ, et al.: Young's syndrome: Obstructive azoospermia and chronic sinopulmonary infections. *N. Engl. J. Med.* 310:3, 1984.

Hughes TM, et al.: Young's syndrome: An often unrecog-

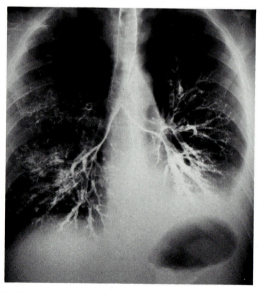

FIG SY−Y−1.
Yellow nail syndrome in a 40-year-old male with a moderate amount of left pleural effusion and bronchiectasis of the left lower lobe, lingula, and anterior segments of the left upper lobe. (From Hiller E, Rosenow EC, Olsen AM: Pulmonary manifestations of yellow nail syndrome. *Chest* 61:452, 1972. Used by permission.)

nized correctable cause of obstructive azoospermia. *J. Urol.* 137:1238, 1987.

Lau K-Y, et al.: Young's syndrome. An association between male sterility and bronchiectasis. *West J. Med.* 144:744, 1986.

Young D: Surgical treatment of male infertility. *J. Reprod. Fertil.* 23:541, 1970.

YOUSSEF SYNDROME

Synonyms: Menouria; postcesarean menouria.

Pathology: Communication between the uterus and bladder after a lower-segment cesarean section, etc.

Clinical Manifestations: (a) cyclic hematuria; (b) absence of vaginal bleeding; (c) urinary continence.

Radiological Manifestations: demonstration of uterocystic communication by cystography or hysterosalpingography.

REFERENCES

Nel JT, et al.: Youssef's syndrome: A case report. *J. Urol.* 133:95, 1985.

Medeiros AD, et al.: Youssef's syndrome. *J. Urol.* 109:828, 1973.

Youssef AF: "Menouria" following lower segment caesarean section. A syndrome. *Am. J. Obstet. Gynecol.* 73:759, 1957.

Z

ZIMMERMANN-LABAND SYNDROME

Synonyms: Laband syndrome; gingival fibromatosis—abnormal fingers.

Mode of Inheritance: Autosomal dominant.

Frequency: 16 cases (de Pina Neto et al.)

Clinical and Radiologic Manifestations: (a) *gingival hypertrophy or fibromatosis;* (b) bulbous soft nose, thick floppy ears, absence or dysplasia of the nails, hypertrichosis; (c) *clubbed "tree frog—like" fingers and toes, absence or hypoplasia of the terminal phalanges of the hands and feet, hyperextensibility of the joints;* (d) other reported abnormalities: mental retardation, asymmetry of the limbs, kyphosis, scoliosis, hepatomegaly, splenomegaly, contractures, (hips and knees), soft skin, large tongue, thick lips, etc.

REFERENCES

Chodirker BN, et al.: Zimmermann-Laband syndrome and profound mental retardation. *Am. J. Med. Genet.* 25:543, 1986.

de Pina Neto JM, et al.: A new case of Zimmermann-Laband syndrome with mild mental retardation, asymmetry of limbs, and hypertrichosis. *Am. J. Med. Genet.* 31:691, 1988.

Laband PF, et al.: Hereditary gingival fibromatosis. Report of an affected family with associated splenomegaly and skeletal and soft tissue abnormalities. *Oral Surg.* 17:339, 1964.

Zimmermann: Uber Anomalien des Ektoderms. *Vjschr. Zahnheilk.* 44:419, 1928.

PART II

Metabolic Disorders

Hooshang Taybi, M.D., M.Sc.

ABETALIPOPROTEINEMIA

Synonyms: Bassen-Kornzweig syndrome; acanthocytosis (thorny red cell).

Mode of Inheritance: Autosomal recessive; an autosomal dominant mode of inheritance has also been suggested.

Clinical Manifestations: (a) *degenerative nervous system disease* involving the cerebellum, long tracts, and peripheral nerves with Friedreich-like ataxia; (b) *acanthocytosis (thorny red cells)*; (c) *atypical retinitis pigmentosa*; (d) *steatorrhea, malabsorption of fat and fat-soluble vitamins*; (e) *absent or greatly reduced β-lipoprotein demonstrable by immunoelectrophoresis*; (f) *other reported abnormalities*: cardiac dysrhythmia; paroxysmal tachycardia; fatty liver; association with acrodermatitis enteropathica; reduced serum cholesterol and triglyceride levels; reduced red cell phosphatidyl choline and linoleic acid; increased red cell sphingomyelin; positive red cell peroxide hemolysis test for vitamin E; oxalate urolithiasis (excessive absorption of dietary oxalate related to unabsorbed fatty acids in the bowel lumen and the formation of insoluble calcium oxalate crystals); early occurrence of hemorrhagic, neurological, and hepatic disturbances leading to death.

Radiologic Manifestations: (a) *thickening of small-intestinal folds* (most marked in the duodenum and jejunum), thickening of the colonic haustra and abnormally prominent mucosal folds; (b) *cardiac failure* in advanced cases (interstitial myocardial fibrosis); (c) *urolithiasis*.

REFERENCES

Bassen FA, Kornzweig AL: Malformations of the erythrocytes in a case of atypical retinitis pigmentosa. *Blood* 5:381, 1950.

Dische MR, et al.: The cardiac lesions in Bassen-Kornzweig syndrome. *Am. J. Med.* 49:568, 1970.

Grise P, et al.: Lithiase oxalique associée à une abêtalipoprotéinemie. *Chir. Pediatr.* 24:411, 1983.

Suarex L, et al.: Abetalipoproteinemia associated with hepatic and atypical neurological disorders. *J. Pediatr. Gastroenterol. Nutr.* 6:799, 1987.

Wallis K, et al.: Acrodermatitis enteropathica associated with low density lipoprotein deficiency. *Clin. Pediatr. (Phila.)* 13:749, 1974.

Weinstein MA, et al.: Abetalipoproteinemia. *Radiology* 108:269, 1973.

Wichman A, et al.: Peripheral neuropathy in abetalipoproteinemia. *Neurology* 35:1279, 1985.

ACROMEGALY AND GIGANTISM

Mode of Inheritance: Sporadic nonfamilial; familial occurrence extremely rare: both autosomal recessive and autosomal dominant have been suggested.

Etiology: See Table ME–A–1.

Clinical Manifestations: See Table ME–A–2.

Radiologic Manifestations:

(A) GIGANTISM: (a) *tumor*: sellar contour abnormality; bone erosion, low density and isodensity of the pituitary tumor on computed tomographic (CT) examination, focal areas of hypointensity on T_1-weighted images on magnetic resonance imaging, extrasellar extension; (b) *accelerated skeletal growth*; normal or retarded bone age; *delay in closure of the growth plate*, which may remain open into adult life; (c) increase in width of the tubular bones; (d) osteopenia (probably due to hypercalciuria).

(B) ACROMEGALY: (a) *craniofacial findings*: enlarged sella turcica and bone erosion, enlargement of the paranasal sinuses and mastoid cells, hyperostosis of the calvaria in the frontal and occipital regions, elongation and widening of the

TABLE ME–A–1.
Etiology of Hypersomatotropism*

Pituitary
  Eutopic
    Densely granulated growth hormone cell adenoma
    Sparsely granulated growth hormone cell adenoma
    Mixed growth hormone cell and prolactin cell adenoma
    Mammosomatotrope cell adenoma
    Acidophil stem cell adenoma
    Plurihormonal adenoma
  Ectopic
    Aberrant growth hormone cell adenoma
      Sphenoid sinus
      Parapharyngeal sinuses
Extrapituitary
  Ectopic growth hormone–secreting tumor
    Pancreas
  Excess GHRH† secretion
    Eutopic—hypothalamic hamartoma
    Ectopic—pancreatic islet cell tumors; bronchial and intestinal carcinoid
Acromegaloidism

*From Melamed S, Fagin JA: Acromegaly update—etiology, diagnosis and management. *West J. Med.* 146:328, 1987. Used by permission.
†GHRH = growth hormone-releasing hormone.

mandible, widening of the mandibular angle; (b) *spine:* widening of the atlantoaxial joint, enlargement of vertebrae, scalloping of the posterior border of vertebral bodies, increase in the kyphotic curve of the thoracic spine, osteoporosis, osteophyte formation, spinal canal stenosis; (c) *ribs:* elongation and thickening, enlargement of costochondral junctions, sclerotic costal margins, wavy lower costal borders, calcification and ossification of the costal cartilages; (d) *limbs:* thickening of soft tissue (positive heel pad sign); widening of joint spaces due to cartilage hypertrophy; thickening of the cortex of the shaft of tubular bones, in particular in the hands and feet; spadelike appearance of the distal phalanges of the hands and feet; increase in number and size of the sesamoids of the hands and feet; (e) other reported abnormalities: ecta-

sia of cerebral arteries, prominence of phalangeal arteries, thickening of the bronchial wall, association with polyostotic fibrous dysplasia, partial carpal fusion, Charcot joints, calcification of the pinna, enlarged cavernous portion of the internal carotid arteries with prolapse into the sella turcica ("kissing intrasellar arteries"), metatarsal penciling, association with suprasellar and pulmonary hemangiopericytoma, association with Zollinger-Ellison syndrome, upper airway obstruction due to a significant increase in the thickness of the true and the false cords, extraocular muscle enlargement, proptosis, etc.

Differential Diagnosis: Sotos syndrome (Figs ME–A–1, and ME–A–2).

TABLE ME–A–2.

Acromegaly—Clinical and Metabolic Features*

Local	
Visual field defects; cranial nerve palsy; headache	
Abdominal or chest mass	
Somatic	
Acral enlargement	Increased heel pad thickness, prognathism, hypertrophy of the frontal bones, malocclusion, macroglossia
Musculoskeletal	Arthralgias, hypertrophic arthropathy, carpal tunnel syndrome, acroparesthesias, proximal myopathy
Skin	Hyperhydrosis, skin tags, acanthosis nigricans
Colon	Polyposis, carcinoma
Cardiovascular	Left ventricular hypertrophy, asymmetrical septal hypertrophy, hypertension, congestive heart failure, arrhythmias, myocardial infarction
Sleep disturbances	Sleep apnea, narcolepsy
Visceromegaly	Salivary glands, liver, spleen, kidney
Metabolic and Endocrine	
Carbohydrate	Insulin resistance and hyperinsulinemia, impaired glucose tolerance, diabetes mellitus
Lipids	Hypertriglyceridemia
Mineral	Hypercalciuria, increased 1,25-dihydroxyvitamin D_3, increased urinary hydroxyproline
Electrolyte	Low renin, increased aldosterone
Gonadal	Menstrual abnormalities, galactorrhea, decreased libido, impotence, low testosterone-binding globulin
Thyroid	Thyromegaly, hyperthyroidism, low thyroid-binding globulin
Multiple endocrine neoplasia (I)	Hyperparathyroidism, pancreatic islet cell tumors

*From Melamed S, Fagin JA: Acromegaly update—etiology, diagnosis and management. *West J. Med.* 146:328, 1987. Used by permission.

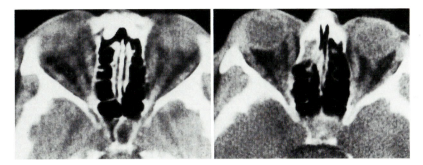

FIG ME–A–1.

Acromegaly: uniform moderate enlargement of the medial and lateral rectus muscles. (From Dal Pozzo G, Boschi MC: Extraocular muscle enlargement in acromegaly. *J. Comput. Assist. Tomogr.* 6:706, 1982. Used by permission.)

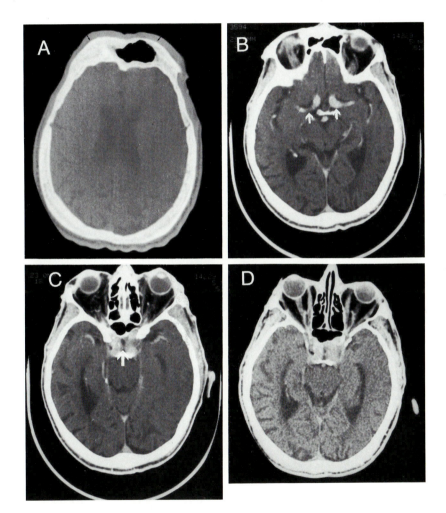

FIG ME–A–2.

Acromegaly in a 70-year-old male: Axial postcontrast CT scans. **A,** thickened calvaria with pronounced bilateral frontal bossing *(arrows)* and marked dilatation of the frontal sinus. **B,** dilation of the middle cerebral arteries *(arrows).* **C** and **D,** dilation of the cavernous portions of the internal carotid arteries. Faint arteriosclerotic calcifications are seen in the wall of the right carotid. Both arteries have prolapsed medially into an enlarged sella turcica with only a small cleft *(arrow,* **C)** remaining between their medial surfaces. There is bilateral proptosis with enlargement of the medial and lateral rectus muscles **(D).** (From Sacher M, Som PM, Shugar JMA, et al.: Kissing intrasellar carotid arteries in acromegaly: CT demonstration. *J. Comput. Assist. Tomogr.* 10:1033, 1986. Used by permission.)

REFERENCES

Abbassioun K, et al.: Familial acromegaly with pituitary adenoma. Report of three affected siblings. *J. Neurosurg.* 64:510, 1986.

Anton HC: Hand measurements in acromegaly. *Clin. Radiol.* 23:445, 1972.

Ardran GM, et al.: The tongue and mouth in acromegaly. *Clin. Radiol.* 23:434, 1972.

Doppman JL, et al.: Metatarsal pencilling in acromegaly: A proposed mechanism based on CT findings. *J. Comput. Assist. Tomogr.* 12:708, 1988.

Duncan TR: Validity of the sesamoid index in the diagnosis of acromegaly. *Radiology* 115:617, 1975.

Efird TA, et al.: Pituitary gigantism with cervical spinal stenosis. *A.J.R.* 134:171, 1980.

Epstein N, et al.: Acromegaly and spinal stenosis. *J. Neurosurg.* 56:145, 1982.

Gebarski SS, et al.: Prominent internal occipital protuberance misdiagnosed as fourth ventricular mass. *J. Comput. Assist. Tomogr.* 8:780, 1984.

Hatam A, et al.: Ectasia of cerebral arteries in acromegaly. *Acta Radiol.* 12:410, 1972.

Laws ER, et al.: The pathogenesis of acromegaly. Clinical and immunocytochemical analysis in 75 patients. *J. Neurosurg.* 63:35, 1985.

Lin SR, et al.: Widening of the median atlanto-axial joint in acromegaly. *J. Can. Assoc. Radiol.* 24:36, 1973.

Melmed S, et al.: Acromegaly update—etiology, diagnosis and management. *West. J. Med.* 146:328, 1987.

Morewood DJW, et al.: The extrathoracic airway in acromegaly. *Clin. Radiol.* 37:243, 1986.

Paisey R, et al.: Is soft tissue radiology useful in acromegaly? *Br. J. Radiol.* 57:561, 1984.

Pozzo GD, et al.: Extraocular muscle enlargement in acromegaly. *J. Comput. Assist. Tomogr.* 6:706, 1982.

Ritter MM, et al.: Acromegaly and colon cancer. *Ann. Intern. Med.* 106:636, 1987.

Sacher M, et al.: Kissing intrasellar carotid arteries in acromegaly: CT demonstration. *J. Comput. Assist. Tomogr.* 10:1033, 1986.

Scurry MT, et al.: Polyostotic fibrous dysplasia and acromegaly. *Arch. Intern. Med.* 114:40, 1964.

Shapiro JH, et al.: Skeletal changes of acromegaly. *Radiology* 125:830, 1977.

Steinbach HL, et al.: Acromegaly. *Radiology* 72:535, 1959.

Thorner MO, et al.: Extrahypothalamic growth-hormone–releasing factor (GRF) secretion is a rare cause of acromegaly: Plasma GRF levels in 177 acromegalic patients. *J. Clin. Endocrinol. Metab.* 59:846, 1984.

Wilson DM, et al.: Acromegaly and Zollinger-Ellison syndrome secondary to an islet cell tumor: Characterization and quantification of plasma and tumor human growth hormone-releasing factor. *J. Clin. Endocrinol. Metab.* 59:1002, 1984.

Yokota M, et al.: Acromegaly associated with suprasellar and pulmonary hemangiopericytomas. *J. Neurosurg.* 62:767, 1985.

ADDISON DISEASE

Synonym: Adrenal cortical insufficiency.

Etiology: (a) primary: infarction associated with infection; hemorrhage; withdrawal from chronic glucocorticoid therapy; tuberculosis; fungal infections; sarcoidosis; hemochromatosis; amyloidosis; congenital and familial Addison disease; idiopathic; metastatic lesions from the lung, kidney, colon, etc.; lymphoma; melanoma; acquired immune deficiency syndrome; etc.; (b) secondary (pituitary): Sheehan syndrome, neoplasms, tuberculosis, sarcoidosis, hemochromatosis, trauma, surgery, postirradiation, etc.; (c) autoimmune Addison disease (association with chronic mucocutaneous candidiasis, acquired hypoparathyroidism, pernicious anemia, insulin-requiring diabetes mellitus, primary hypogonadism, immunoglobulin abnormalities, chronic active hepatitis, alopecia, vitiligo, spontaneous myxedema, Graves disease, chronic lymphocytic thyroiditis); (d) other: association with adrenoleukodystrophy, osteoporosis, hyperthyroidism, myotonic dystrophy, achalasia, and alacrimation (Addison-achalasia-alacrimation syndrome).

Clinical Manifestations: Chronic primary adrenal insufficiency (Addison disease); (a) *weakness and fatigability, weight loss*; (b) *digestive disorders* (anorexia, abdominal pain, vomiting, diarrhea, or constipation); (c) *hyperpigmentation of the skin*; (d) pigmentation in the mucosa of the mouth, vagina, and rectum; (e) salt craving; (f) anemia; (g) irritability, confusion, delusion; (h) very low levels of plasma cortisol, hyponatremia, hyperkalemia, little or no increase in plasma cortisol in response to adrenocorticotropic hormone infusion, elevated percentage of circulating la-positive T cells; (i) triad of Addison-hypoparathyroidism-moniliasis, association with different polyglandular autoimmune (PGA) syndromes; (j) other reported abnormalities: flexion contracture, sciatic-like pain, cardiac failure.

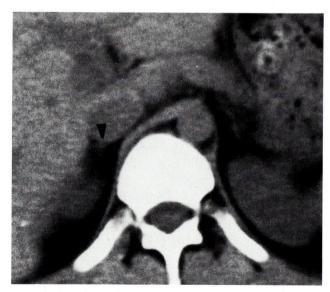

FIG ME–A–3.
Addison disease: small adrenal glands in a patient with idiopathic adrenal atrophy. (From Doppman JL, Gill JR Jr, Nienthius AW, et al.: CT findings in Addison's disease. *J. Comput. Assist. Tomogr.* 6:757, 1982. Used by permission.)

Radiologic Manifestations: (a) adrenal calcification (in about half of the patients with tuberculosis); (b) *microcardia;* (c) other reported associated abnormalities: reduction in kidney size; splenomegaly; *calcification or ossification in the external ear;* increased incidence of gallbladder disease, dental caries, and perialveolar bone resorption; pituitary gland enlargement related to end-organ failure; (d) computed tomography: various presentations including inflammatory space-occupying lesions with central hypodensity and peripheral enhancement after contrast injection; partial or total calcified degeneration of the infected atrophied gland or enlarged gland showing irregular calcified degeneration and parenchymal caseation; small adrenal glands in disease of autoimmune origin, idiopathic, and the pituitary form (the typical shape and density of the organ maintained); neoplasm; hemorrhage; necrosis (Fig ME–A–3).

Differential Diagnosis: Pseudo-Addison disease (isolated corticotropin deficiency associated with hyporeninemic hypoaldosteronism).

REFERENCES

Addison T: Anaemia: Disease of the suprarenal capsules. *London Hosp. Gaz.* 43:517, 1849.

Carey RW, et al.: Addison's disease secondary to lymphomatous infiltration of the adrenal glands. *Cancer* 59:1087, 1987.

Chaussain J-L: La maladie d'Addison de l'enfant. Etiologie et acquisitions physiopathologiques. *Presse Med.* 16:9, 1987.

Doppman JL, et al.: CT findings in Addison's disease. *J. Comput. Assist. Tomogr.* 6:757, 1982.

Ebinger G, et al.: Flexion contractures: A forgotten symptom in Addison's disease and hypopituitarism. *Lancet* 2:858, 1986.

Guenthner EE, et al.: Primary Addison's disease in a patient with acquired immunodeficiency syndrome. *Ann. Intern. Med.* 100:847, 1984.

Hay ID, et al.: Familial cytomegalic adrenocortical hypoplasia: An X-linked syndrome of pubertal failure. *Arch. Dis. Child.* 56:715, 1981.

Huebener K-H, et al.: Adrenal cortex dysfunction: CT findings. *Radiology* 150:195, 1984.

Kalifa, G, et al.: La maladie d'Addison chez l'enfant: Anomalies associées. *Ann. Radiol. (Paris)* 29:327, 1986.

Knowlton AI, et al.: Cardiac failure in Addison's disease. *Am. J. Med.* 74:829, 1983.

Maclaren MK, et al.: Inherited susceptibility to autoimmune Addison's disease is linked to human leukocyte antigen-DR3 and/or DR4, except when associated with type I autoimmune polyglandular syndrome. *J. Clin. Endocrinol. Metab.* 62:455, 1986.

Manser TJ, et al.: Pseudo-Addison's disease. Isolated corticotropin deficiency associated with hyporeninemic hypoaldosteronism. *Arch. Intern. Med.* 146:996, 1986.

Marilus R, et al.: Addison's disease associated with precocious sexual development in a boy. *Acta Paediatr. Scand.* 70:587, 1981.

Martin MM: Familial Addison's disease. *Birth Defects* 7(6):98, 1971.

McMurry JF Jr, et al.: Addison's disease with adrenal enlargement on computed tomographic scanning. *Am. J. Med.* 77:365, 1984.

Mineura K, et al.: Pituitary enlargement associated with Addison's disease. *Clin. Radiol.* 38:435, 1987.

Neufeld M, et al.: Two types of autoimmune Addison's disease associated with different polyglandular autoimmune (PGA) syndromes. *Medicine (Baltimore)* 60:355, 1981.

O'Neill BP, et al.: Familial X-linked Addison disease as an expression of adrenoleukodystrophy (ALD): Elevated C_{26} fatty acid in cultured skin fibroblasts. *Neurology* 32:543, 1982.

Pagliara S, et al.: Hyperthyroidism and Addison's disease in a patient with myotonic dystrophy. *Arch. Intern. Med.* 145:919, 1985.

Rabinowe SL, et al.: Ia-positive T lymphocytes in recently diagnosed idiopathic Addison's disease. *Am. J. Med.* 77:597, 1984.

Rzymski K, et al.: Computed tomography of the adrenal glands in Addison's disease. *Fortsch. Rontgenstr.* 140:48, 1984.

Seidenwurm DJ, et al.: Metastases to the adrenal glands and the development of Addison's disease. *Cancer* 54:552, 1984.

Vita JA, et al.: Clinical clues to the cause of Addison's disease. *Am. J. Med.* 78:461, 1985.

Wakefield MA, et al.: X-linked congenital Addison's disease. *Arch. Dis. Child.* 56:73, 1981.

Wittenberg DF: Familial X-linked adrenocortical hypoplasia: Association with androgenic precocity. *Arch. Dis. Child.* 56:633, 1981.

Zaleske DJ, et al.: Association of sciatica-like pain and Addison's disease. *J. Bone Joint Surg. [Am.]* 66:297, 1984.

ADRENAL HYPERPLASIA (CONGENITAL)

Synonyms: Congenital adrenal hyperplasia; adrenogenital syndrome.

Mode of Inheritance: Autosomal recessive in 21-hydroxylase deficiency; close genetic linkage of 21-hydroxylase deficiency and human leukocyte antigens (HLA) encoded on the short arm of chromosome 6; genetic differences exist between the salt-wasting, simple virilizing, and nonclassic (late onset of clinical symptom or cryptic) types of the disease; combined 21- and 11β-hydroxylase deficiency reported in families.

Frequency: Incidence of 1 in 5,000 to 1 in 25,000 in the Caucasian population (Editorial: *Lancet* 2:663, 1987).

Clinical Manifestations: (a) the classic form recognized at birth or in early childhood: *virilization* (precocious pseudopuberty), *adrenal insufficiency;* (b) late onset: *hirsutism and/or menstrual irregularity;* (c) *prenatal diagnosis of the salt-losing variant of 21-hydroxylase deficiency by amniotic fluid steroid analysis;* (d) some children may also develop true precocious puberty (testicular enlargement in the boys, breast development in the girls, progressive pubic hair development, rapid growth); (e) other reported abnormalities: low fertility rate in women with congenital adrenal hyperplasia,

TABLE ME–A–3.

Defects of Adrenal Steroidogenesis*

Deficiency	Syndrome	Ambiguous Genitalia	Postnatal Virilization	Salt Metabolism	Steroids Increased	Steroids Decreased	Enzyme	Chromosome	Frequency†
Cholesterol desmolase	Lipoid hyperplasia	Males	No	Salt wasting	None	All	P450scc	15	Rare
3β-OH-steroid dehydrogenase	Classic	Males and ? females	Yes	±Salt wasting	DHEA‡ 17-OH-pregnenolone	Aldo‡ cortisol, T	3β-OH-steroid dehydrogenase	?	Rare
	Nonclassic	No	Yes	Normal	DHEA, 17-OH-pregnenolone	—	3β-OH-steroid dehydrogenase	?	? Frequent
17-Hydroxylase	—	Males	No	Hypertension	DOC‡ corticosterone	Cortisol, T	P450c17	10	Rare
17,20-Lyase§	—	Males	No	Normal	—	DHEA, T, androstenedione	P450c17	10	Rare
21-Hydroxylase	Salt wasting	Females	Yes	Salt wasting	17-OHP‡, androstenedione	Aldo, cortisol	P450c21	6p (HLA)	1/10,000
	Simple virilizing	Females	Yes	Normal	17-OHP, androstenedione	Cortisol	P450c21	6p (HLA)	1/20,000
	Nonclassic	No	Yes	Normal	17-OHP, androstenedione	—	p450c21	6p (HLA)	0.1-1% (3% in European Jews)
11-Hydroxylase	Classic	Females	Yes	Hypertension	DOC, 11-deoxycortisol	Cortisol, ±Aldo	P450c11	8q	1/100,000
	Nonclassic	No	Yes	Normal	11-Deoxycortisol, ±DOC	—	P450c11	8q	? Frequent
Corticosterone methyl oxidase II	—	No	No	Salt wasting	18-OH-corticosterone	Aldo	P450c11	8q	Rare (except in Iranian Jews)

*From White PC, New MI, Dupont B: Congenital adrenal hyperplasia. *N. Engl. J. Med.* 316:1580, 1987. Used by permission.
†*Rare* denotes a syndrome accounting for less than 1% of the reported cases of congenital adrenal hyperplasia, which has an overall frequency of about 1 in 5,000 births. *? Frequent* syndromes may occur at frequencies similar to that of nonclassic 21-hydroxylase deficiency, but prevalence data are not available.
‡DHEA = dehydroepiandrosterone; Aldo = aldosterone; T = testosterone; DOC = deoxycorticosterone; 17-OHP = 17-hydroxyprogesterone.
§Deficiency of 17,20-lyase is expressed in the gonads but is included here because it apparently involves the same gene as 17-hydroxylase deficiency.

vaginal introitus inadequate for intercourse, girls diagnosed later in childhood may have unusual muscle strength, bilateral testicular hypertrophy (11β-hydroxylase deficiency), hyperphosphatemic rickets, congenital hypothyroidism, web neck, shield chest, short and curved fingers, syndactyly, hypertelorism, hydrocephalus, craniosynostosis, renal anomalies, etc.

Radiologic Manifestations:

(A) SIMPLE VIRILISM: (a) *advanced skeletal maturation;* (b) advanced pneumatization of the mastoids and paranasal sinuses; (c) premature calcification of the cartilage of the ribs and larynx; (d) *advanced tooth development;* (e) premature muscular development and osseous prominences; (f) premature development of skull diploë; (g) *genitography in females: different degrees of deviation from normal including that of pseudohermaphroditism and true hermaphroditism;* (h) normal topography of the internal genitalia, small uterus, and normal or enlarged ovaries, urinoma of the fallopian tube related to a common urogenital sinus; (i) enlargement of the adrenals with preservation of the usual echo pattern (echo-poor cortex and echo-dense medulla), enlargement predominantly cortical.

(B) ADRENAL INSUFFICIENCY: (a) reduction in soft-tissue thickness due to dehydration; (b) hyperlucent lungs; (c) *microcardia;* (d) paucity or absence of gastrointestinal gas simulating high gastrointestinal obstruction; (e) cardiomegaly and even congestive heart failure (rare).

Differential Diagnosis: Adrenal tumor.

Note: The report of shock following excretory urography in patients with congenital adrenal hyperplasia should be

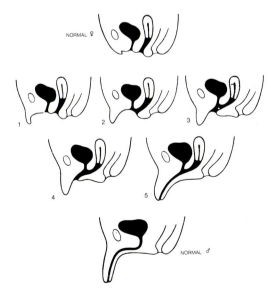

FIG ME−A−4.
Adrenogenital syndrome: five different forms of genital malformations encountered in the female with congenital adrenogenital syndrome. (From Kurlander GJ: Roentgenology of the congenital adrenogenital syndrome. *A.J.R.* 95:189, 1965. Used by permission.)

taken into consideration when using intravascular contrast media (Fig ME−A−4; Table ME−A−3).

REFERENCES

Baskin HJ: Screening for late-onset congenital adrenal hyperplasia in hirsutism or amenorrhea. *Arch. Intern. Med.* 147:847, 1987.

Börger D, et al.: Dermatoglyphics in congenital adrenal hyperplasia (CAH). *Clin. Genet.* 20:173, 1986.

Boué A: Génétique du déficit en 21-hydroxylase. *Arch. Fr. Pediatr.* 44:75, 1987.

Cahen LA, et al.: Congenital hypothyroidism and congenital adrenocortical hyperplasia in an infant. *J. Pediatr.* 90:77, 1977.

Couillin P: Le conseil génétique et le diagnostic prénatal de l'hyperplasie des surrénales par déficit en 21-hydroxylase. *Presse Med.* 13:1087, 1984.

Duck S: Malignancy associated with congenital adrenal hyperplasia. *J. Pediatr.* 99:423, 1981.

Dumas R, et al.: Congenital adrenal hyperplasia associated with hyperphosphatemic rickets. *Clin. Pediatr. (Phila.)* 27:276, 1988.

Ghiacy S, et al.: Ultrasound demonstration of congenital adrenal hyperplasia. *J. Clin. Ultrasound* 13:419, 1985.

Höller W, et al.: Genetic differences between the salt-wasting, simple virilizing, and nonclassical types of congenital adrenal hyperplasia. *J. Clin. Endocrinol. Metab.* 60:757, 1985.

Hughes IA, et al.: Prenatal diagnosis of congenital adrenal hyperplasia: Reliability of amniotic fluid steroid analysis. *J. Med. Genet.* 24:344, 1987.

Hurwitz A, et al.: Combined 21- and 11β-hydroxylase deficiency in familial congenital adrenal hyperplasia. *J. Clinic. Endocrinol. Metab.* 60:631, 1985.

Kaufman FR, et al.: Urinoma of the fallopian tube in virilizing congenital adrenal hyperplasia. *J. Pediatr.* 109:495, 1986.

Khaldi F, et al.: Hypertrophie testiculaire bilatérale et hyperplasie congénitale des surrénales par déficit en 11β-hydroxylase. *Arch. Fr. Pediatr.* 44:513, 1987.

Kirkland RT, et al.: The incidence of associated anomalies in 105 patients with congenital adrenal hyperplasia. *Pediatrics* 49:608, 1972.

Kirkland RT, et al.: Upper urinary tract anomalies in congenital adrenal hyperplasia. *Pediatrics* 59:639, 1977.

Kurlander GJ: Roentgenology of the congenital adrenogenital syndrome. *A.J.R.* 95:189, 1965.

McMillan DD, et al.: Upper urinary tract anomalies in children with adrenogenital syndrome. *J. Pediatr.* 89:953, 1976.

Miller WL, et al.: Molecular and clinical advances in congenital adrenal hyperplasia. *J. Pediatr.* 111:1, 1987.

Mulaikal RM, et al.: Fertility rates in female patients with congenital adrenal hyperplasia due to 21-hydroxylase deficiency. *N. Engl. J. Med.* 316:178, 1987.

Pang S, et al.: Adrenocortical tumor in a patient with congenital adrenal hyperplasia due to 21-hydroxylase deficiency. *Pediatrics* 68:242, 1981.

Pang S, et al.: Worldwide experience in newborn screening for classical congenital adrenal hyperplasia due to 21-hydroxylase deficiency. *Pediatrics* 81:866, 1988.

Pescovitz OH, et al.: True precocious puberty complicating congenital adrenal hyperplasia: Treatment with a luteinizing hormone-releasing hormone analog. *J. Clin. Endocrinol. Metab.* 58:857, 1984.

Peterson RE, et al.: Male pseudohermaphroditism due to multiple defects in steroid-biosynthetic microsomal mixed-function oxidases. A new variant of congenital adrenal hyperplasia. *N. Engl. J. Med.* 313:1182, 1985.

Rodda C, et al.: Muscle strength in girls with congenital adrenal hyperplasia. *Acta Paediatr. Scand.* 76:495, 1987.

Strachan T, et al.: Prenatal diagnosis of congenital adrenal hyperplasia. *Lancet* 2:1272, 1987.

White PC, et al.: Congenital adrenal hyperplasia. *N. Engl. J. Med.* 316:1182, 1580, 1987.

ADRENOLEUKODYSTROPHY AND ADRENOMYELONEUROPATHY

Mode of Inheritance: X-linked recessive in the classic, most common childhood form of adrenoleukodystrophy (ALD) and adrenomyeloneuropathy (AMN); autosomal recessive in the neonatal form of ALD (NALD); male or female phenotype heterogeneity among hemizygotes; female carriers may be symptomatic; ALD and AMN have been reported within the same kindred.

Pathophysiology: Accumulation of a very long chain of saturated fatty acids with carbon length greater than C22 (from C24 to C30 with a peak of C26) in tissues and body fluids, in particular, the nervous system white matter and the adrenal cortex; considered to be due to defective peroxisomal function; widespread demyelination of cerebral white matter, inflammatory reaction, and atrophy of zona reticularis and fasciculata of the adrenal gland with ballooned, striated cells in the adrenal cortex.

Frequency: Uncommon.

Clinical Manifestations: (a) *childhood form (classic X-linked ALD): mild to moderate adrenal insufficiency that may be partially limited to elevation of adrenocorticotropic hormone levels only;* (b) *neonatal form (NALD): hypotonia, poor feeding, failure to thrive, etc.;* (c) *adrenoleukomyeloneuropathy (ALMN) with symptoms usually presenting in young adult period: spastic paraplegia, distal symmetrical peripheral neuropathy, adrenal insufficiency, testicular insufficiency, etc.;* (d) *symptomatic heterozygote: chronic nonprogressive spinal cord syndrome: spastic paraparesis, peripheral neuropathy;* (e) other reported abnormalities: abnormal electroencephalographic findings, increased intracranial pressure (cerebral edema), Addison disease (males), elevated cerebrospinal fluid protein, pipecolic acidemia in NALD, carrier detection by a determination of very long chain fatty acids in plasma and cultured skin fibroblasts, encephalopathy preceding adrenal insufficiency, megaloencephaly, insulin-dependent diabetes mellitus, seizures, coma, frontal lobe syndromes, frequent alterations of visual pigment genes.

Radiologic Manifestations: (a) computed tomography (CT): *low-density white matter lesion originating in the occip-*

TABLE ME–A–4.

Adrenoleukodystrophy: Clinical Spectrum of Phenotypes*

Disease	Phenotype
"Typical" ALD†	Males
	Progressive cerebral syndrome
	Mild to moderate adrenal insufficiency
AMN†	Males
	Spastic paraparesis, peripheral neuropathy
	Moderate adrenal and testicular insufficiency
"Variant" ALD	Present report
Neonatal ALD	Males or females
	"Failure to thrive"
Addison disease	Males
	Moderate adrenal insufficiency
Symptomatic heterozygote	Females
	Spastic paraparesis, peripheral neuropathy

*From Marler JR, O'Neill BP, Forbes GS, et al.: Adrenoleukodystrophy (ALD): Clinical and CT features of a childhood variant. *Neurology* 33:1203, 1983. Used by permission.
†ALD = adrenoleukodystrophe; AMN = adrenomyeloneuropathy.

ital region and migrating forward into the temporal, parietal, and frontal lobes and cerebellum; continuation of the process across the midline; sparing of gray matter; indistinctness of the ventricular wall due to low brain density; rim of enhancement at the periphery of the lesions on a contrast study, pro-gression to generalized central and cortical atrophy; atypical CT presentations such as unilateral lesions in the early phase of the disease, lesions without opacification at the periphery after contrast enhancement, early frontal lobe involvement, ventricular and parietal lobe distortion suggestive of mass effect, cerebellar involvement, central calcifications within the low attenuation lesions of white matter; (b) *magnetic resonance imaging: more sensitive than CT in the early phase of development of demyelination; high signal intensity on T_2-weighted spin-echo sequences (this corresponds to the low attenuation seen on CT examination); prolonged T_1 and T_2 values in the corpus callosum, around the trigones of the lateral ventricles, in the internal capsules, in the pons, and in the cervical spinal cord (ALMN);* auditory pathway disease (lateral lemniscus and medial geniculate body involvement); visual pathway disease (lateral geniculate body, Meyer loop, and optic radiation involvement); (c) *radioisotope brain scan (^{99m}Tc pertechnetate): increased uptake in the involved brain regions;* (d) arteriography: prominent veins in the white matter (Table ME–A–4).

REFERENCES

Aubourg P, et al.: Adrénoleucodystrophie chez l'enfant. A-propos de 20 observations. *Arch. Fr. Pédiatr.* 39:663, 1982.

Aubourg PR, et al.: Frequent alterations of visual pigment

genes in adrenoleukodystrophy. *Am. J. Hum. Genet.* 42:408, 1988.

Bewermeyer H, et al.: MR imaging in adrenoleukomyeloneuropathy. *J. Comput. Assist. Tomogr.* 9:793, 1985.

Chaves-Carballo E, et al.: Increased intracranial pressure in adrenoleukodystrophy. *Arch. Neurol.* 41:339, 1984.

Cotrufo R, et al.: Phenotype heterogeneity among hemizygotes in a family biochemically screened for adrenoleukodystrophy. *Am. J. Med. Genet.* 26:833, 1987.

Davis LE, et al.: Adrenoleukodystrophy and adrenomyeloneuropathy associated with partial adrenal insufficiency in three generations of a kindred. *Am. J. Med.* 66:342, 1979.

Di Chiro G, et al.: A new CT pattern in adrenoleukodystrophy. *Radiology* 137:687, 1980.

Dubois PJ, et al.: Atypical findings in adrenoleukodystrophy. *J. Comput. Assist. Tomogr.* 5:888, 1981.

Ferro JM, et al.: Demonstration of cerebellar involvement in adrenoleucodystrophy by CT. *Neuroradiology* 27:185, 1985.

Furuse M, et al.: Adrenoleukodystrophy: A correlative analysis of computed tomography and radionuclide studies. *Radiology* 126:707, 1978.

Hong-Magno ET, et al.: Atypical CT scans in adrenoleukodystrophy. *J. Comput. Assist. Tomogr.* 11:333, 1987.

Huckman MS, et al.: Magnetic resonance imaging compared with computed tomography in adrenoleukodystrophy. *Am. J. Dis. Child.* 140:1001, 1986.

Inoue Y, et al.: Adrenoleukodystrophy: New CT findings. *A.J.N.R.* 4:951, 1983.

Kelley RI, et al.: Hyperpipecolic acidemia in neonatal adrenoleukodystrophy. *Am. J. Med. Genet.* 19:791, 1984.

Kelley RI, et al.: Neonatal adrenoleukodystrophy. *Am. J. Med. Genet.* 23:869, 1986.

Kodama S, et al.: Childhood form of adrenoleukodystrophy in the sucking infant. *Pediatr. Neurosci.* 12:256, 1985.

Kolodny EH: The adrenoleukodystrophy-adrenomyeloneuropathy complex: Is it treatable? *Ann. Neurol.* 21:230, 1987.

Kumar AJ, et al.: Adrenoleukodystrophy: Correlating MR imaging with CT. *Radiology* 165:497, 1987.

Lenard HG: Adrenoleukodystrophy. *Neuropediatrics* 15(suppl.):16, 1984.

MacDonald JT, et al.: Adrenoleukodystrophy: Early frontal lobe involvement on computed tomography. *J. Comput. Assist. Tomogr.* 8:128, 1984.

Marler JR, et al.: Adrenoleukodystrophy (ALD): Clinical and CT features of a childhood variant. *Neurology* 33:1203, 1983.

Moser HW, et al.: Identification of female carriers of adrenoleukodystrophy. *J. Pediatr.* 103:54, 1983.

Noetzel MJ, et al.: Adrenoleukodystrophy carrier state presenting as a chronic non-progressive spinal cord disorder. *Arch. Neurol.* 44:566, 1987.

O'Neill BP, et al.: Adrenoleukodystrophy: Clinical and biochemical manifestations in carriers. *Neurology* 34:798, 1984.

O'Neill BP, et al.: Familial X-linked Addison disease as an expression of adrenoleukodystrophy (ALD): Elevated C_{26} fatty acid in cultured skin fibroblasts. *Neurology* 32:543, 1982.

Rosen NL, et al.: Adrenoleukomyeloneuropathy with onset in early childhood. *Ann. Neurol.* 17:311, 1985.

Touati G, et al.: Adrénoleucodystrophie et diabète sucré par deficit en recepteurs a l'insuline. *Arch. Fr. Pediatr.* 39:441, 1982.

Young RSK, et al.: Adrenoleukodystrophy. Unusual computed tomographic appearance. *Arch. Neurol.* 39:782, 1982.

AFIBRINOGENEMIA (CONGENITAL)

Mode of Inheritance: Probably autosomal recessive.

Clinical Manifestations: (a) provoked or spontaneous external or visceral *hemorrhages;* (b) *absence of fibrinogen in plasma confirmed by chemical and immunoelectrophoresis,* normal or increased bleeding time, failure of blood clotting.

Radiologic Manifestations: (a) hemarthrosis and "bone cysts" due to bleeding (rare); (b) visceral hemorrhage, pericardial hemorrhage, constrictive pericarditis (Fig ME—A—5).

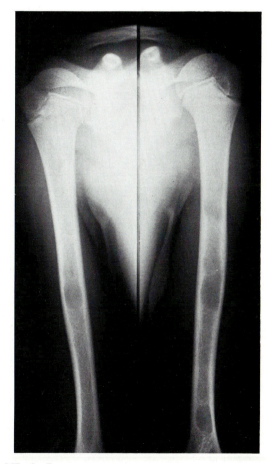

FIG ME—A—5.

Afibrinogenemia (congenital) in a boy aged 12 years and 3 months with multiple radiolucencies located within the medullary cavity of the humeri (From Zenny JC, Chevrot A, Sultan Y, et al.: Lésion hémorrhagiques intra-osseuses des afibrinogénémies congénitales: A propos d'un nouveau cas. *J. Radiol.* 62:263, 1981. Used by permission.)

REFERENCES

Boniske CH, et al.: Spontaneous severe constrictive pericarditis in congenital afibrinogenemia: Mechanism, evaluation, and successful surgical treatment. *Am. Heart J.* 101:503, 1981.

Lagier, R, et al.: Skeletal changes in congenital fibrinogen abnormalities. *Skeletal Radiol.* 5:233, 1980.

Lemoine P, et al.: Afibrinémie congénitale chez deux frères avec lésions osseuses et hepatiques. *Arch. Fr. Pediatr.* 20:463, 1963.

Zenny JC, et al.: Lésions hemorragiques intraosseuses des afibrinogénies congénitales. *J. Radiol.* 62:23, 1981.

AGAMMAGLOBULINEMIA, X-LINKED

Synonyms: Bruton disease; X-linked agammaglobulinemia (XLA); hypogammaglobulinemia (X-linked).

Mode of Inheritance: X-linked recessive, males only affected; an intrinsic defect in B-cell development; in a single eight-generation pedigree the XLA was mapped to the $X_q21.3-X_q22$ area of the X chromosome (Mensink et al.).

Clinical Manifestations: (a) World Health Organization criteria: *onset in infancy or early childhood, serum IgG ≤ 200 mg/dL with IgA and IgM markedly reduced for age, absence of functional serum antibody, normal cell-mediated immunity (positive delayed-type hypersensitivity skin test and/or normal T-cell mitogen stimulation in vitro)*; (b) *deficiency of antibody-producing B-lymphocyte system, paucity of plasma cells and germinal centers in lymph nodes*; (c) *recurrent infections* (bacterial, viral): respiratory, gastrointestinal, skin, central nervous system, skeletal system, hepatic, etc.; (d) rheumatoid-like arthritis; (e) dermatomyositis-like syndrome; (f) other reported abnormalities: neutropenia (associated with infections), thrombocytopenia, Coombs-positive hemolytic anemia, transient lymphopenia, defective platelet aggregation, giardiasis.

Radiologic Manifestations: (a) *recurrent pneumonia* associated with lobar or segmental atelectasis and bronchiectasis, tracheomegaly; (b) *absence of lymphoid tissue in the nasopharynx*, absence of hilar adenopathy; (c) small-bowel pattern suggesting edema or malabsorption; (d) synovial thickening without bone lesions (Fig ME−A−6).

REFERENCES

Bruton OC: Agammaglobulinemia. *Pediatrics* 9:722, 1952.

Conley ME, et al.: Carrier detection in typical and atypical X-linked agammaglobulinemia. *J. Pediatr.* 112:688, 1988.

Conley ME, et al.: Expression of the gene defect in X-linked agammaglobulinemia. *N. Engl. J. Med.* 315:564, 1986.

Fearon ER, et al.: Carrier detection in X-linked agammaglobulinemia by analysis of X-chromosomal inactivation. *N. Engl. J. Med.* 316:427, 1987.

Herman TE, et al.: Radiology of immunodeficiency syndromes. *Postgrad. Radiol.* 1:99, 1981.

Kim HC, et al.: Defective platelet aggregation in congenital agammaglobulinemia. *J. Pediatr.* 98:780, 1981.

Lallemand D, et al.: Trachéomégaly et déficit immunitaire chez l'enfant. *Ann. Radiol. (Paris)* 24:67, 1981.

Lau YL, et al.: Genetic prediction in X-linked agammaglobulinaemia. *Am. J. Med. Genet.* 31:437, 1988.

Lederman HM, et al.: X-linked agammaglobulinemia: An analysis of 96 patients. *Medicine (Baltimore)* 64:145, 1985.

Mensink EJBM, et al.: Genetic hetergeneity in X-linked agammaglobulinemia complicates carrier detection and prenatal diagnosis. *Clin. Genet.* 31:91, 1987.

Norton KI, et al.: Computed tomography findings in a case of hypogammaglobulinemia. *J. Comput. Tomogr.* 10:41, 1986.

Schuurman RKB, et al.: Early diagnosis in X-linked agammaglobulinaemia. *Eur. J. Pediatr.* 147:93, 1988.

ALDOSTERONISM (PRIMARY)

Synonyms: Hyperaldosteronism; Conn syndrome; primary hyperaldosteronism.

Types: (a) adrenal adenoma or carcinoma (about 60% of cases); (b) idiopathic (about 40% of cases): adrenal hyperplasia; (c) adrenal hyperplasia with clinical and chemical responses to glucocorticoid treatment (rare, familial).

Clinical Manifestations: (a) *systemic arterial hypertension*, without edema; (b) *hyperaldosteronism* that is not sup-

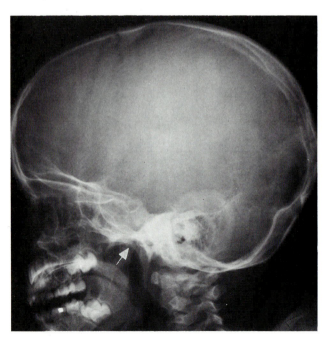

FIG ME−A−6.
Agammaglobulinemia, X-linked, in a 3-year-old male with recurrent infections from early infancy. Laboratory studies revealed gamma globulin level of 0.2 gm/mL; total protein, 5.1 gm; albumin, 3.8 gm; globulin, 1.3 gm. Note the absence of adenoid tissues in the nasopharynx *(arrow)*.

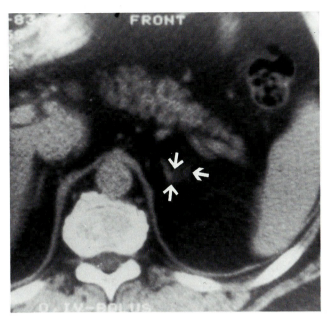

FIG ME–A–7.
Aldosteronoma in a 25-year-old man with hyperaldosteronism. A small nodule is seen in the left adrenal gland *(arrows)*. (From Shirkhoda A: Current diagnostic approach to adrenal abnormalities. *J. Comput. Tomogr.* 8:277, 1984. Used by permission.)

pressed appropriately during volume expansion; (c) *depression of plasma renin activity;* (d) *hypokalemic alkalosis* with muscular weakness and polydipsia; (e) other reported abnormalities: subarachnoid hemorrhage, postural hypotension, bradycardia, etc.

Radiologic Manifestations: (a) *aldosterone assay of adrenal vein;* (b) selective retrograde epinephrophlebography of the adrenal veins demonstrating the *tumor displacing surrounding adrenal veins* (circumferential veins outlining the tumor); (c) arteriographic demonstration of a *sharply delineated avascular area within a densely opacified adrenal cortex,* faint homogeneous blush in some; (d) computed tomography: more reliable for lesions over 10 mm in diameter; (e) magnetic resonance imaging: low-intensity mass; (f) scintigraphy with ^{131}I-6β-iodomethyl-19-norcholesterol (NP59): increased uptake in the abnormal gland; (g) other reported abnormalities: adrenal myelolipoma.

Differential Diagnosis: Secondary hyperaldostronism (extra-adrenal stimulus) resulting from hyperreninemia; pseudohyperaldosteronism (Liddle syndrome) (Fig ME–A–7).

REFERENCES

Banks WA, et al.: Primary adrenal hyperplasia: A new subset of primary hyperaldosteronism. *J. Clin. Endocrinol. Metab.* 58:783, 1984.
Biglieri EG: The pituitary and idiopathic hyperaldostronism. *N. Engl. J. Med.* 311:120, 1984.
Bravo EL, et al.: The changing clinical spectrum of primary aldosteronism. *Am. J. Med.* 74:641, 1983.
Bryer A, et al.: Conn's syndrome presenting as a subarachnoid haemorrhage. *S. Afr. Med. J.* 62:249, 1982.
Carey RM, et al.: Idiopathic hyperaldosteronism. A possible role for aldosterone-stimulating factor. *N. Engl. J. Med.* 311:94, 1984.
Conn JW: Primary aldosteronism: A new clinical syndrome. *J. Lab. Clin. Med.* 45:3, 1955.
Danforth DN, et al.: Renal changes in primary aldosteronism. *J. Urol.* 117:140, 1977.
Dunnick NR, et al.: Preoperative diagnosis and localization of aldosteronomas by measurement of corticosteroids in adrenal venous blood. *Radiology* 133:331, 1979.
Farge D, et al.: Isolated clinical syndrome of primary aldosteronism in four patients with adrenocortical carcinoma. *Am. J. Med.* 83:635, 1987.
Filiatrault D, et al.: CT localization of an aldostronoma in a 10-year-old boy. *Pediatr. Radiol.* 16:85, 1986.
Geisinger MA, et al.: Primary hyperaldostronism: Comparison of CT, adrenal venography, and venous sampling. *A.J.R.* 141:299, 1983.
Gross MD, et al.: Scintigraphic localization of adrenal lesions in primary aldostronism. *Am. J. Med.* 77:839, 1984.
Mutoh S, et al.: Pseudohyperaldosteronism (Liddle's syndrome): A case report. *J. Urol.* 135:557, 1985.
Velchik MG, et al.: Primary aldostronism: CT, MRI, scintigraphic correlation. *Invest. Radiol.* 20:237, 1985.
Whaley D, et al.: Adrenal myelolipoma associated with Conn syndrome: CT evaluation. *J. Comput. Assist. Tomogr.* 9:959, 1985.

ALKAPTONURIA

Synonym: Alcaptonuria.

Etiology: *Absence of homogentisic acid oxidase enzyme leading to an accumulation of homogentisic acid in various tissues.*

Clinical Manifestations: Onset of symptoms usually in adult life. (a) *ochronosis:* brown or black pigmentation of the skin, oral mucosa, sclera, conjunctiva, limbic cornea, tendons, cartilages, cerumen, sweat, etc.; (b) *chronic arthropathy,* in particular, in the shoulder, hip, and knee joints; limitation of spinal motion; loss of height; etc.; (c) *alkaptonuria:* discoloration of the urine to brown or black on standing or on alkalinization; (d) renal stones, decreased kidney function, prostatitis, prostatic enlargement; (e) cardiovascular diseases: mitral and aortic valvular disease, arteriosclerosis, myocardial infarction; (f) upper respiratory symptoms (dryness of the pharynx, hoarseness), dyspnea, restriction of thoracic cage motions, gray airways (vocal cord, tracheal rings, and bronchial cartilage) seen on endoscopy; (g) other reported abnormalities: association with diabetes mellitus, Addison disease, polycythemia vera, hyperuricemia, ankylosing spondylitis, etc.

Radiologic Manifestations: (a) *spinal manifestations:* loss of lumbar lordosis, kyphosis, scoliosis, osteoporosis, narrow-

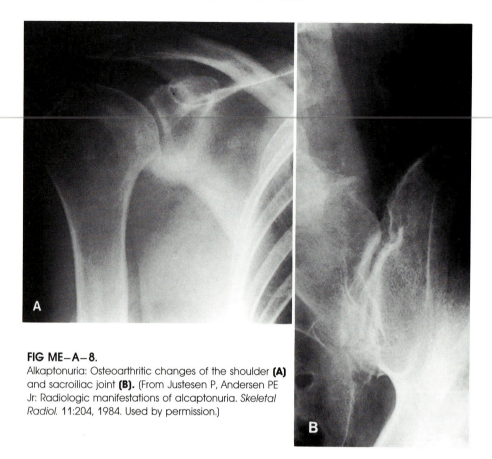

FIG ME—A—8.
Alkaptonuria: Osteoarthritic changes of the shoulder **(A)** and sacroiliac joint **(B)**. (From Justesen P, Andersen PE Jr: Radiologic manifestations of alcaptonuria. *Skeletal Radiol.* 11:204, 1984. Used by permission.)

ing of disk spaces, "vacuum" phenomena, disk calcification and ossification, ruptured intervertebral disks, osteophyte formation, calcification of the interspinous ligament, vertebral fusion, etc.; (b) *extraspinal arthropathy* (sacroiliac joints, symphysis pubis, peripheral joints): cartilage calcification, effusion, loose joint bodies, articular and para-articular calcification (ligaments, tendon sheath, bursal sacs, synovial membrane), joint narrowing, sclerosis, osteophytes, destruction of humeral and femoral heads, rupture of the Achilles tendon, etc.; (c) *renal calculi, nephrocalcinosis,* prostatic calculi; (d) calcification of ear cartilages; (e) calcification of aortic and mitral valves (Fig ME—A—8).

REFERENCES

Christensen K, et al.: Alkaptonuria and ochronosis. *Hum. Hered.* 33:140, 1983.

Gaines JJ, et al.: Cardiovascular ochronosis. *Arch. Pathol. Lab. Med.* 111:991, 1987.

Goldberg BH, et al.: Alkaptonuria with nephrocalcinosis. *J. Pediatr.* 88:518, 1976.

Hartman AR, et al.: Alkaptonuria and aortic stenosis. *Ann. Intern. Med.* 104:446, 1986.

Justesen P, et al.: Radiologic manifestations in alcaptonuria. *Skeletal Radiol.* 11:204, 1984.

Kampik A, et al.: Ocular ochronosis: Clinicopathological, histochemical and ultrastructural studies. *Arch Ophthalmol.* 98:1441, 1980.

Lurie DP, et al.: Knee arthropathy in ochronosis: Diagnosis by arthroscopy with ultrastructural features. *J. Rheumatol.* 11:101, 1984.

Rebuck AS, et al.: Gray airways in ochronosis. *N. Engl. J. Med.* 304:1367, 1981.

Simon G, et al.: The radiographic changes in alkaptonuric ochronosis. *Radiology* 37:295, 1941.

Young H: Calculi of the prostate associated with ochronosis and alkaptonuria. *J. Urol.* 51:48, 1944.

α_1-ANTITRYPSIN DEFICIENCY

Mode of Inheritance: Many genetic variants; inherited via two codominant autosomal alleles; PiM the most common genotype.

Frequency: Estimated to be 1 in 2,000 to 1 in 7,700 in the white population (Cox et al., 1987).

Clinical Manifestations:

(A) Infants and children: (a) *prolonged obstructive jaundice in infancy, liver cirrhosis, hepatosplenomegaly*; (b) pulmonary disease (rare);

(B) Adults: onset of symptoms often prior to 40 years of age: (a) chronic bronchitis, *wheezing, progressive dyspnea, respiratory failure*; (b) *cor pulmonale*; (c) liver cirrhosis; (d) asthenia, malnourished appearance;

(C) Other reported abnormalities: association with other

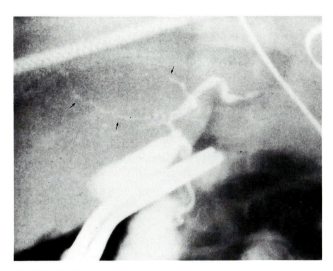

FIG ME–A–9.
α₁-Antitrypsin deficiency in a neonate with obstructive jaundice. Preoperative cholecystography showing hypoplasia of the intrahepatic bile ducts *(arrows).* (From Vandenplas Y, Franckx J, Liebaers I, et al.: Neonatal hepatitis with obstructive jaundice in an SZ heterozygous alpha 1-antitrypsin–deficient boy and destructive lung disease in his SZ mother. *Eur. J. Pediatr.* 144:391, 1985. Used by permission.)

diseases: membranous glomerulopathy, rheumatoid arthritis, fibrosing alveolitis, panniculitis, uveitis, peptic ulcer, recurrent pancreatitis, hepatic tumors, various intra- and extrahepatic biliary anomalies (paucity of the interlobular bile ducts, extrahepatic bile duct hypoplasia, biliary atresia, bile plug), development of liver disease in adults (men more than women), fatty liver, neonatal hepatitis, progressive bronchiectasis without evidence of emphysema, vasculitis (skin, kidney, colon), cystic degeneration of the lung in infancy, immune deficiency, neonatal convulsions due to intracranial hemorrhage associated with cholestatic hepatopathy, etc.

Laboratory Manifestations: (a) *almost complete absence of* α₁-*globulin, very low serum trypsin inhibitory capacity;* (b) *Pi typing: ZZ phenotype shown on crossed immunoelectrophoresis.*

Radiologic Manifestations:

(A) INFANTS AND CHILDREN: hepatosplenomegaly, gastroesophageal varices, ascites, abnormal liver ultrasonogram (focal areas of heterogeneity simulating mass lesions, increased periportal echogenicity, gallbladder enlargement in the neonatal period.

(B) ADULTS: (a) *hyperlucent lungs with or without bullae, emphysema more pronounced in the lower parts of the lungs,* bronchiectasis, flaccid lung syndrome; (b) *marked homogeneous decrease in perfusion at the lung bases with increased flow in the upper portions of the lobes;* (c) cardiomegaly, cor pulmonale with a dilated pulmonary artery and the proximal branches (Figs ME–A–9 and ME–A–10).

REFERENCES

Bell RS: The radiographic manifestations of alpha-1 antitrypsin deficiency: An important recognizable pattern of chronic obstructive pulmonary disease (COPD). *Radiology* 95:19, 1970.
Blane CE, et al.: Sonographic features of hepatocellular disease in neonates and infants. *A.J.R.* 141:1313, 1983.

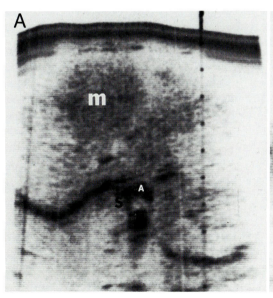
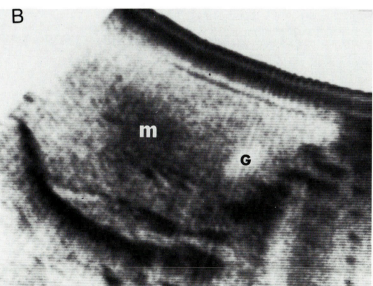

FIG ME–A–10.
α₁-Antitrypsin deficiency in a newborn infant. Transverse **(A)** and sagittal **(B)** sonograms show a focal hyperechoic mass *(m)* cephalad to the gallbladder *(G)* that is simulating a liver tumor. (From Blane CE, et al.: Sonographic features of hepatocellular disease in neonates and infants. *A.J.R.* 141:1313, 1983. Used by permission.)

Brantly M, et al.: Molecular basis of alpha-1-antitrypsin deficiency. *Am. J. Med.* 84(suppl. 6A):13, 1988.

Claque HW, et al.: Lung imaging in alpha-$_1$ antitrypsin deficiency. *J. Can. Assoc. Radiol.* 32:242, 1981.

Cox DW, et al.: Prenatal diagnosis of alpha-$_1$ antitrypsin deficiency and estimates of fetal risk for disease. *J. Med. Genet.* 24:52, 1987.

Cox DW, et al.: Risk for liver disease in adults with alpha-$_1$ antitrypsin deficiency. *Am. J. Med.* 74:221, 1983.

Dorney SFA, et al.: SZ phenotype alpha-$_1$ antitrypsin deficiency with paucity of the intralobular bile ducts. *Aust. Paediatr. J.* 23:55, 1987.

Eriksson S: Alpha 1-antitrypsin deficiency and chronic obstructive bronchopulmonary disease. *Acta Med. Scand.* 177(suppl.):41, 1965.

Fidalgo I, et al.: Serum levels of alpha 1-antitrypsin and Pi types in children with bronchiolitis. *Helv. Paediatr. Acta* 35:471, 1980.

Ghishan FK, et al.: Pyloric stenosis and direct hyperbilirubinemia with alpha-1-antitrypsin deficiency. *Clin. Pediatr. (Phila.)* 19:293, 1980.

Gishen P, et al.: Alpha$_1$-antitrypsin deficiency: The radiological features of pulmonary emphysema in subjects of Pi type Z and Pi type SZ: A survey by the British thoracic association. *Clin. Radiol.* 33:371, 1982.

Gremse DA, et al.: Neonatal gallbladder enlargement and α$_1$-antitrypsin deficiency. *J. Pediatr. Gastroenterol. Nutr.* 6:977, 1987.

Jones DK, et al.: Alpha-$_1$-antitrypsin deficiency presenting as bronchiectasis. *Br. J. Dis. Chest* 79:301, 1985.

Kalsheker NA, et al.: Heterozygosity and localisation of normal allelic fragments for an alpha$_1$-antitrypsin homologous sequence. *Hum. Genet.* 80:108, 1988.

Kennedy JD, et al.: Severe pancreatitis and fatty liver progressing to cirrhosis associated with Coxsackie B4 infection in a three year old with alpha-1-antitrypsin deficiency. *Acta Paediatr. Scand.* 75:336, 1986.

Laros KD, et al.: The flaccid lung syndrome and α$_1$-protease inhibitor deficiency. *Chest* 93:831, 1988.

Lewis M, et al.: Severe deficiency of alpha$_1$-antitrypsin associated with cutaneous vasculitis, rapidly progressive glomerulonephritis, and colitis. *Am. J. Med.* 79:489, 1985.

Lieberman J, et al.: Serum angiotensin converting enzyme levels in patients with alpha$_1$-antitrypsin variants. *Am. J. Med.* 81:821, 1986.

Newman SL, et al.: Cystic degeneration of the lung in an infant with alpha$_1$-antitrypsin deficiency. *Clin. Pediatr. (Phila.)* 22:830, 1983.

Nord KS, et al.: Concurrence of α$_1$-antitrypsin deficiency and biliary atresia. *J. Pediatr.* 111:416, 1987.

Østergaard PA: Combined IgA and alpha-1-antitrypsin deficiency in a boy with severe respiratory tract infections and asthma. *Eur. J. Pediatr.* 138:83, 1982.

Pottage JC, et al.: Panniculitis associated with histoplasmosis and alpha$_1$-antitrypsin deficiency. *Am. J. Med.* 75:150, 1983.

Radetti G, et al.: Neonatale Krämpfe infolge einer Hirnblutung bei alpha-1-antitrypsin-Mangel. *Helv. Paediatr. Acta* 40:173, 1985.

Resendes M: Association of α$_1$-antitrypsin deficiency with lung and liver diseases. *West. J. Med.* 147:48, 1987.

Scott JH, et al.: Alpha 1-antitrypsin deficiency with diffuse bronchiectasis and cirrhosis of the liver. *Chest* 71:535, 1977.

Tobin MJ, et al.: An overview of the pulmonary features of α$_1$-antitrypsin deficiency. *Arch. Intern. Med.* 142:1342, 1982.

ALPHA-CHAIN DISEASE

Synonym: IgA heavy-chain disease.

Pathology: Diffuse lymphoma-type proliferation with involvement of the mesentery and small bowel (peroral jejunal biopsy showing abnormal plasma cells).

Clinical Manifestations: (a) *chronic diarrhea, malabsorption, progressive weight loss;* (b) *impaired absorption of vitamin B$_{12}$, glucose, lactose, and fat;* (c) *heavy-chain fragments of IgA; free of light chains in serum, in urine, and in jejunal fluid.*

Radiologic Manifestations: *Small bowel: thick circular folds, pseudostricture, pseudodiverticula, nodular mucosal pattern with a spiky and scalloped contour, segmental dilatation.*

REFERENCES

Bowie MD, et al.: α-Chain disease in children. *J. Pediatr.* 112:46, 1988.

Doe WF, et al.: Radiological and histological findings in six patients with alpha-chain disease. *Br. J. Radiol.* 49:3, 1976.

Mougenot JF, et al.: Maladie des chaînes lourdes alpha. *Arch. Fr. Pediatr.* 38:431, 1981.

Rambaud J-C, et al.: Alpha-chain disease without qualitative serum IgA abnormality: Report of two cases, including a "nonsecretory" form. *Cancer* 51:686, 1983.

Seligman M.: Alpha chain disease: Immunoglobulin abnormalities, pathogenesis and current concepts. *Br. J. Cancer* 31:356, 1975.

ALUMINUM INTOXICATION

Synonyms: Aluminum-induced bone disease; aluminum-related osteodystrophy; pseudohyperparathyroidism.

Etiology: (a) chronic renal failure and hemodialysis-related disease: aluminum administered as a phosphate binder to uremic patients, aluminum containing dialysate owing to improper water treatment, aluminum in the diet or water supply; (b) aluminum hydroxide antacid.

Clinical Manifestations: (a) *myopathy, muscle weakness;* (b) *bone pain,* (c) *poor response to vitamin D therapy;* (d) *encephalopathy (dialysis dementia);* (e) *microcytic anemia not caused by iron deficiency;* (f) *normal to elevated serum calcium levels, normal or relatively low levels of immunoreactive parathyroid hormone and alkaline phosphatase activity;* (g) *bone histology: deposition of aluminum at the bone-osteoid junction, osteomalacia without features of osteitis fi-*

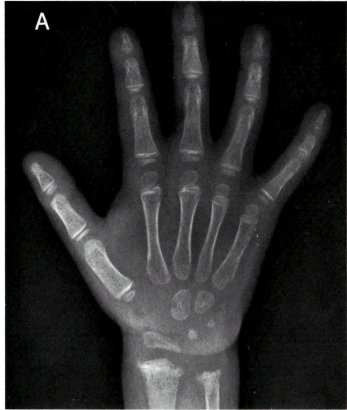
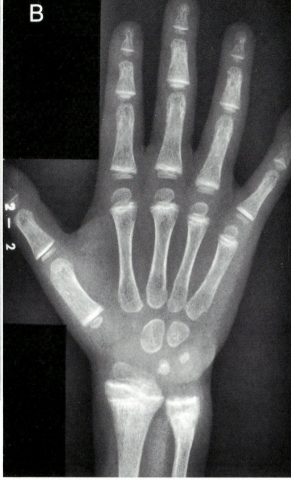

FIG ME—A—11.
Aluminum-induced bone disease in a 7½-year-old boy with a history of chronic renal failure as a result of hemolytic-uremic syndrome and treatment with aluminum hydroxide for control of hyperphosphatemia of several years' duration. **A,** fraying of the radius and ulna, widening of the physis, and osteopenia are present. **B,** 5 weeks after the beginning of chelation therapy, healing in the metaphyseal regions of radius, ulna, and other bones is seen. (From Andreoli SP, Smith JA, Bergstein JM: Aluminum bone disease in children. *Radiology* 156:663, 1985. Used by permission.)

brosa, severe mineralization defect (considered to be the result of the high rate of total-body aluminum accumulation); (h) response to treatment: cessation of exposure to aluminum, deferoxamine chelation (used in some cases).

Radiologic Manifestations: (a) *osteoporosis, osteomalacia, rachitic bone changes;* (b) *fractures* (Fig ME—A—11).

REFERENCES

Adreoli SP, et al.: Aluminum bone disease in children: Radiographic features from diagnosis to resolution. *Radiology* 156:663, 1985.
Andress DL, et al.: Osteomalacia and aplastic bone disease in aluminum-related osteodystrophy. *J. Clin. Endocrinol. Metab.* 65:11, 1987.
Carmichael KA, et al.: Osteomalacia and osteitis fibrosa in a man ingesting aluminum hydroxide antacid. *Am. J. Med.* 76:1137, 1984.
Polinsky MS, et al.: Aluminum toxicity in children with chronic renal failure. *J. Pediatr.* 105:758, 1984.
Sebes JI, et al.: Radiographic manifestations of aluminum-induced bone disease. *A.J.R.* 142:424, 1984.
Sherrard DJ, et al.: Pseudohyperparathyroidism syndrome associated with aluminum intoxication in patients with renal failure. *Am. J. Med.* 79:127, 1985.
Wills MR, et al.: Aluminum poisoning: Dialysis encephalopathy, osteomalacia, and anaemia. *Lancet* 2:29, 1983.

AMYLOIDOSIS

Mode of Inheritance: Autosomal dominant in the familial form.

Clinical Manifestations: (a) *general symptoms:* weight loss, fatigue, dizziness, dyspnea, edema, etc.; (b) *musculoskeletal system:* arthropathy with limitation of joint motion, enlarged soft tissues around joints, muscle stiffness, carpal tunnel syndrome, respiratory muscle weakness, etc.; (c) *urinary system:* renal insufficiency, nephrotic syndrome, etc.; (d) *cardiovascular system:* congestive heart failure, restrictive cardiomyopathy, decreased pulse pressure, arrhythmias, hypertension, orthostatic hypotension, clinical manifestations simulating constrictive pericarditis, low electrocardiographic voltage, conduction defects, etc.; (e) *nervous system:* various motor and sensory deficits, autonomic nervous system symptoms, cranial nerve involvement, intracerebral hemorrhage, etc; (f) *skin:* scleroderma-like skin changes, hemorrhage, etc.; (g) *alimentary system:* anorexia, abdominal pain, dysphagia, salivary gland involvement, changes in taste sensation, xerostomia, diarrhea, constipation, malabsorption, bleeding, esophageal motor dysfunction, gastroparesis, etc.; (h) hepatomegaly, progressive hepatic failure, splenomegaly; (i) upper and low respiratory system: amyloidosis of the nasopharynx, larynx, tracheobronchial tree, and lung (submucosal plaques, parenchymal), pulmonary hemorrhage; (j) laboratory findings: (1) *Congo red test;* (2) *tissue biopsy:* rectum (involvement of arterioles of the rectal mucosa), gingiva, skin, muscle, kidney, liver, spleen, heart, etc.; (3) albuminuria, cylindruria; (4) hypoalbuminemia, hypercholesterolemia; (5) *electrophoresis and immunoelectrophoresis of serum and urine;* (6) bone marrow biopsy (plasma cell dyscrasia). (k) other reported abnormalities: macroglossia (dysarthria, dysphagia), lymphadenopathy, carpal tunnel syndrome, breast mass, Sjögren syndrome, association with hypogammaglobulinemia, hypersplenism, bleeding problems, etc.

Radiological Manifestations: (a) *bone and joint manifestations:* para-articular soft-tissue nodules and swelling; joint subluxation; neuroarthropathy; subchondral cysts; avascular necrosis; osteoporosis; pathological fractures; collapse of vertebral bodies; lytic lesions, in particular, the humeri, femora, ribs, and skull; etc.; (b) *renal manifestations:* enlarged, small, or normal-sized kidneys; irregular renal contour in the con-

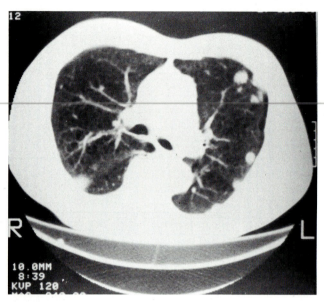

FIG ME—A—12.
Amyloidosis: multiple subpleural nodules approximately 1 to 2 cm in diameter. (From Savader SJ, Nokes SR, Chappel G: Case report and review: Computed tomography of multiple nodular pulmonary amyloidosis. *Comput. Radiol.* 11:111, 1987. Used by permission.)

tracted type of kidneys; reduced renal function on excretory urography; nephroangiographic abnormalities (normal or slightly decreased renal artery size; irregular narrowing and tortuosity of the interlobar arteries; nonvisualization of the interlobular arteries; indistinctness of the corticomedullary

TABLE ME—A—5.

Clinical Classification of Amyloidosis*

Classification†	Amyloid Type	Major Protein Component
1. Primary amyloidosis: no evidence of preceding or coexisting disease except multiple myeloma	AL‡	Ig-V$_L$‡
2. Secondary amyloidosis: coexistence of other conditions such as rheumatoid arthritis or chronic infection	AA‡	Protein A
3. Localized amyloidosis: involvement of a single organ without evidence of generalized involvement	AL	Ig-V$_L$
4. Familial amyloidosis	AF	
Portuguese	AF$_P$	Prealbumin
Japanese	AF$_J$	Prealbumin
Swedish	AF$_S$	Prealbumin
Familial Mediterranean fever	AA	Protein A
5. Senile amyloidosis	AS	
Senile cardiac amyloid	AS$_{C1}$	Prealbumin
Isolated atrial amyloid	IAA	—
Brain	AS$_b$	—

*From Kyle RA, Greipp PR: Amyloidosis (AL). Clinical and laboratory features in 229 cases. *Mayo Clin. Proc.* 58:665, 1983. Used by permission.
†Third International Symposium on Amyloidosis.
‡AL = amyloid light chain, may be κ or λ; Ig-V$_L$ = variable portion of immunoglobulin; AA = amyloid, protein A.

junction; nonvisualization of the cortical arteries, prominent extrarenal arteries, renal vein thrombosis frequently involving the segmental or interlobar veins; asymmetrical and uneven involvement of kidneys); sonographic demonstration of marked echogenicity of the cortex as compared with the liver and spleen; localized amyloidosis of the renal pelvis, ureters, bladder, prostate, seminal vesicles, vas deferens, testes, penis, and urethra that mimics neoplastic lesions; (c) *cardiac manifestations:* radiological manifestations of congestive heart failure, impaired left ventricular systolic contraction, prominence of the papillary muscles, highly refractile granular sparkling myocardial echoes on two-dimensional echocardiography, computed tomography (CT) showing low myocardial density on precontrast tomograms and diffuse myocardial thickening on postcontrast tomograms, abnormal myocardial uptake of bone-seeking radiopharmaceuticals thickening of the myocardium shown by magnetic resonance imaging, luminal irregularity and abrupt arterial caliber changes; (d) *alimentary system manifestations:* dilatation of the intestine, thickening of mucosal folds, slow transit time, pseudo-obstruction, bowel ischemia with ulceration, stricture, bowel perforation, mesenteric amyloidosis mimicking an abdominal tumor (stellate appearance on CT), nodular wall lesions mimicking neoplasms, thumb printing, ileocecal valve enlargement, pneumatosis cystoides intestinalis, pneumoperitoneum, ascites associated with portal hypertension, cardiac or renal disease; (e) lymphadenopathy, filling defect of the nodes shown by lymphangiography; (f) *hepatomegaly, splenomegaly,* and space-occupying lesions in the liver demonstrated by radionuclide, ultrasonographic, and computed imaging techniques; low density that becomes more clearly visible on postcontrast injection CT examination; uptake of bone-seeking radiopharmaceuticals such as technetium 99m methylene diphosphonate and technetium 99m pyrophosphate; (g) central nervous system: cerebral amyloid angiopathy (deposition of amyloid in medium and small arteries of the cerebral cortex and leptomeninges) causing intracerebral hemorrhage at atypical sites (cortical, multiple, bilateral), repeated episodes of bleeding, amyloidoma as a space-occupying lesion, vascular wall irregularity, and vascular occlusion shown by angiography; (h) respiratory system: laryngotracheobronchial lesions (CT: soft-tissue thickening, plaques, amyloidoma, obstruction), pulmonary lesions in many forms (honeycomb, miliary, single or multiple nodules, diffuse alveolar septal, calcification, etc.), pulmonary edema (heart failure) (Fig ME–A–12; Table ME–A–5).

REFERENCES

Allen HA III, et al.: Diffuse mesenteric amyloidosis: CT, sonographic, and pathologic findings. *J. Comput. Assist. Tomogr.* 9:196, 1985.

Benson L, et al.: Magnetic resonance imaging in primary amyloidosis. *Acta Radiol.* 28:13, 1987.

Gertz MA, et al.: Utility of technetium Tc 99m pyrophosphate bone scanning in cardiac amyloidosis. *Arch. Intern. Med.* 147:1039, 1987.

Gil R, et al.: Amylose avec gastroparésie. Amélioration par le dompéridone. *Presse Med.* 13:564, 1984.

Gilles C, et al.: Cerebral amyloid angiopathy as a cause of multiple intracerebral hemorrhages. *Neurology* 34:730, 1984.

Gogel HK, et al.: Primary amyloidosis presenting as Sjögren's syndrome. *Arch. Intern. Med.* 143:2325, 1983.

Goldman AB, et al.: Case report 137 (primary amyloidosis involving the skeletal system). *Skeletal Radiol.* 6:69, 1981.

Ikeda SI, et al.: Hereditary generalized amyloidosis with polyneuropathy. *Brain* 110:315, 1987.

Jacobson I, et al.: Amyloidosis and hyposplenism with leukocytosis and thrombocytosis. *Ann. Intern. Med.* 99:573, 1983.

Kyle RA, et al.: Amyloidosis (AL) clinical and laboratory features in 229 cases. *Mayo Clin. Proc.* 58:665, 1983.

Lee VW, et al.: Amyloidosis of heart and liver: Comparison of Tc-99m pyrophosphate and Tc-99m methylene diphosphonate for detection. *Radiology* 148:239, 1983.

Leekam RN, et al.: Gastric amyloidosis simulating antral malignancy on ultrasound. *J. Clin. Ultrasound* 13:485, 1985.

Legge DA, et al.: Intestinal pseudo-obstruction in systemic amyloidosis. *Gut* 11:764, 1970.

Manco LG, et al.: Computed tomography of macroglossia secondary to amyloidosis. *J. Comput. Assist. Tomogr.* 8:659, 1984.

Marsot-Dupuch K, et al.: L'amylose laryngée et trachéobronchique, cause rare de dyspnée. *Ann. Radiol. (Paris)* 30:347, 1987.

Matsumoto T, et al.: Amyloidomas in the cerebellopontine angle and jugular foramen. *J. Neurosurg.* 62:592, 1985.

Maule WF, et al.: Primary cardiac amyloidosis: An angiocardiographic clue to early diagnosis. *Ann. Intern. Med.* 98:177, 1983.

Nakazato M, et al.: Biochemical and genetic characterization of type I familial amyloidotic polyneuropathy. *Ann. Neurol.* 21:596, 1987.

Neils EW, et al.: Radiologic manifestations of amyloidosis (A reverse gamut). *Semin. Roentgenol.* 21:99, 1986.

Nicolosi GL, et al.: Prospective identification of patients with amyloid heart disease by two-dimensional echocardiography. *Circulation* 70:432, 1984.

O'Connor CR, et al.: Primary (AL) amyloidosis as a cause of breast masses. *Am. J. Med.* 77:981, 1984.

Rauschmeier F, et al.: Amyloidosis of the renal pelvis with ossification (abstract). *Radiology* 152:550, 1984.

Rubinow A, et al.: Esophageal manometry in systemic amyloidosis. A study of 30 patients. *Am. J. Med.* 75:951, 1983.

Santiago RM, et al.: Respiratory muscle weakness and ventilatory failure in AL amyloidosis with muscular pseudohypertrophy. *Am. J. Med.* 83:175, 1987.

Savader SJ, et al.: Case report and review: Computed tomography of multiple nodular pulmonary amyloidosis. *Comput. Radiol.* 11:111, 1987.

Sekiya T, et al.: Computed tomographic appearances of cardiac amyloidosis. *Br. Heart J.* 51:519, 1984.

Simpson GT, et al.: Localized amyloidosis of the head and neck and upper aerodigestive and lower respiratory tracts. *Otol. Rhinol. Laryngol.* 93:374, 1984.

Smith TJ, et al.: Clinical significance of histopathologic patterns of cardiac amyloidosis. *Mayo Clin. Proc.* 59:547, 1984.

Sobel DF, et al.: Cerebral amyloid angiopathy associated with massive intracerebral hemorrhage. *Neuroradiology* 27:318, 1985.

Suzuki S, et al.: CT findings in hepatic and splenic amyloidosis. *J. Comput. Assist. Tomogr.* 10:332, 1986.

Thompson PJ, et al.: Amyloid and the lower respiratory tract. *Thorax* 38:84, 1983.

Wagle WA, et al.: Intracerebral hemorrhage caused by cerebral amyloid angiopathy: Radiographic-pathologic correlation. *A.J.N.R.* 5:171, 1984.

Walzer Y, et al.: Localized amyloidosis of urethra. *Urology* 21:406, 1983.

Yood RA, et al.: Bleeding manifestations in 100 patients with amyloidosis. *J.A.M.A.* 249:1322, 1983.

ASPARTYLGLUCOSAMINURIA

Synonym: Aspartylglycosaminuria.

Mode of Inheritance: Autosomal recessive; high frequency in individuals of Finnish origin.

Enzyme abnormality: Deficiency of the lysosomal enzyme aspartylglucosaminidase (AAD Gase, E.C.3.5.1.26).

Clinical Manifestations: Onset of symptoms at about 2 to 6 years of age: (a) *progressive psychomotor retardation;* (b) *facial dysmorphism,* very mild in early childhood, becoming more apparent at school age: gargoylelike features with a broad face, wide mouth, thick lips, large tongue, low nasal bridge, anteverted nostrils; (c) short neck, prominent thoracic kyphosis, scoliosis, bulging abdomen, hernias, poorly developed sex characteristics, hoarse voice, recurrent respiratory infections, recurrent diarrhea, malabsorption, systolic murmur, mitral insufficiency, joint hyperflexibility, muscular hypotonia, lens opacities, etc.; (d) *multivacuolated lymphocytes in the peripheral blood and bone marrow, increased urinary excretion of aspartylglycosamine, demonstration of enzyme defect (aspartylglucosaminidase) in leukocytes and cultured fibroblasts,* reduced number of neutrophils, decreased prothrombin activity, prenatal diagnosis by demonstrating enzyme deficiency on cultured cells from a midterm amniotic fluid sample, abnormal enzyme assays on cord blood lymphocyts, cultured cells from skin biopsy specimens and placental villi; (e) macro-orchidism.

Radiologic Manifestations: (a) thick calvaria, microcephaly, underdeveloped frontal sinuses, small sella turcica; (b) osteochondrotic vertebral changes, flattening and anterior beaking of some vertebral bodies, spondylolysis and spondylolisthesis in early childhood; (c) cortical thinning of the tubular bones, osteoporosis, pathological fractures, skeletal maturation retardation.

REFERENCES

Aula P, et al.: Prenatal diagnosis and fetal pathology of aspartylglucosaminuria. *Am. J. Med. Genet.* 19:359, 1984.

Borud O, et al.: Aspartylglycosaminuria in northern Norway. *Lancet* 1:1082, 1976.

Chitayat D, et al.: Aspartylglucosaminuria in a Puerto Rican family: Additional features of a panethnic disorder. *Am. J. Med. Genet.* 31:527, 1988.

Gehler J, et al.: Clinical and biochemical delineation of aspartyl-glycosaminuria as observed on two members of an Italian family. *Helv. Paediatr. Acta* 36:179, 1981.

Hreidarsson S, et al.: Aspartylglucosaminuria in the United States. *Clin. Genet.* 23:427, 1983.

Jenner FA, et al.: Large quantities of 2-acetamido-l-(β-L-aspartamido)-1,2-dideoxyglucose in the urine of mentally retarded siblings. *Biochem. J.* 103:48, 1967.

BIOTINIDASE DEFICIENCY

Synonym: Late-onset multiple carboxylase deficiency (MCD).

Clinical Manifestations: Biotinidase deficiency results in reduced activities of biotin-dependent carboxylases with symptoms presenting in infancy: (a) alopecia; (b) conjunctivitis, mucositis, erythematous rash; (c) neurological problems, psychomotor regression; (d) lactic acidemia, a diagnostic urinary metabolite pattern of organic acids; (d) favorable response to pharmacological doses of biotin.

Radiologic Manifestations: Diffuse cortical atrophy of the brain.

Differential Diagnosis: Leigh disease; pyruvate dehydrogenase deficiency; cytochrome C oxidase deficiency; type I glutaric acidemia; etc.

REFERENCES

Mitchell G, et al.: Neurological deterioration and lactic acidemia in biotinidase deficiency. A treatable condition mimicking Leigh's disease. *Neuropediatrics* 17:129, 1986.

Wolf B, et al.: Deficient biotinidase activity in late onset multiple carboxylase deficiency. *N. Engl. J. Med.* 308:161, 1983.

Wolf B, et al.: Phenotypic variation in biotinidase deficiency. *J. Pediatr.* 103:233, 1983.

BLUE DIAPER SYNDROME

Synonyms: Tryptophan malabsorption; familial hypercalcemia with nephrocalcinosis and indicanuria.

Mode of Inheritance: Autosomal recessive or X-linked recessive.

Etiology: *Defect in intestinal absorption of L-tryptophan in association with increased tryptophan in feces and increased tryptophan derivatives in urine.*

Clinical Manifestations: (a) failure to thrive, recurrent fever, irritability, constipation, susceptibility to infections; (b) *blue discoloration of diapers* (indican oxidized to indican blue on exposure to air); (c) *hypercalcemia.*

Radiologic Manifestations: *Nephrocalcinosis.*

REFERENCES

Drummond KN, et al.: The blue diaper syndrome: Familial hypercalcemia with nephrocalcinosis and indicanuria. *Am. J. Med.* 37:928, 1964.

Libit SA, et al.: *Pseudomonas* as a cause of the blue diaper syndrome. *J. Pediatr.* 81:546, 1972.

CALCIUM PYROPHOSPHATE DIHYDRATE DEPOSITION DISEASE

Synonyms: CPPD; pseudogout; pyrophosphate arthropathy; calcium pyrophosphate arthropathy; calcium gout.

Mode of Inheritance: Autosomal dominant (incomplete penetrance, variable expressivity) with an onset in young adults; sporadic cases with an onset usually in middle-aged and older patients.

Clinical Manifestations: (a) *episodic acute or subacute arthralgia with soft-tissue swelling* (knee, hip, shoulder, elbow, wrist, ankle, acromioclavicular, talocalcaneal, metatarsophalangeal), *pseudorheumatoid arthritis or pseudo-osteoarthritis symptoms*; (b) *CPPD crystals within the joint and surrounding tissues*; (c) other reported abnormalities: cervical myelopathy, pseudotumoral lesions.

Radiologic Manifestations: (a) *chondrocalcinosis*; (b) *para-articular tendon and bursal calcification*; (c) *discrete subchondral rarefaction, articular space narrowing, bone sclerosis*; (d) spine and paraspinal soft-tissue CPPD crystal deposition (intervertebral disk, apophyseal and sacroiliac joints, posterior longitudinal ligament, interspinous and supraspinous ligaments, ligamentum flavum, interosseous sacroiliac ligament, transverse atlas ligament, posterior median atlantoaxial joint), spinal stenosis, atlantoaxial subluxation, calcification within soft tissues; (e) other reported abnormalities: massive soft-tissue calcification adjacent to the joint (tumorous form containing CPPD), destructive wrist arthropathy, Charcot-like joints (destructive arthropathy).

Differential Diagnosis: Hemochromatosis; hyperparathyroidism; diabetes mellitus; rheumatoid arthritis; gout.

REFERENCES

Adamson TC III, et al.: Hand and wrist arthropathies of hemochromatosis and calcium pyrophosphate deposition disease: Distinct radiographic features. *Radiology* 147:377, 1983.

Berghausen EJ, et al.: Cervical myelopathy attributable to pseudogout. Case report with radiologic, histologic, and crystallographic observations. *Clin. Orthop.* 214:217, 1987.

Bjelle A, et al.: Hereditary pyrophosphate arthropathy (familial articular chondrocalcinosis) in Sweden. *Clin. Genet.* 21:174, 1982.

Braunstein EM, et al.: Radiologic features of a pyrophosphate-like arthropathy associated with long-term dialysis. *Skeletal Radiol.* 16:437, 1987.

Dalinka MK, et al.: Calcium deposition diseases. *Semin. Roentgenol.* 17:39, 1982.

Dirheimer Y, et al.: Calcification of the transverse ligament in calcium dihydrate deposition disease (CPPD). *Neuroradiology* 27:87, 1985.

El-Khoury GY, et al.: Massive calcium pyrophosphate dihydrate crystal deposition disorder (MCPDD) involving thumb. Case report 364. *Skeletal Radiol.* 15:313, 1986.

Helms CA, et al.: Charcot-like joints in calcium pyrophosphate dihydrate deposition disease. *Skeletal Radiol.* 7:55, 1981.

Leisen J: Calcium pyrophosphate dihydrate deposition disease: Tumorous form. *A.J.R.* 138:962, 1982.

Resnick D, et al.: Vertebral involvement in calcium pyrophosphate dihydrate crystal deposition disease. Radiographic-pathological correlation. *Radiology* 153:55, 1984.

Smathers RL, et al.: The destructive wrist arthropathy of pseudogout. *Skeletal Radiol.* 7:255, 1982.

CARBONIC ANHYDRASE II DEFICIENCY

Synonym: Marble brain disease.

Mode of Inheritance: Autosomal recessive.

Clinical Manifestations: (a) *physical and mental development retardation*; (b) *characteristic facial appearance* (broad face, overhanging forehead, narrow nose, epicanthal fold, thin upper lip, poorly developed philtrum, everted lower lip, micrognathia, abnormal dentition); (c) *renal tubular acidosis*.

Radiologic Manifestations: (a) *osteopetrosis*; (b) *cerebral calcification*: basal ganglia, periventricular white matter.

REFERENCES

Cumming WA, et al.: Intracranial calcification in children with osteopetrosis caused by carbonic anhydrase II deficiency. *Radiology* 157:325, 1985.

Ohlsson A, et al.: Marble brain disease. Recessive osteopetrosis, renal tubular acidosis and cerebral calcification in three Saudi Arabian families. *Dev. Med. Child Neurol.* 22:72, 1980.

Ohlsson A, et al.: Carbonic anhydrase II deficiency syndrome: Recessive osteopetrosis with renal tubular acidosis and cerebral calcification. *Pediatrics* 77:371, 1986.

CARNITINE DEFICIENCY

Classification: (a) primary: (1) systemic: low levels of muscle, blood, and liver carnitine; (2) myopathic: muscle carnitine deficiency; (b) secondary: inadequate intake, inadequate biosynthesis, loss of carnitine (renal failure, Fanconi syndrome, etc.), pregnancy, some endocrine disorders, etc.

Mode of Inheritance: Often sporadic, heterogeneity; autosomal recessive most likely; parental consanguinity has been reported.

Clinical and Radiologic Manifestations: (a) systemic: usually affecting infants and children, *progressive muscle weakness, severe nonketotic hypoglycemia, hepatic encephalopathy, cardiomyopathy, congestive heart failure, ventilatory failure,* death in early childhood in untreated cases; (b) *myopathic*: onset of symptoms in older children and young adults, *slowly progressive muscular weakness, cardiorespiratory as late manifestation*; (c) other reported abnormalities: hypoprothrombinemia, hyperammonemia, elevated levels of liver and muscle enzymes in serum, lipid excess in hepatocytes during the encephalopathic attacks (similar to Reye syndrome), muscle cartinine deficiency presenting as familial fatal cardiomyopathy.

REFERENCES

Colin AA, et al.: Muscle carnitine deficiency presenting as familial fatal cardiomyopathy. *Arch. Dis. Child.* 62:1170, 1987.

Ino T, et al.: Dilated cardiomyopathy with neutropenia, short stature, and abnormal carnitine metabolism. *J. Pediatr.* 113:511, 1988.

Rebouche CJ, et al.: Carnitine metabolism and deficiency syndromes. *Mayo Clin. Proc.* 58:533, 1983.

Reuschenbach C, et al.: Mutant carnitine palmitoyltransferase associated with myoadenylate deaminase deficiency in skeletal muscle. *J. Pediatr.* 112:600, 1988.

CELIAC DISEASE

Synonyms: Gluten-induced enteropathy; celiac sprue; Gee-Herter-Heubner syndrome; Gee-Thaysen disease.

Pathology: Flattening of the jejunal mucosa (villous atrophy, loss of microvilli), increased depth of crypts, cuboid deformation of enterocytes, lymphocyte infiltration between enterocytes, decreased number of mast cells and increased number of eosinophils in the lamina propria, low diamine oxidase activities in the small intestinal biopsy specimen and in the serum.

Pathogenesis: Gluten intolerance resulting in malabsorption; gliadin, a component of wheat gluten, is responsible for the mucosal abnormalities.

Clinical Manifestations: Onset in early life to adulthood: (a) *pale, bulky, loose, greasy, foul-smelling stools; distended abdomen; loss of subcutaneous fat; muscular hypotonia and wasting; anorexia; irritability;* edema; bleeding tendency (vitamin K deficiency); (b) *celiac crisis* in infants: anorexia, depression, irritability, severe vomiting and diarrhea, dehydration, large and watery stools, shocklike state; (c) *increased amount of fecal fat,* abnormal xylose absorption, *abnormal fat and glucose tolerance test findings, hypoproteinemia (protein-losing enteropathy),* iron deficiency anemia; (d) *clinical and histological recovery on a gluten-free diet;* (e) immunologic abnormalities: high levels of IgA and IgG antibodies against gliadin in the patients on a gluten-containing diet, reduced number of T-lymphocytes, etc.; (f) association with other diseases: dermititis herpetiformis, chronic urticaria, cutaneous vasculitis, polyarteritis, glomerulonephritis, chronic liver disease, polymyositis, pericarditis, diabetes mellitus, cystic fibrosis, sarcoidosis, asthma, chronic cough and airway obstruction, intraocular inflammation, transient hypoparathyroidism, Graves disease, fetal alcohol syndrome, malignant tumors, intestinal lymphoma, fibrosarcoma and IgA deficiency, gastrointestinal carcinoma, aneurysmal bone cyst, etc; (g) other reported abnormalities: short stature, obesity, constipation, rectal prolapse, megacolon, bone pain, various nutritional deficiencies (hypozincemia, vitamin D deficiency rickets, scurvy, copper deficiency), tetany, occurrence in monozygotic twin, etc.

Radiologic Manifestations: (a) *abnormal intestinal motor functions:* dilatation (width of the jejunum greater than 65% of the width of the third lumbar vertebra), transient small-bowel intussusception, delay in mouth-to-cecum transit time; (b) *clumping and flocculation of barium in the small bowel, coarsening of mucosal folds,* jejunal fold separation, "bubbly" duodenal bulb (1 to 4 mm filling defects on air-contrast study); (c) mesenteric and para-aortic adenopathy with regression of the findings with clinical improvement; (d) non-

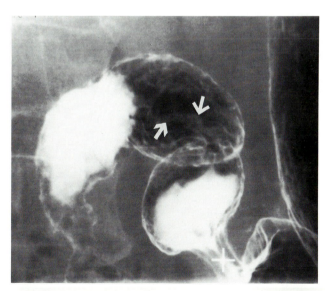

FIG ME–C–1.
Duodenal bulb in celiac disease. Several discrete nodules *(arrows)* are clustered together while other nodules are scattered throughout bulb. (From Jones B, Bayless TM, Hamilton SR, et al.: "Bubbly" duodenal bulb in celiac disease: Radiologic pathology correlation. *A.J.R.* 142:119, 1984. Used by permission.)

specific intestinal ulceration (rare); (e) bone demineralization, rickets, fractures, skeletal maturation retardation (Fig ME–C–1).

REFERENCES

Ashkenazi A, et al.: Cellular immunity in children with coeliac disease. *Eur. J. Pediatr.* 138:250, 1982.

Brocchi E, et al.: Endoscopic demonstration of loss of duodenal folds in the diagnosis of celiac disease. *N. Engl. J. Med.* 319:741, 1988.

De Sousa JS, et al.: Late onset coeliac disease in the monozygotic twin of a coeliac child. *Acta Paediatr. Scand.* 76:172, 1987.

Douglas JG, et al.: Sarcoidosis and coeliac disease: An association? *Lancet* 2:13, 1984.

Forget P, et al.: Diamine oxidase in serum and small intestinal biopsy tissue in childhood celiac disease. *J. Pediatr. Gastroenterol. Nutr.* 5:379, 1986.

Foulston C, et al.: Transient neutral fat steatorrhea, elevated sweat chloride concentration, and hypoparathyroidism in a child with celiac disease. *J. Pediatr. Gastroenterol. Nutr.* 4:143, 1985.

Goyens P, et al.: Copper deficiency in infants with active celiac disease. *J. Pediatr. Gastroenterol. Nutr.* 4:677, 1985.

Hautekeete ML, et al.: Chronic urticaria associated with coeliac disease. *Lancet* 1:157, 1987.

Henker J, et al.: Serumzinkspiegel bei Kindern mit Zöliakie. *Helv. Paediat. Acta* 40:47, 1985.

Herlinger H, et al.: Jejunal fold separation in adult celiac disease: Relevance of enteroclysis. *Radiology* 158:605, 1986.

Høgh B, et al.: Coeliac disease coexistent with fetal alcohol syndrome. *Eur. J. Pediatr.* 143:74, 1984.

Hosker HSR, et al.: Adult coeliac disease presenting with symptoms of worsening asthma. *Lancet* 2:1157, 1986.

Jones B, et al.: "Bubbly" duodenal bulb in celiac disease: Radiologic-pathologic correlation. *A.J.R.* 142:119, 1984.

Jones B, et al.: Lymphadenopathy in celiac disease: Computed tomographic observations. *A.J.R.* 142:127, 1984.

Kappelman NB, et al.: Megacolon associated with celiac sprue: Report of four cases and review of the literature. *A.J.R.* 128:65, 1977.

Kosnai I, et al.: Mast cells and eosinophils in the jejunal mucosa of patients with intestinal cow's milk allergy and celiac disease of childhood. *J. Pediatr. Gastroenterol. Nutr.* 3:368, 1984.

Kumar V, et al.: Are antigliadin antibodies specific for celiac disease? *J. Pediatr. Gastroenterol. Nutr.* 3:815, 1984.

Loughran TP, et al.: T-cell intestinal lymphoma associated with celiac sprue. *Ann. Intern. Med.* 104:44, 1986.

Lowe G, et al.: Sarcoidosis and coeliac disease. *Lancet* 2:637, 1984.

Maggiore G, et al.: Celiac disease presenting as chronic hepatitis in a girl. *J. Pediatr. Gastroenterol. Nutr.* 5:501, 1986.

Masterson JB, et al.: The role of small bowel follow-through examination in the diagnosis of celiac disease. *Br. J. Radiol.* 49:660, 1976.

Naveh Y, et al.: A prospective study of serum zinc concentration in children with celiac disease. *J. Pediatr.* 102:734, 1983.

Nibali SC, et al.: Obesity in a child with untreated coeliac disease. *Helv. Paediatr. Acta* 42:45, 1987.

Osman MZ, et al.: Celiac disease (gluten-induced enteropathy). *Semin. Roentgenol.* 8:243, 1973.

Ross JR, et al.: Gluten enteropathy and skeletal disease. *J.A.M.A.* 196:270, 1966.

Ruch W, et al.: Coexistent coeliac disease, Graves' disease and diabetes mellitus type 1 in a patient with Down syndrome. *Eur. J. Pediatr.* 144:89, 1985.

Ruddy RM, et al.: Abnormal sweat electrolytes in a case of celiac disease and a case of psychosocial failure to thrive. Review of other reported causes. *Clin. Pediatr. (Phila.)* 26:83, 1987.

Saari KM, et al.: Immunological disorders of the eye complicating coeliac disease. *Lancet* 1:968, 1984.

Sarles J, et al.: Subcellular localization of class I (A,B,C) and class II (DR and DQ) MHC antigens in jejunal epithelium of children with coeliac disease. *J. Pediatr. Gastroenterol. Nutr.* 6:51, 1987.

Savilahti E, et al.: Celiac disease in insulin-dependent diabetes mellitus. *J. Pediatr.* 108:690, 1986.

Shanahan F, et al.: Extending the scope in celiac disease. *N. Engl. J. Med.* 319:782, 1988.

Similä S, et al.: Cutaneous vasculitis as a manifestation of coeliac disease. *Acta Paediatr. Scand.* 71:1051, 1982.

Stenhammar L, et al.: Coeliac disease in children of short stature without gastrointestinal symptoms. *Eur. J. Pediatr.* 145:185, 1986.

Stenhammar L: Coeliac disease presenting as vitamin D deficiency rickets in a vegetarian child. *Acta Paediatr. Scand.* 74:972, 1985.

Stenhammar L, et al.: Aneurysmal bone cyst of the femur in a child with celiac disease. *J. Pediatr. Gastroenterol. Nutr.* 5:814, 1986.

Stenhammar L, et al.: Serum gliadin antibodies for detection and control of childhood coeliac disease. *Acta Paediatr. Scand.* 73:657, 1984.

Tarlo M, et al.: Association between celiac disease and lung disease. *Chest* 80:715, 1981.

Verkasalo M, et al.: Fibrosarcoma in a girl with celiac disease and IgA deficiency. *J. Pediatr. Gastroenterol. Nutr.* 4:839, 1985.

Zultak M, et al.: Scorbut révélant une maladie coeliaque. *Presse Med.* 15:1730, 1986.

CEROID LIPOFUSCINOSIS (NEURONAL)

Synonym: Neuronal ceroid lipofuscinosis.

Mode of Inheritance: Autosomal recessive.

Pathology: A lipid metabolic disease characterized by widespread neural and visceral storage of ceroid lipofuscin; neural destruction and gliosis in the cerebral cortical gray matter; characteristic cytoplasmic inclusion (rectal mucosa, skin, peripheral blood).

Classification: (a) infantile (first year of life); (b) late infantile (1 to 4 years of age); (c) juvenile (5 to 8 years); (d) adult (after 20 years of age).

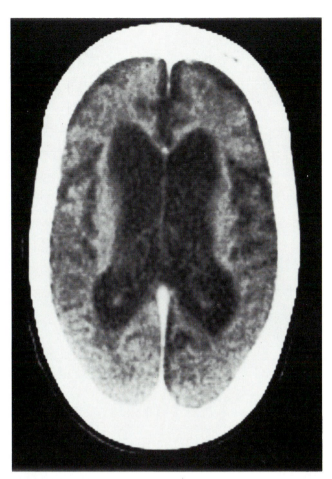

FIG ME–C–2.
Ceroid lipofuscinosis. Ventricular dilatation and cortical brain atrophy are shown. (From Savolaine ER, Voeller K, Gunning W, et al.: Computed tomography in neuronal ceroid lipofuscinosis: Four case reports. *J. Comput. Tomogr.* 11:73, 1987. Used by permission.)

Clinical Manifestations: (a) progressive deterioration of motor and intellectual capabilities, seizures; (b) progressive visual loss; (c) speech disorders; (d) extrapyramidal, pyramidal, and cerebellar signs.

Radiologic Manifestations: Progressive cerebral cortical and cerebellar atrophy (ventricular dilatation, increased extra-axial space); marked enlargement of the fourth ventricle and cerebellar atrophy without concomitant cerebral atrophy (Fig ME–C–2).

REFERENCES

Dunn DW: CT in ceroid lipofuscinosis. *Neurology* 37:1025, 1987.
Lagenstein I, et al.: Neuronal ceroid lipofuscinosis: CT findings in fourteen patients. *Acta Paediatr. Scand.* 70:857, 1981.
Savolaine ER, et al.: Computed tomography in neuronal ceroid lipofuscinosis: Four case reports. *J. Comput. Tomogr.* 11:73, 1987.
Valavanis A, et al.: Computed tomography in neuronal ceroid lipofuscinosis. *Neuroradiology* 19:35, 1980.

CHOLESTEROL ESTER STORAGE DISEASE

Synonyms: Cholesteryl ester storage disease; CESD.

Mode of Inheritance: Autosomal recessive.

Enzyme Deficiency: Lysosomal acid lipase (acid cholesteryl ester hydrolase)

Clinical Manifestations: Onset in childhood to adulthood: (a) *elevated plasma concentration of cholesterol, premature atherosclerosis;* (b) *hyperlipidemia;* (c) *hepatomegaly* (deposition of cholesteryl esters and triglycerides in the hepatocytes and Kupffer cells; periportal infiltration by lymphocytes, plasma cells, and foamy macrophages; septal fibrosis), micronodular cirrhosis and portal hypertension; (d) splenomegaly.

Radiologic Manifestations: (a) *hepatomegaly, splenomegaly, portal hypertension,* esophageal varices; (b) faint adrenal calcification (rare).

Note: Presumably CESD is allelic to Wolman disease with similar genetic and enzymatic defects but has a distinctive clinical course and biochemical findings (enzyme activity reduced 50- to 100-fold in CESD fibroblasts as compared with a 200-fold reduction in cells with Wolman disease).

REFERENCES

Hill SC, et al.: CT findings in acid lipase deficiency: Wolman disease and cholesteryl ester storage disease. *J. Comput. Assist. Tomogr.* 7:815, 1983.
Hoeg JM, et al.: Cholesteryl ester storage disease and Wolman disease: Phenotypic variants of lysosomal acid cholesteryl ester hydrolase deficiency. *Am. J. Hum. Genet.* 36:1190, 1984.
Schiff L, et al.: Hepatic cholesterol ester storage disease, a familial disorder. I. Clinical aspects. *Am. J. Med.* 44:538, 1968.

CHRONIC GRANULOMATOUS DISEASE OF CHILDHOOD

Synonyms: Neutrophil dysfunction syndrome; granulomatous disease of childhood; phagocyte oxidase deficiency syndrome; fatal granulomatous disease of childhood; Bridges-Good syndrome.

Mode of Inheritance: X-linked recessive (in the typical form, about 85% of the patients are males); transmission in females presumed to be autosomal recessive.

Etiology: *Inability of peripheral blood neutrophils and monocytes to kill certain phagocytized and opsonized bacterial species; lack of leukocystic oxidase enzyme.*

Clinical Manifestations: (a) *chronic and recurrent severe suppurative infections* in the lungs, lymph nodes, bones, spleen, liver, etc., caused by catalase-positive, e.g., staphylococci, *Serratia, Klebsiella-Aerobacter, Pseudomonas, Escherichia coli, Proteus, and Salmonella,* fungi, and *Pneumocystis carinii;* (b) eczematoid dermatitis; (c) granulocytes fail to reduce nitroblue tetrazolium to blue formazin, antenatal diagnosis by fetal blood testing: cytochemical reduction of nitroblue tetrazolium, chemiluminescence after activation by opsonized zymosan or phorbol myristate acetate, and production of superoxide anion (O_2^-); (d) other reported manifestations: rhinitis, conjunctivitis, stomatitis, vomiting, intestinal obstruction, cystitis, unexplained fever, diarrhea, malabsorption, perianal abscesses, pericarditis, anemia, leukocytosis, elevated sedimentation rate, association with McLeod syndrome, ascites (peritonitis) as a presenting sign, absence

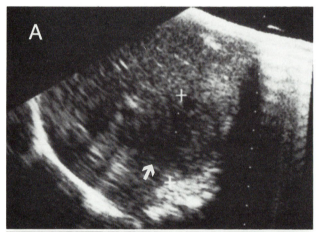

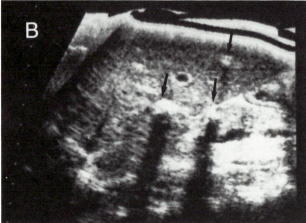

FIG ME–C–3.
Chronic granulomatous disease. Longitudinal ultrasonograms show two poorly marginated, hypoechoic areas *(arrow)* in the right lobe of the liver **(A)**. Calcifications with distal acoustic shadowing *(arrows)* are visible on the longitudinal scan along the aorta and suggest previous chronic granulomatous disease involvement of the left lobe **(B)**. (From Garel LA, et al.: Liver involvement in chronic granulomatous disease: The role of ultrasound in diagnosis and treatment. *Radiology* 153:117, 1984. Used by permission.)

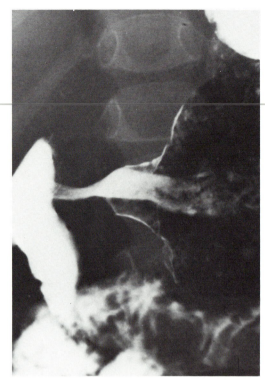

FIG ME–C–4.
Chronic granulomatous disease of childhood in a 6-year-old boy with a known diagnosis of chronic granulomatous disease since the age of 2 years and a recent history of vomiting and heartburn after the ingestion of solid foods. A concentric funnel-shaped narrowing of the gastric antral lumen is shown. (From Bowen A III, Gibson MD: Chronic granulomatous disease with gastric antral narrowing. *Pediatr. Radiol.* 10:119, 1980. Used by permission.)

of cytochrome b_{-245}, selective IgA deficiency, association with chronic glomerulonephritis, short stature.

Radiologic Manifestations: (a) *chronic and recurrent pneumonia;* persistent pneumatocele; honeycomb lung; *hilar adenopathy;* emphysema; mediastinitis; pericarditis; cardiac failure in children with mediastinitis; stenosis of the aorta and brachiocephalic vessels, mycotic pseudoaneurysm of the internal mammary artery; diffusion of mediastinitis into the vertebrae, ribs, and spinal canal; (b) fungus infections; (c) hepatic granuloma (hypoechoic, poorly marginated areas without posterior enhancement), hepatosplenomegaly; (d) subdiaphragmatic and visceral abscesses, suppurative retroperitoneal lymphadenopathy, scrotal abscess; (e) *speckled calcific densities in the lungs, liver, spleen, and lymph nodes;* (f) osteomyelitis, sequestra formation rare, small bones of the hands and feet often involved; (g) esophageal obstruction, focal or diffuse gastric wall involvement (contrast study, computed tomography [CT], echography), annular stenosis of the gastric outlet, intestinal obstruction, enterocolitis mimicking Crohn disease, progressive esophageal dysfunction, functional gastrointestinal obstruction; (h) hydronephrosis, destruction of papillae, abscess formation in the kidneys, cystitis, bullous edema of the bladder in association with reduced

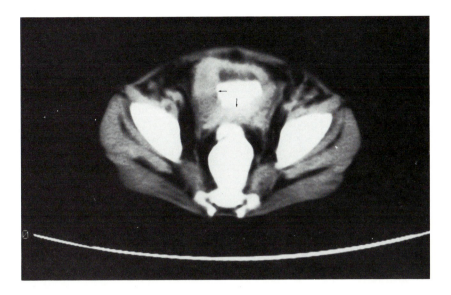

FIG ME–C–5.
Cystitis in chronic granulomatous disease. Axial CT of the pelvis demonstrates bladder wall thickening *(arrows)*. (From Hassel DR, Glassier CM, McDonnell JR: Granulomatous cystitis in chronic granulomatous disease: Ultrasound diagnosis. *Pediatr. Radiol.* 17:254, 1987. Used by permission.)

bladder capacity; (i) subsidence of obstructive lesions of the esophagus, gastrointestinal tract, and genitourinary tract with corticosteroid treatment (Figs ME–C–3 to ME–C–5).

REFERENCES

Azimi P, et al.: Chronic granulomatous disease in three female siblings. *J.A.M.A.* 206:2865, 1968.

Bowen A III, Gibson MD: Chronic granulomatous disease with gastric antral narrowing. *Pediatr. Radiol.* 10:119, 1980.

Bridges RA, et al.: A fatal granulomatous disease of childhood: The clinical, pathological and laboratory features of a new syndrome. *Am. J. Dis. Child.* 97:387, 1959.

Buescher ES, et al.: Stature and weight in chronic granulomatous disease. *J. Pediatr.* 104:911, 1984.

Chin TW, et al.: Corticosteroids in treatment of obstructive lesions of chronic granulomatous disease. *J. Pediatr.* 111:349, 1987.

Chusid MJ, et al.: Pulmonary aspergillosis appearing as chronic nodular disease in a chronic granulomatous disease. *Pediatr. Radiol.* 18:232, 1988.

Ezekowitz RAB, et al.: Partial correction of the phagocyte defect in patients with X-linked chronic granulomatous disease by subcutaneous interferon gamma. *N. Engl. J. Med.* 319:146, 1988.

Fikrig SM, et al.: Chronic granulomatous disease and McLeod syndrome in a black child. *Pediatrics* 66:403, 1980.

Fleming GM, et al.: Chronic granulomatous disease of childhood: An unusual cause of honeycomb lung. *Chest* 68:834, 1975.

Forbes GS, et al.: Genitourinary involvement in chronic granulomatous disease of childhood. *A.J.R.* 127:683, 1976.

Frifelt JJ, et al.: Chronic granulomatous disease associated with chronic glomerulonephritis. *Acta. Paediatr. Scand.* 74:152, 1985.

Garel LA, et al.: Liver involvement in chronic granulomatous disease: The role of ultrasound in diagnosis and treatment. *Radiology* 153:117, 1984.

Gerba WM, et al.: Chronic granulomatous disease and selective IgA deficiency. *Am. J. Pediatr. Hematol. Oncol.* 4:155, 1982.

Granot E, et al.: Functional gastrointestinal obstruction in a child with chronic granulomatous disease. *J. Pediatr. Gastroenterol. Nutr.* 5:321, 1986.

Hartenberg MA, et al.: Chronic granulomatous disease of childhood. Probable diffuse gastric involvement. *Pediatr. Radiol.* 14:57, 1984.

Hassel DR, et al.: Granulomatous cystitis in chronic granulomatous disease: Ultrasound diagnosis. *Pediatr. Radiol.* 17:254, 1987.

Hitzig WH, et al.: Chronic granulomatous disease, a heterogeneous syndrome. *Hum. Genet.* 64:207, 1983.

Huu TP, et al.: Diagnostic anténatal d'exclusion de la granulomatose septique chronique familiale. *Arch. Fr. Pediatr.* 42:103, 1985.

Isaacs D, et al.: Chronic granulomatous disease mimicking Crohn's disease. *J. Pediatr. Gasteroenterol. Nutr.* 4:498, 1985.

Kenney PJ, et al.: Gastric involvement in chronic granulomatous disease of childhood: Demonstration by computed tomography and upper gastrointestinal studies. *J. Comput. Assist. Tomogr.* 9:563, 1985.

Kopen PA, et al.: Upper gastrointestinal and ultrasound examinations of gastric antral involvement in chronic granulomatous disease. *Pediatr. Radiol.* 14:91, 1984.

Lindahl JA, et al.: Small bowel obstruction in chronic granulomatous disease. *J. Pediatr. Gastroenterol. Nutr.* 3:637, 1984.

Markowitz JF, et al.: Progressive esophageal dysfunction in chronic granulomatous disease. *J. Pediatr. Gastroenterol. Nutr.* 1:145, 1982.

Mizuno Y, et al.: Classification of chronic granulomatous disease on the basis of monoclonal antibody–defined surface cytochrome b deficiency. *J. Pediatr.* 113:458, 1988.

Rossi TM, et al.: Ascites as a presenting sign of peritonitis in chronic granulomatous disease of childhood. *Clin. Pediatr. (Phila.)* 26:544, 1987.

Sanchez FW, et al.: Embolotherapy of a mycotic pseudoaneurysm of the internal mammary artery in chronic granulomatous disease. *Cardiovasc. Intervent. Radiol.* 8:43, 1985.

Segal AW, et al.: Absence of cytochrome b$_{-245}$ in chronic granulomatous disease: A multicenter European evaluation of its incidence and relevance. *N. Engl. J. Med.* 308:245, 1983.

Southwick FS, et al.: Recurrent cystitis and bladder mass in two adults with chronic granulomatous disease. *Ann. Intern. Med.* 109:118, 1988.

Stricof DD, et al.: Chronic granulomatous disease: Value of the newer imaging modalities. *Pediatr. Radiol.* 14:328, 1984.

Tauber AI, et al.: Chronic granulomatous disease: A syndrome of phagocyte oxidase deficiencies. *Medicine (Baltimore)* 62:286, 1983.

Vichi GF, et al.: Unusual evolution of chronic granulomatous disease with mediastinum localization and diffusion into vertebrae, ribs and vertebral canal. *Fortschr. Rontgenstr.* 145:109, 1986.

Wood BP, et al.: Persistent pneumatoceles associated with systemic leukocyte abnormalities. *Pediatr. Radiol.* 5:10, 1976.

Young AK, et al.: Urologic manifestations of chronic granulomatous disease of infancy. *J. Urol.* 123:119, 1980.

COPPER DEFICIENCY

Etiology: Chronic diarrhea; chronic intestinal malabsorption; infants and adults receiving total parenteral nutrition treatments; infants with prolonged liver damage; chronic draining biliary or enteric fistulas; protein loss; use of chelating agents; restricted cow milk feeding in infants; premature babies fed milk formula low in copper.

Clinical Manifestations: (a) *depigmentation of the skin and hair;* (b) *psychomotor retardation, hypotonia;* (c) *swelling of limbs* due to subperiosteal hemorrhage; (d) *distended blood vessels;* (e) association with rickets; (f) *sideroblastic anemia,* vacuolation of erythroid and myeloid bone marrow cells, iron deposition in some mitochondria and the vacuoles, *leukopenia, neutropenia;* (g) *low levels of ceruloplasmin, serum copper,* and urinary copper.

Radiologic Manifestations: (a) *osteoporosis* in the early stage; (b) *irregularity, increased density, and cupping of the provisional zone of calcification; sickle-shaped spur formation in continuity with the provisional zone of calcification;* (c) multiple undisplaced fractures, epiphyseal separation, subperiosteal hemorrhage, periosteal elevation with subperiosteal calcification; (d) soft-tissue calcification; (e) skeletal maturation retardation.

Differential Diagnosis: (a) Menke syndrome; (b) scurvy; (c) hemarthrosis or pyarthrosis (epiphyseal separation with the epiphysis not yet ossified), nonaccidental injury (child abuse).

Note: Copper deficiency has been reported in a boy and his mother (X-linked or autosomal dominant) (Mehes et al.) (Fig ME–C–6).

REFERENCES

Allen TM, et al.: Skeletal changes associated with copper deficiency. *Clin. Orthop.* 168:206, 1982.

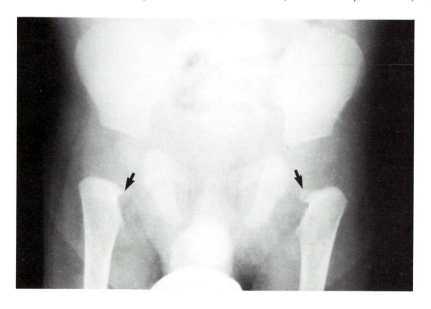

FIG ME–C–6.
Copper deficiency: spur formation *(arrows)* of the femoral necks. (From Levy Y, Zeharia A, Grunebaum M, et al.: Copper deficiency in infants fed cow milk. *J. Pediatr.* 106:786, 1985. Used by permission.)

Becton DL, et al.: Severe neutropenia caused by copper deficiency in a child receiving continuous ambulatory peritoneal dialysis. *J. Pediatr.* 108:735, 1986.

Grünebaum M, et al.: The radiographic manifestations of bone changes in copper deficiency. *Pediatr. Radiol.* 9:101, 1980.

Higuchi S, et al.: Nutritional copper deficiency in severely handicapped patients on a low copper enteral diet for a prolonged period: Estimation of the required dose of dietary copper. *J. Pediatr. Gastroenterol. Nutr.* 7:583, 1988.

Levy J, et al.: Epiphyseal separation simulating pyarthrosis, secondary to copper deficiency, in an infant receiving total parenteral nutrition. *Br. J. Radiol.* 57:636, 1984.

Levy Y, et al.: Copper deficiency in infants fed cow milk. *J. Pediatr.* 106:786, 1985.

McGill LC, et al.: Extremity swelling in an infant with copper and zinc deficiency. *J. Pediatr. Surg.* 15:746, 1980.

Mehes K, et al.: Familial benign copper deficiency. *Arch. Dis. Child.* 57:716, 1982.

Shaw JCL: Copper deficiency and non-accidental injury. *Arch. Dis. Child.* 63:448, 1988.

CUSHING SYNDROME

Etiology: Excessive endogenous excretion of cortisol and other adrenal steroids or corticosteroid therapy: (a) pituitary-dependent adrenal hyperplasia (Cushing disease); (b) adrenal tumors (adenoma, carcinoma); (c) exogenous, naturally oc-

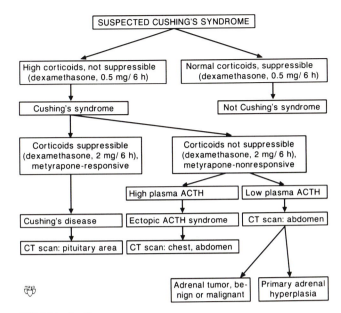

FIG ME–C–8.
Evaluation of patients with suspected Cushing syndrome. Because some medications alter the ACTH production rate, patients should be medication free before the initiation of assessment (ACTH = adrenocorticotropic hormone; CT = computed tomography). (From Carpenter PC: Cushing's syndrome: Update of diagnosis and management. *Mayo Clin. Proc.* 61:49, 1986. Used by permission.)

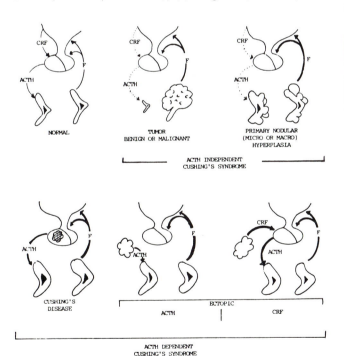

FIG ME–C–7.
Roles of adrenocorticotropic hormone *(ACTH)*, corticotropin-releasing factor *(CRF)*, and blood cortisol *(F)* in normal function and in ACTH-independent and ACTH-dependent Cushing syndrome. (From Carpenter PC: Cushing's syndrome: Update of diagnosis and management. *Mayo Clin. Proc.* 61:49, 1986. Used by permission.)

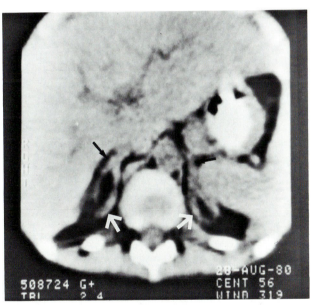

FIG ME–C–9.
Cushing syndrome: bilateral adrenal hyperplasia in a 10-year-old girl. Both adrenals are diffusely enlarged *(arrows)*. (From Shirkhoda A: Current diagnostic approach to adrenal abnormalities. *J. Comput. Tomogr.* 8:277, 1984. Used by permission.)

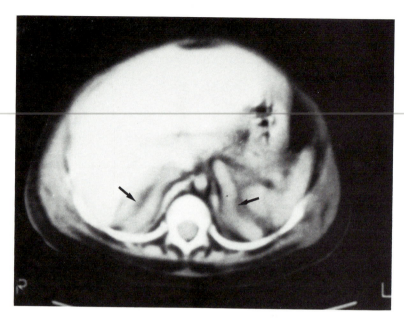

FIG ME−C−10.
Cushing syndrome in a 7-month-old male with infantile spasms, pancytopenia, and Cushing syndrome secondary to ACTH administration. Marked enlargement of the adrenal glands is present.

(Courtesy of Ronald A. Cohen, M.D., Children's Hospital Medical Center, Oakland, Calif.)

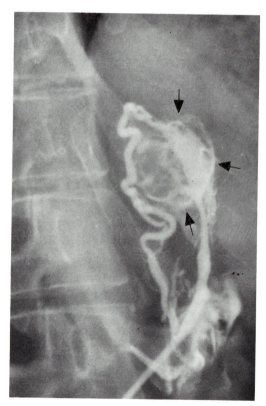

FIG ME−C−11.
Cushing syndrome. An adrenal venogram in a 32-year-old female demonstrates a tumor *(arrows)*. Left adrenalectomy was performed for an adrenal cortical adenoma. (Courtesy of Dr. Jalil Farah, Royal Oak, Mich.)

curring: secretions of adrenocorticotropic hormone (ACTH) by benign or malignant tumors of nonendocrine origin (ectopic ACTH syndrome)—tumors of the thymus, pancreas, thyroid, and ovaries; Wilms tumor; neuroblastoma; bronchogenic carcinoma or adenoma; carcinoid tumor; adrenal rest tumor of the liver; metastatic medullary carcinoma of the thyroid containing corticotropin-releasing factor; etc.; (d) iatrogenic: corticosteroid therapy, triamcinolone injection for urethral strictures, etc.

Clinical Manifestations: (a) *moon face;* (b) *buffalo hump;* (c) *thinning of the skin;* (d) *wasting and muscle weakness;* (e) *fragility of blood vessels* and a tendency to bruise; (f) headaches; (g) back pain; (h) mental changes; (i) *excessive endogenous excretion of cortisol and other adrenal steroids;* (j) growth failure in juvenile Cushing syndrome; (k) other reported abnormalities: association with craniopharyngioma, Zollinger-Ellison syndrome, menstrual changes, opportunistic infections, hypoadrenalism following venography in Cushing disease, cyclic Cushing syndrome (fluctuation of adrenal steroid production), rupture of the Achilles tendon, etc.

Radiologic Manifestations: (a) *osteoporosis, pathological fractures,* heavy callus formation at the site of fractures (ribs, pelvis), cystic changes of the skeleton, aseptic necrosis of the epiphyses with secondary arthropathy, *compression fractures of the vertebrae* with marginal condensation of bodies; (b) enlargement and erosion of the sella turcica (in a few), empty sella turcica, pituitary imaging demonstrating the microadenoma or macroadenoma, petrosal sinus sampling for differentiation between pituitary and ectopic-ACTH Cushing syndromes; (c) adrenal neoplasm, accuracy of computed tomography in diagnosis near 100%; (d) adrenal hyperplasia: the glands may be enlarged without a change in shape; (e) radionuclide scanning (19-iodo-cholesterol ^{131}I) helpful in evaluation of the physiology of the glands and differential diagnosis of the neoplasm and hyperplasia; (f) other reported abnormalities: adrenal calcification, advanced or retarded skeletal maturation, muscle atrophy, loss of the lamina dura, lipomatosis (mediastinal, cavernous sinus, episternal, presacral, intrahepatic, intraspinal causing spinal canal stenosis), nephrocalcinosis, increased echogenicity of the pancreas (after ACTH therapy), rebound thymic hyperplasia after treatment of the Cushing syndrome, failure of bone scanning to detect fracture, cortical atrophy of cerebral and cerebellar hemispheres, ectopic pituitary adenoma within the sphenoid sinus, etc.

Notes: Ruder syndrome represents adrenal hyperfunction (bilateral micronodular adrenal hyperplasia) associated with severe osteoporosis in young adults; the typical symptoms and signs of Cushing syndrome are minimal or absent (Figs ME−C−7 to ME−C−11).

REFERENCES

Ackland FM, et al.: Cushing's disease and craniopharyngioma. *Arch. Dis. Child.* 62:1077, 1987.

Augspurger RR, et al.: Cushing's syndrome: Complication of triamcinolone injection for urethral strictures in children. *J. Urol.* 123:932, 1980.

Bachow TB, et al.: Fat deposition in the cavernous sinus in Cushing disease. *Radiology* 153:135, 1984.

Belsky JL, et al.: Cushing's syndrome due to ectopic production of corticotropin-releasing factor. *J. Clin. Endocrinol. Metab.* 60:496, 1985.

Bien ME, et al.: Computed tomography in the evaluation of mediastinal lipomatosis. *J. Comput. Assist. Tomogr.* 2:379, 1978.

Burch W, et al.: Cushing's disease caused by an ectopic pituitary adenoma within the sphenoid sinus. *N. Engl. J. Med.* 312:587, 1985.

Carey RM, et al.: Ectopic secretion of corticotropin-releasing factor as a cause of Cushing's syndrome. *N. Engl. J. Med.* 311:13, 1984.

Carpenter PC: Cushing's syndrome: Update of diagnosis and management. *Mayo Clin. Proc.* 61:49, 1986.

Christian CD, et al.: Fatty tumor of the liver in a patient with Cushing's syndrome. *Arch. Intern. Med.* 143:1605, 1983.

Contreras P, et al.: Adrenal rest tumor of the liver causing Cushing's syndrome: Treatment with ketoconazole preceding an apparent surgical cure. *J. Clin. Endocrinol. Metab.* 60:21, 1985.

Cryer PE, et al.: Vertebral compression fractures with accelerated bone turnover in a patient with Cushing's disease. *Am. J. Med.* 68:932, 1980.

Cummins GE, et al.: Cushing's syndrome secondary to ACTH-secreting Wilms tumor. *J. Pediatr. Surg.* 9:535, 1974.

Cushing HW: The basophil adenomas of the pituitary body and their clinical manifestations (pituitary basophilism). *Bull. Johns Hopkins Hosp.* 50:137, 1932.

Darling DB, et al.: The roentgenographic manifestations of Cushing's syndrome in infancy. *Radiology* 96:503, 1970.

Doppman JL, et al.: Macronodular adrenal hyperplasia in Cushing disease. *Radiology* 166:347, 1988.

Doppman JL, et al.: Petrosal sinus sampling for Cushing syndrome: Anatomical and technical considerations. *Radiology* 150:99, 1984.

Doppman JL, et al.: Rebound thymic hyperplasia after treatment of Cushing's syndrome. *A.J.R.* 147:1145, 1986.

Dwyer AJ, et al.: Pituitary adenomas in patients with Cushing disease: Initial experience with Gd-DTPA-enhanced MR Imaging. *Radiology* 163:421, 1987.

Eastridge CE, et al.: Cushing's syndrome associated with bronchial adenoma. *Am. J. Surg.* 133:236, 1977.

Felson B, et al.: Cushing syndrome associated with mediastinal mass. *A.J.R.* 138:815, 1982.

Foley LC, et al.: Nephrocalcinosis: Sonographic detection in Cushing syndrome. *A.J.R.* 139:610, 1982.

Gemme G, et al.: Cushing's syndrome due to topical corticosteroids. *Am. J. Dis. Child.* 138:987, 1984.

George WE, et al.: Medical management of steroid-induced epidural lipomatosis. *N. Engl. J. Med.* 308:316, 1983.

Góth M, et al.: Hypoadrenia following adrenal venography in Cushing's disease. *Eur. J. Radiol.* 4:68, 1984.

Graham BS, et al.: Opportunistic infections in endogenous Cushing's syndrome. *Ann. Intern. Med.* 101:334, 1984.

Guegan Y, et al.: Spinal cord compression by extradural fat after prolonged corticosteroid therapy. *J. Neurosurg.* 56:267, 1982.

Herreman G, et al.: Rupture bilaterale du tendon d'Achille au cours d'un syndrome de Cushing. *Presse Med.* 14:1972, 1985.

Hodge BO, et al.: Familial Cushing's syndrome. Micronodular adrenocortical dysplasia. *Arch. Intern. Med.* 148:1133, 1988.

Howland WJ Jr, et al.: Roentgenologic changes of the skeletal system in Cushing's syndrome. *Radiology* 71:69, 1958.

Jex RK, et al.: Ectopic ACTH syndrome. Diagnostic and therapeutic aspects. *Am. J. Surg.* 149:276, 1985.

Kaplan FS, et al.: Multiple pathologic fractures of the appendicular skeleton in a patient with Cushing's disease. *Clin. Orthop.* 216:171, 1987.

Laissy JP, et al.: Intérêt et limites de la tomodensitométrie dans les masses surrénaliennes sécrétantes de l'adulte. *Ann. Radiol. (Paris)* 30:255, 1987.

Landis B, et al.: Ruder syndrome. Clinical and pathologic correlation. *Urology* 22:200, 1983.

Larsen JL, et al.: Primary adrenocortical nodular dysplasia, a distinct subtype of Cushing's syndrome. Case report and review of the literature. *Am. J. Med.* 80:976, 1986.

Lipkin EW, et al.: Cushing's syndrome in a patient with suppressible hypercortisolism and an empty sella. *West J. Med.* 140:613, 1984.

Madell SH, et al.: Avascular necrosis of bone in Cushing's syndrome. *Radiology* 83:1068, 1964.

Maehara T, et al.: Medically treated steroid-induced epidural lipomatosis. *Neuroradiology* 30:281, 1988.

Maton PN, et al.: Cushing's syndrome in patients with the Zollinger-Ellison syndrome. *N. Engl. J. Med.* 315:1, 1986.

Mitty HA, et al.: Adrenal venography: Clinical-roentgenographic correlation in 80 patients. *A.J.R.* 119:564, 1973.

Momose KJ, et al.: High incidence of cortical atrophy of the cerebral and cerebellar hemispheres in Cushing's disease. *Radiology* 99:341, 1971.

Pojunas KW, et al.: Pituitary and adrenal CT of Cushing syndrome. *A.J.R.* 146:1235, 1986.

Rausch HP, et al.: Medullary nephrocalcinosis and pancreatic calcifications demonstrated by ultrasound and CT in infants after treatment with ACTH. *Radiology* 153:105, 1984.

Sakiyama R, et al.: Cyclic Cushing's syndrome. *Am. J. Med.* 77:944, 1984.

Santelices R, et al.: Cushing's syndrome due to ectopic ACTH production by a carcinoid tumor not producing serotonin. *N. Engl. J. Med.* 308:463, 1983.

Saris SC, et al.: Cushing syndrome: Pituitary CT scanning. *Radiology* 162:775, 1987.

Scott S, et al.: Failure of bone scanning to detect fractures in a woman on chronic steroid therapy. *Skeletal Radiol.* 12:204, 1984.

Shirkhoda A: Current diagnostic approach to adrenal abnormalities. *J. Comput. Tomogr.* 8:277, 1984.

Smals AGH, et al.: Macronodular adrenocortical hyperplasia in long-standing Cushing's disease. *J. Clin. Endocrinol. Metab.* 58:25, 1984.

Solomon IL, et al.: Juvenile Cushing syndrome manifested primarily by growth failure. *Am. J. Dis. Child.* 130:200, 1976.

Streiter ML, et al.: Steroid-induced thoracic lipomatosis: Paraspinal involvement. *A.J.R.* 139:679, 1982.

Taillefer R, et al.: ^{131}I-iodocholesterol (NP-59) scintigraphy in adrenocortical diseases. *J. Can. Assoc. Radiol.* 34:120, 1983.

CYSTINOSIS

Synonyms: Lignac-Fanconi syndrome; Lignac–de Toni–Fanconi syndrome; cystine storage disease; nephropathic cystinosis.

Mode of Inheritance: Autosomal recessive.

Pathophysiology: (a) cystine accumulation within the lysosomes of the cells in various tissues: reticuloendothelial cells, meninges, choroid plexus, pineal gland, kidneys, ocular tissues, bone marrow, circulating leukocytes, pancreas, intestine, thyroid, etc.; (b) deficiency of tubular reabsorption of water, glucose, amino acids, phosphate, sodium, potassium, bicarbonate, etc.

Classification: Considerable clinical heterogeneity: infantile, nephropathic, adolescent, and adult types; severe renal tubular and glomerular dysfunction in the infantile form; kidneys usually not affected in the adult form.

Clinical Manifestations: (a) *failure to thrive;* (b) dehydration; (c) polyuria, polydipsia; (d) renal tubular acidosis, rickets, hypophosphatemia; (e) hypokalemia; (f) renal glycosuria, chronic renal failure; (g) hepatosplenomegaly; (h) cystine crystals in eyes (conjunctiva, cornea, slit-lamp examination), bone marrow, leukocytes, intestinal mucosa, lymph nodes, etc; (i) heterozygote detection for cystinosis with measure-

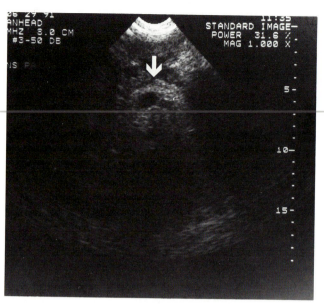

FIG ME–C–12.
Cystinosis. An ultrasound examination of the pancreas *(arrow)* shows diminished size with a marked increase in echogenicity. (From Fivush B, Flick JA, Gahl WA, et al.: Pancreatic exocrine insufficiency in a patient with nephropathic cystinosis. *J. Pediatr.* 112:49, 1988. Used by permission.)

ment of the cystine content of purified preparations of polymorphonuclear leukocytes; (j) other reported abnormalities: blond hair sometimes in contrast to the other members of the family, photophobia, retinal depigmentation, hypohidrosis, hypothyroidism, pancreatic endocrine insufficiency (insulin-dependent diabetes mellitus), pancreatic exocrine insufficiency, seizures, coma, hypothyroidism, decreased visual acuity, corneal ulcerations, hepatomegaly, splenomegaly, inflammatory bowel disease, neurological deficits (motor incoordination, hypotonia, etc.).

Radiologic Manifestations: (a) *severe resistant rickets;* (b) secondary hyperparathyroidism; (c) skeletal maturation retardation; (d) other reported abnormalities: thyroid atrophy, manifestations of hypothyroidism, hydrocephalus, subcortical and cortical atrophy, radiolucent urinary stone(s), diminished pancreatic size with increased echogenicity consistent with chronic pancreatitis (Fig ME–C–12).

REFERENCES

Ammenti A, et al.: Infantile cystinosis and insulin-dependent diabetes mellitus. *Eur. J. Pediatr.* 145:548, 1986.

Black J, et al.: Varied types of urinary calculi in a patient with cystinosis without renal tubular acidosis. *Pediatrics* 78:295, 1986.

Ehrich JHH, et al.: Evidence for cerebral involvement in nephropathic cystinosis. *Neuropaediatrie* 10:128, 1979.

Fanconi G: Die nicht diabetischen Glycosurien und Hyperglykämien des lateren Kindes. *Jb. Kinderheilkd.* 133:257, 1931.

Fivush B, et al.: Pancreatic endocrine insufficiency in post-transplant cystinosis. *Am. J. Dis. Child.* 141:1087, 1987.

Fivush B, et al.: Pancreatic exocrine insufficiency in a patient with nephropathic cystinosis. *J. Pediatr.* 112:49, 1988.

Gahl WA, et al.: Course of nephropathic cystinosis after age 10 years. *J. Pediatr.* 109:605, 1986.

Gahl WA, et al.: Cystamine therapy for children with nephropathic cystinosis. *N. Engl. J. Med.* 316:971, 1987.

Gahl WA, et al.: Decreased sweat production in cystinosis. *J. Pediatr.* 104:904, 1984.

Grünebaum M, et al.: Hypothyroidism in cystinosis. *A.J.R.* 129:629, 1977.

Iancu TC, et al.: Intestinal mucosa in nephropathic cystinosis. *J. Pediatr. Gastroenterol. Nutr.* 6:359, 1987.

Jonas AJ, et al.: Cystinosis in a black child. *J. Pediatr.* 100:934, 1982.

Lignac GOE: Ueber Störung des cystinoffwechsel bei Kindern. *Dtsch. Arch. Klin. Med.* 145:139, 1924.

Ross DL, et al.: Nonabsorptive hydrocephalus associated with nephropathic cystinosis. *Neurology* 32:1330, 1982.

Smolin LA, et al.: An improved method for heterozygote detection of cystinosis, using polymorphonuclear leukocytes. *Am. J. Hum. Genet.* 41:266, 1987.

Trauner DA, et al.: Neurologic and cognitive deficits in children with cystinosis. *J. Pediatr.* 112:912, 1988.

Treem WR, et al.: Inflammatory bowel disease in a patient with nephropathic cystinosis. *Pediatrics* 81:584, 1988.

CYSTINURIA

Mode of Inheritance: Autosomal recessive with heterogeneity; three mutant alleles (I, II, and III): (a) homozygotes (I/I, II/II, and III/III) and compound heterozygotes (I/II, I/III, II/III) with high urinary excretion of cystine, lysine, arginine, and ornithine are prone to cystine stone formation; (b) heterozygotes: +/II and +/III (detectable with a variable increase in urinary cystine, lysine, and arginine excretion.

Etiology: *Inborn error of membrane transport of cystine, lysine, ornithine, and arginine in the intestinal tract and renal tubules.*

Clinical Manifestations: Onset of symptoms in childhood or young adult life: (a) *nephrolithiasis:* abdominal colic, dysuria; (b) recurrent urinary tract infections; (c) hyperuricemia; (d) *cystine crystal in the urine, positive nitroprusside test reaction, thin-layer chromatography or high-voltage electrophoresis for the identification of urinary amino acids,* intestinal transport defect demonstrated by oral loading tests and by intestinal perfusion studies, renal tubular transfer defects demonstrated by clearance studies (cystine, lysine, arginine, and ornithine); (e) other reported abnormalities: slight shortness of stature, association with congenital myotonic dystrophy, anuria due to bilateral cystine urolithiasis.

Radiologic Manifestations: *Urolithiasis:* single, multiple, staghorn configuration.

REFERENCES

Brown RC, et al.: Cystine calculi are radiopaque. *A.J.R.* 135:565, 1980.

Carpentier PJ, et al.: Heterozygous cystinuria and calcium oxalate urolithiasis. *J. Urol.* 130:302, 1983.

Dahlberg PJ, et al.: Clinical features and management of cystinuria. *Mayo Clin. Proc.* 52:533, 1977.

Giugliani R, et al.: Heterozygous cystinuria and urinary lithiasis. *Am. J. Med. Genet.* 22:703, 1985.

Kimura S, et al.: Cystinuria with congenital myotonic dystrophy. *Pediatr. Neurol.* 3:233, 1987.

Martini A, et al.: Anuria due to bilateral cystine urolithiasis in an infant. *Helv. Paediatr. Acta* 41:545, 1986.

Reander A: The roentgen density of the cystine calculus; a roentgenographic and experimental study including a comparison with more common uroliths. *Acta Radiol.* 41(suppl.):1, 1944.

Scriver CR: Cystinuria. *N. Engl. J. Med.* 315:1155, 1986.

D

DEPRIVATION DWARFISM

Synonym: Psychological dwarfism.

Clinical Manifestations: (a) *adverse family environment, emotional and behavioral disorders, developmental delay;* (b) *short stature;* (c) *small head size, rapid increase in head circumference on restoration of adequate nutrition* (catch-up growth) associated with widening of cranial sutures but without evidence of increased intracranial pressure; (d) hormonal abnormalities (pituitary, thyroid, adrenal); (e) other reported abnormalities: elevated levels of sweat electrolytes, acute gastric dilatation, etc.

Radiologic Manifestations: (a) *widening of cranial sutures during treatment;* (b) *computed tomography:* prominent cortical and interhemispheric sulci suggestive of mild cerebral atrophy before treatment; obliteration of sulci and various cisternae following treatment; (c) *demineralization;* (d) *skeletal maturation retardation.*

REFERENCES

Afshani E, et al.: Widening of cranial sutures in children with deprivation dwarfism. *Radiology* 109:141, 1973.

Berdon WE, et al.: Radiographic and computed tomographic demonstration of pseudotumor cerebri due to rapid weight gain in a child with pelvic rhabdomyosarcoma. *Radiology* 143:679, 1982.

Capitanio MA, et al.: Widening of the cranial sutures: A roentgen observation during periods of accelerated growth in patients treated for deprivation dwarfism. *Radiology* 92:53, 1969.

Dobbing J: CT brain scans following undernutrition in infancy. *Br. J. Radiol.* 55:168, 1982.

Franken EA Jr, et al.: Acute gastric dilatation in neglected children. *A.J.R.* 130:297, 1978.

Gloebl HJ, et al.: Radiographic findings in children with psychosocial dwarfism. *Pediatr. Radiol.* 4:83, 1976.

Marks HG, et al.: Catch-up brain growth-demonstration by CAT scan. *J. Pediatr.* 93:254, 1978.

Neufeld ND: Endocrine abnormalities associated with deprivational dwarfism and anorexia nervosa. *Pediatr. Clin. North Am.* 26:199, 1979.

Ruddy RM, et al.: Abnormal sweat electrolytes in a case of celiac disease and a case of psychosocial failure to thrive. Review of other reported causes. *Clin. Pediatr. (Phila.)* 26:83, 1987.

Sarr M, et al.: Les retards de croissance psychogènes. Etude critique des élements de diagnostic. *Arch. Fr. Pediatr.* 44:331, 1987.

DIABETES INSIPIDUS

Classification:

(A) CENTRAL DIABETES INSIPIDUS (NEUROHYPOPHYSEAL): (a) primary: (1) *idiopathic;* (2) *defective synthesis or secretion of antidiuretic hormone (ADH):* tumor, postsurgical, trauma, histiocytosis X, leukemic infiltration, infections, intracranial birth defect, vascular abnormalities, sarcoidosis, dysplastic pancytopenia, carbon monoxide poisoning, after an aortocoronary bypass operation, brain death, etc.; (b) *familial, autosomal dominant, and X-linked recessive.*

(B) NEPHROGENIC DIABETES INSIPIDUS (ADH-RESISTANT DIABETES INSIPIDUS): failure of response of the distal nephron cells to normal amounts of circulatory ADH (vasopressin-resistant hyposthenuria): pharmacologically induced (lithium carbonate, demeclocycline, methoxyflurane), electrolyte disorders (hypercalcemia, chronic hypokalemia), chronic renal insufficiency, adult polycystic disease, medullary cystic disease, obstructive uropathy, chronic pyelonephritis, sickle cell disease, Sjögren syndrome, etc.

Clinical Manifestations: (a) *polyuria, polydipsia, nocturia, failure to thrive, vomiting, constipation, excessive crying in infants, dehydration, intermittent fever;* (b) *hypotonic urine, normal or elevated serum osmolarity;* (c) *unresponsiveness to ADH in the nephrogenic type;* (d) association with other conditions and diseases: (1) central diabetes insipidus: Wolfram or DIDMOAD syndrome (association of diabetes insipidus, diabetes mellitus, optic atrophy, and deafness), dysplastic pancytopenia, anterior pituitary dysfunction in the idiopathic form, amenorrhea-galactorrhea (post-traumatic after pituitary stalk rupture), etc.; (2) nephrogenic diabetes insipidus: central nervous system disorder, including hydrocephalus, cystinosis, trans-sphenoidal meningoencephalocele, etc.

Radiologic Manifestations: (a) *intracranial lesion* evaluated by neuroradiological procedures, empty sella; (b) *hydronephrosis, hydroureter, megalocystis;* (c) absence of the normal high signal (T_1-weighted image) of the posterior lobe of the pituitary gland on magnetic resonance examination, pituitary stalk rupture (post-traumatic), etc. (Fig ME–D–1).

REFERENCES

Aggarwal R, et al.: Nephrogenic diabetes insipidus in a female infant with hydrocephalus. *Am. J. Dis. Child.* 140:1095, 1986.

Czernichow P, et al.: Diabetes insipidus in children. III. Anterior pituitary dysfunction in idiopathic types. *J. Pediatr.* 106:41, 1985.

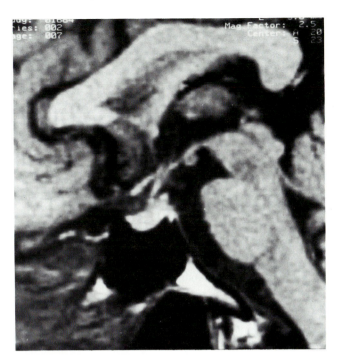

FIG ME–D–1.
Diabetes insipidus (idiopathic) in a 48-year-old female with a history of polyuria and polydipsia of 3 months' duration and hyposecretion of ADH with normal function of the anterior lobe of the pituitary gland. A T_1-weighted image demonstrates no space-occupying lesion, and the normally high signal of the posterior lobe is absent in the posterior part of the pituitary fossa. (From Fujisawa I, Nishimura K, Asato R, et al.: Posterior lobe of the pituitary in diabetes insipidus: MR findings. *J. Comput. Assist. Tomogr.* 11:221, 1987. Used by permission.)

Friedman E, et al.: A variant of the "DIDMOAD" syndrome (diabetes insipidus, diabetes mellitus, optic atrophy and deafness). *Clin. Genet.* 29:79, 1986.

Fujisawa E, et al.: Posterior lobe of the pituitary in diabetes insipidus: MR findings. *J. Comput. Assist. Tomogr.* 11:221, 1987.

Greger NG, et al.: Central diabetes insipidus. 22 years' experience. *Am. J. Dis. Child.* 140:551, 1986.

Hadani M, et al.: Unusual delayed onset of diabetes insipidus following closed head trauma. *J. Neurosurg.* 63:456, 1985.

Halebian P, et al.: Diabetes insipidus after carbon monoxide poisoning and smoke inhalation. *J. Trauma* 25:662, 1985.

Halimi Ph, et al.: Post-traumatic diabetes insipidus: MR demonstration of pituitary stalk rupture. *J. Comput. Assist. Tomogr.* 12:135, 1988.

Katzir Z, et al.: Nephrogenic diabetes insipidus, cystinosis, and vitamin D. *Arch. Dis. Child.* 63:548, 1988.

Knoers N, et al.: Nephrogenic diabetes insipidus: Close linkage with markers from the distal long arm of the human X chromosome. *Hum. Genet.* 80:31, 1988.

Kuan P, et al.: Transient central diabetes insipidus after aortocoronary bypass operations. *Am. J. Cardiol.* 52:1181, 1983.

Manelfe C, et al.: Computed tomography in diabetes insipidus. *J. Comput. Assist. Tomogr.* 3:309, 1979.

Marano GD, et al.: Computed tomography in diabetes insipidus: Posterior empty sella. *Br. J. Radiol.* 54:263, 1981.

Massol J, et al.: Post-traumatic diabetes insipidus and amenorrhea-galactorrhea syndrome after pituitary stalk rupture. *Neuroradiology* 29:299, 1987.

Najjar SS, et al.: Association of diabetes insipidus, diabetes mellitus, optic atrophy, and deafness. The Wolfram or DIDMOAD syndrome. *Arch. Dis. Child.* 60:823, 1985.

Nishi Y, et al.: Hypopituitarism associated with transsphenoidal meningoencephalocele. *Eur. J. Pediatr.* 139:81, 1982.

Ohzeki T, et al.: Familial cases of congenital nephrogenic diabetes insipidus type II: Remarkable increment of urinary adenosine 3',5'-monophosphate in response to antidiuretic hormone. *J. Pediatr.* 104:593, 1984.

Rockoff MA: Central diabetes insipidus caused by brain death. *Am. J. Dis. Child.* 140:1093, 1986.

Sherwood MC, et al.: Diabetes insipidus and occult intracranial tumours. *Arch. Dis. Child.* 61:1222, 1986.

Tank ES, et al.: Polyuric megalocystis. *J. Urol.* 124:692, 1980.

Zijlstra F, et al.: Diabetes insipidus associated with dysplastic pancytopenia. *Am. J. Med.* 82:339, 1987.

DIABETES MELLITUS

Classification:

(A) IDIOPATHIC: (a) type 1: insulin dependent, familial occurrence in some; (b) type 2: non–insulin dependent, more common in males, strong family history of diabetes mellitus.

(B) SECONDARY DIABETES: (a) pancreatic disease: congenital pancreatic hypoplasia, pancreatectomy, pancreatitis, hemochromatosis, neoplasms, etc; (b) insulin receptor abnormalities; (c) hormonal disorders: acromegaly, Cushing syndrome, primary aldostronism, pheochromocytoma, glucagonoma, etc.; (d) drugs: diuretics, oral contraceptives, glucocorticoids, phenytoin, phenothiazines, tricyclic antidepressants, etc; (e) pregnancy; (f) genetic syndromes: Prader-Willi syndrome, myotonic dystrophy, hyperlipemias, leprechaunism, Friedreich ataxia, etc.

Clinical Manifestations: (a) *polyuria, polydipsia, polyphagia, weight loss, lethargy, leg cramps, etc.*; (b) *hyperglycemia* (increased hepatic glucogenesis and reduced tissue uptake), *glycosuria, elevated fasting blood glucose level, ketosis, acidosis, hyperlipoproteinemia, etc.*; (c) *complications: ocular* (blurring of vision, myopia, weakness of accommodation, cataract, lipemia retinalis, diabetic retinopathy, blue-yellow vision deficits, etc.), *renal* (pyelonephritis, nodular glomerulosclerosis, tubular dysfunction, hypernatremia, hematuria, hypercalciuria, erectile dysfunction, penile necrosis, etc.), *dermal* (infections; eruptive xanthomatosis; necrobiosis lipoidica diabeticorum; thickening, tightening, and/or waxy quality of the skin; etc., *digestive* (motility disorders, vomiting, constipation, diarrhea, fecal incontinence, megacolon, esophageal dysfunction), *neurological* (peripheral neuropathy, cranial nerve dysfunction, autonomic nervous system dysfunction manifested by orthostatic hypotension, decreased sweating, hyperhidrosis, delayed gastric emptying, bowel and bladder distension), *cardiovascular* (hypertension, myocardial infarction, atherosclerosis, peripheral vascular disease), *infections, male impotence;* (d) *Rosenbloom syndrome:* flexion contracture as a consequence of rigidity of connective tissue, small stature, and diabetes mellitus; (e) other reported abnormalities: amyotrophy, impaired respiratory function, abnormal zinc metabolism, hypomagnesemia, Wolfram or DIDMOAD syndrome (diabetes insipidus, diabetes mellitus, optic atrophy, and deafness), association with gouty arthritis, calcium pyrophosphate dihydrate (CPPD) crystal deposition disease, ankylosing hyperostosis of the spine, etc.

Radiologic Manifestations: (a) *bones, joints, and soft tissues:* osteoporosis, glenohumeral periarthritis, flexor tenosynovitis, Dupuytren contracture, carpal tunnel syndrome, osteomyelitis, septic arthritis, neuroarthropathy, forefoot osteolysis, diabetic cheiroarthropathy (joint contractures of the fingers and some other joints associated with thickening of the skin), less-than-normal thickness of the heel soft tissues (ultrasonography); (b) three-phase scintigraphy demonstrating increased activity in both infected and noninfected diabetic osteopathy, leukocyte imaging (indium 111 labeled) helpful in excluding infection, *scintigraphy in osteoarthropathy* of the ankle and foot: combination of diffuse and focal uptake, usually more extensive than detectable by radiographic examination; (c) *arterial calcification* (soft tissues, visceral), arterial wall stiffness in insulin-dependent diabetes mellitus, narrowing and rugosities of the leg arteries; (d) abnormal esophageal function, gastric dilatation with impaired peristalsis, gastric

retention, gastric bezoar, retained gastric contrast material on delayed radiographic examination; (e) bilateral renal enlargement, "upside-down" contrast-urine level in glycosuria; (f) cerebral edema with increased intracranial pressure associated with diabetic ketoacidosis, intracerebral hematoma; high-risk for metrizamide myelography.

Notes: (a) Mendenhall syndrome: insulin-resistant diabetes mellitus associated with dysmorphism, dental precocity, hirsutism, acanthosis nigrans, abdominal protuberance, and phallic enlargement; (b) Wolcott-Rallison syndrome: infancy-onset diabetes mellitus and multiple epiphyseal dysplasia (Fig ME–D–2).

REFERENCES

Atluru VL: Spontaneous intracerebral hematomas in juvenile diabetic ketoacidosis. *Pediatr. Neurol.* 2:167, 1986.

Barta L: Flexion contractures in a diabetic child (Rosenbloom syndrome). *Eur. J. Pediatr.* 135:101, 1980.

Borgström PS, et al.: Pharyngeal and oesophageal function in patients with diabetes mellitus and swallowing complaints. *Br. J. Radiol.* 61:817, 1988.

Bour J, et al.: Penile necrosis in patients with diabetes mellitus and end stage renal disease. *J. Urol.* 132:560, 1984.

Buckingham B, et al.: Skin, joint, and pulmonary changes in type I diabetes mellitus. *Am. J. Dis. Child.* 140:420, 1986.

Christensen T, et al.: Arterial wall stiffness in insulin-dependent diabetes mellitus. An in vivo study. *Acta Radiol.* 28:207, 1987.

Christensen T, et al.: Internal diameter of the common femoral artery in patients with insulin-dependent diabetes mellitus. *Acta Radiol.* 29:423, 1988.

Edidin DV: Cutaneous manifestations of diabetes mellitus in children. *Pediatr. Dermatol.* 2:161, 1985.

Editorial: DIDMOAD (Wolfram) syndrome. *Lancet* 1:1075, 1986.

Ewald U, et al.: Hypomagnesemia in diabetic children. *Acta. Paediatr. Scand.* 72:367, 1983.

Eymontt MJ, et al.: Bone scintigraphy in diabetic osteoarthropathy. *Radiology* 140:475, 1981.

Friedman E, et al.: A variant of the "DIDMOAD" syndrome (diabetes insipidus, diabetes mellitus, optic atrophy and deafness). *Clin. Genet.* 29:79, 1986.

Flatow EL, et al.: Diabetic amyotrophy. *J. Bone Joint Surg. [Am.]* 67:1132, 1985.

Genuth S: Classification and diagnosis of diabetes mellitus. *Med. Clin. North Am.* 66:1191, 1982.

Gooding GAW, et al.: Sonography of the sole of the foot. Evidence for loss of foot pad thickness in diabetes and its relationship to ulceration of the foot. *Invest. Radiol.* 21:45, 1986.

Harati Y, et al.: Diabetic thoracoabdominal neuropathy. A cause for chest and abdominal pain. *Arch. Intern. Med.* 146:1493, 1986.

Heer M, et al.: Diabetic megacolon—a rare late complication. *Radiologe* 23:233, 1983.

Hoffman WH, et al.: Cranial CT in children and adolescents with diabetic ketoacidosis. *A.J.N.R.* 9:733, 1988.

Käär ML, et al.: Peripheral neuropathy in diabetic children

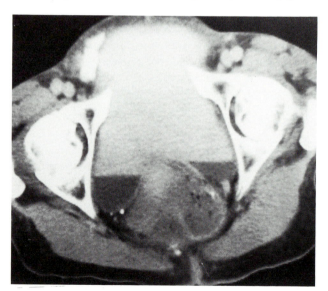

FIG ME–D–2.

A computed tomographic scan at the level of the acetabula shows inverted contrast-urine levels in the bladder (considered to be related to glycosuria with a very high specific gravity of the urine already in the bladder prior to the administration of contrast material. (From Savit RM, Udis DS: "Upside-down" contrast-urine levels in glycosuria: CT features. *J. Comput. Assist. Tomogr.* 11:911, 1987. Used by permission.)

and adolescents. A cross-sectional study. *Acta Paediatr. Scand.* 72:373, 1983.

Kennedy WR, et al.: Quantitation of the sweating deficiency in diabetes mellitus. *Ann. Neurol.* 15:482, 1984.

Kereiakes DJ, et al.: The heart in diabetes. *West J. Med.* 140:583, 1984.

Kinlaw WB, et al.: Abnormal zinc metabolism in type II diabetes mellitus. *Am. J. Med.* 75:273, 1983.

Loo D, et al.: Gastric emptying in patients with diabetes mellitus. *Gastroenterology* 86:485, 1984.

Maatman TJ, et al.: Erectile dysfunction in men with diabetes mellitus. *Urology* 24:589, 1987.

Malone JI, et al.: Hematuria and hypercalciuria in children with diabetes mellitus. *Pediatrics* 79:756, 1987.

Maurer AH, et al.: Infection in diabetic osteoarthropathy: Use of indium-labeled leukocytes for diagnosis. *Radiology* 161:221, 1986.

Miltényi M, et al.: Tubular dysfunction in type I diabetes mellitus. *Arch. Dis. Child.* 60:929, 1985.

Najjar SS, et al.: Association of diabetes insipidus, diabetes mellitus, optic atrophy, and deafness. The Wolfram or DIDMOAD syndrome. *Arch. Dis. Child.* 60:823, 1985.

Neubauer B, et al.: Calcifications, narrowing and rugosities of the leg arteries in diabetic patients. *Acta Radiol.* 24:401, 1983.

Niakan E, et al.: Silent myocardial infarction and diabetic cardiovascular autonomic neuropathy. *Arch. Intern. Med.* 146:2229, 1986.

Rittey CDC, et al: Melatonin state in Mendenhall's syndrome. *Arch. Dis. Child.* 63:852, 1988.

Rockett M, et al.: Blue-yellow vision deficits in patients with diabetes. *West J. Med.* 146:431, 1987.

Rosenbloom AL, et al.: Limited joint mobility and diabetic retinopathy demonstrated by fluorescein angiography. *Eur. J. Pediatr.* 141:163, 1984.

Russell COH, et al.: Relationship among esophageal dysfunction, diabetic gastroenteropathy, and peripheral neuropathy. *Dig. Dis. Sci.* 28:289, 1983.

Sartoris DJ, et al.: Plantar compartmental infection in the diabetic foot. The role of computed tomography. *Invest. Radiol.* 20:772, 1985.

Sato M, et al.: Exocrine pancreatic function in diabetic children. *J. Pediatr. Gastroenterol. Nutr.* 3:415, 1984.

Savit RM, et al.: "Upside-down" contrast—urine level in glycosuria: CT features. *J. Comput. Assist. Tomogr.* 11:911, 1987.

Segel MC, et al.: Diabetes mellitus: The predominant cause of bilateral renal enlargement. *Radiology* 153:341, 1984.

Soejima K, et al.: Osteoporosis in juvenile-onset diabetes mellitus: Morphometric and comparative studies. *Pediatr. Pathol.* 6:289, 1986.

Steiner E, et al.: Neurologic complications in diabetics after metrizamide lumbar myelography. *A.J.N.R.* 7:323, 1986.

Stöss H, et al: Wolcott-Rallison syndrome: Diabetes mellitus and spondyloepiphyseal dysplasia. *Eur. J. Pediatr.* 138:120, 1982.

Walters EG, et al.: Hyponatraemia in diabetes without ketoacidosis. *Arch. Dis. Child.* 59:785, 1984.

Winter W, et al.: Congenital pancreatic hypoplasia; a syndrome of exocrine and endocrine pancreatic insufficiency. *J. Pediatr.* 109:465, 1986.

Zlatkin MB, et al.: The diabetic foot. *Radiol. Clin. North Am.* 25:1095, 1987.

DIABETES MELLITUS (INFANTS BORN TO DIABETIC MOTHERS)

Synonyms: Infant of a diabetic mother; IDM.

Clinical Manifestations: Usually infants born to insulin-dependent diabetic mothers: (a) *high birth weight or small for gestational age,* more than normal subcutaneous fat; (b) *tachypnea, diabetes-related idiopathic lung disease;* (c) *cardiomyopathy* (obstructive and nonobstructive), *congestive heart failure,* congenital heart defects, persistence of fetal circulation, thrombosis at various sites, gangrene; (d) seizures, neurological instability; (e) *organomegaly;* (f) polycythemia and hyperviscosity, hypocalcemia, hypoglycemia, hypomagnesemia, hyperbilirubinemia, transient hematuria, increased blood volume, uremia; (g) congenital anomalies: branchial arch malformations, central nervous system anomalies, micrognathia, genitourinary anomalies, diastasis recti, thin abdominal muscles, Potter facies, various limb anomalies in-

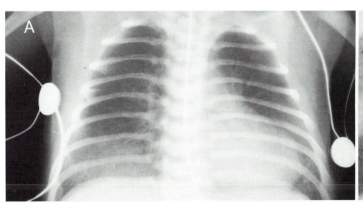
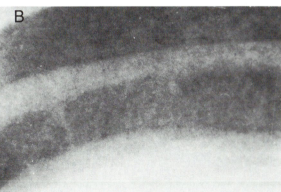

FIG ME–D–3.
Infant born to a diabetic mother. **A,** a chest radiograph at 12 hours shows a hazy density of the right base and a large lung volume. **B,** a magnified view of the area shows a granular quality of the densities. (From Duara S, Spachman TJ, Boutwell WC, et al.: A newly recognized profile in neonatal lung disease with maternal diabetes. *A.J.R.* 144:529, 1985. Used by permission.)

cluding femoral hypoplasia and digital anomalies, spinal deformities, hearing disorders, absence of the pituitary gland, tracheal stenosis; (h) other reported abnormalities: asphyxia neonatorum, birth injury, hepatic erythropoiesis, permanent neonatal diabetes, arthrogryposis, etc.

Radiologic Manifestations: *(a) greater than normal amounts of subcutaneous fat for gestational age; (b) cardiomegaly, cardiac failure; (c) hepatomegaly; (d) small−left colon syndrome; (e) skeletal anomalies: vertebrae (caudal regression syndrome, hemivertebrae, spina bifida, meningocele), etc.; (f) respiratory distress with a radiographic pattern distinct from hyaline membrane disease and transient tachypnea of the newborn: regional distribution of reticulogranular densities, increased lung volume, gradual improvement over a period of about 2 weeks. (g) holoprosencephaly, neural tube defects, spontaneous resolution of the fetal ventriculomegaly (second trimester), microcephaly, hydrocephaly, intracranial hemorrhage; (h) genitourinary anomalies, renal vein thrombosis, renal hemorrhage; (i) other reported abnormalities: visceral situs inversus, poor mineralization of primary teeth, adrenal hemorrhage, etc.* (Fig ME−D−3).

REFERENCES

Anderton JM, et al.: Absence of the pituitary gland in a case of congenital sacral agenesis. *J. Bone Joint Surg. [Br.]* 65:182, 1983.

Barr M, et al.: Holoprosencephaly in infants of diabetic mothers. *J. Pediatr.* 102:565, 1983.

Cowett RM, et al.: The infant of the diabetic mother. *Pediatr. Clin. North Am.* 29:1213, 1982.

Duara S, et al.: A newly recognized profile in neonatal lung disease with maternal diabetes. *A.J.R.* 144:529, 1985.

Dunn V, et al.: Infants of diabetic mothers: Radiographic manifestations. *A.J.R.* 137:123, 1981.

Grix A Jr: Malformations in infants of diabetic mothers. *Am. J. Med. Genet.* 13:131, 1982.

Hsi AC, et al.: Neonatal gangrene in the newborn infant of a diabetic mother. *J. Pediatr. Orthop.* 5:358, 1985.

Johnson JP, et al.: Branchial arch malformations in infants of diabetic mothers: Two case reports and a review. *Am. J. Med. Genet.* 13:125, 1982.

Johnson JP, et al.: Femoral hypoplasia—unusual facies syndrome in infants of diabetic mothers. *J. Pediatr.* 102:866, 1983.

Kuhn LR, et al.: Fat thickness in the newborn infant of a diabetic mother. *Radiology* 111:665, 1974.

Miller JM Jr, et al.: Fetal overgrowth. Diabetic versus nondiabetic. *J. Ultrasound Med.* 7:577, 1988.

Mimouni F, et al.: Polycythemia, hypomagnesemia, and hypocalcemia in infants of diabetic mothers. *Am. J. Dis. Child.* 140:798, 1986.

Morville P, et al.: La cardiomyopathie de l'enfant de mère diabétique. Hyperinsulinisme foetal et cardiomyopathie. *Ann. Pediatr. (Paris)* 32:363, 1985.

Moya FR, et al.: Fetal-neonatal uremia in advanced maternal diabetes. *Clin. Pediatr. (Phila.)* 23:229, 1984.

Nelson M, et al.: Optic nerve hypoplasia and maternal diabetes mellitus. *Arch. Neurol.* 43:20, 1986.

Singer DB: Hepatic erythropoiesis in infants of diabetic mothers: A morphometric study. *Pediatr. Pathol.* 5:471, 1986.

Swenne I: The fetus of the diabetic mother: Growth and malformations. *Arch. Dis. Child.* 63:1119, 1988.

Tack E, et al.: Tracheal stenosis. Lethal malformation in two infants of diabetic mothers. *Am. J. Dis. Child.* 141:77, 1987.

Toi A: Spontaneous resolution of fetal ventriculomegaly in a diabetic patient. *J. Ultrasound Med.* 6:37, 1987.

Trowitzsch E, et al.: Echocardiographic profile of infants of diabetic mothers. *Eur. J. Pediatr.* 140:311, 1983.

Violaris K, et al.: Increased blood viscosity and tachypnoea in infants of diabetic mothers. *Arch. Dis. Child.* 61:910, 1986.

West DL, et al.: Maternal diabetes and neonatal macrosomia. Dynamic skinfold thickness measurements. *Am. J. Perinatol.* 3:9, 1986.

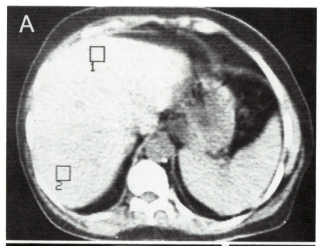

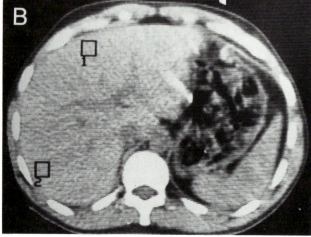

FIG ME−D−4.
Abdominal CT in a patient with Dubin-Johnson syndrome **(A)** and a control patient **(B)**. Note the clearly higher liver density in the Dubin-Johnson syndrome. (From Rubinstein ZJ, Seligsohn U, Modan M, et al.: Hepatic computerized tomography in Dubin-Johnson syndrome: Increased liver density as a diagnostic aid. *Comput. Radiol.* 9:315, 1985. Used by permission.)

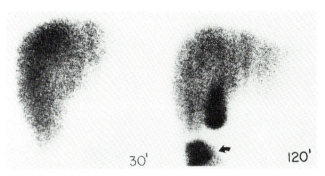

FIG ME–D–5.
Child with Dubin-Johnson syndrome. A 30-minute image shows the characteristic persistent hemogeneous concentration of the ⁹⁹ᵐTc-HIDA without any concentration in the intrahepatic biliary tree. The 120-minute image shows the delayed filling of the gall-bladder with some clearance to the intestines *(arrow)* but still no visualization of the biliary ducts. (From Bujanover Y, Bar-Meir S, Hayman I, et al.:⁹⁹ᵐTc-HIDA cholescintigraphy in children with Dubin-Johnson syndrome. *J. Pediatr. Gastroenterol. Nutr.* 2:311, 1983. Used by permission.)

Widness JA, et al.: Permanent neonatal diabetes in an infant of an insulin-dependent mother. *J. Pediatr.* 100:926, 1982.

DUBIN-JOHNSON SYNDROME

Synonyms: Black liver–jaundice syndrome; icterus–hepatic pigmentation syndrome.

Mode of Inheritance: Autosomal recessive.

Clinical Manifestations: (a) chronic or intermittent hyperbilirubinemia (conjugated types predominating), *persistent nonhemolytic hyperbilirubinemia;* (b) *a black liver, lip-ochrome-like pigmentation of liver cells;* (c) elevated sulfobromophthalein (Bromsulphalein) level after 2 hours; (d) urinary excretion of coproporphyrin; mostly (80%) as isomer I instead of isomer III, normal total urinary coproporphyrin.

Radiological Manifestations: (a) nonvisualization of the gallbladder on oral cholecystography; (b) computed tomography (CT): increased liver density; (c) ⁹⁹ᵐTc-HIDA cholescintigraphy: delayed visualization or nonvisualization of the gallbladder and bile duct in association with a prolonged, intense, and homogeneous visualization of the liver (Figs ME–D–4 and ME–D–5).

REFERENCES

Bar-Meir S., et al.:⁹⁹ᵐTc-HIDA cholecintigraphy in Dubin-Johnson and Rotor syndromes. *Radiology* 142:743, 1982.

Bremmelgaard A, et al.: Congenital intrahepatic cholestasis with pigment deposits and abnormal bile acid metabolism. A variant of Dubin-Johnson's syndrome. *Liver* 7:31, 1987.

Bujanover Y, et al.:⁹⁹ᵐTc-HIDA cholescintigraphy in children with Dubin-Johnson syndrome. *J. Pediatr. Gastroenterol. Nutr.* 2:311, 1983.

Cohen C, et al.: Porphobilinogen deaminase and the synthesis of porphyrin isomers in the Dubin-Johnson syndrome. *S. Afr. Med. J.* 70:36, 1986.

Dubin IN, Johnson FB: Chronic idiopathic jaundice with unidentified pigment in liver cells: A new clinicopathologic entity with a report of 12 cases. *Medicine (Baltimore)* 33:155, 1954.

Nakata F, et al.: Dubin-Johnson syndrome in a neonate. *Eur. J. Pediatr.* 132:299, 1979.

Rubinstein ZJ, et al.: Hepatic computerized tomography in the Dubin-Johnson syndrome: Increased liver density as a diagnostic aid. *Comput. Radiol.* 9:315, 1985.

ERDHEIM-CHESTER DISEASE

Synonym: *Chester-Erdheim disease.*

Pathology: *Lipogranulomatous lesion* in the skeletal system, visceral organs, retroperitoneal, etc.; bone biopsy: granular lipid-laden histiocytes in the bone marrow, thickened bony trabeculae, extraosseous discharge of xanthomatous marrow

Clinical Manifestations: Onset of symptoms often in the fifth to seventh decade of life; (a) xanthomatous patches of the eyelids, bone pain, chest pain, cough, sinus discharge, secondary infection, etc.; (b) cardiac failure, myocardial infiltration, pericardial infiltration, pulmonary infiltration, etc.; (c) other reported abnormalities: hepatosplenomegaly, proptosis, diabetes insipidus, fever, weight loss, renal disease.

Radiologic Manifestations: Appendicular skeleton often involved: (a) *progressive and widespread irregular patchy sclerosis of the medullary region, obliteration of the corticomedullary junction, thick cortices, coarse trabecular architecture,* subperiosteal reaction, epiphyses usually uninvolved or minimally involved, minimal vertebral changes, focal rib lesions (lipid granulomatosis of the ribs); (b) augmented uptake of ^{99m}Tc in the skeletal system at various sites; (c) retroperitoneal and visceral infiltration shown on computed tomographic examination; (d) cardiomegaly, pulmonary infiltration, pleural effusion; (e) retro-orbital masses due to diffuse infiltration, proptosis (Figs ME−E−1 and ME−E−2).

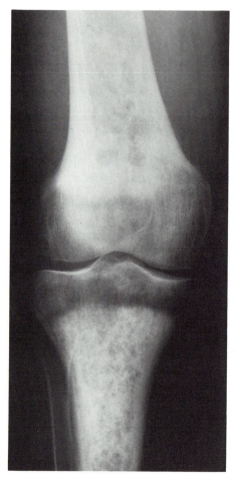

FIG ME−E−1.
Erdheim-Chester disease in a 57-year-old male with bilateral proptosis and a dense infiltrative process sheathing both optic nerves and deforming the inner orbital walls. (From Rozenberg I, Pinaudeau Y, Coscas G: Erdheim-Chester disease presenting as malignant exophthalmos. *Br. J. Radiol.* 59:173, 1986. Used by permission.)

FIG ME−E−2.
Erdheim-Chester disease in a 78-year-old patient. Dense metaphyseal sclerosis is present. (From Dee P, Westgaard T, Langholm R, Erdheim-Chester disease: Case with chronic discharging sinus from bone. *A.J.R.* 134:837, 1980. Used by permission.)

REFERENCES

Bohne WHO, et al.: Case report 96 (Chester-Erdheim disease). *Skeletal Radiol.* 4:164, 1979.

Chester W: Uber Lipoidgranulomatose. *Virchows Arch. [A]* 279:561, 1930.

Dalinak MK, et al.: Lipid granulomatosis of the ribs: Focal Erdheim-Chester disease. *Radiology* 142:297, 1982.

Dee P, et al.: Erdheim-Chester disease: Case with chronic discharging sinus from bone. *A.J.R.* 134:837, 1980.

Miller RL, et al.: Erdheim-Chester disease. Case report and review of the literature. *Am. J. Med.* 80:1230, 1986.

Resnick D, et al.: Erdheim-Chester disease. *Radiology* 142:289, 1982.

Rozenberg I, et al.: Erdheim-Chester disease presenting as malignant exophthalmos. *Br. J. Radiol.* 59:173, 1986.

Sherman JL, et al.: Erdheim-Chester disease: Computed tomography in two cases. *A.J.N.R.* 6:444, 1985.

Simpson FG: Erdheim-Chester disease associated with retroperitoneal xanthogranuloma. *Br. J. Radiol.* 52:232, 1979.

ETHANOLAMINOSIS

Clinical Manifestations: (a) physical and mental retardation; (b) hepatosplenomegaly; (c) cardiomegaly; (d) abnormal storage of ethanolamine, high ethanolamine activity in the liver and urine, reduced ethanolamine kinase activity in the liver; (e) death in childhood (reported in a brother and sister).

Radiologic Manifestations: (a) cardiomegaly; (b) esophageal ectasia; (c) hydrocephalus.

REFERENCE

Vietor KW, et al.: Aethanolaminose, eine generalisierte Speicherkrankheit mit Kardiomegalie, zerebraler Dysfunktion und frühem Tod. *Monatsschr. Kinderheilkd.* 125:470, 1977.

F

FABRY DISEASE

Synonyms: Angiokeratoma corporis diffusum universalis; glycosphingolipidosis; Fabry-Anderson syndrome; etc.

Mode of Inheritance: X-linked.

Pathology: Disorder of glycolipid metabolism due to a deficiency of the enzyme α-galactosidase that results in an accumulation of ceramide trihexoside in many tissues (kidney, skin, heart, neural tissues, leukocytes, etc.): intracellular deposits of ceramide trihexoside forming lamellar structures arranged either concentrically or in a parallel stack.

Clinical Manifestations: Onset of symptoms in childhood or at puberty: (a) *pain in the hands and feet, etc.*; (b) *angiokeratoma of the skin;* (c) fever, nausea, vomiting, abdominal pain; (d) progressive azotemia and renal failure; (e) varicosities, hemorrhoids; (f) corneal opacities, aneurysmal dilatation and tortuosity of conjunctival and retinal vessels, haziness or whorled streaks in the corneal epithelium; (g) recurrent hemoptysis, bronchitis, asthmatic wheezing; (h) renovascular hypertension, mitral valve prolapse, left ventricular hypertrophy, myocardial infarction or ischemia, abnormal electrocardiographic findings (short PR interval, giant negative T waves, high-voltage QRS complexes in the left precordial leads), thromboembolism; (i) cerebrovascular disease, dizziness, sensory deficits, aphasia, convulsions, cerebral hemorrhage, autonomic and sensory nerve involvement (painful neuropathy, acroparesthesia, altered vasomotor activity, loss of the ability to sweat, etc.); (j) priapism; (k) laboratory findings: anemia; proteinuria; azotemia; elevation of the erythrocyte sedimentation rate; urinary sediment containing casts, red cells, and glycolipids; enzyme deficiency in fibroblasts, kidney, heart, etc.; prenatal diagnosis by a demonstration of deficient α-galactosidase in cultured cells from amniotic fluid.

Radiologic Manifestations: (a) *cardiomegaly,* congestive heart failure, highly refractile myocardial echoes that are very similar to those reported in amyloidosis; (b) hypertensive heart disease; (c) *poor renal function* on excretory urography and isotope studies; (d) bowel involvement resulting in thickened mucosal folds of the small bowel and a lack of normal colonic haustration, spasticity, dilatation of the bowel, granular pattern of the ileum; (e) chronic airflow obstruction, pulmonary ventilation and perfusion defects, hyperaeration, bullae; (f) deformities of the hands, wrists, ankles, and feet due to joint involvement; limitation of joint motions; avascular necrosis, in particular, the femoral head and talus.

REFERENCES

Cable WJL, et al.: Fabry disease: Detection of heterozygotes by examination of glycolipids in urinary sediment. *Neurology* 32:1139, 1982.

Cable WJL, et al.: Fabry disease: Significance of ultrastructural localization of lipid inclusions in dermal nerves. *Neurology* 32:347, 1982.

Cohen IS, et al.: Two dimensional echocardiographic similarity of Fabry's disease to cardiac amyloidosis: A function of ultrastructural analogy? *J. Clin. Ultrasound* 11:437, 1983.

Dubost JJ, et al.: La maladie de Fabry. *Ann. Med. Interne (Paris)* 139:265, 1988.

Fabry J: Ein Beitrag zur Kenntnis der Purpura haemorrhagica nodularis. *Arch. Dermatol. Syph.* 43:187, 1898.

Herve J-P, et al.: Maladie de Fabry. Intérêt diagnostique de la ponction biopsie rénale dans les formes paucisymptomatiques. *Presse Med.* 12:1874, 1983.

Jongkind JF, et al.: Detection of Fabry's disease heterozygotes by enzyme analysis in single fibroblasts after cell sorting. *Clin. Genet.* 23:261, 1983.

Kaye EM, et al.: Nervous system involvement in Fabry's disease: Clinicopathological and biochemical correlation. *Ann. Neurol.* 23:515, 1988.

Rosenberg DM, et al.: Chronic airflow obstruction in Fabry's disease. *Am. J. Med.* 68:898, 1980.

Rowe JW, et al.: Intestinal manifestations of Fabry's disease. *Ann. Intern. Med.* 81:628, 1974.

Sakuraba H, et al.: Cardiovascular manifestations in Fabry's disease. A high incidence of mitral valve prolapse in hemizygotes and heterozygotes. *Clin. Genet.* 29:276, 1986.

Seino Y, et al.: Peripheral hemodynamics in patients with Fabry's disease. *Am. Heart J.* 105:783, 1983.

Sheth KJ, et al.: Heterozygote detection in Fabry disease utilizing multiple enzyme activities. *Am. J. Med. Genet.* 10:141, 1981.

Wilson SK, et al.: A new etiology of priapism: Fabry's disease. *J. Urol.* 109:646, 1973.

Yokoyama A, et al.: A case of heterozygous Fabry's disease with a short PR interval and giant negative T waves. *Br. Heart J.* 57:296, 1987.

FAHR DISEASE

Synonyms: Fahr syndrome; ferrocalcinosis.

Mode of Inheritance: Autosomal recessive.

Pathology: Cerebral and cerebellar calcification in the vessel walls and in the perivascular spaces of arterioles, capillaries, and veins (basal ganglia, periventricular white matter of the cerebral hemispheres, dentate nuclei of the cerebellum); laser spectroscopy shows in addition to calcium the

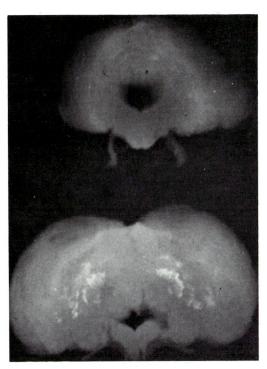

FIG ME—F—1.
Fahr syndrome. A postmortem roentgenogram of a section through the cerebellum demonstrates extensive calcification of the dentate nucleus and adjacent areas. (From Babbitt DP, Tang T, Dobb J, et al.: Idiopathic familial cerebrovascular ferrocalcinosis (Fahr disease) and review of differential diagnosis of intracranial calcification in children. *A.J.R.* 105:352, 1969. Used by permission.)

presence of mucopolysaccharides, zinc, phosphorus, chlorine, iron, aluminum, magnesium, and potassium.

Clinical Manifestations: (a) seizures, tetany, rigidity, tremors; (b) physical retardation; (c) mental deterioration; (d) *progressive development of spasticity and sometimes athetosis,* progression to a decerebrate state; (e) coincidence with phenylketonuria.

Radiologic Manifestations: (a) widespread *intracranial calcification* having an irregular, punctate, and occasionally dustlike appearance that is *densest in the basal ganglia region* and usually symmetrical; (b) magnetic resonance imaging: *varying degrees of signal intensity from the calcified regions* ("black to white") probably reflecting the different stages of the disease or different metabolic states at the sites of calcium deposition, (Fig ME—F—1).

REFERENCES

Babbitt DP, et al.: Idiopathic familial cerebrovascular ferro-calcinosis (Fahr's disease) and review of differential diagnosis of intracranial calcification in children. *A.J.R.* 105:352, 1969.

Fahr T: Idiopathische Verkalkung der Hirngefässe. *Zentralbl. Allg. Pathol.* 50:129, 1930.

Parker CE, et al.: Coincidence of Fahr disease and phenylketonuria. *J. Pediatr.* 91:273, 1977.

Scotti G, et al.: MR imaging in Fahr disease. *J. Comput. Assist. Tomogr.* 9:790, 1985.

Turpin JC, et al.: Rubrique iconographique. *Arch. Fr. Pediatr.* 41:653, 1984.

FANCONI SYNDROME

Synonym: de Toni-Debré-Fanconi syndrome.

Classification: (a) *idiopathic;* (b) *genetic diseases:* cystinosis, tyrosinemia, Lowe syndrome, galactosemia, fructose intolerance, Wilson disease, glycogen storage disease, familial nephrosis; (c) *acquired diseases:* amyloidosis, nephrotic syndrome, multiple myeloma, Sjögren syndrome, renal transplantation, drugs, heavy metals (mercury, lead, etc.), malignant neoplasms, etc.

Clinical Manifestations: Triad of *glycosuria, generalized aminoaciduria, and hypophosphaturia* (due to a defect in phosphate reabsorption and phosphaturia): (a) dwarfism; (b) muscle weakness; (c) anorexia; (d) vomiting; (e) inanition; (f) photophobia with cystine deposits in the cornea; (g) chronic acidosis; (h) uremia; (i) hypouricemia; (j) hypokalemia; (k) other reported abnormalities: occurrence of diabetes mellitus with idiopathic Fanconi syndrome, hypercalciuria, familial Fanconi syndrome with malabsorption and galactose intolerance, elevated serum 1,25-dihydroxyvitamin D concentration, acute neurological deterioration resembling Leigh syndrome, muscle cytochrome c oxidase deficiency, mitochondrial myopathy with lactic acidemia, etc.

Radiologic Manifestations: *Rickets or osteomalacia resistant to vitamin D in the usual dose.*

REFERENCES

Aperia A, et al.: Familial Fanconi syndrome with malabsorption and galactose intolerance, normal kinase and transferase activity: A report of two siblings. *Acta Paediatr. Scand.* 70:527, 1981.

Baran DT, et al.: Evidence for a defect in vitamin D metabolism in a patient with incomplete Fanconi syndrome. *J. Clin. Endocrinol. Metab.* 59:998, 1984.

Chesney RW, et al.: Metabolic abnormalities in the idiopathic Fanconi syndrome: Studies of carbohydrate metabolism in two patients. *Pediatrics* 67:113, 1981.

Debré R, et al.: Rachidisme tardif coexistent avec une néphrite chronique et une glycosurie. *Arch. Med. Enf.* 37:597, 1934.

de Toni G: Remarks on the relations between renal rickets (renal dwarfism) and renal diabetes. *Acta Paediatr.* 16:479, 1933.

Dumas R, et al.: Glomerulonéphrite extra-membraneuse chez deux frères associée dans un cas à une néphropathie tubulo-interstitielle avec syndrome de Fanconi et anticorp antimembrane basale tubulaire. *Arch. Fr. Pediatr.* 39:75, 1982.

Fanconi G: Die nicht diabetischen Glykosurien und Hyperglykamien des älteren Kindes. *Jb. Kinderheilkd.* 133:257, 1931.

Morris RC: The clinical spectrum of Fanconi's syndrome. *Calif. Med.* 108:225, 1968.

Ogier H, et al.: de Toni-Fanconi-Debré syndrome with Leigh syndrome revealing severe muscle cytochrome c oxidase deficiency. *J. Pediatr.* 112:734, 1988.

Russo JC, et al.: Gentamicin-induced Fanconi syndrome. *J. Pediatr.* 96:151, 1980.

Schwartz JH, et al.: Fanconi syndrome associated with cephalothin and gentamicin therapy. *Cancer* 41:769, 1978.

Sperl W, et al.: Mitochondrial myopathy with lactic acidaemia, Fanconi-de Toni-Debré syndrome and a disturbed succinate: cytochrome c oxidoreductase activity. *Eur. J. Pediatr.* 147:418, 1988.

Tieder M, et al.: Elevated serum 1,25-dihydroxyvitamin D concentrations in siblings with primary Fanconi's syndrome. *N. Engl. J. Med.* 319:845, 1988.

FARBER DISEASE

Synonyms: Lipogranulomatosis; Farber lipogranulomatosis.

Mode of Inheritance: Autosomal recessive.

Frequency: 28 published cases to 1985 (Burck et al.).

Etiology: Deficiency of lysosomal acid ceramidase resulting in tissue storage of ceramide (subcutaneous, kidney, brain, etc.).

Clinical Manifestations: Symptomatic in the first few months of life: (a) failure to thrive, cachexia; (b) projectile vomiting; (c) cutaneous pigmented lesions over bony promi-nences, xanthoma-like lesions on the face and hands; (d) *nodular masses mainly over the wrist and ankles;* (e) *hoarse-ness* and later laryngeal obstruction; (f) hyperesthesia; (g) *joint swelling and contracture;* (h) hepatosplenomegaly; (i) *mental and neurological deterioration;* (j) ceramidase activity assay in various tissues (skin, fibroblasts, white blood cells, liver, etc.) showing deficiency.

Radiologic Manifestations: (a) generalized demineraliza-tion; (b) muscle atrophy; (c) *nodular tumefaction about the peripheral joints;* (d) *joint capsular distension;* (e) subluxation of hip joints due to distension; (f) *juxta-articular bone ero-sions;* (g) flaring of costochondral junctions; (h) *pulmonary interstitial finely nodular infiltrates;* (i) internal hydroceph-alus.

Notes: Three types according to symptomatology and course (severe, intermediate, and mild); death in the first 4 years of life in the majority, survival into the second decade in about one third of the patients (Fig ME−F−2).

REFERENCES

Antonarakis SE, et al.: Phenotypic variability in siblings with Farber disease. *J. Pediatr.* 104:406, 1984.

Burck U, et al.: A case of lipogranulomatosis Farber: Some clinical and ultrastructural aspects. *Eur. J. Pediatr.* 143:206, 1985.

Dihlmann W: Richtungweisende Röntgenzichen bei der dis-seminierten Lipogranulomatose (Morbus Farber). *Fortschr. Rontgenstr.* 117:47, 1972.

Farber S: A lipid metabolic disorder-disseminated "lipogran-ulomatosis": A syndrome with similarity to, and important difference from Niemann-Pick and Hand-Schüller-

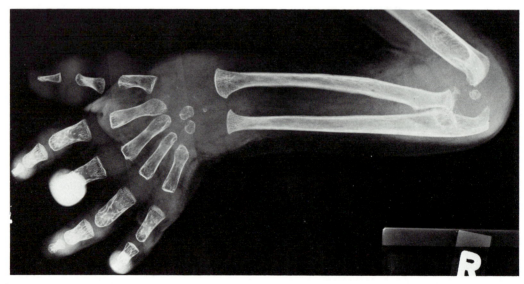

FIG ME−F−2.
Farber disease: marked capsular distension of the elbow, wrist, and interphalangeal joints by a substance of soft-tissue density. Note the subluxation of the elbow joint and grotesque deformity of the soft tissues of the thumb. (From Schultze G, Lang EK: Dissem-inated lipogranulomatosis: Report of a case. *Radiology* 74:428, 1960. Used by permission.)

Christian disease, (abstracted). *Am. J. Dis. Child.* 84:499, 1952.

Fensom AH, et al.: Prenatal diagnosis of Farber's disease. *Lancet* 2:990, 1979.

Schultz G, Lang EK: Disseminated lipogranulomatosis: Report of a case. *Radiology* 74:428, 1960.

Toppet M, et al.: Farber's disease as a ceramidosis: Clinical, radiological and biochemical aspects. *Acta Paediatr. Scand.* 67:113, 1978.

FLUOROSIS

Etiology: Chronic exposure to cryolite or rock phosphate dust containing fluoride salts or excess fluorides in the water supply; iatrogenic.

Clinical Manifestations: (a) *painful limbs, joint deformities,* knock-knee, bowlegs, saber shins, limitation of joint motions; (b) *stiffness and rigidity of the spine,* thoracic kyphosis; (c) *myelopathy* caused by compression of the spinal cord; (d) *dental mottling,* etc.; (e) increased total-body calcium (neutron activation analysis).

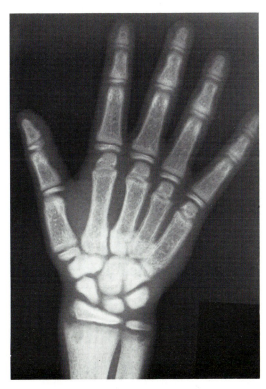

FIG ME−F−3.
Fluorosis. A radiogram of the hand and wrist of child with fluorosis shows eccenteric rachitic-like changes in the metaphyses of the radius and ulna. The carpal bones are sclerotic; the metacarpals are widened and lack modeling. The cortices are thinned and poorly defined. Periosteal changes are present, but without typical changes of subperiosteal resorption of hyperparathyroidism. (From Christie DP: The spectrum of radiographic bone changes in children with fluorosis. *Radiology* 136:85, 1980. Used by permission.)

Radiologic Manifestations: (a) children: *ground-glass density of the calvaria; lack of a normal distinct diploic space; sharp borders of the cranial sutures; absence of the lamina dura; wide vertebral bodies and dense end plates;* relative thickening of intervertebral disk spaces; a combination of a radiological picture of osteomalacia, osteoporosis, and osteosclerosis; *thickened ribs; serrations along the iliac crests;* etc.; (b) adults: *thickened and dense skull, in particular, at the base; irregularity and hypercementosis of dental roots; resorption of periodontal bone, sclerosis of the vertebrae; calcification of the spinous ligaments; osteophytosis of vertebral bodies, generalized skeletal sclerosis* associated with narrowing of thickened bony trabeculae; *periostitis deformans;* needlelike calcific projections at sites of attachment of the intercostal muscles; *calcification of the interosseous ligaments* and joint capsules; etc.; (c) osteoporosis as the earliest detectable radiographic change; (d) intense skeletal uptake of ^{99}Tc-MDP (Fig ME−F−3).

REFERENCES

Azar HA, et al.: Skeletal sclerosis due to chronic fluoride intoxication: Cases from endemic area of fluorosis in region of Persian Gulf. *Ann. Intern. Med.* 55:193, 1961.

Christie DP: The spectrum of radiographic bone changes in children with fluorosis. *Radiology* 136:85, 1980.

El-Khoury GY, et al.: Sodium fluoride treatment of osteoporosis: Radiologic findings. *A.J.R.* 139:39, 1982.

Hummel P, et al.: A propos d'un cas d'ostéopathie fluorée induite par l'acide niflumique. *Ann. Radiol. (Paris)* 26:687, 1983.

Jimenez LE, et al.: Total body calcium in skeletal fluorosis. *Lancet* 1:1443, 1983.

Leone NC, et al.: A roentgenologic study of a human population exposed to high-fluoride domestic water: A ten-year study. *A.J.R.* 74:874, 1955.

Morris JW: Skeletal fluorosis among Indians of the American Southwest. *A.J.R.* 94:608, 1965.

Thivolle P, et al.: Bone imaging in a case of chronic fluorine intoxication with mineral water. *Clin. Nucl. Med.* 11:771, 1986.

Zong-Cheng L, et al.: Osteoporosis—an early radiographic sign of endemic fluorosis. *Skeletal Radiol.* 15:350, 1986.

FUCOSIDOSIS

Mode of Inheritance: Autosomal recessive.

Etiology: Deficiency of α-L-fucosidase enzyme leading to an accumulation of fucosyl compounds (glycolipids, lipoproteins, oligosaccharides, and polysaccharide) in almost all organs.

Types: *Type I* with an onset of symptoms in the first few months of life, a fast progression of symptoms, and death in early childhood; *type II* with an onset of symptoms in the second year of life, a moderate rate of progression of symptoms, and death in childhood; *type III* with a later onset of symptoms and slow progression of the disease.

Clinical Manifestations: (a) *Hurler-like clinical features* with a coarse facies, prominent forehead, hypertelorism, broad and flattened nose, heavy eyebrows, large tongue, thick lips, broad thorax, lumbar hyperlordosis, hepatosplenomegaly, recurrent respiratory infections; (b) *deteriorating psychomotor achievements, peripheral neuropathy,* amyotrophy, muscular weakness, hypotonia changing to hypertonia, spastic quadriplegia, decorticate and/or decerebrate rigidity; (c) *angiokeratoma corporis diffusum,* thick skin, thin dry skin; (d) histochemical and ultrastructural abnormalities on the biopsy specimens (skin, conjunctiva, rectal mucosa): abnormal macrophages filled with fucose-rich granules; characteristic inclusions in the endothelial cells, fibroblasts, and Schwann cells; etc.

Radiologic Manifestations: (a) *skull:* progressive thickening of the diploic spaces, particularly over the frontal and supraorbital region; early synostosis of one or more cranial sutures, absent or poorly developed paranasal sinuses; (b) *spine:* short odontoid, cervical platyspondyly, kyphosis at the thoracolumbar junction, anterior beaking of the lower thoracic and lumbar vertebrae, small fifth lumbar vertebra, vacuum disks, short sacrum with square-shaped vertebrae, absent or rudimentary coccyx; (c) *chest:* medial widening and slight shortening of the clavicles, slight expansion of the ribs, slightly widened and poorly developed glenoids; (d) *pelvis and limbs:* sclerosis, scalloping and widening of the acetabular roofs, flattening and irregularity of the femoral heads, coxa valga, widening of the shaft of long bones; (e) *skeletal maturation retardation;* (f) cerebral atrophy (Fig ME−F−4).

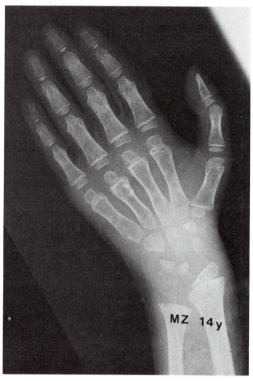

FIG ME−F−4.
Fucosidosis in a 14-year-old boy with markedly retarded bone age, a V-shaped distal radio-ulnar configuration, deformed carpal bones, sclerotic epiphyses, and bilateral notching of the proximal metacarpals and distal ends of the proximal phalanges. (From Lee FA, Donnell GN, Gwinn JL: Radiographic features of fucosidosis. *Pediatr. Radiol.* 5:204, 1977. Used by permission.)

REFERENCES

Brill, PW et al.: Roentgenographic findings in fucosidosis type 2. *A.J.R.* 124:75, 1975.
Christomanou H, et al.: Absence of α-fucosidase activity in two sisters showing a different phenotype. *Eur. J. Pediatr.* 140:27, 1983.
Durand P, et al.: New mucopolysaccharide lipid-storage disease? *Lancet* 2:1313, 1966.
Hoof FV, et al.: Mucopolysaccharidosis by absence of α-fucosidase. *Lancet* 1:1198, 1968.
Ikeda S-I, et al.: Adult fucosidosis: Histochemical and ultrastructural studies of rectal mucosa biopsy. *Neurology* 34:451, 1984.
Kessler RM, et al.: Cranial CT in fucosidosis. *A.J.N.R.* 2:591, 1981.
Lee FA, et al.: Radiographic features of fucosidosis. *Pediatr. Radiol.* 5:204, 1977.

GALACTOSEMIA

Mode of Inheritance: Autosomal recessive.

Etiology: Cellular deficiency of either galactokinase or galactose-1-phosphate uridyl transferase.

Clinical Manifestations:

(A) NEONATE: *symptoms develop with milk feeding:* (a) *lethargy, hypotonia;* (b) *vomiting, diarrhea;* (c) *failure to thrive;* (d) *jaundice, hepatomegaly;* (e) *susceptibility to infection;* (f) *signs of increased intracranial pressure (cerebral edema).*

(B) CHILDHOOD (untreated patients, occasionally also in treated patients): (a) *mental retardation;* (b) *tremor, cerebellar dysfunction;* (c) *cataracts;* (d) *liver cirrhosis;* (e) *other reported abnormalities: ovarian hypofunction, galactosuria.*

Radiologic Manifestations: (a) neonate: brain edema; (b) childhood: brain atrophy (Fig ME–G–1).

REFERENCES

Belman AL, et al.: Computed tomographic demonstration of cerebral edema in a child with galactosemia. *Pediatrics* 78:606, 1986.
Berlier P, et al.: Insuffisance ovarienne et galactosemie congénitale. *Ann. Pediatr. (Paris)* 34:75, 1987.
Böhles H, et al.: Progressive cerebellar and extrapyramidal motor disturbances in galactosaemic twins. *Eur. J. Pediatr.* 145:413, 1986.
Welch RJ, et al.: Cerebral edema and galactosemia. *Pediatrics* 80:598, 1987.

GALACTOSIALIDOSIS

Enzyme Deficiencies: Combined β-galactosidase and *N*-acetyl-neuraminidase.

Mode of Inheritance: Autosomal recessive.

Clinical Manifestations: Phenotypic variations: (a) early infantile form: *edema, ascites, cherry-red macular spot,* early death; (b) late infantile form (onset at 6 to 12 months of age): *dysmorphism, organomegaly, cherry-red spot, mental retardation;* (c) childhood-adulthood presentation: *corneal clouding, cherry-red spot, various neurological symptoms, mental retardation;* (d) other reported abnormalities: coarse facial features, joint movement limitation, cardiomyopathy, kidney enlargement, hernias, hypotonia, anemia, proteinuria, Hurler-like picture.

Radiologic Manifestations: (a) organomegaly, increased renal echogenicity; (b) various skeletal manifestations (generally less pronounced as compared with sialidosis); dysostosis multiplex.

Note: The terms *Goldberg syndrome* and *Goldberg-Wenger syndrome* refer to the childhood-adult form of this metabolic disorder (Fig ME–G–2).

REFERENCES

Goldberg M, et al.: Macular cherry-red spot, corneal clouding and β-galactosidase deficiency. *Arch. Intern. Med.* 128:387, 1971.
Loonen MCB, et al.: Combined sialidase (neuraminidase) and β-galactosidase deficiency. Clinical, morphological and enzymological observations in a patient. *Clin. Genet.* 26:139, 1984.
Okada S, et al.: A case of neuraminidase deficiency associated with a partial β-galactosidase defect. Clinical, biochemical and radiological studies. *Eur. J. Pediatr.* 130:239, 1979.
Sewell AC, et al.: Clinical heterogeneity in infantile galactosialidosis. *Eur. J. Pediatr.* 146:528, 1987.
Spranger J: Mini review: Inborn errors of complex carbohydrate metabolism. *Am. J. Med. Genet.* 28:489, 1987.
Wenger DA, et al.: Macular cherry-red spot and myoclonus with dementia: coexistent neuraminidase and β-galactosidase deficiencies. *Biochem. Biophys. Res. Commun.* 82:589, 1978.

GAUCHER DISEASE

Synonym: Cerebroside lipidosis.

Mode of Inheritance: Autosomal recessive; genetic heterogeneity within and among subtypes.

Pathogenesis: Absence or severe deficiency of glucosylceramide β-glucosidase activity in various body tissues.

Classification: (a) type 1 ("adult form"): chronic nonneuropathic most common type, clinical presentation at any age, skin pigmentation, bone lesions, hypersplenism, and pingueculae; (b) type 2 (the acute neuropathic form): onset of symptoms in infancy and the clinical picture of "pseudo-bulbar palsy"; (c) type 3 (the subacute neuropathic, juvenile form): onset usually in childhood, slow and progressive neurological manifestations (hypertonicity, seizures, gait problems, mental retardation, etc.).

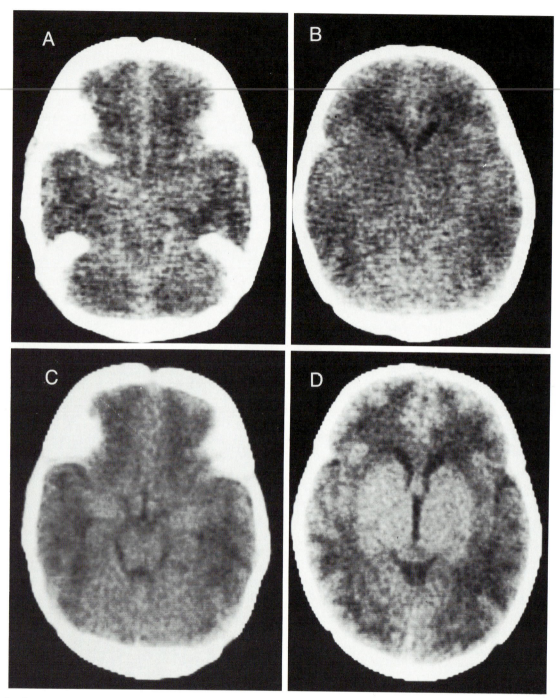

FIG ME–G–1.

Galactosemia in a newborn infant. **A** and **B,** note the diffuse cerebral edema manifested by severe hypodensity of the brain with compression of the ventricles and obliteration of the subarachnoid spaces. The dura and vasculatures are relatively dense as compared with the adjacent hypodense, edematous brain. **C** and **D,** a repeat computed tomographic scan 12 days later reveals a dramatic decrease in edema. Ventricles are now normal in size for age *(right),* and subarachnoid spaces (sylvian fissures, suprasellar and circum-mesencephalic cisterns) are now visible. The gray matter (cortex and basal ganglia) has normal density and is easily distinguished from the white matter, which has residual hypodensity due to persistent white matter edema. (From Belman AL, Moshe SL, Zimmerman RD: Computed tomographic demonstration of cerebral edema in a child with galactosemia. *Pediatrics* 78:606, 1986. Used by permission.)

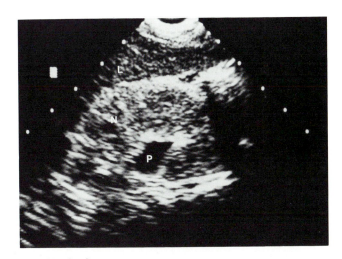

FIG ME–G–2.
Galactosialidosis. Note the marked increase in renal echogenicity (*L* = liver; *N* = renal parenchymal tissue; *P* = renal pelvis. (From Sewell AC, Pontz BF, Weitzel D, et al.: Clinical heterogeneity in infantile galactosialidosis. *Eur. J. Pediatr.* 146:528, 1987. Used by permission.)

Clinical Manifestations: (a) bone and joint pain, bone tenderness; (b) fever; (c) purpura, epistaxis, hemorrhagic infarcts, hematuria; (d) conjunctival pigmentation, abnormal skin pigmentations; (e) abdominal fullness, *hepatosplenomegaly*, hypersplenism; (f) anemia, thrombocytopenia, leukopenia; (g) Gaucher cells in the bone marrow, acid β-glucosidase activity deficiency in fibroblasts and circulating white blood cells, elevated non–tartarate-inhibitable acid phosphatase activity; (h) other reported abnormalities: elevation of serum angiotensin-converting enzyme levels; cardiac, renal, and pulmonary involvement; pulmonary hypertension; white spots in the fundi; neonatal ascites; "collodion baby" (collodion skin).

Radiologic Manifestations: (a) skeletal manifestations: (1) plain radiography: *resorption of bone trabeculae, coarse foamlike appearance, moth-eaten pattern, pathological sclerotic changes, expansion of bones (Erlenmeyer flask deformity of the femora)*, pathological fractures, collapse of the femoral head, collapse of the vertebrae, periosteal reaction with a solid or lacelike type of *subperiosteal new bone formation*, degenerative articular changes, rare involvement of the skull, enlarged phalangeal nutrient foramina, accelerated skeletal deterioration after splenectomy, acute hematogenous osteomyelitis, findings simulating sacroiliitis, small tubular hands and feet involvement similar to those of thalassemia major (osteoporosis, reticulated trabecular pattern, widening of the medullary cavity, thinned cortex), bone lesion mimicking osteosarcoma, regression of the skeletal changes following a bone marrow transplant (type 1 Gaucher), thinning and deformity of the ribs and slender long bones in neonatal disease; (2) computed tomography (CT) in type 1: abnormal cortical density, expansion of the marrow space, abnormal attenuation of the marrow cavity, calcification in the marrow

cavity, (3) technetium 99m sulfur colloid bone marrow useful in determination of the extent and severity of skeletal involvement: peripheral expansion of normal marrow, greater marrow expansion with patchy areas lacking uptake, or a greater loss of uptake with retention of the nuclide in other reticuloendothelioid organs and circulation; (4) magnetic resonance imaging (MRI): more sensitive than CT is in evaluation of the extent of abnormalities, low-intensity signals (longer than normal T_1 and shorter T_2 values) in the bone marrow; (b) *hepatosplenomegaly*, shorter-than-normal T_1 values of the spleen (MRI imaging) compatible with fibrosis, increased echogenicity of the liver, lobulation of the liver surface, central areas of decreased attenuation (CT), hypoechoic splenic lesions (focal homogeneous clusters of Gaucher cells), hyperechoic splenic lesion (Gaucher cells, fibrosis, infarction); (c) lung involvement; (d) other reported abnormalities: combined portal and vena caval hypertension, exaggerated anterior vertebral notching, central depression of multiple vertebral endplates, bone lesions simulating osteomyelitis (Figs ME–G–3 and ME–G–4).

REFERENCES

Beaudet AL: Gaucher's disease. *N. Engl. J. Med.* 316:619, 1987.

Bell RS, et al.: Osteomyelitis in Gaucher disease. *J. Bone Joint Surg. [Am.]* 68:1380, 1986.

Choulot JJ, et al.: Hypertension portale au cours d'une maladie de Gaucher. *Arch. Fr. Pediatr.* 38:267, 1981.

Choy FYM, et al.: Gaucher disease: Accurate identification of asymptomatic French-Canadian carrier using nonlabeled authentic sphingolipid substrate *N*-palmitoyl dihydroglucocerebroside. *Am. J. Med. Genet.* 27:895, 1987.

Choy FYM: Intrafamilial clinical variability of type I Gaucher disease in a French-Canadian family. *J. Med. Genet.* 25:322, 1988.

Cogan DG, et al.: Fundal abnormalities of Gaucher's disease. *Arch. Ophthalmol.* 98:2202, 1980.

Daneman A, et al.: Neonatal ascites due to lysosomal storage disease. *Radiology* 149:463, 1983.

Fabbro D, et al.: Gaucher disease: Genetic heterogeneity within and among subtypes detected by immunoblotting. *Am. J. Hum. Genet.* 40:15, 1987.

Fink IJ, et al.: Enlarged phalangeal nutrient foramina in Gaucher disease and β-thalassemia major. *A.J.R.* 143:647, 1984.

Gaucher P: *De l'épithelioma primitif de la rate: Hypertrophie Idiopathique de la Rate Sans Leucémie* (thesis). Paris, 1882.

Glass RBJ, et al.: Gaucher disease of the liver: CT appearance. *Pediatr. Radiol.* 17:417, 1987.

Goldblatt J: Type I Gaucher disease. *J. Med. Genet.* 25:415, 1988.

Grafe M, et al.: Infantile Gaucher's disease: A case with neuronal storage. *Ann. Neurol.* 23:300, 1988.

Hermann G, et al.: Gaucher's disease type 1: Assessment of bone involvement by CT and scintigraphy. *A.J.R.* 147:943, 1986.

Hill SC, et al.: Gaucher disease: Sonographic appearance of the spleen. *Radiology* 160:631, 1986.

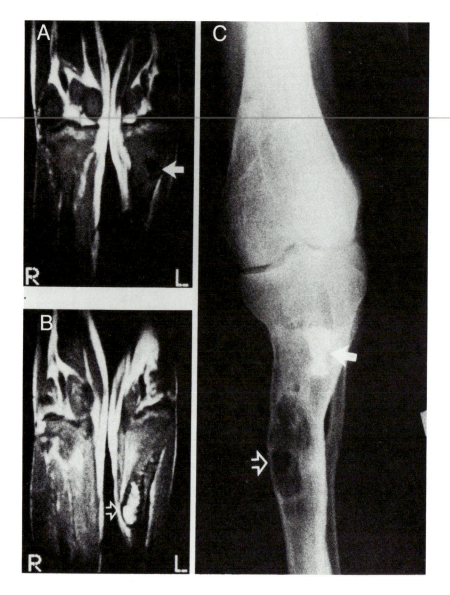

FIG ME–G–3.
Gaucher disease. **A,** coronal MRI (2.0 T, SE 600/28.5) of a 31-year-old man. The upper portion of the shaft of the tibia shows a low signal from marrow infiltration. The absence of a signal on MRI *(arrow)* corresponds to a sclerotic area *(white arrow)* in upper part of the shaft of the tibia on the radiograph. **B,** MRI of the midshaft of the tibia shows an area of intense signal surrounded by a black line *(open arrow)* that corresponds to the lucent defect *(open arrow)* surrounded by dense cortical type bone seen in **C.** The intense signal is related to fat in normal marrow that has formed after osteotomy. (From Lanir A, Hadar H, Cohen I, et al.: Gaucher disease: Assessment with MR imaging. *Radiology* 161:239, 1986. Used by permission.)

Katz K, et al.: Fractures in children who have Gaucher disease. *J. Bone Joint Surg.* [Am.] 69:1361, 1987.

Lanir A, et al.: Gaucher disease: Assessment with MR imaging. *Radiology* 161:239, 1986.

Lieberman J, et al.: Elevation of serum angiotensin-converting enzyme in Gaucher's disease. *N. Engl. J. Med.* 294:1442, 1976.

Lui K, et al.: Collodion babies with Gaucher's disease. *Arch. Dis. Child.* 63:854, 1988.

Matoth Y, et al.: Frequency of carriers of chronic (type I) Gaucher disease in Ashkenazi Jews. *Am. J. Med. Genet.* 27:561, 1987.

Miller JH, et al.: Juvenile Gaucher disease simulating osteomyelitis. *A.J.R.* 137:880, 1981.

Nishimura RN, et al.: Neurologic complications of Gaucher's disease, type 3. *Arch. Neurol.* 37:92, 1980.

Pastakia B, et al.: Skeletal manifestations of Gaucher's disease. *Semin. Roentgenol.* 21:264, 1986.

Rose JS, et al.: Accelerated skeletal deterioration after splenectomy in Gaucher type I disease. *A.J.R.* 139:1202, 1982.

Schoenfeld A, et al.: Ultrasonographic aspects of Gaucher's disease: Report of a patient during three pregnancies. *J. Clin. Ultrasound* 15:207, 1987.

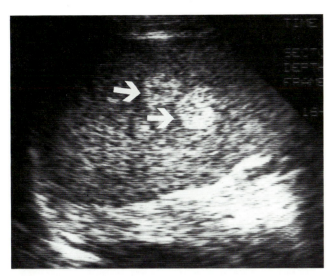

FIG ME–G–4.
Gaucher disease. A sagittal image of the spleen shows two hyperechoic masses *(arrows)*. (From Hill SC, Reinig JW, Barranger JA, et al.: Gaucher disease: Sonographic appearance of the spleen. *Radiology* 160:631, 1986. Used by permission.)

Schubiner H, et al.: Pyogenic osteomyelitis versus pseudo-osteomyelitis in Gaucher's disease. *Clin. Pediatr. [Phila.]* 20:667, 1981.
Smith RL, et al.: Unusual cardiac, renal and pulmonary involvement in Gaucher's disease: Interstitial glucocerebroside accumulation, pulmonary hypertension and fatal bone marrow embolization. *Am. J. Med.* 65:352, 1980.
Starer F, et al.: Regression of the radiological changes of Gaucher's disease following bone marrow transplantation. *Br. J. Radiol.* 60:1189, 1987.
Stevens PG, et al.: Splenic involvement in Gaucher's disease: Sonographic findings. *J. Clin. Ultrasound* 15:397, 1987.
Svennerholm L, et al.: Prenatal diagnosis of Gaucher disease: Assay of the beta-glucosidase activity in amniotic fluid cells cultivated in two laboratories with different cultivation conditions. *Clin. Genet.* 19:16, 1981.
Tibblin E, et al.: Hematological findings in the Norrbottnian type of Gaucher disease. *Eur. J. Pediatr.* 139:187, 1982.

GEOPHAGIA

Synonym: Earth-eating syndrome.

Clinical Manifestations: (a) *geophagia*; (b) *iron deficiency with microcytic anemia*; (c) hepatosplenomegaly; (d) *short stature*; (e) *delay in puberty*.

Radiologic Manifestations: (a) skeletal maturation retardation; (b) *radiopaque materials within the digestive tract*; (c) hepatosplenomegaly; (d) cardiomegaly; (e) thick calvaria due to anemia.

REFERENCES

Clayton RS, et al.: The roentgenographic diagnosis of geophagia (dirt eating). *A.J.R.* 73:203, 1955.
Courbon B, et al.: "Geophagie au plâtre" chez un enfant maghrébin transplanté. *Arch. Fr. Pediatr.* 44:145, 1987.
Parsad AS, et al.: Syndrome of iron deficiency anemia, hepatosplenomegaly, hypogonadism, dwarfism and geophagia. *Am. J. Med.* 31:532, 1961.
Perrimond H, et al.: Géophagie et syndromes apparentés. *Ann. Pediat.* 29:273, 1982.
Ronaghy HA, et al.: A six-year follow-up of Iranian patients with dwarfism, hypogonadism and iron deficiency anemia. *Am. J. Clin. Nutr.* 21:709, 1968.

GILBERT SYNDROME

Mode of Inheritance: Autosomal dominant; isolated sporadic cases.

Frequency: Affecting 2% to 5% of the population.

Clinical Manifestations: (a) vague symptoms: fatigue, weakness, abdominal pain; (b) *jaundice due to low-grade unconjugated hyperbilirubinemia*, normal liver biopsy findings; (c) immunohemolytic anemia (a case report).

Radiologic Manifestations: Normal cholecystographic findings in the presence of jaundice.

REFERENCES

Berk PD, et al.: Inborn errors of bilirubin metabolism. *Med. Clin. North Am.* 59:803, 1975.
Bloch HS, et al.: Oral cholecystography in Gilbert's syndrome and diagnostics of jaundice. *J.A.M.A.* 218:1302, 1971.
Gilbert NA, Lereboullet P: La cholémie simple familiale. *Sem. Med.* 11:241, 1901.
Lake AM, et al.: Marked hyperbilirubinemia with Gilbert syndrome and immunohemolytic anemia. *J. Pediatr.* 93:812, 1978.
McColl KEL, et al.: Porphyrin metabolism and haem biosynthesis in Gilbert's syndrome. *Gut* 28:125, 1987.

GLUCAGONOMA SYNDROME

Pathology: Pancreatic alpha-cell tumor (glucagonoma).

Clinical Manifestations: (a) *necrolytic migratory erythematous rash*; (b) *angular stomatitis, painful glossitis*; (c) *normochromic normocytic anemia*; (d) *mild diabetes mellitus*; (e) *tendency to thrombosis*; (f) *weight loss*; (g) *neuropsychiatric disorders*; (h) *high plasma glucagon concentration*; (i) *tumor identification: immunocytochemistry with glucagon antibodies*.

Radiologic Manifestations: *Pancreatic tumor;* metastases.

REFERENCES

Assaad SN, et al.: Glucagonoma syndrome. Rapid response following arterial embolization of glucagonoma metastatic to the liver. *Am. J. Med.* 82:533, 1987.

Bloom SR, et al.: Glucagonoma syndrome. *Am. J. Med.* 82(suppl. 5B):25, 1987.

Breatnach ÉS, et al.: CT evaluation of glucagonomas. *J. Comput. Assist. Tomogr.* 9:25, 1985.

Fujita J, et al.: A functional study of a case of glucagonoma exhibiting typical glucagonoma syndrome. *Cancer* 57:860, 1986.

GLYCOGENOSIS, TYPE I

Synonyms: Glycogen storage disease, type I; von Gierke disease.

Classification: (a) type Ia (von Gierke disease): deficiency of the microsomal enzyme glucose-6-phosphatase in the liver, kidney, and small bowel mucosa; (2) type Ib: deficiency of the transport of glucose-6-phosphate into hepatic endoplasmic reticulum (translocase deficiency), the clinical features similar to type Ia, glucose-6-phosphatase activity is almost normal in biopsy specimen of the liver.

Mode of Inheritance: Autosomal recessive.

Clinical Manifestations: Onset of symptoms in infancy: (a) failure to thrive; (b) *massive hepatomegaly;* (c) convulsions; (d) repeated episodes of *hypoglycemia* and acidosis; (e) hyperlipidemia; (f) hyperuricemia; (g) gouty arthritis; (h) nephritis (persistent proteinuria, hematuria, altered creatinine clearance, hypertension, progressive renal insufficiency, death from renal failure); (i) other reported abnormalities: hemorrhagic pancreatitis, increased incidence of urolithiasis, uric acid nephropathy, familial bleeding tendency, recurrent infections, inflammatory bowel disease indistinguishable from Crohn disease, neutropenia, neutrophil dysfunction, oral mucosal lesions.

Radiologic Manifestations: (a) *hepatomegaly,* variable attenuation coefficient of liver on computed tomographic (CT) examination (13 to 80 Hounsfield units [HU] in one report) depending on simultaneous glycogen deposition and fatty infiltration (the CT attenuation coefficient of glycogen is in the 50- to 70-HU range), liver tumor (adenoma, carcinoma, hepatoblastoma); (b) *progressive enlargement of the kidneys,* CT demonstration of an increased attenuation coefficient of the renal cortex due to glycogen deposition; (c) *osteoporosis;* (d) pathological fracture; (e) retarded bone maturation; (f) gouty changes; (g) multiple growth lines; (h) renal calculi; (i) radionuclide study: hepatomegaly with diminished radionuclide accumulation, splenomegaly with increased uptake; (j) barium enema: smooth-walled, slightly narrow co-

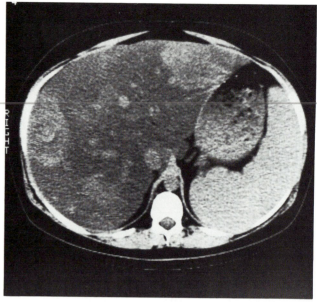

FIG ME–G–5.
Glycogenosis (type I) in a 21-year-old man with hepatomegaly and extensive nonhomogeneous fatty replacement of the liver. (From Doppman JL, Cornblath M, Dwyer AJ, et al.: Computed tomography of the liver and kidneys in glycogen storage disease. *J. Comput. Assist. Tomogr.* 6:67, 1982. Used by permission.)

lon; absence of haustrations; normal colonic length; moyamoya (Fig ME–G–5).

REFERENCES

Bowerman RA, et al.: Ultrasonographic features of hepatic adenomas in type I glycogen storage disease. *J. Ultrasound Med.* 2:51, 1983.

Brunelle F, et al.: Liver adenomas in glycogen storage disease in children. Ultrasound and angiographic study. *Pediatr. Radiol.* 14:94, 1984.

Chen Y-T, et al.: Renal disease in type I glycogen storage disease. *N. Engl. J. Med.* 318:7, 1988.

Doppman JL, et al.: Computed tomography of the liver and kidneys in glycogen storage disease. *J. Comput. Assist. Tomogr.* 6:67, 1982.

Fellows RA, et al.: Barium enema in type I hepatorenal glycogen storage disease. *Pediatr. Radiol.* 3:75, 1975.

Gahr M, et al.: Impaired metabolic function of polymorphonuclear leukocytes in glycogen storage disease Ib. *Eur. J. Pediatr.* 140:329, 1983.

Gierke E, von: Hepato-nephromegalia glycogenica (Glycogenspeicherkrankheit der Leber und Nieren). *Beitr. Pathol. Anat.* 82:497, 1929.

Heyne K, et al.: Glycogen storage disease type Ib: Familial bleeding tendency. *Eur. J. Pediatr.* 143:7, 1984.

Ito E, et al.: Type Ia glycogen storage disease with hepatoblastoma in siblings. *Cancer* 59:1776, 1987.

Michels VV, et al.: Hemorrhagic pancreatitis in a patient with glycogen storage disease type I. *Clin. Genet.* 17:220, 1980.

Miller JH, et al.: Radiography of glycogen storage disease. *A.J.R.* 132:379, 1979.

Miller JH, et al.: Scintigraphic abnormalities in glycogen storage disease. *J. Nucl. Med.* 19:354, 1978.

Preger L, et al.: Roentgenographic skeletal changes in the glycogen storage diseases. *A.J.R.* 107:840, 1969.

Roe TF, et al.: Inflammatory bowel disease in glycogen storage disease type Ib. *J. Pediatr.* 109:55, 1986.

Sunder TR: Moyamoya disease in patient with type I glycogenosis. *Arch. Neurol.* 38:251, 1981.

GLYCOGENOSIS, TYPE II

Synonyms: Pompe disease; acid maltase deficiency; glycogen storage disease, type II.

Mode of Inheritance: Autosomal recessive.

Enzyme Defect: Lysosomal α-1,4-glucosidase (acid maltase), demonstrable in the liver, muscle, fibroblast, chorionic villi.

Classification: According to the age of onset, extent of organ involvement, and life expectancy there are three clinical forms: (a) type IIa: classic or infantile form; (b) type IIb: juvenile form; (c) type IIc: adult form.

Pathology: Generalized involvement, in particular, the heart, nerves, and muscles.

Clinical Manifestations:

(A) TYPE IIa (INFANTILE FORM): (a) hypotonicity, difficulty in sucking, dyspnea, circumoral cyanosis, irritability, failure to thrive, macroglossia; (b) cardiac involvement: (left-axis deviation, short PR interval, huge QRS complexes, T-wave inversion, left ventricular outflow obstruction, pronounced systolic anterior motion of the anterior mitral valve leaflet (echocardiography); (c) rapid progression of disease with the development of firm muscles, loss of deep tendon reflexes, respiratory infections, and cardiac failure; (d) death in the first year of life in most cases.

(B) TYPE IIb (JUVENILE FORM): (a) muscular involvement (weakness with a clinical picture similar to pseudohypertrophic muscular dystrophy, firm muscles); (b) intercostal muscle disease predisposing to recurrent pneumonia; (c) death in the first decade of life.

(C) TYPE IIc (ADULT FORM): progressive myopathy (striated muscles).

Radiologic Manifestations: (a) *moderate to massive cardiomegaly* with normal pulmonary vasculature or vascular congestion in some; (b) marked thickening of the ventricular wall, significant obstruction of the left ventricular outflow tract (echocardiography, cardioangiography, magnetic resonance imaging [MRI]); (c) irregular inhomogeneous appearance of the myocardium (MRI); (d) radionuclide evaluation of heart: muscular hypertrophy, hypokinesis of the ventricles.

Differential Diagnosis: Muscular dystrophy (type IIb, IIc); cardiomyopathies (type IIa) (Fig ME–G–6).

REFERENCES

Besançon A-M, et al.: Prenatal diagnosis of glycogenosis type II (Pompe's disease) using chorionic villi biopsy. *Clin. Genet.* 27:479, 1985.

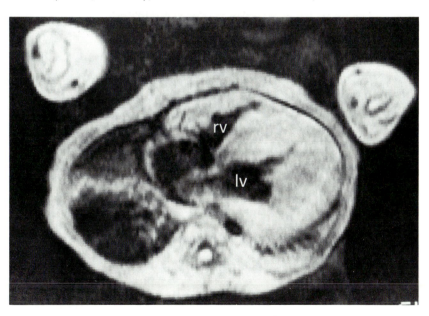

FIG ME–G–6.
Glycogenosis, type II: Axial MRI at the base of the left ventricle *(lv)*. There is enchrochment on the ventricular cavity by hypertrophy of all walls of the left ventricle, most marked in the anteroseptal and anterolateral regions *(rv* = right ventricle). (From Boxer RA, Fishman M, LaCorte MA, et al.: Cardiac MR imaging in Pompe disease. *J. Comput. Assist. Tomogr.* 10:857, 1986. Used by permission.)

Bonnici F, et al.: Angiographic and enzyme studies in a patient with type II glycogenosis (Pompe's disease). *S. Afr. Med. J.* 58:860, 1980.

Boxer RA, et al.: Cardiac MR imaging in Pompe disease. *J. Comput. Assist. Tomogr.* 10:857, 1986.

Bulkley BH, et al.: Pompe's disease presenting as hypertrophic myocardiopathy with Wolff-Parkinson-White syndrome. *Am. Heart J.* 96:246, 1978.

Dickinson DF, et al.: Unusual angiographic appearances of the left ventricle in 2 cases of Pompe's disease (glycogenosis type II). *Br. Heart J.* 41:238, 1979.

Grubisic A, et al.: First trimester diagnosis of Pompe's disease (glycogenosis type II) with normal outcome: Assay of acid α-glucosidase in chorionic villous biopsy using antibodies. *Clin. Genet.* 30:298, 1986.

Iancu TC, et al.: Juvenile acid maltase deficiency presenting as paravertebral pseudotumour. *Eur. J. Pediatr.* 147:372, 1988.

Lorber A, et al.: Radionuclide evaluation of a patient with neonatal presentation of Pompe's disease. *Clin. Nucl. Med.* 12:972, 1987.

Miller JH, et al.: Radiography of glycogen storage disease. *A.J.R.* 132:379, 1979.

Pompe JC: Over idiopatsche hypertrophie van het hart. *Ned. Tijdschr. Geneeskd.* 76:304, 1932.

Rees A, et al.: Echocardiographic evidence of outflow tract obstruction in Pompe's disease (glycogen storage disease of the heart). *Am. J. Cardiol.* 37:1103, 1976.

Ruttenberg HD, et al.: Glycogen-storage disease of the heart: Hemodynamic and angiocardiographic features in two cases. *Am. Heart. J.* 67:469, 1964.

Temple JK, et al.: The "muscular variant" of Pompe disease: Clinical, biochemical and histologic characteristics. *Am. J. Med. Genet.* 21:597, 1985.

GLYCOGENOSIS, TYPE III

Synonyms: Glycogen storage disease, type III; Cori disease; Forbes disease; debranching enzyme deficiency (liver, muscle, red and white blood cells, fibroblast, etc.).

Enzyme Defect: Amylo-1,6-glucosidase.

Mode of Inheritance: Autosomal recessive.

Clinical and Radiologic Manifestations: (a) short stature; (b) protuberant abdomen; (c) hepatomegaly, hepatic cirrhosis (rare), splenomegaly; (d) hypoglycemia with a failure to respond to glucagon, ketoacidosis, hyperlipidemia; (e) myopathic pattern, "mixed" (neuromyopathic) pattern, peripheral neuropathy, cardiomyopathy; (f) deficiency of amylo-1,6-glucosidase (debrancher deficiency) demonstrated by liver biopsy.

REFERENCES

Miller JH, et al.: Radiography of glycogen storage diseases. *A.J.R.* 132:379, 1979.

Moses SW et al.: Neuromuscular involvement in glycogen

storage disease type III. *Acta Paediatr. Scand.* 75:289, 1986.

Rossignol A-M, et al.: La myocardiopathie de la glycogenose type III. *Arch. Fr. Pediatr.* 36:303, 1979.

Ugawa Y, et al.: Accumulation of glycogen in sural nerve axons in adult-onset type III glycogenosis. *Ann. Neurol.* 19:294, 1986.

GLYCOGENOSIS, TYPE IV

Synonyms: Andersen disease; glycogen storage disease, type IV; amylopectinosis.

Enzyme Deficiency: α-1,4-Glucan; α-1,4-glucan-6-glucosyltransferase.

Clinical and Radiologic Manifestations: Onset in early infancy, death usually before the fourth year of life: (a) *progressive hepatic cirrhosis*, portal hypertension, ascites, esophageal varices; (b) *failure to thrive*; (c) *enzyme deficiency* demonstrable in cultured skin fibroblasts and leukocytes.

REFERENCES

Andersen DH: Familial cirrhosis of the liver with storage of abnormal glycogen. *Lab. Invest.* 5:11, 1956.

Greene HL, et al.: Hypoglycemia in type IV glycogenosis: Hepatic improvement in two patients with nutritional management. *J. Pediatr.* 112:55, 1988.

Guerra AS, et al.: A juvenile variant of glycogenosis IV (Andersen disease). *Eur. J. Pediatr.* 145:179, 1986.

GLYCOGENOSIS, TYPE V

Synonyms: Glycogen storage disease, type V; McArdle disease.

Enzyme Deficiency: Myophosphorylase.

Mode of Inheritance: Autosomal recessive.

Clinical Manifestations: (a) *severe muscle cramps, inability to sustain exercise*; (b) *muscle wasting*; (c) *acute oliguric renal failure, myoglobulinuria and creatinuria after vigorous exercise*; (d) *failure of venous lactate to increase after exercise*; (e) *muscle biopsy: excess glycogen, decreased muscle phosphorylase activity*; (f) ^{31}P nuclear magnetic resonance test: absence of a drop in intramuscular pH, excessive reduction in phosphocreatine in response to exercise, failure of a breakdown of glycogen and the formation of lactic acid.

Radiologic Manifestations: Renal angiography: preferential diffuse reduction in cortical perfusion, attenuation of distal interlobar and arcuate arteries, absence of cortical nephrogram, delay in the clearing of contrast medium through the renal parenchyma.

REFERENCES

Argov Z, et al.: Muscle energy metabolism in McArdle's syndrome by in vivo phosphorus magnetic resonance spectroscopy. *Neurology* 37:1720, 1987.

Heller SL, et al.: 2,4-Dinitrophenol, muscle biopsy, and McArdle's disease. *Neurology* 38:15, 1988.

Layzer RB: McArdle's disease in the 1980s. *N. Engl. J. Med.* 312:370, 1985.

McArdle B: Myopathy due to a defect in muscle glycogen breakdown. *Clin. Sci.* 10:13, 1951.

Miller JH, et al.: Radiography of glycogen storage diseases. *A.J.R.* 132:379, 1979.

Paster SB, et al.: Acute renal failure in McArdle's disease and myoglobulinuric states. *Radiology* 114:567, 1975.

Ross BD, et al.: Examination of a case of suspected McArdle's syndrome by ^{31}P nuclear magnetic resonance. *N. Engl. J. Med.* 304:1338, 1981.

Williams J, et al.: Type V glycogen storage disease. *Arch. Dis. Child.* 60:1184, 1985.

GM₁ GANGLIOSIDOSIS

Synonyms: Gangliosidose GM_1; Norman-Landing disease; Landing disease.

Mode of Inheritance: Autosomal recessive, phenotype variation within a family.

Enzyme Deficiency: A generalized sphingolipidosis; storage of GM_1 ganglioside and oligosaccharides in the brain and viscera; β-gangliosidase deficiency.

Classification: (a) infantile; (b) juvenile; (c) variant juvenile or adult forms: spectrum of phenotypes variable, clinical picture ranging from the severe infantile type to the mild adult type.

Clinical Manifestations:

(A) GM₁ GANGLIOSIDOSIS, TYPE 1: (a) *retarded psychomotor development from birth;* (b) *abnormal facial features* (frontal bossing, depression of the nasal bridge, large low-set ears and a long upper lip); (c) *hepatosplenomegaly;* (d) *dorsal kyphoscoliosis;* (e) enlargement and stiffness of the wrist and ankle joints; (f) *short and stubby fingers with flexion contracture;* (g) cherry-red macular changes; (h) vacuolized lymphocytes and marrow cells; normal levels of urinary mucopolysaccharide; GM_1 ganglioside increase in the brain and increased ganglioside and mucopolysaccharide levels in the viscera; deficiency of β-galactosidase activity in leukocytes, urine, brain, liver, or cultured skin fibroblasts; enzyme assays of cultured amniotic fluid cells; detection of galactosyl-oligosaccharides in amniotic fluid with high-performance liquid chromatography; anomalous eosinophil granulocytes in the blood and bone marrow; (i) other reported abnormalities: (a) infantile cardiomyopathy, neuromyopathy (muscular weakness, hypotonia), neonatal ascites; (j) death in infancy.

(B) GM₁ GANGLIOSIDOSIS, TYPE 2 (JUVENILE): Onset of symptoms in the first 2 years of life, (a) mental and motor retarda-

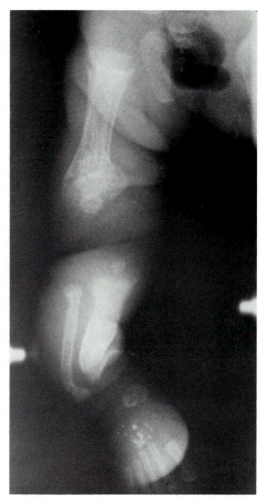

FIG ME–G–7.
GM₁ gangliosidosis I in a 1-week-old female. Her tubular bones are short, wide, and deformed. Thin cortices, a coarse trabecular pattern, flaring and cupping of the metaphyses, and medullary cavity expansion are present. Note the stippled calcification in the sacral and ankle regions. (Courtesy of Dr. Virgil R. Condon, Salt Lake City.)

tion, spasticity, ataxia, seizures, dementia, absence of Hurler-like features, slight to moderate organomegaly; (b) foam cells in the bone marrow; vacuolated cells in the liver, spleen, and glomeruli; deficient β-galactosidase activity in leukocytes, brain, liver, and cultured fibroblasts; (c) death in childhood.

(C) ADULT GM₁ GANGLIOSIDOSIS: Onset of clinical manifestations in the teen years; wide range of clinical manifestations: (a) seizures, near-normal intellect to severe intellectual impairment, extrapyramidal signs, pyramidal signs, dementia, dysarthria, dystonia, etc.

Radiologic Manifestations:

(A) GM₁ GANGLIOSIDOSIS, TYPE 1: (a) *gibbus deformity, beaking and hypoplasia of the vertebral bodies;* (b) *thin cortices of the tubular bones, coarse trabecular pattern, marked*

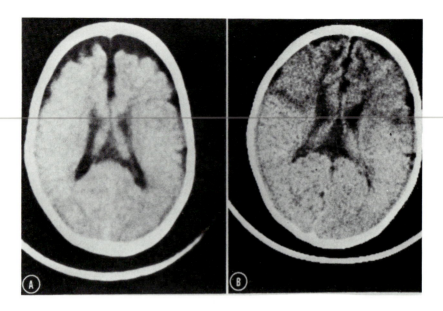

FIG ME–G–8.
GM$_1$ gangliosidosis. A noncontrast CT scan in a 13-month-old girl shows large extra-axial space and frontal white matter lucencies.

(From Curless RG: Computed tomography of GM$_1$ gangliosidosis. *J. Pediatr.* 105:964, 1984. Used by permission.)

subperiosteal new bone formation of the humeri and medullary expansion, widened ribs, flaring and cupping of the metaphyses (wrists, knees, and ankles in particular), stippled calcific densities in the ankle and some other joint regions; (c) neonatal ascites: (d) brain atrophy, areas of decreased attenuation in the white matter (computed tomography [CT]).

(B) GM$_1$ GANGLIOSIDOSIS (JUVENILE AND ADULT TYPES): Variable skeletal abnormalities, normal or dysplastic; cortical thinness of the long bones, dysplasia of the femoral head, hypoplasia of the vertebral bodies, flatness of the vertebral bodies, osteosclerosis of the skull, etc. (Figs ME–G–7 to ME–G–9).

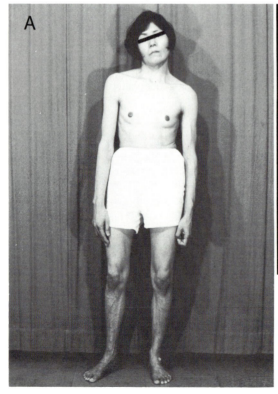

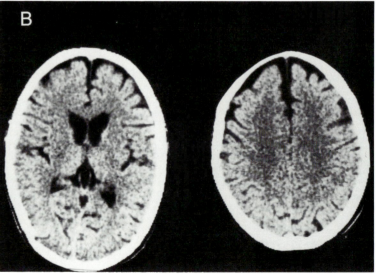

FIG ME–G–9.
GM$_1$ gangliosidosis (adult) in a 38-year-old woman. **A,** note the dystonic torticollis. **B,** CT. Note the shrinkage of both caudate nuclei with dilatation of the bilateral frontal horns and atrophy of the frontal lobes. (From Nakano T, Ikeda S-I, Kondo K, et al.: Adult GM$_1$-gangliosidosis: Clinical patterns and rectal biopsy. *Neurology* 35:875, 1985. Used by permission.)

REFERENCES

Charrow J, et al.: Cardiomyopathy and skeletal myopathy in an unusual variant of GM$_1$ gangliosidosis. *J. Pediatr.* 108:729, 1986.

Curless RG: Computed tomography of GM$_1$ gangliosidosis. *J. Pediatr.* 105:964, 1984.

Daneman A, et al.: Neonatal ascites due to lysosomal storage disease. *Radiology* 149:463, 1983.

Farrell DF, et al.: Gm$_1$ gangliosidosis: Enzymatic variation in a single family. *Ann. Neurol.* 9:232, 1981.

Farrell DF, et al.: Gm$_1$ gangliosidosis: Phenotype variation in a single family. *Ann. Neurol.* 9:225, 1981.

Gitzelmann R, et al.: Anomalous eosinophil granulocytes in blood and bone marrow: A diagnostic marker for infantile GM$_1$-gangliosidosis? *Eur. J. Pediatr.* 144:82, 1985.

Landing BH, et al.: Familial neurovisceral lipidosis. *Am. J. Dis. Child.* 108:503, 1964.

Mutoh T, et al.: A family with β-galactosidase deficiency: Three adults with atypical clinical patterns. *Neurology* 36:54, 1986.

Nakano T, et al.: Adult GM$_1$-gangliosidosis: Clinical patterns and rectal biopsy. *Neurology* 35:875, 1985.

O'Brien J: Generalized gangliosidosis. *J. Pediatr.* 75:167, 1969.

Ohta K, et al.: Type 3 (adult) GM$_1$ gangliosidosis: Case report. *Neurology* 35:1490, 1985.

Ponet D, et al.: La maladie de Landing ou gangliosidose généralisée à GM1, type I. A propos de deux cas dans la même fratrie. *Ann. Pediatr. (Paris)* 29:691, 1982.

Robinowitz JG, et al.: Gangliosidosis (Gm$_1$): A reevaluation of the vertebral deformity. *A.J.R.* 121:155, 1974.

Warner TG, et al.: Prenatal diagnosis of GM$_1$ gangliosidosis by detection of galactosyl-oligosaccharides in amniotic fluid with high performance liquid chromatography. *Am. J. Hum. Genet.* 35:1034, 1983.

GM$_2$ GANGLIOSIDOSES

Synonyms: Gangliosidoses (GM$_2$); hexosaminidase deficiency disease.

Clinical Manifestations: (a) Tay-Sachs disease (late infantile): hexosaminidase A deficiency, autosomal recessive, onset of symptoms in early infancy, apathy, hypotonia, "doll-like" appearance, delayed psychomotor development, exaggerated startle response to noise, blindness, cherry-red macular spot, optic atrophy after the first year, usually fatal within 5 years, prenatal diagnosis in the first trimester by chorionic villi sampling; (b) Sandhoff disease: hexosaminidase A and B deficiency, onset of symptoms in early infancy, visceromegaly; (c) juvenile GM$_2$ gangliosidosis with hexosaminidase A deficiency: onset of symptoms between 2 and 6 years of age, anterior horn cell disease, ataxia, spasticity, loss of speech, athetoid posturing of the extremities, psychomotor deterioration, decerebrate rigidity, blindness in the late stage, death between 5 and 15 years of age; (d) juvenile Sandhoff disease: hexosaminidase A and B deficiency: cerebellar ataxia, cherry-red maculae, intact mentation; (e) others (hexosaminidase A deficiency): adult type with the clinical features of amyotrophic lateral sclerosis; chronic type with spinocerebellar degeneration, muscle wasting dystonia, and intact mentation.

Radiologic Manifestations: (a) Tay-Sachs disease: macrocephaly, increased thickness of the cerebral cortex; (b) Sandhoff disease: occasionally bone deformities resembling those seen in infantile GM$_1$ gangliosidosis (O'Brien).

REFERENCES

Argov Z, et al.: Clinical and genetic variations in the syndrome of adult GM$_2$ gangliosidosis resulting from hexosaminidase A deficiency. *Ann. Neurol.* 16:14, 1984.

Bolhuis PA, et al.: Ganglioside storage, hexosaminidase lability, and urinary oligosaccharides in adult Sandhoff's disease. *Neurology* 37:75, 1987.

Budde-Steffen C: Presence of β-hexosaminidase. A α-chain mRNA in two different variants of GM$_2$-gangliosidosis. *Neuropediatrics* 19:59, 1988.

Cantor RM, et al.: Sandhoff disease heterozygote detection: A component of population screening for Tay-Sachs disease carriers. II. Sandhoff disease gene frequencies in American Jewish and non-Jewish populations. *Am. J. Hum. Genet.* 41:16, 1987.

Conzelmann E, et al.: Ganglioside GM$_2$ N-acetyl-β-D-galactosaminidase activity in cultured fibroblasts of late-infantile and adult GM$_2$ gangliosidosis patients and of healthy probands with low hexosaminidase level. *Am. J. Hum. Genet.* 35:900, 1983.

Kotagal S, et al.: AB variant GM$_2$ gangliosidosis: Cerebrospinal fluid and neuropathologic characteristics. *Neurology* 36:438, 1986.

O'Brien JS: The gangliosidoses, in Stanbury JB, et al. (eds.): *The Metabolic Basis of Inherited Disease*, ed 5. New York, McGraw-Hill International Book Co., 1983, pp. 945–969.

Pergament E, et al.: Prenatal Tay-Sachs diagnosis by chorionic villi sampling. *Lancet* 2:286, 1983.

Sachs B: On arrested cerebral development, with special reference to its cortical pathology. *J. Nerv. Ment. Dis.* 14:541, 1887.

Tay W: Symmetrical changes in the region of the yellow spot in each eye of an infant. *Trans. Ophthalmol. Soc. U.K.* 1:55, 1881.

Willner JP, et al.: Chronic GM$_2$ gangliosidosis masquerading as atypical Friedreich ataxia: Clinical, morphologic and biochemical studies of nine cases. *Neurology* 31:787, 1981.

GOUT

Classification: (a) idiopathic; (b) associated with other metabolic disorders; (c) drug induced.

Mode of Inheritance (Primary): Polygenic (genetic and nongenetic factors); in some familial cases autosomal dominant factors and in others sex-linked factors have been suggested.

Clinical Manifestations: Acute gouty arthritis or chronic tophaceous gout: (a) *arthritis* involving various joints with a predilection for joints of the lower limbs, soft-tissue swelling and nodular masses in the para-articular regions; (b) *hyperuricemia, deposition of monosodium urate crystals in joints and periarticular tissues;* (c) *gouty renal disease,* renal failure, nephrolithiasis; (d) other reported abnormalities: the majority of gouty arthritis in women is postmenopausal and often associated with renal insufficiency, neuropathy, carpal tunnel syndrome (gouty tenosynovitis).

Radiologic Manifestations: (a) *soft-tissue swelling, nodular para-articular densities, calcification or ossification of tophi;* (b) *arthritis:* preservation of the articular space in the early stage of disease, narrowing of joints in the advanced stage; bone erosions in articular and/or periarticular regions; expansile bone lesions with bony spurs extending into periosseous soft tissues; osteophytosis; cystlike or punched-out bone lesions with minimal sclerotic changes surrounding the

bone lesions; enlarged ulnar styloid process; club-shaped deformity of the metacarpal, metatarsal, and phalangeal heads; thickening of the diaphyses; intra-articular milk of calcium in saturnine gout; pseudotumor of the outer end of the clavicle (saturnine gout); pathological fracture of the patella; intraosseous calcification in tophaceous gout; etc.; (c) narrowing of intervertebral disk spaces, erosion of end plates, erosion of the odontoid process, subluxation of the atlas, sacroiliac joint lesions with bone erosion; (d) osteoporosis (Fig ME–G–10).

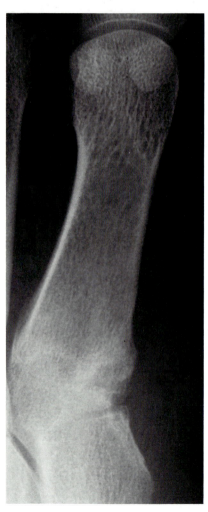

FIG ME–G–10.
Arthritic gout in a 31-year-old male with glycogen storage disease, type I. Clinical gout started at the age of 26 years. Erosive and cystic changes at the base of the first metatarsal are shown. (From Preger L, Sanders GW, Gold RH, et al.: Roentgenographic skeletal changes in the glycogen storage diseases. *A.J.R.* 107:840, 1969. Used by permission.)

REFERENCES

Barthelemy CR, et al.: Gouty arthritis: A prospective radiographic evaluation of sixty patients. *Skeletal Radiol.* 11:1, 1984.

Daniel WW, et al.: Intra-articular milk of calcium in saturnine gout. *Radiology* 137:389, 1983.

Delaney P: Gouty neuropathy. *Arch. Neurol.* 40:823, 1983.

Foucar E, et al.: Gout presenting as a femoral cyst. *J. Bone Joint Surg. [Am.]* 66:294, 1984.

Gottlieb NL, et al.: Allopurinol-associated hand and foot deformities in chronic tophaceous gout. *J.A.M.A.* 238:1663, 1977.

Greenberg DC: Pathological fracture of the patella secondary to gout. *J. Bone Joint Surg. [Am.]* 68:1286, 1986.

Jajić I: Gout in the spine and sacro-iliac joints: Radiological manifestations. *Skeletal Radiol.* 8:209, 1982.

Janssen T, et al.: Gouty tenosynovitis and compression neuropathy of the median nerve. *Clin. Orthop.* 216:204, 1981.

Lally EV, et al.: The clinical spectrum of gouty arthritis in women. *Arch. Intern. Med.* 146:2221, 1986.

Lambeth JT, et al.: Sacroiliac gout associated with hemoglobin E and hypersplenism. *Radiology* 95:413, 1970.

Pennes DR, et al.: Hyperuricemia and gout. *Semin. Roentgenol.* 21:245, 1986.

Podgorski MR, et al.: Bilateral acromioclavicular gouty arthritis with pseudotumor of the outer end of the right clavicle: Saturnine gout. *Skeletal Radiol.* 16:589, 1987.

Preger L, et al.: Roentgenographic skeletal changes in the glycogen storage disease. *A.J.R.* 107:840, 1969.

Reif MC, et al.: Chronic gouty nephropathy: A vanishing syndrome? *N. Engl. J. Med.* 304:535, 1981.

Resnick D: Crystal-induced arthropathy: Gout and pseudogout. *J.A.M.A.* 242:2440, 1979.

Resnick D, et al.: Early-onset gouty arthritis. *Radiology* 114:67, 1975.

Resnick D, et al.: Intraosseous calcifications in tophaceous gout. *A.J.R.* 137:1157, 1981.

Schabel SI, et al.: Bone infarction in gout. *Skeletal Radiol.* 3:42, 1978.

Seegmiller JE: Diseases of purine and pyrimidine metabolism, in Bondy PK, Rosenberg LE (eds.): *Metabolic Control and Disease,* ed. 8. Philadelphia, W.B. Saunders Co., 1980, p. 778.

Vinstein AL, et al.: Involvement of the spine in gout: A case report. *Radiology* 103:311, 1972.

Warren DJ, et al.: Familial gout and renal failure. *Arch. Dis. Child.* 56:699, 1981.

Yarom A, et al.: Juvenile gouty arthritis. *Am. J. Dis. Child.* 138:955, 1984.

H

HALLERVORDEN-SPATZ DISEASE

Mode of Inheritance: Autosomal recessive.

Pathology: A degenerative disorder with excess deposition of iron-containing pigments within the globus pallidus, pars reticularis of the substantia nigra, and red nuclei; pallidal demyelination and focal axonal swellings in the pallidonigral system and the cortex.

Clinical Manifestations: Onset often in adolescence; onset in childhood and adulthood less common: (a) progressive pyramidal and extrapyramidal signs, predominantly in the lower limbs; (b) mental deterioration; (c) progressive loss of verbal communication; (d) death within few years after onset.

Radiologic Manifestations: (a) computed tomography: infratentorial atrophy, symmetrical areas of increased density in the globus pallidus, basal ganglia mineralization; (b) magnetic resonance imaging (MRI): marked symmetrical hypointensity related to abnormal iron deposits (T_2-weighted spin-echo sequence) (Fig ME–H–1).

REFERENCES

Boltshauser E, et al.: Computed tomography in Hallervorden-Spatz disease. *Neuropediatrics* 18:81, 1987.

Eidelberg D, et al.: Adult onset Hallervorden-Spatz disease with neurofibrillary pathology. A discrete clinicopathological entity. *Brain* 110:993, 1987.

Hallervorden J, Spatz H: Eigenartige Erkrankung im extrapyramidalen System mit besonderer Beteiligung des Globus pallidus und der Substantia nigra. Ein Beitrag zu den Beziehungen zwischen diesen beiden Zentren. *Z. Neurol.* 79:254, 1922.

Littrup PJ, et al.: MR imaging of Hallervorden-Spatz disease. *J. Comput. Assist. Tomogr.* 9:491, 1985.

Mutoh K, et al.: MR imaging of a group I case of Hallervorden-Spatz disease. *J. Comput. Assist. Tomogr.* 12:851, 1988.

Tanfani G, et al.: MR imaging in a case of Hallervorden-Spatz disease. *J. Comput. Assist. Tomogr.* 11:1057, 1987.

Tennison MB, et al.: Mineralization of the basal ganglia detected by CT in Hallervorden-Spatz syndrome. *Neurology* 38:154, 1988.

HEMOCHROMATOSIS

Classification: (a) *primary (hereditary hemochromatosis)*: four types: (1) classic type with elevated transferrin saturation, serum ferritin levels, and liver iron content; (2) severe iron overload presenting at an early age; (3) elevated total-body iron stores, normal serum ferritin levels and transferrin saturation; (4) markedly elevated transferrin saturation and serum ferritin levels, minimal elevation in total-body iron stores; (b) *secondary*: multiple blood transfusions, refractory anemia, liver cirrhosis, chronic excessive iron intake, portal-to-systemic venous shunts.

Mode of Inheritance (Primary Hematochromatosis): Autosomal recessive; genetic heterogeneity; tight linkage with HLA (types A3, B7, and B14) on the short arm of chromosome 6; frequency of the gene 3 to 8 per 1,000 population with a carrier rate (heterozygosity) of about 10% in the population; clinical manifestations more common in males.

Pathophysiology: Gradual absorption of excessive amounts of iron from the digestive tract and deposition in various body organs (liver, pancreas, spleen, heart, kidneys, endocrine glands, gastrointestinal tract).

Clinical Manifestations: Onset of symptoms in primary hemochromatosis usually between 40 and 60 years of age, rarely onset in childhood or young adulthood: (a) *bronze pigmentation of the skin;* (b) *liver cirrhosis,* hepatomegaly, splenomegaly; (c) diabetes mellitus (bronze diabetes); (d) *cardiac arrhythmias,* congestive heart failure, cardiac dysfunction as a presenting manifestation of the disease in some cases, ventricular abnormality on echocardiography and blood pool imaging (ventricular size and function), early death due to cardiac dysfunction; (e) *arthralgia,* in particular, of the second and third metacarpophalangeal joints; (f) hypogonadotropic hypogonadism: loss of libido, impotence, amenorrhea, absence of spermatozoa in the seminal fluid, impairment of spermatogenesis shown by testicular biopsy; (g) *increased serum iron levels, almost complete saturation of iron-binding capacity,* transferrin saturation index (plasma iron concentration/total iron-binding capacity) over 50% (in the 70% range in advanced cases), liver biopsy (estimation of the iron content, iron-related liver damage); (h) other reported manifestations: abdominal pain, weight loss, decreased hearing, confusion, dementia, rigidity, myoclonic jerks, ataxia, peripheral neuropathy, syndrome of hepatocerebral degeneration, hypothyroidism, association with Turner syndrome, presentation as acute hepatitis in a child, jaundice, ascites, spider angiomas, loss of body hair.

Radiologic Manifestations: (a) *generalized arthropathy* (metacarpophalangeal, proximal interphalangeal, and radiocarpal joints most commonly involved): thinning of cartilage, subchondral sclerosis, and cyst formation; (b) *fibrocartilage calcification:* chondrocalcinosis (shoulder, elbow, wrist, sym-

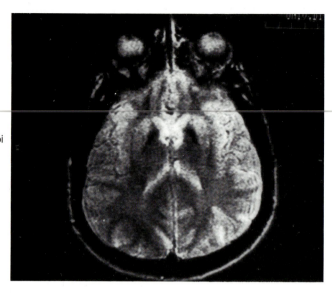

FIG ME–H–1.
Hallervorden-Spatz disease: Axial MRI through the basal ganglia (SE:TR, 1600; TE, 100 ms). Note the marked hypointensity of the globi pallidi. (From Tanfani G, Mascalchi M, Dal Pozzo GC, et al.: MR imaging in a case of Hallervorden-Spatz disease. *J. Comput. Assist. Tomogr.* 11:1057, 1987. Used by permission.)

physis pubis, hip, intervertebral disk, etc.), tendon calcification (Achilles, plantar fascia, ligamentum flavum, etc.); (c) *osteoporosis:* may cause vertebral collapse; (d) *cardiomegaly,* congestive heart failure, "restrictive" type of cardiomyopathy; (e) liver neoplasm as a complication: hepatoma, cholangiocarcinoma, tumors of mixed elements; (f) *computed tomography* of the abdomen: increased attenuation (liver, spleen, lymph nodes) due to iron deposition; (g) magnetic resonance imaging (MRI): short T_1 and T_2 values; T_2 relaxation time in the 15–30 ms range (normal, 52 ± 8 ms) resulting in the image-labeled "black" liver.

Notes: (a) a few cases of a distinct neonatal iron storage have been reported with iron deposition in many organs (heart, endocrine and exocrine glands, etc.), liver fibrosis, hepatic dysfunction; (b) a diffusely increased attenuation of

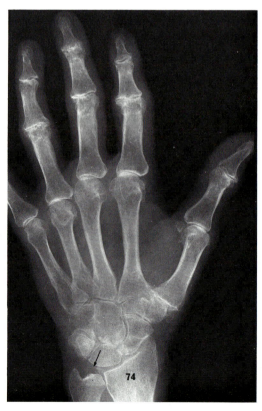

FIG ME–H–2.
Hemochromatosis (idiopathic) with metacarpophalangeal joint narrowing, bony enlargement of the metacarpal heads, nonuniform carpal joint narrowing and cartilage calcification *(arrow),* joint narrowing, and hypertrophic osteophyte formation involving the proximal and distal interphalangeal joints. (From Jensen PS: Hemochromatosis: A disease often silent but not invisible. *A.J.R.* 126:343, 1976. Used by permission.)

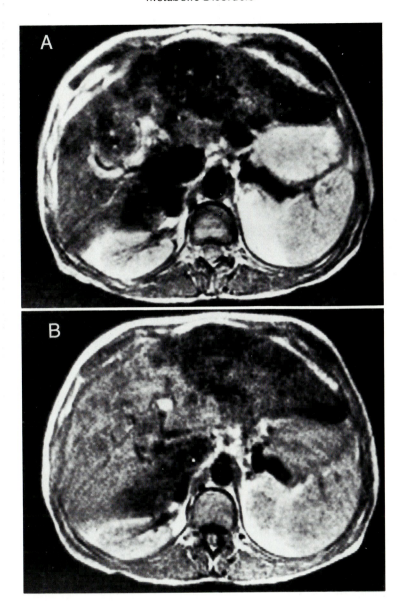

FIG ME–H–3.
Hemochromatosis. **A,** MRI of the liver shows focal areas of low signal in the left lobe, right lobe, and caudate lobe. Note the region of relatively normal signal in the lateral aspect of the posterior portion of the right lobe (SE:TE 50, TR 2000). **B,** MRI at a different level than **A** again shows regional abnormalities (SE:TE 30, TR 900). (From Murphy FB, Bernardino ME: MR imaging of focal hemochromatosis. *J. Comput. Assist. Tomogr.* 10:1044, 1986. Used by permission.)

the liver in the presence of an elevated serum ferritin level indicates iron overload; a normal hepatic density does not exclude iron overload (Figs ME–H–2 and ME–H–3).

REFERENCES

Adamson TC, et al.: Hand and wrist arthropathies of hemochromatosis and calcium pyrophosphate deposition disease: Distinct radiographic features. *Radiology* 147:377, 1983.

Colletti RB, et al.: Familial neonatal hemochromatosis with survival. *J. Pediatr. Gastroenterol. Nutr.* 7:39, 1988.

Crosby WH: Hemochromatosis. The missed diagnosis. *Arch. Intern. Med.* 146:1209, 1986.

Dabestani A, et al.: Primary hemochromatosis: Anatomic and physiologic characteristics of the cardiac ventricles and their response to phlebotomy. *Am. J. Cardiol.* 54:153, 1984.

DeBont B, et al.: Idiopathic hemochromatosis presenting as acute hepatitis. *J. Pediatr.* 110:431, 1987.

De Jonge-Bok JM, et al.: The articular diversity of early haemochromatosis. *J. Bone Joint Surg. [Br.]* 69:41, 1987.

Dreyfuss AI, et al.: Hemochromatosis simulating hepatoma by computed tomography. *J. Comput. Tomogr.* 8:13, 1984.

Edwards CQ, et al.: Thyroid disease in hemochromatosis. Increased incidence in homozygous men. *Arch. Intern. Med.* 143:1890, 1983.

Escobar GJ, et al.: Primary hemochromatosis in childhood. *Pediatrics* 80:549, 1987.

Fairbanks VF, et al.: Hemochromatosis: The neglected diagnosis. *Mayo Clin. Proc.* 61:296, 1986.

Fujisawa I, et al.: Hemochromatosis of the pituitary gland: MR imaging. *Radiology* 168:213, 1988.

Goldschmidt H, et al.: Idiopathic hemochromatosis presenting as amenorrhea and arthritis. *Am. J. Med.* 82:1057, 1987.

Haddy TB, et al.: Hereditary hemochromatosis in children, adolescents, and young adults. *Am. J. Pediatr. Hematol. Oncol.* 10:23, 1988.

Howard JM, et al.: Diagnostic efficacy of hepatic computed tomography in the detection of body iron overload. *Gastroenterology* 84:209, 1983.

Jensen PS: Hemochromatosis: A disease often silent but not invisible. *A.J.R.* 126:343, 1976.

Jonas MM, et al.: Neonatal hemochromatosis: Failure of deferoxamine therapy. *J. Pediatr. Gastroenterol. Nutr.* 6:984, 1987.

Jones HR, et al.: Idiopathic hemochromatosis (IHC): Dementia and ataxia as presenting signs. *Neurology* 33:1479, 1983.

Kaloustian E, et al.: Survenue d'une hémochromatose primitive au cours d'un syndrome de Turner. *Presse Med.* 13:1962, 1984.

Mitnick JS, et al.: CT in β-thalassemia: Iron deposition in the liver, spleen and lymph nodes. *A.J.R.* 136:1191, 1981.

Muir WA, et al.: Evidence for heterogeneity in hereditary hemochromatosis. Evaluation of 174 persons in nine families. *Am. J. Med.* 76:806, 1984.

Murphy FB, et al.: MR imaging of focal hemochromatosis. *J. Comput. Assist. Tomogr.* 10:1044, 1986.

Noma S, et al.: MR imaging of thyroid hemochromatosis. *J. Comput. Assist. Tomogr.* 12:639, 1988.

Siemons LJ, et al.: Hypogonadotropic hypogonadism in hemochromatosis: Recovery of reproductive function after iron depletion. *J. Clin. Endocrinol. Metab.* 65:585, 1987.

HEMOPHILIA

Mode of Inheritance: X-linked recessive (hemophilia A and B).

Clinical Manifestations: (a) *bleeding at various sites:* joints, periarticular, subcutaneous, intramuscular, gastrointestinal wall, central nervous system, urinary tract, etc.; (b) *deficiency of factors VIII (hemophilia A) or IX (hemophilia B, Christmas disease),* prenatal diagnosis by an examination of fetal plasma and by the study of DNA polymorphic markers genetically linked to the hemophilia locus (hemophilia A); (c) other abnormalities: acquired immunodeficiency syndrome (AIDS), leukemia, Burkitt lymphoma, generalized lymphadenopathy and T-cell abnormalities), septic arthritis, progressive liver disease (in the patients having received factor VIII or IX concentrates (chronic active hepatitis, cirrhosis), association with pulmonary valve stenosis, coronary artery disease, acquired hemophilia due to the production of antibody against factor VIII coagulant activity.

Radiologic Manifestations: (a) *skeletal system: joint distension* with active bleeding episodes; *cartilage and subchondral bone erosions; subchondral cysts; narrowing of joint spaces; synovial irregularities (arthrogram);* chondrocalcinosis; increased articular and periarticular tissue density; epiphyseal necrosis; *premature closure of the growth plates;*

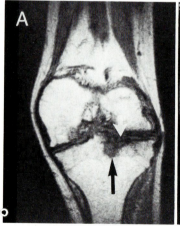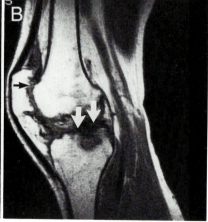

FIG ME–H–4.
Hemophilic arthropathy. **A,** a relatively T_1 weighted (SE 700/17) coronal image of the knee in a patient with severe hemophilia shows marked disorganization of the joint with enlarged epiphyses, a subchondral cyst of the tibia *(black arrow)*, material of low and intermediate signal intensity within the joint consistent with a hypertrophic synovium *(white arrow)*, and marked destruction of articular cartilage and menisci. **B,** a relatively T_1 weighted (SE 700/ 17) sagittal image shows the subchondral cyst in the tibia, a hypertrophic synovium within the joint *(white arrows)*, erosions of the posterior portion of the patella, and a loss of the posterior patellar cartilage *(black arrow)*. The lack of a large effusion may indicate that this joint is fibrotic and contracted. (From Yulish BS, Lieberman JM, Strandjord SE, et al.: Hemophilic arthropathy: Assessment with MR imaging. *Radiology* 164:759, 1987. Used by permission.)

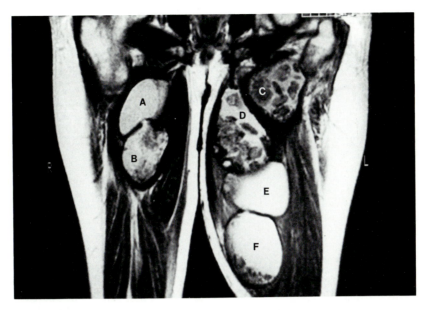

FIG ME–H–5.
Hemophilic pseudotumor. A T$_1$-weighted coronal MR image (TR, 250 ms; TE, 30 ms) of both thighs shows two pseudotumors on the right **(A** and **B)** and four pseudotumors on the left **(C** to **F). (From

Wilson DA, Prince JR: MR imaging of hemophilic pseudotumors. *A.J.R.* 150:349, 1988. Used by permission.)

limb shortening, *accelerated growth maturation; epiphyseal overgrowth;* slipped epiphysis, widening of the radial notch of the ulna; widening of the femoral intercondylar notch; flattening of the inferior border of the patella; *squared appearance of the patella;* patellar ratio (length to width) over 2; *pseudotumor* at sites of tendinous attachments, in muscles with large periosteal attachment, in subperiosteal or intraosseous locations (hematoma with thick fibrous capsule, filled with coagulum, calcified or ossified, bone erosion or destruction with periosteal elevation and new bone formation, intraosseous cyst); osteopenia; bony ankylosis; hip joint dislocation complicating repeated hemarthrosis; joint contractures (ankle, knee, elbow); cervical spine abnormalities in adults (cystic changes or end-plate irregularity within one or more vertebral bodies, increased atlantodens interval of 5 mm); gradual resolution of myositis ossificans (case report); etc.; (b) gastrointestinal system: *intramural hemorrhage,* thickening and shortening of small-bowel mucosal folds, thickening of the bowel wall, pseudotumor of the stomach; (c) urinary system: filling defects due to blood clots, nonfunctioning kidney, chronic obstructive renal enlargement, distorted upper collecting system due to compression, calculus, renal papillary necrosis, hemorrhage into the bladder wall; (d) chest: hemopneumothorax, hemomediastinum, pulmonary scarring and fibrosis, pleural thickening, hyperinflation; (e) *central nervous system: intracranial hemorrhage,* intraspinal bleeding, congenital intracranial hemorrhage, intraspinal bleeding (intra-axial or extra-axial); (f) other reported sites of bleeding: sublingual, laryngeal, pharyngeal, peritoneal, retroperitoneal, splenic (calcifying hematoma), perineal; (g) cholelithiasis; CT changes of liver disease (chronic active hepatitis, cirrhosis) (Figs ME–H–4 and ME–H–5).

Notes: Ultrasonography and computed tomography (CT) comparable in the diagnosis of soft-tissue hemorrhage, the extent of bleeding, the effect on the neighboring organs, and in the follow-ups after treatment; computed tomography the most efficient tool in the detection of bone destruction associated with a hemophilic pseudotumor, magnetic resonance imaging (MRI) very accurate in demonstrating the soft-tissue and articular cartilage damage of hemophilic arthropathy.

REFERENCES

Ackerman Z, et al.: Pulmonary valve stenosis and hemophilia A. Report of three cases and discussion of a possible genetic linkage. *Arch. Intern. Med.* 146:2233, 1986.

Altay C, et al.: Acute leukemia in two patients with hemophilia. *Cancer* 55:510, 1985.

Antonarakis SE, et al.: Prenatal diagnosis of haemophilia A by factor VIII gene analysis. *Lancet* 1:1407, 1985.

Atkins RM, et al.: Joint contractures in the hemophilias. *Clin. Orthop.* 219:97, 1987.

Baker SR, et al.: Radiographic abnormalities in coagulation factor VII deficiency. *J. Can. Assoc. Radiol.* 38:64, 1987.

Bloom AL: Acquired immunodeficiency syndrome and other possible immunological disorders in European haemophiliacs. *Lancet* 1:1452, 1984.

Bray G, et al.: Hemorrhage involving the upper airway in hemophilia. *Clin. Pediatr. (Phila.)* 25:436, 1986.

Burke JF, et al.: Spontaneous hemopneumothorax in a hemophiliac. *J.A.M.A.* 169:1623, 1959.

Chlosta EM, et al.: The "patellar ratio" in hemophilia and juvenile rheumatoid arthritis. *Radiology* 116:137, 1975.

Coblentz CL, et al.: Resolution of myositis ossificans in a hemophiliac. *J. Can. Assoc. Radiol.* 36:161, 1985.

Dodds WJ, et al.: Gastrointestinal roentgenographic manifestations of hemophilia. *A.J.R.* 110:413, 1970.

Floman Y, et al.: Dislocation of the hip joint complicating repeated hemarthrosis in hemophilia. *J. Pediatr. Orthop.* 3:99, 1983.

Franze I, et al.: Sonographic diagnosis of a subdural hematoma as the initial manifestation of hemophilia in a newborn. *J. Ultrasound Med.* 7:149, 1988.

Gerlock AJ, et al.: Angiography of the hemophilic joint. *Radiology* 130:627, 1979.

Gill JC, et al.: Generalized lymphadenopathy and T cell abnormalities in hemophilia A. *J. Pediatr.* 103:18, 1983.

Gordon EM, et al.: Burkitt lymphoma in a patient with classic hemophilia receiving factor VIII concentrates. *J. Pediatr.* 103:75, 1983.

Gordon RA, et al.: Intramural gastric hematoma in a hemophiliac with an inhibitor. *Pediatrics* 67:417, 1981.

Graif M, et al.: Sonographic localization of hematomas in hemophilic patients with positive iliopsoas sign. *A.J.R.* 148:121, 1987.

Hamel J, et al.: Radiological evaluation of chronic hemophilic arthropathy by the Pettersson score: Problems in correlation in adult patients. *Skeletal Radiol.* 17:32, 1988.

Hermann G, et al.: Computed tomography and ultrasonography of the hemophilic pseudotumor and their use in surgical planning. *Skeletal Radiol.* 15:123, 1986.

Högh J, et al.: Hemophilic arthropathy of the upper limb. *Clin. Orthop.* 218:225, 1987.

Iannaccone G, et al.: Calcifying splenic hematoma in a hemophilic newborn. *Pediatr. Radiol.* 10:183, 1981.

Johnson RJ, et al.: Computed tomography: Qualitative and quantitative recognition of liver disease in haemophilia. *J. Comput. Assist. Tomogr.* 7:1000, 1983.

Levine PH: The acquired immunodeficiency syndrome in persons with hemophilia. *Ann. Intern. Med.* 103:723, 1985.

Lottenberg R, et al.: Acquired hemophilia. A natural history study of 16 patients with factor VIII inhibitors receiving little or no therapy. *Arch. Intern. Med.* 147:1077, 1987.

Markowitz RI, et al.: Retropharyngeal bleeding in haemophilia. *Br. J. Radiol.* 54:521, 1981.

Pettersson H, et al.: Intracranial hemorrhage in hemophilic children. CT follow-up. *Acta Radiol.* 25:161, 1984.

Putman CE, et al.: Radiographic chest abnormalities in adult hemophilia. *Radiology* 118:41, 1976.

Ragni MV, et al.: Recurrent infections and lymphadenopathy in the child of a hemophiliac: A survey of children of hemophiliacs positive for human immunodeficiency virus antibody. *Ann. Intern. Med.* 105:886, 1986.

Roberts GM, et al.: Renal papillary necrosis in haemophilia and Christman disease. *Clin. Radiol.* 34:201, 1983.

Romeyn RL, et al.: The cervical spine in hemophilia. *Clin. Orthop.* 210:113, 1986.

Rose JS, et al.: Duodenal radiographic findings in hemophilia. *Am. J. Gastroenterol.* 76:160, 1981.

Scott JP, et al.: Septic arthritis in two teenaged hemophiliacs. *J. Pediatr.* 107:748, 1985.

Shaw PJ, et al.: Extrahepatic biliary obstruction due to stone. *Arch. Dis. Child.* 59:896, 1984.

Shirkhoda A, et al.: Soft-tissue hemorrhage in hemophiliac patients. *Radiology* 147:811, 1983.

Small M, et al.: Coronary artery disease in severe haemophilia. *Br. Heart J.* 49:604, 1983.

Stanley P, et al.: Chronic spinal epidural hematoma in hemophilia A in a child. *Pediatr. Radiol.* 13:241, 1983.

Stoker DJ, et al.: Skeletal changes in hemophilia and other bleeding disorders. *Semin. Roentgenol.* 9:185, 1974.

Sumer T, et al.: Severe congenital factor X deficiency with intracranial haemorrhage. *Eur. J. Pediatr.* 145:119, 1986.

Weintraub PS, et al.: Immunologic abnormalities in patients with hemophilia A. *J. Pediatr.* 103:692, 1983.

Whitelaw A, et al.: Factor V deficiency and antenatal intraventricular haemorrhage. *Arch. Dis. Child.* 59:997, 1984.

Wilson DA, et al.: MR imaging of hemophilic pseudotumors. *A.J.R.* 150:349, 1988.

Wilson DJ, et al.: Diagnostic ultrasound in haemophilia. *J. Bone Joint Surg. [Br.]* 69:103, 1987.

Wisoff JH, et al.: Spontaneous hematomyelia secondary to factor XI deficiency. *J. Neurosurg.* 63:293, 1985.

Yulish BS, et al.: Hemophilic arthropathy: Assessment with MR imaging. *Radiology* 164:759, 1987.

HEMOSIDEROSIS (IDIOPATHIC PULMONARY)

Synonyms: Idiopathic pulmonary hemosiderosis; pulmonary hemosiderosis (idiopathic); childhood idiopathic pulmonary hemosiderosis.

Mode of Inheritance: Some familial cases have been reported (mother and son, siblings).

Pathology: (a) *recurrent intrapulmonary bleeding with hemosiderin deposition in the lungs;* (b) pulmonary fibrosis in the late stage.

Clinical Manifestations: Onset of symptoms in infancy or childhood: (a) *cough, dyspnea, hemoptysis,* fever during acute attacks; (b) *remissions* lasting months to years; (c) *microcytic hypochromic anemia;* (d) *hemosiderin-laden macrophages in sputum and gastric washings;* (e) other reported abnormalities: decreased dismutase activity of erythrocytes in association with easy peroxidability of the erythrocytes, association with enteropathy and jejunal villous atrophy, etc.; (f) lung biopsy needed for a definitive diagnosis (recurrent intrapulmonary bleeding with hemosiderin deposition in the lungs; pulmonary fibrosis in the late stage), increase in the numbers of mast cells in the lung.

Radiologic Manifestations: Findings most marked in perihilar and basilar regions: (a) *small nodules, diffuse ground-glass infiltrates, fine patchy stippling;* (b) marked clearing and *changing pattern* during periods of clinical recovery; (c) reticulostriate pattern of *interstitial fibrosis* after subsidence of recurrent episodes of acute hemorrhages; (d) cor pulmonale with cardiomegaly in some cases; (e) hilar lymphadenopathy; (f) accumulation of radio-labeled red cells in the lung on a scan image.

Differential Diagnosis: Pulmonary hemosiderosis associated with renal disease (Goodpasture syndrome, immune complexes, diabetes mellitus), chemicals, multisystem vasculitis (systemic lupus erythematosus, microangiopathic hemolytic anemia and pulmonary vasculitis), lymphangiomyomatosis, small-bowel disease (celiac disease), autoimmune hemolytic anemia, etc.

REFERENCES

Beckerman RC, et al.: Familial idiopathic pulmonary hemosiderosis. *Am. J. Dis. Child.* 133:609, 1979.

Breckenridge RL Jr, et al.: Idiopathic pulmonary hemosiderosis: A report of familial occurrence. *Chest* 75:636, 1979.

Chryssanthopoulos CH, et al.: Prognostic criteria in idiopathic pulmonary hemosiderosis in children. *Eur. J. Pediatr.* 140:123, 1983.

Dolan J, et al.: Mast cells in pulmonary haemosiderosis. *Arch. Dis. Child.* 59:276, 1984.

Kobayashi Y, et al.: Significance of erythrocyte lipid peroxidation and superoxide dismutase activity in a patient with idiopathic pulmonary haemosiderosis. *Eur. J. Pediatr.* 143:64, 1984.

Kurzweil PR, et al.: Use of sodium chromate Cr 51 in diagnosing childhood idiopathic pulmonary hemosiderosis. *Am. J. Dis. Child.* 138:746, 1984.

Miller T, et al.: Nuclear scan of pulmonary hemorrhage in idiopathic pulmonary hemosiderosis. *A.J.R.* 132:120, 1979.

Nomura S, et al.: Association of idiopathic pulmonary haemosiderosis with IgA monoclonal gammopathy. *Thorax* 42:697, 1987.

Rafferty JR, et al.: Idiopathic pulmonary haemosiderosis with autoimmune haemolytic anaemia. *Br. J. Dis. Chest* 78:282, 1984.

Rieu D, et al.: Hémosidérose pulmonaire idiopathique et maladie coeliaque chez l'enfant. *Presse Med.* 12:2931, 1983.

Soergel KH, et al.: Idiopathic pulmonary hemosiderosis and related syndromes. *Am. J. Med.* 32:499, 1962.

Thaell JF, et al.: Idiopathic pulmonary hemosiderosis: Two cases in a family. *Mayo Clin. Proc.* 53:113, 1978.

Turner-Warwick M, et al.: Pulmonary haemorrhage and pulmonary haemosiderosis. *Clin. Radiol.* 33:361, 1982.

Wright PH, et al.: Adult idiopathic pulmonary haemosiderosis: A comparison of lung function changes and the distribution of pulmonary disease in patients with and without coeliac disease. *Br. J. Dis. Chest* 77:282, 1983.

HERMANSKY-PUDLAK SYNDROME

Synonyms: Delta-storage pool disease.

Mode of Inheritance: Autosomal recessive.

Frequency: Approximately 1:2,000 Puerto Ricans in the northern part of the island (Witkop et al.).

Clinical Manifestations: (a) *oculocutaneous tyrosinase-positive albinism;* (b) *platelets lacking dense bodies, bleeding disorder;* (c) *deposition of ceroidlike material in tissues:* granulomatous colitis, cardiomyopathy, restrictive lung disease, kidney failure; (d) increased urinary excretion of dolichols in

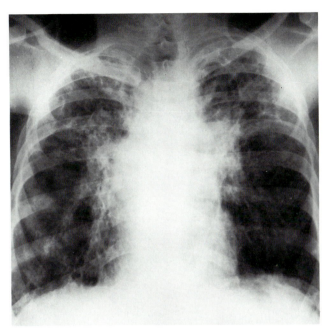

FIG ME–H–6.
Hermansky-Pudlak syndrome. The chest radiograph of a 46-year-old man shows extensive fibrosis with volume loss in the upper portions of the lobes as well as bulbous spaces and bronchiectatic areas bilaterally. (From Leitman BS, Balthazar EJ, Garay SM, et al.: The Hermansky-Pudlak syndrome: Radiographic features. *J. Can. Assoc. Radiol.* 37:42, 1986. Used by permission.)

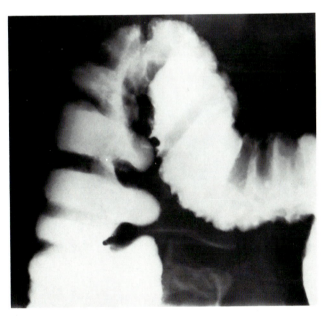

FIG ME–H–7.
Hermansky-Pudlak syndrome. A barium enema shows asymmetrical focal mucosal irregularities and ulceration in the transverse colon. (From Leitman BS, Balthazar EJ, Garay SM, et al.: The Hermansky-Pudlak syndrome: Radiographic features. *J. Can. Assoc. Radiol.* 37:42, 1986. Used by permission.)

the patients with evidence of ceroid storage in the kidneys; (e) other reported abnormalities: recurrent bacterial pharyngitis and otitis, anergy to commonly occurring antigens.

Radiologic Manifestations: (a) progressive, diffuse, bilateral interstitial fibrosis; honeycomb cystic lung pattern; bullous lung changes; (b) diffuse colitis: asymmetrical pattern of focal, superficial, and deep ulcerations (Figs ME–H–6 and ME–H–7).

REFERENCES

Depinho RA, et al.: The Hermansky-Pudlak syndrome. Report of three cases and review of pathophysiology and management considerations. *Medicine (Baltimore)* 64:192, 1985.

Hermansky F, Pudlak P: Albinism associated with hemorrhagic diathesis and unusual pigmented reticular cells in the bone marrow: Report of two cases with histochemical studies. *Blood* 14:162, 1959.

Leitman BS, et al.: The Hermansky-Pudlak syndrome: Radiographic features. *J. Can. Assoc. Radiol.* 37:42, 1986.

White DA, et al.: Hermansky-Pudlak syndrome and interstitial lung disease: Report of a case with lavage findings. *Am. Rev. Respir. Dis.* 130:138, 1984.

Witkop CJ, et al.: Elevated urinary dolichol excretion in the Hermansky-Pudlak syndrome. Indicator of lysosomal dysfunction. *Am. J. Med.* 82:463, 1987.

HOMOCYSTINURIA (CYSTATHIONINE SYNTHASE DEFICIENCY)

Mode of Inheritance: Autosomal recessive.

Frequency: Estimated at 1 in 35,000 to 1 in 300,000 (Wichernik-Bol et al.).

Clinical Manifestations: (a) marfanoid features (in one third); (b) *cutaneous malar flush*, patchy erythematous blotches; (c) fine, sparse, dry, fair hair; (d) miscellaneous ocular abnormalities (cataract, optic atrophy, cystic degeneration of the retina, retinal detachment, glaucoma, dislocation of the ocular lenses); (e) *subluxation of the ocular lens*; (f) hepatomegaly; (g) hernia; (h) mental retardation (in one third to one half), seizures, stroke, psychiatric problems (predisposition to schizophrenia, episodic depression, chronic disorders of behavior, chronic obsessive-compulsive disorder, personality disorders); (i) high levels of plasma homocystine and methionine, homocysteine, and a mixed disulfide of cysteine and homocysteine; persistent urinary excretion of homocystine; raised levels of homocystine and methionine in amniotic fluid (amniocentesis); (j) other reported abnormalities: abnormal clotting tendency, homocysteine-induced epithelial damage with platelet involvement, cerebral and cardiovascular atherosclerosis and thromboses, factor VII deficiency.

Radiologic Manifestations: (a) *osteoporosis*; (b) "codfish" vertebrae, scoliosis, kyphosis; (c) *dolichostenomelia with a tendency to bowing or fracture*; (d) humerus varus, bowed radius and ulna, enlarged carpal bones, accelerated skeletal maturation, genu valgum, short fourth metacarpal; (e) microcephaly, overdevelopment of the paranasal sinuses, thick calvaria, hyperostosis frontalis interna, wide diploic space, dural calcification, prognathism; (f) pectus carinatum or excavatum; (g) vascular abnormalities: calcification, intimal striation of the arteries with a rippled appearance on arteriography, thromboembolic episodes, atheromatous lesion, vascular narrowing or total obstruction, saccular expansion, etc. (Fig ME–H–8).

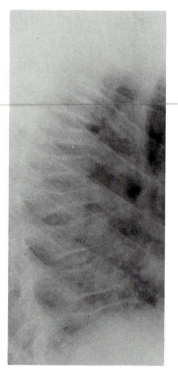

FIG ME–H–8.
Homocystinuria: poor mineralization and flattening of the thoracic vertebral bodies. (Courtesy of J.M.T. MacCarthy, Dublin, Ireland.)

REFERENCES

Abbott MH, et al.: Psychiatric manifestations of homocystinuria due to cystathionine β-synthase deficiency: Prevalence, natural history, and relationship to neurologic impairment and vitamin B$_6$-responsiveness. *Am. J. Med. Genet.* 26:959, 1987.

Arbour L, et al.: Postoperative dystonia in a female patient with homocystinuria. *J. Pediatr.* 113:863, 1988.

Ben Dridi MF, et al.: L'homocystinurie. Forme avec thrombose vasculaire et déficit en facteur VII. *Arch. Fr. Pediatr.* 43:41, 1986.

Boers GHJ, et al.: Heterozygosity for homocystinuria: A risk factor of occlusive cerebrovascular disease? *Clin. Genet.* 24:300, 1983.

Kurczynski TW, et al.: Maternal homocystinuria: Studies of an untreated mother and fetus. *Arch. Dis. Child.* 55:721, 1980.

MacCarthy JMT, Carey MC: Bone changes in homocystinuria. *Clin. Radiol.* 19:128, 1968.

Palareti G, et al.: Blood coagulation changes in homocystinuria: Effects of pyridoxine and other specific therapy. *J. Pediatr.* 109:1001, 1986.

Rosenblatt DS, et al.: Vitamin B$_{12}$ responsive homocystinuria and megaloblastic anemia: Heterogeneity in methylcobalamin deficiency. *Am. J. Med. Genet.* 26:377, 1987.

Schedewie H, et al.: Skeletal findings in homocystinuria: A collaborative study. *Pediatr. Radiol.* 1:12, 1973.

Schwab FJ, et al.: CT of cerebral venous sinus thrombosis in a child with homocystinuria. *Pediatr. Radiol.* 17:244, 1987.

Sensenbrenner JA, et al.: Homocystinuria with hyperostosis frontalis interna. *Birth Defects* 9(4):359, 1974.

Skovby F: Homocystinuria. Clinical, biochemical and genetic aspects of cystathionine β-synthase and its

deficiency in man. *Acta Paediatr. Scand. Suppl.* 321:7, 1985.

Tamburrini O, et al.: Short fourth metacarpal in homocystinuria. *Pediatr. Radiol.* 15:209, 1985.

Watanabe T, et al.: Urinary homocystine levels in a newborn infant with cystathionine synthase deficiency. *Eur. J. Pediatr.* 146:436, 1987.

Wicherink-Bol HF, et al.: Angiographic findings in homocystinuria. *Cardiovasc. Intervent. Radiol.* 6:125, 1983.

HYDROXYAPATITE DEPOSITION DISEASE

Synonyms: HADD; calcium hydroxyapatite crystal deposition disease; hydroxyapatite rheumatism, etc.

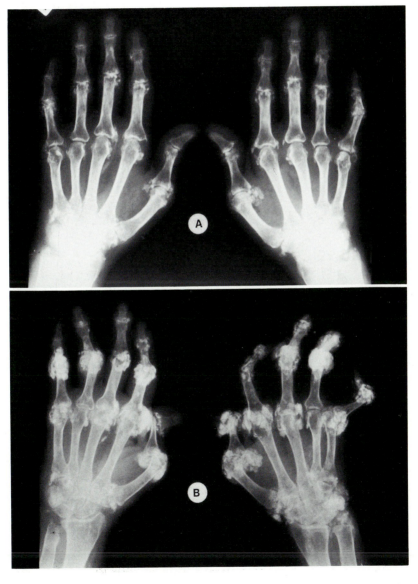

FIG ME–H–9.
Hydroxyapatite deposition disease in a 46-year-old woman. **A,** periarticular calcification. **B,** radiography taken about 3 years later shows progression of the disease with deformity, erosions, and increased periarticular calcification. Aspiration of the fourth metacarpophalangeal joint of the left hand yielded a chalky deposit of hydroxyapatite crystals. (From Nguyen VD, London J: Hydroxyapatite deposition disease. *Orthop. Rev.* 14:503, 1985. Used by permission.)

Etiology: *Calcium hydroxyapatite crystal deposition in periarticular tissue,* in some cases associated with intra-articular deposition of the crystals.

Clinical Manifestations: Onset of symptoms usually between the ages of 40 and 70 years; acute chronic or intermediate presentation: (a) *monoarticular or polyarticular pain;* (b) *limitation of joint motion;* (c) *swelling,* tenderness; (d) other reported abnormalities: tender nodule(s), mild fever, elevated sedimentation rate, association with renal failure and hemodialysis, etc.

Radiologic Manifestations: (a) *periarticular calcification (tendon, capsule, bursa);* shoulder joint, especially at the site of the insertion of the supraspinatus tendon, the lateral epicondyle of the humerus, the flexor carpi ulnaris, flexor carpi radialis and extensor carpi ulnaris tendons of the wrist, the metacarpophalangeal joints, the greater trochanter, the medial and lateral compartments of the knee, and the metatarsophalangeal joints; (b) *abnormality of adjacent osseous structures (osteoporosis, osteosclerosis, cystic lesions, irregularity of the bony contour)* (Fig ME–H–9).

REFERENCES

Bonavita JA, et al.: Hydroxyapatite deposition disease. *Radiology* 134:621, 1980.
Doherty M, et al.: Crystal deposition disease in the elderly. *Clin. Rheum. Dis.* 12:97, 1986.
Nguyen VD, et al.: Hydroxyapatite deposition disease. *Orthop. Rev.* 14:503, 1985.
Resnick D, et al.: Rheumatoid arthritis and pseudo-rheumatoid arthritis in calcium pyrophosphate dihydrate crystal deposition disease. *Radiology* 140:615, 1981.
Rush PJ, et al.: Hydroxyapatite deposition disease presenting as calcific periarthritis in a 14-year-old girl. *Pediatr. Radiol.* 16:169, 1986.

HYPERAMMONEMIC DISORDERS

Enzyme Deficiencies: See Table ME–H–1.

Clinical Manifestations: Symptoms progressively related to the level of ammonia: (a) neonates: Onset of symptoms hours or days after birth: lethargy, poor feeding, vomiting, hyperventilation, grunting respiration, seizures, diaphoresis, coma; (b) children: anorexia, vomiting, irritability, ataxia, hyperactivity, combativeness, stupor, delirium, coma, increased intracranial pressure; (c) other manifestations: less severe signs or symptoms than the aforementioned, cyclic vomiting, migrainous headaches, cognitive impairment, mental retardation, etc.

Radiologic Manifestations: Cerebral atrophy; delayed myelination; etc.

Note: Other disorders with hyperammonemia include acute or chronic liver disease, drug-induced conditions, Reye syndrome, hepatotoxity, primary systemic carnitine deficiency, HHH-syndrome (hyperammonemia, hyperornithinemia, homocitrullinuria), etc. (Table ME–H–1).

REFERENCES

Batshaw ML, et al.: Risk of serious illness in heterozygotes for ornithine transcarbamylase deficiency. *J. Pediatr.* 108:236, 1986.
Breningstall GN: Neurologic syndromes in hyperammonemic disorders. *Pediatr. Neurol.* 2:253, 1986.
Harding BN, et al.: Ornithine carbamoyl transferase deficiency: A neuropathological study. *Eur. J. Pediatr.* 141:215, 1984.
Hommes FA, et al.: Studies on a case of HHH-syndrome (hyperammonemia, hyperornithinemia, homocitrullinuria). *Neuropediatrics* 17:48, 1986.

HYPERIMMUNOGLOBULINEMIA E SYNDROME

Synonyms: Hyper-IgE syndrome; Job syndrome; Buckley syndrome; HIE syndrome.

Mode of Inheritance: Autosomal recessive.

Clinical Manifestations: (a) *eczematoid dermatitis;* (b) *recurrent "cold" suppurative skin infections, usually by pyogenic staphylococci;* (c) *chronic purulent sinusitis and otitis media, chronic pulmonary infections;* (d) *cellular defect in chemotaxis;* (e) *high levels of serum IgE (at least ten times normal: 2,000 IU/mL), depressed specific cell-mediated immune responses, deficient antibody-forming capacity;* (f) other reported findings: hyperkeratotic nails, hyperextensible joints, periodontal disease, cranial synostosis, coarse facies, mild eosinophilia, mucocutaneous candidiasis, neutrophil chemotactic defect (variable), esophageal cryptococcosis, systemic mastocytosis, short stature, cyclic eosinophilic myositis, membranoproliferative glomerulonephritis, etc.

Radiologic Manifestations: (a) sinusitis, mastoidis; (b) recurrent pneumonias, pneumatocele formation with variable persistence and expansion; (b) osteoporosis, recurrent fractures; (c) craniosynostosis (Figs ME–H–10 and ME–H–11).

REFERENCES

Brestel EP, et al.: Osteogenesis imperfecta tarda in a child with hyper-IgE syndrome. *Am. J. Dis. Child.* 136:774, 1982.
Buckley RH, et al.: Extreme hyperimmunoglobulinemia E and undue susceptibility to infection. *Pediatrics* 49:59, 1972.
Davis SD, et al.: Job's syndrome: Recurrent "cold" staphylococcal abscesses. *Lancet* 1:1013, 1966.
Donabedian H, et al.: The hyperimmunoglobulin E recurrent-infection (Job's) syndrome. A review of the NIH

TABLE ME–H–1.

Inherited Organic Acidemias Associated With Hyperammonemia*

Disorder	Enzyme Defect	Laboratory Findings	Associated Features	Treatment
Propionic acidemia	Propionyl-CoA carboxylase	Serum: ↑Glycine, propionate Urine: ↑Glycine, methylcitrate, β-hydroxypropionate	Neutropenia, thrombocytopenia	Dietary protein restriction, some forms biotin responsive
Methylmalonic acidemia	Methylmalonyl-CoA mutase, racemase, cobalamin metabolism defect	Serum: ↑Glycine, methylmalonate Urine: ↑Glycine, methylmalonate	Neutropenia, thrombocytopenia	Dietary protein restriction, cobalamin supplementation
Isovaleric acidemia	Isovaleryl-CoA dehydrogenase	Serum: ↑Lactate, isovaleric acid Urine: ↑Isovaleric acid, isovalerylglycine	Cheese or sweaty feet odor	Dietary protein restriction, glycine administration
Multiple carboxylase deficiency	Holocarboxylase synthetase or biotin transport defect, biotinidase deficiency	Serum: ↑Glycine, propionate lactate, pyruvate Urine: ↑Glycine, methylcitrate, β-hydroxyisovalerate, β-methylcrotonylglycine, β-hydroxypropionate	Alopecia, erythematous or eczematous skin rash, unusual odor	Dietary protein restriction, biotin supplementation
Glutaric acidemia II	Multiple acyl-CoA dehydrogenases	Serum: ↑Lactate, glutarate, butyrate, isobutyrate, 2-methylbutyrate, isovalerate Urine: ↑Dicarboxylic and hydroxyacids	Hepatomegaly, fatty infiltration of the liver	Dietary protein restriction, riboflavin
β-Ketothiolase deficiency	β-Ketothiolase	Serum: ↑Glycine Urine: ↑Methylacetoacetate, butanone, tiglic acid	—	Dietary protein restriction

*From Breningstall GN: Neurologic syndromes in hyperammonemic disorders. *Pediatr. Neurol.* 2:253, 1986. Used by permission.

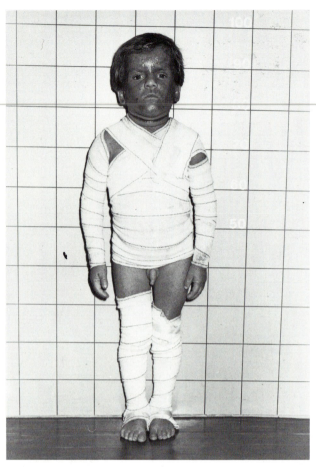

FIG ME−H−10.
Hyperimmunoglobulin E syndrome in a 5¾-year-old boy with short stature, severe eczematous dermatitis (note the facial manifestation), and a history of recurrent *Staphylococcus aureus* superinfection. (From Massa G, De Swert L, Vanderschueren-Lodeweyckx M: Short stature in a "hyperimmunoglobulin E syndrome". *Helv. Paediatr. Acta* 41:531, 1986. Used by permission.)

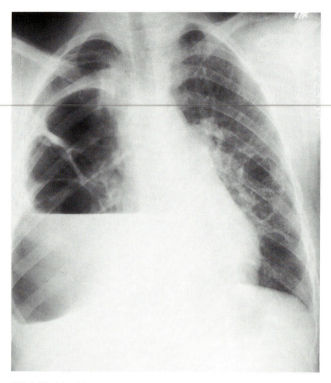

FIG ME−H−11.
Hyperimmunoglobulinemia E syndrome. A posteroanterior chest radiograph demonstrates multiple pneumatoceles. The right lung is more severely affected. An air-fluid level is noted in a large pneumatocele in the lower part of the right lobe. (From Fitch SJ, Magill HL, Herrod HG, et al.: Hyperimmunoglobulinemia E syndrome: Pulmonary imaging considerations. *Pediatr. Radiol.* 16:285, 1986. Used by permission.)

experience and the literature. *Medicine (Baltimore)* 62:195, 1983.

Fitch SJ, et al.: Hyperimmunoglobulinemia E syndrome: Pulmonary imaging considerations. *Pediatr. Radiol.* 16:285, 1986.

Gahr M, et al.: A boy with recurrent infections, impaired PMN-chemotaxis, increased IgE concentrations and cranial synostosis—a variant of the hyper-IgE syndrome? *Helv. Paediatr. Acta* 42:185, 1987.

Höger PH, et al.: Craniosynostosis in hyper-IgE-syndrome. *Eur. J. Pediatr.* 144:414, 1985.

Jacobs DH, et al.: Esophageal cryptococcosis in a patient with the hyperimmunoglobulin E-recurrent infection (Job's) syndrome. *Gastroenterology* 87:201, 1984.

Jaramillo D, et al.: Demonstration of a cold abscess by gallium-67 imaging in a patient with Job syndrome. *A.J.R.* 147:610, 1986.

Kamei R, et al.: Neonatal Job's syndrome featuring a vesicular eruption. *Pediatr. Dermatol.* 5:75, 1988.

Kirchner SG, et al.: Hyperimmunoglobulinemia E syndrome:

Association with osteoporosis and recurrent fractures. *Radiology* 156:362, 1985.

Lagrue G, et al.: Glomérulonephrite membrano-proliférative associée a un syndrome de Buckley traitée par la ciclosporine. *Presse Med.* 16:619, 1987.

Lebranchu Y, et al.: Syndrome hyper-IgE et infections récidivantes (syndrome de Buckley). Association à un genu varum. *Ann. Pediatr. (Paris)* 33:109, 1986.

Massa G, et al.: Short stature in the "hyperimmunoglobulin E syndrome. *Helv. Paediatr. Acta* 41:531, 1986.

Meyers DA, et al.: The inheritance of immunoglobulin E: Genetic linkage analysis. *Am. J. Med. Genet.* 16:575, 1983.

Symmans WA, et al.: Cyclic eosinophilic myositis and hyperimmunoglobulin-E. *Ann. Intern. Med.* 104:26, 1986.

HYPERINSULINISM

Mode of Inheritance (nesidioblastosis): Autosomal recessive.

Etiology: Nesidioblastosis, beta-cell hyperplasia, beta-cell adenoma, Beckwith-Wiedemann syndrome, leucine sensitivity.

Clinical Manifestations: (a) transient hypoglycemia in the infants of diabetic mothers and infants with erythroblastosis fetalis; (b) nesidioblastosis, adenoma: (1) persistent hypoglycemia, elevated plasma insulin levels, intravenous glucose infusion rate of more than 15 mg/kg/min to maintain a blood glucose level over 2 mmol/L, low blood ketones, a glycemic response to glucagon; (2) clinical manifestation of hypoglycemia (tremors, jitteriness, apnea, cyanosis, seizures, central nervous system damage; (3) abnormal fat thickness (above normal) in the neonates with nesidioblastosis.

Radiologic Manifestations: (a) noninvasive imaging techniques (ultrasound, computed tomography, magnetic resonance imaging); (b) arteriography for localization of islet cell adenomas; (c) measurement of insulin concentration in the pancreatic venous effluent.

REFERENCES

Cho KJ, et al.: Localization of the source of hyperinsulinism: Percutaneous transhepatic portal and pancreatic vein catheterization with hormone assay. *A.J.R.* 139:237, 1982.

Gough MH: The surgical treatment of hyperinsulinism in infancy and childhood. *Br. J. Surg.* 71:75, 1984.

Gorman B, et al.: Benign pancreatic insulinoma: Preoperative and intraoperative sonographic localization. *A.J.R.* 147:929, 1986.

Gould VE, et al.: Nesidiodysplasia and nesidioblastosis of infancy: Structural and functional correlations with the syndrome of hyperinsulinemic hypoglycemia. *Pediatr. Pathol.* 1:7, 1983.

Günther RW, et al.: Islet-cell tumors: Detection of small lesions with computed tomography and ultrasound. *Radiology* 148:485, 1983.

Moulopoulou A, et al.: Intra-arterial digital subtraction angiography in the diagnosis of insulinomas. *J. Med. Imag.* 2:98, 1988.

Oestreich AE, et al.: Abnormal fat thickness in newborns with nesidioblastosis. *Radiology* 141:679, 1981.

Rossi P, et al.: CT of functioning tumors of the pancreas. *A.J.R.* 144:57, 1985.

Telander RL, et al.: Endocrine disorders of the pancreas and adrenal cortex in pediatric patients. *Mayo Clin. Proc.* 61:459, 1986.

HYPERLIPOPROTEINEMIAS

Synonym: Hyperlipidemia.

Clinical and Radiologic Manifestations:

(A) Type i—hyperlipoproteinemia (chylomicrons): Eruptive xanthomas, autosomal recessive transmission.

(B) Type ii—hyperlipoproteinemia (β lipoprotein): Also known as familial hypercholesterolemia: (a) eruptive xanthomas, migratory arthritis, increased incidence of cholecystitis/cholelithiasis, premature corneal arcus, gout, markedly elevated serum cholesterol level, elevated plasma triglyceride levels, hyperuricemia, clear serum; (b) tuberous xanthomas: subcutaneous water density masses over the extensor sur-

faces, in particular, in the elbow, hand, buttocks, knee, and ankle regions; rare occurrence of soft-tissue calcification; (c) tendinous xanthomas: most common sites: elbow, palm and dorsum of the hand, Achilles tendon, peroneal tendons, plantar tendons; calcification may be present; intracranial xanthoma with stippled calcification (computed tomographic examination); (d) bone involvement either by an extrinsic effect of xanthomas (multiple well-defined periarticular cortical erosions with intact cortices, most common in the small bones of the hands and feet) or primary bone lesions due to subperiosteal xanthomas and intramedullary lesions (scalloping of the external cortical surface, small and round or oval lytic medullary defects, honeycomb appearance, endosteal erosion, subchondral collapse, juxta-articular defects, pathological fractures), increased uptake on bone scan using ^{99m}Tc pyrophosphate; (e) coronary artery disease, calcific atherosclerosis of the aortic root, calcification of the aortic arch, narrowing of the ascending aorta, left ventricular outflow obstruction, aortic valve stenosis; (f) autosomal dominant transmission, onset of symptoms in childhood in homozygotes.

(C) Type iii—hyperlipoproteinemia (β/pre-β-lipoprotein): (a) eruptive xanthomas, yellowish elevation on the palmar aspect of the hand, coronary and peripheral vascular disease,

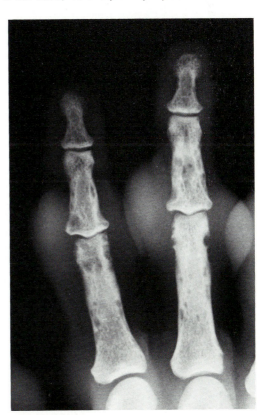

FIG ME–H–12.
Hyperlipoproteinemia, type III, in a 25-year-old man. Multiple tendon xanthomatoses as well as extrinsic and intrinsic bone involvement is present. (From Yaghmai I: Intra- and extraosseous xanthoma associated with hyperlipidemia. *Radiology* 128:49, 1978. Used by permission.)

corneal arcus, opalescent serum, hypercholesterolemia, hyperlipoproteinemia, hyperuricemia; (b) tuberous, tendinous, and osseous xanthomas similar to those in type II; (c) autosomal dominant, usually diagnosed in the fourth to sixth decades of life.

(D) Type IV—HYPERLIPOPROTEINEMIA (PRE-β-LIPOPROTEIN): (a) eruptive xanthomas (osseous), coronary artery disease common, peripheral vascular disease uncommon, arthralgia, arthritis, hepatosplenomegaly (occasionally), opalescent serum, hyperlipoproteinemia, normal or elevated serum cholesterol levels, hyperuricemia; (b) tuberous and osseous xanthomas; (c) coronary artery calcification; (d) possibly autosomal dominant, often diagnosed after the second decade of life.

(E) Type V—HYPERLIPOPROTEINEMIA (PRE-β-LIPOPROTEIN, CHYLOMICRONS): (a) eruptive xanthomas, coronary artery disease, abdominal pain, hepatosplenomegaly, lipemia retinalis, paresthesias, opalescent plasma, elevated serum cholesterol levels,

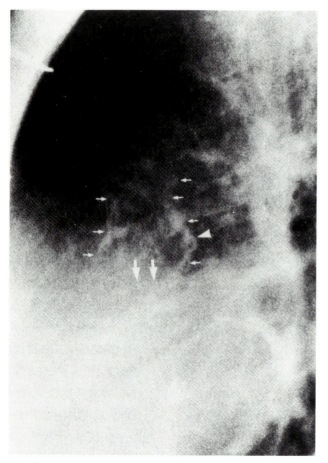

FIG ME—H—13.
Hyperlipoproteinemia in a 56-year-old woman with homozygous type II hyperlipoproteinemia and valvar aortic stenosis. Extensive calcification of the aortic sinuses, lower ascending aorta (small arrows), aortic valve (large arrows) and left coronary artery (arrowhead) is present. (From Dinsmore RE, Lees RS: Vascular calcification in type II and IV hyperlipoproteinemia: Radiographic appearance and clinical significance. A.J.R. 144:895, 1985. Used by permission.)

hyperlipoproteinemia, hyperuricemia; (b) possibly autosomal dominant transmission, usually detected in the third decade of life (Figs ME—H—12 and ME—H—13).

REFERENCES

Akazawa S, et al.: Familial type IIa hyperlipoproteinemia associated with a huge intracranial xanthoma. *Arch. Neurol.* 41:793, 1984.

Bjersand AJ: Bone changes in hypercholesterolemia. *Radiology* 130:101, 1979.

Brown MS, et al.: Familial hypercholesterolemia: Genetic, biochemical and pathophysiologic considerations. *Adv. Intern. Med.* 20:273, 1975.

Dinsmore RE, et al.: Vascular calcification in types II and IV hyperlipoproteinemia: Radiographic appearance and clinical significance. *A.J.R.* 144:895, 1985.

Francois JL, et al.: Genetic study of hyperlipoproteinemia type IV and V. *Clin. Genet.* 12:202, 1977.

Fredrickson DS, et al.: Type III hyperlipoproteinemia: An analysis of two contemporary definitions. *Ann. Intern. Med.* 82:150, 1975.

Inserra S, et al.: Intraosseous xanthoma associated with hyperlipoproteinemia. *Clin. Orthop.* 187:218, 1984.

Kovac A, et al.: Radiographic and radioisotope evaluation of intra-osseous xanthoma. *Br. J. Radiol.* 49:281, 1976.

Lindner MA, et al.: Expression of type III hyperlipoproteinemia in an adolescent patient with hypothyroidism. *J. Pediatr.* 113:86, 1988.

Yaghmai I: Intra-extraosseous xanthoma associated with hyperlipidemia. *Radiology* 128:49, 1978.

HYPERPARATHYROIDISM (NEONATAL)

Mode of Inheritance: Sporadic; familial (hypocalciuric hypercalcemia present in the majority of the familial cases).

Classification: (a) primary type; (b) infant born to a mother with poorly controlled hypoparathyroidism.

Clinical Manifestations: (a) *respiratory difficulty, poor feeding, hypotonia, failure to thrive, seizures, polydipsia, polyuria, constipation,* vomiting, swallowing difficulty; (b) splenomegaly, hepatomegaly; (c) *hypercalcemia, hypophosphatemia, hypercalciuria, hyperphosphaturia, aminoaciduria, normal levels of serum alkaline phosphatase, elevated levels of serum immunoreactive parathormone,* anemia; (d) other reported abnormalities: association with familial hypocalciuric hypercalcemia, association with alkaptonuria, occurrence in twins, chest wall deformity, limb deformity, craniotabes, facial dysmorphism, bulging fontanelle, absent reflexes, hyperreflexia, heart murmur, etc.

Radiologic Manifestations: (a) *severe generalized bone demineralization, coarse bony trabeculae, subperiosteal bone resorption, metaphyseal cupping, periodontal osteoporosis, osteitis fibrosa cystica;* (b) *pathological fractures;* (c) renal calcinosis (Fig ME—H—14).

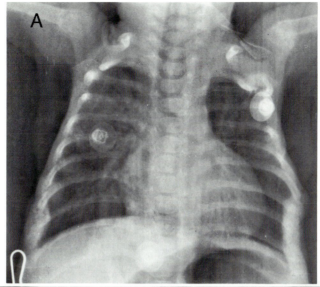

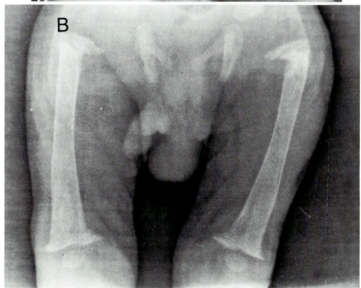

FIG ME–H–14.

Hyperparathyroidism (primary infantile) in a 37-day-old infant. **A** and **B,** "rachitic changes," pathological fractures, and subperiosteal bone erosion. (From Eftekhari F, Yousefzadeh DK: Primary in- fantile hyperparathyroidism: Clinical, laboratory, and radiographic features in 21 cases. *Skeletal Radiol.* 8:201, 1982. Used by permission.)

REFERENCES

Cooper L, et al.: Severe primary hyperparathyroidism in a neonate with two hypercalcemic parents: Management with parathyroidectomy and heterotopic autotransplantation. *Pediatrics* 78:263, 1986.

Eftekhari F, et al.: Primary infantile hyperparathyroidism: Clinical, laboratory, and radiographic features in 21 cases. *Skeletal Radiol.* 8:201, 1982.

Gilsanz V, et al.: Nephrolithiasis in premature infants. *Radiology* 154:107, 1985.

Glass EJ, et al.: Transient neonatal hyperparathyroidism secondary to maternal pseudohypoparathyroidism. *Arch. Dis. Child.* 56:565, 1981.

Just J, et al.: L'hyperparathyroïdie primitive néonatale chez deux jumelles dizygotes. Importance de la parathyroïdectomie en urgence. *Ann. Pediatr. (Paris)* 33:217, 1986.

Marcombes F, et al.: Hyperparathyroïdie congénitale. Trois observations. *Ann. Med. Interne (Paris)* 137:401, 1986.

Page LA, et al.: Self-limited neonatal hyperparathyroidism in familial hypocalciuric hypercalcemia. *J. Pediatr.* 111:261, 1987.

Schonwetter BS, et al.: Hypertension in neonatal hyperthyroidism. *Am. J. Dis. Child.* 137:954, 1983.

Spiegel AM, et al.: Neonatal primary hyperparathyroidism with autosomal dominant inheritance. *J. Pediatr.* 90:269, 1977.

Steinmann B, et al.: Neonatal severe primary hyperparathyroidism and alkaptonuria in a boy born to related parents with familial hypocalciuric hypercalcemia. *Helv. Paediatr. Acta* 39:171, 1984.

HYPERPARATHYROIDISM (PRIMARY)

Mode of Inheritance: Sporadic; familial (autosomal dominant) with and without other components of the multiple endocrine neoplasia syndromes.

Etiology: Parathyroid adenoma; parathyroid hyperplasia; parathyroid carcinoma; multiple endocrine neoplasia, type II; nonparathyroid tumors secreting a parathormone-like substance.

Clinical Manifestations: (a) *bone and joint pain and tenderness;* (b) *symptoms related to hypercalcemia:* psychological disorders, hypotonicity of smooth and skeletal muscles, nausea, vomiting, polyuria, polydipsia, abnormal electrocardiographic findings; (c) *renal stones,* terminal uremia; (d) *systemic hypertension;* (e) *limb deformities,* decrease in stature, finger clubbing; (f) *high levels of serum calcium, depressed serum phosphate levels, elevated urine calcium and phosphate levels, elevated serum alkaline phosphatase levels, elevated circulating parathyroid hormone levels, positive phosphate resorption and calcium infusion tests;* (g) other reported abnormalities: anemia, pancreatitis, peptic ulcer disease, thymic carcinoid tumors, thyroid carcinoma, induction by radioactive iodine, induction by neck irradiation, Graves disease, familial hyperparathyroidism caused by solitary adenomatosis, pancytosis, colonic carcinoma, myotonic dystrophy, hypertrophic cardiomyopathy, etc.

Radiologic Manifestations: (a) *renal calculi, nephrocalcinosis;* (b) *demineralization, brown tumor* (sharply marginated bone lesion that may expand the cortex, single or multiple, increased ^{99m}Tc pyrophosphate uptake, hypervascularity on arteriography and computed tomography), bone resorption (particularly in the radial margin of the middle phalanges, medial and lateral ends of the clavicle, ribs, sacroiliac joint, tarsal bones, ischial tuberosity, humerus, iliac crest, scapula, and lamina dura), erosive arthritis, demineralization of calvaria (homogeneous, mottled, granular, or ground-glass patterns), patchy sclerosis of the calvaria, basilar invagination, biconcave deformity of the vertebral bodies, kyphosis, scoliosis, deformed pelvis, pathological fractures, osteosclerosis (rare); (c) *pathological calcifications:* vessels, articular cartilages, periarticular soft tissues, lung, prostate, pancreas, salivary glands, conjunctiva, etc.; (d) peptic ulcer, pancreatitis, gallstones; (e) *parathyroid mass.*

Note: Hypohyperparathyroidism refers to a disorder with the following features: (a) *renal resistance to exogenous parathyroid hormone;* (b) *hypocalcemia, hyperphosphatemia, elevated serum alkaline phosphatase levels, elevated level of serum parathyroid hormone;* (c) no evidence of renal disease or malabsorption; (d) *subperiosteal bone resorption, metaphyseal changes, epiphyseal displacement* (particularly slipped capital femoral epiphysis), brown tumor; (e) bone biopsy finding of hyperparathyroidism.

REFERENCES

Arem R, et al.: Concomitant Graves' disease and primary hyperparathyroidism. Influence of hyperthyroidism on serum calcium and parathyroid hormone. *Am. J. Med.* 80:693, 1986.

Bennett JT, et al.: Parathyroid adenoma presenting as a pathologic fracture of the femoral neck in an adolescent. *J. Pediatr. Orthop.* 6:473, 1986.

Benson L, et al.: Hyperparathyroidism presenting as the first lesion in multiple endocrine neoplasia type I. *Am. J. Med.* 82:731, 1987.

Birnberg FA, et al.: Thymic carcinoid tumors with hyperparathyroidism. *A.J.R.* 139:1001, 1982.

Bone LB, et al.: Slipped capital femoral epiphysis associated with hyperparathyroidism. *J. Pediatr. Orthop.* 5:589, 1985.

Brasier AR, et al.: Hungry bone syndrome: Clinical and biochemical predictors of its occurrence after parathyroid surgery. *Am. J. Med.* 84:654, 1988.

Connors MH, et al.: Hypo-hyperparathyroidism: Evidence for a defective parathyroid hormone. *Pediatrics* 60:343, 1977.

Ellis K, et al.: The skull in hyperparathyroid bone disease. *A.J.R.* 83:732, 1960.

Feig DS, et al.: Familial hyperparathyroidism in association with colonic carcinoma. *Cancer* 60:429, 1987.

Genant HK, et al.: Primary hyperparathyroidism: A comprehensive study of clinical, biochemical and radiographic manifestations. *Radiology* 109:513, 1973.

Harada SI, et al.: Association of primary hyperparathyroidism with myotonic dystrophy in two patients. *Arch. Intern. Med.* 147:777, 1987.

Hedman I, et al.: Associated hyperparathyroidism and nonmedullary thyroid carcinoma: The etiologic role of radiation. *Surgery* 95:392, 1984.

Higashihara E, et al.: Medullary sponge kidney and hyperparathyroidism. *Urology* 31:155, 1988.

Holsbeeck MV, et al.: Osteosclerosis in primary hyperparathyroidism. *Fortschr. Rontgenstr.* 147:690, 1987.

Krudy AG, et al.: Hyperfunctioning cystic parathyroid glands: CT and sonographic findings. *A.J.R.* 142:175, 1984.

Mallette LE, et al.: Familial cystic parathyroid adenomatosis. *Ann. Intern. Med.* 107:54, 1987.

Naiman J, et al.: Brown tumor of the orbit associated with primary hyperparathyroidism. *Am. J. Ophthalmol.* 90:565, 1980.

Obley DL, et al.: Parathyroid adenomas studied by digital subtraction angiography. *Radiology* 153:449, 1984.

Patten BM, et al.: Severe neurological disease associated with hyperparathyroidism. *Ann. Neurol.* 15:453, 1984.

Peck WW, et al.: Hyperparathyroidism: Comparison of MR imaging with radionuclide scanning. *Radiology* 163:415, 1987.

Pont A, et al.: Hyperparathyroidism in twins. *Ann. Intern. Med.* 97:721, 1982.

Rapaport D, et al.: Primary hyperparathyroidism in children. *J. Pediatr. Surg.* 21:395, 1986.

Reading CC, et al.: Postoperative parathyroid high-frequency sonography: Evaluation of persistent or recurrent hyperparathyroidism. *A.J.R.* 144:399, 1985.

Resnick DL: Erosive arthritis of the hand and wrist in hyperparathyroidism. *Radiology* 110:263, 1974.

Rosen IB, et al.: Induction of hyperparathyroidism by radioactive iodine. *Am. J. Surg.* 148:441, 1984.

Spritzer CE, et al.: Abnormal parathyroid glands: High-resolution MR imaging. *Radiology* 162:487, 1987.

Steinbach HL, et al.: Primary hyperparathyroidism: A correlation of roentgen, clinical, and pathologic features. *A.J.R.* 86:329, 1961.

Sundaram MI, et al.: Primary hyperparathyroidism presenting with acute paraplegia. *A.J.R.* 128:674, 1977.

Symons C, et al.: Cardiac hypertrophy, hypertrophic cardiomyopathy, and hyperparathyroidism—an association. *Br. Heart J.* 54:539, 1985.

Teplick JG, et al.: Erosion of the sternal ends of the clavicles: A new sign of primary and secondary hyperparathyroidism. *Radiology* 113:323, 1974.

Tisell LE, et al.: Hyperparathyroidism subsequent to neck irradiation. Risk factors. *Cancer* 56:1529, 1985.

Tsang RC, et al.: Pediatric parathyroid disorders. *Pediatr. Clin. North Am.* 26:223, 1979.

Ziv Y, et al.: Primary hyperparathyroidism associated with pancytosis. *N. Engl. J. Med.* 313:187, 1985.

HYPERPARATHYROIDISM (SECONDARY)

Synonyms: Osteitis fibrosa cystica; renal osteodystrophy.

Clinical Manifestations: (a) pronounced parathyroid hyperplasia secondary to chronic renal disease, common occurrence in hemodialysis patients; (b) other etiologic factors: long-term furosemide therapy in infants, oral contraceptives, idiopathic hypercalciuria, gluten enteropathy; (c) *elevated serum phosphate levels, low ionized serum calcium levels.*

Radiologic Manifestations: (a) *bone resorption;* (1) *subperiosteal* (phalangeal tufts; radial aspect of the proximal and

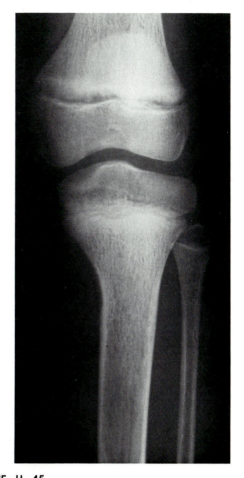

FIG ME–H–15.
Hyperparathyroidism (secondary) in a 10-year-old girl with chronic renal disease. Coarse bone trabeculae, metaphyseal irregularities, and subperiosteal bone resorption in the medial margin of the proximal part of the shaft of the tibia are present.

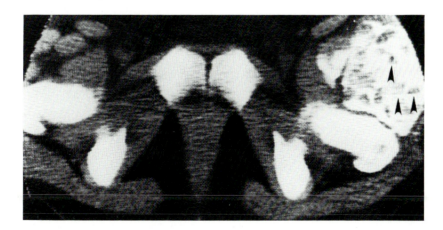

FIG ME–H–16.
Soft-tissue calcification layering *(arrowheads)* in a 27-year-old woman with chronic renal failure and secondary hyperparathyroidism. (From Gordon LF, Arger PH, Dalinka MK, et al.: Computed tomography in soft tissue calcification layering. *J. Comput. Assist. Tomogr.* 8:71, 1984. Used by permission.)

middle phalanges of the fingers; margins of the ribs; lamina dura; and medial margin of the proximal segment of the humerus, femur, and tibia); (2) *intracortical* (cortex of the metacarpals); (3) *endosteal* (phalanges of the digits), (4) *subligamentous* (humeral and ischial tuberosities, trochanters, inferior margin of the distal portion of the clavicle, inferior surface of the calcaneus); (5) *subchondral* (sternoclavicular, acromioclavicular, and sacroiliac joints; discovertebral junctions; pubic symphysis; shoulder), erosive arthropathy; (6) distal phalangeal brachydactyly secondary to healed renal osteodystrophy; (b) *brown tumor*, vertebral brown tumor as an expansive mass in association with paraplegia, sellar and parasellar destructive lesions; (c) *epiphyseal displacement* due to metaphyseal fracture (most common sites—distal part of the radius, proximal portion of the humerus, distal aspect of the femur, and heads of the metacarpal and metatarsal bones); (d) *osteosclerosis:* spine (rugger-jersey pattern), pelvis, ribs, epiphyses, etc.; (e) *periosteal neostosis* (most common sites—metatarsals, femora, and pelvis); (f) osteoporosis, osteomalacia; (g) chondrocalcinosis (pyrophosphate dihydrate crystal deposition), vascular calcification, pulmonary calcified nodule (increased radionuclide uptake using ^{99m}Tc methylene diphosphate, and chest radiography), cerebral subcortical calcification, soft-tissue calcification layering, cardiac calcification, breast calcification; (h) increased bone radiotracer uptake; (i) enlarged parathyroid glands (ultrasonography) (Figs ME–H–15 and ME–H–16).

REFERENCES

Andresen J, et al.: Renal osteodystrophy in nondialysed patients with chronic renal failure. *Acta Radiol.* 21:803, 1980.

Beerman PJ, et al.: Metastatic pulmonary calcification from chronic renal failure. *Am. J. Dis. Child.* 137:1120, 1983.

Bohlman ME, et al.: Brown tumor in secondary hyperparathyroidism causing acute paraplegia. *Am. J. Med.* 81:545, 1986.

Day D, et al.: Musculoskeletal case of the day. *A.J.R.* 148:1048, 1987.

D'Cruz IA: Mitral anulus calcification in patients with chronic renal failure. *Chest* 86:507, 1984.

deGraaf P, et al.: Increased bone radiotracer uptake in renal osteodystrophy: Clinical evidence of hyperparathyroidism as the major cause. *Eur. J. Nucl. Med.* 7:152, 1982.

de Moraes CR: Calcification of the heart: A rare manifestation of chronic renal failure. *Pediatr. Radiol.* 16:422, 1986.

Ehrlich GW, et al.: Secondary hyperparathyroidism and brown tumors in a patient with gluten enteropathy. *A.J.R.* 141:381, 1983.

Garver P, et al.: Epiphyseal sclerosis in renal osteodystrophy simulating osteonecrosis. *A.J.R.* 136:1239, 1981.

Gordon LF, et al.: Computed tomography in soft tissue calcification layering. *J. Comput. Assist. Tomogr.* 8:71, 1984.

Hooge WA, et al.: CT of sacroiliac joints in secondary hyperparathyroidism. *J. Can. Assoc. Radiol.* 31:42, 1981.

Johannsen A, et al.: Bone maturation in children with chronic renal failure. *Acta Radiol.* 20:193, 1978.

Kattan KR, et al.: Brown tumor of the right seventh rib with

osteomalacia and secondary hyperparathyroidism. *Skeletal Radiol.* 10:47, 1983.

Kricum ME, et al.: Patellofemoral abnormalities in renal osteodystrophy. *Radiology* 143:667, 1982.

Meema HE, et al.: The mode of progression of subperiosteal resorption in the hyperparathyroidism of chronic renal failure. *Skeletal Radiol.* 10:157, 1983.

Moore ES, et al.: Secondary hyperparathyroidism in children with symptomatic idiopathic hypercalciuria. *J. Pediatr.* 103:932, 1983.

Moses AM, et al.: Secondary hyperparathyroidism caused by oral contraceptives. *Arch. Intern. Med.* 142:128, 1982.

Nixon JR, et al.: Bilateral slipping of the upper femoral epiphysis in end-stage renal failure. *J. Bone Joint Surg. [Br.]* 62:18, 1980.

Nussbaum AJ, et al.: Shoulder arthropathy in primary hyperparathyroidism. *Skeletal Radiol.* 9:98, 1982.

Resnick D, et al.: Renal osteodystrophy: Magnification radiography of target sites of absorption. *A.J.R.* 136:711, 1981.

Sanders C, et al.: Metastatic calcification of the heart and lungs in end-stage renal disease: Detection and quantification by dual-energy digital chest radiography. *A.J.R.* 149:881, 1987.

Schwartz EE, et al.: Erosion of the inferior aspect of the clavicle in secondary hyperparathyroidism. *A.J.R.* 129:291, 1977.

Shenker Y, et al.: Ectopic prolactinoma in a patient with hyperparathyroidism and abnormal sellar radiography. *J. Clin. Endocrinol. Metab.* 62:1065, 1986.

Sommer G, et al.: Breast calcifications in renal hyperparathyroidism. *A.J.R.* 148:855, 1987.

Steadman C, et al.: Painful bone and sclerosis. Variant of renal osteodystrophy simulating osteonecrosis. *Am. J. Med.* 82:171, 1987.

Sundaram M, et al.: Erosive azotemic osteodystrophy. *A.J.R.* 136:363, 1981.

Swartz JD, et al.: CT demonstration of cerebral subcortical calcifications. *J. Comput. Assist. Tomogr.* 7:476, 1983.

Takebayashi S, et al.: Sonography for early diagnosis of enlarged parathyroid glands in patients with secondary hyperparathyroidism. *A.J.R.* 148:911, 1987.

Venkataraman PS, et al.: Secondary hyperparathyroidism and bone disease in infants receiving long-term furosemide therapy. *Am. J. Dis. Child.* 137:1157, 1983.

Watanabe T, et al.: Pleural calcification: A type of "metastatic calcification" in chronic renal failure. *Br. J. Radiol.* 56:93, 1983.

Wu AC, et al.: Distal phalangeal brachydactyly secondary to healed renal osteodystrophy. *Skeletal Radiol.* 16:312, 1987.

Ziter FMH Jr: Central vertebral end-plate depression in chronic renal disease: report of two cases. *A.J.R.* 132:809, 1979.

HYPERPHOSPHATASEMIA

Synonyms: Hyperphosphatasia; osteoectasia; juvenile Paget disease; familial osteoectasia; osteochalasia desmalis familiaris; etc.

Mode of Inheritance: Autosomal recessive.

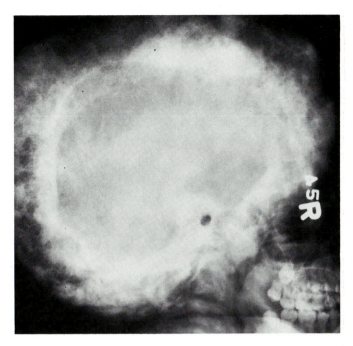

FIG ME–H–17.
Hyperphosphatasemia in a 9-year-old male who has a thickened calvaria with numerous round whitish patches and an uneven outer border. (From Caffey J: *Progress in Pediatric Radiology.* Basel, S. Karger AG, 1973, vol. 4, p. 438. Used by permission.)

Frequency: Over 20 published cases (Döhler et al.).

Clinical Manifestations: Onset of symptoms in infancy or early childhood: (a) dwarfism; (b) *progressive enlargement of the head,* saddle nose, short neck; (c) bowed limbs; (d) pigeon breast deformity; (e) muscular weakness; (f) swelling of the extremities; (g) premature shedding of deciduous teeth; (h) *high levels of serum acid and alkaline phosphatases,* high levels of urinary excretion of hydroxyproline; elevated activity of serum aminopeptidase, increased uric acid levels in serum and urine; (i) improvement in the clinical and roentgenographic picture after treatment with calcitonin; (j) other reported abnormalities: association with salt-losing congenital adrenal hyperplasia, cardiomegaly, angioid streaks of the retina, macular atrophy, optic atrophy, hearing loss, systemic vascular hypertension, skin pigmentation, subclinical hearing loss, pathological fracture.

Radiologic Manifestations: *Progressive skeletal deformities:* (a) enlargement and *thickening of the skull,* widening of the diploic space, indistinct outer table, uneven mineralization of the calvaria; (b) platyspondyly, kyphoscoliosis, biconcave vertebral bodies, enlarged disk spaces; (c) osteomalacic type of deformity of the pelvis, protrusio acetabuli, coxa vara; (d) long-bone deformities: curved, thickened, cylindrical transverse trabeculae, narrowed or dilated medullary cavity, meshed radiolucent bone texture; (e) thickened metacarpals, metatarsals, and phalanges; (f) scintigraphy: intense uptake of radionuclide by the skeleton.

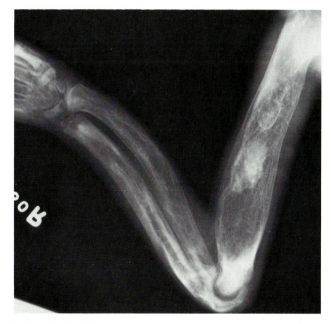

FIG ME–H–18.
Hyperphosphatasemia. The bones of the upper limb at 19 years of age are malformed and have streaky and rarefied cortices and dilated medullary cavities. (From Caffey J: *Progress in Pediatric Radiology.* S. Karger AG, Basel, 1973, vol. 4. p. 438. Used by permission.)

Differential Diagnosis: Diaphyseal dysplasia (Camurati-Engelmann); Paget disease; transient hyperphosphatasemia (Figs ME−H−17 and ME−H−18).

REFERENCES

Bakwin H, Eiger MS: Fragile bones and macrocranium. *J. Pediatr.* 49:558, 1956.

Caffey J: Familial hyperphosphatasemia with ateliosis and hypermetabolism of growing membranous bones: Review of the clinical, radiographic and chemical features, in Kaufmann HJ (ed.): *Progress in Pediatric Radiology.* Basel, S. Karger AG, 1973, vol. 4, p. 438.

Döhler JR, et al.: Idiopathic hyperphosphatasia with dermal pigmentation. A twenty-year follow-up. *J. Bone Joint Surg. [Br.]* 68:305, 1986.

Dunn V, et al.: Familial hyperphosphatasemia: Diagnosis in early infancy and response to human thyrocalcitonin therapy. *A.J.R.* 132:541, 1979.

Einhorn TA, et al.: Hyperphosphatasemia in an adult. Clinical, roentgenographic and histomorphometric findings and comparison to classical Paget's disease. *Clin. Orthop.* 204:253, 1986.

Eroglu M, et al.: Congenital hyperphosphatasia (juvenile Paget's disease). Eleven years follow-up of three sisters. *Ann. Radiol. (Paris)* 20:145, 1977.

Kraut JR, et al.: Isoenzyme studies in transient hyperphosphatasemia of infancy. Ten new cases and a review of the literature. *Am. J. Dis. Child.* 139:736, 1985.

Whalen JP, et al.: Calcitonin treatment in hereditary bone dysplasia with hyperphosphatasemia: A radiographic and histologic study of bone. *A.J.R.* 129:29, 1977.

HYPERTHYROIDISM

Etiology: Congenital; Graves disease (diffusely enlarged gland); thyroid nodule; thyroiditis; chorionic TSH; ovarian carcinoma.

Clinical Manifestations: (a) newborn: *hyperactivity, irritability, tachycardia, tachypnea, vomiting, diarrhea, hypertension, delayed cerebral development, periorbital edema, exophthalmos, high-output cardiac failure,* association with hyperviscosity syndrome, *abnormally high levels of long-acting thyroid-stimulating hormone (LATS);* (b) children and adults: *weight loss, increased appetite, muscular weakness, tremor, nervousness, palpitation, intolerance to heat, sweating, menstrual irregularities, decreased libido, impotence, arrhythmias, angina, congestive heart failure, swelling of the extremities, skin changes, diarrhea, ophthalmopathy (exophthalmos, subconjunctival edema, extraocular muscle paralysis, lid lag),* psychiatric problems, thyroid acropachy (soft-tissue swelling of the hands and feet, digital clubbing, active or treated hyperthyroidism), goiter, thyroid bruit, tumor of the thyroid gland; (c) other reported abnormalities: cardiac tamponade, corticospinal tract disease in thyrotoxicosis, association with myasthenia gravis, micturition frequency, nocturia, adult enuresis, rapid gastrointestinal transit time, thyroid-related coronary artery spasm, mitral valve prolapse, gyneco-

mastia, Plummer nails (onycholysis), rhabdomyolysis in thyroid storm, Graves disease in a patient with the del(18p) syndrome, etc.

Laboratory Findings: (a) *elevated thyroxine (T$_4$) levels, elevated levels of triiodothyronine (T$_3$);* (b) *radioactive iodine (^{131}I) uptake test;* (c) *T$_3$ suppression test;* (d) leukopenia, lymphocytosis, anemia, thrombocytopenia; (e) elevated alkaline phosphatase levels, hypercalcemia.

Radiologic Manifestations: (a) *skeletal system:* (1) infants and children: advanced skeletal maturation, premature closure of cranial sutures, cone-shaped epiphyses, brachydactyly, asymmetrical shortening of the metacarpals and phalanges, osteopenia, early costochondral calcification in adolescents; (2) adults: osteoporosis, in particular, involving the spine and pelvis; spontaneous fractures following minor traumas; thyroid acropachy (periosteal new bone formation in the diaphyses of tubular bones, in particular, involving the metacarpals, metatarsals, and proximal and middle phalanges, having a "bubbly" or "lacy" appearance); anterior marginal osteophytes of the cervical vertebrae and straightening or reversal of cervical lordosis; (b) chest: cardiomegaly, thymic enlargement; (c) ophthalmic Graves disease (unilateral or bilateral): swelling of the extrocular muscles sparing the tendons, proptosis, bowing of the medial lamina papyracea, venous engorgement (compression of orbital venous drainage), conjunctival and eyelid swelling, enlargement of the lacrimal gland, enlargement of the optic nerve with compression at the orbital apex causing vision decrease, enlargement of the fat compartment; (d) evaluation of the thyroid gland: scintigraphy (high sensitivity, specificity, and accuracy), mag-

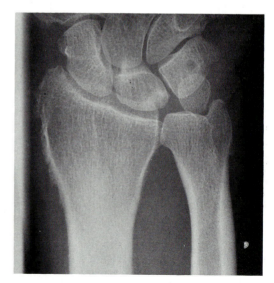

FIG ME−H−19.
Hyperthyroidism: periosteal new bone of the radius and ulna in a 72-year-old woman with clinical manifestations of thyroid acropachy. (From Torres-Reyes E, Staple TW: Roentgenographic appearance of thyroid acropachy. *Clin. Radiol.* 21:95, 1970. Used by permission.)

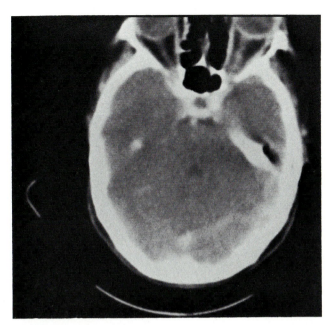

FIG ME−H−20.
Hyperthyroidism (thyroid ophthalmopathy): proptosis of the right globe and enlargement of right lateral rectus as well as enlargement of the right optic nerve sheath complex in a 50-year-old female. (From Healy JF, Rosenkrantz H: Enlargement of optic nerve sheath complex in thyroid ophthalmopathy. *J. Comput. Tomogr.* 5:8, 1981. Used by permission.)

netic resonance imaging (moderate to marked diffuse increase in signal intensity), computed tomography (a complementary procedure, intrathoracic goiter); (e) other reported abnormalities: cerebral development abnormalities (ventriculomegaly, increased space in the interhemispheric fissure, exaggerated gyral pattern) (Figs ME−H−19 and ME−H−20).

REFERENCES

Adrouny A, et al.: Variable presentation of thrombocytopenia in Graves' disease. *Arch. Intern. Med.* 142:1460, 1982.

Andersen LF, et al.: Micturition pattern in hyperthyroidism and hypothyroidism. *Urology* 29:223, 1987.

Bennett WR, et al.: Rhabdomyolysis in thyroid storm. *Am. J. Med.* 77:733, 1984.

Bonakdarpour A, et al.: Skeletal changes in neonatal thyrotoxicosis. *Radiology* 102:149, 1972.

Brauman A, et al.: Mitral valve prolapse in hyperthyroidism of two different origins. *Br. Heart J.* 53:374, 1985.

Bussman YL, et al.: Neonatal thyrotoxicosis associated with the hyperviscosity syndrome. *J. Pediatr.* 90:266, 1977.

Charkes ND, et al.: MR imaging in thyroid disorders: Correlation of signal intensity with Graves disease activity. *Radiology* 164:491, 1987.

Coupe B, et al.: Myasthénie et hyperthyroïdie basedowienne. *Arch. Fr. Pediatr.* 41:341, 1984.

Featherstone HJ, et al.: Angina in thyrotoxicosis. Thyroid-related coronary artery spasm. *Arch. Intern. Med.* 143:554, 1983.

Forbes G, et al.: Ophthalmopathy of Graves' disease: Computerized volume measurements of the orbital fat and muscle. *A.J.N.R.* 7:651, 1986.

Ford HC, et al.: Anterior mediastinal mass and Graves's disease. *Thorax* 40:469, 1985.

Healy JF, et al.: Enlargement of the optic nerve sheath complex in thyroid ophthalmopathy. *J. Comput. Tomogr.* 5:8, 1981.

Johnsonbaugh RE, et al.: Premature craniosynostosis: A common complication of juvenile thyrotoxicosis. *J. Pediatr.* 93:188, 1978.

Jones KL, et al.: Graves disease in a patient with the del(18p) syndrome. *Am. J. Med. Genet.* 11:449, 1982.

Komolafe F: Cervical spine changes in goitres. *Clin. Radiol.* 33:25, 1982.

Kopelman AE: Delayed cerebral development in twins with congenital hyperthyroidism. *Am. J. Dis. Child.* 137:842, 1983.

Landier F, et al.: Pathologie thyroïdienne des nouveau-nés de mères basedowiennes. *Arch. Fr. Pediatr.* 41:163, 1984.

Léger J, et al.: Ostéopénie grave chez de jeunes enfants atteints d'hyperthyroïdie. *Arch. Fr. Pediatr.* 43:123, 1986.

Lentino W, et al.: The roentgen manifestations of Plummer's nails (onycholysis) in hyperthyroidism. *A.J.R.* 84:941, 1960.

Lester LA, et al.: Cardiac abnormalities in children with hyperthyroidism. *Pediatr. Cardiol.* 2:215, 1982.

Meema HE, et al.: Simple radiologic demonstration of cortical bone loss in thyrotoxicosis. *Radiology* 97:9, 1970.

Mitchell I, et al.: Neonatal thyrotoxicosis associated with transplacental passage of human thyroid stimulating immunoglobulin (HTSI). *Arch. Dis. Child.* 51:565, 1976.

Newcomer J, et al.: Coma and thyrotoxicosis. *Ann. Neurol.* 14:689, 1983.

Nicholson RL: Thymic hyperplasia in thyrotoxicosis. *J. Can. Assoc. Radiol.* 29:264, 1978.

Park H-M, et al.: Efficacy of thyroid scintigraphy in the diagnosis of intrathoracic goiter. *A.J.R.* 148:527, 1987.

Riggs W Jr, et al.: Neonatal hyperthyroidism with accelerated skeletal maturation, craniosynostosis, and brachydactyly. *Radiology* 105:621, 1972.

Sadeghi-Nejad A, et al.: Hypercalcemia: An unusual complication of hyperthyroidism in a child. *Acta Paediatr. Scand.* 75:504, 1986.

Senac MO, et al.: Early costochondral calcification in adolescent hyperthyroidism. *Radiology* 156:375, 1985.

Shafer RB, et al.: Gastrointestinal transit in thyroid disease. *Gastroenterology* 86:852, 1984.

Silverman PM, et al.: Computed tomography in the evaluation of thyroid disease. *A.J.R.* 141:897, 1984.

Thomas J, et al.: Thyroid acropachy. *Am. J. Dis. Child.* 125:745, 1973.

Tourniaire J, et al.: Tamponnade par péricardite subaiguë au cours de la maladie de Basedow. *Presse Med.* 12:1989, 1983.

Trokel SL, et al.: Correlation of CT scanning and pathologic features of ophthalmic Graves' disease. *Ophthalmology* 88:553, 1981.

Uretsky S, et al.: Graves' ophthalmopathy in childhood and adolescence. *Arch. Ophthalmol.* 98:1963, 1980.

Walter S, et al.: Adult enuresis and hyperthyroidism. *Urology* 22:151, 1983.

Willinsky RA, et al.: Ultrasonic B-scan measurement of the

extra-ocular muscles in Graves' orbitopathy. *J. Can. Assoc. Radiol.* 35:171, 1984.

HYPOPARATHYROIDISM

Classification: (a) *idiopathic,* more common in females; (b) *secondary:* postoperative, hypomagnesemia, iron overloading (particularly with hemolytic anemias); (c) *neonatal:* maternal hyperparathyroidism, transient neonatal hypoparathyroidism (premature infants, infants of diabetic mothers, infants with birth asphyxia), DiGeorge syndrome; (d) *familial* (X-linked, autosomal recessive, autosomal dominant); (e) in conjunction with other hypofunction endocrinopathies (adrenocortical insufficiency, hypothyroidism, diabetes mellitus), considered to be an autoimmune disorder; association with other manifestations of the syndrome: mucocutaneous candidiasis, vitiligo, alopecia; (f) associated with other diseases and syndromes: pernicious anemia, steatorrhea, Kearns-Sayre syndrome, Wilson syndrome, hemochromatosis, tumor metastasis to the parathyroids, rickets, congenital lymphedema, nephropathy, etc.

Clinical Manifestations: (a) *neuromuscular hyperirritability:* carpopedal spasms, tetany, paresthesia of the limbs and/or around the mouth, laryngeal stridor, hyperreflexia, positive Chvostek and Trousseau signs; (b) *seizures, psychosis, parkinsonism, mental retardation;* (c) *diarrhea, steatorrhea;* (d) dental defects; (e) cataract; (f) congestive heart failure, prolonged QT interval; (g) ectodermal disorders: eczema, alopecia, skin moniliasis, etc.; (h) short stature; (i) *hypocalcemia, hyperphosphatemia, phosphate diuresis following the administration of parathyroid hormone, low or undetectable serum immunoreactive parathyroid hormone level;* (j) other reported abnormalities: hypocalcemic myopathy, partial monosomy 10p, dementia, congenital pulmonary valve defects, pseudotumor cerebri, etc.

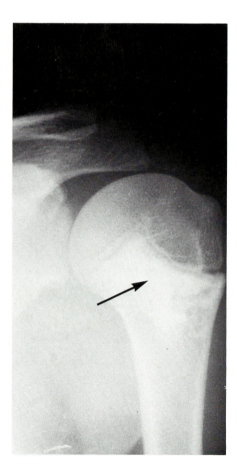

FIG ME–H–21.
Hypoparathyroidism in an 11-year-old female with a history of seizures and typical chemical manifestations of hypoparathyroidism. There is a marked increase in density of the proximal metaphyseodiaphyseal region of the humerus *(arrow).* A similar increased density was noted in the portions of the distal radii, ulnae, and femora and the proximal segments of the tibias. (From Taybi H, Keele D: Hypoparathyroidism: A review of literature and report of two cases in sisters, one with steatorrhea and intestinal pseudoobstruction. *A.J.R.* 88:432, 1962. Used by permission.)

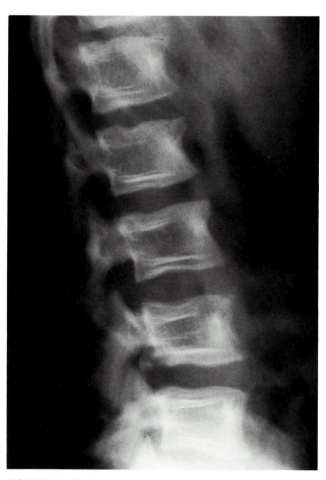

FIG ME–H–22.
Hypoparathyroidism: growth arrest recovery lines of the vertebrae in an 18-year-old boy with symptoms since birth. (From Rosen RA, Deshmukh SM: Growth arrest recovery lines in hypoparathyroidism. *Radiology* 155:61, 1985. Used by permission.)

Radiologic Manifestations: (a) *head:* thickening of calvarial tables, homogeneous thickening of petrous bones, thickening of facial bones, widening of sutures due to increased intracranial pressure, brain edema associated with a clinical picture of pseudotumor cerebri, intracranial calcification (basal ganglia, cerebellum, choroid plexus, vascular and perivascular in the white matter of the cerebral and cerebellar hemispheres, depth of the sulci), hypoplasia of enamel and dentine, blunting of dental roots, delayed or failure of eruption, thickening of the lamina dura, prominence of the dental membrane; (b) *bones:* generalized or focal areas of an increase in bone density; demineralization (very rare); premature closure of the epiphyseal growth plates; undertubulation of the metacarpals; bandlike irregular area of increased density in the metaphyseal regions, iliac crest, and vertebral bodies; spinal changes simulating those of ankylosing spondylitis; periosteal reaction; (c) soft-tissue calcification (skin, muscle); (d) gastrointestinal system: hypersecretion, spasm, pseudoobstruction; (e) cardiomegaly, congestive heart failure (Figs ME-H-21 and ME-H-22).

REFERENCES

Ahn TG, et al.: Familial isolated hypoparathyroidism: A molecular genetic analysis of 8 families with 23 affected persons. *Medicine (Baltimore)* 65:73, 1986.

Aryanpur I, et al.: Congestive heart failure secondary to idiopathic hypoparathyroidism. *Am. J. Dis. Child.* 127:738, 1974.

Bainbridge R, et al.: Transient congenital hypoparathyroidism: How transient is it? *J. Pediatr.* 111:866, 1987.

Barakat AY, et al.: Familial nephrosis, nerve deafness, and hypoparathyroidism. *J. Pediatr.* 91:61, 1977.

Bhimani S, et al.: Computed tomography of cerebrovascular calcifications in postsurgical hypoparathyroidism. *J. Comput. Assist. Tomogr.* 9:121, 1985.

Carpenter TO, et al.: Hypoparathyroidism in Wilson's disease. *N. Engl. J. Med.* 309:873, 1983.

Dahlberg PJ, et al.: Autosomal or X-linked recessive syndrome of congenital lymphedema, hypoparathyroidism, nephropathy, prolapsing mitral valve, and brachytelephalangy. *Am. J. Med. Genet.* 16:99, 1983.

DeCarvalho A, et al.: Idiopathic hypoparathyroidism (IHP). *Skeletal Radiol.* 15:52, 1986.

Duran MJ, et al.: Concurrent renal hypomagnesemia and hypoparathyroidism with normal parathormone responsiveness. *Am. J. Med.* 76:151, 1984.

Hanukoglu A, et al.: Late-onset hypocalcemia, rickets, and hypoparathyroidism in an infant of a mother with hyperparathyroidism. *J. Pediatr.* 112:751, 1988.

Illum F, et al.: Prevalences of CT-detected calcification in the basal ganglia in idiopathic hypoparathyroidism and pseudohypoparathyroidism. *Neuroradiology* 27:32, 1985.

Koening R, et al.: Hypoparathyroidism with partial monosomy 10p. *J. Pediatr.* 111:310, 1987.

Kruse K, et al.: Hypocalcemic myopathy in idiopathic hypoparathyroidism. *Eur. J. Pediatr.* 138:280, 1982.

Lyles KW, et al.: The concurrence of hypoparathyroidism provides new insights to the pathophysiology of X-linked hypophosphatemic rickets. *J. Clin. Endocrinol. Metab.* 60:711, 1985.

Mallette LE, et al.: Transient congenital hypoparathyroidism: Possible association with anomalies of the pulmonary valve. *J. Pediatr.* 101:928, 1982.

Martins L, et al.: Asymptomatic autosomal dominant hypoparathyroidism in six family members of a symptomatic infant. *J. Pediatr.* 106:167, 1985.

Mateo D, et al.: Dementia in idiopathic hypoparathyroidism. Rapid efficacy of alfacalcidol. *Arch. Neurol.* 39:424, 1982.

Mor F, et al.: Evidence on computed tomography of pseudotumour cerebri in hypoparathyroidism. *Br. J. Radiol.* 61:158, 1988.

Nusynowitz ML, et al.: The spectrum of the parathyroid states: A classification based on physiologic principles. *Medicine (Baltimore)* 55:105, 1976.

Rosen RA, et al.: Growth arrest recovery lines in hypoparathyroidism. *Radiology* 155:61, 1985.

Schutt-Aîné JC, et al.: Hypoparathyroidism: A possible cause of rickets. *J. Pediatr.* 106:255, 1985.

Taybi H, Keele D: Hypoparathyroidism: A review of the literature and report of two cases in sisters, one with steatorrhea and intestinal pseudo-obstruction. *A.J.R.* 88:432, 1962.

Tsang RC, et al.: Pediatric parathyroid disorders. *Pediatr. Clin. North Am.* 26:223, 1979.

Winter WE, et al.: Autosomal dominant hypoparathyroidism with variable, age-dependent severity. *J. Pediatr.* 103:387, 1983.

HYPOPHOSPHATASIA

Synonym: Rathbun disease.

Mode of Inheritance: Autosomal dominant (adult form); autosomal recessive (infantile and childhood forms).

Clinical Manifestations: (a) *severe congenital form:* manifestations present at birth: *globular "boneless" skull, severe deformities and shortness of the limbs,* skin dimple over the sites of angulation of the long bones, blue sclerae, *stillborn or often death soon after birth,* some may survive and fall into the pattern of group b; (b) *infantile form:* onset of symptoms after the first month of life: *anorexia, vomiting, constipation, failure to thrive, fever of unknown origin, irritability, convulsions, cyanotic episodes, loud cries, dehydration, wide cranial sutures, bulging fontanelle, angulation of limbs;* (c) *childhood form:* often discovered in early childhood—*delayed onset of walking, weakness, painful limbs, dental caries, premature loss of deciduous teeth;* (d) *adult form:* bone pain, tendency to fractures.

Laboratory Findings: (a) low or absent serum alkaline phosphate activity (total and bone fraction); (b) increased blood and urine levels of phosphoethanolamine and inorganic pyrophosphate; (c) hypercalcemia in severe forms; (d) prenatal diagnosis: first trimester diagnosis with a monoclonal antibody to the liver/bone/kidney isoenzyme of alkaline phos-

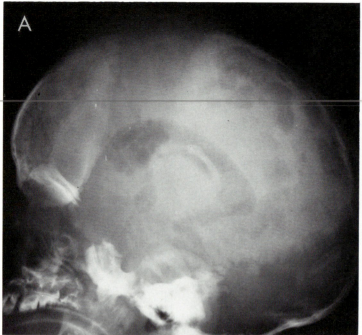
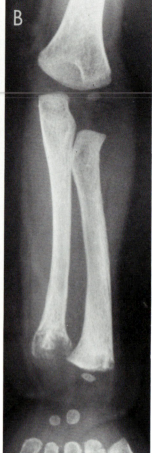

FIG ME—H—23.
Hypophosphatasia. **A,** wide sutures, irregular mineralization of the calvaria, and normal ventricular size in a 6½-month-old girl who had a bulging fontanelle. Her serum phosphorus concentration was 4.6 mg/dL; calcium, 10.5 mg/dL and alkaline phosphatase, 1.0 Bodansky units. **B,** coarse trabecular pattern, irregular ossification of the metaphyseal regions, and a deep cup-shaped defect of ossification in the ulnar metaphysis noted at 14 months of age. (From Taybi H, Kane P: Hypophosphatasia and hyperphosphatasia, In Newton TH, Potts DG (eds.): *Radiology of the Skull and Brain.* St. Louis, C.V. Mosby Co., 1971, vol. 1, p. 674. Used by permission.)

phatase (chorionic villus sample), alkaline phosphatase in amniotic fluid cell culture.

Radiologic Manifestations: (a) prenatal: failure to observe a fetal head by 16 weeks' gestation, increased echogenicity of the falx cerebri in association with poor mineralization of the skull, shortness and bowing of the poorly mineralized tubular bones, fractures, increased amniotic fluid volume; (b) *severe congenital form: marked retardation of skeletal ossification,* partial or complete absence of calcium deposits in the cranial vault, partial ossification of the base of the skull and facial bones, poor and irregularly ossified skeleton with some bones not ossified at all, *multiple fractures;* (c) *infantile form: defective skeletal mineralization,* in particular, in the growing ends of bones with *irregular ossification of the metaphyses* and a coarse trabecular pattern; *wide cranial sutures;* may develop premature closure of cranial sutures; (d) *childhood form:* mild to moderate *rachitic changes,* premature closure of sutures rare; (e) *adult form: osteoporosis;* (f) other reported abnormalities: slender bones, defect in the central metaphyseal region of the distal segments of the femora, epiphyseal defects, S-shaped configuration of the tibias, abnormal configuration of the distal phalanges, partial pre-

mature fusion of the epiphyses, wedging of the lower thoracic and upper lumbar vertebrae, premature closure of cranial sutures (early scintigraphic detection by a demonstration of increased abnormal activity along the suture lines), loss of the lamina dura, premature tooth loss, nephrocalcinosis, articular chondrocalcinosis, calcification of the ligaments and intervertebral disks (Fig ME—H—23).

REFERENCES

Currarino G: Hypophosphatasia, in Kaufmann HJ (ed.): *Progress in Pediatric Radiology.* Basel, S. Karger AG, 1973, vol. 4, p. 469.

Fallon MD, et al.: Hypophosphatasia: Clinicopathologic comparison of the infantile, childhood, and adult forms. *Medicine (Baltimore)* 63:12, 1984.

Kozlowski K, et al.: Hypophosphatasia: Review of 24 cases. *Pediatr. Radiol.* 5:103, 1976.

Laughlin CL, et al.: The prominent falx cerebri: New ultrasonic observation in hypophosphatasia. *J. Clin. Ultrasound* 10:37, 1982.

Pinquier JL, et al.: Hypophosphatasie de l'adulte révélée par une chondrocalcinose articulaire isolée. *Presse Med.* 15:1976, 1986.

Rathbun JC: "Hypophosphatasia," new developmental anomaly. *Am. J. Dis. Child.* 75:822, 1948.

Royce PM, et al.: Lethal osteogenesis imperfecta: Abnormal collagen metabolism and biochemical characteristics of hypophosphatasia. *Eur. J. Pediatr.* 147:626, 1988.

Sty JR, et al.: Skull scintigraphy in infantile hypophosphatasia. *J. Nucl. Med.* 20:305, 1979.

Warren RC, et al.: First trimester diagnosis of hypophosphatasia with a monoclonal antibody to the liver/bone/kidney isoenzyme of alkaline phosphatase. *Lancet* 2:856, 1985.

Whyte MP, et al.: Infantile hypophosphatasia: Normalization of circulating bone alkaline phosphatase activity followed by skeletal remineralization. *J. Pediatr.* 108:82, 1986.

Wolff C, et al.: Hypophosphatasia congenita letalis. *Eur. J. Pediatr.* 138:197, 1982.

Yagel S, et al.: Imaging case of the month. *Am. J. Perinatol.* 2:261, 1985.

HYPOPITUITARISM (ANTERIOR LOBE)

Classification: (a) hypothalamic lesions; (b) destruction of the gland (trauma, surgery, tumor, infection, granulomas, irradiation), amyloidosis, hemochromatosis (hypogonadotropic hypogonadism); (c) vascular diseases: infarction, postpartum necrosis, diabetes mellitus, collagen vascular lesions, sickle cell disease, aneurysm of the internal carotid artery; (d) idiopathic; (e) familial (autosomal recessive and X-linked recessive); (f) congenital absence of pituitary gland.

Hormonal Deficiencies: (a) somatotrope (growth hormone); (b) lactotrope (prolactin); (c) thyrotrope (thyroid-stimulating hormone); (d) gonadotrope: follicle-stimulating hormone, luteinizing hormone; (e) corticotrope: adrenocorticotropic hormone (ACTH), β-lipotropin, β-endorphin.

Clinical Manifestations: Various combinations of hormonal deficiencies may be present with corresponding clinical manifestations:

(A) *Congenital absence of the pituitary gland:* (a) *apnea, cyanosis, prolonged hypoglycemia,* microphthalmos, micropenis, cryptorchidism; (b) absence or hypoplasia of the sella turcica; (c) hyperbilirubinemia.

(B) *Prepubertal (Lorain-type dwarfism):* (a) *short stature, normal body proportions, infantile cranial proportions;* (b) *high-pitched voice;* (c) *poor dentition, crowding and impaction of teeth;* (d) *underdevelopment of secondary sex characteristics.*

(C) *Adults:* (a) ACTH deficiency: weakness, weight loss, dizziness, headaches, hair loss, hypotension, dehydration, hypoglycemia, etc.; (b) thyroid-stimulating hormone (TSH) deficiency: tiredness, paresthesia of the extremities, hair loss, dry skin, constipation, etc.; (c) gonadotropins: amenorrhea, decreased libido, impotence, skin wrinkles, hair loss, etc.; (d) pituitary apoplexy: symptoms simulating meningitis or subarachnoid hemorrhage.

(D) *Association with conditions:* Sensorineural deafness in congenital hypopituitarism; postaxial polydactyly; dental

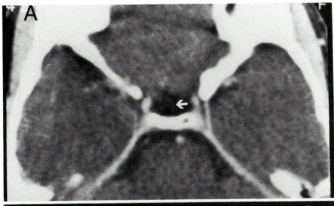

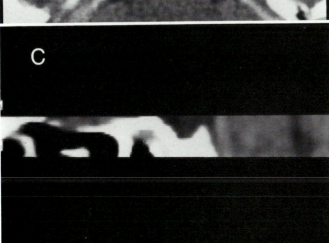

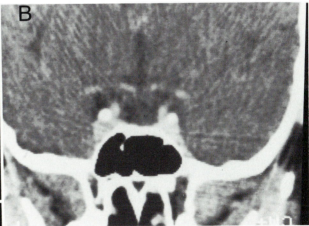

FIG ME–H–24.
Hypopituitarism (pituitary dwarfism): axial **(A)**, coronal **(B)**, and reformed sagittal **(C)** computed tomographic scans. The pituitary gland cannot be seen, but a faint stalk *(arrow)* is evident. (From Inoue Y, Nemoto Y, Fujita K, et al.: Pituitary dwarfism: CT evaluation of the pituitary gland. *Radiology* 159:171, 1986. Used by permission.)

malformations (upper incisors); midline facial anomalies; de Morsier syndrome; cleft palate/lip; holoprosencephaly; Rothmund-Thomson syndrome; primary empty-sella syndrome; Turner syndrome; Silver-Russell syndrome; Reiger syndrome; Pallister-Hall syndrome; acquired anhaptoglobinemia in panhypopituitarism (Sheehan syndrome); X-linked hypogammaglobulinemia and isolated growth hormone deficiency (Fleischer syndrome); etc.

Radiologic Manifestations:

(A) Prepubertal: (a) *relatively large cranial vault in relation to the facial bones,* small sella turcica volume, large sellar volume (empty sella), lack of demonstration of the pituitary gland or stalk or a small gland in pituitary dwarfism (computed imaging); (b) *marked delay in eruption of teeth;* (c) *skeletal maturation retardation,* with more severe retardation seen in carpal bones than in the epiphyses of the tubular bones; (d) absence of growth lines in the tubular bones; (e) osteoporosis (in growth hormone deficiency); (f) delayed ossification of the marginal epiphyses of the vertebrae, relative platyspondyly, slipped capital femoral epiphysis; (g) craniopharyngioma, cyst, etc.

(B) *Adults:* (a) pituitary stone, enlarged sella turcica related to a tumor; (b) calcification of the auricular cartilage; (c) neuroradiological investigations of intrasellar and parasellar lesions (Fig ME–H–24).

REFERENCES

Abboud CF: Laboratory diagnosis of hypopituitarism. *Mayo Clin. Proc.* 61:35, 1986.

Ahmadi J, et al.: Ischemic chiasmal syndrome and hypopituitarism associated with progressive cerebrovascular occlusive disease. *A.J.N.R.* 5:367, 1984.

Barkan A, et al.: Calcification of auricular cartilages in patients with hypopituitarism. *J. Clin. Endocrinol. Metab.* 55:354, 1982.

Boudailliez B, et al.: Panhypopituitarisme (révélé par une hyponatrémie) dans les suites immediates d'un traumatisme crânien. *Ann. Pediatr. (Paris)* 32:461, 1985.

Cazzola M, et al.: Juvenile idiopathic haemochromatosis: A life-threatening disorder presenting as hypogonadotropic hypogonadism. *Hum. Genet.* 65:149, 1983.

Culler FL, et al.: Hypopituitarism in association with postaxial polydactyly. *J. Pediatr.* 104:881, 1984.

Delcros B, et al.: Déficit en hormone de croissance et selle turcique vide primitive chez l'enfant. *Ann. Pediatr. (Paris)* 35:123, 1988.

De Luca F, et al.: Sensorineural deafness in congenital hypopituitarism with severe hypothyroidism. *Acta Paediatr. Scand.* 74:148, 1985.

Fitz-Patrick D, et al.: Pituitary apoplexy: The importance of skull roentgenograms and computerized tomography in diagnosis. *J.A.M.A.* 244:59, 1980.

Fleischer TA, et al.: X-linked hypogammaglobulinemia and isolated growth hormone deficiency. *N. Engl. J. Med.* 302:1457, 1980.

Hernandez R, et al.: Hand radiographic measurements in growth hormone deficiency before and after treatment. *A.J.R.* 129:487, 1977.

Hernandez RJ, et al.: Size and skeletal maturation of the hand in children with hypothyroidism and hyperpituitarism. *A.J.R.* 133:405, 1979.

Hernandez RJ, et al.: Incidence of growth lines in psychosocial dwarfs and idiopathic hypopituitarism. *A.J.R.* 131:477, 1978.

Inoue Y, et al.: Pituitary dwarfism: CT evaluation of the pituitary gland. *Radiology* 159:171, 1986.

Kaufmann S, et al.: Growth hormone deficiency in the Rothmund-Thomson syndrome. *Am. J. Med. Genet.* 23:861, 1986.

Kuriyama M, et al.: Acquired anhaptoglobinemia in panhypopituitarism. *Am. J. Med.* 78:850, 1985.

Laron Z: Pituitary insufficiency in cleft palate or lip (letter). *Am. J. Med. Genet.* 24:547, 1986.

Las MS, et al.: Hypopituitarism associated with systemic amyloidosis. *N.Y. State Med.* 83:1183, 1983.

LeMay M: The radiologic diagnosis of pituitary disease. *Radiol. Clin. North Am.* 5:303, 1967.

Liapi CH, et al.: Les malformations dentaires et faciales associées à l'insuffisance hypophysaire en hormone de croissance. *Arch. Fr. Pediatr.* 42:829, 1985.

McArthur RG, et al.: The natural history of familial hypopituitarism. *Am. J. Med. Genet.* 22:553, 1985.

Omar FB, et al.: Nanismes hypophysaires de types familiaux. A propos de 7 familles en Algérie Ouest. *Helv. Paediat. Acta* 41:31, 1986.

Rappaport EB, et al.: Slipped capital femoral epiphysis in growth hormone–deficient patients. *Am. J. Dis. Child.* 139:396, 1985.

Rappaport R, et al.: Aspects radiologiques irreguliers des métaphyses des doigts chez des enfants atteints d'insuffisance hypothalamo-hypophysaires. *Arch. Fr. Pediatr.* 26:1135, 1969.

Shulman DI, et al.: Hypothalamic-pituitary dysfunction in primary empty sella syndrome in childhood. *J. Pediatr.* 108:540, 1986.

Smith SP, et al.: Value of computed tomographic scanning in patients with growth hormone deficiency. *Pediatrics* 78:601, 1986.

Snyder PJ, et al.: Hypopituitarism following radiation therapy of pituitary adenomas. *Am. J. Med.* 81:457, 1986.

Taylor HC, et al.: Pituitary stones and associated hypopituitarism. *J.A.M.A.* 242:751, 1979.

Van den Broeck J, et al.: Prediction of final height in boys with non-tumorous hypopituitarism. *Eur. J. Pediatr.* 147:245, 1988.

van Gelderen HH, et al.: Familial isolated growth hormone deficiency. *Clin. Genet.* 20:173, 1981.

HYPOTHYROIDISM (ADULTS)

Clinical Manifestations: (a) *neuropsychiatric symptoms;* (b) *myxedema;* (c) *gastrointestinal symptoms:* bloating, flatulence, constipation, paralytic ileus, pseudo-obstruction; (d) heart: pericardial effusion, cardiac tamponade, myocardiopathy (abnormal left ventricular function, low cardiac output, reduced stroke volume, depressed contractility, reduced left ventricular ejection time and prolonged pre-ejection period, abnormal echocardiographic findings, e.g., asymmetrical thickening or hypertrophy of the interventricular septum, reduced left ventricular internal dimensions and outflow dimensions, reduced systolic septal excursion, etc.); (e) *myopathy of various severity* (delay in tendon reflexes, respiratory muscle weakness), Hoffmann syndrome (increased muscle mass, muscle stiffness, muscle weakness, low levels of serum thyroxine); (f) *joint effusion* with rheumatic signs, viscous joint fluid containing calcium pyrophosphate crystals; (g) *low levels of serum thyroxine, high levels of thyroid-stimulating hormone*, increased levels of serum creatinine phosphokinase; (h) other reported abnormalities: restless leg syndrome, urticaria in association with hypothyroidism, anemia (normochromic normocytic, hypochromic microcytic, or macrocytic), pseudotumor cerebri, abnormal gonadal function (infertility, impotence, etc.), myxedema coma, hyponatremia, increased plasma arginine vasopressin level, reduced micturition frequency, etc.

Radiologic Manifestations: (a) *skeletal system:* no significant bone changes with an onset in adulthood, joint effusion, chondrocalcinosis, popliteal cyst, rheumatoid manifestations, radiographic findings similar to juvenile hypothyroidism in adult cretinism; (b) *gastrointestinal system:* hypotonicity; acute or chronic paralytic ileus; loss of colonic haustrations (smooth colon); pseudo-obstruction, in particular, of the colon; cholestasis; biliary cirrhosis; (c) *ascites, pleural effusion, pericardial effusion, cardiac tamponade;* (d) pituitary hyperplasia secondary to thyroid failure; (e) cerebellar calcification.

HYPOTHYROIDISM (JUVENILE)

Clinical Manifestations: (a) sluggish behavior, growth retardation, infantile appearance, myxedema, recurrent respiratory infections; (b) head and neck: small face, large fontanelle, relative macrocephaly, widely separated eyes, puffy face, prognathism, underdeveloped jaw, delay in shedding primary teeth and in eruption of permanent teeth, macroglossia, thick neck; (c) failure of development of secondary sex characteristics or precocious sexual development, vaginal bleeding, adnexal masses (cystic ovaries), irregular menses, galactorrhea, gynecomastia, bloody discharge from breasts, testicular enlargement, apparent "ambiguous genitalia"; (d) hypersensitivity to vitamin D, increased calcium absorption from the gastrointestinal tract, hypercalcemia, nephrocalcinosis, dystrophic calcium deposits; (e) pericardial effusion, cardiomyopathy, asymmetrical septal hypertrophy, myocardial dysfunction (echocardiography); (f) neurological disorders, ataxic syndrome, mental retardation; (g) secondary to or associated with other diseases: chronic lymphocytic thyroiditis, cystinosis (due to an accumulation of cystine crystals in the thyroid gland and tissue atrophy), Down syndrome, genetic factor in a limited number of familial cases, reversible hypocalciuric hypercalcemia associated with hypothyroidism, sensorineural hearing loss in sporadic congenital hypothyroidism, association with acquired von Willebrand disease; (h) Kocher-Debré-Sémélaigne syndrome (cretinism with muscular hypertrophy); (i) low levels of T_4 and T_3, high levels of thyroid-stimulating hormone (TSH), elevated cholesterol level, carotenemia, flat glucose tolerance curve, anemia, de-

pressed renal function; (j) ectopic thyroid tissue detected on an isotope study (in the midline of the neck, between the base of the tongue and aortic arch) in a high percentage of infants and children with hypothyroidism; (k) other reported abnormalities: transient hypothyroidism in infants following contrast angiocardiography, vasculitis associated with anemia and pulmonary cavitation during antithyroid drug therapy, pseudotumor cerebri following treatment of hypothyroidism, hypertrichosis, etc.

Radiologic Manifestations: (a) head: brachycephaly; flat forehead; wide sutures; late appearance of the diploic space and vascular markings; large fontanelle in infants; multiple wormian bones; short base of the skull; dense skull, in particular, at the base; sclerosis in the periorbital region; diminished angle between the nasal bones and frontal bone; enlarged sella turcica, often with a round appearance and well-defined margins ("cherry" sella); truncated anterior clinoid processes; vertical clivus; delayed closure of the synchondrosis at the base; delayed development of sinuses and pneumatization of the mastoids; premature craniosynostosis (a complication of thyroid replacement therapy); prominent obtuse mandibular angle; hyperplasia or microadenoma of the pituitary gland (computed tomography, magnetic resonance imaging), empty sella, cerebral atrophy in young congenital hypothyroid subjects; (b) trunk: flattened and hypoplastic vertebral bodies, wide disk spaces, dorsolumbar kyphosis, gibbus deformity associated with beaking of the lower dorsal and upper lumbar vertebrae, persistent segmentation of the sternum into adulthood, narrow pelvis with decreased pubic angle, vertical iliac wing, wide acetabular roof corresponding to a deformed femoral head; (c) limbs: delayed appearance and retarded growth of secondary ossification centers; "cretinoid epiphyseal dysgenesis" (irregular granular pattern of ossification, widening and flattening of the epiphyses); delayed closure of the growth plates; osteochondroses; slipping of the

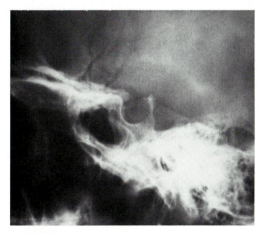

FIG ME–H–25.
Hypothyroidism: very round appearance of the sella ("cherry" sella) in an 8-year-old patient with untreated primary hypothyroidism from birth. (From Swischuk LE, Sarwar M: The sella in childhood hypothyroidism. *Pediatr. Radiol.* 6:1, 1977. Used by permission.)

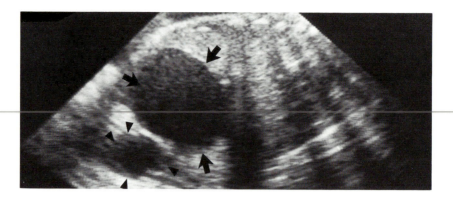

FIG ME–H–26.
Fetal ovarian cysts associated with hypothyroidism. A longitudinal sonogram of the fetus shows an 8 × 5-cm fluid-filled lower abdominal mass *(arrows)* separate from the fetal urinary bladder *(arrowheads)*. A serum thyroid screening profile drawn on the third day of life revealed a serum T₄ level of 8.4 μg/dL (normal, 15 to 16 μg/dL) and a serum TSH level of 54 μg/dL (normal, 20 μg/dL). (From Jafri SZH, Bree RL, Silver TM, et al.: Fetal ovarian cysts: Sonographic detection and association with hypothyroidism. *Radiology* 150:809, 1984. Used by permission.)

femoral head; shortening of long bones; associated thickening of the cortex and narrowing of the medullary canal; thick transverse bands in the shaft and metaphyses of long bones; increased density of the provisional zone of calcification; humerus varus; normal, stubby, or slender tubular bones of the hand; distal extension of an osseous projection from the midportion of the metaphyses of the distal phalanges; irregular ossification and fragmentation of the femoral head; short femoral neck; coxa vara; low calcaneal arch; shortened calcaneus; changes in the tubular bones of the foot similar to the hand; (d) nephrocalcinosis; (e) ovarian cysts with resolution in response to treatment of hypothyroidism; (f) teeth: primary teeth less affected, delay in shedding of primary teeth, delay in formation of secondary teeth, multiple dental caries; (g) heart: pericardial effusion, dilatation of the cardiac chambers, muscular hypertrophy.

HYPOTHYROIDISM (INFANTS)

Etiology: Thyroid agenesis or dysgenesis; congenital goiter due to maternal drug ingestion; genetic defects in thyroid hormone synthesis or metabolism; abnormal thyroxine-

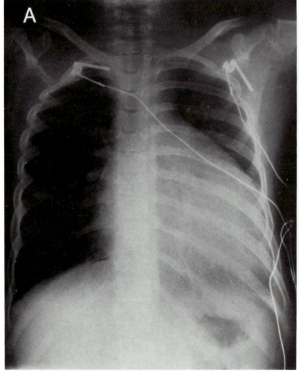

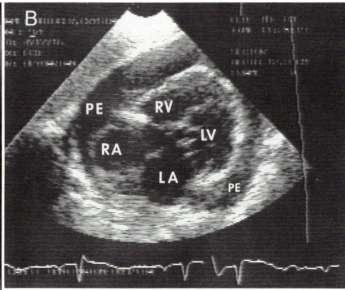

FIG ME–H–27.
A and **B** hypothyroidism, cardiac tymponade, and Down syndrome. The two-dimensional echocardiogram shows massive pericardial effusion *(PE)*. The patient also has an ostium primum atrial septal defect. Five hundred fifty milliliters of straw-colored fluid was drained. There was an excellent response to thyroid replacement therapy *(RV = right ventricle; LV = left ventricle; RA = right atrium; LA = left atrium)*. (From Heydarian M, Kelly PJ: Radiological case of the month. *AJDC* 141:641, 1987. Used by permission.)

binding globulin synthesis; congenital endemic goiter; familial transient hypothyroidism secondary to transplacental thyrotropin-blocking antibodies; transient primary hypothyroidism in sick premature newborns.

Clinical Manifestations: (a) *lethargy, respiratory distress, nasal stuffiness, noisy respiration, hoarse cry, feeding problems, constipation, intermittent cyanosis, persistent neonatal jaundice, distended abdomen, umbilical hernia;* (b) *facial features:* narrow forehead, puffy eyes, puffy cheeks, depressed nasal bridge, pug nose, protruding tongue, small mandible, delayed fontanelle closure, sparse hair, thick neck, redundancy of the skin of the neck; (c) *bradycardia;* hypotension; congenital heart block; increased circulation time; heart murmur; diminished T, P, and R waves; asymmetrical septal hypertrophy; (d) *hyponia,* hyporeflexia, persistent infantile reflexes, organic brain damage; (e) *myxedema, hair and nail abnormalities;* (f) *depressed basal metabolic rate;* (g) *low levels of T_4 and T_3 and high levels of thyroid-stimulating hormone in cord serum,* serum thyroglobulin assay (good correlation with thyroid scintigraphy and ultrasonography) in athyroid infants; (h) other reported abnormalities: hypercalcemia, polycythemia, galactorrhea, infantile hypothyroidism in siblings (an unusual presentation of pseudohypoparathyroidism, type Ia), spiky-hair syndrome in brothers (spiky hair, cleft lip and palate, choanal atresia, hypoplastic epiglottis and larynx, long tortuous eyelashes, and undetectable thyroid tissue on an ^{132}I scan), chromosome abnormalities (trisomy 9, trisomy 21), congenital heart disease, meningocele, etc.

Radiologic Manifestations: (a) normal or slightly retarded bone age at birth, *delayed skeletal maturation and long bone growth in the postnatal period;* (b) *epiphyseal dysgenesis, increased bone density, poor cortical bone differentiation,* congenital vertebral anomalies (partial absence of the vertebral bodies, hemivertebrae, abnormal rib-vertebral articulations), abnormal segmentation of the ribs; (c) thickening of precervical soft tissues; (d) mild cardiomegaly; (e) thyroid ultrasonography: accurate in the absence of the thyroid from the normal site, not accurate in ectopic thyroid tissue detection; (f) thyroid scintigraphy: localization of ectopic tissue, absence of thyroid activity, etc; (g) sonographic detection of fetal ovarian cysts (Figs ME–H–25 to ME–H–27).

REFERENCES

Altman DI, et al.: Asymmetric septal hypertrophy and hypothyroidism in children. *Br. Heart J.* 54:533, 1985.
Andersen LF, et al.: Micturition pattern in hyperthyroidism and hypothyroidism. *Urology* 29:223, 1987.
Archambeaud-Mouveroux F, et al.: Coma myxoedémateux avec hypervasopressinisme. Deux observations. *Ann. Med. Interne. (Paris)* 138:114, 1987.
Ariza CR, et al.: Hypothyroidism-associated cholestasis. *J.A.M.A.* 252:2392, 1984.
Bamforth JS, et al.: Congenital anomalies associated with hypothyroidism. *Arch. Dis. Child.* 61:608, 1986.
Barnett SH, et al.: Redundancy of the skin of the neck as a sign of congenital hypothyroidism. *Am. J. Dis. Child.* 141:477, 1987.
Bellini MA, et al.: The skull in childhood myxedema: Its roentgen appearance. *A.J.R.* 76:495, 1956.
Borg SA, et al.: Roentgenologic aspects of adult cretinism: Two case reports and review of the literature. *A.J.R.* 123:820, 1975.
Burke JW, et al.: "Idiopathic" cerebellar calcifications: Association with hypothyroidism? *Radiology* 167:533, 1988.
Burrell M, et al.: Myxedema megacolon. *Gastrointest. Radiol.* 5:181, 1980.
Burt L, et al.: Head circumference in children with short stature secondary to primary hypothyroidism. *Pediatrics* 59:628, 1977.
Cassorla FG, et al.: Vasculitis, pulmonary cavitation, and anemia during antithyroid drug therapy. *Am. J. Dis. Child.* 137:118, 1983.
Contis G, et al.: Cardiac manifestations of congenital hypothyroidism in infants. *Pediatrics* 38:452, 1966.
Dalton RG, et al.: Hypothyroidism as a cause of acquired von Willebrand's disease. *Lancet* 1:1007, 1987.
Dammacco F, et al.: Serum thyroglobulin and thyroid ultrasound studies in infants with congenital hypothyroidism. *J. Pediatr.* 106:451, 1985.
Daudet M, et al.: Les lésions de la hanche au cours du myxoedème congénital chez l'enfant. *Chir. Pediatr.* 27:94, 1986.
Dorwart BB, et al.: Joint effusion, chondrocalcinosis and other rheumatoid manifestations in hypothyroidism. A clinicopathologic study. *Am. J. Med.* 59:780, 1975.
Elta GH, et al.: Increased incidence of hypothyroidism in primary biliary cirrhosis. *Dig. Dis. Sci.* 28:971, 1983.
Farooki ZQ, et al.: Myocardial dysfunction in hypothyroid children. *Am. J. Dis. Child.* 137:65, 1983.
Floyd JL, et al.: Pituitary hyperplasia secondary to thyroid failure: CT appearance. *A.J.N.R.* 5:469, 1984.
Francis G, et al.: Congenital familial transient hypothyroidism secondary to transplacental thyrotropin-blocking autoantibodies. *Am. J. Dis. Child.* 141:1081, 1987.
Grünebaum M, et al.: Hypothyroidism in cystinosis. *A.J.R.* 129:629, 1977.
Hagberg B, et al.: Ataxic syndrome in congenital hypothyroidism. *Acta Paediatr. Scand.* 59:323, 1970.
Hennessy MJ, et al.: Slipped capital femoral epiphysis in a hypothyroid adult male. *Clin. Orthop.* 165:204, 1982.
Hernandez RJ, et al.: Distinctive appearance of the distal phalanges in children with primary hypothyroidism. *Radiology* 132:83, 1979.
Heydarian M, et al.: Cardiac tamponade heralding hypothyroidism in Down's syndrome. *Am. J. Dis. Child.* 141:642, 1987.
Ichiya Y, et al.: Coexistence of a nonfunctioning thyroid nodule in Plummer's disease demonstrated by thallium-201 imaging. *Clin. Nucl. Med.* 13:117, 1988.
Jafri SZH, et al.: Fetal ovarian cysts: Sonographic detection and association with hypothyroidism. *Radiology* 150:809, 1984.
Jawadi MH, et al.: Primary hypothyroidism and pituitary enlargement. *Arch. Intern. Med.* 138:1555, 1978.
Kaplan M, et al.: Hypothyroidism due to ectopy in siblings. *Am. J. Dis. Child.* 131:1264, 1977.
Klein I, et al.: Hypothyroidism presenting as muscle stiffness and pseudohypertrophy: Hoffmann's syndrome. *Am. J. Med.* 70:891, 1981.

Klein I, et al.: Unusual manifestations of hypothyroidism. *Arch. Intern. Med.* 144:123, 1984.

Klein RZ: Infantile hypothyroidism then and now: The results of neonatal screening. *Curr. Probl. Pediatr.* 15:5, 1985.

Kulaylat NA, et al.: Transient primary hypothyroidism in prematures. *Clin. Pediatr.* 26:339, 1987.

Lanigan SW, et al.: Association between urticaria and hypothyroidism. *Lancet* 1:1476, 1984.

Laron Z, et al.: Juvenile hypothyroidism with testicular enlargement. *Acta Paediatr. Scand.* 59:317, 1970.

Léger J, et al.: Hypothyroïdie congénitale ou néonatale avec ≪TSH papier de dépistage≫ inférieur a 50 µU/mL. *Arch. Fr. Pediatr.* 44:13, 1987.

Levine MA, et al.: Infantile hypothyroidism in two sibs: An unusual presentation of pseudohypoparathyroidism type Ia. *J. Pediatr.* 107:919, 1985.

Lintermans JP, et al.: Hypothyroidism and vertebral anomalies. A new syndrome? *A.J.R.* 109:294, 1970.

Macaron C: Galactorrhea and neonatal hypothyroidism. *J. Pediatr.* 101:576, 1982.

Manolis AS, et al.: Hypothyroid cardiac tamponade. *Arch. Intern. Med.* 147:1167, 1987.

McVie R: Abnormal TSH regulation, pseudotumor cerebri, and empty sella after replacement therapy in juvenile hypothyroidism. *J. Pediatr.* 105:768, 1984.

Nishi Y, et al.: Pituitary abnormalities detected by high resolution computed tomography with thin slices in primary hypothyroidism and Turner syndrome. *Eur. J. Pediatr.* 142:25, 1984.

Nishi Y, et al.: Primary hypothyroidism associated with pituitary enlargement, slipped capital femoral epiphysis and cystic ovaries. *Eur. J. Pediatr.* 143:216, 1985.

Penfold JL, et al.: Premature craniosynostosis—a complication of thyroid replacement therapy. *J. Pediatr.* 86:360, 1975.

Pöyhönen L, et al.: Ultrasonography in congenital hypothyreosis. *Acta Paediatr. Scand.* 73:523, 1984.

Press OW, et al.: Pseudotumor cerebri and hypothyroidism. *Arch. Intern. Med.* 143:167, 1983.

Puri R, et al.: Slipped upper femoral epiphysis and primary juvenile hypothyroidism. *J. Bone Joint Surg. [Br.]* 67:14, 1985.

Ramayya MV, et al.: Hypothyroidism and apparent 'ambiguous genitalia.' *Am. J. Dis. Child.* 136:464, 1982.

Richard GE, et al.: Combined hypothyroidism and hypoparathyroidism in an infant after maternal ^{131}I administration. *J. Pediatr.* 99:141, 1981.

Riddlesberger MM Jr, et al.: The association of juvenile hypothyroidism and cystic ovaries. *Radiology* 139:77, 1981.

Rohn R: Pseudotumor cerebri following treatment of hypothyroidism. *Am. J. Dis. Child.* 139:752, 1985.

Röhner G, et al.: Transient hypothyroidism in infants following contrast angiocardiography. *Rontgenpraxis* 36:301, 1983.

Santos AD, et al.: The cardiomyopathy of hypothyroidism revisited: Are children different than adults? *Am. J. Dis. Child.* 134:547, 1980.

Schlienger JL: Syndrome des membres inférieurs impatients dû à une hypothyroïdie modérée. *Presse Med.* 14:791, 1985.

Smith DW, et al.: Congenital hypothyroidism—signs and symptoms in the newborn period. *J. Pediatr.* 87:958, 1975.

Stern SR, et al.: Hypertrichosis due to primary hypothyroidism. *Arch. Dis. Child.* 60:763, 1985.

Swischuk LE, et al.: The sella in childhood hypothyroidism. *Pediatr. Radiol.* 6:1, 1977.

Tau C, et al.: Hypercalcemia in infants with congenital hypothyroidism and its relation to vitamin D and thyroid hormones. *J. Pediatr.* 109:808, 1986.

Thévenon A, et al.: Le retentissement osseux de l'hypothyroïdie chez l'adulte. A propos de 20 patients. *Ann. Med. Interne (Paris)* 137:212, 1986.

Tomei E, et al.: La diagnostica per immagini nello studio dell'ipofisi nell' ipotiroidismo congenito. *Radiol. Med.* 74:39, 1987.

Tümay SB, et al.: Skeletal changes and nephrocalcinosis in a case of athyreosis. *Arch. Dis. Child.* 37:543, 1962.

Vanderschueren-Lodeweyckx M, et al.: Sensorineural hearing loss in sporadic congenital hypothyroidism. *Arch. Dis. Child.* 58:419, 1983.

Virtanen M: Manifestations of congenital hypothyroidism during the 1st week of life. *Eur. J. Pediatr.* 147:270, 1988.

Walmsley D, et al.: Pituitary size in hypothyroidism as determined by computed tomography. *Br. J. Radiol.* 60:935, 1987.

Weinblatt ME, et al.: Polycythemia in hypothyroid infants. *Am. J. Dis. Child.* 141:1121, 1987.

Weiner M, et al.: Reversible respiratory muscle weakness in hypothyroidism. *Br. J. Dis. Chest* 80:391, 1986.

Wells RG, et al.: Technetium 99m pertechnetate thyroid scintigraphy: Congenital hypothyroid screening. *Pediatr. Radiol.* 16:368, 1986.

Wietersen FK, et al.: The radiologic aspects of thyroid disease. *Radiol. Clin. North Am.* 5:255, 1967.

Williams LHP, et al.: Massive pericardial effusion in a hypothyroid child. *Br. Heart J.* 51:231, 1984.

Wortsman J, et al.: Abnormal testicular function in men with primary hypothyroidism. *Am. J. Med.* 82:207, 1987.

Zaloga G, et al.: Reversible hypocalciuric hypercalcemia associated with hypothyroidism. *Am. J. Med.* 77:1101, 1984.

IMMUNE DISORDERS

Immune Disorders and the Syndromes Associated With Them: See Tables ME–I–1 and ME–I–2.

Clinical and Radiologic Manifestations:

(A) Skeletal system: (a) immune deficiency and short-limb dwarfism: bowing of the long bones, autosomal recessive, recurrent pulmonary infections, diarrhea, moniliasis, lymphopenia, reduced immunoglobulin concentrations, flaring of rib ends, metaphyseal chondrodysplasia, short and stubby pelvic bones, flat acetabular roofs, decrease in the vertical height of vertebral bodies, etc.; (b) severe combined immunodeficiency and adenosine deaminase deficiency: autosomal recessive, recurrent infections, irregularity of the metaphyseal ends of long bones, splayed metaphyses, metaphyseal spurs perpendicular to the long axis of bones, short ribs, cup-shaped costochondral junctions, "bone-within-bone" appearance of the vertebral bodies, central beaking of the lower thoracic vertebrae, mild platyspondyly, square-shaped iliac wings, flat acetabular roofs, irregular iliac crests, narrow sciatic notches, absence of a thymic shadow on chest roentgenogram.

(B) Alimentary system: intestinal nodular lymphoid hyper-

TABLE ME–I–1.

Classification of Primary Immunodeficiency Diseases (Lymphocyte Abnormalities Only)*

Disorder	Functional Deficiencies	Presumed Cellular Level of Defect
X-linked agammaglobulinemia	Antibody	Pre-B cell
Common variable (acquired) hypogammaglobulinemia	Antibody	B lymphocyte
Selective IgA deficiency	IgA antibody	IgA B lymphocyte
Secretory component deficiency	Secretory IgA	Mucosal epithelium
Selective IgM deficiency	IgM antibody	T-helper cells
Immunodeficiency with elevated IgM levels	IgG and IgA antibodies	IgG, IgA B lymphocytes; "switch" T cells
Transient hypogammaglobulinemia of infancy	None; immunoglobulin levels low but antibodies present	Unknown
Antibody deficiency with near-normal immunoglobulin levels	Antibody	Unknown; B cell?
X-linked lymphoproliferative disease	Anti–Epstein-Barr virus nuclear antigen antibody	B cell; also T cell?
DiGeorge syndrome	T cellular; some antibody	Dysmorphogenesis of 3rd and 4th branchial pouches
Nezelof syndrome (including purine nucleoside phosphorylase deficiency)	T cellular; some antibody	Unknown; thymus?; T-cell metabolic defects?
Severe combined immunodeficiency syndromes (autosomal recessive adenosine deaminase deficiency, X-linked recessive, defective expression of HLA antigens, reticular dysgenesis)	Antibody and T cellular; phagocytic in reticular dysgenesis	Unknown; metabolic defect(s); T cell?; stem cell?; thymus?; regulatory gene defects
Wiskott-Aldrich syndrome	Antibody; T cellular	Unknown
Ataxia-telangiectasia	Antibody; T cellular	B lymphocyte; helper T lymphocyte
Cartilage-hair hypoplasia	T cellular	G_1 cycle of many cells
Immunodeficiency with thymoma	Antibody; some T cellular	B lymphocyte; excessive T-suppressor cells
Hyperimmunoglobulinemia E	Specific immune responses; excessive IgE	Unknown
Lymphocyte function antigen 1 deficiency	Cytotoxic cells; phagocytic cells	95-kilodalton molecular weight β-chain of lymphocyte function antigen 1, complement receptor type 3, and p150,95

*From Buckley RH: Immunodeficiency diseases. *J.A.M.A.* 258:2841, 1987. Used by permission.

TABLE ME−I−2.

Immunodeficiency Syndromes *Sensu Strictu* and Syndromes With Immunodeficiency

Immunodeficiency syndromes
    X-linked agammaglobulinemia
    X-linked agammaglobulinemia with hyper-IgE
    Late-onset agammaglobulinemia
    Transient hypogammaglobulinemia of infancy
    Deficiency of C1 esterase inhibitor
    Deficiency of "late" complement components
    Selective IgA deficiency
    "Lazy leukocyte" syndrome
    Duncan syndrome
Immunodeficiency syndromes/syndromes with
    immunodeficiency
    Chronic granulomatous disease
    Chronic mucocutaneous candidiasis
    Severe combined immunodeficiency
Syndromes with immunodeficiency
    DiGeorge syndrome
    Wiskott-Aldrich syndrome
    Ataxia-telangiectasia (Louis-Bar syndrome)
    Short-limbed dwarfism
    Cartilage-hair hypoplasia
    Chédiak-Higashi syndrome
    Hyper-IgE syndrome
    Acrodermatitis enteropathica
    Protein-losing enteropathy
    Whittaker syndrome
    Transcobalamin II deficiency
    Defects of "early" complement components
    Down syndrome
    Bloom syndrome
    Malnutrition
    Wiedemann-Beckwith syndrome
    Shwachman syndrome
    Menkes syndrome
    Xeroderma pigmentosum

*Modified from Burgio GR, Ugazio AG: Immunodeficiency and syndromes: A nosographic approach. *Eur. J. Pediatr.* 138:288, 1982. Used by permission.

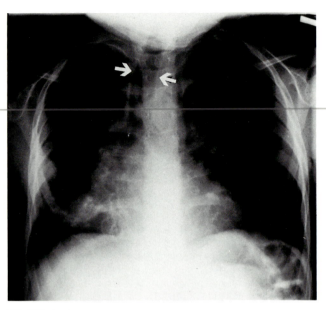

FIG ME−I−1.
Severe combined immune deficiency in a 7-year-old female. Note the tracheomegaly *(arrows).* (Courtesy of George R. Barnes, M.D., Tucson.)

syndrome, cartilage-hair hypoplasia (metaphyseal chondrodysplasia—McKusick), chronic granulomatous disease, DiGeorge syndrome, hyperimmunoglobulin E syndrome, Whittaker syndrome, Wiskott-Aldrich syndrome (Fig ME−I−1).

REFERENCES

Ammann AJ, et al.: Antibody-mediated immunodefiency in short-limbed dwarfism. *J. Pediatr.* 84:200, 1974.

Beall GN: Immunologic aspects of endocrine diseases. *J.A.M.A.* 258:2952, 1987.

Bersani D, et al.: Hyperplasie lymphoïde nodulaire. Forme diffuse étendue du bulbe duodénal au rectum, associée a une agammaglobulinémie. *J. Radiol.* 65:863, 1984.

Buckley RH: Immunodeficiency diseases. *J.A.M.A.* 258:2841, 1987.

Burgio GR, et al.: Immunodeficiency and syndromes: A nosographic approach. *Eur. J. Pediatr.* 138:288, 1982.

Chandra RK, et al.: Severe combined immunodeficiency associated with adenosine deaminase deficiency. *Am. J. Dis. Child.* 132:621, 1978.

Garel L, et al.: Dilatation biliaire et deficit immunitaire chez l'enfant. Une série de quatre cas. *Ann. Radiol. (Paris)* 28:249, 1985.

Hass A, et al.: Hoarseness in immunocompromised children: Association with invasive fungal infection. *J. Pediatr.* 111:731, 1987.

Hausser C, et al.: Common variable hypogammaglobulinemia in children. Clinical and immunologic observations in 30 patients. *Am. J. Dis. Child.* 137:833, 1983.

Herman TE, et al.: Radiology of immunodeficiency syndromes. *Postgrad. Radiol.* 1:99, 1981.

Lallemand D, et al.: Trachéomégalie et déficit immunitaire chez l'enfant. *Ann. Radiol. (Paris)* 24:67, 1981.

plasia, chronic atrophic gastritis, partial villous atrophy, malabsorption, diarrhea, protein-losing enteropathy, various infections (fungi, protozoa, viruses, atypical mycobacteria), bile duct dilatation, primary sclerosing cholangitis, hepatocellular disease.

(C) RESPIRATORY SYSTEM: recurrent respiratory tract infections and pneumonias, hoarseness (invasive fungal infection), tracheomegaly, bronchiectasis, absence of lymphoid tissues in the nasopharynx, etc.

(D) OTHER REPORTED ABNORMALITIES: aortic calcification in hypogammaglobulinemia, absent thymic shadow, cardiovascular anomalies, chromosomal abnormalities, endocrinopathies, anemia, renopathies, arthritis, endocarditis, etc.

Note: For a more complete description of the following immune disorders please refer to the page under the corresponding titles: acquired immunodeficiency syndrome, agammaglobulinemia (X-linked), ataxia-telangiectasia, Bloom

Levy Y, et al.: Adenosine deaminase deficiency with late onset of recurrent infections: Response to treatment with polyethylene glycol–modified adenosine deaminase. *J. Pediatr.* 113:312, 1988.

Naveh Y, et al.: Primary sclerosing cholangitis associated with immunodeficiency. *Am. J. Dis. Child.* 137:114, 1983.

Nockler IB, et al.: Calcification of the thoracic aorta in a child. *Br. J. Radiol.* 58:1008, 1985.

Rose JS, et al.: Unusual radiographic presentations of immuno-deficiency disorders. *Ann. Radiol. (Paris)* 25:415, 1982.

Rosen FS, et al.: The primary immunodeficiencies. *N. Engl. J. Med.* 311:235, 300, 1984.

Sauerbrei E, et al.: Hypogammaglobulinemia and nodular lymphoid hyperplasia of the gut. *J. Can. Assoc. Radiol.* 30:362, 1979.

Stricker RB, et al.: Pernicious anemia, 18q deletion syndrome, and IgA deficiency. *J.A.M.A.* 248:1359, 1982.

Strober W, et al.: The immunopathogenesis of gastrointestinal and hepatobiliary diseases. *J.A.M.A.* 258:2962, 1987.

Taalman RDFM, et al.: Chromosome studies in IgA-deficient patients. *Clin. Genet.* 32:81, 1987.

Valkova G, et al.: Centromeric instability of chromosomes 1, 9 and 16 with variable immune deficiency. Support of a new syndrome. *Clin. Genet.* 31:119, 1987.

Vossen J: Classification des déficits immunitaires congénitaux. *Arch. Fr. Pediatr.* 39:539, 1982.

Walters MDS, et al.: Obstructive endocarditis in an immunodeficient infant. *Eur. J. Pediatr.* 145:553, 1986.

Watts WJ, et al.: Respiratory dysfunction in patients with common variable hypogammaglobulinemia. *Am. Rev. Respir. Dis.* 134:699, 1986.

Wilson CB: Immune aspects of renal diseases. *J.A.M.A.* 258:2957, 1987.

Zweiman B, et al.: Immunologic aspects of neurological and neuromuscular diseases. *J.A.M.A.* 258:2970, 1987.

IRON DEFICIENCY ANEMIA

Stages in the Development of Iron Deficiency: Stage 1, depletion of iron stores; stage 2, decrease in transport iron resulting in an inhibition of the production of metabolically active compounds requiring iron; stage 3, hypochromic, microcytic anemia.

Clinical Manifestations: (a) tiredness, easy fatigability, palpitations, dyspnea, irritability, headache, light-headedness, numbness, tingling, poor development, difficulty in feeding, etc.; (b) pallor, angular stomatitis, glossitis, gastritis, nail abnormalities (thinning, brittleness, longitudinal ridging, spoon nails, etc.); (c) hemic murmurs, cardiomegaly, cardiac hypertrophy, congestive heart failure; (d) hepatosplenomegaly; (e) papilledema associated with increased intracranial pressure; (f) hypochromic microcytic anemia, anisocytosis, poikilocytosis, low serum iron levels, increased iron-binding capacity, erythroid hyperplasia detected on bone marrow studies; (g) other reported abnormalities: blue sclerae, susceptibility to infections, thrombocytosis, hypoproteinemia, anemia caused by an antibody against the transferrin receptor.

Radiologic Manifestations: (a) skull: widening of the diploic space (frontal, parietal, occipital), thinning of the outer table, vertical striation, small sella turcica; (b) hands: widening of tubular bones due to expansion of the medullary space, thin cortices; (c) osteoporosis; (d) association with a syndrome of geophagia, hypogonadism, dwarfism, and hepatosplenomegaly.

REFERENCES

Agarwal KN, et al.: Roentgenographic changes in iron deficiency anemia. *A.J.R.* 110:635, 1970.

Eng LI: Chronic iron deficiency anemia with bone changes resembling Cooley's anemia. *Acta Haematol.* 19:263, 1958.

Kalra L, et al.: Blue sclerae: A common sign of iron deficiency? *Lancet* 2:1267, 1986.

Lanzkowsky PH: Radiological features of iron deficiency anemia. *Am. J. Dis. Child.* 116:16, 1968.

Larrick JW, et al.: Acquired iron-deficiency anemia caused by an antibody against the transferrin receptor. *N. Engl. J. Med.* 311:214, 1984.

Lundström U, et al.: Iron deficiency anaemia with hypoproteinaemia. *Arch. Dis. Child.* 58:438, 1983.

Reeves JD, et al.: Iron deficiency in health and disease. *Adv. Pediatr.* 30:281, 1983.

Rossi MA, et al.: Norepinephrine and cardiac hypertrophy in iron deficiency anemia. *Am. Heart J.* 105:874, 1983.

Say B, et al.: Geophagia associated with iron-deficiency anemia, hepatosplenomegaly, hypogonadism and dwarfism. A syndrome probably associated with zinc deficiency. *Clin. Pediatr. (Phila.)* 8:661, 1969.

KEARNS-SAYRE SYNDROME

Synonyms: Oculocraniosomatic syndrome; ophthalmoplegia-plus syndrome; mitochondrial cytopathy; oculocranial disease; oculocraniosomatic neuromuscular disease with mitochondrial myopathy.

Frequency: 70 published cases to 1983 (Rowland et al.).

Pathology: *Mitochondrial and muscle fiber abnormalities ("ragged-red" fibers); spongiform degeneration of white matter; fibrotic lesions in the His bundle and proximal bundle branches;* progressive cytochome c oxidase deficiency; fatty infiltration of the pancreas.

Clinical Manifestations: Onset of symptoms often before the age of 20 years: (a) *progressive external ophthalmoplegia;* (b) *retinitis pigmentosa;* (c) *cardiac conduction defects* (heart block), cardiovascular dysfunction resulting in death; (d) other reported manifestations: cerebellar ataxia, somnolence, lethargy, neurosensory hearing loss, short stature, delayed sexual maturation, muscle weakness, mental retardation or dementia, endocrine disorders (diabetes mellitus, pseudohypoparathyroidism, hypoparathyroidism), seizures, elevated cerebrospinal fluid protein levels, corneal clouding, reduced plasma and cerebrospinal fluid folate, reduced levels of coenzyme Q_{10} in serum and in the mitochondrial fraction of skeletal muscle, occurrence in twins, etc.; (e) abnormal electroencephalographic findings.

Radiologic Manifestations: (a) *microcephaly;* (b) *cerebral calcification* (basal ganglia, thalami, cerebral hemispheres), *cerebellar hypoplasia,* scattered areas of decreased attenuation within the parietocentral white matter (on computed tomography [CT]) (Figs ME−K−1 and ME−K−2).

REFERENCES

Allen RJ, et al.: Kearns-Sayre syndrome with reduced plasma and cerebrospinal fluid folate. *Ann. Neurol.* 13:679, 1983.

Boltshauser E, et al.: Diabetes mellitus in Kearns-Sayre syndrome. *Am. J. Dis. Child.* 132:321, 1978.

Bresolin N, et al.: Progressive cytochrome oxidase deficiency in a case of Kearns-Sayre syndrome: Morphological, immunological, and biochemical studies in muscle biopsies and autopsy tissues. *Ann. Neurol.* 21:564, 1987.

Byrne E, et al.: Mitochondrial studies in Kearns-Sayre syndrome: Normal respiratory chain function with absence of a mitochondrial translation product. *Neurology* 37:1530, 1987.

Channer KS, et al.: Cardiomyopathy in the Kearns-Sayre syndrome. *Br. Heart J.* 59:486, 1988.

Curless RG, et al.: Fatal metabolic acidosis, hyperglycemia, and coma after steroid therapy for Kearns-Sayre syndrome. *Neurology* 36:872, 1986.

Gallastegui J, et al.: Cardiac involvement in the Kearns-Sayre syndrome. *Am. J. Cardiol.* 60:385, 1987.

Kearns TP, Sayre GP: Retinitis pigmentosa, external ophthalmoplegia, and complete heart block. *Arch. Ophthalmol.* 60:280, 1958.

Kotagal S, et al.: Hypersomnia, bithalamic lesions, and altered sleep architecture in Kearns-Sayre syndrome. *Neurology* 35:574, 1985.

Ogasahara S, et al.: Treatment of Kearns-Sayre syndrome with coenzyme Q_{10}. *Neurology* 36:45, 1986.

Rheuban KS, et al.: Near-fatal Kearns-Sayre syndrome. A case report and review of clinical manifestations. *Clin. Pediatr. (Phila.)* 22:822, 1983.

Robain O, et al.: Syndrome de Kearns et Sayre avec hypoparathyroïdie et diabète. *Ann. Pediatr. (Paris)* 27:305, 1980.

Rowland LP, et al.: Kearns-Sayre syndrome in twins: Lethal dominant mutation or acquired disease? *Neurology* 38:1399, 1988.

Zeviani M, et al.: Deletions of mitochondrial DNA in Kearns-Sayre syndrome. *Neurology* 38:1339, 1988.

KOCHER-DEBRÉ-SÉMÉLAIGNE SYNDROME

Synonym: Cretinism with muscular hypertrophy.

Clinical Manifestations: (a) *myxedema,* retarded intellectual, physical, osseous, and dental development, constipation, bradycardia, peculiar facies, large tongue, coarse hair and skin; (b) *generalized increase in muscular mass* ("Herculean appearance," "prizefighter," "athletic appearance," "pseudoathletic"); (c) other reported abnormalities: congenital nystagmus.

Radiologic Manifestations: (a) *retarded skeletal and dental maturation;* (b) *large muscle mass.*

REFERENCES

Debré R, Sémélaigne G: Hypertrophie musculaire generalisée du petit enfant. *Bull. Soc. Pediatr. (Paris)* 32:699, 1934.

Hopwood NJ, et al.: Acquired hypothyroidism with muscular hypertrophy and precocious testicular enlargement. *J. Pediatr.* 85:233, 1974.

Kocher T: Zur Verhutüng der Cretinismus und cretinoider Zustände nach neuen Forschungen. *Dtsch. Z. Chir.* 34:556, 1892.

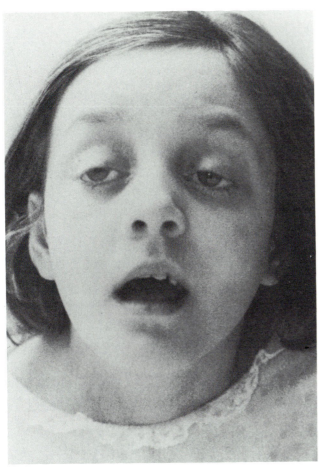

FIG ME–K–1.
Kearns-Sayre syndrome in a 13-year-old female. Note the ptosis, ophthalmoplegia, and facial weakness. (From Rheuban KS, Ayres NA, Sellers TD, et al.: Near-fatal Kearns-Sayre syndrome. *Clin. Pediatr.* (Phila.) 22:822, 1983. Used by permission.)

Radhakrishnan K, et al.: Kocher-Debré-Sémélaigne syndrome and congenital nystagmus. *Postgrad. Med. J.* 58:307, 1982.

Yeshwanth M, et al.: Kocher Debré Sémélaigne syndrome. *Indian Pediatr.* 24:346, 1987.

KRABBE DISEASE

Synonyms: Globoid cell leukodystrophy; galactosylceramide β-galactosidase deficiency.

Mode of Inheritance: Autosomal recessive.

Frequency: Marked difference between ethnic groups; incidence in Sweden: 1:25,000 to 1:50,000 (Hagberg et al.).

Etiology: A progressive degenerative disease of the central and peripheral nervous system (leukodystrophy) due to a deficiency of β-galactocerebrosidase activity (reflected in serum, leukocytes, cultured skin fibroblasts, and amniotic fluid).

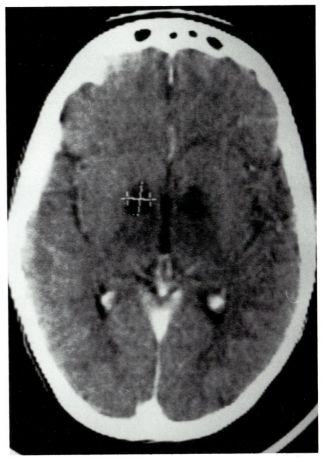

FIG ME–K–2.
Kearns-Sayre syndrome. Contrast CT of the head in a 10-year-old boy shows "mirror-image," nonenhancing, hypodense lesions in the thalami. (From Kotagal S, Archer CR, Walsh JK, et al.: Hypersomnia, bithalamic lesions, and altered sleep architecture in Kearns-Sayre syndrome. *Neurology* 35:574, 1985. Used by permission.)

Histology: Severe degree of a loss of oligodendroglia; marked demyelination in the cerebral hemispheres, cerebellum, brain stem, and spinal cord; segmental demyelination of the peripheral nerves; presence of globoid cells (considered to be macrophages containing galactocerebroside).

Clinical Manifestations: (a) infantile type (onset in the first year of life): unexplained fever, irritability, hypertonia, feeding problems, myoclonic seizure, quadriparesis, progression to a decerebrate state, early slowing and arrest of growth, failure to thrive, microcephaly, protruding ears, death within the first 2 years of life; (b) late onset (late infantile-juvenile): visual failure, cerebellar ataxia, spasticity, polyneuropathy, dementia, psychosis.

Radiologic Manifestations: (a) computed tomography (CT): (1) increased attenuation in the thalami, caudate nuclei, corona radiata, brain stem, and cerebellum; (2) decreased attenuation of white matter; (3) brain atrophy at the late stage

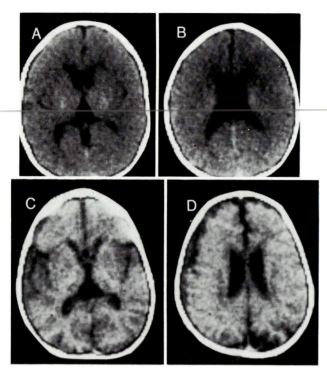

FIG ME–K–3.
Krabbe disease in a 5-month-old girl. Nonenhanced scans **(A** and **B)** show a symmetrical, increased density in the thalami, body of the caudate nuclei, and corona radiata. CT, 6 months later **(C** and **D),** shows rapidly progressive atrophy and symmetrical, abnormal low attenuation in the corona radiata. (From Kwan E, Drace J, Enzmann D: Specific CT findings in Krabbe disease. *A.J.R.* 143:665, 1984. Used by permission.)

of the disease; (1) is present before or in conjunction with (2); (b) magnetic resonance imaging: (1) early: decreased T_1 values and normal or slightly decreased T_2 values in the areas of the lesions, high T_1 and T_2 values in the white matter of the centrum ovale; (2) late: reduction in white and gray matter.

Notes: The infantile type has been subdivided into classic irritative-hypertonic, neonatal feeding abnormality variant, infantile spasm variant, hemiplegic variant, and prolonged floppy variant; the late-onset (late infantile-juvenile) has been subdivided into visual failure variant, cerebellar ataxia variant, spastic-onset variant, acute polyneuropathy variant, and dementia-psychosis variant (Fig ME–K–3).

REFERENCES

Baram TZ, et al.: Krabbe disease: Specific MRI and CT findings. *Neurology* 36:111, 1986.
Cavanagh N, et al.: High density on computed tomography in infantile Krabbe's disease: A case report. *Dev. Med. Child Neurol.* 28:799, 1986.
Hagberg B: Krabbe's disease: Clinical presentation of neurological variants. *Neuropediatrics* 15:11, 1984.
Kurokawa T, et al.: Late infantile Krabbe leukodystrophy: MRI and evoked potentials in a Japanese girl. *Neuropediatrics* 18:182, 1987.
Kwan E, et al.: Specific CT findings in Krabbe disease. *A.J.R.* 143:665, 1984.
Naidu S, et al.: Galactosylceramide-β-galactosidase deficiency in association with cherry red spot. *Neuropediatrics* 19:46, 1988.
Zlotogora J, et al.: Growth pattern in Krabbe's disease. *Acta Paediatr. Scand.* 75:251, 1986.
Zlotogora J, et al.: Krabbe disease and protruding ears (letter). *Am. J. Med. Genet.* 28:759, 1987.

KWASHIORKOR

Clinical Manifestations: (a) *failure to thrive (usually after weaning)*, mental apathy, weak cry; (b) diarrhea; (c) skin pigmentation and dryness; (d) change of color of the hair from black to brown and then to red; (e) edema; (f) *hypokalemia, hyponatremia, hypochloremia, low serum albumin levels, mild anemia*, endotoxemia (the lipopolysaccharide toxic component of the cell wall of gram-negative bacteria); (g) abnormal brain stem auditory evoked potentials; (h) vitamin A deficiency (conjunctival xerosis, Bitot spot, corneal xerosis, keratomalacia).

Radiologic Manifestations: (a) *markedly abnormal motor function of the intestine:* abnormal transit time, temporary stoppage of barium suspension, uneven diameter of the intestinal lumen; (b) brain atrophy (protein energy malnutrition); (c) small heart size due to decreased muscle mass (echocardiography); (d) osteoporosis.

REFERENCES

Bartel PR, et al.: Brainstem auditory evoked potentials in severely malnourished children with kwashiorkor. *Neuropediatrics* 17:178, 1986.
Bergman JW, et al.: Effect of kwashiorkor on the cardiovascular system. *Arch. Dis. Child.* 63:1359, 1988.
Berlin CM, et al.: Kwashiorkor in a child in central Pennsylvania. A seven-year follow-up. *Am. J. Dis. Child.* 136:822, 1982.
Finberg L: Kwashiorkor. *Am. J. Dis. Child.* 129:665, 1975.
Hendrickse RG: Kwashiorkor and aflatoxins. *J. Pediatr. Gastroenterol. Nutr.* 7:633, 1988.
Klein K, et al.: Endotoxemia in protein-energy malnutrition. *J. Pediatr. Gastroenterol. Nutr.* 7:225, 1988.
Kowalski R: Roentgenologic studies of the alimentary tract in kwashiorkor. *A.J.R.* 100:100, 1967.
McLaren DS: Aetiology of kwashiorkor. *Lancet* 1:55, 1985.

LACTASE DEFICIENCY

Mode of Inheritance: Autosomal recessive; most common in American Indians, black Americans, and Asians; less common in Caucasians.

Frequency: 5% to 15% of Americans of Scandinavian or northern European origin; over two thirds of randomly selected American blacks, Mexican Americans, Orientals, and Ashkenazi Jews (Bayless et al.).

Classification: (a) primary: may not manifest itself until adulthood; (b) secondary: caused by diseases damaging the enterocytes.

Clinical Manifestations: *Intolerance to milk-containing foods:* (a) abdominal cramps, bloating, diarrhea due to a shift of water into the intestinal tract; (b) positive lactose-H_2 breath test.

Radiologic Manifestations: *Stress test with the use of lactose* produces symptoms and radiological abnormalities of *barium dilution, bowel dilatation, and an extremely rapid transit time.*

REFERENCES

Bayless TM, et al: Lactose and milk intolerance: Clinical implications. *N. Engl. J. Med.* 292:1156, 1975.

Ceriani R, et al.: Lactose malabsorption and recurrent abdominal pain in Italian children. *J. Pediatr. Gastroenterol. Nutr.* 7:852, 1988.

Howell JM, et al.: Population screening for human adult lactase phenotypes with a multiple breaths version of the breath hydrogen test. *Hum. Genet.* 57:276, 1981.

Kolars JC, et al.: Yogurt—An autodigesting source of lactose. *N. Engl. J. Med.* 310:1, 1984.

Morrison WJ, et al.: Low lactase levels: Evaluation of the radiologic diagnosis. *Radiology* 111:513, 1974.

Ting CW, et al.: Developmental changes of lactose malabsorption in normal Chinese children: A study using breath hydrogen test with a physiological dose of lactose. *J. Pediatr. Gastroenterol. Nutr.* 7:848, 1988.

LARON DWARFISM

Synonyms: Pituitary dwarfism II; Laron-type pituitary dwarfism; Laron syndrome.

Mode of Inheritance: Autosomal recessive.

Clinical Manifestations: (a) *proportionate dwarfism resembling a clinical picture of growth hormone deficiency,* relative prominence of the calvaria in relation to facial structures, saddle nose, sparse hair, small genitalia, delayed puberty and maturity; (b) *elevated basal plasma immunoreactive growth hormone levels, low levels of circulating somatomedins, resistance to the effects of endogenous or exogenous growth hormone,* abnormal glucose metabolism (hypoglycemia, hypersensitivity to insulin, insulinopenia).

Radiologic Manifestations: (a) *skeletal maturation retardation;* (b) craniofacial disproportion.

REFERENCES

Eshet R, et al.: Defect of human growth hormone receptors in the liver of two patients with Laron-type dwarfism. *Isr. J. Med. Sci.* 20:8, 1984.

Geffner ME, et al.: Tissues of the Laron dwarf are sensitive to insulin-like growth factor I but not to growth hormone. *J. Clin. Endocrinol. Metab.* 64:1042, 1987.

Golde DW, et al.: Peripheral unresponsiveness to human growth hormone in Laron dwarfism. *N. Engl. J. Med.* 303:1156, 1980.

Laron Z, et al.: Genetic pituitary dwarfism with high serum concentration of growth hormone: A new inborn error of metabolism? *Isr. J. Med. Sci.* 2:152, 1966.

Mariani P, et al.: Nanism sévère avec taux sériques d'hormone de croissance élevée et activité somatomédine nulle: Syndrome de Laron. *Ann. Pediatr. (Paris)* 27:42, 1980.

Saldanha PH, et al.: Familial dwarfism with high IR-GH: Report of two affected sibs with genetic and epidemiologic considerations. *Hum. Genet.* 59:367, 1981.

LEAD INTOXICATION

Etiology: Pica; industrial exposure; drinking moonshine liquor; inhalation; gunshot wound with retained lead particles; Mexican folk remedy (lead tetroxide—azarcón), herbal medicinals, inadequately fired ceramics, indoor firing ranges, cosmetics, etc.

Clinical Manifestations: (a) *encephalopathy* associated with increased intracranial pressure, mild pleocytosis, and a moderate increase in protein content of the cerebrospinal fluid; (b) *neurological sequelae:* mental retardation, weakness, hemiparesis, recurrent seizures, optic atrophy; (c) anemia; (d) higher than the control blood lead levels in some cases of sudden infant death.

Radiologic Manifestations: (a) *widening of cranial sutures; cerebral edema; focal abnormality with a gyrate pattern of enhancement* (as shown by computed tomography); *brain* atrophy; dense calvaria (congenital lead poisoning); intracranial calcifications (punctiform, curvilinear, specklike and diffuse) in the subcortical area, basal ganglia, vermis, and cerebellum in chronic adult lead exposure associated with non-specific neurological manifestations such as dementia, diminished visual acuity, peripheral neuropathy, etc.; presentation as a posterior fossa "mass" (swollen vermis); (b) *lead lines in the metaphyses of tubular bones* (increased relative density of the proximal metaphysis of the fibula in particular), *iliac crest, scapulae, costochondral junctions;* separation of lead lines from the zone of provisional calcification within 4 weeks at sites of rapid growth; spontaneous disappearance of lead lines within 4 years; (c) *lead density of ingested material on abdominal roentgenograms;* (d) other reported abnormalities: saturnine gout associated with intra-articular milk of calcium (coexistence of saturnine gout and calcium pyrophosphate dihydrate deposition disease), thrombosis of the superior sagittal sinus.

REFERENCES

Bellinger D, et al.: Longitudinal analyses of prenatal and postnatal lead exposure and early cognitive development. *N. Engl. J. Med.* 316:1037, 1987.

Benson MD, et al.: Cerebellar calcification and lead. *J. Neurol. Neurosurg. Psychiatry* 48:814, 1985.

Blickman JG, et al.: The radiologic "lead band" revisited. *A.J.R.* 146:245, 1986.

Bose A, et al.: Azarcón por empacho—Another cause of lead toxicity. *Pediatrics* 72:106, 1983.

Cohen AR, et al.: Reassessment of the microcytic anemia of lead poisoning. *Pediatrics* 67:904, 1981.

Daniel WW, et al.: Intra-articular milk of calcium in saturnine gout. *Radiology* 137:389, 1983.

Drasch GA, et al.: Lead and sudden infant death. Investigations on blood samples of SID babies. *Eur. J. Pediatr.* 147:79, 1988.

Ghafour SY, et al.: Congenital lead intoxication with seizures due to prenatal exposure. *Clin. Pediatr. (Phila.)* 23:282, 1984.

Goldman RH, et al.: Lead poisoning in automobile radiator mechanics. *N. Engl. J. Med.* 317:214, 1987.

Harrington JF, et al.: Lead encephalopathy presenting as a posterior fossa mass. Case report. *J. Neurosurg.* 65:713, 1986.

Lightfoote J, et al.: Lead intoxication in an adult caused by Chinese herbal medication. *J.A.M.A.* 238:1539, 1977.

Pearl M, et al.: Radiographic findings in congenital lead poisoning. *Radiology* 136:83, 1980.

Reyes PF, et al.: Intracranial calcification in adults with chronic lead exposure. *A.J.R.* 146:267, 1986.

Sachs HK: The evolution of the radiologic lead line. *Radiology* 139:81, 1981.

Selbst SM, et al.: Lead poisoning in a child with a gunshot wound. *Pediatrics* 77:413, 1986.

Smulewicz JJ: Lead line at the iliac crest and "early" diagnosis of lead poisoning. *Am. J. Med. Sci.* 267:49, 1974.

Viader F, et al.: Encéphalopathie saturnine avec thrombose du sinus longitudinal supérieur. *Ann. Med. Interne (Paris)* 136:401, 1985.

LESCH-NYHAN SYNDROME

Mode of Inheritance: X-linked recessive trait.

Etiology: Absence of the enzyme hypoxanthine guanine phosphoribosyltransferase (PRT-ase) resulting in the *overproduction of purine and consequently uric acid.*

Frequency: Approximately 200 published cases (Mizuno et al.).

Clinical Manifestations: (a) *self-mutilation,* probably caused by dopaminergic denervation; altered central nervous system dopamine metabolism; (b) *mental and growth retardation;* (c) *motor dysfunction,* spasticity, choreoathetosis; (d) *microcephaly;* (e) *cerebral palsy;* (f) *tophaceous gout;* (g) *high concentration of uric acid in blood and urine,* low dopamine β-hydroxylase activity and diminished sympathetic response to stress and posture, detection of carriers by an analysis of hair roots for enzyme activity (agarose gel electrophoresis and autoradiography), first-trimester diagnosis by chorionic biopsy (radiochemical assay of hypoxanthine phosphoribosyltransferase activity and fetal sexing), reduced enzyme activity in cultured amniotic fluid cells, detection of the carrier state by the use of lymphocytic cloning; (h) *mild anemia;* (i) *nephropathy and nephrolithiasis* (manifestations of gout); (j) *partial deficiency of the enzyme hypoxanthine-guanine phosphoribosyl transferase: renal failure, failure to thrive, hyperuricemia.*

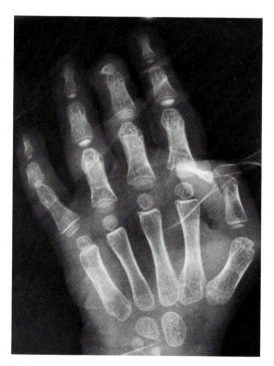

FIG ME–L–1.
Lesch-Nyhan syndrome: destruction of soft tissues and the distal phalanx of the middle finger. (Courtesy of Dr. Melvin H. Becker, New York.)

Radiologic Manifestations: (a) changes secondary to self-mutilation: *amputation of fingertips and phalanges;* (b) *radiolucent urinary stones* (hypoxanthine, xanthine, and uric acid); (c) *microcephaly;* (d) brain atrophy (mild); (e) bone erosions; (f) calcareous deposits of gout; (g) skeletal maturation retardation; (h) peripheral manifestations of cerebral palsy (coxa valga, hip subluxation or dislocation) (Fig ME−L−1).

REFERENCES

Bakay B, et al.: Detection of Lesch-Nyhan syndrome carriers: Analysis of hair roots for HPRT by agarose gel electrophoresis and autoradiography. *Clin. Genet.* 17:369, 1980.

Becker MH, et al.: Congenital hyperuricosuria: Associated radiologic features. *Radiol. Clin. North Am.* 6:239, 1968.

Brock WA, et al.: Xanthine calculi in the Lesch-Nyhan syndrome. *J. Urol.* 130:157, 1983.

Dempsey JL, et al.: Detection of the carrier state for an X-linked disorder, the Lesch-Nyhan syndrome, by the use of lymphocyte cloning. *Hum. Genet.* 64:288, 1983.

Gibbs DA, et al.: First-trimester diagnosis of Lesch-Nyhan syndrome. *Lancet* 2:1180, 1984.

Goldstein M, et al.: Self-mutilation in Lesch-Nyhan disease is caused by dopaminergic denervation. *Lancet* 1:338, 1985.

Holdeigel M: Craniales computertomogramm bei inkomplettem Lesch-Nyhan-Syndrom. *Radiologe* 27:127, 1987.

Jankovic J, et al.: Lesch-Nyhan syndrome: A study of motor behavior and cerebrospinal fluid neurotransmitters. *Ann. Neurol.* 23:466, 1988.

Kopin IJ: Neurotransmitters and the Lesch-Nyhan syndrome. *N. Engl. J. Med.* 305:1148, 1981.

Lake CR, et al.: Lesch-Nyhan syndrome: Low dopamine-beta-hydroxylase activity and diminished sympathetic response to stress and posture. *Science* 196:905, 1977.

Lesch M, Nyhan WL: A familial disorder of uric acid metabolism and central nervous system function. *Am. J. Med.* 36:561, 1964.

Lorentz WB, et al.: Failure to thrive, hyperuricemia, and renal insufficiency in early infancy secondary to partial hypoxanthine-guanine phosphoribosyl transferase deficiency. *J. Pediatr.* 104:94, 1984.

Mizuno T: Long-term follow-up of ten patients with Lesch-Nyhan syndrome. *Neuropediatrics* 17:158, 1986.

Nyhan WL: Clinical features of Lesch-Nyhan syndrome. *Arch. Intern. Med.* 130:186, 1972.

Riley JD: Gout and cerebral palsy in three-year-old boy. *Arch. Dis. Child.* 35:293, 1960.

Silverstein FS, et al.: Lesch-Nyhan syndrome: CSF neurotransmitter abnormalities. *Neurology* 35:907, 1985.

LIPODYSTROPHY

Synonym: Lipoatrophy (partial or total absence of subcutaneous fat).

Classification and Mode of Inheritance: (a) progressive partial lipodystrophy (Barraquer-Simons syndrome): usually sporadic, familial incidence rare, strong predilection for females (4:1); (b) familial partial lipodystrophy (Köbberling-Dunnigan syndrome): a dominant mode of transmission has been suggested; (c) congenital total lipodystrophy with a loss of subcutaneous fat within the first 2 years of life (Bernardinelli-Seip syndrome): consanguinity of parents common, autosomal recessive, sexes equally affected; (d) acquired lipoatrophic diabetes (Lawrence): sporadic, predominantly in females.

Clinical Manifestations:

(A) PROGRESSIVE PARTIAL LIPODYSTROPHY (Barraquer-Simons): Onset of symptoms usually between 5 and 15 years of age: (a) fat loss from the face, arms, and trunk; normal or excessive fat deposition on the pelvic girdle and lower limbs; (b) other reported abnormalities (in a minority of the patients): glomerulonephritis, hepatomegaly, diabetes, hyperlipidemia, mental retardation.

(B) FAMILIAL PARTIAL LIPODYSTROPHY (Köbberling-Dunnigan syndrome): Two types: (a) limb lipodystrophy: loss of subcutaneous fat confined to the limbs and sparing the face and trunk; (b) limb and trunk lipodystrophy: the trunk affected with the exception of the vulva (pseudolabial hypertrophy); diabetes mellitus, hyperlipoproteinemia, acanthosis nigricans present in some patients.

(C) CONGENITAL TOTAL LIPODYSTROPHY (Bernardinelli-Seip syndrome, lipoatrophic diabetes): (a) *hirsutism;* (b) *acanthosis nigricans;* (c) *generalized absence of adipose tissue;* (d) large hands and feet; (e) large penis or clitoris in infancy; (f) *accelerated growth and maturation;* (g) prominent musculature; (h) phlebomegaly; (i) hepatosplenomegaly with cirrhosis; (j) mental retardation; (k) *insulin-resistant diabetes mellitus* not associated with ketosis, hypertriglyceridemia, elevated basal metabolic rate, decreased binding of insulin to its receptor, oligomenorrhea, polycystic ovarian disease, hirsutism; (l) functional and morphological abnormalities of the heart muscle and chambers (muscular hypertrophy, increased chamber size and myocardial indentation, systolic anterior movement of the mitral valve, wall motion abnormalities).

(D) ACQUIRED LIPOATROPHIC DIABETES (Lawrence): Associated in some cases with infective processes (mumps, pertussis), difficult labor and delivery, etc.

Radiologic Manifestations (Congenital Total Lipodystrophy): (a) *absence of fat in soft tissues,* difficulty in abdominal organ delineation by computed tomography due to a paucity of fat, fatty liver (low computed tomographic [CT] attenuation, hyperechoic pattern on sonography), abnormally low or absent signal on magnetic resonance imaging evaluation of the bone marrow (atrophy of fatty tissue); (b) *increased bone density;* (c) *thickened cortex of tubular bones;* (d) *prominent and hypertrophic epiphyses,* scattered areas of radiodensity and cystic changes in periarticular regions; (e) *advanced skeletal maturation;* (f) *thick calvaria,* calcification of the falx cerebri, excessive pneumatization of sinuses and mastoids; (g) *dense transverse bands in the vertebrae;* (h) *nephromegaly* with splaying of calices and infundibula; (i) *hepatosplenomegaly;* (j) *advanced dentition;* (k) other reported abnormalities: enlargement of basal cisterns and the third ventricle with

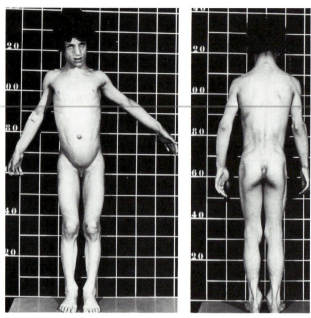

FIG ME–L–2.
Lipodystrophy (lipoatrophic diabetes) in a 13-year-old girl with muscular hypertrophy of the android type, facial dysmorphism, and hypertrophy of the clitoris. (From Lestradet C, Massol J, Plouvier E, et al.: Lipodystrophie généralisée congénitale. *Arch. Fr. Pediatr.* 42:705, 1985. Used by permission.)

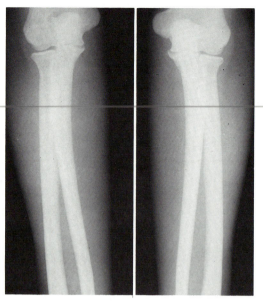

FIG ME–L–3.
Lipoatrophic diabetes in a 19-year-old male with an absence of fat in the subcutaneous tissue and between muscle bundles. Muscles are prominent. (From Gold RH, Steinback HL: Lipoatrophic diabetes mellitus (generalized lipodystrophy): Roentgen findings in two brothers with congenital disease. *A.J.R.* 101:884, 1967. Used by permission.)

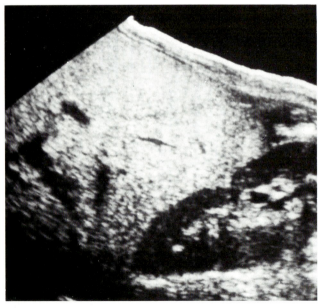

FIG ME–L–4.
Congenital generalized lipodystrophy. An ultrasound image of a 29-year-old woman shows a bright liver pattern compatible with fatty infiltration of the liver parenchyma. Marked differences in echogenicity between the liver and the kidney are evident. (From Smevik B, Swensen T, Kolbenstvedt A, et al.: Computed tomography and ultrasonography of the abdomen in congenital generalized lipodystrophy. *Radiology* 142:687, 1982. Used by permission.)

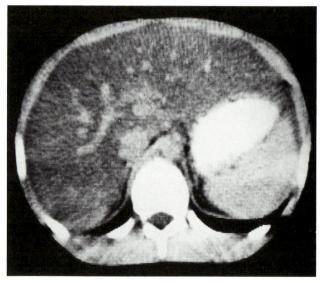

FIG ME–L–5.
Congenital generalized lipodystrophy. CT of a 15-year-old boy shows an enlarged liver with dense vascular structures contrasting with the less-dense liver parenchyma. The following attenuation values were found: liver, 10 Hounsfield units (HU); spleen, 53 HU. (From Smevik B, Swensen T, Kolbenstvedt A, et al.: Computed tomography and ultrasonography of the abdomen in congenital generalized lipodystrophy. *Radiology* 142:687, 1982. Used by permission.)

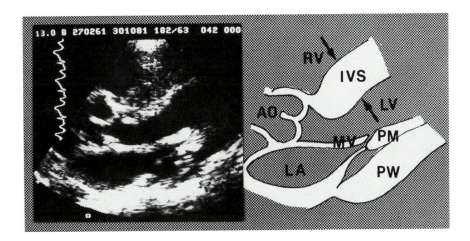

FIG ME—L—6.
Generalized lipodystrophy in a 20-year-old female. A long-axis echocardiogram shows a very thick interventricular septum (*AO* = aorta; *IVS* = interventricular septum; *LA* = left atrium; *LV* = left ventricle; *MV* = mitral valve; *PM* = papillary muscle, *PW* = posterior wall). (From Bjørnstad PG, Semb BKH, Trygstad O, et al.: Echocardiographic assessment of cardiac function and morphology in patients with generalized lipodystrophy. *Eur. J. Pediatr.* 144:355, 1985. Used by permission.)

or without enlargement of the lateral ventricles, narrowing of interpediculate distances, polycystic ovarian disease.

Differential Diagnosis: Leprechaunism (may represent a lethal form of lipoatrophic diabetes); diencephalic syndrome; lipoatrophy associated with hyperthyroidism, tubular acidosis, malnutrition, anorexia nervosa, progeria, etc.

Note: AREDYLD refers to a syndrome combining an acrorenal field defect, ectodermal dysplasia, lipoatrophic diabetes, etc. (Pinheiro et al.) (Figs ME—L—2 to ME—L—6).

REFERENCES

Arico M, et al.: Insulin receptor evaluation in congenital generalized lipodystrophy. *Helv. Paediatr. Acta* 42:167, 1987.

Barraquer L: Histoire clinique d'un cas d'atrophie du tissue cellulo-adipeux. Barcelona, 1906.

Berardinelli W: An undiagnosed endocrinometabolic syndrome: Report of two cases. *J. Clin. Endocrinol.* 14:193, 1954.

Bjørnstad PG, et al: Echocardiographic assessment of cardiac function and morphology in patients with generalized lipodystrophy. *Eur. J. Pediatr.* 144:355, 1985.

Gold RH, Steinbach HL: Lipoatrophic diabetes mellitus (generalized lipodystrophy): Roentgen findings in two brothers with congenital disease. *A.J.R.* 101:884, 1967.

Holländer E: Ueber einen Fall von fortschreitendem Schwund des Fettgewebes und seinen kosmetischen Ersatz durch Menschenfett. *Munch. Med. Wochenschr.* 57:1794, 1910.

Köbberling J, Dunnigan MG: Familial partial lipodystrophy: Two types of an X linked dominant syndrome, lethal in the hemizygous state. *J. Med. Genet.* 23:120, 1986.

Lawrence RD: Lipodystrophy and hepatomegaly with diabetes, lipaemia, and other metabolic disturbances: Case throwing new light on action of insulin. *Lancet* 1:724, 1946.

Lestradet C, et al.: Lipodystrophie généralisée congénitale. *Arch. Fr. Pediatr.* 42:705, 1985.

Mitchell SW: Singular case of absence of adipose matter in upper half of the body. *Am. J. Med. Sci.* 90:105, 1885.

Pinheiro M, et al.: AREDYLD: A syndrome combining an acrorenal field defect, ectodermal dysplasia, lipoatrophic diabetes, and other manifestations. *Am. J. Med. Genet.* 16:29, 1983.

Poley JR, et al.: Progressive lipodystrophy: A clinical study of 50 patients. *Am. J. Dis. Child.* 106:356, 1963.

Sebrechts CH, et al.: Lipoatrophic diabetes mellitus (generalized lipodystrophy) *Skeletal Radiol.* 16:320, 1987.

Seip M: Lipodystrophy and gigantism with associated endocrine manifestation: A new diencephalic syndrome. *Acta Paediatr. Scand.* 48:555, 1959.

Simons A: Eine seltene Trophoneurose ("Lipodystrophia progressiva"). *Z. Ges. Neurol. Psychiatr.* 5:29, 1911.

Smevik B, et al.: Computed tomography and ultrasonography of the abdomen in congenital generalized lipodystrophy. *Radiology* 142:687, 1982.

Wesenberg RL, et al.: The roentgenographic findings in total lipodystrophy. *A.J.R.* 103:154, 1968.

Wilson TA, et al.: Cerebral computed tomography in lipodystrophy. *Arch. Neurol.* 39:733, 1982.

LIPOID PROTEINOSIS

Synonyms: Lipoglycoproteinosis; Urbach-Wiethe disease; hyalinosis cutis et mucosae.

Mode of Inheritance: Autosomal recessive.

Pathology: *Infiltration of various tissues (skin, mucosa, central nervous system, respiratory system, gastrointestinal tract, lymph nodes, and striated muscles) by a complex glycolipoprotein.*

Clinical Manifestations: Onset of symptoms often at birth: (a) *mucosal involvement* of the oropharynx, larynx, and nose: diminished gustation, cracked lips, pale irregular buccopharyngeal mucosa, diminished gag reflex, tethering of the tongue, limited tongue motility, dysphagia, hoarseness with an onset in as early as neonatal, thickened epiglottis, thickened aryteroepiglottic folds, thickened irregular false vocal cords, swollen arythenoids, plaquelike excrescence of the laryngeal mucosa; (b) skin infiltration: yellow or brown papules on the face giving a waxy look to the skin, beaded papules along the eyelids, nodular lesions on the elbows and knees, nonscarring alopecia; (c) *neuropsychiatric disorders:* seizures, mental retardation, choreoathetosis, paresthesia of the fingers, indifference to pain, behavior problems; (d) eye lesions: retinal degeneration, etc.; (e) abnormal dentition; (f) elevated lipid levels in the blood.

Radiologic Manifestations: (a) *intracranial calcifications in the hippocampal gyri* that are located superolateral to dorsum sella and project over the medial aspect of the orbits in

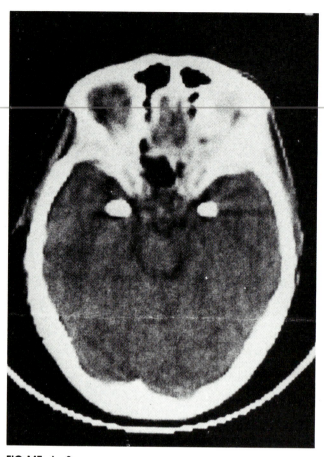

FIG ME–L–8.
Lipoid proteinosis. Note the bilateral temporal lobe calcification. (From Leonard JN, Ryan TJ, Sheldon PWE: CT scan appearance in a patient with lipoid proteinosis. *Br. J. Radiol.* 54:1098, 1981. Used by permission.)

the frontal view (bean-shaped, inverted commas), areas of lucency within the calcification; (b) *vocal cord thickening* (diffuse or nodular); (c) reticular and nodular densities in the lung (Figs ME–L–7 and ME–L–8).

REFERENCES

Francis RS: Lipoid proteinosis: A case report. *Radiology* 117:301, 1975.

Friedman L, et al.: Radiographic and computed tomographic findings in lipoid proteinosis. *S. Afr. Med. J.* 65:734, 1984.

Gurecki H: *Maladie de Urbach-Wiethe et Indifférence Congénitale à la douleur* (thesis). Nancy, 1966.

Harper JI, et al.: Oropharyngeal and laryngeal lesions in lipoid proteinosis. *J. Laryngol. Otol.* 97:877, 1983.

Leonard JN, et al.: CT scan appearances in a patient with lipoid proteinosis. *Br. J. Radiol.* 54:1098, 1981.

Singh G, et al.: Lipoid proteinosis. *Int. J. Dermatol.* 27:344, 1988.

Urbach E, Wiethe C: Lipoidosis cutis et mucosae. *Virchows Arch. [A]* 273:285, 1929.

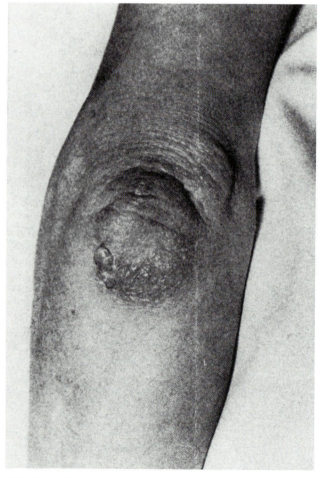

FIG ME–L–7.
Lipoid proteinosis: warty plaque on the elbow (From Leonard JN, Ryan TJ, Sheldon PWE: CT scan appearances in a patient with lipoid proteinosis. *Br. J. Radiol.* 54:1098, 1981. Used by permission.)

Yakout YM, et al.: Radiological findings in lipoid proteinosis. *J. Laryngol. Otol.* 99:259, 1985.

LOWE SYNDROME

Synonym: Oculocerebrorenal syndrome.

Mode of Inheritance: X-linked.

Clinical Manifestations: Onset of symptoms in early infancy: (a) *mental retardation;* (b) *growth retardation;* (c) *cataract, glaucoma;* (d) *progressive renal tubular dysfunction* (decreased ability to secrete hydrogen ions and to produce ammonia, hyperaminoaciduria, proteinuria, hyperchloremic acidosis, phosphaturia, hypophosphatemia); (e) other reported abnormalities: episodes of fever, *hypotonia,* joint hypermobility, diminished or absent deep tendon reflexes, hyperactivity, muscular hypoplasia, cryptorchidism, buphthalmos, corneal scarring, superficial granulations of the eyes, nystagmus, seizures, high-pitched cry, hematuria, granular casts, anemia, hyperhemolysis, tenosynovitis, joint effusion, manifestations of the syndrome in a girl with no family history of the disorder who had a de novo balanced X/3 translocation with a breakpoint at Xq25 and inheritance of a balanced $^{14}/_{17}$ translocation from her father, lenticular opacities in females heterozygous for this X-linked condition.

Radiologic Manifestations: (a) *rickets and/or osteoporosis;* (b) pathological fracture through the shafts of long bones, healing with large callus formation; (c) frontal bossing, scoliosis, kyphosis, platyspondyly, cervical spine anomalies (increased motion at the C_1–C_2 level, fusion of C_1 and the occiput, basilar impression), hip dislocation or subluxation; (d) computed tomography: diffuse scalloping of the calvarial bones, ventricular dilatation, periventricular decrease in density, diffuse low-absorption areas in the cortical white matter; (e) magnetic resonance imaging: nonhomogeneous areas of increased T_2-weighted signal intensity in the centrum semiovale, abnormal areas of high signal intensity in the periventricular white matter.

REFERENCES

Bailey RR, et al.: Homozygous cystinuria and the oculo-cerebro-renal dystrophy of Lowe in the same family. *Arch. Dis. Child.* 51:558, 1976.

Charnas L, et al.: MRI findings and peripheral neuropathy in Lowe's syndrome. *Neuropediatrics* 19:7, 1988.

Gobernado JM, et al.: Mitochondrial defects in Lowe's oculocerebrorenal syndrome. *Arch. Neurol.* 41:208, 1984.

Hodgson SV, et al.: A balanced de novo X/autosome translocation in a girl with manifestations of Lowe syndrome. *Am. J. Med. Genet.* 23:837, 1986.

Holtgrewe JL, et al.: Orthopedic manifestations of the Lowe (oculocerebrorenal) syndrome. *J. Pediatr. Orthop.* 6:165, 1986.

Lachaux A, et al.: Le syndrome oculo-cérébro-rénal chez une fille. Réévaluation clinique, génétique et biologique a l'âge de 10 ans. *Arch. Fr. Pediatr.* 43:67, 1986.

Lowe CU, et al.: Organic aciduria, decreased renal ammonia production, hydrophthalmos, and mental retardation. *Am. J. Dis. Child.* 83:164, 1952.

O'Tuama LA, et al.: Oculocerebrorenal syndrome: Case report with CT and MR correlates. *A.J.N.R.* 8:555, 1987.

Pavone L, et al.: Haematogical studies in a case of oculocerebro-renal syndrome. *Helv. Paediatr. Acta* 31:509, 1976.

MANNOSIDOSIS

Synonym: Lysosomal α-ᴅ-mannosidose deficiency.

Classifications: Type I homozygotes with severe disease, gross psychomotor retardation, hepatosplenomegaly, recurrent infections, short stature, dysostosis multiplex, and early death; type II homozygotes with moderate retardation, deafness, near-normal stature, milder dysostosis multiplex, and survival to adult life.

Mode of Inheritance: Autosomal recessive with considerable variation in clinical manifestations within the family.

Frequency: Over 60 published cases (Patton et al. and others).

Clinical Manifestations: Clinical features become apparent in about 1 to 3 years of life: (a) *craniofacial dysmorphism:* macrocephaly, coarse and puffy facial features, high frontal region, slight flattening of the nasal root, flat face, prominent mandible, macroglossia, large ears, widely spaced teeth; (b) *psychomotor retardation,* normal or accelerated early growth followed by *growth arrest, hypotonia, hyperreflexia;* (c) *corneal clouding, cataract, ptosis,* wheel-like or spoke-shaped opacities in the lens; (d) *high-frequency mixed hearing loss* (common); (e) deficiency of α-mannosidase leading to an accumulation of mannose-rich glycoproteins in tissues, excretion of glycoproteins in urine, abnormal α-mannosidase activity demonstrable in cultured skin fibroblasts, hypogammaglobulinemia, vacuolized peripheral lymphocytes, coarse and dark granules in neutrophils, reduced α-mannosidase in cultured amniotic fluid cells; etc.; (f) other reported abnormalities: frequent upper respiratory infections, protuberant abdomen, testicular hydrocele, gibbus deformity, umbilical hernia, vomiting, large hands and feet, autoimmune pancytopenia.

Radiologic Manifestations: *Dysostosis multiplex* of varying severity: (a) skull: thick calvaria, dolichocephaly or brachycephaly, partial craniosynostosis; (b) widening of the ribs; (c) mild flattening of the vertebrae, trapezoid-shaped vertebrae with anterior wedging or anterior beaking at the thoracolumbar junction; (d) expansion of the diaphyses of tubular bones, mild bowing of long bones, slight irregularity of metaphyses, narrow basilar segment of the iliac wings, coxa valga; (e) osteoporosis, coarse bone trabeculae; (f) communicating hydrocephalus associated with a gait disorder Fig ME–M–1).

REFERENCES

Aylsworth AS, et al.: Mannosidosis: Phenotype of a severely affected child and characterization of alpha/mannosidose activity in cultured fibroblasts from the patient and his parents. *J. Pediatr.* 88:814, 1976.

Farriaux J-P, et al.: La mannosidose: Un diagnostic simple. *Arch. Fr. Pediatr.* 33:11, 1976.

Halperin JJ, et al.: Communicating hydrocephalus and lysosomal inclusions in mannosidosis. *Arch. Neurol.* 41:777, 1984.

Mitchell ML, et al.: Mannosidosis: Two brothers with different degrees of disease severity. *Clin. Genet.* 20:191, 1981.

Öckerman PA: A generalized storage disease resembling Hurler's syndrome. *Lancet* 2:239, 1967.

Patton MA, et al.: Mannosidosis in two brothers: Prolonged survival in the severe phenotype. *Clin. Genet.* 22:284, 1982.

Press OW, et al.: Pancytopenia in mannosidosis. *Arch. Intern. Med.* 143:1266, 1983.

Spranger J, et al.: The radiographic features of mannosidosis. *Radiology* 119:401, 1976.

Will A, et al.: Bone marrow transplantation in the treatment of α-mannosidosis. *Arch. Dis. Child.* 62:1044, 1987.

MAPLE SYRUP URINE DISEASE

Synonyms: MSUD; branched-chain ketoaciduria.

Mode of Inheritance: Autosomal recessive; genetic heterogeneity.

Etiology and Pathology: (a) *decreased activity of branched-chain ketoacid decarboxylase leading to elevation of branched-chain amino acid or ketoacid levels in blood and excretion of same in urine;* (b) *pathological cerebral changes:* cerebral edema, cystic degeneration, gliosis, decreased myelination.

Classification: Five different clinical forms: classic, intermittent, intermediate, thiamine-responsive, and E_3 deficiency.

Clinical Manifestations: (a) symptoms often occurring in the first postnatal days: *vomiting, feeding difficulty, neurological manifestations* (lethargy, shrill cry, hypotonicity, opisthotonos, convulsions, pseudotumor cerebri, respiratory difficulties, coma), mental retardation in surviving children; (b) urine with characteristic odor (sweet, malty, or caramel-like); (c) hypoglycemia (in some in the acute phase); (d) prenatal diagnosis with evaluation of the enzyme activity in cultured amniotic fluid cells; (e) postnatal diagnostic tests: plasma and urine assays for increased amino acids (leucine,

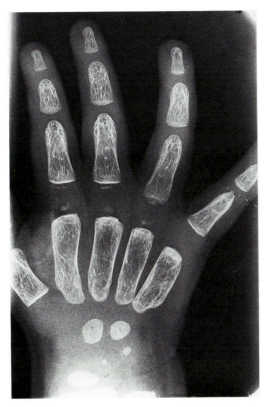

FIG ME–M–1.
Mannosidosis in a 1-year-old child. Shafts of tubular bones are slightly expanded with a loss of diaphyseal constriction. The second to fifth metacarpals are proximally pointed. Bone trabeculation is prominent. (From Spranger J, Gehler J, Cantz M: The radiographic features of mannosidosis. *Radiology* 119:401, 1976. Used by permission.)

isoleucine, valine); ferric chloride test (gray-blue color); 2,4-dinitrophenylhydrazine test (heavy yellow precipitate).

Radiologic Manifestations: (a) *brain edema in infants,* subsidence of edema with the institution of appropriate therapy; (b) progressive global (end-stage) brain atrophy over a period of several years in a missed or delayed diagnosis; (c) scoliosis (Fig ME–M–2).

REFERENCES

DiGeorge AM, et al.: Prospective study of maple-syrup-urine disease for the first four days of life. *N. Engl. J. Med.* 207:1492, 1982.

Frézal J, et al.: Maple syrup urine disease: Two different forms within a single family. *Hum. Genet.* 71:89, 1985.

Gonzalez-Rios MDC, et al.: A distinct variant of intermediate maple syrup urine disease. *Clin. Genet.* 27:153, 1985.

Herndon WA: Scoliosis and maple syrup urine disease. *J. Pediatr. Orthop.* 4:126, 1984.

Indo Y, et al.: Maple syrup urine disease: A possible biochemical basis for the clinical heterogeneity. *Hum. Genet.* 80:6, 1988.

Irnberger Th, et al.: Die kraniale Computertomographie bei der Ahornsiruperkrankung. *Fortschr. Rontgenstr.* 144:413, 1986.

Jinno Y, et al.: Complementation analysis in lymphoid cells from five patients with different forms of maple syrup urine disease. *Hum. Genet.* 68:54, 1984.

Mantovani JF, et al.: MSUD: Presentation with pseudotumor cerebri and CT abnormalities. *J. Pediatr.* 96:279, 1980.

Menkes JH, et al.: A new syndrome: Progressive familial cerebral dysfunction with an unusual urinary substance. *Pediatrics* 14:462, 1954.

Romero FJ, et al.: Cerebral computed tomography in maple

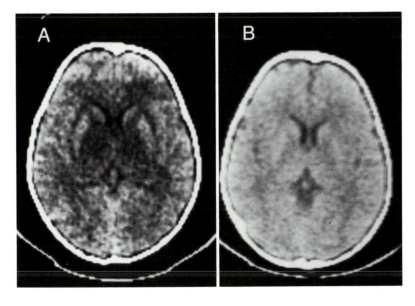

FIG ME–M–2.
Maple syrup urine disease: cranial computed tomography in an 18-month-old infant. **A,** a scan before treatment shows decreased density in the cerebral white matter. **B,** a scan after 6 months of dietary treatment shows normal white matter density. (From Verdu

A, Lopez-Herce J, Pascual-Castroviejo I, et al.: Maple syrup urine disease variant form: Presentation with psychomotor retardation and CT scan abnormalities. *Acta Paediatr. Scand.* 74:815, 1985. Used by permission.)

syrup urine disease. *J. Comput. Assist. Tomogr.* 8:410, 1984.

Suzuki S, et al.: Cranial computed tomography in a patient with a variant form of maple syrup urine disease. *Neuropediatrics* 14:102, 1983.
Verdu A, et al.: Maple syrup urine disease variant form: Presentation with psychomotor retardation and CT scan abnormalities. *Acta Paediatr. Scand.* 74:815, 1985.

MAURIAC SYNDROME

Etiology: *Diabetic children treated with insufficient insulin and diet.*

Clinical Manifestations: (a) *dwarfism;* (b) *protuberant abdomen, moon-shaped face, cushinoid fat deposition;* (c) *hepatomegaly,* glycogen infiltration of the liver; (d) other reported abnormalities: *retarded sexual maturation,* malnutrition, edema, transient false sweat test (elevated sweat chloride level), subtotal villous atrophy of the jejunum.

Radiologic Manifestations: (a) *skeletal maturation retardation;* (b) osteoporosis.

REFERENCES

Dorchy H, et al.: Cause of dwarfism in Mauriac syndrome. *J. Pediatr.* 98:857, 1981.
Mauriac P: Gros ventre, hépatomégalie, troubles de la croissance chez les enfants diabétiques: Traités depuis plusieurs années par l'insuline, *Gaz. Hebl. Sci. Med.* 26:402, 1930.
Rosenfeld R, et al.: False positive sweat test, malnutrition, and the Mauriac syndrome. *J. Pediatr.* 94:240, 1979.
Traisman HS, et al.: Mauriac's syndrome revisited. *Eur. J. Pediatr.* 142:296, 1984.

MELAS SYNDROME

Synonym: Mitochondrial myopathy, encephalopathy, lactic acidosis, and stroke-like episodes.

Mode of Inheritance: Unknown, very few familial cases have been reported.

Clinical Manifestations: Variability in expression; onset in childhood or adulthood: (a) episodic vomiting, headache, sensorineural hearing loss, seizures, *recurrent cerebral strokes* (hemiparesis, hemianopia, cortical blindness); (b) dwarfism; (c) *lactic acidosis;* (d) pathology: *myopathy, ragged red fibers.*

Radiologic Manifestations: (a) computed tomography (CT): focal low-attenuation areas in the temporal and occipital regions, ventricular dilatation, basal ganglia calcification, cortical enhancement on postcontrast scans; development of brain atrophy in the low-attenuation regions; (b) magnetic resonance imaging (T$_2$ weighted): high signal at various sites,

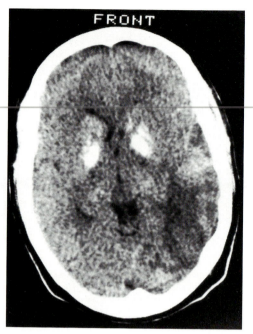

FIG ME–M–3.
MELAS syndrome in a 25-year-old male. A CT scan of the head after a first stroke event shows bilateral basal ganglia calcifications and a left parietal-occipital infarction. The CT scan of the patient's mother also showed bilateral basal ganglia calcification. (From Driscoll PF, Larsen PD, Gruber AB: MELAS syndrome involving a mother and two children. *Arch. Neurol.* 44:971, 1987. Used by permission.)

in particular, in the occipital and temporal lobes; (c) cerebral angiography: capillary blush and early venous filling without occlusive changes in the affected areas.

Differential Diagnosis: Kearns-Sayre syndrome; myoclonus epilepsy, ragged red fiber syndrome (MERRE); multi-infarct dementia; postinflammatory or post-traumatic change; anoxic injury; vasculitis; Cockayne syndrome; Canavan sclerosis; Wilson disease; Leigh disease; Alper disease; Lafora disease; Krabbe disease; Fahr disease; ceroid lipofuscinosis; adrenoleukodystrophy; progressive multifocal encephalopathy.

Notes: MELAS represents an acronym: Mitochondrial myopathy, Encephalopathy, Lactic Acidosis, and Stroke-like episodes (Fig ME–M–3).

REFERENCES

Allard JC, et al.: CT and MR of MELAS syndrome. *A.J.N.R.* 9:1234, 1988.
Driscoll PF, et al.: MELAS syndrome involving a mother and two children. *Arch. Neurol.* 44:971, 1987.
Hasuo K, et al.: Computed tomography and angiography in MELAS (mitochondrial myopathy, encephalopathy, lactic

acidosis and stroke-like episodes); report of 3 cases. *Neuroradiology* 29:393, 1987.

Kabayashi M, et al.: Two cases of NADH—coenzyme Q reductase deficiency: Relationship to MELAS syndrome. *J. Pediatr.* 110:223, 1987.

Pavlakis SG, et al.: Mitochondrial myopathy, encephalopathy, lactic acidosis, and strokelike episodes: A distinctive clinical syndrome. *Ann. Neurol.* 16:481, 1984.

MEMBRANOUS LIPODYSTROPHY

Synonyms: Lipomembranous polycystic osteodysplasia; polycystic lipomembranous osteodysplasia with sclerosing leukoencephalopathy; hereditary angionecrotic polyostotic osteodysplasia.

Mode of Inheritance: Autosomal recessive.

Histology: Convoluted membranes interlaced with lipoid structures; leukodystrophy, general diffuse atrophy, and sclerosis of the white matter, especially in the frontal lobes.

Clinical Manifestations: Onset of symptoms often in adolescence or young adult life: (a) *swelling and pain in joints,* fractures with minor trauma; (b) *neuropsychiatric symptoms* with an onset in middle age: impairment of memory, euphoria, indifference, impotence or frigidity, ataxia, tremor, urinary incontinence, exaggerated deep tendon reflexes, pathological reflexes, abnormal electroencephalographic findings

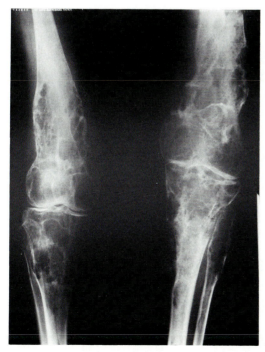

FIG ME—M—4.
Membranous lipodystrophy: multiple symmetrical radiolucent defects in the femora and tibias of a 32-year-old man. (From Akai M, Tatcishi A, Cheng CH, et al.: Membranous lipodystrophy. *J. Bone Joint Surg. [Am.]* 59:802, 1977. Used by permission.)

(slow activity, spike and wave complexes, and spike discharges), frontal syndrome, epileptic convulsions; (c) other reported abnormalies: leukemia, disorder of intestinal motility; (d) death: 40 to 60 years of age.

Radiologic Manifestations: (a) *osteopenia; thin cortices; pathological fractures; radiolucent cystic areas with irregular borders involving the ends of the carpal and tarsal bones and the shafts, metaphyses, and epiphyses of tubular bones symmetrically;* skull and vertebrae not involved; Erlenmeyer deformity of the long bones with scalloping of the endosteal aspect of the cortex; (b) *brain atrophy* associated with ventricular dilatation, basal ganglia calcification.

Differential Diagnosis: Alzheimer disease; Pick disease; polyostotic fibrous dysplasia; multiple intraosseous lipomas; multifocal cystic angiomatosis; hyperparathyroidism; histiocytosis X; multiple benign cysts; etc. (Fig ME—M—4).

REFERENCES

Akai M, et al.: Membranous lipodystrophy: A clinicopathological study of six cases. *J. Bone Joint Surg. [Am.]* 59:802, 1977.

Bird TD, et al.: Lipomembranous polycystic osteodysplasia (brain, bone and fat disease): A genetic cause of presenile dementia. *Neurology* 33:81, 1983.

Hakola HPA, et al.: Osteodysplasia polycystica hereditaria combined with sclerosing leucoencephalopathy. A new entity of the dementia praesenilis group. *Acta Neurol. Scand. Suppl.* 43:79–80, 1970.

Hasegawa Y, et al.: Membranous lipodystrophy (lipomembranous polycystic osteodysplasia) Two case reports. *Clin. Orthop.* 181:229, 1983.

Järvi OH, et al.: A new entity of phacomatosis; a. Bone lesions (hereditary angionecrotic polycystic osteodysplasia). *Acta Pathol. Microbiol. Scand. Suppl.* 215:27, 1970.

Järvi OH, et al.: Membranous reticulin dysplasia of bones. Probably a new disease entity, in *Proceedings of the 14th Scandinavian Congress of Pathology and Microbiology.* Oslo, Universitetsforlaget, 1964, p. 51.

Mäkelä P, et al.: Radiologic bone changes of polycystic lipomembranous osteodysplasia with sclerosing leukoencephalopathy. *Skeletal Radiol.* 8:51, 1982.

Nasu T, et al.: A lipid metabolic disease—"Membranous lipodystrophy"—An autopsy case demonstrating numerous peculiar membrane structures composed of compound lipid in bone and bone marrow and various adipose tissues. *Acta Pathol. Jpn.* 23:539, 1973.

Pazzaglia UE, et al.: Case report 381. *Skeletal Radiol.* 15:474, 1986.

MENKES SYNDROME

Synonyms: Kinky-hair syndrome; trichopoliodystrophy; steely hair disease; copper transport disease.

Mode of Inheritance: X-linked recessive; gene defect located near Xcen.

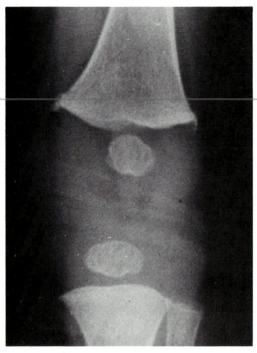

FIG ME–M–5.
Menkes syndrome: metaphyseal spurs on the lower end of the femur in a month-old male infant. (From Danks DM, Campbell PE, Stevens BJ, et al.: Menkes' kinky-hair syndrome: An inherited defect in copper absorption with widespread effects. *Pediatrics* 50:188, 1972. Used by permission.)

Frequency: Approximately 150 published and unpublished cases (Sander et al.).

Clinical Manifestations: (a) *sparse, stubby, twisted, and fractured hairs; variation in diameter of the hair shaft;* (b) *developmental regression, mental retardation, seizures, ataxia, irritability, hypothermia,* intracranial hemorrhage, death in early infancy; (c) laboratory findings: *low level of copper in plasma, urine, and hair; low level of plasma ceruloplasmin;* an increased number of free sulfhydryl groups and decreased number of disulfide bonds in hairs; cultured fibroblasts containing four to six times higher concentrations of copper than control cells; postmortem diagnosis by copper measurement in the muscle tissue (high); copper measurement in the chorionic villi of the affected fetus in the first trimester (high); (d) *malabsorption and maldistribution of copper in body organs;* (e) other reported abnormalities: cryptorchidism, cataracts, atypical form (hypotonicity, fine myoclonic movements, ataxia, delayed psychomotor development, pili torti, etc.), etc.

Radiologic Manifestations: (a) bilateral symmetrical *metaphyseal spurring* of long bones in infancy; (b) flaring of ribs; (c) osteoporosis, fracture(s); (d) *diaphyseal periosteal reaction of long bones;* (e) thickening of scapulae and clavicles; (f) *microcephaly,* excessive wormian bones in the posterior fontanelle region; (g) computed tomography (CT): *progressive development of diffuse cortical brain atrophy,* subdural accumulation of fluid, multifocal areas of ischemic infarction; (h) *widespread arterial changes:* narrowing of the lumen, dilatation, tortuosity, elongation; (i) *cerebral arteriogram,* CT: *loop-the-loop appearance,* supernumerary serpentine branches,

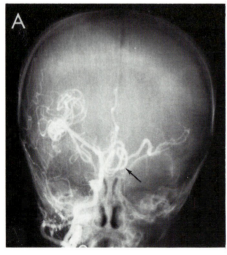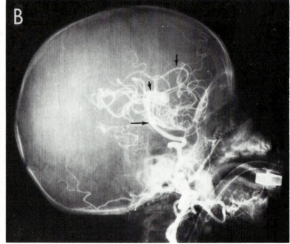

FIG ME–M–6.
Menkes syndrome: right carotid arteriogram of a 5-month-old child. **A,** marked tortuosity of the superior aspect of the cervical portion of the internal carotid artery. Note the "loop-the-loop" appearance of the left anterior cerebral artery *(arrow)* and supernumerary, serpentine branches in the region of the insula. **B,** super-numerary arteries, marked tortuosity of vessels, and abnormal position of vessels *(arrows).* (From Wesenberg RL, Gwinn JL, Barnes CR: Radiological findings in the kinky-hair syndrome. *Radiology* 92:500, 1969. Used by permission.)

marked tortuosity; (j) other reported abnormalities: hydronephrosis, hydroureter, bladder diverticula, polypoid lesion in stomach, emphysema, round lumbar and thoracic vertebral bodies, ureteropelvic junction obstruction, vesicoureteral reflux, urinary tract infection.

Differential Diagnosis: Battered-child syndrome, scurvy, nutritional copper deficiency, late form of argininosuccinic aciduria (trichorrhexis nodosa, seizures, mental retardation), occipital horn syndrome (lysyl oxidase deficiency), etc.

Notes: The serum copper and ceruloplasmin levels are higher than normal in the cord blood of the affected newborn and fall gradually; the levels are within the normal range in the first week of life; in suspected cases the measurements should be made after the first month of life (Figs. ME–M–5 and ME–M–6).

REFERENCES

Adams PC, et al.: Kinky hair syndrome: Serial study of radiological findings with emphasis on the similarity to the battered child syndrome. *Radiology* 112:401, 1974.

Daly WJ, et al.: Urologic abnormalities in Menkes' syndrome. *J. Urol.* 126:262, 1981.

Farrelly C, et al.: CT manifestations of Menkes' kinky hair syndrome (trichopoliodystrophy). *J. Can. Assoc. Radiol.* 35:406, 1984.

Gunn TR, et al.: Difficulties in the neonatal diagnosis of Menkes' kinky hair syndrome—trichopoliodystrophy. *Clin. Pediatr.* 23:514, 1984.

Harcke HT, et al.: Bladder diverticula and Menkes' syndrome. *Radiology* 124:459, 1977.

Hoeldtke RD, et al.: Catecholamine metabolism in kinky hair disease. *Pediatr. Neurol.* 4:23, 1988.

Inagaki M, et al.: Atypical form of Menkes kinky hair disease with mitochondrial NADH-CoQ reductase deficiency. *Neuropediatrics* 19:52, 1988.

Kozlowski K, et al.: Early osseous abnormalities in Menkes' kinky hair syndrome. *Pediatr. Radiol.* 8:191, 1979.

Menkes JH, et al.: A sex-linked recessive disorder with retardation of growth, peculiar hair and focal cerebral and cerebellar degeneration. *Pediatrics* 29:764, 1962.

Nadal D, et al.: Menkes' disease: Long-term treatment with copper and D-penicillamine. *Eur. J. Pediatr.* 147:621, 1988.

Onishi T, et al.: Abnormal copper metabolism in Menkes cultured fibroblasts. *Eur. J. Pediatr.* 134:205, 1980.

Procopis P, et al.: A mild form of Menkes steely hair syndrome. *J. Pediatr.* 98:97, 1981.

Sakano T, et al.: A case of Menkes syndrome with cataracts. *Eur. J. Pediatr.* 138:357, 1982.

Sander C, et al.: Life-span and Menkes kinky hair syndrome: Report of a 13-year course of this disease. *Clin. Genet.* 33:228, 1988.

Seay AR, et al.: CT scans in Menkes disease. *Neurology* 29:304, 1979.

Stanley PH, et al.: The osseous abnormalities in Menkes' syndrome. *Ann. Radiol. (Paris)* 19:167, 1976.

Tønnesen T, et al.: Copper-measurement in a muscle-biopsy. A possible method for postmortem diagnosis of Menkes disease. *Clin. Genet.* 29:258, 1986.

Tønnesen T, et al.: Measurement of copper in chorionic villi for first-trimester diagnosis of Menkes' disease. *Lancet* 1:1038, 1985.

Tønnesen T, et al.: Postmortem Menkes diagnosis from carrier testing of female relatives. *Clin. Genet.* 32:393, 1987.

Von Wendler H, et al.: Menkes-Syndrome mit exzessiven Skelettveränderungen. *Fortschr. Rontgenstr.* 143:351, 1985.

Wesenberg RL, et al.: Radiological findings in the kinky-hair syndrome. *Radiology* 92:500, 1969.

Westman JA, et al.: Atypical Menkes' steely hair disease. *Am. J. Med. Genet.* 30:853, 1988.

Wienker TF, et al.: Evidence that the Menkes locus maps on proximal Xp. *Hum. Genet.* 65:72, 1983.

METACHROMATIC LEUKODYSTROPHIES

Synonyms: Sulfatide lipidosis; cerebroside sulfatidosis; mucosulfatidosis; MLD.

Mode of Inheritance: Autosomal recessive; genetic heterogeneity.

Frequency: 3 to 5:100,000 (Schipper et al.).

Classification: Congenital, late infantile, juvenile, and adult forms.

Enzymatic Deficiency: Failure of the catabolism of sulfatide (the sulfate ester of galactose cerebroside); *accumulation of sulfatides in various tissues; deficient activity of type A arylsulfatase (ASA, arylsulfate sulfohydrolase, EC 3.1.6.1.) in most patients;* variant O (Austin disease) due to multiple enzyme deficiencies (all three arylsulfatases—types A, B, and C, steroid sulfatase, etc.).

Pathology: Accumulation of cerebroside sulfate (sulfatide) in the central nervous system and peripheral nerves (symmetrical demyelination in the cerebral and cerebellar hemispheres, basal ganglia, brain stem and long tracts of the spinal cord), gallbladder wall, epithelial cells of the renal tubules, etc.

Clinical Manifestations: Depend on the age of onset: (a) late infantile form: *difficulty in walking, ataxia, defect in coordination of movement of the limbs, difficulty in swallowing, physical and mental deterioration, decerebrate posture,* abnormalities on evoked potential studies (somatosensory, visual, brain stem auditory); (2) *severe constipation;* (3) *ichthyosis;* (4) *metachromatic granules in the urine, demonstration of various forms of arylsulfatase deficiency in leukocytes by electrophoretic techniques and cultured skin fibroblasts,* absence of arylsulfatase in amniotic fluid (chromatography), assay of chorionic villi for enzyme deficiency; (b) juvenile form: often seen initially with ataxia, progression slower than

TABLE ME−M−1.

Metachromatic Leukodystrophy: Symptoms, Signs, and Course*

Type	Early Clinical Symptoms	Late Clinical Symptoms	Motor Signs	Clinical Course
1. Late infantile: onset, ½−2 yr	Gait disorder Ataxia Hypotonia	Mental regression Loss of language Seizures (25%) Optic atrophy	Pyramidal and cerebellar Decreased DTRs,† particularly AJs† Extensor plantars Peripheral neuropathy may dominate	Predictable in most Unable to sit, feed, or speak by the age of 3 yr Death usually by 5 yr after onset
2. Early juvenile: onset, 4−6 yr	Gait disorder Intellectual deterioration	Loss of speech Loss of motor function Seizures (50%) Optic atrophy	Extrapyramidal postural abnormalities Increased tone tremor Cerebellar ataxia Gait abnormalities Pyramidal signs DTRs increased Extensor plantars	Variable 75% unable to walk or talk 3 yr after diagnosis Death usually within 6 yr of diagnosis, but patients may live 15+ years.
3. Juvenile: onset, 6−16 yr	School difficulties Behavioral disorders	Motor dysfunction Emotional lability Seizures (60%) Mental deterioration Optic atrophy	Extrapyramidal Cerebellar DTRs increased Extensor plantars	Variable Motor deterioration 4−5 yr after onset, may be rapid Death usually 5−10 yr after onset
4. Adult: onset, 16−60 yr	Behavioral abnormalities Poor work performance Emotional lability Schizophrenia-like psychosis Dementia Defective visual-spatial discrimination	Further loss of mentation Motor dysfunction: Clumsiness—early Spastic tetraparesis—late Optic atrophy	Choreiform movements Dystonia DTRs increased Increased plantars	Variable Rapid deterioration in some Most progress slowly—over years

*From McKhann GM: Metachromatic leukodystrophy: Clinical and enzymatic parameters. *Neuropediatrics* 15(suppl):4, 1984. Used by permission.
†DTR = deep tendon reflex; AJ = ankle jerk.

TABLE ME−M−2.

Metachromatic Leukodystrophy: Laboratory Characterization of Clinical Forms*

Type	Arylsulfatase A	Urinary Sulfatide Excretion	Fibroblast Sulfatide Catabolism	Nerve Conduction	CSF Protein
1. Late infantile	Decreased 0−15% normal	Increased	Very low	Decreased early	Elevated
2. Early infantile	Decreased 0−15% normal	Increased	Very low	Decreased later	Elevated
3. Juvenile	Decreased 0−15% normal	Increased	Low	Decreased later	Elevated (not in all)
4. Adult	Decreased	Increased (not as much as other forms)	Decreased	Decreased later (not in all)	Elevated (not in all)
5. MLD heterozygote	Decreased 30−50%	Normal	Normal	Normal	Normal
6. Pseudodeficient	Decreased 10−50%	Normal	Normal	Normal	Normal
7. Activator deficient	Normal	Increased	Low	Decreased	?

*From McKhann GM: Metachromatic leukodystrophy: Clinical and enzymatic parameters. *Neuropediatrics* 15 (suppl.):4, 1984. Used by permission.

in the late infantile form; (c) adult form: often seen initially with progressive dementia and behavior disorders.

Radiologic Manifestations: (a) progressive inability of the gallbladder to concentrate bile: resulting in poor or nonvisualization of the gallbladder in roentgenologic studies, a thick gallbladder wall due to sulfatide deposition, intraluminal filling defects (globules of sulfatide or papillomatosis), very echogenic gallbladder wall, very echogenic material within the gallbladder and common bile duct; (b) megacolon; (c) computed tomography: degenerative disease with diminished attenuation in the brain tissue and a progressive increased difference in attenuation values between the white and gray matter, with changes most marked in the white matter; ventricular dilatation; brain atrophy; (d) other reported abnormalities: lumbar kyphosis, wide ribs, irregular metaphyses, epiphyseal dysgenesis, narrowing of the base of the iliac wings, wide acetabular angles, osteopenia, epiphyseal dysgenesis/chondrodystrophia punctata, hypoplastic vertebral bodies, spondylolisthesis of D_{12} on L_1, butterfly vertebral deformity, etc.

Note: Several cases of combination of MLD and mucopolysaccharidosis have been reported (with skeletal changes of mucopolysaccharidosis in early infancy) (Tables ME–M–1 and ME–M–2).

REFERENCES

Bach G, et al.: Diagnosis of arylsulfatase A deficiency in intact cultured cells using a fluorescent derivative of cerebroside sulfate. *Clin. Genet.* 31:211, 1987.

Burch M, et al.: Multiple sulphatase deficiency presenting at birth. *Clin. Genet.* 30:409, 1986.

Burk RD, et al.: Early manifestations of multiple sulfatase deficiency. *J. Pediatr.* 104:574, 1984.

Carlin L, et al.: Juvenile metachromatic leukodystrophy: Evoked potentials and computed tomography. *Ann. Neurol.* 13:105, 1983.

Eto Y, et al.: Prenatal diagnosis of metachromatic leukodystrophy. A diagnosis by amniotic fluid and its confirmation. *Arch. Neurol.* 39:29, 1982.

Fensom AH, et al.: First trimester diagnosis of metachromatic leucodystrophy. *Clin. Genet.* 34:122, 1988.

Finelli PF: Metachromatic leukodystrophy manifesting as a schizophrenic disorder: Computed tomographic correlation. *Ann. Neurol.* 18:94, 1985.

Greenfield JG: Form of progressive cerebral sclerosis in infants associated with primary degeneration of the interfascicular glia. *J. Neurol. Psychopathol.* 13:289, 1933.

Heier L, et al.: Biliary disease in metachromatic leukodystrophy. *Pediatr. Radiol.* 13:313, 1983.

Kihara H: Genetic heterogeneity in metachromatic leukodystrophy. *Am. J. Hum. Genet.* 34:171, 1982.

MacFaul R, et al.: Metachromatic leucodystrophy: Review of 38 cases. *Arch. Dis. Child.* 57:168, 1982.

McKhann GM: Metachromatic leukodystrophy: Clinical and enzymatic parameters. *Neuropediatrics* 15:4, 1984.

Perlmutter-Cremer N, et al.: Unusual early manifestation of multiple sulfatase deficiency. *Ann. Radiol. (Paris)* 24:43, 1981.

Rodriguez-Soriano J, et al.: Proximal renal tubular acidosis in metachromatic leukodystrophy. *Helv. Paediatr. Acta* 33:45, 1978.

Schipper HE, et al.: Computed tomography in late-onset metachromatic leucodystrophy. *Neuroradiology* 26:39, 1984.

MEVALONIC ACIDURIA

Mode of Inheritance: Autosomal recessive.

Etiology: An inborn error of cholesterol and nonsterol isoprene biosynthesis due to a deficiency of mevalonate kinase activity.

Clinical Manifestations: (a) failure to thrive, mental retardation; (b) cataract; (c) high concentration of mevalonic acid in plasma, urine, and amniotic fluid; (d) severe deficiency of mevalonate kinase activity in fibroblasts, lymphocytes, and lymphoblasts.

Radiologic Manifestation: Generalized brain atrophy (a case report of a child with a history of being born prematurely and developing intraventricular hemorrhage in the perinatal period).

REFERENCE

Hoffmann G, et al.: Mevalonic aciduria—an inborn error of cholesterol and nonsterol isoprene biosynthesis. *N. Engl. J. Med.* 314:1610, 1986.

MILK-ALKALI SYNDROME

Etiologic Factors: (a) hypercalcemia secondary to high calcium intake and excessive gastrointestinal calcium absorption; hypercalcemia maintained at high levels because of impaired renal calcium excretion (alkalosis, renal insufficiency, thiazide diuretics); (b) development of alkalosis secondary to the intake of absorbable alkali and maintenance of alkalosis related to impaired renal bicarbonate excretion (calcium ingestion, parathyroid hormone suppression, hypercalcemia, renal insufficiency); (c) development of renal dysfunction: hypercalcemia, hyperphosphatemia, alkalosis, dehydration.

Clinical Manifestations: (a) nausea, vomiting, weakness, headache, dizziness, ataxia, mental confusion, toxic psychosis, etc.; (b) *hyperazotemia, hypercalcemia*.

Radiologic Manifestations: (a) *deposits of calcium in different body tissues* (nephrocalcinosis, soft-tissue calcification, corneal calcification); (b) ^{99m}Tc uptake in nonosseous lesions.

Note: Alkalosis and hypercalcemia have also been reported after cardiac transplantation (long-term calcium carbonate antacid therapy to aid in the prevention of peptic ulcer disease and osteoporosis associated with glucocorticoid immunosuppressive therapy).

Differential Diagnosis: Primary hyperparathyroidism.

REFERENCES

Burnett CH, et al.: Hypercalcemia without hypercalciuria or hypophosphatemia, calcinosis and renal insufficiency: A syndrome following prolonged intake of milk and alkali. *N. Engl. J. Med.* 240:787, 1949.

Carroll PR, et al.: Milk-alkali syndrome: Does it exist and can it be differentiated from primary hyperparathyroidism? *Ann. Surg.* 197:427, 1983.

Cope CL: Base changes in the alkalosis produced by the treatment of gastric ulcer with alkalies. *Clin. Sci.* 2:287, 1936.

Desai A, et al.: ^{99m}Tc-MDP uptake in nonosseous lesions. *Radiology* 135:181, 1980.

Hardt LL, et al.: Toxic manifestations following the alkaline treatment of peptic ulcer. *Arch. Intern. Med.* 31:171, 1923.

Kapsner P, et al.: Milk-alkali syndrome in patients treated with calcium carbonate after cardiac transplantation. *Arch. Intern. Med.* 146:1965, 1986.

Orwoll ES: The milk-alkali syndrome: Current concepts. *Ann. Intern. Med.* 97:242, 1982.

MUCOLIPIDOSES, MUCOPOLYSACCARIDOSES, AND OTHER ERRORS OF COMPLEX CARBOHYDRATE METABOLISM

Classification and Defective Enzyme: See Table ME–M–3.

REFERENCES

Eggli KD, Dorst JP: The mucopolysaccharidoses and related conditions. *Semin. Roentgenol.* 21:275, 1986.

Mueller OT, et al.: I-cell disease and pseudo-Hurler polydystrophy: Heterozygote detection and characteristics of the altered N-acetyl-glucosamine-phosphotransferase in genetic variants. *Clin. Chim. Acta* 150:175, 1985.

Spranger J: Mini review: Inborn errors of complex carbohydrate metabolism. *Am. J. Med. Genet.* 28:489, 1987.

Wraith JE, et al.: The mucopolysaccharidoses. *Aust. Paediatr. J.* 23:329, 1987.

MUCOLIPIDOSIS II

Synonyms: I-cell disease; Leroy I-cell disease.

Mode of Inheritance: Autosomal recessive; genetic heterogeneity.

Enzyme Deficiency: N-acetylglucosaminylphosphotransferase.

Clinical Manifestations: Onset of symptoms in the first few months of life—may be evident from birth: (a) *abnormal facies* with a high forehead, flat bridge of the nose, anteverted nostrils, increased distance between the upper lip and nares, puffy eyelids, prominent epicanthal folds, increased length of the filtrum, the cornea usually clear, fine granularity on slit-lamp examination, corneal opacity (uncommon), increased corneal diameter; (b) *Hurler-like body configuration;* (c) *marked psychomotor and growth retardation;* (d) thickened skin, especially over the joints; thick and firm earlobes; (e) restricted motion of joints; (f) hypertrophied gingiva; (g) widely spaced nipples; (h) hepatomegaly; (i) recurrent respiratory infections; (j) hoarse voice, narrow trachea (storage material accumulation); (k) hypertrophic cardiomyopathy; (l) *fibroblasts grown from skin biopsy specimens containing large number of dark inclusions in the cytoplasm (I cell),* high lipid content of I cells, *elevated activities of acid hydrolase in serum and culture medium, decreased acid hydrolase activities in cultured fibroblasts, normal or decreased activity in leukocytes, abnormal storage of glycoproteins and glycolipids,* impaired neutrophil chemotaxis; (m) first trimester prenatal evaluation by N-acetylglucosamine-1-phosphotransferase assay (chorionic villi and in the cultured trophoblasts); amniotic fluid and maternal serum: abnormally increased levels of lysosomal enzymes; (n) death between 2 and 8 years of life.

Radiologic Manifestations:

(A) Early infancy: (a) osteopenia; *subperiosteal diaphyseal bone deficiency; multiple areas of bone destruction, especially in the metaphyses of long bones; cortical bone erosion, in particular, in the medial aspects of the proximal parts of the femora; pathological fractures; congenital angulated fracture; modeling abnormalities of metacarpals and metatarsals; brachyphalangia; stippled calcification of the calcaneus;* (b) *ovoid vertebral bodies, narrowness of interpediculate distances in the lower thoracic regions,* intervertebral disk calcification; (c) *flared iliac wings, horizontal acetabular roofs, supra-acetabular constriction.*

(B) Early childhood: (a) craniomegaly, thickened cranium (in some), normal or enlarged sella turcica, (b) *shortness of the long bones with abnormal tubulation, irregularity in ossification and widening of the metaphyses, varus deformity of the humeral neck,* tilted distal ends of the radius and ulna, (c) extreme hypoplasia of carpal bones, short metacarpals with rudimentary distal epiphyses and conical tapering to the base of the second through fifth metacarpals, *hypoplasia of the epiphyses of the phalanges at the base and conical bullet-shaped distal ends,* relatively normal-appearing tarsals, metatarsals, and phalanges of the feet, (d) short anteroposterior diameter of the thoracolumbar vertebrae, inferior *beaking of the vertebral bodies at* T_{12} *through* L_3, (e) broad and spatulate-appearing ribs, (f) hypoplasia of the scapula, (g) *wide iliac flare with hypoplasia of the base, irregular contours of the pubis and ischium, hip dislocation.*

Differential Diagnosis (Neonate, Early Infancy): Hyperparathyroidism; rickets; congenital syphilis; GM_1 gangliosidosis (Fig ME–M–7).

TABLE ME−M−3.

Synopsis of Inborn Errors of Complex Carbohydrate Metabolism*

Name	Defective Enzyme
Mucopolysaccharidosis I†	α-L-Iduronidase
I-H (Hurler)	
I-S (Scheie)	
I-HS (Compound)	
Others	
Mucopolysaccharidosis II‡	Iduronate sulfate sulfatase
Hunter, severe	
Hunter, mild	
Mucopolysaccharidosis III	
Sanfilippo A†	Heparan-N-sulfatase
Sanfilippo B†	α-N-acetylglucosaminidase
Sanfilippo C†	Acetyl-CoA: α-glucosaminide-N-acetyl-transferase
Sanfilippo D†	N-acetylglucosaminide-6-sulfatase
Mucopolysaccharidosis IV	
Morquio A, severe†	Galactosamine-6-sulfate sulfatase
Morquio A, intermediate†	
Morquio A, mild†	
Morquio B†	β-Galactosidase
Other form(s)	Unknown
Mucopolysaccharidosis VI†	N-acetylgalactosamine-4-sulfate sulfatase
Maroteaux-Lamy, severe	
Maroteaux-Lamy, mild	
Mucopolysaccharidosis VII†	β-Glucuronidase
Severe	
Mild	
Fucosidosis†	α-Fucosidase
I	Defective enzyme synthesis
II	Defective enzyme processing
Mannosidosis†	α-Mannosidase
Severe	Low residual enzyme activity
Mild	Higher residual enzyme activity
Aspartylglucosaminuria†	Aspartamido-N-acetylglucosamine-amidohydrolase
GM₁ gangliosidosis†	β-Galactosidase
I, Infantile	
II, Juvenile	
III, Adult	
Sialidosis†	Glycoprotein-specific N-acetylneuraminidase
I, Early infantile	
II, Late infantile (nephrosialidosis)	
III, Juvenile (mucolipidosis I)	
IV, Adult (cherry-red macular spot−myoclonus syndrome)	
Sialic acid storage disease	Unknown
I, Early form	
II, Salla disease†	
Galactosialidosis†	β-Galactosidase and N-acetylneuraminidase
I, Early infantile	Low synthesis of protective protein (PP) precursor
II, Late infantile	Low conversion of PP precursor
III, Juvenile	Slightly low synthesis of PP precursor
Mucosulfatidosis†	Multiple sulfatases
Mucolipidoses II and III†	
Complementation groups (Mueller et al., 1985)	Phosphotransferase
A Mucolipidosis II (I-cell disease)	
Mucolipidosis III (pseudo-Hurler polydystrophy)	
B Mucolipidosis III (pseudo-Hurler polydystrophy)	
C Mucolipidosis III (pseudo-Hurler polydystrophy)	
Mucolipidosis IV	Ganglioside-specific N-acetylneuraminidase?

*From Spranger J: Mini review: Inborn errors of complex carbohydrate metabolism. *Am. J. Med. Genet.* 28:489, 1987. Used by permission.

†Autosomal recessive.

‡X-chromosomal recessive.

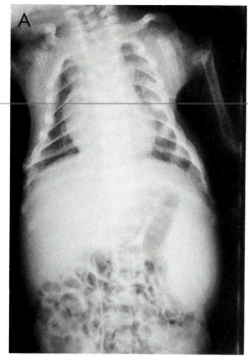

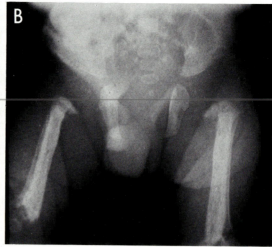

FIG ME–M–7.
Mucolipidosis II in a newborn male with hepatosplenomegaly. **A** and **B,** subperiosteal new bone formation and resorption, multiple areas of "bone destruction" in the metaphyseal regions, cortical bone erosion in the medial aspects of the proximal segments of the femora, and widening and deformity of the ribs and clavicles.

Notes: (a) the "I cell" refers to the cytoplastic granular inclusions (lysosomes containing heterogenous material secondary to an absence or deficiency of most lysosomal acid hydrolases); (b) bone dysplasia present in early fetal life (decreased bone mineralization; coarse, lacy, trabecular pattern; shortness and undermodeling of the tubular bones; subperiosteal deficiency of bone formation; abnormal formation and poor ossification of the vertebrae; etc.).

REFERENCES

Babcock DS, et al.: Fetal mucolipidosis II (I-cell disease): Radiologic and pathologic correlation. *Pediatr. Radiol.* 16:32, 1986.

Ben-Yoseph Y, et al.: First trimester prenatal evaluation for I-cell disease by *N*-acetyl-glucosamine 1-phosphotransferase assay. *Clin. Genet.* 33:38, 1988.

Colome MF, et al.: Observation d'une mucolipidose de type II a revelation neonatal (cas radiologique du mois). *Arch. Fr. Pediatr.* 42:539, 1985.

Lemaitre L, et al.: Radiological signs of mucolipidosis II or I-cell disease: A study of nine cases. *Pediatr. Radiol.* 7:97, 1978.

Leroy JG, et al.: I-cell disease: A clinical picture. *J. Pediatr.* 79:360, 1971.

Michels VV, et al.: Mucolipidosis II: Unusual presentation with a congenital angulated fracture. *Clin. Genet.* 21:225, 1982.

Mogle P, et al.: Calcification of intervertebral disks in I-cell disease. *Eur. J. Pediatr.* 145:226, 1986.

Okada S, et al.: I-cell disease: Clinical studies of 21 Japanese cases. *Clin. Genet.* 28:207, 1985.

Patriquin HB, et al.: Neonatal mucolipidosis II (I-cell disease): Clinical and radiologic features in three cases. *A.J.R.* 129:37, 1977.

Peters ME, et al.: Narrow trachea in mucopolysaccharidoses. *Pediatr. Radiol.* 15:225, 1985.

Sakaguchi T, et al.: Impaired neutrophil chemotaxis in two patients with mucolipidosis II. *Acta Paediatr. Scand.* 77:609, 1988.

Shows TB, et al.: Genetic heterogeneity of I-cell disease is demonstrated by complementation of lysosomal enzyme processing mutants. *Am. J. Med. Genet.* 12:343, 1982.

Whelan DT, et al.: Mucolipidosis II. The clinical, radiological and biochemical features in three cases. *Clin. Genet.* 24:90, 1983.

MUCOLIPIDOSIS III

Synonym: Pseudo-Hurler polydystrophy.

Mode of Inheritance: Autosomal recessive.

Enzyme Deficiency: *N*-acetylglucosaminyl-phosphotransferase; closely related to mucolipidosis II (I-cell disease).

Clinical Manifestations: Onset of clinical manifestations usually in late infancy: (a) *short stature*; (b) *coarse facies*; (c) *joint stiffness*; (d) *mild corneal clouding*; (e) *mild mental retardation*; (f) *valvular heart disease*; (g) *abnormal storage of glycoproteins and glycolipids*; (h) *normal levels of urinary acid mucopolysaccharides, marked decrease in activities of several lysosomal hydrolases in cultured fibroblasts with concomitant elevated activity of these hydrolases in serum and elevated activities in urine, coarse perinuclear refractile inclusions in cultured fibroblasts.*

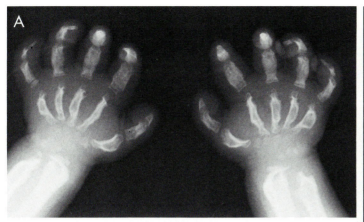

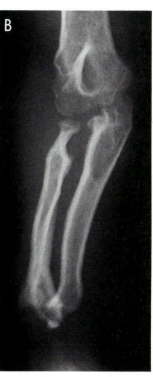

FIG ME–M–8.
Mucolipidosis, type III, in a 16-year-old female. **A,** the radius and ulna are broad in their shaft and tapered in the metaphyseal regions, with an angulated obliquity of the growth plates. **B,** ossification of the carpal bones and epiphyses is retarded; the metacarpals are centrally thickened, and the second to fifth are proximally pointed. Note the tapering of the distal phalanges and tilting of the lower ends of the radius and ulna toward each other. (From Herd JK, Dvorak AD, Wiltse HE, et al.: Mucolipidosis type III. *Am. J. Dis. Child.* 132:1181, 1978. Used by permission.)

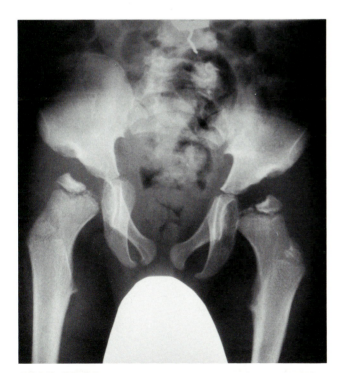

FIG ME–M–9.
Mucolipidosis III in a 3-year-old male with flaring of the iliac wings, constriction of the iliac bodies, shallow and deformed acetabular fossae, broad femoral necks, and dysgenesis of the femoral epiphysis.

Radiologic Manifestations: *Changes similar to those of Hurler and Hunter syndromes:* (a) premature closure of the cranial sutures (in older cases), J-shaped sella turcica, mandibular prognathism; (b) short and thick clavicles; (c) wide and slightly short ribs; (d) beaking of some vertebrae (upper lumbar), absence of a dens; (e) flaring of the iliac wings; (f) constriction of the iliac bodies; (g) shallow acetabular fossae; (h) shortening and poor tubulation of long bones; (i) broad metaphyses and small and flat epiphyses; (j) proximal pointing of metacarpals; (k) clawhand deformity; (l) soft-tissue swelling around the interphalangeal joints; (m) smallness and irregularity of carpal bones; (n) mild to moderate delay in skeletal maturation (Figs ME–M–8 to ME–M–10).

REFERENCES

Aviad I, et al.: Roentgen findings of pseudo-Hurler polydystrophy in the adult with a note on cephalometric changes. *A.J.R.* 122:56, 1974.

Eggli KD, et al.: The mucopolysaccharidoses and related conditions. *Semin. Roentgenol.* 21:275, 1986.

Herd JK, et al.: Mucolipidosis type III: Multiple elevated serum and urine enzyme activities. *Am. J. Dis. Child.* 132:1181, 1978.

Maroteaux P, et al.: La pseudo-polydystrophie de Hurler. *Presse Med.* 74:2889, 1966.

Melhem R, et al.: Roentgen findings in mucolipidosis III (pseudo-Hurler polydystrophy). *Radiology* 106:153, 1973.

Nolte K, et al.: Early skeletal changes in mucolipidosis III. *Ann. Radiol. (Paris)* 19:151, 1976.

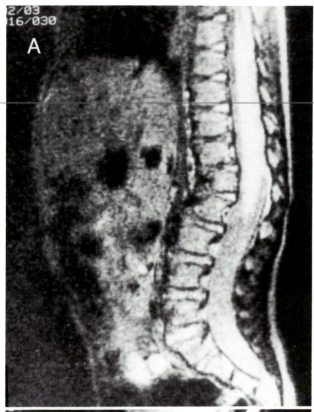

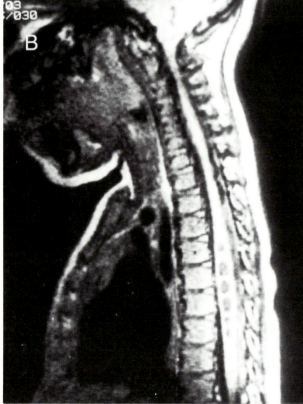

MUCOLIPIDOSIS IV

Mode of Inheritance: Autosomal recessive.

Clinical Manifestations: Onset of symptoms in infancy: (a) mild to severe psychomotor retardation; (b) early or congenital corneal cloudiness, retinal degeneration; (c) corneal and conjunctival biopsy specimens, cultured amniotic fluid cells, and fibroblast culture: lysosomal inclusions; (d) tissue accumulation of gangliosides, phospholipids, and acidic mucopolysaccharides; (e) electron microscopy: typical abnormal inclusion bodies in various organ tissues (corneal and conjunctival biopsy material, chorionic cells, cultured amniotic fluid cells, and cultured fetal skin fibroblasts); (f) the enzyme deficiency not definitely determined, ganglioside-specific N-acetylneuraminidase has been suggested.

Radiologic Manifestations: No skeletal changes; no organomegaly.

REFERENCES

Amir N, et al.: Mucolipidosis type IV: Clinical spectrum and natural history. *Pediatrics* 79:953, 1987.
Ben-Yoseph Y, et al.: Catalytically defective ganglioside neuraminidase in mucolipidosis IV. *Clin. Genet.* 21:374, 1982.
Crandall BF, et al.: Mucolipidosis IV. *Am. J. Med. Genet.* 12:301, 1982.
Kohn G, et al.: Prenatal diagnosis of mucolipidosis IV by electron microscopy. *J. Pediatr.* 90:62, 1977.
Merin S, et al.: Mucolipidosis IV: Ocular, systemic, and ultrastructural findings. *Invest. Ophthalmol.* 14:437, 1975.
Ornoy A, et al.: Early prenatal diagnosis of mucolipidosis IV (letter). *Am. J. Med. Genet.* 27:983, 1987.

MUCOPOLYSACCHARIDOSIS I-H

Synonym: Hurler syndrome.

Mode of Inheritance: Autosomal recessive.

Frequency: 1:100,000 births (Eggli et al.).

Enzyme Deficiency: α-L-Iduronidase.

Clinical Manifestations: Onset of detectable clinical findings by 1 to 2 years of age; fully developed picture: (a) *grotesque facial features* (scaphocephalic large head, protruding eyes, patulous lips, thick cheeks and jaw, low nasal bridge, flared nostrils, enlarged protruding tongue, small

FIG ME—M—10.
Mucolipidosis III in a 4-year-old male. Magnetic resonance imaging of the cervical, thoracic, and lumbosacral regions shows a gibbous deformity at the L₁ level **(A)** and a multiloculated syrinx **(B).** (Courtesy of Bent Kjos, M.D., Magnetic Imaging Affiliates, Oakland, Calif.)

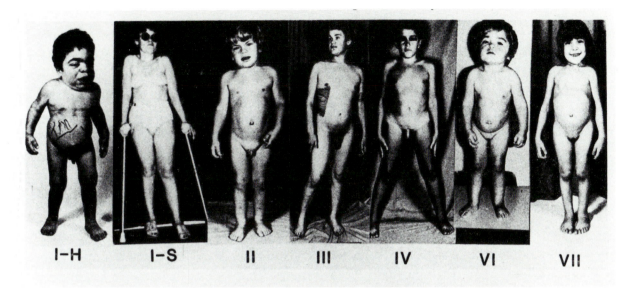

I-H   I-S   II   III   IV   VI   VII

FIG ME–M–11.
Mucopolysaccharidoses: Clinical appearance of patients with various mucopolysaccharidoses. **I-H,** 8 years of age, Hurler disease. **I-S,** adult, Scheie disease. **II,** 3 years old, Hunter disease. **III,** 18 years of age, Sanfilippo A disease. **IV,** 12 years of age, Morquio A disease (the patient standing with spread legs in order to prevent

the femoral heads from slipping out of the acetabular fossae). **VI,** 4 years of age, Maroteaux-Lamy disease. **VII,** 8 years of age, mucopolysaccharidosis VII. (From Spranger J: Mini Review: Inborn errors of complex carbohydrate metabolism. *Am. J. Med. Genet.* 28:489, 1987. Used by permission.)

malaligned teeth); (b) *severe mental retardation;* (c) coarse hair, hirsutism; (d) *corneal opacification,* glaucoma; (e) *dwarfism;* (f) thoracolumbar *gibbus;* (g) protuberant abdomen, hernias; (h) *flexion contracture* of all joints, claw-hand deformity; (i) harsh voice; (j) *hepatosplenomegaly,*

hepatic fibrosis, nephrotic syndrome and hypertension; (k) rhinitis, deafness; (l) death occurring usually in childhood; (m) *excess storage of acid mucopolysaccharides in tissues and excess excretion in urine:* dermatan sulfate and heparan sulfate.

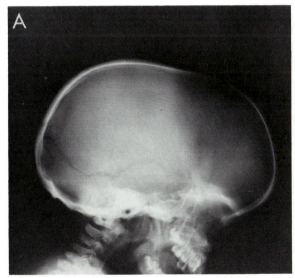
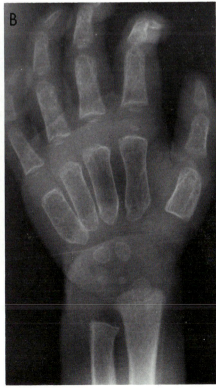

FIG ME–M–12.
Mucopolysaccharidosis I (Hurler) in a 2-year-old female. **A,** large and dense dolichocephalic skull, J-shaped sella turcica, and enlarged soft tissues of the nasopharynx causing upper airway obstruction. **B,** lateral tilt of the distal part of the ulna, widening of the diaphyseals of the metacarpals and phalanges, and pointed proximal ends of the second through fifth metacarpals.

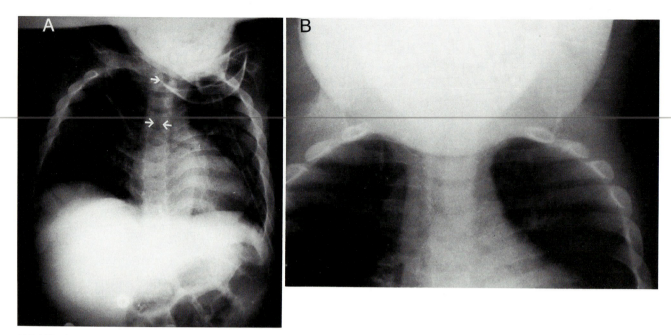

FIG ME–M–13.
Mucopolysaccharidosis I-H (Hurler syndrome): narrowing of the trachea at 8 years of age **(A)** as compared with the normal tracheal width at 2 years of age **(B)**.

Radiologic Manifestations: (a) *craniofacial:* large neurocranium, premature closure of the sagittal and lambdoid sutures; thick calvaria, in particular, at the base; shallow orbits with vertically oriented roofs; enlarged J-shaped sella turcica; calcified stylohyoid ligament thicker than normal; short and wide mandible with obtuse angle; short rami and flat or concave condyle; abnormally directed molar teeth; dentigerous cysts; hyperplasia of dental follicles; (b) *vertebrae:* moderate dorsolumbar gibbus, hooklike dysplasia of the vertebrae at the apex of the gibbus, decreased anteroposterior diameters of vertebral bodies, biconvex vertebral bodies, relatively long pedicles, failure of development of the dens with resultant subluxation of C_1 on C_2, subluxation of C_3 on C_4; (c) *thorax:* wide oar-shaped ribs, short and thick clavicles, thick elevated scapulae with poorly formed glenoid fossae; (d) *long bones:* widening of the midshaft, in particular, that of humerus; varus deformity of the humeral neck; tilt of the distal parts of the radius and ulna toward each other; (e) *pelvis and hips:* flared small iliac wings, steep acetabular roofs, poorly formed and thickened ischial and pubic bones, coxa valga, subluxation of the femoral heads; (f) *hands:* widening of the diaphyses of metacarpals and proximal and middle phalanges ("sugarloaf" metacarpals), shortness of the phalanges, smallness and irregularity of the carpal bones, pointed proximal end of the second to fifth metacarpals; (g) *feet:* less severe deformities of the tarsals, metatarsals, and phalanges as compared with the hands and wrists; (h) cardiomegaly, echocardiographic demonstration of abnormal thickening of the valves, calcification of the mitral annulus, mitral stenosis, mitral regurgitation, coronary artery narrowing, myocardial involvement, etc.; (i) narrow trachea, recurrent pneumonia and atelectasis; (j) central nervous system: hydrocephalus (acute,

chronic), leptomeningeal cysts, computed tomographic abnormalities (symmetrical low attenuation in the white matter, enlargement of the cortical sulci and interhemispheric fissures), magnetic resonance image (MRI) abnormalities (reduced gray-white matter contrast, ventricular and cortical sulcal enlargement, prolonged periventricular T_2), improved MRI findings after bone marrow transplant (improvement in gray-white matter contrast, progressive increase in myelination, and less prominent periventricular increase of T_2) (Figs ME–M–11 to ME–M–13).

REFERENCES

Brodius FC, et al.: Coronary artery disease in the Hurler syndrome. *Am. J. Cardiol.* 47:649, 1981.
Eggli KD, et al.: The mucopolysaccharidoses and related conditions. *Semin. Roentgenol.* 21:275, 1986.
Gardner DG: The oral manifestations of Hurler's syndrome. *Oral Surg.* 32:46, 1971.
Hurler G: Ueber einen Typ multipler Abartungen, vorwiegend am Skelettsystem. *Z. Kinderheilkd.* 24:220, 1919.
Johnson GL, et al.: Echocardiographic mitral valve deformity in the mucopolysaccharidoses. *Pediatrics* 67:401, 1981.
Johnson MA, et al.: Magnetic resonance imaging of the brain in Hurler syndrome. *A.J.N.R.* 5:8, 1984.
Mueller OT, et al.: Apparent allelism of the Hurler, Scheie, and Hurler/Scheie syndromes. *Am. J. Med. Genet.* 18:547, 1984.
Muller VJ, et al.: α-L-Iduronidase deficiency in mucopolysaccharidosis type I against a radiolabelled sulfated disaccharide substrate derived from dermatan sulfate. *Clin. Genet.* 26:414, 1984.

Nowaczyk, MJ, et al.: Glaucoma as an early complication of Hurler's disease. *Arch. Dis. Child.* 63:1091, 1988.

Oestreich AE: The stylohyoid ligament in Hurler syndrome and related conditions: Comparison with normal children. *Radiology* 154:665, 1985.

Peters ME, et al.: Narrow trachea in mucopolysaccharidoses. *Pediatr. Radiol.* 15:225, 1985.

Schochet SS Jr, et al.: Pituitary gland in patients with Hurler syndrome. *Arch. Pathol.* 97:96, 1974.

Semenza GL, et al.: Airway narrowing in mucopolysaccharide storage disorders, Presented at the Birth Defect Meeting, Baltimore, 1988.

Shinnar S, et al.: Acute hydrocephalus in Hurler's syndrome. *Am. J. Dis. Child.* 136:556, 1982.

Spranger J: Mini review: Inborn errors of complex carbohydrate metabolism. *Am. J. Med. Genet.* 28:489, 1987.

Storme B, et al.: Allogreffe de moelle dans une maladie de Hurler. Résultats clinique et biologique après un an d'évolution. *Ann. Pediatr. (Paris)* 35:117, 1988.

Taylor J, et al.: Nephrotic syndrome and hypertension in two children with Hurler syndrome. *J. Pediatr.* 108:726, 1986.

Thomas SL, et al.: Hypoplasia of the odontoid with atlanto-axial subluxation in Hurler's syndrome. *Pediatr. Radiol.* 15:353, 1985.

Watts RWE, et al.: Computed tomography studies on patients with mucopolysaccharidoses. *Neuroradiology* 21:9, 1981.

MUCOPOLYSACCHARIDOSIS I-H/S

Synonym: Hurler-Scheie compound.

Mode of Inheritance: Autosomal recessive.

Frequency: 1:500,000 births (Eggli et al.).

Enzyme Deficiency: α-L-Iduronidase.

Clinical Manifestations: A phenotype intermediate between that of Hurler and Scheie compound; appearance of clinical signs between 1 and 2 years of age: (a) excessive birth weight and infantile growth, ultimate short height; (b) normal to mild retardation of intelligence; (c) *moderate joint stiffness and limitation of motion;* (d) *hepatosplenomegaly;* (e) *neurological symptoms related to spinal cord compression;* (f) *corneal clouding;* (g) *thickened skin, hirsuitism;* (h) hernias; (i) echocardiography: myocardial dysfunction, mitral valvular disease; (j) psychosis; (k) *urinary excretion of dermatan sulfate and heparan sulfate;* (l) *impaired mucopolysaccharide degradation and correction by Hurler factor.*

Radiologic Manifestations: (a) *mild to moderate dysostosis multiplex;* (b) cardiomegaly, calcific mitral stenosis; (c) concentric impingement on the subarachnoid space, cord compression, hydrocephalus; low white matter density (computed tomography); (d) dentigerous cysts.

Note: Hurler-Scheie genetic compound: one Hurler gene and one Scheie gene present at the affected gene locus (Figs ME–M–14 and ME–M–15).

REFERENCES

Colavita N, et al.: A further contribution to the knowledge of mucopolysaccharidosis I H/S compound. Presentation of two cases and review of the literature. *Australas. Radiol.* 30:142, 1986.

Dugas M, et al.: Symptomatologie psychotique au cours de l'evolution dementielle d'une mucopolysaccharidose de phenotype Hurler-Scheie. *Arch. Fr. Pediatr.* 42:373, 1985.

Eggli KD, et al.: The mucopolysaccharidoses and related conditions. *Semin. Roentgenol.* 21:275, 1986.

Lorincz AE, et al.: Mucopolysaccharidosis (type 1 Hurler-Scheie compound). *J. Cutan. Pathol.* 2:214, 1975.

Schieken RM, et al.: Cardiac manifestations of the mucopolysaccharidoses. *Circulation* 52:700, 1975.

Schmidt H, et al.: Radiological findings in patients with mucopolysaccharidosis I H/S (Hurler-Scheie syndrome). *Pediatr. Radiol.* 17:409, 1987.

Sostrin RD, et al.: Myelographic features of mucopolysaccharidoses: A new sign. *Radiology* 125:421, 1977.

Stevenson RE, et al.: The iduronidase-deficient mucopolysaccharidoses: Clinical and roentgenographic features. *Pediatrics* 57:111, 1976.

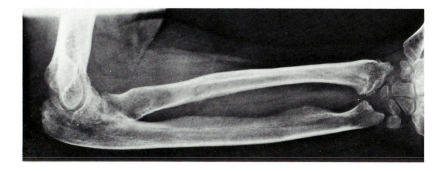

FIG ME–M–14.
Mucopolysaccharidosis I-H/S (Hurler-Scheie compound) in a 20-year-old female. Thickening and irregularity of both the ulna and radius, a V-shaped configuration of the distal parts of the ulna and radius, and small carpal bones with irregular margins are present.

(From Stevenson RE, Howell R, McKusick VA, et al.: The iduronidase-deficient mucopolysaccharidoses: Clinical and roentgenographic features. *Pediatrics* 57:111, 1976. Used by permission.)

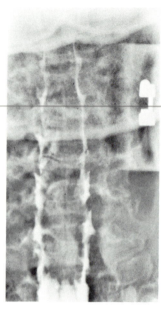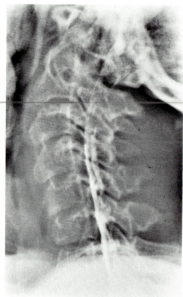

FIG ME—M—15.
Mucopolysaccharidosis I-H/S (Hurler-Scheie compound) in a 22-year-old man with a history of progressive weakness of all extremities of 4 years' duration. An oil contrast myelogram in the lateral projection shows cord compressed in the sagittal plane, with marked separation of spinal structures from the ventral surface of the bony canal. (From Sostrin RD, Hasse AN, Peterson DI, et al.: Myelographic features of mucopolysaccharidoses: A new sign. *Radiology* 125:421, 1977. Used by permission.)

Watts RWE, et al.: Computed tomography studies on patients with mucopolysaccharidoses. *Neuroradiology* 21:9, 1981.

MUCOPOLYSACCHARIDOSIS I-S

Synonym: Scheie disease.

Mode of Inheritance: Autosomal recessive.

Enzyme Deficiency: α-L-Iduronidase.

Clinical Manifestations: Abnormalities usually appear in childhood: (a) *corneal clouding,* retinitis pigmentosa; (b) broad mouth, full lips; (c) *joint stiffness;* (d) clawhand, genu valgum, carpal tunnel syndrome; (e) heart murmur, often aortic valvular disease; (f) normal intelligence or mild mental retardation, psychotic episodes; (g) excessive dermatan sulfate and heparan sulfate excretion in urine; (h) impaired mucopolysaccharide degradation and correction by Hurler factor (see Fig ME—M—11).

Radiologic Manifestations: (a) *deformities and cystic changes in the carpals and metacarpals, tarsals and metatarsals, and some other bones;* femoral head dysplasia; (b) *widening of the clavicles and ribs;* (c) aortic valvular disease.

REFERENCES

Dekaban AS, et al.: Mucopolysaccharidosis type V (Scheie syndrome). *Arch. Pathol. Lab. Med.* 100:237, 1976.

Grossman H, et al.: The mucopolysaccharidoses and mucolipidoses, in Kaufmann HJ (ed.): *Progress in Pediatric Radiology.* Basel, S. Karger AG, 1973, vol. 4, p. 495.

Lamon JM, et al.: Bone cysts in mucopolysaccharidosis I S (Scheie syndrome). *Johns Hopkins Med. J.* 146:73, 1980.

McKusick VA, et al.: Allelism, non allelism and genetic compounds among the mucopolysaccharidoses. *Lancet* 1:993, 1972.

Scheie HG, et al.: A newly recognized forme fruste of Hurler's disease (gargoylism). *Am. J. Ophthalmol.* 53:753, 1962.

Watts RWE, et al.: Computed tomography studies on patients with mucopolysaccharidoses. *Neuroradiology* 21:9, 1981.

MUCOPOLYSACCHARIDOSIS II

Synonym: Hunter disease.

Mode of Inheritance: X-linked recessive; localization of the gene on the long arm of the X chromosome; clinical and genetic heterogeneity; heterozygote detection with the use of serum and lymphocyte extract for the determination of enzyme levels (iduronate sulfate sulfatase).

Frequency: 0.6:100,000 births (Eggli et al.).

Enzyme Deficiency: Iduronate sulfate sulphatase.

Clinical Manifestations: Wide clinical spectrum ranging from normal intelligence to marked mental retardation; onset of clinically detectable findings between the ages of 2 and 4

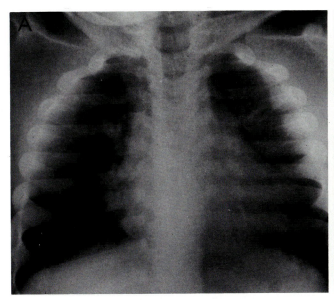
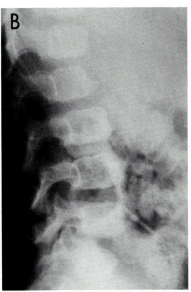

FIG ME—M—16.
Mucopolysaccharidosis II (Hunter): One of three male siblings affected by the disease. **A,** chest at 4 years of age: wide ribs, thick scapulae, and cardiomegaly. **B,** a hooklike deformity of the second lumbar vertebra is seen at 2 years and 8 months of age.

years; physical features similar but usually milder than in Hurler disease: (a) *coarse facies, prominent lips, protruding tongue, large scaphoid head, widely spaced teeth, short neck, etc.;* (b) *mental retardation,* destructive behavior, seizures; (c) *hepatosplenomegaly;* (d) hirsutism, thick skin, *firm ivory-white papules and nodules that may coalesce to form ridges or a reticular pattern;* (e) clear or cloudy cornea, papilledema, retinal pigmentation; (f) mild dwarfism; (g) *flexion contractures* (flexed knees and elbows, prominent buttocks, clawhand); (h) *dorsolumbar kyphosis;* (i) *progressive deafness;* (j) protuberant abdomen, hernias, mucoid diarrhea; (k) echocardiographic and electrocardiographic evidence of impaired left ventricular function suggesting the presence of myocardial damage; (l) life span may extend into adulthood; (m) *excess storage of acid mucopolysaccharides in tissues and excess excretion of dermatan sulfate and heparan sulfate in urine;* hair root and serum enzyme studies, chorion biopsy, and amniotic fluid enzyme assay for prenatal diagnosis; enzyme determination in the serum of pregnant heterozygote women; (n) pink rings lymphocyte.

Radiologic Manifestations: (a) dysostosis multiplex *similar to Hurler syndrome with findings being less severe and more slowly progressive;* (b) narrow trachea; (c) low white matter density (computed tomography) (Fig ME—M—16).

REFERENCES

Eggli KD, et al.: The mucopolysaccharidoses and related conditions. *Semin. Roentgenol.* 21:275, 1986.

Grossman H, et al.: The mucopolysaccharidoses and mucolipidoses, in Kaufmann HJ (ed.): *Progress in Pediatric Radiology.* Basel, S. Karger AG, 1973, vol. 4, p. 495.

Harper PS, et al.: Chorion biopsy for prenatal testing in Hunter's syndrome. *Lancet* 2:812, 1984.

Hunter CA: A rare disease in two brothers. *Proc. R. Soc. Med.* 10:104, 1917.

Maier-Redelsperger M, et al.: Pink rings lymphocyte: A new cytologic abnormality characteristic of mucopolysaccharidosis type II (Hunter disease). *Pediatrics* 82:286, 1988.

Peters ME, et al.: Narrow trachea in mucopolysaccharidoses. *Pediatr. Radiol.* 15:225, 1985.

Prystowsky SD, et al.: Cutaneous marker in the Hunter syndrome: Report of 4 cases. *Arch. Dermatol.* 113:602, 1977.

Schiavulli E, et al.: La diagnosi di malattia di Hunter. *Minerva Pediatr.* 29:1937, 1977.

Schieken RM, et al.: Cardiac manifestations of the mucopolysaccharidoses. *Circulation* 52:700, 1975.

Spranger J, et al.: Mucopolysaccharidosis II (Hunter disease) with corneal opacities: Report on two patients at the extremes of a wide clinical spectrum. *Eur. J. Pediatr.* 129:11, 1978.

Upadhyaya M, et al.: Localisation of the gene for Hunter syndrome on the long arm of X chromosome. *Hum. Genet.* 74:391, 1986.

Wakai S, et al.: Skeletal muscle involvement in mucopolysaccharidosis type II A: Severe type of Hunter syndrome. *Pediatr. Neurol.* 4:178, 1988.

Watts RWE, et al.: Computed tomography studies on patients with mucopolysaccharidoses. *Neuroradiology* 21:9, 1981.

Young ID, et al.: A clinical and genetic study of Hunter's syndrome. 1 Heterogeneity. *J. Med. Genet.* 19:401, 1982.

Young ID, et al.: Long term complications in Hunter's syndrome. *Clin. Genet.* 16:125, 1979.

Zlotogora J, et al.: Heterozygote detection in Hunter syndrome. *Am. J. Med. Genet.* 17:661, 1984.

Zlotogora J, et al.: Hunter syndrome: Prenatal diagnosis in maternal serum. *Am. J. Hum. Genet.* 38:253, 1986.

MUCOPOLYSACCHARIDOSIS III

Synonym: Sanfilippo disease, types A, B, C, and D.

Mode of Inheritance: Autosomal recessive; genetic heterogeneity.

Frequency: 1:200,000 births (Eggli et al.).

Enzyme Deficiency: Type A, heparan *N*-sulfatase; type B, *N*-acetyl-α-D-glucosaminidase; type C, acetyl-CoA: α-glucosaminide-*N*-acetyltransferase; type D, *N*-acetylglucosaminide-6-sulfate sulfatase.

Clinical Manifestations: Onset of detectable abnormalities in early childhood: (a) *mild coarsening of facial features;* (b) normal height or mild dwarfism; (c) *minimal corneal clouding;* (d) *mild joint stiffness and clawhand deformity;* (e) *mental and motor deterioration,* behavior disorders, sleep disturbances, hyperactivity, insomnia, aggressive reactions to fear, dementia; (f) hepatosplenomegaly; (g) *excessive amount of heparan sulfate in the urine;* (h) prenatal diagnosis: chorionic biopsy and enzyme assay, cultured amniotic fluid cell test, increased level of heparan sulfate in amniotic fluid (two-dimensional electrophoresis of glycosaminoglycans).

Radiologic Manifestations: Much milder skeletal deformities than Hurler syndrome: (a) *marked thickening of the posterior aspect of the calvaria* in association with mild thickening of the base, underdevelopment of mastoid cells; (b) *ovoid or rectangular appearance of the thoracic and lumbar vertebrae;* (c) *thickened ribs;* (d) broad iliac wings, steep acetabular roofs, small femoral heads; (e) poor modeling of the tubular bones of the hand, tilt of the distal part of the radius toward the ulna; (f) thick cortex of long bones and coarse trabeculae; (g) ventricular dilatation and wide subarachnoid space, low white matter density (computed tomography).

Note: Clinical intertype and intratype variability; the patients with type A are more severely affected and have an earlier onset of symptoms and more rapid progression as compared with type B; type C is intermediate in severity between types A and B (see Fig ME−M−11).

REFERENCES

Eggli KD, et al.: The mucopolysaccharidoses and related conditions. *Semin. Roentgenol.* 21:275, 1986.

Gatti R, et al.: Sanfilippo type D disease: Clinical findings in two patients with a new variant of mucopolysaccharidosis III. *Eur. J. Pediatr.* 138:168, 1982.

Grossman H, et al.: The mucopolysaccharidoses and mucolipidoses, in Kaufmann HJ (ed.): *Progress in Pediatric Radiology*. Basel, S. Karger AG, 1973, vol. 4, p. 495.

Kaplan P, et al.: Sanfilippo syndrome type D. *J. Pediatr.* 110:267, 1987.

Kleijer WJ, et al.: First-trimester diagnosis of mucopolysaccharidosis IIIA (Sanfilippo A disease). *N. Engl. J. Med.* 314:185, 1986.

Kleijer WJ, et al.: Prenatal diagnosis of Sanfilippo disease type B. *Hum. Genet.* 66:287, 1984.

Sanfilippo SJ, et al.: Mental retardation associated with acid mucopolysacchariduria (heparitin sulfate type). *J. Pediatr.* 63:837, 1963.

Sewell AC, et al.: Mucopolysaccharidosis type III C (Sanfilippo): Early clinical presentation in a large Turkish pedigree. *Clin. Genet.* 34:116, 1988.

Uvebrant P: Sanfilippo type C syndrome in two sisters. *Acta Paediatr. Scand.* 74:137, 1985.

van de Kamp JJP, et al.: Genetic heterogeneity and clinical variability in the Sanfilippo syndrome (types A, B, and C). *Clin. Genet.* 20:152, 1981.

Van Schrojenstein−de Valk HMJ, et al.: Follow-up on seven adult patients with mild Sanfilippo B-disease. *Am. J. Med. Genet.* 28:125, 1987.

Watts RWE, et al.: Computed tomography studies on patients with mucopolysaccharidoses. *Neuroradiology* 21:9, 1981.

MUCOPOLYSACCHARIDOSIS IV A

Synonyms: Morquio disease, type A; MPS IVA; Brailsford-Morquio syndrome; Morquio-Ulrich syndrome; Morquio-Brailsford syndrome; etc.

Mode of Inheritance: Autosomal recessive.

Frequency: 1:100,000 births (Eggli et al.).

Classification: Clinical heterogeneity: (a) Morquio A, severe ("classic" type); (b) Morquio A, intermediate; (c) Morquio A, mild.

Enzyme Deficiency: Galactosamine-6-sulfate sulfatase.

Clinical Manifestations: The disease usually becomes detectable between the first and third year of age; fully developed clinical picture: (a) *short-trunk dwarfism;* (b) mildly coarse facial features, broad mouth, short nose; (c) *abnormal posture* (kyphosis at the thoracolumbar junction, prominent buttocks, pectus carinatum, severe knock-knee); (d) misshapen hands and feet; (e) hyperextensible joints; (f) spinal cord compression due to atlantoaxial dislocation, chronic myelopathy with a slow or rapid rate of progression, quadriparesis, sudden death by respiratory arrest; (g) minimal corneal clouding; (h) *normal intelligence;* (i) progressive deafness; (j) recurrent or chronic pneumonia, cardiac failure secondary to thoracic cage deformities, restricted pattern on ventilatory studies, hypoxemia due to right-to-left shunting (probably caused by microatelectasis); (k) aortic regurgitation in the advanced stage, mitral stenosis; (l) dental abnormalities: thin enamel layers, smallness, more opaque than normal, pointed cusps of the permanent posterior teeth (concave and saucer-shaped biting surface, concave buccal surface), pitting of the buccal surfaces of the permanent posterior teeth, spade-shaped and spaced permanent maxillary incisors and deciduous teeth; (m) *excess keratan sulfate excretion in the urine,* most marked in childhood, decreasing and becoming normal in adults; some cases with keratosulfaturia absent in childhood; two-dimensional electrophoresis of urine glycosaminoglycans; enzyme deficiency in fibroblasts.

Radiologic Manifestations:

(A) Skeletal system: (a) mildly dolichocephalic skull, underdevelopment of mastoid cells, flat or concave mandibular condyles; (b) *universal platyspondyly, small or disappearing odontoid process* of the axis, *atlantoaxial subluxation* resulting in narrowing of the spinal canal, irregular margins of the vertebral bodies; (c) *flaring of ribs, pectus carinatum,* shortness of superoinferior height and an increase in anteroposterior diameter of the thorax, premature fusion of ossification centers of the sternum; (d) *constricted iliac wings, steeply ob-*

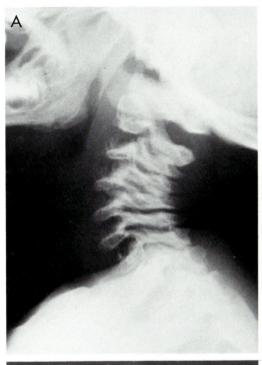

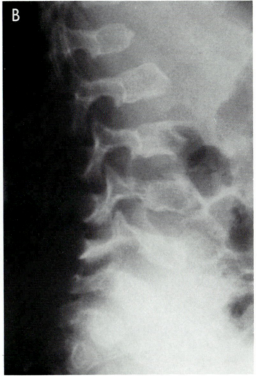

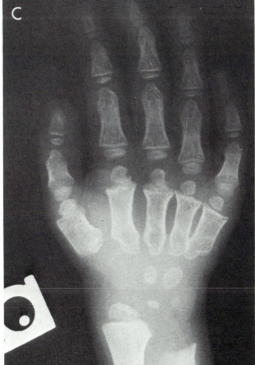

FIG ME–M–17.
Mucopolysaccharidosis IV A in a 3-year-old girl. **A,** platyspondyly of the cervical vertebrae, underdevelopment of the odontoid process of the axis, and atlantoaxial subluxation in the extension position. **B,** universal platyspondyly of the lumbar vertebrae and a central beak protruding from the vertebral bodies. **C,** marked irregularity of the distal metaphysis of the radius and ulna, pointed proximal end of the second through fifth metacarpals, shortness of the metacarpals, and pointed distal end of the middle and distal phalanges.

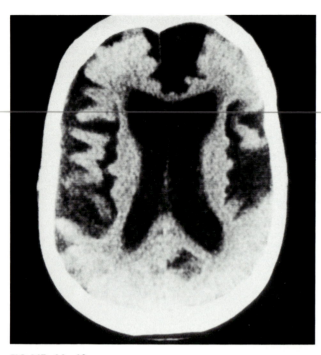

FIG ME–M–18.
Mucopolysaccharidosis IV A. A noncontrast CT of a male aged 36 years, 7 months shows marked dilatation of the ventricles and subarachnoid spaces. (From Nelson J, Grebbell FS: The value of computed tomography in patients with mucopolysaccharidosis. *Neuroradiology* 29:544, 1987. Used by permission.)

lique acetabular roofs, coxa valga, gradual disappearance of the ossified femoral head (aseptic necrosis); (e) slight to moderate widening of the diaphyses and irregularity of the epiphyses and metaphyses of long bones in the advanced stage of the disease; (f) *small and irregular carpal bones, pointed proximal end of the second through fifth metacarpals*, relatively wide first and fifth metacarpals and phalanges; (g) irregular contour and delay in ossification of the tarsal bones, central constriction and shortness of the metatarsals and phalanges.

(B) Dental abnormalities: thinness of the enamel with enamel not extending as far down the neck of the tooth (thin enamel cap), widely spaced teeth, dental caries.

(C) Central nervous system: white matter low density (computed tomography [CT]), ventriculomegaly and dilatation of the basal cisterns and subarachnoid space may be associated with increasing age; narrow craniospinal canal with or without instability at the C_1–C_2 level, spinal cord compression.

(D) Airway obstruction: narrow trachea, collapse of trachea during head flexion.

Differential Diagnosis: Legg-Calvé-Perthes disease; spondyloepiphyseal dysplasia; multiple epiphyseal dysplasia; non-keraan sulfate–excreting Morquio syndrome (Figs ME–M–17 and ME–M–18).

REFERENCES

Beck M, et al.: Heterogeneity of Morquio disease. *Clin. Genet.* 29:325, 1986.

Brailsford JF: Chondro-osteo-dystrophy. *Am. J. Surg.* 7:404, 1929.

Buhain WJ, et al.: Pulmonary function in Morquio's disease: A study of two siblings. *Chest* 68:41, 1975.

Driscoll DJ, et al.: Mild MPS IV A in an extended inbred Mennonite family. Presented at the Birth Defect Meeting, Baltimore, 1988.

Eggli KD, et al.: The mucopolysaccharidoses and related conditions. *Semin. Roentgenol.* 21:275, 1986.

Fujimoto A, et al.: Biochemical defect of non-keratan-sulfate–excreting Morquio syndrome. *Am. J. Med. Genet.* 15:265, 1983.

Grossman H, et al.: The mucopolysaccharidoses and mucolipidoses, in Kaufmann HJ (ed.): *Progress in Pediatric Radiology.* Basel, S. Karger AG, 1973, vol. 4, p. 495.

Hecht JT, et al.: Mild manifestations of the Morquio syndrome (letter). *Am. J. Med. Genet.* 18:369, 1984.

Ireland MA, et al.: Mucopolysaccharidosis type IV as a cause of mitral stenosis in an adult. *Br. Heart J.* 46:113, 1981.

Morquio L: Sur une forme de dystrophie osseuse familiale. *Arch. Med. Enf.* 32:129, 1929.

Nelson J, et al.: Clinical findings in 12 patients with MPS IV A (Morquio's disease). Further evidence for heterogeneity. Part I: Clinical and biochemical findings. *Clin. Genet.* 33:111, 1988.

Nelson J, et al.: Clinical findings in 12 patients with MPS IV A (Morquio's disease) Further evidence for heterogeneity. Part II: Dental findings. *Clin. Genet.* 33:121, 1988.

Nelson J, et al.: Clinical findings in 12 patients with MPS IV A (Morquio's disease) Further evidence for heterogeneity. Part III: Ondontoid dysplasia. *Clin. Genet.* 33:126, 1988.

Nelson J, et al.: The value of computed tomography in patients with mucopolysaccharidosis. *Neuroradiology* 29:544, 1987.

Peters ME, et al.: Narrow trachea in mucopolysaccharidoses. *Pediatr. Radiol.* 15:225, 1985.

Pouliquen JC, et al.: Charnière cranio-rachidienne et maladie de Morquio. A propos de 6 observations. *Chir. Pediatr.* 23:247, 1982.

Pritzker MR, et al.: Upper airway obstruction during head flexion in Morquio's disease. *Am. J. Med.* 69:467, 1980.

Roach JW, et al.: Atlanto-axial instability and spinal cord compression in children—diagnosis by computerized tomography. *J. Bone Joint Surg. [Am.]* 66:708, 1984.

Voisin J, Voisin R: Un cas d'achondroplasie. *Encephale* 4:221, 1909.

Watts RWE, et al.: Computed tomography studies on patients with mucopolysaccharidoses. *Neuroradiology* 21:9, 1981.

MUCOPOLYSACCHARIDOSIS IV B

Synonyms: Morquio syndrome B; β-galactosidase deficiency Morquio syndrome; Morquio-B disease.

Mode of Inheritance: Autosomal recessive.

Enzyme Deficiency: β-Galactosidase.

Clinical Manifestations: Similar to Morquio disease: (a) short stature; (b) corneal clouding; (c) chest deformity; (d) normal intelligence; (e) normal enamel; (f) excess keratan sulfate excretion in the urine, oligosacchariduria; (g) other reported abnormalities: cervical myelopathy, progressive mental handicap.

Radiologic Manifestations: Skeletal abnormalities similar to Morquio disease, but with milder deformities (progressive spondyloepiphyseal dysplasia).

REFERENCES

Arbisser AI, et al.: Morquio-like syndrome with beta-galactosidase deficiency and normal hexosamine sulfate activity: Mucopolysaccharidosis IV B. *Am. J. Med. Genet.* 1:195, 1977.

Eggli KD, et al.: The mucopolysaccharidoses and related conditions. *Semin. Roentgenol.* 21:275, 1986.

Giugiani R, et al.: Progressive mental regression in siblings with Morquio disease type B (mucopolysaccharidosis IV B). *Clin. Genet.* 32:313, 1987.

Guibaud P, et al.: Syndrome de Morquio modéré par déficit en bêta-galactosidase. Mucopolysaccharidose (type IV B ou oligosaccharidose). *Ann. Pediatr. (Paris)* 30:681, 1983.

O'Brien JS, et al.: Spondylo-epiphyseal dysplasia, corneal clouding, normal intelligence and acid beta-galactosidase deficiency. *Clin. Genet.* 9:495, 1976.

Van der Horst GTJ, et al.: Morquio B syndrome: A primary defect in β-galactosidase. *Am. J. Med. Genet.* 16:261, 1983.

MUCOPOLYSACCHARIDOSIS VI

Synonym: Maroteaux-Lamy syndrome.

Mode of Inheritance: Autosomal recessive.

Genetic Heterogeneity: severe (A) and mild (B) forms.

Enzyme Deficiency: Arylsulfatase B (*N*-acetylgalactosamine 4-sulfatase).

Clinical Manifestations: (a) prominent forehead, sternal protrusion, and *joint stiffness* may be present at birth; (b) growth arrest at about 2 to 4 years of age; (c) *coarse facies,* usually less grotesque than in Hurler syndrome; (d) *corneal opacity;* (e) normal mental development; (f) hearing defect; (g) hepatosplenomegaly; (h) hernias; (i) hydrocephalus, optic atrophy, progressive hearing loss, myelopathy (gait disturbances, pain, paresthesia, urinary and fecal incontinence, etc.); (j) aortic and mitral valve involvement, cardiac and respiratory failure, endocardial fibroelastosis; (k) excess excretion of dermatan sulfate in the urine; (l) improvement of symptoms following bone marrow transplantation (see Fig ME−M−11).

Radiologic Manifestations:

(A) Skeletal changes: quite variable in severity and extent: (a) *large dolichocephalic skull, large omega-shaped sella turcica, thick calvaria, premature closure of cranial sutures,* large foramina for the emissary veins, short mandibular rami; (b) oval or bullet-shaped vertebral bodies, kyphosis at the lower thoracic or upper lumbar regions with a wedged-shaped vertebra at the center of the curve, hypoplasia of the odontoid; (c) *canoe paddle appearance of the ribs,* small and highly located scapulae, hypoplastic glenoid fossae, widening of the medial aspect of the clavicles; (d) irregularity and underdevelopment of the acetabular roofs, fragmentation of the femoral head (aseptic necrosis); (e) *widening of the diaphyses of long bones and constriction of metaphyseal regions, hatchet-shaped proximal portions of the humeri,* bowed radii and ulnae, irregularity of metaphyses and deformity of epiphyses, pointed base of metacarpals and widening of the shafts of short tubular bones.

(B) Central nervous system: (a) hydrocephalus internus, symmetrically low attentuation in the white matter on computed tomographic examination, empty sella; (b) narrowing of the cervical spinal canal, concentric impingement of the subarachnoid space and cord compression due to dural thickening in the cervical region, narrowing of the subarachnoid space in the occipitocervical junction, dysplastic arch of C_1 protruding dorsally into the foramen magnum, displacement of the cervical cord.

(C) Airway obstruction: retropharyngeal and retrotracheal swelling, narrowing of the upper airways, narrow trachea.

REFERENCES

Black SH, et al.: Maroteaux-Lamy syndrome in a large consanguineous kindred: Biochemical and immunological studies. *Am. J. Med. Genet.* 25:273, 1986.

Eggli KD, et al.: The mucopolysaccharidoses and related conditions. *Semin. Roentgenol.* 21:275, 1986.

Goldberg MF, et al.: Hydrocephalus and papilledema in Maroteaux-Lamy syndrome (mucopolysaccharidosis type VI). *Am. J. Ophthalmol.* 69:969, 1970.

Grossman H, et al.: The mucopolysaccharidoses and mucolipidoses, in Kaufmann HJ (ed.): *Progress in Pediatric Radiology.* Basel, S. Karger AG, 1973, vol. 4, p. 495.

Keller Ch, et al.: Mukopolysaccharidose Typ VI-A (Morbus Maroteaux-Lamy): Korrelation der klinischen und pathologisch-anatomischen Befunde bei einem 27 jährigen Patienten. *Helv. Paediatr. Acta.* 42:317, 1987.

Krivit W, et al.: Bone-marrow transplantation in the Maroteaux-Lamy syndrome (mucopolysaccharidosis type VI). Biochemical and clinical status 24 months after transplantation. *N. Engl. J. Med.* 311:1606, 1984.

Maroteaux P, Levêque B, Marie J, Lamy, M: Une nouvelle dysostose avec élimination urinaire de chondroitine sulfate B. *Presse Med.* 71:1849, 1963.

Miller G, et al.: Mucopolysaccharidosis type VI presenting in infancy with endocardial fibroelastosis and heart failure. *Pediatr. Cardiol.* 4:61, 1983.

Mühlendahl, KEV, et al.: Empty sella syndrome in a boy

with mucopolysaccharidosis type VI (Maroteaux-Lamy). *Helv. Paediatr. Acta* 30:185, 1975.

Paterson DE, et al.: Maroteaux-Lamy syndrome, mild form—MPS vi b. *Br. J. Radiol.* 55:805, 1982.

Rampini S, et al.: Mukopolysaccharidose VI-A (Morbus Maroteaux-Lamy, schwere Form): beginnende kompressive Myelopathie, Liquorfestel und Trachealstenose bei einem erwachsenen Patienten. *Helv. Paediatr. Acta* 41:515, 1986.

Schieken R, et al.: Cardiac manifestations of the mucopolysaccharidoses. *Circulation* 52:700, 1975.

Sostrin RD, et al.: Myelographic features of mucopolysaccharidoses: A new sign. *Radiology* 125:421, 1977.

Van Bierviet JPGM: Un cas de maladie de Maroteaux-Lamy découvert précocement. *Arch. Fr. Pediatr.* 34:362, 1977.

Vestermark S, et al.: Mental retardation in a patient with Maroteaux-Lamy. *Clin. Genet.* 31:114, 1987.

Watts RWE, et al.: Computed tomography studies on patients with mucopolysaccharidoses. *Neuroradiology.* 21:9, 1981.

Young R, et al.: Compressive myelopathy in Maroteaux-Lamy syndrome: Clinical and pathological findings. *Ann. Neurol.* 8:336, 1980.

MUCOPOLYSACCHARIDOSIS VII

Synonyms: Sly syndrome; β-glucuronidase deficiency.

Mode of Inheritance: Autosomal recessive.

Enzyme Deficiency: β-Glucuronidase.

Clinical Manifestation: *Considerable phenotype variation with minimal to marked clinical abnormalities;* onset of symptoms in early infancy and childhood: (a) *craniofacial dysmorphism:* large skull, coarsened facies, hypertelorism, gingivitis; (b) short neck; (c) *corneal clouding;* (d) *short stature, protruding sternum, kyphosis, kyphoscoliosis;* (e) hepatosplenomegaly; (f) subnormal intelligence; (g) *excessive excretion of dermatan sulfate and heparan sulfate;* (h) other reported abnormalities: hypertrichosis, hernia, arterial fibromuscular dysplasia, aortic regurgitation, left-sided heart failure, frequent respiratory infections, dislocated hips, joint contracture, hydrocephalus, presentation as nonimmune hydrops fetalis, Alder-Reilly granulations in polymorphonuclear neutrophils, etc.; (i) death in early childhood in the severe form.

Radiologic Manifestations: (a) *dysostosis multiplex with various degrees of bone deformities* (J-shaped sella, platyspondyly, vertebral beaking, broadening of tubular bones, defective ossification of carpal and tarsal bones, hip dislocation, metatarsus adductus, etc.) (see Fig ME–M–11).

REFERENCES

Capdeville R, et al.: Un nouveau cas de mucopolysaccharidose de type VII, avec importantes anomalies squelettiques. *Ann. Pediat. (Paris)* 30:689, 1983.

Eggli KD, et al.: The mucopolysaccharidoses and related conditions. *Semin. Roentgenol.* 21:275, 1986.

Hoyme HE, et al.: Presentation of mucopolysaccharidosis VII (β-glucuronidase deficiency) in infancy. *J. Med. Genet.* 18:237, 1981.

Lee JES, et al.: β-Glucuronidase deficiency. A heterogeneous mucopolysaccharidosis. *Am. J. Dis. Child.* 139:57, 1985.

Nelson A, et al.: Mucopolysaccharidosis VII (β-glucuronidase deficiency) presenting as nonimmune hydrops fetalis. *J. Pediatr.* 101:574, 1982.

Sly WS, et al.: Beta-glucuronidase deficiency: Report of clinical, radiologic, and biochemical features of a new mucopolysaccharidosis. *J. Pediatr.* 82:249, 1973.

NIEMANN-PICK DISEASE

Synonym: Sphingomyelin lipidoses.

Mode of Inheritance: Autosomal recessive.

Pathology: Accumulation of sphingomyelin (ceramide phosphorylcholine) in different tissues; hepatosplenomegaly; foam cells in the bone marrow; pulmonary infiltration; varying degrees of nervous system involvement.

Enzyme Deficiency: *Sphinogomyelinase deficiency* (in types A, B, and C) shown by tissue assays: leukocyte extracts, cultured skin fibroblasts, ^{14}C-labeled sphingomyelin or a chromogenic analogue of sphingomyelin, 2-hexadecanoyl-4-nitrophenyl phosphorylcholine (HNP) assays; quantitative evaluation in biopsy materials (liver, lymph node); radioactive sphinogomyelin or HNP assays for prenatal diagnosis.

Clinical Classification and Manifestations:

(A) TYPE A (ACUTE NEURONOPATHIC FORM): Onset of symptoms in infancy (a) *feeding difficulties;* (b) *weight loss, cachexia;* (c) *regressive intellectual capabilities, hypotonia, flaccidity;* (d) *hepatosplenomegaly, protuberant abdomen;* (e) brownish yellow skin discoloration; (f) ocular manifestations: *cherry-red spots* (50% of patients), corneal opacification, retinal opacification, brownish discoloration of the anterior lens capsule; (f) *foamy histiocytes* in the bone marrow, spleen, lymph nodes, adrenal medulla, and the alveoli of the lungs; (g) death by the third year of life.

(B) TYPE B (CHRONIC FORM WITHOUT CENTRAL NERVOUS SYSTEM INVOLVEMENT): Onset of symptoms in infancy (a) *hepatosplenomegaly;* (b) recurrent pneumonias; (c) *delayed in growth and height;* (d) anemia; (e) *foam cells in the bone marrow;* (f) polyglandular involvement; (g) first trimester prenatal diagnosis (chorionic villi and chemical study).

(C) TYPE C (CHRONIC NEURONOPATHIC FORM, JUVENILE FORM): Onset of symptoms in infancy or early childhood (a) *hepatosplenomegaly;* (b) *progressive neurological manifestations:* regressive intellectual capabilities, ataxia, seizures, loss of coordination, hypertonia, hyperactive reflexes; (c) cholestasis; (d) *foamy macrophages in the bone marrow;* (e) death in childhood or adolescence; (f) other reported abnormalities: biliary atresia and meconium ileus, presentation as "neonatal hepatitis," clinical heterogenity in a sibship, cataplexy (abrupt loss of muscle tone, reversible).

(D) TYPE D (NOVA SCOTIA VARIANT): Onset of symptoms in early childhood with a *clinical picture similar to type C* but lacking evidence of sphingomyelinase deficiency; patients with a common ancestry from the coastal area in western Nova Scotia.

(E) TYPE E (ADULT, NONNEURONOPATHIC FORM): (a) *moderate hepatosplenomegaly;* (b) *foam cells in the bone marrow;* (c) biochemically closely related to type C.

(F) TYPE F: Onset in childhood: (a) *splenomegaly;* (b) *diminished activity of a thermolabile sphingomyelinase;* (c) *"sea-blue" histiocytes;* (d) lack of neurological involvement; (e) pulmonary involvement, cor pulmonale.

Radiologic Manifestations: (a) *widening of the medullary cavities of the ribs and long bones, thinning of the cortices and expansion of the shafts of tubular bones,* Erlenmeyer-flask deformity of distal portions of the femora, anterior notching of the vertebrae at the thoracolumber junction; (b) *osteoporosis;* (c) spontaneous fractures; (d) coxa valga; (e) notch defects in the proximal humeral diaphysis and metaphysis of older children (also noted in normal children); (f) *miliary, nodular, or reticular infiltration of the lung;* (g) ?adrenal calcification; (h) diffuse lung and liver calcifications; (i) *hepatosplenomegaly,* renomegaly; (j) punctate calcific deposits inferior to the sacrum and coccyx, in the hips and feet (in two infants); (k) small-bowel changes (in type A): dilatation, delayed transit time, loss of normal mucosal pattern.

Note: There is considerable variability of clinical manifestations, some of which have been reported to be quite inconsistent with the classifications generally used in this metabolic disorder (Fig ME−N−1).

REFERENCES

Adam G, et al.: Biliary atresia and meconium ileus associated with Niemann-Pick disease. *J. Pediatr. Gastroenterol. Nutr.* 7:128, 1988.

Alexander WS: Niemann-Pick disease: Report of case showing calcification in the adrenal glands. *N.Z. Med. J.* 45:43, 1946.

Barness LA, et al.: One-year-old infant with hepatosplenomegaly and developmental delay. *Am. J. Med. Genet.* 28:411, 1987.

Ceuterick C, et al.: Neimann-Pick disease type C. Skin biopsies in parents. *Neuropediatrics* 17:111, 1986.

Elleder M, et al.: International symposium on Niemann-Pick disease. *Eur. J. Pediatr.* 140:90, 1983.

Elleder M, et al.: Niemann-Pick disease (variation in the sphingomyelinase deficient group). Neurovisceral phenotype (A) with an abnormally protracted clinical course and variable expression of neurological symptomatology in three siblings. *Eur. J. Pediatr.* 140:323, 1983.

Grünebaum M: The roentgenographic findings in acute neuronopathic forms of Niemann-Pick disease. *Br. J. Radiol.* 49:1018, 1976.

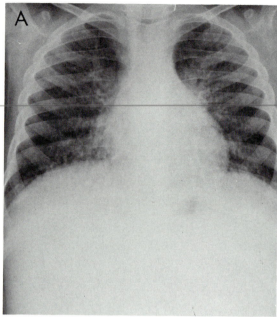

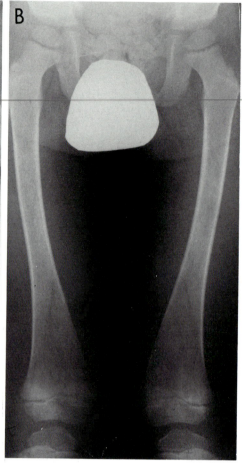

FIG ME–N–1.
Niemann-Pick disease in a 5½-year-old boy with a history
of recurrent epistaxis, abdominal pain, and marked
hepatosplenomegaly. **A,** widening of the ribs and
extensive reticular lung infiltration. **B,** expansion of the
distal shaft and metaphysis of the femora and widening
of medullary cavities.

Kandt RS, et al.: Cataplexy in variant forms of Niemann-Pick
   disease. *Ann. Neurol.* 12:284, 1982.
Lachman R, et al.: Radiological findings in Niemann-Pick
   disease. *Radiology* 108:659, 1973.
Lever A, et al.: Cor pulmonale in an adult secondary to
   Niemann-Pick disease. *Thorax* 38:873, 1983.
Niemann A: Ein unbekanntes Krankheitsbild. *Jb.
   Kinderheilkd.* 79:1, 1914.
Özsoylu S, et al.: Pseudo-osteomyelitis in Niemann-Pick
   disease. *Clin. Pediatr. (Phila.)* 27:394, 1988.
Pick L: Der morbus Gaucher und die ihm ähnlichen
   Krankheiten (die lipoidzellige Splenohepatomegalie Typus
   Niemann und die diabetische Lipoidzellenhypoplasie der
   Milz). *Ergeb. Inn. Med.* 29:519, 1926.
Poulos A, et al.: Sphingomyelinase in cultured skin fibro-
   blasts from normal and Niemann-Pick type C patients.
   Clin. Genet. 24:225, 1983.
Semeraro LA, et al.: Niemann-Pick variant lipidosis present-
   ing as "neonatal hepatitis." *J. Pediatr. Gastroenterol. Nutr.*
   5:492, 1986.

Strisciuglio P, et al.: Evidence of polyglandular involvement
   in Niemann-Pick disease type B. *Eur. J. Pediatr.* 146:431,
   1987.
Vanier MT, et al.: Biochemical studies in Niemann-Pick disease. III. In vitro and in vivo assays of sphingomyelin degradation in cultured skin fibroblasts and amniotic fluid
   cells for the diagnosis of the various forms of the disease.
   Clin. Genet. 27:20, 1985.
Vanier MT, et al.: Niemann-Pick disease group C: Clinical
   variability and diagnosis based on defective cholesterol
   esterification. A collaborative study on 70 patients. *Clin.
   Genet.* 33:331, 1988.
Vanier MT, et al.: Niemann-Pick disease type B: First trimester prenatal diagnosis on chorionic villi and biochemical
   study of a foetus at 12 weeks of development. *Clin.
   Genet.* 28:348, 1985.
Yatziv S, et al.: Clinical heterogeneity in a sibship with
   Niemann-Pick disease type C. *Clin. Genet.* 23:125, 1983.

O

OCCIPITAL HORN SYNDROME

Synonym: Cutis laxa, X-linked.

Mode of Inheritance: X-linked.

Enzyme Deficiency: Lysyl oxidase; abnormal copper metabolism.

Clinical Manifestations: (a) peculiar facies (high forehead, narrow face), occipital exostosis (horn); (b) soft and lax skin, recurrent inguinal hernias; (c) coarse and abundant hair; (d) chronic diarrhea and malabsorption; (e) syncopal episodes; (f) low-normal intelligence; (g) respiratory and urinary tract infections; (h) reduced activity of lysyl oxidase in the skin fibroblasts, abnormal concentrations of copper in the patients and in the cultured fibroblasts.

Radiologic Manifestations: (a) bilateral, symmetrical, occipital, bony protuberance ("occipital horns"); (b) capitate-hamate fusion, mild platyspondyly, flattened acetabular roofs, coxa valga, dislocated radial head, widening and bowing of multiple long bones at tendinous and ligamentous insertion sites, deformed clavicles ("hammer shaped"), wavy appearance of the cortices of the tubular bones, etc.

Note: Formerly this syndrome was known as "occipital horn–type Ehlers-Danlos syndrome (Ehlers-Danlos type IX)" (Fig ME–O–1).

REFERENCES

Blackston RD, et al.: Ehlers-Danlos syndrome (EDS), type IX: Biochemical evidence for X-linkage (abstract). *Am. J. Hum. Genet.* 41:49, 1987.
Kuivaniemi H, et al.: Abnormal copper metabolism and deficient lysyl oxidase activity in a heritable connective tissue disorder. *J. Clin. Invest.* 69:730, 1982.
Kuivaniemi H, et al.: Type IX Ehler-Danlos syndrome and Menkes syndrome: the decrease in lysyl oxidase activity is associated with a corresponding deficiency in the enzyme protein. *Am. J. Hum. Genet.* 37:798, 1985.
Lazoff SG, et al.: Skeletal dysplasia, occipital horns, diarrhea and obstructive uropathy—A new hereditary syndrome. *Birth Defects* 11(5):71, 1975.
Sartoris DJ, et al.: The horn: A pathognomonic feature of paediatric bone dysplasias. *Aust. Paediatr. J.* 23:347, 1987.
Sartoris DJ, et al.: Type IX Ehlers-Danlos syndrome. A new variant with pathognomonic radiographic features. *Radiology* 152:665, 1984.

ORNITHINE TRANSCARBAMYLASE DEFICIENCY

Synonym: Ornithine carbamoyl transferase deficiency.

Mode of Inheritance: X-linked, variable expression in females and fatal in males.

Frequency: The overall prevalence of five enzymes of the urea cycle: 1 in 30,000 live births (Msall et al.).

Clinical Manifestations: An inborn error of the urea cycle with a postnatal onset of symptoms and fluctuating course: (a) vomiting, lethargy, feeding difficulties, grunting, tachypnea, respiratory aklalosis; (b) seizures, hypertonicity or hypotonicity, abnormal electroencephalographic findings, coma; (c) hyperammonemia, elevated levels of glutamine and alanine, orotic aciduria after a standard protein load; (d) other reported abnormalities: hemorrhagic diathesis (pulmonary hemorrhage, intracranial hemorrhage); (d) neuropathologic changes acquired in utero.

Radiologic Manifestations: Computed tomography: cerebral swelling, diffuse low attenuation changes in the cerebral white and gray matters followed by cerebral atrophy (symmetrical or asymmetrical), cavitation at the base of the sulci (Fig ME–O–2).

REFERENCES

Amir J, et al.: Intracranial haemorrhage in siblings and ornithine transcarbamylase deficiency. *Acta Paediatr. Scand.* 71:671, 1982.
Drogari E, et al.: Late onset ornithine carbamoyl transferase deficiency in males. *Arch. Dis. Child.* 63:1363, 1988.
Filloux F, et al.: Ornithine transcarbamylase deficiency: Neuropathologic changes acquired in utero. *J. Pediatr.* 108:942, 1986.
Kendall BE, et al.: Neurological features and computed tomography of the brain in children with ornithine carbamoyl transferase deficiency. *J. Neurol. Neurosurg. Psychiatry* 46:28, 1983.
Largilliere C, et al.: Ornithine transcarbamylase deficiency in a boy with long survival. *J. Pediatr.* 113:952, 1988.
Msall M, et al.: Neurologic outcome in children with inborn errors of urea synthesis. Outcome of urea-cycle enzymopathies. *N. Engl. J. Med.* 310:1500, 1984.

OXALOSIS

Synonym: Hyperoxaluria.

Mode of Inheritance: Autosomal recessive, heterozygous carriers, genetic heterogeneity.

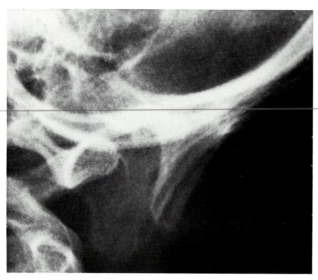

FIG ME–O–1.
Occipital horn syndrome in an 11-year-old boy. A coned-down view of the occipital bone shows bilaterally symmetrical bony protuberances ("occipital horns"). (From Lazoff SG, Ryback JJ, Parker BR, et al.: Skeletal dysplasia, occipital horns, diarrhea, and obstructive uropathy—A new hereditary syndrome, in Bergsma D (ed.): *New Chromosomal and Malformation Syndromes.* New York, Stratton Intercontinental Medical Book Corp., 1975, p. 71. Used by permission.)

Classification:

(A) PRIMARY: A defect in glyoxylate metabolism resulting in an increased synthesis of oxalic acid: (a) type 1—glycolic aciduria due to a defect of α-ketoglutarate-glyoxylate carboligase, deficiency of peroxisomal enzyme alanine: glyoxylate aminotransferase (liver specimen); (b) type 2—L-glyceric aciduria due to a defect of D-glyceric dehydrogenase.

(B) SECONDARY: Ethylene glycol ingestion, pyridoxine deficiency, ileal resection, excess ingestion of oxalate or its precursors, methoxyflurane anesthesia, liver cirrhosis, renal failure, renal tubular acidosis, sarcoidosis, long-term hemodialysis (hemodialysis oxalosis synovitis), intravenous xylitol treatment (renocerebral oxalosis), small-bowel bypass for morbid obesity, steatorrhea.

Pathology: High urinary oxalate excretion; deposition of calcium oxalate crystals in bones, skin, muscles, eyes, kidneys, and other organs; renal calculi, nephrocalcinosis, pyelonephritis, progressive renal destruction, and atrophy.

Clinical Manifestations: Heterogenous presentation and clinical course ranging from the malignant neonatal form causing death in infancy to the milder form in which the patient may not become symptomatic until adulthood: (a) *urinary calculi,* urinary tract infections, *renal failure;* (b) *growth delay;* (c) other reported abnormalities: acute arthritis, cardiac arrhythmias, bulbous enlargement of the tips of the fingers and extrusion of calcium oxalate from nail beds, pancytopenia (related to bone marrow obliteration by calcium oxalate crystals), hepatosplenomegaly; (d) hyperoxalemia; hypercalcemia; high levels of serum parathyroid hormone (secondary hyperparathyroidism); excessive excretion of oxalate, glycolic acid, and glycoxylic acid in urine; (e) symptoms often before 5 years of age, death often before the age of 15 years (primary oxalemia), prolongation of survival to adulthood with regular dialysis treatment.

Radiologic Manifestations: (a) *increased kidney radiopacity, closely packed marked increased echogenicity of the renal parenchyma as compared with renal sinus fat; computed tomography: uniformly dense cortex and medulla and parenchymal loss in the later stage of the disease; renal scin-*

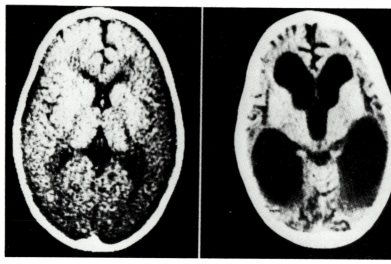

FIG ME–O–2.
Ornithine transcarbamylase deficiency, hyperammonemia: computed tomography at 3 years of age **(A)** and at 4½ years **(B)** after an episode of hyperammonemic coma. Note the evidence of mild cortical atrophy in the first scan and severe cortical atrophy with ventricular dilatation after hyperammonemic coma. (From Batshaw ML, Msall M, Beaudet AL, et al.: Risk of serious illness in heterozygotes for ornithine transcarbamylase deficiency. *J. Pediatr.* 108:236, 1986. Used by permission.)

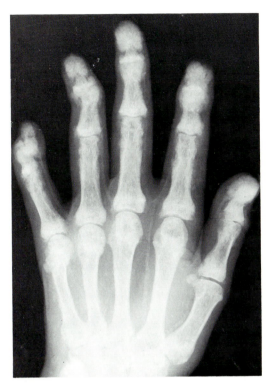

FIG ME–O–3.
Oxalosis in a 38-year-old man: soft-tissue deposition of calcium oxalate in the fingers in association with uremic bone lesions due to secondary hyperparathyroidism and vascular calcification. (From Brancaccio D, Poggi A, Ciccarelli C, et al.: Bone changes in end-stage oxalosis. *A.J.R.* 136:935, 1981. Used by permission.)

tigram: *poor perfusion and function,* (b) *radiopaque renal calculi;* (c) *nephrocalcinosis;* (d) *marked increase in bone density,* in particular, in the metaphyses and adjacent diaphyses of tubular bones (calcium oxalate crystal deposition); (e) renal osteodystrophy; (f) soft-tissue and vascular calcifications; (g) pathological fractures (Fig ME–O–3).

REFERENCES

Billimoria PE, et al.: Acquired renal oxalosis. *J. Comput. Assist. Tomogr.* 7:158, 1983.

Brancaccio D, et al.: Bone changes in end-stage oxalosis. *A.J.R.* 136:935, 1981.

Breed A, et al.: Oxalosis-induced bone disease: A complication of transplantation and prolonged survival in primary hyperoxaluria. *J. Bone Joint Surg. [Am.]* 63:310, 1981.

Brennan JN, et al.: Ultrasonic diagnosis of primary hyperoxaluria in infancy. *Radiology* 145:147, 1982.

Carsen GM, et al.: Calcium oxalosis: A case report. *Radiology* 113:165, 1974.

Danpure CJ, et al.: Enzymological diagnosis of primary hyperoxaluria type 1 by measurement of hepatic alanine: glyoxylate aminotransferase activity. *Lancet* 1:289, 1987.

Day DL, et al.: Radiological aspects of primary hyperoxaluria. *A.J.R.* 146:395, 1986.

Gilboa N, et al.: Primary oxalosis presenting as anuric renal failure in infancy: Diagnosis by x-ray diffraction of kidney tissue. *J. Pediatr.* 103:88, 1983.

Glickstein ME, et al.: Vascular and soft tissue calcification in systemic oxalosis: CT diagnosis. *J. Comput. Assist. Tomogr.* 10:691, 1986.

Hricik DE, et al.: Pancytopenia and hepatosplenomegaly in oxalosis. *Arch. Intern. Med.* 144:167, 1984.

Hug IV, et al.: Die primäre oxalosis. *Fortschr. Rontgenstr.* 123:154, 1975.

Jones DP, et al.: Urolithiasis and enteric hyperoxaluria in a child with steatorrhea. *Clin. Pediatr. (Phila.)* 26:304, 1987.

Kalifa G, et al.: Aspects radiologiques de l'oxalose. *J. Radiol.* 60:45, 1979.

Ludwig B, et al.: Reno-cerebral oxalosis induced by xylitol. *Neuroradiology* 26:517, 1984.

Luers PR, et al.: CT demonstration of cortical nephrocalcinosis in congenital oxalosis. *Pediatr. Radiol.* 10:116, 1980.

Martijn A, et al.: Radiologic findings in primary hyperoxaluria. *Skeletal Radiol.* 8:21, 1982.

Morris MC, et al.: Oxalosis in infancy. *Arch. Dis. Child.* 57:224, 1982.

Reginato AJ, et al.: Arthropathy and cutaneous calcinosis in hemodialysis oxalosis. *Arthritis Rheum.* 29:1387, 1986.

Rotenberg B, et al.: Manifestation osseuse de l'oxalose (cas radiologique du mois). *Arch. Fr. Pediatr.* 45:53, 1988.

Wiggelinkhuizen J, et al.: Radiologic case of the month: Nephroxalosis. *Am. J. Dis. Child.* 132:517, 1978.

PARANEOPLASTIC SYNDROMES

Synonyms: Humoral syndromes; tumor and humor syndromes.

Definition: Remote effect of neoplasia due to known hormone production in some cases and unknown mechanism in others.

Clinical and Radiologic Manifestations:

A. ENDOCRINE DISORDERS:
1. *Cushing syndrome* (production of adrenocorticotropic hormone by neoplasm): carcinoma of the lung, malignant epithelial thymoma, islet cell carcinoma, small-cell carcinoma, carcinoids, carcinomas of the larynx and salivary glands, medullary thyroid carcinoma, ovarian carcinoma, pheochromocytoma, etc; most of amine precursor uptake and decarboxylation (APUD) series origin.
2. *Hypoglycemia* (associated with non–islet cell neoplasms): fibrosarcomas, other sarcomas, benign fibromas, mesotheliomas, adrenal cortical carcinoma, lymphomas, gastrointestinal carcinomas.
3. *Hyperglycemia:* glucagon-producing islet cell neoplasms, enteroglucagon-producing renal carcinoma, somatostatin-containing islet cell neoplasm.
4. *Hypercalcemia:* osseous metastases, elevated levels of parathormone and hypercalcemia (carcinomas of the lung, esophageal neoplasms with ectopic hyperparathyroidism, squamous carcinomas of the head and neck region, carcinomas in other locations, lymphomas, and leukemias).
5. *Hypocalcemia and osteomalacia:* hypocalcemia very rarely associated with neoplasia; rickets and osteomalacia have been reported with various "tumors" (hemangiomas of bones or soft tissues, hemangiopericytoma, giant-cell tumor, osteoblastoma, fibrous dysplasia, malignant neurinoma, sarcoma, epidermal nevus syndrome, nonosteogenic fibroma, etc.).
6. *Inappropriate secretion of antidiuretic hormone:* lung cancer, digestive system cancer, lymphoma.
7. *Carcinoid syndrome* associated with noncarcinoid neoplasms: adenocarcinoma of the pancreas, islet cell neoplasms, small-cell carcinoma of the lung, medullary carcinoma of the thyroid; most of APUD series origin.
8. *Gynecomastia:* nonseminomatous carcinomas of the testis, liver cell and renal carcinomas, lung carcinomas, etc.
9. *Hyperthyroidism:* hydatidiform mole or choriocarcinoma, nonseminomatous testicular carcinoma.
10. *Hypertension:* pheochromocytoma, neuroblastoma, aldosteronoma, renal tumors (Wilms, renal cell carcinoma, hemangiopericytoma, etc.).

B. HEMATOLOGIC DISORDERS:
1. *Polycythemia:* renal tumors (Wilms, renal cell carcinoma), liver cell carcinoma, cerebellar hemangioblastoma, leiomyomas of the uterus, renal cystic disease, hydronephrosis, etc.
2. *Erythroid aplasia:* thymoma, cancer of the lung, stomach, or thyroid; lymphoid neoplasia.
3. *Hemolytic anemia:* lymphoid malignancies; carcinomas of the ovary, stomach, colon, lung, cervix, breast.
4. *Thrombocytosis and leukocytosis:* metastatic lesions, especially with marrow involvement.

C. COAGULOPATHIES:
1. *Intravascular coagulation:* acute progranulocytic leukemia, carcinoma of the prostate, mucin-producing adenocarcinomas.
2. *Venous thrombosis:* neoplasms of the stomach, pancreas, ovary, lung, colon, etc.
3. *Sterile endocarditis:* mucinous adenocarcinomas, etc.
4. *Dysfibrinogenemia:* liver cell carcinoma, metastatic liver tumors, etc.

D. PROTEIN DISORDERS:
1. *Amyloidosis:* myeloma, macroglobulinemia, lymphomas, renal cell and gastric carcinomas.
2. *Paraproteinemia* (monoclonal gammopathy): plasmacytic neoplasms, carcinomas, sarcomas, lymphomas, and leukemias.

E. DIGESTIVE DISORDERS:
1. *Zollinger-Ellison syndrome:* non–beta cell adenomas or carcinomas of the pancreas or duodenum, mucinous adenocarcinoma of the ovary, ductal adenocarcinoma of the pancreas.
2. *Multiple endocrine neoplasia* (MEN):
   a. MEN-1: gastrinomas or insulinomas, parathyroid and pituitary neoplasms.
   b. MEN-2a: medullary carcinoma of the thyroid, pheochromocytoma, and parathyroid neoplasm.
   c. MEN-2b: medullary carcinoma of the thyroid, pheochromocytoma, and dermal or mucosal neuromas.
3. *Diarrhea and tumors:* Zollinger-Ellison syndrome, carcinoid syndrome, "pancreatic cholera" (non–beta islet cell neoplasm, vasoactive intestinal polypeptide production).

F. NEPHROGENIC HEPATIC DYSFUNCTION SYNDROME: liver dysfunction associated with renal cell carcinoma.

G. Renal dysfunction:

1. *Nephrotic syndrome:* lymphomas; carcinomas of the lung, stomach, colon, or ovary.
2. *Tubular dysfunction:* multiple myeloma, idiopathic light-chain proteinuria, acute nonlymphocytic leukemia.

H. Musculoskeletal disorders:

1. *Hypertrophic osteoarthropathy:* malignant (primary or secondary) or benign lung tumors, intraabdominal cancers.
2. Dermatomyositis: carcinoma of the breast, lung, ovary, or stomach; leukemias; lymphomas; sarcomas.

I. Skin disorders:

1. *Acanthosis nigricans:* adenocarcinomas (stomach, etc.).
2. *Miscellaneous dermatoses:* pellagra-like lesions (carcinoid syndrome), porphyria cutanea tarda (liver cell carcinoma or adenoma), pemphigus vulgaris or bullous pemphigoid, nodular panniculitis (adenocarcinoma of the pancreas), acquired hypertrichosis lagunosa, erythema gyratum repens, acquired ichthyosis, hyperkeratosis of the palms and soles, sebaceous adenomas, cutaneous angiitis and arthritis associated with myeloproliferative disorders (myelofibrosis, myelogenous leukemia).

J. Neurological disorders:

1. *Progressive multifocal leukoencephalopathy:* leukemia, lymphoma, myeloma, carcinomas, polycythemia vera.
2. *Limbic encephalopathy:* carcinomas of the lung, uterus, breast, etc.
3. *Pontine lesions* (central pontine myelinolysis): leukemia, etc.
4. *Cerebellar atrophy:* carcinomas of the lung, breast, ovary, and kidney; lymphomas.
5. *Myelopathy:* visceral carcinomas.
6. *Neuropathy* (cranial, peripheral): epithelial and lymphoid neoplasms.
7. *Myasthenia gravis:* thymoma, thymic hyperplasia.
8. *Myasthenic syndrome:* nonthymic neoplasms, especially small-cell carcinoma of the lung (Lambert-Eaton syndrome).

REFERENCES

Abeloff MD: Paraneoplastic syndromes. A window on the biology of cancer. *N. Engl. J. Med.* 217:1598, 1987.

Broadus AE, et al.: Humoral hypercalcemia of cancer. Identification of a novel parathyroid hormone-like peptide. *N. Engl. J. Med.* 319:556, 1988.

Carrasco CH, et al.: Apudomas metastatic to the liver: Treatment by hepatic artery embolization. *Radiology* 149:79, 1983.

Fiedler V, et al.: Radiologische Tumorsuche bei Hautveränderungen. Paraneoplastische Syndrom und hereditäre Erkrankungen mit erhöhtem Tumorrisiko. *Radiologe* 28:300, 1988.

Friesen SR: APUD: Dogma defended. *Lancet* 1:350, 1983.

Grajower M: Ectopic hyperparathyroidism (pseudohyperparathyroidism) in esophageal malignancy. *Am. J. Med.* 61:134, 1976.

Guillon JM: Les syndromes paranéoplasiques endocriniens des cancers bronchiques primitifs. *Ann. Med. Interne (Paris)* 137:420, 1986.

Lips CJM, et al.: Common precursor molecules as origin for the ectopic-hormone-producing-tumour syndrome. *Lancet* 1:16, 1978.

Longley S, et al.: Paraneoplastic vasculitis. Unique syndrome of cutaneous angiitis and arthritis associated with myeloproliferative disorders. *Am. J. Med.* 80:1027, 1986.

Mundy GR, et al.: The hypercalcemia of cancer. Clinical implications and pathogenic mechanisms. *N. Engl. J. Med.* 310;1718, 1984.

Nausieda PA, et al.: Opsoclonic cerebellopathy. A paraneoplastic syndrome responsive to thiamine. *Arch. Neurol.* 38:780, 1981.

Palma G: Paraneoplastic syndromes of the nervous system. *West. J. Med.* 142:787, 1985.

Shiel WC, et al.: Palmar fasciitis and arthritis with ovarian and non-ovarian carcinomas. New syndrome. *Am. J. Med.* 79:640, 1985.

Stolinsky DC: Paraneoplastic syndromes. *West. J. Med.* 132:189, 1980.

PAROXYSMAL NOCTURNAL HEMOGLOBINURIA

Clinical Manifestations: (a) *chronic intravascular hemolysis, recurrent thrombotic episodes;* (b) *hemolytic anemia, pancytopenia, iron deficiency, acholuric jaundice;* (c) *hemoglobulinuria, hemosiderinuria;* (d) Ham test (use of acidified serum to enhance hemolysis); (e) abdominal pain, peptic ulcer, *cholecystitis, cholelithiasis, bowel hemorrhage;* (f) other reported abnormalities: association with Evans syndrome (association of autoimmune hemolytic anemia and autoimmune thrombocytopenia), association with acquired immunodeficiency syndrome.

Radiologic Manifestations: (a) *venous thrombosis (hepatic, intestinal, cerebral, etc.);* (b) scintigraphy: focal hot spots in the liver on sulfur colloid testing as well as IDA imaging; hot kidneys on bone imaging; (c) magnetic resonance imaging of the kidneys: *diffuse bilateral depression of renal cortical signal intensity due to massive renal cortical hemosiderosis* (Fig ME−P−1).

REFERENCES

Baumann MA, et al.: Paroxysmal nocturnal hemoglobinuria associated with the acquired immunodeficiency syndrome. *Arch. Intern. Med.* 148:212, 1988.

Birgens HS, et al.: Ultrasonic demonstration of clinical and subclinical hepatic venous thrombosis in paroxysmal nocturnal haemoglobinuria. *Br. J. Haematol.* 64:737, 1986.

Blum SF, et al.: Intestinal infarction in paroxysmal nocturnal hemoglobinuria. *N. Engl. J. Med.* 274:1137, 1966.

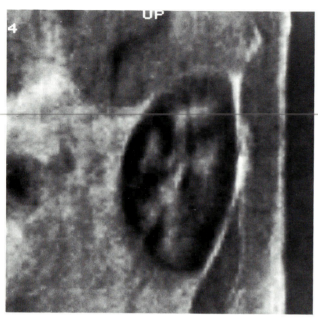

FIG ME—P—1.
Paroxysmal nocturnal hemoglobinuria: T_2 sagittal section of the right kidney (TR = 2.1 seconds, TE = 70 ms). Reverse corticomedullary differentiation is present. Note the relatively higher signal intensity of the liver in comparison to the renal cortex, which excludes the possibility of significant intrahepatic iron overload. (From Lupetin AR: Magnetic resonance appearance of the kidneys in paroxysmal nocturnal hemoglobinuria. *Urol. Radiol.* 8:101, 1986. Used by permission.)

Conti L, et al.: Evans' syndrome in paroxysmal nocturnal hemoglobinuria. *Acta Haematol (Basel)* 73:210, 1985.

Hertz IH, et al.: Paroxysmal nocturnal hemoglobinuria: Small-bowel findings. *A.J.R.* 136:204, 1981.

Lee BCP, et al.: Paroxysmal nocturnal hemoglobinuria presenting as an acute abdominal emergency. *Br. J. Radiol.* 46:467, 1973.

Lupetin AR: Magnetic resonance appearance of the kidneys in paroxysmal nocturnal hemoglobinuria. *Urol. Radiol.* 8:101, 1986.

Valla D, et al.: Hepatic vein thrombosis in paroxysmal nocturnal hemoglobinuria. A spectrum from asymptomatic occlusion of hepatic venules to fatal Budd-Chiari syndrome. *Gastroenterology* 93:569, 1987.

Van Vleymen B, et al.: Cerebral venous thrombosis in paroxysmal nocturnal haemoglobinuria. *Acta Neurol. Belg.* 87:80, 1987.

Wilansky DL, et al.: Renal and hepatic scintigraphy in paroxysmal nocturnal hemoglobinuria (PNH). *Clin. Nucl. Med.* 10:369, 1985.

PELIZAEUS-MERZBACHER DISEASE

Mode of Inheritance: X-linked recessive.

Clinical Manifestations: Onset within the first few months of life, a form of sudanophilic leukodystrophy: (a) early nystagmoid movements; (b) progressive pyramidal, dys-tonic, and cerebellar signs; (c) precocious psychomotor deterioration; (d) laryngeal stridor.

Radiologic Manifestations: (a) Magnetic resonance imaging (MRI): reversal of the normal gray/white matter signal relationship (dysmyelination), low-intensity lentiform nuclei and thalami; (b) computed tomography (abnormalities reported in adolescent or young adults): decreased density in white matter, cerebellar atrophy, ventricular dilatation.

Notes: (a) the term *Pelizaeus-Merzbacher disease* includes several types of sudanophilic leukodystrophy with similar clinical manifestations but different ages of onset and rate of progression of degenerative disease: type I (classic) has its onset within the first few months of life; Connatal Pelizaeus-Merzbacher disease (Steitselberger type, type II) has a neonatal onset of developmental failure, seizures, visual impairment, nystagmus, spasticity and abnormal movements,

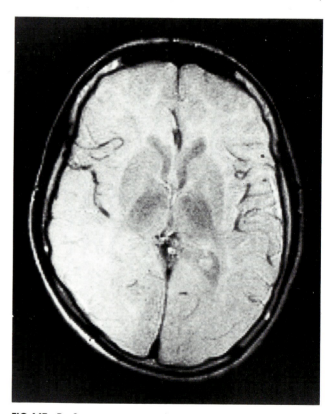

FIG ME—P—2.
Pelizaeus-Merzbacher disease: Axial MRI of the head (TR, 2000 ms; TE, 60 ms). The white matter is more intense than the gray matter is. This is the reverse of the normal relationship at 15 years of age. This signal aberration suggests a decreased lipid content and increased water content in the white matter. The homogeneous, symmetrical signal favors dysmyelinating rather than demyelinating disease. Low-intensity lentiform nuclei and thalami are present. This signal aberration could be secondary to disordered myelination of the interdigitating white matter. Pathological ferric iron deposition is another possibility. (From Penner MW, Li KC, Gerbaski SS, et al.: MR imaging of Pelizaeus-Merzbacher disease. *J. Comput. Assist. Tomogr.* 11:591, 1987. Used by permission.)

and a recessive inheritance is very likely; autosomal dominant Pelizaeus-Merzbacher disease is a multiple sclerosis–like disorder with adult onset; (b) the MRI findings are nonspecific, and pathological investigation is necessary to confirm tigroid demyelination; (c) identification of heterozygotes by MRI is possible (Fig ME–P–2).

REFERENCES

Boltshauser E, et al.: Pelizaeus-Merzbacher disease: Identification of heterozygotes with magnetic resonance imaging? *Helv. Paediatr. Acta* 42:337, 1987.

Boulloche J, et al.: Pelizaeus-Merzbacher disease: Clinical and nosological study. *J. Child Neurol.* 1:233, 1986.

Cassidy SB, et al.: Connatal Pelizaeus-Merzbacher disease: An autosomal recessive form. *Pediatr. Neurol.* 3:300, 1987.

Eldridge R, et al.: Hereditary adult-onset leukodystrophy simulating chronic progressive multiple sclerosis. *N. Engl. J. Med.* 311:948, 1984.

Iyoda K, et al.: Histopathologic and biochemical analysis of classic Pelizaeus-Merzbacher disease. *Pediatr. Neurol.* 4:252, 1988.

Journel H, et al.: Magnetic resonance imaging in Pelizaeus-Merzbacher disease. *Neuroradiology* 29:403, 1987.

Merzbacher L: Weitere Mitteilungen über eine eigenartige hereditär-familiäre Erkrankung des Zentralnervensystems. *Med. Klin. Berlin* 4:1952, 1908.

Pelizaeus F: Ueber eine eigentümliche Form spastischer Lähmung mit Cerebralerscheinungen auf hereditärer Grundlage (multiple Sklerose). *Arch. Psychiatr. Nervenkr.* 16:698, 1885.

Penner MW, et al.: MR imaging of Pelizaeus-Merzbacher disease. *J. Comput. Assist. Tomogr.* 11:591, 1987.

Sano N, et al.: Infantile sudanophilic leukodystrophy: Computed tomography demonstration. *Neuroradiology* 28:170, 1986.

Shimomura C, et al.: Magnetic resonance imaging in Pelizaeus-Merzbacher disease. *Pediatr. Neurol.* 4:124, 1988.

Zebrin-Rubin E, et al.: Ein genetischer Beitrag zur Frage der Spaetform der Pelizaeus-Merzbacherschen Krankheit. *Humangenetik* 1:107, 1964.

PHENYLKETONURIA

Mode of Inheritance: Autosomal recessive.

Frequency: 1 in 10,000 births in the population of western European origin (Scott, 1983).

Enzyme Deficiency: Deficiency of hepatic phenylalanine hydroxylase (faulty conversion of phenylalanine to tyrosine).

Clinical Manifestations: (a) *usually fair-skinned child with blond hair and blue eyes;* (b) *neurological symptoms:* poor coordination, tremor, dystonia, athetoid movements, hyperactivity; (c) *mental retardation;* (d) *seizures* (in some); (e) *eczema;* (f) *urinary excretion of phenylpyruvic acid, persistent blood phenylalanine levels above 6 mg/100 mL (posi-*

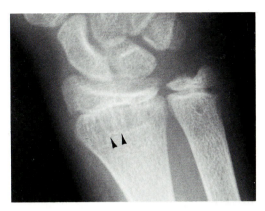

FIG ME–P–3.
Phenylketonuria: buried metaphyseal spicules *(arrowheads)* in a mentally retarded 12-year-old girl with untreated phenylketonuria. (From Woodring JH, Rosenbaum HD: Bone changes in phenylketonuria reassessed. *A.J.R.* 137:241, 1981. Used by permission.)

tive urinary ferric chloride test), prenatal diagnosis by means of a cloned human phenylalanine hydroxylase gene probe (analysis of DNA isolated from cultured amniotic fluid cells); (g) abnormal electroencephalographic findings (single repetitive or multiple spikes and/or sharp waves, focal or scattered) in some infants; (h) growth and developmental retardation in children born to mothers with phenylketonuria, premature closure of cranial sutures in some of these children; (i) other reported abnormalities: vomiting in infancy, unusual odor, association with myotonic dystrophy in an infant, occurrence of phenylketonuria and galactosemia within the same family, etc.

Radiologic Manifestations: (a) widening and cupping of the metaphysis (wrist); (b) calcified spicules of cartilage projecting into the growth cartilage from the metaphyses of growing bones in infants, incorporation of calcified cartilage into the metaphysis with progression of bone growth; (c) skeletal maturation retardation; (d) growth arrest lines.

Notes: (a) the phenylalanine hydroxylate gene is part of chromosome 12 and is located in all nucleated cells in the organism; (b) in addition to classic phenylketonuria, variants have been recognized, and various terminologies have been used: "phenylalaninemia, type II to IV"; "mild hyperphenylalaninemia"; "Mediterranean type"; "hyperphenylalaninemia without PKU"; "atypical PKU"; "non-PKU hyperphenylalaninemia"; "atypical phenylketonuria" due to tetrahydrobiopterin deficiency; (c) the development of dense bony spicules projecting into the growth cartilage has been prevented; this is apparently related to a special liberal diet (Woodring and Rosenbaum) (Fig ME–P–3).

REFERENCES

Blaskovics M, et al.: EEG pattern in phenylketonuria under early initiated dietary treatment. *Am. J. Dis. Child.* 135:802, 1981.

Crosley CJ, et al.: Phenylketonuria and neonatal myotonic dystrophy. *Clin. Pediatr. (Phila.)* 21:56, 1982.

Dhondt J-L, et al.: Atypical cases of phenylketonuria *Eur. J. Pediatr.* 146(suppl. 1):A38, 1987.

Endres W, et al.: Atypical phenylketonuria due to biopterin deficiency. *Helv. Paediatr. Acta* 37:489, 1982.

Feinberg SB, et al.: Bone changes in untreated neonatal phenylketonuric patients: A new radiographic observation and interpretation. *J. Pediatr.* 81:540, 1972.

Fisch RO, et al.: The occurrence of phenylketonuria and galactosemia within the same family. *Clin. Pediatr. (Phila.)* 24:456, 1985.

Fölling A: Ueber Ausscheidung von Phenylbenztraubensäure in den Harn als Stoffwechselanomalie in Verbindung mit Imbezilität. *Z. Physiol. Chem.* 227:169, 1934.

Güttler F, et al.: Molecular biology of phenylketonuria (abstract). *Eur. J. Pediatr.* 146(suppl. 1):5, 1987.

Herrmann FH, et al.: Haplotype analysis of classical and mild phenotype of phenylketonuria in the German Democratic Republic. *Clin. Genet.* 34:176, 1988.

Houston CS, et al.: Cranial growth retardation from maternal phenylketonuria. *A.J.R.* 122:33, 1974.

Ledley FD, et al.: Phenylalanine hydroxylase expression in liver of a fetus with phenylketonuria. *J. Pediatr.* 113:463, 1988.

Lidsky AS, et al.: Prenatal diagnosis of classic phenylketonuria by DNA analysis. *Lancet* 1:549, 1985.

Murdoch MM, et al.: Roentgenologic bone changes in phenylketonuria. *Am. J. Dis. Child.* 107:523, 1964.

Scott CR: Disorders of amino acid metabolism, in Emery AH, Rimoin DL (eds): *Principles and Practice of Medical Genetics.* New York, Churchill Livingston, 1983.

Waisbren SE, et al.: Intelligence and personality characteristics in adults with untreated atypical phenylketonuria and mild hyperphenylalaninemia. *J. Pediatr.* 105:955, 1984.

Woodring JH, Rosenbaum HD: Bone changes in phenylketonuria reassessed. *A.J.R.* 137:241, 1981.

POLYCYSTIC OVARY SYNDROME

Pathogenesis: Heterogenous endocrine disorders (congenital adrenal hyperplasia, Cushing syndrome, hyperprolactinemia, insulin-resistant states, etc.) with a similar clinical presentation; classic Stein-Leventhal syndrome (*amenorrhea, hirsutism, sterility, and obesity*) represents a subgroup of polycystic ovary syndrome.

Clinical Manifestations: (a) ovulatory dysfunction: oligomenorrhea or amenorrhea, infertility, dysfunctional uterine bleeding; (b) hyperadrenogenism (excessive androgen production): hirsutism, acne, excessive sebaceous gland secretions; (c) anabolic state: obesity, difficulty in losing weight; (d) other reported abnormalities: occurrence in several members of some families, an increased occurrence of tetraploidy in two sisters and their mother, etc.

Radiologic Manifestations: (a) *enlarged ovaries in 70% of cases;* (b) *polycystic ovaries with varous ultrasonographic patterns:* discretely resolved cysts, hypoechoic, and isoechoic to the uterus; magnetic resonance imaging (MRI) more accurate in demonstrating the characteristic small peripheral ovarian cysts; (c) mammography: decrease in glandular parenchyma; (d) scintigraphic evidence of adrenal cortical dysfunction (Fig ME−P−4).

REFERENCES

Balcar V, et al.: Soft tissue radiography of the female breast and pelvic pneumoperitoneum in the Stein-Leventhal syndrome. *Acta Radiol.* 12:353, 1972.

Gross MD, et al.: Scintigraphic evidence of adrenal cortical dysfunction in the polycystic ovary syndrome. *J. Clin. Endocrinol. Metab.* 62:197, 1986.

Hann LE, et al.: Polycystic ovarian disease: Sonographic spectrum. *Radiology* 150:531, 1984.

McKenna TJ: Pathogenesis and treatment of polycystic ovary syndrome. *N. Engl. J. Med.* 318;558, 1988.

Mitchell DG, et al.: Polycystic ovaries: MR imaging. *Radiology* 160:425, 1986.

Pang S, et al.: Hirsutism, polycystic ovarian disease, and ovarian 17-keto-steroid reductase deficiency. *N. Engl. J. Med.* 316:1295, 1987.

Rochiccioli P, et al.: Syndrome de Stein-Leventhal de l'adolescente. Etude d'une série de trente-quatre observations. *Ann. Pediatr. (Paris)* 31:225, 1984.

Rojanasakul A, et al.: Tetraploidy in two sisters with the polycystic ovary syndrome. *Clin. Genet.* 27:167, 1985.

Stein IF, et al.: Amenorrhea associated with bilateral polycystic ovaries. *Am. J. Obstet. Gynecol.* 29:181, 1935.

Wajchenberg B, et al.: Determination of the source(s) of androgen overproduction in hirsutism associated with polycystic ovary syndrome by simultaneous adrenal and ovarian venous catheterization. Comparison with the dexamethasone suppression test. *J. Clin. Endocrinol. Metab.* 63:1204, 1986.

Waldstreicher J, et al.: Hyperfunction of the hypothalamic-pituitary axis in women with polycystic ovarian disease: Indirect evidence for partial gonadotroph desensitization. *J. Clin. Endocrinol. Metab.* 66:165, 1988.

Yeh HC, et al.: Polycystic ovarian disease: US features in 104 patients. *Radiology* 163:111, 1987.

POLYGLANDULAR AUTOIMMUNE DISEASE

Synonyms: Autoimmune polyglandular syndrome; Whitaker syndrome; Schmidt syndrome.

Classification and Mode of Inheritance: (a) type I, *at least two of the three conditions must be present: Addison disease, hypoparathyroidism, chronic mucocutaneous moniliasis;* autosomal recessive transmission; associated immune disorders may be present; (b) type II (Schmidt syndrome), *Addison disease plus one or both of the following two conditions: autoimmune thyroid disease* (chronic lymphocytic thyroiditis, Graves disease or spontaneous myxedema), *insulin-requiring diabetes;* autosomal dominant trait with variable expressivity has been reported; associated immune disorders may be present; (c) type III, *autoimmune thyroid disease without Addison disease but with one of the following: insu-*

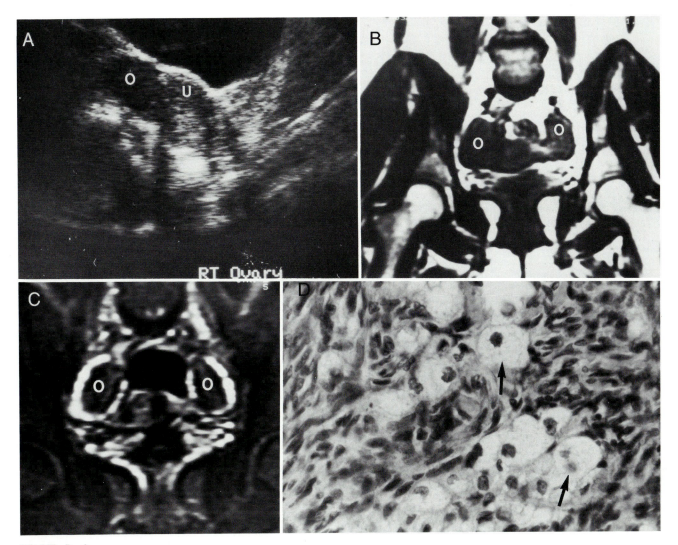

FIG ME–P–4.
Polycystic ovary syndrome. **A,** an oblique sonogram shows the right ovary *(O),* which is hypoechoic when compared with the uterus *(U).* No discrete cysts are resolved. **B,** coronal spin-echo (SE) 600/25 (TR ms/TE ms) MRI. The ovaries *(O)* are larger than the uterus is and are of similar signal intensity. **C,** MRI (2500/80) shows multiple, high-intensity cysts less than 1 cm in diameter surrounding low-intensity ovaries *(O).* **D,** histologic section from a wedge biopsy. The ovarian stroma is hypertrophied, and there are several enlarged, luteinized cells *(arrows)* (hematoxylin-eosin, ×400). (From Mitchell DG, Gefter WB, Spritzer CE, et al.: Polycystic ovaries: MR imaging. *Radiology* 160:425, 1986. Used by permission.)

lin-requiring diabetes with or without other immune disease, pernicious anemia, vitiligo, and/or alopecia.

Clinical and Radiologic Manifestations: (a) *mucocutaneous:* alopecia, dry skin, brittle and rigid nails, chronic moniliasis, vitiligo; (b) *endocrine:* acquired primary hypogonadism, chronic lymphocystic thyroiditis, Graves disease, hypophysitis, insulin-requiring diabetes, myasthenia gravis, nontuberculous Addison disease, spontaneous acquired hypoparathyroidism; (c) malabsorption syndrome, atrophic gastritis; (d) chronic active hepatitis, primary biliary cirrhosis; (e) pernicious anemia; (f) quantitative immunoglobulin abnormalities; (g) other reported abnormalities: keratoconjunctivitis, Sjögren syndrome, exophthalmos, dental abnormalities (chalky teeth, pitted crowns, transverse grooves), intracranial calcification, etc.

REFERENCES

Breynaert R, et al.: Une observation familiale de syndrome de Whitaker. *Arch. Fr. Pediatr.* 31:426, 1974.
Butler MG, et al.: Linkage analysis in a large kindred with autosomal dominant transmission of polyglandular autoimmune disease type II (Schmidt syndrome). *Am. J. Med. Genet.* 18:61, 1984.

Castells S, et al.: Familial moniliasis, defective delayed hypersensitivity and adrenocorticotrophic hormone deficiency. *J. Pediatr.* 79:72, 1971.

Gass JD: The syndrome of keratoconjunctivitis, superficial moniliasis, idiopathic hypoparathyroidism and Addison's disease. *Am. J. Ophthalmol.* 54:660, 1962.

Kenny FM, et al.: Hypoparathyroidism, moniliasis, Addison's and Hashimoto's disease. *N. Engl. J. Med.* 271:708, 1964.

Neufeld M, et al.: Autoimmune polyglandular syndromes. *Pediatr. Ann.* 9:154, 1980.

Neufeld M, et al.: Two types of autoimmune Addison's disease associated with different polyglandular autoimmune (PGA) syndrome. *Medicine (Baltimore)* 60:355, 1981.

Saenger P, et al.: Progressive adrenal failure in polyglandular autoimmune disease. *J. Clin. Endocrinol. Metab.* 54:863, 1982.

Whitaker J, et al.: The syndrome of familial juvenile hypoadrenocortism, hypoparathyroidism and superficial moniliasis. *J. Clin. Endocrinol.* 16:1374, 1956.

Wirfalt A: Genetic heterogeneity in autoimmune polyglandular failure. *Acta Med. Scand.* 210:7, 1981.

PORPHYRIAS

Classification and Clinical Manifestations:

A. Erythropoietic:
1. Congenital erythropoietic porphyria (Gunther disease): autosomal recessive, uroporphyrinogen III cosynthetase deficiency, *photosensitivity, hemolytic anemia,* splenomegaly.
2. Erythropoietic protoporphyria: autosomal dominant, ferrochelatase deficiency, *sunlight-induced edema and scarring,* liver failure.

B. Hepatic:
1. Acute intermittent porphyria: autosomal dominant, uroporphyrinogen I synthetase deficiency, *drug-induced visceral pain, muscle group or respiratory paralysis, behavior problems ("peculiar," depressed, hysterical, etc.).*
2. Hereditary coproporphyria: autosomal dominant, coproporphyrinogen oxidase deficiency, photosensitivity (rare), *drug-induced visceral pain, paralysis,* etc.
3. Variegata porphyria: autosomal dominant, protoporphyrinogen oxidase or ferrochelatase deficiency, *light-induced blisters, hyperpigmentation, hirsutism, neuropathy,* etc.
4. Porphyria cutanea tarda: autosomal dominant (in some families), uroporphyrinogen decarboxylase deficiency, *light-induced blisters, hyperpigmentation, hirsutism, epidermal inclusion cysts,* diabetes, liver tumor (rare).

Radiologic Manifestations: (a) congenital erythropoietic porphyria: *scleroderma-like cutaneous and subcutaneous calcifications, osteopenia, fractures related to osteopenia, acroosteolysis, imperfect modeling of the bones, delayed epiphysiometaphyseal fusion, shortening of fingers, atrophy of soft tissues,* sunray spiculation and diploic widening, dura mater and calvarium calcification (a case report); (b) acute intermittent porphyria: *pseudo-obstruction of the alimentary tract* (autonomic dysfunction) (Figs ME–P–5 and ME–P–6).

REFERENCES

Bundino S, et al.: Hepatoerythropoietic porphyria. *Pediatr. Dermatol.* 4:229, 1987.

Levesque M, et al.: Radiological features in congenital erythropoietic porphyria (Gunther's disease). *Pediatr. Radiol.* 18:62, 1988.

Roberts AG, et al.: Heterogeneity of familial porphyria cutanea tarda. *J. Med. Genet.* 25:669, 1988.

Srugo I, et al.: Acute intermittent porphyria—an unusual cause of "surgical" abdomen. Response to propranolol therapy. *Eur. J. Pediatr.* 146:305, 1987.

A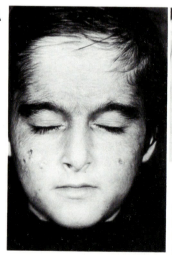

B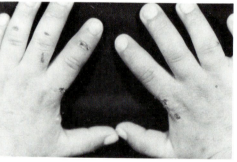

FIG ME–P–5.
Porphyria (hepatoerythropoietic) in a 10-year-old boy. **A,** hypertrichosis, erosions, and scars on the patient's face. **B,** bullous and erosive lesions on the backs of his hands. (From Bundino S, Topi GC, Zina AM, et al.: Hepatoerythropoietic porphyria. *Pediatr. Dermatol.* 4:229, 1987. Used by permission.)

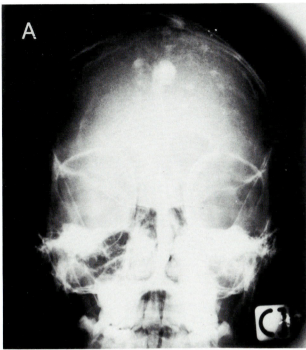

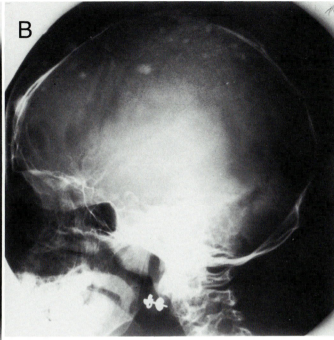

FIG ME–P–6.
Porphyria (erythropoietic) in an 8-year-old girl with Calvarial and meningeal calcification not present on previous radiograms taken at 3 years of age. Note the widening of the diploic space in the frontal and occipital areas. (From Levesque M, Legmann P, LeCloirec A, et al.: Radiological features in congenital erythropoietic porphyria (Gunther's disease). *Pediatr. Radiol.* 18:62, 1988. Used by permission.)

PROLACTIN-SECRETING PITUITARY ADENOMA

Synonyms: Galactorrhea-amenorrhea syndrome; prolactinoma.

Clinical Manifestations: Usually in young women; may or may not be associated with pregnancy: (a) *galactorrhea;* (b) *amenorrhea,* delayed puberty or very rarely precocious puberty in males; (c) *elevated prolactin levels* that fail to respond to phenothiazines, thyrotropin-releasing hormone, or hypoglycemia; normal or more often low plasma gonadotropin levels.

Radiologic Manifestations: More than half of tumors are *microadenomas* (less than 1 cm in diameter): (a) normal sella turcica size in most cases, abnormal sellar contour (asymmetry and erosion of sellar floor) (b) computed tomography: focal hypodense lesion, sellar floor erosion, infundibulum displacement, gland height greater than 8 mm, abnormal diaphragm sellae configuration (these signs are not present in all cases of microadenoma and missed diagnosis possible); (c) magnetic resonance imaging (thin sections, short TR sequence): upward convexity of a pituitary gland containing a low-intensity lesion, contralateral deviation of the stalk.

Notes: (a) some tumors may be the source of ectopic production of prolactine; (b) invasive prolactinoma may cause marked destruction of the base of the skull and various soft-tissue structures.

REFERENCES

Daunt N, et al.: Computed tomographic appearances and clinical features of prolactin-secreting pituitary adenomas in young male patients. *Clin. Radiol.* 36:227, 1985.

Davis PC, et al.: Prolactin-secreting pituitary microadenomas: Inaccuracy of high-resolution CT imaging. *A.J.R.* 144:151, 1985.

Hardy M, et al.: Precocious puberty associated with hyperprolactinemia in a male patient. *J. Pediatr.* 113:508, 1988.

Marcovitz S, et al.: Diagnostic accuracy of preoperative CT scanning of pituitary prolactinomas. *A.J.N.R.* 9:13, 1988.

Murphy FY, et al.: Giant invasive prolactinomas. *Am. J. Med.* 83:995, 1987.

Ozarda AT: Prolactin-secreting tumors. *J. Surg. Oncol.* 22:9, 1983.

Virapongse C, et al.: Prolactin-secreting pituitary adenomas: CT appearance in diffuse invasion. *Radiology* 152:447, 1984.

PSEUDOHYPOPARATHYROIDISM AND PSEUDOPSEUDOHYPOPARATHYROIDISM (TYPE I)

Synonyms: Albright hereditary osteodystrophy; PHP; PPHP.

Mode of Inheritance: X-linked dominant most likely; sex-influenced autosomal transmission possible; autosomal recessive transmission in some cases.

Clinical Manifestations: (a) *short stature;* (b) *round face, depressed nasal bridge;* (c) *obesity;* (d) seizures, *mental retardation;* (e) short fingers and/or toes, *positive "knuckle sign";* (f) cataract; (g) *abnormal dentition;* (h) *hypocalcemia and hyperphosphatemia that do not respond adequately to parathormone in pseudohypoparathyroidism, normal calcium and phosphorus in pseudopseudohypoparathyroidism,* lack of an increase in urinary excretion of cyclic adenosine monophosphate in response to parathormone injections, increased serum parathormone levels; (i) other reported abnormalities: cardiac failure, hypothyroidism due to thyroid-stimulating hormone deficiency, various unusual dermatoglyphic patterns, association with anticonvulsant rickets, progressive paraparesis with ossification of the posterior longitudinal ligament (C_4 to T_5), etc.

Radiologic Manifestations: (a) thick calvaria (in about one third of cases); (b) *intracranial calcification;* (c) *soft-tissue calcification or ossification;* (d) *disproportionate shortness and/or deformity of the metacarpals, metatarsals, and phalanges;* (e) premature fusion of the epiphyses of the hands, cone-shaped epiphyses of the hands, a typical pattern profile (Poznanski) but similar to acrodysostosis; (f) other reported abnormalities: bowing of long bones, coxa vara or valga, syndactyly, osteochondromas, spinal cord compression due to a narrowing of the spinal canal, association with hyperparathyroid bone disease, spinal cord compression (osseous tubercle on the anterolateral margin of the foramen magnum), subperiosteal bone resorption, radiolucent lesions caused by either brown tumors or bone cysts, slipped capital femoral epiphyses, focal areas of osteosclerosis, periosteal neo-ostosis, osteopenia.

Notes: (a) the major clinical features of the originally reported cases by Albright et al. included short stature, brachydactyly, mental retardation, obesity, hypocalcemia, and hyperphosphatemia; since the original description many patients with biochemical findings of *pseudohypoparathyroidism* but without somatic features enumerated above have been reported; some of the reported cases with clinical and radiological evidence of bone responsiveness to parathyroid hormone have shown no renal responsiveness to parathyroid hormone; (b) It has been suggested that the term *normocalcemic pseudohypoparathyroidism* be used rather than pseudopseudohypothyroidism; (c) type II pseudohypoparathyroidism: the phosphaturic effects of parathormone are decreased but urinary levels of cyclic adenosine monophosphate are normal or elevated (Figs ME–P–7 and ME–P–8).

REFERENCES

Albright F, et al.: Pseudo-hyperparathyroidism: Example of "Seabright-Bantam syndrome"; report of 3 cases. *Endocrinology* 30:922, 1942.

Albright F, et al.: Pseudo-pseudohypoparathyroidism. *Trans. Assoc. Am. Physicians* 65:337, 1952.

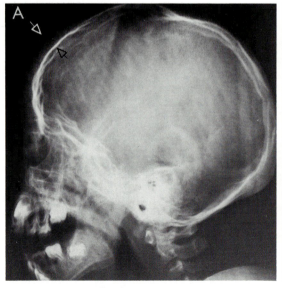 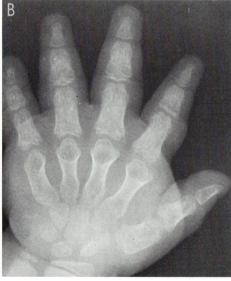

FIG ME–P–7.
Pseudohypoparathyroidism in a 4-year-old, short, obese girl with mental and motor retardation and a round face. **A,** extremely thick calvaria *(arrows).* **B,** short metacarpals and phalanges and cone-shaped epiphyses. (From Taybi H: Pseudo-hypoparathyroidism (PH). *Semin. Roentgenol.* 8:214, 1973. Used by permission.)

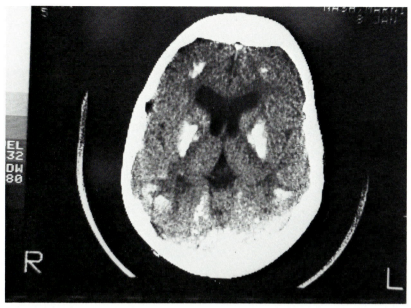

FIG ME−P−8.
Pseudohypoparathyroidism in a 12-year-old girl. Computed tomography of the head shows a thick calvaria, hydrocephalus, and extensive intracerebral calcification at various sites.

Burnstein MI, et al.: Metabolic bone disease in pseudohypoparathyroidism: Radiologic features. *Radiology* 155:351, 1985.

Dabbagh S, et al.: Renal-nonresponsive, bone-responsive pseudohypoparathyroidism. A case with normal vitamin D metabolite levels and clinical features of rickets. *Am. J. Dis. Child.* 138:1030, 1984.

Firooznia H, et al.: Case report 312. Diagnosis: Progressive paraparesis in a woman with pseudohypoparathyroidism (PHP) with ossification of the posterior longitudinal ligament from C4 to T5. *Skeletal Radiol.* 13:310, 1985.

Fitch N: Albright's hereditary osteodystrophy: A review. *Am. J. Med. Genet.* 11:11, 1982.

Frech RS, et al.: Radiological case of the month: Pseudohypoparathyroidism (infant) and pseudopseudohypoparathyroidism (mother). *Am. J. Dis. Child.* 119:447, 1970.

Hall FM, et al.: Pseudohypoparathyroidism presenting as renal osteodystrophy. *Skeletal Radiol.* 6:43, 1981.

Matsuda I, et al.: Pseudohypoparathyroidism type II and anticonvulsant rickets. *Eur. J. Pediatr.* 132:303, 1979.

Miano A: Cardiac failure in pseudohypoparathyroidism. *Helv. Paediatr. Acta* 36:191, 1981.

Poznanski AK, et al.: The pattern of shortening of the bones of the hand in PHP and PPHP—A comparison with brachydactyly E, Turner syndrome, and acrodysostosis. *Radiology* 123:707, 1977.

Radeke HH, et al.: Multiple pre- and postreceptor defects in pseudohypoparathyroidism (a multicenter study with twenty four patients). *J. Clin. Endocrinol. Metab.* 62:393, 1986.

Silve C, et al.: Selective resistance to parathyroid hormone in cultured skin fibroblasts from patients with pseudohypoparathyroidism type Ib. *J. Clin. Endocrinol. Metab.* 62:640, 1986.

Talon PH, et al.: Pseudo-pseudo-hypoparathyroïdie. A propos d'une observation familiale. *Ann. Pediatr. (Paris)* 32:295, 1985.

Tsang RC, et al.: The development of pseudohypoparathyroidism. Involvement of progressively increasing serum parathyroid hormone concentrations, increased 1,25-dihydroxyvitamin D concentrations, and 'migratory' subcutaneous calcifications. *Am. J. Dis. Child.* 138:654, 1984.

Van Dop C, et al.: Pseudopseudohypoparathyroidism with spinal cord compression. *Pediatr. Radiol.* 18:429, 1988.

White BJ, et al.: Dermatoglyphic and radiographic findings in a mother and daughter with pseudohypoparathyroidism. *Clin. Genet.* 13:359, 1978.

Williams AJ, et al.: Pseudohypoparathyroidism: Variable manifestations within a family. *Arch. Dis. Child.* 52:798, 1977.

PYRUVATE DEHYDROGENASE COMPLEX DEFICIENCY

Mode of Inheritance: Autosomal recessive.

Clinical Manifestations: Variable presentations (severe lactic acidosis in the neonatal period, recurrent episodes of lactic acidosis and associated neurological disorders, chronic acidosis throughout childhood): (a) *slow mental and physical development, microcephaly, cerebellar ataxia, seizures, spasticity,* etc.; (b) *lactic acidemia;* (c) deficient pyruvate dehydrogenase activity in cultured fibroblasts; (d) elevated levels of lactate and pyruvate in the cerebrospinal fluid and blood.

Radiologic Manifestations: Brain atrophy with grossly dilated ventricles and a reduction in the cerebral mantle.

Differential Diagnosis: Hydrocephaly of other causes and hydranencephaly.

REFERENCES

Aleck KA, et al.: In utero central nervous system damage in pyruvate dehydrogenase deficiency. *Arch. Neurol.* 45:987, 1988.

Brown GK, et al.: "Cerebral" lactic acidosis: Defects in pyruvate metabolism with profound brain damage and minimal systemic acidosis. *Eur. J. Pediatr.* 147:10, 1988.

Chow CW, et al.: Neuropathology in cerebral lactic acidosis. *Acta Neuropathol. (Berl.)* 74:393, 1987.

Robinson BH, et al.: The genetic heterogeneity of lactic acidosis: Occurrence of recognisable inborn errors of metabolism in a pediatric population with lactic acidosis. *Pediatr. Res.* 14:956, 1985.

PYRUVATE KINASE DEFICIENCY HEMOLYTIC ANEMIA

Mode of Inheritance: Autosomal recessive.

Clinical Manifestations: Onset usually in infancy: (a) *hemolytic anemia*, jaundice; (b) low hemoglobin levels, macrocytosis, normochromic erythrocytes, slight anisocytosis and poikilocytosis, *deficiency of glycolytic enzyme pyruvate kinase;* (c) *splenomegaly, hepatomegaly;* (d) other reported abnormalities: frontal bossing, chronic leg ulcer, hemolytic anemia and functional abnormality of pyruvate kinase in the presence of elevated red blood cell enzyme activity.

Radiologic Manifestations: (a) *skull: widened diploic space, vertical striations, atrophy of the outer table;* (b) mild demineralization of long bones, thinning of cortices, failure of tubulation; (c) cardiomegaly; (d) cholelithiasis.

Note: Acquired decreased enzyme activity may be associated with various myeloproliferative disorders, myeloblastic leukemia, and preleukemia; there is a concurrent development of hemolytic anemia with pyruvate kinase deficiency and preleukemia.

REFERENCES

Becker MH et al.: Roentgenographic manifestations of pyruvate kinase deficiency hemolytic anemia. *A.J.R.* 113:491, 1971.

Beutler E, et al.: Elevated pyruvate kinase activity in patients with hemolytic anemia due to red cell pyruvate kinase "deficiency." *Am. J. Med.* 83:899, 1987.

Kornberg A, et al.: Preleukemia manifested by hemolytic anemia with pyruvate-kinase deficiency. *Arch. Intern. Med.* 146:785, 1986.

Valentine WN, et al.: A specific erythrocyte glycolytic enzyme defect (pyruvate kinase) in three subjects with congenital non-spherocytic hemolytic anemia. *Trans. Assoc. Am. Physicians* 74:100, 1961.

R

REFSUM DISEASE

Synonyms: Phytanic acid storage disease; heredopathia atactica polyneuritiformis.

Mode of Inheritance: Autosomal recessive.

Enzyme Defect: Absence of the enzyme phytanic acid α-hydroxylase, resulting in an accumulation of C20 branched fatty acid (phytanic acid) in various tissues (liver, kidney, heart, peripheral nerves, etc.).

Clinical Manifestations: (a) *neurological manifestations*: cerebellar ataxia, polyneuropathy, enlargement of peripheral nerves, hyposmia, nerve deafness; (b) *ocular manifestations*: progressive visual deterioration, night blindness, optic atrophy, pigmentary retinal degeneration; (c) *ichthyosis*; (d) raised phytanic acid value in plasma, in utero diagnosis by a determination of phytanic acid oxidase activity and very long chain fatty acids in cultured amniotic cells; (e) impaired renal hemodynamic and tubular function (vacuolization and mitochondrial changes of tubular epithelial cells, vacuolization of the visceral epithelial cells of the glomeruli, mesangial sclerosis).

Radiologic Manifestations: (a) symmetrical epiphyseal dysplasia, in particular, at the knees: flattening and irregularity of the subchondral bone, marginal osteophytes, etc.; (b) shortening and deformity of the tubular bones in the hands and feet; (c) osteopenia in the infantile Refsum disease.

Notes: (a) Infantile Refsum disease with an onset in the first year of life is clinically characterized by psychomotor retardation, transient jaundice, hepatomegaly, neurosensory deafness, retinitis pigmentosa, and the biochemical changes present in classic Refsum disease (elevation of the phytanic acid concentration in plasma in combination with a tissue phytanic acid oxidase deficiency) in addition to the biochemical abnormalities present in adrenoleukodystrophy (ALD), adrenomyeloneuropathy (AMN), and Zellweger syndrome (elevated levels of plasma and skin fibroblast C24 and C26 fatty acids); abnormal bile acid metabolites and accumulation of very long chain fatty acids (pipecolic acid) similar to that seen in Zellweger syndrome; deficiency of catalase-containing particles (peroxisomes), alkyl dihydroxyacetone phosphate synthase, and acyl-CoA oxidase protein (deficiency of peroxisomes as in Zellweger syndrome); abnormal bile acids in plasma; impaired plasmogen metabolism; (b) failure to detect high levels of plasma phytanic acid may not necessarily indicate normal fibroblast phytanic acid oxidase activity.

REFERENCES

Pabico RC, et al.: Renal involvement in Refsum's disease. *Am. J. Med.* 70:1136, 1981.

Poll-Thé BT, et al: Impaired plasmalogen metabolism in infantile Refsum's disease. *Eur. J. Pediatr.* 144:513, 1986.

Poll-Thé BT, et al.: Infantile Refsum disease: An inherited peroxisomal disorder. Comparison with Zellweger syndrome and neonatal adrenoleukodystrophy. *Eur. J. Pediatr.* 146:477, 1987.

Poulos A, et al.: Infantile Refsum's disease (phytanic acid storage disease): a variant of Zellweger's syndrome? *Clin. Genet.* 26:579, 1984.

Poulos A, et al.: Patterns of Refsum's disease. Phytanic acid oxidase deficiency. *Arch. Dis. Child.* 59:222, 1984.

Refsum S: Heredoataxia hemeralopica-polyneuritiformis et tidligere ikke beskrevet familiaert syndrom? *Nord. Med.* 28:2682, 1945.

Roels F, et al.: Hepatic peroxisomes are deficient in infantile Refsum disease: A cytochemical study of 4 cases. *Am. J. Med. Genet.* 25:257, 1986.

Wall WJH, et al.: Skeletal changes in Refsum's disease. *Clin. Radiol.* 30:657, 1979.

Wanders RJA, et al.: Infantile Refsum disease: Deficiency of catalase-containing particles (peroxisomes), alkyldihydroxyacetone phosphate synthase and peroxisomal β-oxidation enzyme proteins. *Eur. J. Pediatr.* 145:172, 1986.

RENAL TUBULAR ACIDOSIS

Synonym: RTA.

Pathophysiology: Disorder of renal acidification leading to metabolic acidosis often without a reduction in renal mass.

Classification:

(A) TYPE 1 (DISTAL) RENAL TUBULAR ACIDOSIS: inappropriately high pH of urine in association with persistent hyperchloremic acidosis, absence of glycosuria, hyperphosphaturia, or excessive bicarbonate excretion; autosomal dominant inheritance in some cases; occurrence with the use of certain drugs and in various autoimmune disorders; etc.

(B) TYPE 2 (PROXIMAL) RENAL TUBULAR ACIDOSIS (Butler-Albright distal tubular acidosis): defect in acidification in the proximal tubule leading to alkali loss, high pH of urine, heavy bicarbonaturia; occurrence in association with various drugs, amyloidosis, multiple myeloma, Sjögren syndrome, medullary cystic disease, vitamin D deficiency, genetic disorders (cystinosis, Wilson disease, fructose intolerance, Lowe syndrome, tyrosinemia, etc.); primary inherited (autosomal recessive) or sporadic.

(C) TYPE 3 (HYBRID): formerly used in reference to infants

TABLE ME—R—1.

Clinical and Laboratory Characteristics of the Various Types of Renal Tubular Acidosis in Children*

Characteristic	Type 1 (Classic, Distal)	Type 2 (Proximal)	Type 3 (Hybrid)	Type 4 (Aldosterone Deficiency)
Growth failure	+++†	++†	++	+++
Hypokalemic muscle weakness	++	+†	+	Hyperkalemia
Nephrocalcinosis	Frequent	Rare	±	Rare
Low citrate excretion	+++	±†	±	±
Fractional excretion of filtered HCO_3 at normal serum bicarbonate levels (%)	<5	>15	5–15	<15
Glycosuria and aminoaciduria	Absent	Present	±	±
Daily alkali treatment (mEq/kg body weight)	2–4	2–14	2–14	2–3
Daily potassium requirement	Decreases with correction	Increases with correction	±	±

*From Chan JCM: Renal tubular acidosis. *J. Pediatr.* 102:327, 1983. Used by permission.
†+ = present; ++ = common; +++ = very common; − = not present; ± = variable.

with renal bicarbonate wasting associated with a distal acidification disorder and inappropriately high urinary pH; it is considered to be a variant of type 1.

(D) TYPE 4 RENAL TUBULAR ACIDOSIS: metabolic acidosis, hyperkalemia, decrease in the glomerular filtration rate.

Clinical Manifestations: (a) "rheumatic" complaints: arthralgia, myalgia, low back pain; (b) muscle weakness; (c) growth retardation; (d) recurrent nephrolithiasis; (e) other reported abnormalities: type 1 RTA associated with Shwachman syndrome; type 4 in association with diabetes mellitus (diabetic nephropathy), chronic renal parenchymal damage, and interstial nephritis; association of proximal renal tubular acidosis and glycogen storage diseases; distal renal tubular acidosis in polyarteritis nodosa.

Radiologic Manifestations: (a) *nephrocalcinosis;* (b) nephrolithiasis; (c) generalized skeletal demineralization of mild to marked severity; (d) pathological fractures; (e) skeletal maturation retardation.

Notes: (a) skeletal abnormalities are often limited to patients with type 2 or azotemic individuals; (b) nephrocalcinosis common in distal RTA, rare in proximal RTA, and usually absent in type 4; (c) a sibship with neuroaxonal dystrophy, renal tubular acidosis and hyperdense lesions in the thalamus and basal ganglia (computed tomography) has been reported (Maccario, et al.); (d) renal tubular acidosis in association with sensorineural hearing loss or deafness is considered to be a distinct syndrome (Table ME—R—1).

REFERENCES

Anai T, et al.: Siblings with renal tubular acidosis and nerve deafness. The first family in Japan. *Hum. Genet.* 66:282, 1984.

Breedveld FC, et al.: Distal renal tubular acidosis in polyarteritis nodosa. *Arch. Intern. Med.* 146:1009, 1986.

Brenner RJ, et al.: Incidence of radiographically evident bone disease, nephrocalcinosis, and nephrolithiasis in various types of renal tubular acidosis. *N. Engl. J. Med.* 307:217, 1982.

Butler AM, et al.: Dehydration and acidosis with calcification at renal tubules. *J. Pediatr.* 8:489, 1936.

Chan JCM: Renal tubular acidosis. *J. Pediatr.* 102:327, 1983.

Courey WR, et al.: The radiographic findings in renal tubular acidosis: Analysis of 21 cases. *Radiology* 105:497, 1972.

Donckerwolcke RA, et al.: The syndrome of renal tubular acidosis with nerve deafness. *Acta Paediatr. Scand.* 65:100, 1976.

Harrington TM, et al.: Renal tubular acidosis. A new look at treatment of musculoskeletal and renal disease. *Mayo Clin. Proc.* 58:354, 1983.

Hassan M, et al.: Detection echographique neonatale de la nephrocalcinose medullaire associee a l'acidose tubulaire distale de Butler-Albright. *J. Radiol.* 66:689, 1985.

Lightwood R: Calcium infarction of the kidneys in infants. *Arch. Dis. Child.* 10:205, 1935.

Maccario M, et al.: A sibship with neuroaxonal dystrophy and renal tubular acidosis: A new syndrome? *Ann. Neurol.* 13:608, 1983.

Marra G, et al.: Renal tubular acidosis in a case of Shwachman's syndrome. *Acta Paediatr. Scand.* 75:682, 1986.

Matsuo N, et al.: Proximal renal tubular acidosis in a child with type 1 glycogen storage disease. *Acta Paediatr. Scand.* 75:332, 1986.

Morris RC Jr: Renal tubular acidosis. *N. Engl. J. Med.* 304:418, 1981.

Nagai T, et al.: Proximal renal tubular acidosis associated with glycogen storage disease, type 9. *Acta Paediatr. Scand.* 77:460, 1988.

Pohlman T, et al.: Renal tubular acidosis. *J. Urol.* 132:431, 1984.

Sluysmans T, et al.: Growth failure associated with medullary sponge kidney, due to incomplete renal tubular acidosis type 1. *Eur. J. Pediatr.* 146:78, 1987.

RICKETS/OSTEOMALACIA

Classification:

(A) TYPE I: Abnormality of vitamin D metabolism resulting in a deficiency of active vitamin D: (a) inadequate exposure to sunlight; (b) deficient intake of vitamin D; (c) malabsorption of fat-soluble vitamins (cystic fibrosis, etc.); (d) liver disease: failure of 25-hydroxylation and/or malabsorption; (e) renal glomerular destruction (depressed vitamin D activation); (f) increased hepatic metabolism (anticonvulsant therapy); (g) vitamin D–dependent rickets (pseudo–vitamin D-deficient rickets): functional reduction in the concentration of kidney "1α-hydroxylase enzyme."

(B) TYPE II: Target cell abnormalities (renal tubular disorders leading to decreased reabsorption of phosphate and reduced serum phosphate levels): (a) primary renal hypophosphatemic rickets (vitamin D–resistant rickets); (b) renal tubular acidosis; (c) Fanconi–de Toni syndrome.

(C) TYPE III: Tumor-induced rickets and osteomalacia: hemangiomas of bones or soft tissues, hemangiopericytoma, giant-cell tumor, osteoblastoma, fibrous dysplasia, malignant neurinoma, sarcoma, epidermal nevus syndrome, nonosteogenic fibroma, etc.

Clinical Manifestations:

(A) TYPE I: (a) muscle weakness, waddling gait, bone pain, growth failure, irritability, sweating, respiratory distress

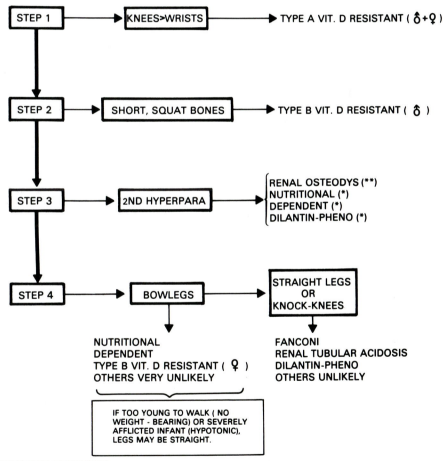

(*) A FEW SEVERE CASES ONLY
(**) ACCOUNT FOR MOST CASES

FIG ME–R–1.
Rickets: roentgenographic scheme for diagnosis. (From Swischuk LE, Hayden CK Jr: Rickets: A roentgenographic scheme for diagnosis. *Pediatr. Radiol.* 8:203, 1979. Used by permission.)

in small preterm infants; (b) skeletal deformities: frontal and parietal bossing; pigeon breast; Harrison groove; rachitic rosaries; enlarged costochondral junctions; kyphoscoliosis; pelvic deformity; knobby joints, particularly in the wrist and ankle regions; abnormal limb curvatures; etc.; (c) normal or decreased serum calcium level, decreased serum phosphate level, increased alkaline phosphatase level, increased aminoaciduria; (d) autosomal recessive and autosomal dominant (in some families) in vitamin D−dependent rickets; (e) pseudotumor cerebri in association with nutritional rickets.

(B) Type II: (a) *vitamin D−resistant rickets:* (1) X-linked dominant mode of inheritance; (2) dwarfism, growth retardation; (3) bowleg; (4) waddling gait; (5) rachitic rosary of the rib ends; (6) protuberant abdomen; (7) hypophosphatemia associated with diminished tubular resorption of inorganic phosphate; (8) rickets unresponsive to usual amounts of vitamin D; (9) elevated serum alkaline phosphatase levels; (b) renal tubular acidosis—distal type: (1) primary (with an onset of symptoms often in infancy or early childhood, sporadic or autosomal dominant), secondary (drugs, autoimmune disorders, nephrocalcinosis from a variety of causes, sickle cell anemia, pyelonephritis, obstructive uropathy, renal transplantation, hepatic cirrhosis); (2) anorexia, vomiting, hyperpnea, polyuria, constipation, failure to thrive, rickets, symptoms related to renal calculi; (3) low plasma concentration of bicarbonate, potassium, and calcium; high plasma concentration of chloride; low plasma pH; relatively high urine pH; hypercalciuria. (c) renal tubular acidosis—proximal type: (1) primary (familial or sporadic) or in association with various etiologic factors (drugs, amyloidosis, multiple myeloma, Sjögren syndrome, medullary cystic disease, cystinosis, Wilson disease, fructose intolerance, Lowe syndrome, tyrosinemia, etc.); (2) growth failure, malnutrition, muscle weakness, polyuria, polydipsia, metabolic acidosis, secondary hyperaldosteronism, rickets; (3) hypokalemia, hypocalcemia, hypophosphatemia, hypouricemia, aminoaciduria, increased phosphate and uric clearance, increased sodium and potassium loss, Fanconi syndrome (hyperaminoaciduria, glucosuria, increased phosphaturia, uricosuria).

Radiologic Manifestations:

(A) Osteomalacia: Skeletal deformities (limbs, spine, thorax, pelvis), diminished bone density, coarsened trabeculae, mottled bone texture; cortical thinning, intercortical striations, pseudofractures (Looser lines), sclerosis at the sites of pseudofractures, plantar fasciitis as a presenting manifestation, spinal stenosis, tumorlike bone lesion as a manifestation of vitamin D−resistant hypophatemic osteomalacia.

(B) Rickets: demineralization, widening of the epiphyseal plates, metaphyseal cupping, irregularity and indistinctness of the provisional zone of calcification, poorly ossified epiphyses with indistinct borders, coarsened trabeculae, lack of a normal sharp border of the inferior scapular angle and iliac crest, poor subperiosteal new bone formation of mandible, pathological fractures, skeletal deformities, premature closure of cranial sutures, increased metacarpal diameter associated with decreased combined cortical thickness, calcification of entheses (exuberant calcification of tendon and ligament in-

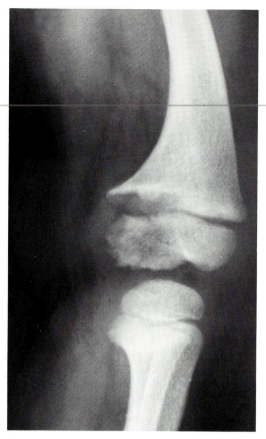

FIG ME−R−2.
Vitamin D−resistant rickets in a 2½-year-old female with bowed legs and hypophosphatemia. Abnormal mineralization and fraying of the medial aspect of the distal part of the femur are present. The trabeculae are coarse and dense. The optimum vitamin D dosage was in the range of 300,000 units daily, at which level improvement was noted.

sertions and joint capsules) in association with X-linked hypophosphatemic osteomalacia (increased prevalence and extent with age).

Notes: (a) Milkman syndrome: osteomalacia with "pseudofractures"; (b) the roentgenographic scheme for diagnosis reported by Swischuk and Hayden is helpful in the differentiation of rickets in most patients over 6 months of age.

- *Step 1:* Determination of the uniformity of rachitic epiphyseal-metaphyseal changes throughout the skeleton or a preponderance in the lower limbs: changes are most marked in the lower limbs (best assessed by comparing knee and wrist radiograms) in vitamin D−resistant rickets (type I).
- *Step 2:* Presence or absence of generalized modeling error resulting in short, squat bones (type II).
- *Step 3:* Presence of secondary hyperparathyroidism (renal osteodystrophy).
- *Step 4:* Presence of bowleg, knock-knee, or straight leg.

(c) radiographic examinations in patients with X-linked hypophosphatemic osteomalcia and hearing loss have shown generalized osteosclerosis and thickening of the petrous bone, with some narrowing of the internal auditory meatus, particularly in its midportion; (d) association with achalasia-adrenal-alacrima syndrome (familial glucocorticoid deficiency); (e) association of congenital adrenal hyperplasia and hyperphosphatemic rickets (Figs ME–R–1 and ME–R–2).

REFERENCES

Alpan G, et al.: Respiratory failure and multiple fractures in vitamin D–dependent rickets. *Acta Paediatr. Scand.* 74:300, 1985.

Andrews WS, et al.: Fat soluble vitamin deficiency in biliary atresia. *J. Pediatr. Surg.* 16:284, 1981.

Binstadt DH, et al.: Rickets as a complication of intravenous hyperalimentation in infants. *Pediatr. Radiol.* 7:211, 1978.

Carey DE, et al.: Hypophosphatemic rickets/osteomalacia in linear sebaceous nevus syndrome: A variant of tumor-induced osteomalacia. *J. Pediatr.* 109:994, 1986.

Clemens P: Premature cranial synostosis and hypophosphatemic rickets. *Acta Paediatr. Scand.* 73:857, 1984.

DeJong AR, et al.: Pseudotumor cerebri and nutritional rickets. *Eur. J. Pediatr.* 143:219, 1985.

Dopplet SH: Vitamin D, rickets, and osteomalacia. *Orthop. Clin. North Am.* 15:671, 1984.

Dumas R, et al.: Congenital adrenal hyperplasia associated with hyperphosphatemic rickets. *Clin. Pediatr. (Phila.)* 27:276, 1988.

Godsall JW, et al.: Vitamin D metabolism and bone histomorphometry in a patient with antacid-induced osteomalacia. *Am. J. Med.* 77:747, 1984.

Harrison HE, et al.: Rickets: Primary hypophosphatemic and vitamin D–dependent varieties. *J. Pediatr.* 99:84, 1981.

Herweijer TJ, et al.: Metacarpal measurements in X-linked hypophosphataemic rickets. *Helv. Paediatr. Acta* 41:331, 1986.

Hunt PA, et al.: Bone disease induced by anticonvulsant therapy and treatment with calcitriol (1,25-dihydroxy-vitamin D₃). *Am. J. Dis. Child.* 140:715, 1986.

Katayama H, et al.: Bone changes in congenital biliary atresia: Radiologic observation of 8 cases. *A.J.R.* 124:107, 1975.

Khajavi A, et al.: The rachitic lung. *Clin. Pediatr. (Phila.)* 16:36, 1977.

Koeger A-C, et al.: Les ostéomalacies tumorales hypophosphorémiques. *Presse Med.* 14:1747, 1985.

Kruger DM, et al.: Vitamin D deficiency rickets. *Clin. Orthop.* 224:277, 1987.

Lever EG, et al.: Albright's syndrome associated with a soft-tissue myxoma and hypophosphataemic osteomalacia. *J. Bone Joint Surg. [Br.]* 65:621, 1983.

Looser E: Ueber Spätrachitis und Osteomalazie. *Dtsch. Ztschr. Chir.* 152:210, 1920.

Lyon AJ, et al.: Radiological rickets in extremely low birth-weight infants. *Pediatr. Radiol.* 17:56, 1987.

Mächler M, et al.: X-linked dominant hypophosphatemia is closely linked to DNA markers DXS41 and DXS43 at Xp22. *Hum. Genet.* 73:271, 1986.

Masel JP, et al.: Hypophosphataemic vitamin D–resistant rickets—a cause of spinal stenosis in adults. *Aust. Radiol.* 25:264, 1981.

McAlister WH, et al.: Tibial bowing exacerbated by partial premature epiphyseal closure in sex-linked hypophosphatemic rickets. *Radiology* 162:461, 1987.

Milgram JW, et al.: Hypophosphatemic vitamin D–refractory osteomalacia with bilateral femoral pseudofractures. *Clin. Orthop.* 160:78, 1981.

Milkman LA: Multiple spontaneous idiopathic symmetrical fractures. *A.J.R.* 32:622, 1934.

Milkman LA: Pseudofractures (hunger osteopathy, late rickets, osteomalacia): Report of case. *A.J.R.* 24:29, 1930.

Miyauchi A, et al.: Hemangiopericytoma-induced osteomalacia: Tumor transplantation in nude mice causes hypophosphatemia and tumor extracts inhibit renal 25-hydroxyvitamin D 1-hydroxylase activity. *J. Clin. Endocrinol. Metab.* 67:46, 1988.

Moorjani R, et al.: Feuerstein and Mims syndrome with resistant rickets. *Pediatr. Radiol.* 5:120, 1976.

O'Malley SP, et al.: The petrous temporal bone and deafness in X-linked hypophosphataemic osteomalacia. *Clin. Radiol.* 39:528, 1988.

Paice EW, et al.: Nutritional osteomalacia presenting with plantar fasciitis. *J. Bone Joint Surg. [Br.]* 69:38, 1987.

Papapoulos SE, et al.: A tumour-like bone lesion as a manifestation of vitamin D–resistant hypophosphataemic osteomalacia. *Br. J. Radiol.* 60:285, 1987.

Park W, et al.: Osteomalacia of the mother—rickets of the newborn. *Eur. J. Pediatr.* 146:292, 1987.

Perry W, et al.: Hereditary hypophosphatemic rickets with autosomal recessive inheritance and severe osteosclerosis. *J. Bone Joint Surg. [Br.]* 60:430, 1978.

Pitt MJ: Rachitic and osteomalacic syndromes. *Radiol. Clin. North Am.* 19:581, 1981.

Polisson RP, et al.: Calcification of entheses associated with X-linked hypophosphatemic osteomalacia. *N. Engl. J. Med.* 313:1, 1985.

Rosen JF, et al.: Rickets with alopecia: An inborn error of vitamin D metabolism. *J. Pediatr.* 94:729, 1979.

Ryan EA, et al.: Oncogenous osteomalacia. Review of the world literature of 42 cases and report of two new cases. *Am. J. Med.* 77:501, 1984.

Saul PD, et al.: The role of bone scanning in neonatal rickets. *Pediatr. Radiol.* 13:89, 1983.

Shah BR, et al.: Familial glucocorticoid deficiency in a girl with familial hypophosphatemic rickets. *Am. J. Dis. Child.* 142:900, 1988.

Siris ES, et al.: Tumor-induced osteomalacia. Kinetics of calcium, phosphorus, and vitamin D metabolism and characteristics of bone histomorphometry. *Am. J. Med.* 82:307, 1987.

Skovby F, et al.: Hypophosphatemic rickets in linear sebaceous nevus sequence. *J. Pediatr.* 111:855, 1987.

Steinbach HL, et al.: Roentgen appearance of the skeleton in osteomalacia and rickets. *A.J.R.* 91:955, 1964.

Steinbach HL, et al.: Unusual roentgen manifestations of osteomalacia. *A.J.R.* 82:875, 1959.

Sudhaker D, et al.: Hypophosphatemic osteomalacia and adult Fanconi syndrome due to light-chain nephropathy. Another form of oncogenous osteomalacia. *Am. J. Med.* 82:333, 1987.

Swischuk LE, et al.: Seizures and demineralization of the skull: A diagnostic presentation of rickets. *Pediatr. Radiol.* 6:65, 1977.

Swischuk LE, Hayden CK Jr: Rickets: A roentgenographic scheme for diagnosis. _Pediatr. Radiol._ 8:203, 1979.

Thomas PS, et al.: The "mandibular mantel"—a sign of rickets in very low birth weight infants. _Br. J. Radiol._ 51:93, 1978.

Toomey F, et al.: Rickets associated with cholestasis and parenteral nutrition in premature infants. _Radiology_ 142:85, 1982.

Touloukian RJ, et al.: Vitamin D deficiency rickets as a late complication of the short gut syndrome during infancy. _J. Pediatr. Surg._ 16:230, 1981.

Weidner N, et al.: Neoplastic pathology of oncogenic osteomalacia/rickets. _Cancer_ 55:1691, 1985.

Weiss A: The scapular sign in rickets. _Radiology_ 98:633, 1971.

Winnacker JL, et al.: Rickets in children receiving anticonvulsant drugs. _Am. J. Dis. Child._ 131:286, 1977.

Zamboni G, et al.: Association of osteopetrosis and vitamin D–resistant rickets. _Helv. Paediatr. Acta_ 32:363, 1977.

ROTOR SYNDROME

Synonym: Hyperbilirubinemia, Rotor type.

Mode of Inheritance: Autosomal recessive.

Clinical Manifestations: (a) _chronic, predominantly conjugated hyperbilirubinemia without evidence of hemolysis;_ (b) _plasma retention of Bromsulphalein 45 minutes after the intravenous injection of a 5 mg/kg dose exceeds 25%;_ (c) _normal liver histology_ (no excess pigmentation); (d) _marked increase in the total coproporphyrin excretion in the urine._

Radiologic Manifestations: (a) oral cholecystography often normal; (b) ^{99m}Tc-HIDA cholescintigraphy: nonvisualization of the bile ducts (case report, Bar-Meir et al.), selective excretion through the kidneys.

REFERENCES

Bar-Meir S, et al.: ^{99m}Tc-HIDA cholescintigraphy in Dubin-Johnson and Rotor syndromes. _Radiology_ 142:743, 1982.

Haverbach BJ, et al.: Familial nonhemolytic jaundice with normal liver histology and conjugated bilirubin. _N. Engl. J. Med._ 262:113, 1960.

Rotor AB, et al.: Familial non-hemolytic jaundice with direct van den Bergh reaction. _Acta Med. Phil._ 5:37, 1948.

SALLA DISEASE

Synonym: Sialuria, Finnish type.

Mode of Inheritance: Autosomal recessive.

Frequency: Over 50 published cases (Ylitalo et al.).

Clinical Manifestations: Onset in infancy or early childhood (a) *mental and physical retardation; (b) neurological abnormalities:* ataxia, athetosis, abnormal deep tendon reflexes, inability to walk, impaired speech, epileptic fits; (c) *moderate to marked increase in the excretion of free N-acetylneuraminic acid (sialic acid) in urine,* prenatal detection (increased free sialic acid in amniocytes); (d) other reported abnormalities: exotropia, hypertelorism, inguinal hernia, abnormal electroencephalographic findings, congenital ascites.

Radiologic Manifestation: Thick calvarium in adult patients; brain atrophy in some.

Note: The eponym *Salla disease* refers to the geographic area in northern Finland from which the patients originated.

REFERENCES

Aula P, et al.: Salla disease: A new lysosomal storage disorder. *Arch. Neurol.* 36:88, 1979.
Echenne B, et al.: Salla disease in one non-Finnish patient. *Eur. J. Pediatr.* 145:320, 1986.
Gillan JE, et al.: Congenital ascites as a presenting sign of lysosomal storage disease. *J. Pediatr.* 104:225, 1984.
Renlund M: Clinical and laboratory diagnosis of Salla disease in infancy and childhood. *J. Pediatr.* 104:232, 1984.
Renlund M, et al.: Prenatal detection of Salla disease based upon increased free sialic acid in amniocytes. *Am. J. Med. Genet.* 28:377, 1987.
Ylitalo V, et al.: Salla disease variants. Sialoylaciduric encephalopathy with increased sialidase activity in two non-Finnish children. *Neuropediatrics* 17:44, 1986.

SCURVY

Synonym: Vitamin C (ascorbic acid) deficiency.

Clinical Manifestations: Onset of symptoms usually between 3 months and 2 years of age: (a) *irritability;* (b) *pain, swelling, tenderness, pseudoparalysis of the legs, frog-leg position, external hemorrhage (skin, mucous membranes);* (c) *swelling of the gums;* (d) *costal rosaries, limb deformities;* (e) adult scurvy: muscle fatigue, subcutaneous and mucosal bleeding, swelling, pain, and discoloration of the lower limbs; decreased range of motion of the ankle and knee joints; petechiae, purpura, and ecchymoses; enlargement and hyperkeratosis of the hair follicles with a red hemorrhagic halo; corkscrew deformity and swan neck deformity of hair; anemia.

Radiologic Manifestations: (a) *generalized osteoporosis, ground-glass appearance, thickening of the provisional zone of calcification (Fränkel sign), white rim about the epiphyseal center (Wimberger sign), metaphyseal zone of demineralization, "corner sign" (subepiphyseal infraction);* (b) *fracture with epiphyseal slipping, subperiosteal hemorrhage, subperiosteal calcifying hematoma;* (c) *metaphyseal cupping, ball-in-socket deformity of the epiphyseal-metaphyseal junction, improvement of the deformity in a long range follow-up.*

Differential Diagnosis: Battered child syndrome; syphilis; copper deficiency; Menkes syndrome; tyrosinosis; etc.

REFERENCES

Carpenter KJ: *The History of Scurvy and Vitamin C.* New York, Cambridge University Press, 1986.
Hallel T, et al.: Epiphyseometaphyseal cupping of the distal femoral epiphysis following scurvy in infancy. *Clin. Orthop.* 153:166, 1980.
Hirsch M, et al.: Neonatal scurvy: Report of a case. *Pediatr. Radiol.* 4:251, 1976.
Quiles M, et al.: Epiphyseal separation in scurvy. *J. Pediatr. Orthop.* 8:223, 1988.
Reuler JB, et al.: Adult scurvy. *J.A.M.A.* 253:805, 1985.
Schiliro G, et al.: Scurvy: Almost historic, but not quite. *Am. J. Dis. Child.* 133:323, 1979.
Silverman FN: Recovery from epiphyseal invagination: Sequel to an unusual complication of scurvy. *J. Bone Joint Surg. [Am.]* 52:384, 1970.

SIALIDOSIS

Definition: A group of inborn errors of metabolism caused by the intracellular accumulation of sialic acid−containing oligosaccharides.

Mode of Inheritance: Autosomal recessive.

Frequency (Infantile): 22 published cases (Pueschel et al.).

Enzyme Deficiency: Glycoprotein-specific N-acetylneuraminidase.

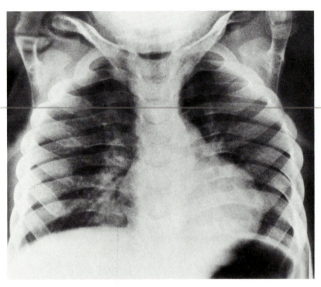

FIG ME–S–1.
Sialidosis in a 2-year-old girl with wide ribs and mild cardiomegaly. (From Kelly TE, Batroshesky L, Harris DJ, et al.: Mucolipidosis I (acid neuroaminidase deficiency). *Am. J. Dis. Child.* 135:703, 1981. Used by permission.)

Clinical Manifestations: Four different clinical phenotypes: (a) the early infantile form: nonimmune hydrops fetalis, ascites, hepatosplenomegaly, failure to thrive, recurrent infections, death usually within the first year of life; (b) the late infantile form: motor retardation, progressive neurological deterioration, axial hypotonia, limb hypertonicity, hepatosplenomegaly, coarse facial features, recurrent infections, death in early childhood; (c) the juvenile form (previously known as "mucolipidosis I"): progressive neurological deterioration, impaired hearing, impaired speech, Hurler-like appearance in early childhood, hernias, myoclonus, ataxia, cherry-red macular spot, mental retardation, hepatosplenomegaly, survival into early adulthood; (d) the adult form ("cherry-red spot–myoclonus syndrome"): onset in adolescence, progressive myoclonus, bilateral macular cherry-red spots, gradual visual loss, normal or near normal intelligence, death in the fourth decade of life.

Radiologic Manifestations: (a) infantile: coarsened bony trabecular pattern mainly in the long bones, metaphyseal irregularity and increased density; (b) juvenile: (1) *mild to moderate dysostosis multiplex:* flat vertebral bodies, beaking of vertebral bodies, irregular vertebral endplates, small and flared iliac wings, shallow acetabular roofs, flat capital femoral epiphyses, coxa valga, thickened calvaria, mandibular prognathism, osteopenia, thin cortex of the tubular bones, cystic-type changes of the phalanges, bifid ossification of the calcaneus; (2) skeletal maturation retardation; (3) cardiomegaly; (4) persistent pulmonary infiltrates (Fig ME–S–1).

REFERENCES

Beck M, et al.: Neuraminidase deficiency presenting as nonimmune hydrops fetalis. *Eur. J. Pediatr.* 143:135, 1984.

Daneman A, et al.: Neonatal ascites due to lysosomal storage disease. *Radiology* 149:463, 1983.

Eggli KD, et al.: The mucopolysaccharidoses and related conditions. *Semin. Roentgenol.* 21:275, 1986.

Kelly TE, et al.: Mucolipidosis I (acid neuraminidase deficiency). *Am. J. Dis. Child.* 135:703, 1981.

Laver J, et al.: Infantile lethal neuraminidase deficiency (sialidosis). *Clin. Genet.* 23:97, 1983.

O'Brien JS, et al.: Sialidosis: Delineation of subtypes by neuraminidase assay. *Clin. Genet.* 17:35, 1980.

Paschke E, et al.: Infantile type of sialic acid storage disease with sialuria. *Clin. Genet.* 417, 1986.

Pueschel SM, et al.: Infantile sialic acid storage disease associated with renal disease. *Pediatr. Neurol.* 4:207, 1988.

Spranger J: Mini review: Inborn errors of complex carbohydrate metabolism. *Am. J. Med. Genet.* 28:489, 1987.

Spranger J, et al.: Mucolipidosis 1—A sialidosis. *Am. J. Med. Genet.* 1:21, 1977.

Staalman CR, et al.: Mucolipidosis I. Roentgenographic follow-up. *Skeletal Radiol.* 12:153, 1984.

Young ID, et al.: Neuraminidase deficiency: Case report and review of the phenotype. *J. Med. Genet.* 24:283, 1987.

SICKLE CELL ANEMIA

Mode of Inheritance: Autosomal recessive; homozygosity for HbS in sickle cell anemia (HbSS); heterozygosity for HbS in sickle cell trait.

Frequency: Sickle cell hemoglobin present in 8% of the black population of the United States; 1 in 625 has sickle cell disease (homozygous for hemoglobin S) (Lande et al.).

Etiology: The presence of abnormal β-chain in HbS (valine substituted for glutamic acid) results in erythrocyte sickling at a reduced oxygen tension; the deformed and fragmented erythrocyte associated with an increase in blood viscosity leads to occlusion of small blood vessels and infarct.

Clinical Manifestations: (a) *anemia;* (b) *jaundice,* liver and biliary tract dysfunction; (c) *splenomegaly* in the early stage, *splenic fibrosis* in a later stage; (d) *hepatomegaly;* (e) *abdominal crisis* (intravascular thrombosis, infarcts): pain, vomiting, distension, splenic sequestration crises, etc.; (f) *painful limbs:* bone infarcts, hand-foot syndrome (swelling, tenderness, fever, and leukocytosis), osteomyelitis (*Salmonella* or staphylococcal infections); (g) arthralgia, arthritis, hemarthrosis; (h) chronic leg ulcers; (i) *pulmonary infarcts, recurrent pneumonias;* (j) *cardiomegaly, congestive heart failure,* abnormal septal Q waves, ventricular dysfunction, pulmonary hypertension, cor pulmonale; (k) neurological complications: seizures, hemiplegia, stupor, coma, cerebral infarction, intracranial hemorrhage, spinal cord infarction, isolated neuropathies due to anatomic proximity to infarcted bones, auditory problems, ocular manifestations, recurrent cerebral ischemia during hypertransfusion therapy; (l) *hematuria;* (m) prenatal diagnosis: first-trimester diagnosis with chorionic villus sampling (enzymatic DNA test), amniocentesis in the second trimester; (n) other reported abnormalities: priapism, lymphadenopathy, growth disturbances, bacteremia, painful crises (acute chest syndrome, abdominal crises), mitral valve prolapse, retinopathy, exophthalmos associated with bone infarction, fat embolism (bone marrow necrosis), abnormal body shape (reduction in weight, height, sitting height, limb length, interacromial and intercristal diameters, and skin fold thickness; increased anteroposterior chest diameter), ischemic colitis, etc.

Radiologic Manifestations:

(A) SKELETAL SYSTEM: (a) *skull: granular pattern, widening of diploic space, decrease in width of the outer table,* hair-on-end appearance, decreased calvarial density, focal radiolucent areas, focal or diffuse osteosclerosis, radiolucency and coarsening of the bony trabeculae of the mandible, prominent lamina dura, orbital bone infarction, calvarial infarction; (b) spine and pelvis: *osteoporosis, depression of end plates with a squared-off appearance of the indentation,* prominent vertical bony trabeculae, increased thoracic kyphosis and lumbar lordosis, prominence and persistence of anterior vascular foramina of the thoracic vertebral bodies in children, pelvic osteomyelitis, osteitis pubis, protrusio acetabuli; (c) thoracic cage: sternal cupping, patchy areas of rarefaction and/or sclerosis of the ribs; (d) *long bones: diaphyseal infarction* (mottled and strandy medullary sclerotic densities, cortex-within-cortex pattern, cortical fissuring, massive infarct of the entire shaft in children, scintigraphic demonstration of infarcted segment), *epiphyseal infarction* (proximal humeral and femoral epiphyses most common sites, osteonecrosis, collapse and disintegration, osteosclerosis), *osteomyelitis,* pathological fractures, "ulcer osteoma" (chronic ulcer in the superficial tissues adjacent to the involved bone); (e) hands and feet: *hand-foot syndrome* in children (most frequent between 6 months and 2 years of age, "dactylitis," soft-tissue swelling, bone resorption in infarcted or infected areas, periosteal elevation and subperiosteal new bone formation), slender marfanoid fingers or brachydactyly associated with cone-shaped epiphyses and concave metaphyses of the metacarpal bones and phalanges, terminal phalangeal sclerosis, erosive disease of the calcaneus (loss of definition of the cortical margin in the superior aspect of the bone); (f) *skeletal maturation retardation;* (g) *arthropathy:* joint effusion (noninflammatory), septic arthritis, hemarthrosis; (h) magnetic resonance imaging (MRI): helpful in the differentiation between acute and chronic marrow infarcts.

(B) CHEST: (a) *pulmonary infarct, pleural effusion;* (b) pulmonary hypertension and cor pulmonale following repeated episodes of pulmonary vascular occlusion, cardiomegaly, congestive heart failure; (c) extramedullary hematopoiesis (masses in the paravertebral region).

(C) URINARY SYSTEM: (a) *renal enlargement, thickening of the renal medulla, focal cortical hypertrophy, caliceal clubbing, papillary necrosis;* (b) pyelonephritis; (c) perirenal hematoma; (d) renal arteriography: focal cortical hypertrophy, "pseudobrain" nephrogram due to a mixture of hypertrophy and scar formation, thinning of the cortex, medullary hypertrophy, pruning of the arterial tree; (e) MRI of sickle-cell nephropathy: decreased relative cortical signals, most evident on T_2-weighted images; (f) renal vein thrombosis.

(D) CENTRAL NERVOUS SYSTEM: (a) *partial or complete vascular occlusion* of major arteries or distal branches, moyamoya, vascular occlusion or stenosis shown by MRI; (b) brain changes, in particular, in the general regions of arterial border zones between the major cerebral arteries and adjacent deep white matter (distal small-vessel disease due to "sludging"); (c) decrease in total, hemispheral, or regional cerebral

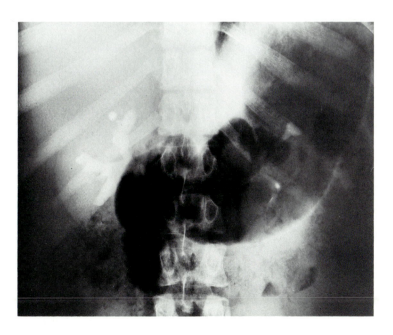

FIG ME−S−2.
Sickle cell anemia: excretory urography in an 18-year-old female with homozygous sickle cell disease. Note the blunting of the calices, in particular, on the right side, and papillary necrosis of one of the calices of the upper pole of the right kidney. (From Taybi H: Urinary tract manifestations of multisystem diseases in children, in Margulis AR, Gooding CA (eds.): *Diagnostic Radiology.* San Francisco, University of California, 1979, p. 141.)

blood flow (xenon 133 inhalation method); (d) intracranial hemorrhage (intracerebral, subarachnoid), intracranial aneurysm(s); retro-orbital and epidural hematoma (associated with bone infarct).

(E) ABDOMEN: (a) *bowel distension related to vascular occlusion;* (b) *cholelithiasis* (calcium bicarbonate); (c) retroperitoneal fibrosis (sickle cell trait), abnormal accumulation of ^{99m}Tc methylene diphosphate in the spleen and kidneys (children); (e) imaging in the sickle cell patients with abdominal pain: splenic abnormalities (low-density infarcts, rupture, hemorrhage, calcification), liver abnormalities (abscess, infarcts, hemochromatosis, gallstones, etc.), appendicitis with abscess formation, hepatic vein thrombosis, abnormal biliary scintigraphy (delayed gallbladder visualization consistent with chronic cholecystitis).

Notes: (a) in vitro studies have shown that nonionic contrast medium causes significantly less sickling than ionic contrast agent does; (b) magnetic fields and radiofrequency (RH) energy affect sickle erythrocytes in vitro; no changes in sickle

blood cell flow have been shown during MRI in vivo; (c) post-transfusion hypertension in association with seizures and intracranial hemorrhage has been reported as a characteristic syndrome in sickle cell disease (Figs ME–S–2 and ME–S–3).

REFERENCES

Alavi A, et al.: Scintigraphic examination of bone and marrow infarcts in sickle cell disorders. *Semin. Roentgenol.* 22:213, 1987.

Amundsen TR, et al.: Osteomyelitis and infarction in sickle cell hemoglobinopathies: Differentiation by combined technetium and gallium scintigraphy. *Radiology* 153:807, 1984.

Balfour IC, et al.: Cardiac size and function in children with sickle cell anemia. *Am. Heart J.* 108:345, 1984.

BenDridi MF, et al.: Radiological abnormalities of the skeleton in patients with sickle-cell anemia. *Pediatr. Radiol.* 17:296, 1987.

Bohrer SP: Bone changes in the extremities in sickle cell anemia. *Semin. Roentgenol.* 22:176, 1987.

Brody AS, et al.: Preservation of sickle cell blood-flow patterns during MR imaging: An in vivo study. *A.J.R.* 151:139, 1988.

Buchanan GR, et al.: Recurrent cerebral ischemia during hypertransfusion therapy in sickle cell anemia. *J. Pediatr.* 103:921, 1983.

Collins FS, et al.: Pulmonary hypertension and cor pulmonale in the sickle hemoglobinopathies. *Am. J. Med.* 73:814, 1982.

D'Alonzo WA, et al.: Biliary scintigraphy in children with sickle cell anemia and acute abdominal pain. *Pediatr. Radiol.* 15:395, 1985.

Davies SC, et al.: Acute chest syndrome in sickle-cell disease. *Lancet* 1:36, 1984.

DeCeulaer K, et al.: Pneumonia in young children with homozygous sickle cell disease: Risk and clinical features. *Eur. J. Pediatr.* 144:255, 1985.

Ebong W, et al.: Bilateral pelvic osteomyelitis in children with sickle-cell anemia. *J. Bone Joint Surg. [Am.]* 64:945, 1982.

ElGammal T, et al.: MR and CT investigation of cerebrovascular disease in sickle cell patients. *A.J.N.R.* 7:1043, 1986.

Embury SH: Advances in the prenatal diagnosis of sickle cell anemia. *West J. Med.* 147:580, 1987.

Fabian RH, et al.: Neurological complications of hemoglobin SC disease. *Arch. Neurol.* 41:289, 1984.

Gage TP, et al.: Ischemic colitis complicating sickle cell crisis. *Gastroenterology* 84:171, 1983.

Gaston MH: Sickle cell disease: An overview. *Semin. Roentgenol.* 22:150, 1987.

Girardet JPh, et al.: Les cardiomégalies drépanocytaires de l'enfant. *Arch. Fr. Pediatr.* 40:525, 1983.

Goldberg HI, et al.: Central nervous system. *Semin. Roentgenol.* 22:205, 1987.

Greene WB, et al.: *Salmonella* osteomyelitis and hand-foot syndrome in a child with sickle cell anemia. *J. Pediatr. Orthop.* 7:716, 1987.

Gumbs RV, et al.: Thoracic extramedullary hematopoiesis in sickle-cell disease. *A.J.R.* 149:889, 1987.

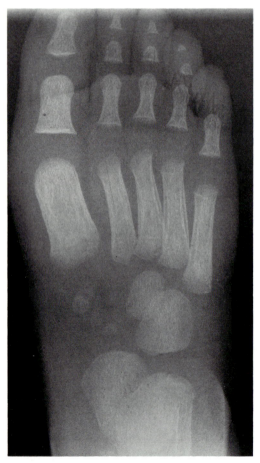

FIG ME–S–3.
Sickle cell anemia (hand-foot syndrome) in a 19-month-old black male with sickle cell anemia (hemoglobin SS) and swelling and tenderness of both hands and feet. Note the periosteal elevation and subperiosteal new bone formation of the metatarsals.

Haupt HM, et al.: The lung in sickle cell disease. *Chest* 81:332, 1981.

Hernandez RJ, et al.: MR evaluation of liver iron overload. *J. Comput. Assist. Tomogr.* 12:91, 1988.

Herrick JB: Peculiar elongated and sickle shaped red blood corpuscles in a case of severe anemia. *Arch. Intern. Med.* 6:517, 1910.

Hill MC, et al.: Abnormal epiphyses in the sickling disorders. *A.J.R.* 124:34, 1975.

Hoff JV, et al.: Intracranial hemorrhage in children with sickle cell disease. *Am. J. Dis. Child.* 139:1120, 1985.

Huttenlocher PR, et al.: Cerebral blood flow in sickle cell cerebrovascular disease. *Pediatrics* 73:615, 1984.

Johnson CS, et al.: Liver involvement in sickle cell disease. *Medicine (Baltimore)* 64:349, 1985.

Khademi M, et al.: Renal arteriography in sickle-cell disease. *Radiology* 107:41, 1973.

Lande IA, et al.: Sickle-cell nephropathy: MR imaging. *Radiology* 158:379, 1986.

Landesman SH, et al.: Infections in children with sickle cell anemia. Special reference to pneumococcal and salmonella infections. *Am. J. Pediatr. Hematol. Oncol.* 4:407, 1982.

Lanzer W, et al.: Avascular necrosis of the lunate and sickle cell anemia. *Clin. Orthop.* 187:168, 1984.

Levine MS, et al.: Sternal cupping: A new finding in childhood sickle cell anemia. *Radiology* 142:367, 1982.

Lippman SM, et al.: Abnormal septal Q waves in sickle cell disease. Prevalence and causative factors. *Chest.* 88:543, 1985.

Lippman SM, et al.: Mitral valve prolapse in sickle cell disease. *Arch. Intern. Med.* 145:435, 1985.

Magid D, et al.: Abdominal pain in sickle cell disease: The role of CT. *Radiology* 163:325, 1987.

Mallouh AA, et al.: Intracranial hemorrhage in patients with sickle cell disease. *Am. J. Dis. Child.* 140:505, 1986.

Mallouh AA, et al.: Proptosis, skull infarction, and retro-orbital and epidural hematomas in a child with sickle cell disease. *Clin. Pediatr. (Phila.)* 26:536, 1987.

Mapp E, et al.: Uroradiological manifestations of S-hemoglobinopathy. *Semin. Roentgenol.* 22:186, 1987.

Martinez S, et al.: Protrusio acetabuli in sickle-cell anemia. *Radiology* 151:43, 1984.

Miller ST, et al.: Cerebrovascular accidents in children with sickle-cell disease and alpha-thalassemia. *J. Pediatr.* 113:847, 1988.

Overby MC, et al.: Multiple intracranial aneurysms in sickle cell anemia. *J. Neurosurg.* 62:430, 1985.

Pavlakis SG, et al.: Brain infarction in sickle cell anemia: Magnetic resonance imaging correlates. *Ann. Neurol.* 23:125, 1988.

Phills JA, et al.: Retroperitoneal fibrosis in three siblings with the sickle cell trait. *Can. Med. Assoc. J.* 108:1025, 1973.

Poncz M, et al.: Acute chest syndrome in sickle cell disease: Etiology and clinical correlates. *J. Pediatr.* 107:861, 1985.

Ransewak W, et al.: Moyamoya in sickle cell disease demonstrated by DSA and hexabrix. *J. Can. Assoc. Radiol.* 36:332, 1985.

Rao KRP: Angiography in hemoglobin S-C disease. *Ann. Intern. Med.* 105:971, 1986.

Rao VM, et al.: Painful sickle cell crisis: Bone marrow patterns observed with MR imaging. *Radiology* 161:211, 1986.

Rao VM, et al.: Radiology of the gastrointestinal tract in sickle cell anemia. *Semin. Roentgenol.* 22:195, 1987.

Rao VM, et al.: The effect of ionic and nonionic contrast media on the sickling phenomenon. *Radiology* 144:291, 1982.

Reynolds J: Radiologic manifestations of sickle cell hemoglobinopathy. *J.A.M.A.* 238:247, 1977.

Reynolds J: The skull and spine. *Semin. Roentgenol.* 22:168, 1987.

Riggs W Jr, et al.: Roentgen chest findings in childhood sickle cell anemia. *A.J.R.* 104:838, 1968.

Rosenberg RF: Priapism and sickle-cell disease. *Radiology* 98:135, 1971.

Roth EF, et al.: Sickle cell anemia (homozygosity for hemoglobin S) affecting the calvaria (case report 391). *Skeletal Radiol.* 14:65, 1985.

Rothchild BM, et al.: Calcaneal abnormalities and erosive bone disease. Associated with sickle cell anemia. *Am. J. Med.* 71:427, 1981.

Saiki RK, et al.: Diagnosis of sickle cell anemia and β-thalassemia with enzymatically amplified DNA and nonradioactive allele-specific oligonucleotide probes. *N. Engl. J. Med.* 319:537, 1988.

Sarnaik S, et al.: Incidence of cholelithiasis in sickle cell anemia using the ultrasonic gray-scale technique. *J. Pediatr.* 96:1005, 1980.

Sarnaik SA, et al.: Neurological complications of sickle cell anemia. *Am. J. Pediatr. Hematol. Oncol.* 4:386, 1982.

Sebes JI, et al.: Terminal phalangeal sclerosis in sickle cell disease. *A.J.R.* 140:763, 1983.

Shapiro MP, et al.: Fat embolism in sickle cell disease. Report of a case with brief review of the literature. *Arch. Intern. Med.* 144:181, 1984.

Shaub MS, et al.: Tibiotalar slant: A new observation in sickle cell anemia. *Radiology* 117:551, 1975.

Sickles EA, et al.: Perirenal hematoma as a complication of renal infarction in sickle-cell trait. *A.J.R.* 122:800, 1974.

Silver L, et al.: Bone scan in the hand-foot syndrome. *Clin. Nucl. Med.* 9:710, 1984.

Smith JA: Cardiopulmonary manifestations of sickle cell disease in childhood. *Semin. Roentgenol.* 22:160, 1987.

Solanki DL, et al.: Acute splenic sequestration crises in adults with sickle cell disease. *Am. J. Med.* 80:985, 1986.

Stevens MCG, et al.: Body shape in young children with homozygous sickle cell disease. *Pediatrics* 71:610, 1983.

Stevens MCG, et al.: Observation on the natural history of dactylites in hemozygous sickle cell disease. *Clin. Pediatr. (Phila.)* 20:311, 1981.

Stevens MCG, et al.: Prepubertal growth and skeletal maturation in children with sickle cell disease. *Pediatrics* 78:124, 1986.

Sty JR, et al.: Abnormal Tc-99m methylene diphosphate accumulation in the kidneys of children with sickle cell disease. *Clin. Nucl. Med.* 5:445, 1980.

Sty JR: Ultrasonography: Hepatic vein thrombosis in sickle cell anemia. *Am. J. Pediatr. Hematol. Oncol.* 4:213, 1982.

Weinberg S: Severe sclerosis of the long bones in sickle cell anemia. *Radiology* 145:41, 1982.

Wiggins T, et al.: "Ulcer osteoma" associated with sickle cell disease. (Case report 379). *Skeletal Radiol.* 15:409, 1986.

Wolff MH, et al.: Orbital infarction in sickle cell disease. *Pediatr. Radiol.* 15:50, 1985.

Zarkowsky HS, et al.: Bacteremia in sickle hemoglobinopathies. *J. Pediatr.* 109:579, 1986.

Zimmerman RA, et al.: MRI of sickle cell cerebral infarction. *Neuroradiology* 29:232, 1987.

SOMATOSTATINOMA SYNDROME

Etiology: Pancreatic tumor producing somatostatin-like immunoreactivity and bioactivity.

Clinical and Radiologic Manifestations: (a) dry mouth, dyspepsia, postprandial fullness, steatorrhea, diabetes mellitus; (b) normocytic, normochromic anemia; (c) cholelithiasis; (d) pancreatic tumor.

REFERENCES

Friesen SR: Update on the diagnosis and treatment of rare neuroendocrine tumors. *Surg. Clin. North Am.* 67:379, 1987.

Krejs GJ, et al.: Somatostatinoma syndrome: Biochemical, morphologic and clinical features. *N. Engl. J. Med.* 301:285, 1979.

Larsson LI, et al.: Pancreatic somatostatinoma: Clinical features and physiological implications. *Lancet* 1:666, 1977.

Stackpoole PW, et al.: Somatostatinoma syndrome: Does a clinical entity exist? *Acta Endocrinol.* 102:80, 1983.

SPHEROCYTOSIS

Synonym: Minkowski-Chauffard disease.

Mode of Inheritance: Autosomal dominant with variable penetrance; less common are cases of autosomal recessive inheritance and sporadic occurrence.

Frequency: 2 to 4 cases per 10,000 population in the United States (Croom et al.).

Pathophysiology: Deficiency of spectrin (a protein of the erythrocyte membrane skeleton) resulting in the formation of spherocytes that lack the normal strength; the spherocytes trapped in the splenic red pulp have a short survival period and are destroyed.

Clinical Manifestations: (a) *jaundice;* (b) *splenomegaly;* (c) *chronic hemolytic anemia* with an onset in childhood or adolescence, *spherocytes in the peripheral blood, increased osmotic fragility of erythrocytes, shortened life span of erythrocytes* from an affected person in a normal recipient, rapid hemolysis of spherocytes in the spleen; (d) diagnosis in newborn infants: increased osmotic fragility of fresh and incubated red blood cells, moderately increased autohemolysis, and partial reduction of autohemolysis by the addition of glucose; (e) other reported abnormalities: atypical hyperbilirubinemia in newborns, aplastic crisis, leg ulcerations.

Radiologic Manifestations: (a) *bilirubin stones;* (b) *osteoporosis, widening of the medullary canal of tubular bone,* widening of the diploic space, hair-on-end appearance of the calvaria; (c) extramedullary hematopoiesis (paravertebral); (d) secondary hemochromatosis (related to repeated transfusions); (e) splenomegaly, usually with a homogeneous increased echogenicity; well-defined focal defects of high echogenicity relative to the normal spleen (soft areas composed of dilated sinuses and extramedullary hemopoiesis), splenic rupture; (f) ischemic cerebral accident.

REFERENCES

Agre P, et al.: Deficient red-cell spectrin in severe, recessively inherited spherocytosis. *N. Engl. J. Med.* 306:1155, 1982.

Bruguier A, et al.: Accident ischémique cérébral et sphérocytose héréditaire. *Arch. Fr. Pediatr.* 40:653, 1983.

Croom RD, et al.: Hereditary spherocytosis. *Ann. Surg.* 203:34, 1986.

Gupta R, et al.: Unusual ultrasound appearance of the spleen—a case of hereditary spherocytosis. *Br. J. Radiol.* 59:284, 1986.

Iwai N, et al.: Cholelithiasis in children with congenital spherocytosis. *Z. Kinderchir.* 41:308, 1986.

Moseley JE: Skeletal changes in the anemias. *Semin. Roentgenol.* 9:169, 1974.

Schröter W, et al: Diagnosis of hereditary spherocytosis in newborn infants. *J. Pediatr.* 103:460, 1983.

Wolfe LC, et al.: A genetic defect in the binding of protein 4.1 to spectrin in a kindred with hereditary spherocytosis. *N. Engl. J. Med.* 307:1367, 1982.

T

TESTICULAR FEMINIZATION

Mode of Inheritance: X-linked recessive or sex-modified autosomal dominant.

Frequency: Approximately 1 in 50,000; syndrome present in 1% to 2% of all females with inguinal hernias.

Clinical Manifestations: (a) *genetic male;* (b) *female phenotype;* (c) *primary amenorrhea, sterility;* (d) *intra-abdominal, inguinal, or intralabial testicular location;* (e) testes secrete androgens; (f) inguinal hernia; (h) *lack of a cytosolic receptor for dihydrotestosterone* in androgen-dependent tissues, plasma testosterone levels in the male range, normal follicle-stimulating hormone concentration, elevated luteinizing hormone levels, XY karyotype; (g) small or absent clitoris, blind-ending vaginal pouch, absent cervix on rectal examination.

Radiologic Manifestations: (a) *absence of uterus and ovaries;* (b) *presence of testes.*

REFERENCES

Hales ED, et al.: Computed tomography of testicular feminization. *J. Comput. Assist. Tomogr.* 8:772, 1984.
Hodgins MB, et al.: Carrier detection in the testicular feminisation syndrome: deficient 5 α-dihydrotestosterone binding in cultured skin fibroblasts from the mothers of patients with complete androgen insensitivity. *J. Med. Genet.* 21:178, 1984.
Nichols MM: Rectal examination in testicular feminization syndrome. *Am. J. Dis. Child.* 140:1101, 1986.
Schwimer SR, et al.: Sonographic evaluation of the testicular feminization syndrome. *J. Ultrasound Med.* 4:503, 1985.
Sheridan-Pereira M, et al.: Testicular feminisation syndrome presenting in the newborn. *Arch. Dis. Child.* 58:380, 1983.
Strickland AL, et al.: Testicular feminization syndrome. *Am. J. Dis. Child.* 140:565, 1986.

THALASSEMIA

Biochemical Classification: (a) α-thalassemia: deficiency of α-globin chain synthesis; (b) β-thalassemia: deficiency of β-globin chain synthesis; (c) others: less common, hemoglobin polypeptide chains (δ, δβ).

Clinical Types: (a) thalassemia major (homozygote): two similar or identical genes for thalassemia; (b) thalassemia minor (heterozygote), mildly affected; (c) thalassemia intermedia (heterozygote), moderately affected.

Frequency: Relatively high incidence in the people of Mediterranean origin.

Clinical Manifestations (thalassemia major): (a) *severe anemia, jaundice;* (b) *hepatosplenomegaly;* (c) *cephalofacial deformities:* prominent parietal and frontal bones, depressed nasal bridge, hypertelorism, prominent maxilla with an overbite on the mandible, retraction of the upper lip, protrusion of the incisors ("rodent facies"); (d) *cardiomegaly,* pericardial effusion, pericarditis, disturbance of conductions and rhythm, right and left ventricular dysfunction (shown by radionuclide angiography) related to excessive iron deposition in the myocardium as a result of recurrent transfusions, congestive heart failure; (e) *endocrine disorders:* hypogonadotropic hypogonadism (retarded sex characteristics), hypoparathyroidism, reduced adrenocorticotropic hormone reserve, reduced growth hormone, reduced thyroid hormone reserve, diabetes mellitus; (f) *iron overload* (liver cirrhosis, myocardial degeneration, endocrinopathies); (g) *bilirubin stones;* (h) dwarfism, adult height deficiency; (i) laboratory findings in Cooley anemia (Mediterranean anemia): *hypochromic microcytic anemia, poikilocytosis, polychromatophilia, target cells, nucleated erythroid precursors, decreased red cell survival, increased serum bilirubin and fecal urobilinogen, elevated serum iron level, excess hemoglobin A_2 (over 3%) and hemoglobin F (50% to 90%), elevated serum iron level;* (j) prenatal diagnosis: chorionic villus sampling and fetal DNA analysis, analysis of amniocyte DNA; (k) other reported abnormalities: scurvy despite a normal intake of vitamin C, gout, arthropathy (secondary to hemochromatosis), osteomyelitis, septic arthritis, association with pyknodysostosis (heterozygous β-thalassemia), mild-to-moderate small-airway obstruction and hyperinflation in homozygous β-thalassemia, deletion of all four α-globin loci (Bart hemoglobin hydrops fetalis syndrome), hypersplenism in thalassemia major, enlargement of the adenoids and tonsils, hypertrophy of the nasal turbinates and hearing deficits associated with changes in the bones of the middle ear, generalized epileptiform seizures due to an extramedullary hematopoietic mass compressing the brain, spinal cord compression due to extramedullary hematopoiesis, etc.

Radiologic Manifestations:

(A) SKELETAL SYSTEM: (a) skull: *osteoporosis with a granular pattern; expansion of the diploic space,* most prominent in the frontal bone; thinning of the outer *table; hair-on-end appearance;* enlarged calvarial vascular markings; circumscribed lytic lesions; *hypertelorism; hypoplasia of the paranasal sinuses due to osseous expansion of the facial bones (mar-*

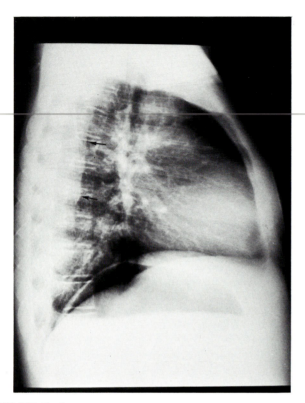

FIG ME–T–1.
Thalassemia: extramedullary hematopoiesis demonstrated in this lateral projection as soft-tissue densities *(arrows)* overlying the spine. (From Lawson JP, Ablow RC, Pearson HA: The ribs in thalassemia. *Radiology* 140:663, 1981. Used by permission.)

row hyperplasia); *malocclusion of the jaws; dental displacement and deformities;* (b) trunk: *osteoporosis, coarse bony trabeculae,* thinning of the cortex, rib-within-rib appearance, *costal widening,* rib notching, *accentuation of vertical bone trabeculae of the vertebrae,* biconcave vertebral configuration ("fish vertebrae"), *medullary hyperplasia of the pelvic bones and clavicles;* (c) tubular bones: *widened medullary cavity, thinning of the cortex, underconstriction,* premature closure of growth plates, pathological fractures, perpendicular periosteal spiculation, enlarged phalangeal nutrient foramina, aseptic necrosis of the femoral head; (d) *skeletal maturation retardation;* (e) avidity of radiogallium for bone (marrow cavity hypertrophy).

(B) Chest and abdomen: (a) *extramedullary hematopoiesis:* multiple lobular intrathoracic masses adjacent to the ribs and thoracic vertebrae, pelvic mass, extradural mass causing cord compression, low-intensity signal similar to marrow on magnetic resonance imaging; (b) *hemochromatosis* (following transfusion and chelation therapy); *increased density of the liver, spleen, and lymph nodes; hepatosplenomegaly;* renal enlargement; *gallstones;* porcelain gallbladder; highly echogenic pancreas (similar to that reported in cystic fibrosis) following repeated transfusions in patients with thalassemia major (Fig ME–T–1).

REFERENCES

Abbassioun K, et al.: Spinal cord compression due to extradural extramedullary hematopoiesis in chronic anemias. *Iranian J. Med. Sci.* 13:21, 1986.

Aksoy M, et al.: "Porcelain gallbladder" in a case of thalassemia intermedia. *Radiology* 95:265, 1970.

Beaudry MA, et al.: Survival of a hydropic infant with homozygous α-thalassemia-1. *J. Pediatr.* 108:713, 1986.

Borgna-Pignatti C, et al.: Growth and sexual maturation in thalassemia major. *J. Pediatr.* 106:150, 1985.

Brasch RC, et al.: Magnetic resonance imaging of transfusional hemosiderosis complicating thalassemia major. *Radiology* 150:767, 1984.

Caffey J: Cooley's anemia: A review of the roentgenographic findings in the skeleton. *A.J.R.* 78:381, 1957.

Cassady JR, et al.: The "typical" spine changes of sickle-cell anemia in a patient with thalassemia major (Cooley's anemia). *Radiology* 89:1065, 1967.

Chao PW, et al.: CT features of presacral mass: An unusual focus of extramedullary hematopoiesis. *J. Comput. Assist. Tomogr.* 10:684, 1986.

Cohen A, et al.: Scurvy and altered iron stores in thalassemia major. *N. Engl. J. Med.* 304:158, 1981.

Colavita N, et al.: Premature epiphyseal fusion and extramedullary hematopoiesis in thalassemia. *Skeletal Radiol.* 16:533, 1987.

Colonna P: Les β-thalassémies. *Ann. Med. Interne (Paris)* 134:147, 1983.

Costin G, et al.: Endocrine abnormalities in thalassemia major. *Am. J. Dis. Child.* 133:497, 1979.

De Luca F, et al.: Adult height in thalassaemia major without hormonal treatment. *Eur. J. Pediatr.* 146:494, 1987.

De Sanctis V, et al.: Insulin dependent diabetes in thalassaemia. *Arch. Dis. Child.* 63:58, 1988.

De Virgillis S, et al.: Deferoxamine-induced growth retardation in patients with thalassemia major. *J. Pediatr.* 113:661, 1988.

Erttmann R, et al.: Pancreatic sonography in thalassemia major. *Klin. Padiatr.* 195:97, 1983.

Fink IJ, et al.: Enlarged phalangeal nutrient foramina in Gaucher disease and β-thalassemia major. *A.J.R.* 143:647, 1984.

Finsterbush A, et al.: Fracture patterns in thalassemia. *Clin. Orthop.* 192:132, 1985.

Freeman AP, et al.: Early left ventricular dysfunction and chelation therapy in thalassemia major. *Ann. Intern. Med.* 99:450, 1983.

Fucharoen S, et al.: Intracranial extramedullary hematopoiesis inducing epilepsy in a patient with β-thalassemia-hemoglobin E. *Arch. Intern. Med.* 145:739, 1985.

Girot R, et al.: Hypersplénisme de la thalassémie majeure. *Presse Med.* 13:1881, 1984.

Gomori JM, et al.: MR relaxation times and iron content of thalassemic spleens: An in vitro study. *A.J.R.* 150:567, 1988.

Grimmond AP, et al.: Avidity of radiogallium for bone in thalassemia. *Clin. Nucl. Med.* 12:758, 1987.

Grossman H, et al.: Renal enlargement in thalassemia major. *Radiology* 100:645, 1971.

Gugliantini P, et al.: Incisure costali nella anemia di Cooley. *Radiol. Med.* 72:173, 1986.

Hazell JWP, et al.: E.N.T. complication in thalassaemia major. *J. Laryngol. Otol.* 90:877, 1979.

Hoyt RW, et al.: Pulmonary function abnormalities in homozygous β-thalassemia. *J. Pediatr.* 109:452, 1986.

Koren (Kurlat) A et al: Right ventricular cardiac dysfunction in β-thalassemia major. *Am. J. Dis. Child.* 141:93, 1987.

Lawson JP, et al.: Calvarial and phalangeal vascular impressions in thalassemia. *A.J.R.* 143:641, 1984.

Lawson JP, Ablow RC, Pearson HA: The ribs in thalassemia: I. The relationship to therapy. *Radiology* 140:663, 1981.

Lawson JP, Ablow RC, Pearson HA: The ribs in thalassemia: II. The pathogenesis of the changes. *Radiology* 140:673, 1981.

Lehmann H: Nomenclature of the α-thalassaemias. *Lancet* 1:552, 1984.

Mandell GA, et al.: Exaggerated anterior vertebral notching. *Radiology* 131:367, 1979.

Mann KS, et al.: Paraplegia due to extramedullary hematopoiesis in thalassemia. *J. Neurosurg.* 66:938, 1987.

Mitnick JS, et al.: CT in β-thalassemia: Iron deposition in the liver, spleen and lymph nodes. *A.J.R.* 136:1191, 1981.

Old JM, et al.: First-trimester fetal diagnosis for haemoglobinopathies: Report on 200 cases. *Lancet* 2:764, 1986.

Orzincolo C, et al.: Aseptic necrosis of femoral head complicating thalassemia. *Skeletal Radiol.* 15:541, 1986.

Orzincolo C, et al.: Circumscribed lytic lesions of the thalassaemic skull. *Skeletal Radiol.* 17:344, 1988.

Özoylu S: Hand-foot syndrome in sickle-cell thalassemia. *N. Engl. J. Med.* 284:219, 1971.

Papavasiliou C, et al.: Magnetic resonance imaging of marrow heterotopia in haemoglobinopathy. *Eur. J. Radiol.* 8:50, 1988.

Sabato AR, et al.: Primary hypothyroidism and the low T3 syndrome in thalassaemia major. *Arch. Dis. Child.* 58:120, 1983.

Scutellari PN, et al.: The incidence of cholelithiasis in beta-thalassemias. *Rays* 7:17, 1982.

Sculellari PN, et al.: Xeroradiography in β-thalassemia. *Skeletal Radiol.* 13:39, 1985.

Sklar CA, et al.: Adrenal function in thalassemia major following long-term treatment with multiple transfusions and chelation therapy. *Am. J. Dis. Child.* 141:327, 1987.

Sinniah D, et al.: Intracranial hemorrhage and circulating coagulation inhibitor in beta-thalassemia major. *J. Pediatr.* 99:700, 1981.

Smithson LV, et al.: Paranasal sinus involvement in thalassemia major: CT demonstration. *A.J.N.R.* 8:564, 1987.

Thein SL, et al.: Feasibility of prenatal diagnosis of β-thalassaemia with synthetic DNA probes in two Mediterranean populations. *Lancet* 2:345, 1985.

Valdez VA, et al.: Visualization of the liver with 99mTc-EHDP in thalassemia major. *Gastrointest. Radiol.* 6:175, 1981.

Yamato M, et al.: Computed tomography of fatty replacement in extramedullary hematopoiesis. *J. Comput. Assist. Tomogr.* 11:541, 1987.

Zamboni G, et al.: Parathyroid hormone, calcitonin and vitamin D metabolites in beta-thalassaemia major. *Eur. J. Pediatr.* 145:133, 1986.

TYROSINEMIA, TYPE I

Synonyms: Hereditary tyrosinemia; congenital tyrosinemia; hepatorenal tyrosinemia; fumarylacetoacetase (FAA) deficiency.

Mode of Inheritance: Autosomal recessive.

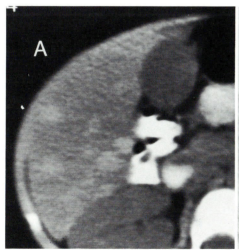
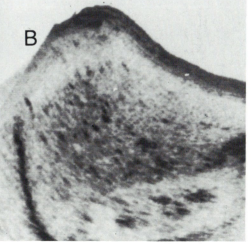

FIG ME—T—2.
Tyrosinemia in a 2½-year-old boy with cirrhosis and multiple regenerating nodules. **A,** an unenhanced upper abdominal computed tomographic scan shows multiple high-attenuation foci (approximately 80 Hounsfield units [HU]) scattered diffusely throughout the lowly dense liver (approximately 60 HU). The lesions became almost isodense with the adjacent hepatic parenchyma after IV contrast administration. **B,** a right parasagittal liver sonogram reveals diffuse increased echogenicity consistent with diffuse fatty infiltration or fibrosis. No focal lesions are evident. (From Day DL, Letourneau JG, Allan BT, et al.: Hepatic regenerating nodules in hereditary tyrosinemia. *A.J.R.* 149:391, 1987. Used by permission.)

Clinical Manifestations:

(A) Acute hereditary tyrosinemia: (a) onset in the first year of life, rapid lethal course; (b) *lethargy, irritability, failure to gain weight, fever, jaundice, diarrhea, ecchymosis, melena;* (c) *ascites, splenomegaly, hepatomegaly, liver failure.*

(B) Chronic hereditary tyrosinemia: (a) *hepatic cirrhosis;* (b) *generalized renal reabsorption defects* (Fanconi renotubular syndrome); (c) other reported abnormalities: hepatoma, neurological disorders, mental retardation.

Laboratory Findings: (a) anemia, coagulation defect due to a combination of deficient hepatic synthesis of clotting factors and a consumption coagulopathy; (b) *persistent elevation of plasma tyrosine levels (above 3 mg/100 mL); increased urinary excretion of tyrosyl compounds;* generalized aminoaciduria; hyperphosphaturia; hypophosphatemia; hypoglycemia; urinary excretion of glucose, fructose, galactose, and lactose; elevated serum methionine levels; (c) prenatal diagnosis: determination of succinylacetone in amniotic fluid supernatant, assay of FAA in cultured amniotic fluid cells; determination of FAA in chorionic villus material.

Radiologic Manifestations: (a) *rickets;* (b) *nephromegaly;* (c) cirrhosis in early childhood, regenerating nodules, hepatocellular carcinoma in about one third of children surviving over 2 years of age (detection by various imaging techniques is difficult in the presence of cirrhosis and the regenerating nodules).

Note: Other disorders of tyrosine metabolism (hypertyrosinemia): (a) tyrosinemia II (Richner-Hanhart syndrome): autosomal recessive inheritance, tyrosine transaminase deficiency, corneal erosions and plaques, palm and sole erosions, and hyperkeratoses; mental retardation in some; (b) neonatal transitory tyrosinemia: *p*-OH-phenylpyruvic acid oxidase deficiency; infants may be lethargic, have difficulty in feeding, impaired motor activity, etc.; (c) "tyrosinosis" in a single patient reported by Medes in 1932, the enzymatic defect not determined; (d) hypertyrosinemia in patients with liver disease; (e) tyrosinemia III (4-hydroxyphenylpyruvic acid oxidase deficiency) (Fig ME−T−2).

REFERENCES

Day DL, et al.: Hepatic regenerating nodules in hereditary tyrosinemia. *A.J.R.* 149:391, 1987.

Driscoll DJ, et al.: Corneal tyrosine crystals in transient neonatal tyrosinemia. *J. Pediatr.* 113:91, 1988.

Emdo F, et al.: Four-hydroxyphenlpyruvic acid oxidase deficiency with normal fumarylacetoacetase: A new variant form of hereditary hypertyrosinemia. *Pediatr. Res.* 17:92, 1983.

Evans DIK, et al.: Coagulation defect of congenital tyrosinaemia. *Arch. Dis. Child.* 59:1088, 1984.

Goldsmith LA: Tyrosinemia II. A large North Carolina kindred. *Arch. Intern. Med.* 145:1697, 1985.

Hervé F, et al.: Keratite "inguérissable" et hyperkératose palmo-plantaire chronique avec hypertyrosinémie. *Arch. Fr. Pediatr.* 43:19, 1986.

Jakobs C, et al.: Prenatal diagnosis of tyrosinaemia type I by use of stable isotope dilution mass spectrometry. *Eur. J. Pediatr.* 144:209, 1985.

Kvittingen EA, et al.: Prenatal diagnosis of hereditary tyrosinaemia type I by determination of fumarylacetoacetase in chorionic villus material. *Eur. J. Pediatr.* 144:597, 1986.

Medes G: A new error of tyrosine metabolism: Tyrosinosis. The intermediary metabolism of tyrosine and phenylalanine. *Biochem. J.* 26:917, 1932.

Tuchman M, et al.: Contribution of extrahepatic tissues to biochemical abnormalities in hereditary tyrosinemia type I: Study of three patients after liver transplantation. *J. Pediatr.* 110:399, 1987.

V

VERNER-MORRISON SYNDROME

Synonyms: WDHA syndrome; pancreatic cholera; watery diarrhea-hypokalemia-achlorhydria syndrome.

Etiology: (a) *pancreatic non−beta islet cell tumor (vipoma)* or hyperplasia; other less common causes: bronchogenic carcinoma, pheochromocytoma, ganglioneuroblastoma, etc.

Clinical Manifestations: (a) *watery diarrhea* (tea-colored watery stool); (b) *hypokalemia;* (c) gastric hypochlorhydria or achlorhydria; (d) *elevated levels of plasma vasoactive intestinal peptide (VIP);* (e) significant weight loss, dehydration, and electrolyte depletion; tetany due to hypomagnesemia.

Radiologic Manifestations: (a) mass with compression of the stomach and/or duodenum; (b) multiple air-fluid levels in the bowel; (c) arteriography: *hypervascular mass with hypertrophied feeding vessels, persistent dense capillary stain;* (d) *computed tomography: pancreatic tumor demonstrable in about one third of WDHA cases;* (e) endoscopic retrograde cholangiopancreatography (ERCP) study showing pancreatic duct distortion by the mass.

Differential Diagnosis: (a) secretory diarrhea: cholera, malignant carcinoid, medullary thyroid carcinoma, systemic mastocytosis, bronchogenic carcinoma, and neural crest tumors; (b) VIP is the major hormone in the pathogenesis of the symptoms, but other polypeptides are also secreted by pancreatic mixed tumors in association with pancreatic cholera.

Notes: (a) WDHA: Watery Diarrhea, Hypokalemia, Achlorhydria; (b) VIP: it was originally isolated from porcine gut and was given this name because it produced systemic vasodilatation in dogs; (c) many patients exhibit hypochlorhydria rather than achlorhydria.

REFERENCES

Brenner RW, et al.: Resection of a vipoma of the pancreas in a 15-year-old girl. *J. Pediatr. Surg.* 21:983, 1986.
deWin von JLM, et al: Radiodiagnostik des Glukagonom und Vipom, zwei seltenen endokrinen Pankreastumoren. *Fortschr. Rontgenstr.* 140:537, 1984.
Dodds WJ, et al.: MEN I syndrome and islet cell lesions of the pancreas. *Semin. Roentgenol.* 20:17, 1985.
Dunnick NR, et al.: Computed tomographic detection of nonbeta pancreatic islet cell tumors. *Radiology* 135:117, 1980.
Dupont C: Les vipomes. *Ann. Med. Interne (Paris)* 135:400, 1984.
Gilbard JP, et al.: Increased tear secretion in pancreatic cholera: A newly recognized symptom in an experiment of nature. *Am. J. Med.* 85:552, 1988.
Gold RP, et al.: Radiologic and pathologic characteristics of the WDHA syndrome. *A.J.R.* 127:397, 1976.
Inamato K, et al.: Angiographic diagnosis of a pancreatic islet tumor in a patient with the WDHA syndrome. *Gastrointest. Radiol.* 5:259, 1980.
Kane MG, et al.: Production of secretory diarrhea by intravenous infusion of vasoactive intestinal polypeptide. *N. Engl. J. Med.* 309:1482, 1983.
Kudo K, et al.: WDHA syndrome caused by VIP-producing ganglioneuroblastoma. *J. Pediatr. Surg.* 17:426, 1982.
Maton PN, et al.: Effect of a long-acting somatostatin analogue (SMS 201-995) in a patient with pancreatic cholera. *N. Engl. J. Med.* 321:17, 1985.
Verner JV, Morrison AB: Islet cell tumor and a syndrome of refractory watery diarrhea and hypokalemia. *Am. J. Med.* 25:374, 1958.
Wall BM, et al.: Chloride-resistant metabolic alkalosis in an adult with congenital chloride diarrhea. *Am. J. Med.* 85:570, 1988.

VITAMIN A DEFICIENCY

Clinical and Radiological Manifestations: (a) growth retardation; (b) anemia; (c) recurrent infections; (d) increased intracranial pressure: bulging fontanelles, widening of sutures.

Note: Many preterm infants are deficient in vitamin A at birth. It has been suggested that the failure to correct this deficiency may contribute to the development of chronic lung disease.

REFERENCES

Abernathy RS: Bulging fontanelle as presenting sign in cystic fibrosis: Vitamin A metabolism and effect on cerebrospinal fluid pressure. *Am. J. Dis. Child.* 130:1360, 1976.
Hustead VA, et al.: Relationship of vitamin A (retinol) status to lung disease in preterm infant. *J. Pediatr.* 105:610, 1984.
Wolf IJ: Vitamin A deficiency in an infant. *J.A.M.A.* 166:1859, 1958.

VITAMIN A INTOXICATION

Etiology: (a) acute poisoning due to a large single dose of 300,000 to 1,000,000 IU, ingestion of polar bear liver or shark liver; (b) chronic poisoning due to intake of 100,000 IU or more per day for 6 months or longer, daily ingestion of

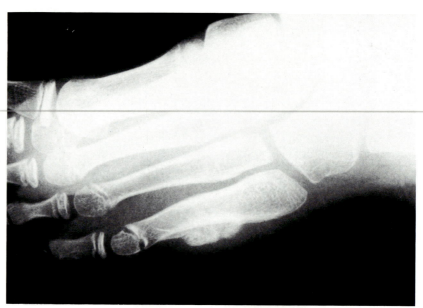

FIG ME–V–1.
Vitamin A intoxication in an 11-year-old male with a very high oral intake of vitamins A and D, hypercalcemia, and a painful foot. There is marked subperiosteal new bone formation.

chicken liver in infancy, long-term paranteral hyperalimentation.

Clinical Manifestations:

(A) ACUTE HYPERVITAMINOSIS A: *Insomnia or irresistible desire to sleep, drowsiness, sluggishness, irritability, headaches, vomiting, peeling of skin, increased intracranial pressure, acute hydrocephalus.*

(B) CHRONIC HYPERVITAMINOSIS A: (a) fetal: malformations of the central nervous system with exposure in early pregnancy; (b) early infancy: *anorexia, hyperirritability, tenderness and swelling of the scalp, bulging fontanelles,* craniotabes; (c) children: *anorexia, hyperesthesia, irritability,* impaired attention span, emotional instability, focal motor seizures, electroencephalographic abnormalities, pseudotumor cerebri, hepatosplenomegaly, *limb pain and swelling, loss of hair, pruritus, rhagades;* (d) adolescents and adults: *skin dryness, maculopapular rash, fissures, desquamation, pigmentation, pruritus, loss of hair, brittle nails, yellow discoloration of the skin, gingivitis, generalized weakness, fatigue, pain in bones and joints, tenderness of limbs, anorexia, headaches, muscle stiffness,* papilledema, diplopia, psychiatric symptoms, insomnia, somnolence, exophthalmos, hepatomegaly, liver cirrhosis, splenomegaly, absent or decreased menorrhea, weight loss, polyuria, polydipsia, edema of the lower limbs, epistaxis, lymphadenopathy, hypercalcemia.

Radiologic Manifestations: (a) early infancy: thinness and poor mineralization of the skull; relative hyperostosis of the sutural margins; hydrocephalus; *osteopenia;* cup-shaped, sharply demarcated, and widened metaphyses; (b) children: *widening of cranial sutures,* hyperostosis of the occipital and temporal bones, normal-appearing or enlarged cerebral ventricles and subarachnoid space, thickening of the mandible, *cortical hyperostosis of the tubular bones,* pleural effusion, ascites, increase in uptake of ^{99m}Tc-pyrophosphate in the diaphyses of long bones (present before the appearance of ra-

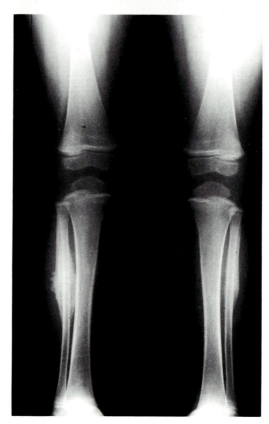

FIG ME–V–2.
Vitamin A intoxication in a 4½-year-old boy with intestinal pseudo-obstruction who had been maintained by parenteral hyperalimentation for 1 year. Classic signs of hypervitaminosis A developed. Serum vitamin A levels were five times normal. Radiograms of the legs show periosteal new bone formation about the proximal portion of both fibulas. (From Seibert JJ, Byrn WJ, Golladay ES: Development of hypervitaminosis A in a patient on long-term parenteral hyperalimentation. *Pediatr. Radiol.* 10:173, 1981. Used by permission.)

diographic manifestations); (c) adolescents and adults: demineralization of the floor of the sella turcica simulating an intrasellar tumor, with return to normal after discontinuation of vitamin A ingestion; wavy and laminated periosteal calcification of the tubular bones; skeletal hyperostoses.

Differential Diagnosis: Osteomyelitis; traumatic periosteal reaction; bone neoplasm; idiopathic skeletal hyperostosis; leukemia; hypertrophic osteoarthropathy; etc.

Note: Variable tolerance has been reported in siblings (Figs ME−V−1 and ME−V−2).

REFERENCES

Baxi SC, et al.: Hypervitaminosis A. A cause of hypercalcemia. *West. J. Med.* 137:429, 1982.

Caffey J: Chronic poisoning due to excess of vitamin A. *A.J.R.* 65:12, 1951.

Carpenter TO, et al.: Severe hypervitaminosis A in siblings: Evidence of variable tolerance to retinol intake. *J. Pediatr.* 111:507, 1987.

Gamble JG, et al.: Hypervitaminosis A in a child from megadosing. *J. Pediatr. Orthop.* 5:219, 1985.

James MB, et al.: Hypervitaminosis A: A case report. *Pediatrics* 69:112, 1982.

Josephs HW: Hypervitaminosis A and carotenemia. *Am. J. Dis. Child.* 67:33, 1944.

Mahoney CP, et al.: Chronic vitamin A intoxication in infants fed chicken liver. *Pediatrics* 65:893, 1980.

Miller JH, et al.: Bone scintigraphy in hypervitaminosis A. *A.J.R.* 144:767, 1985.

Muenter MD, et al.: Chronic vitamin A intoxication in adults: Hepatic, neurologic and dermatologic complications. *Am. J. Med.* 50:129, 1971.

Pennes DR, et al.: Early skeletal hyperostoses secondary to 13-*cis*-retinoic acid. *A.J.R.* 141:979, 1984.

Rosenberg HK, et al.: Pleural effusion and ascites. Unusual presenting features in a pediatric patient with vitamin A intoxication. *Clin. Pediatr. (Phila.)* 21:435, 1982.

Schurr D, et al.: Unusual presentation of Vitamin A intoxication. *J. Pediatr. Gastroenterol. Nutr.* 2:705, 1983.

Seibert JJ, et al.: Development of hypervitaminosis A in a patient on long-term parenteral hyperalimentation. *Pediatr. Radiol.* 10:173, 1981.

VITAMIN B₁ DEFICIENCY

Synonyms: Beriberi; thiamin deficiency.

Clinical and Radiological Manifestations: (a) generalized weakness, anorexia, failure to thrive; (b) tachycardia, arrhythmias, cardiomegaly, heart failure, increased QT interval, in-

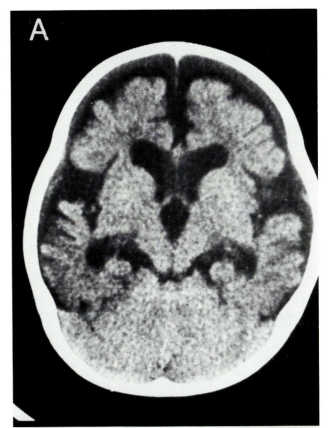

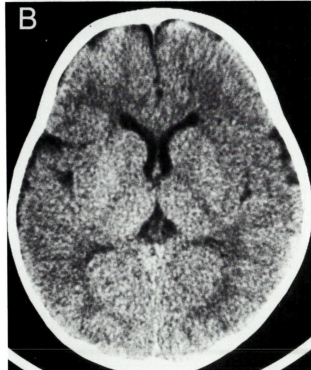

FIG ME−V−3.
Vitamin B₁₂ deficiency in a 1½-year-old male with psychomotor retardation, megaloblastic anemia, and a history of being exclusively breast-fed by his mother who had been a strict vegetarian for more than 4 years before the child was born. A CT scan shows severe brain atrophy before treatment with vitamin B₁₂ **(A)**. After 1 month of vitamin B₁₂ therapy the brain atrophy has improved dramatically **(B)**. (From Stollhoff K, Schulte FJ: Vitamin B₁₂ and brain development. *Eur. J. Pediatr.* 146:201, 1987. Used by permission.)

version of T waves, low voltage; (c) psychiatric disorders, laryngeal nerve paralysis, pain, burning feet, tenderness of the nerve trunks, ataxia, loss of coordination, loss of deep sensation, optic nerve atrophy, increased intracranial pressure, meningism, coma; (d) elevated levels of blood pyruvic acid and lactic acid, low levels of red cell transketolase and high blood and urinary levels of glyoxylate (Fig ME–V–3).

Notes: (a) cardiovascular beriberi may have the following two forms of clinical presentations: (1) predominantly right-sided heart failure associated with a high cardiac output failure (due to peripheral vasodilatation); (2) Shoshin beriberi or acute pernicious beriberi: cardiovascular collapse; (b) thiamine-responsive anemia syndrome: anemia in association with diabetes mellitus and sensorineural deafness; (c) a case of severe iatrogenic infantile beriberi in which the clinical, radiological (computed tomography [CT]), and biochemical findings were indistinguishable from those of Leigh disease has been reported.

REFERENCES

Attas M: Fulminant beriberi heart disease with lactic acidosis: Presentation of a case with evaluation of left ventricular function and review of pathophysiologic mechanisms. *Circulation* 58:566, 1978.

Delorme N, et al.: Shoshin béribéri avec hyponatrémie chez un buveur de bière. *Presse Med.* 15:2005, 1986.

Engbers JG, et al.: Shoshin beriberi: A rare diagnostic problem. *Br. Heart J.* 51:581, 1984.

Mandel H, et al.: Thiamine-dependent beriberi in the "thiamine-responsive anemia syndrome". *N. Engl. J. Med.* 311:836, 1984.

Moran JR, et al.: The B vitamins and vitamin C in human nutrition. *Am. J. Dis. Child.* 133:192, 1979.

Wyatt DT, et al.: Infantile beriberi presenting as subacute necrotizing encephalomyelopathy. *J. Pediatr.* 110:888, 1987.

VITAMIN B₁₂ (COBALAMIN) DEFICIENCY

Etiology: Strictly vegetarian diet; breast-fed infants with the mother on strictly vegetarian diet (Vegan); malabsorption of B_{12} vitamin.

Clinical manifestatons: (a) *progressive neurological disorder clinically resembling leukodystrophy;* (b) *megaloblastic anemia;* (c) diminished plasma level of vitamin B_{12}; (d) dramatic improvement of clinical manifestations with vitamin B_{12} therapy.

Radiologic Manifestations: CT: "brain atrophy" in infancy with improvement during B_{12} therapy (Fig ME–V–3).

REFERENCES

Ashkenazi S, et al.: Vitamin B_{12} deficiency due to a strictly vegetarian diet in adolescence. *Clin. Pediatr.* 26:662, 1987.

Sadowitz PD, et al.: Developmental regression as an early manifestation of vitamin B_{12} deficiency. *Clin. Pediatr.* 25:369, 1986.

Stollhoff K, et al.: Vitamin B_{12} and brain development. *Eur. J. Pediatr.* 146:201, 1987.

Cartlidge PHT, et al.: Specific malabsorption of vitamin B_{12} in Down's syndrome. *Arch. Dis. Child.* 61:514, 1986.

Carmel R: Pernicious anemia. The expected findings of very low serum cobalamine levels, anemia, and macrocytosis are often lacking. *Arch. Intern. Med.* 148:1712, 1988.

VITAMIN D INTOXICATION

Clinical Manifestations: (a) history of excessive intake of vitamin D over a period of a few days to several years; (b) loss of appetite, abdominal cramps, nausea, vomiting, polydipsia, polyuria, seizures, coma; (c) renal insufficiency, impaired ability to concentrate urine; (d) generalized calcinosis; (e) hypercalcemia, hypercalciuria, elevated blood urea nitrogen levels, elevated serum creatinine levels, abnormal urine sediment.

Radiologic Manifestations: (a) generalized calcinosis (falx, tentorium, kidneys, myocardium, lung, gastric wall, adrenal, parathyroid and thyroid glands, pancreas, skin, arteries, joints); (b) dense transverse metaphyseal bands, cortical thickening of tubular bones, bone sclerosis, dense vertebral end plates, thickening of the calvaria; osteoporosis in some adult patients.

Differential Diagnosis: (a) dense metaphyseal band: heavy-metal poisoning, etc; (b) soft-tissue calcification (see Gamut).

REFERENCES

Christensen WR, et al.: Skeletal and periarticular manifestations of hypervitaminosis D. *A.J.R.* 65:27, 1951.

Debré R, et al.: Action toxique de la vitamine D_2 administrée à dose trop forte chez l'enfant. *Ann. Med.* 50:417, 1949.

De Wind LT: Hypervitaminosis D with osteosclerosis. *Arch. Dis. Child.* 36:373, 1961.

Friedman WF: Vitamin D as a cause of the supravalvular aortic stenosis syndrome. *Am. Heart J.* 73:718, 1967.

Holman CB: Roentgenologic manifestations of vitamin D intoxication. *Radiology* 59:805, 1952.

Irnell L: Metastatic calcification of soft tissue on overdosage of vitamin D. *Acta Med. Scand.* 185:147, 1969.

Ross SG: Vitamin D intoxication in infancy. *J. Pediatr.* 41:815, 1952.

Schwartzman MS, et al.: Vitamin D toxicity complicating the treatment of senile, postmenopausal, and glucocorticoid-induced osteoporosis. Four case reports and a critical commentary on the use of vitamin D in these disorders. *Am. J. Med.* 82:224, 1987.

Seelig MS: Vitamin D and cardiovascular, renal and brain damage in infancy and childhood. *Ann. N.Y. Acad. Sci.* 147:539, 1969.

Swoboda W: Die Roentgensymptomatik der Vitamin-

D-Intoxikation im Kindesalter. *Fortschr. Roentgenstr.* 77:534, 1952.

VON WILLEBRAND DISEASE

Mode of Inheritance: Autosomal dominant.

Frequency: 1:10,000 (classic, autosomal dominantly inherited, Kühsel et al.).

Clinical and Radiologic Manifestations: (a) *hemorrhagic disorder:* visceral bleeding (post-traumatic, postsurgical), external bleeding (easy bruising, epistaxis, gingival), rare occurrence of hemarthrosis, etc.; (b) *prolonged bleeding time,* reduced glass bead adherence, reduced factor VIII procoagulant activity (VIII:C), decreased ristocetin-induced platelet aggregation (VIII:RCOF), reduced factor VIII—related antigen (VIII:Ag); (c) high incidence of association with mitral valve prolapse (this has been questioned); (d) association with hereditary hemorrhagic telangiectasia, gastrointestinal angiodysplasia; (e) acquired von Willebrand disease in association with angiodysplasia, hypothyroidism; (f) other reported abnormalities: throbocytopenia, platelet function defect, and an abnormal factor VIII molecule.

REFERENCES

Arkel YS, et al.: Von Willebrand's disease with thrombocytopenia, platelet function defect, and an abnormal factor VIII molecule. *Am. J. Pediatr. Hematol. Oncol.* 4:249, 1982.

Bush RW, et al.: Von Willebrand's disease and severe gastrointestinal bleeding. Report of a kindred. *West J. Med.* 140:781, 1984.

Dalton RG, et al.: Hypothyroidism as a cause of acquired von Willebrand's disease. *Lancet* 1:1007, 1987.

Kühsel LC, et al.: An investigation into the frequency of mitral valve prolapse in von Willebrand disease. *Clin. Genet.* 24:128, 1983.

Pickering NJ, et al.: Von Willebrand syndromes and mitral-valve prolapse: Linked mesenchymal dysplasias. *N. Engl. J. Med.* 305:131, 1981.

Sitbon N: La maladie de Willebrand. *Nouv. Presse Med.* 10:2161, 1981.

Smith SR, et al.: Hypothyroidism and von Willebrand's disease. *Lancet* 1:1314, 1987.

W

WILSON DISEASE

Synonym: Hepatolenticular degeneration.

Mode of Inheritance: Autosomal recessive, genetic expression at a locus on chromosome 13.

Pathophysiology: A disorder of copper metabolism with impairment of the ability of the liver to handle copper and excrete it in the bile, resulting in the excessive accumulation of copper in various organs (central nervous system, kidneys, liver, cornea, etc.); a low serum ceruloplasmin level, and an increased rate of urinary copper excretion.

Clinical Manifestations: Onset in childhood: (a) *neurological symptoms*: lethargy, abdominal pain, malaise, poor coordination, tremor, psychological disorders, drooling, dysphagia, dysarthria, masked face, disturbed locomotion, dystonia and hypertonia, choreoathetosis, blurred vision, headache, seizures, coma; (b) *Kayser-Fleischer ring at the limbus of the cornea*; (c) jaundice, hepatomegaly, liver cirrhosis, splenomegaly; (d) renal dysfunctions: renal tubular acidosis (proximal and distal tubular dysfunctions), decreased renal plasma flow, decreased glomerular filtration rate, aminoaciduria; (e) *cupriuria, elevated "free" copper and deficiency of ceruloplasmin, spectrometric demonstration of high corneal copper content*; (f) subclinical dysfunction in major sensory pathways: somatosensory, brain stem auditory and pattern-reversal visual evoked potentials; (g) other reported abnormalities: hyperpigmentation of the legs, bleeding tendency, edema, arthralgias, ascites, fever, pancreatitis, "uncombable hair syndrome," persistent hypertransaminasemia, hemolytic anemia (which may be the presenting manifestation in response to the ingestion of food with a high copper content), electrocardiographic abnormalities (left ventricular hypertrophy, biventricular hypertrophy, early repolarization, ST depression and T inversion, premature atrial or ventricular contractions, atrial fibrillation, sinoatrial block, Mobitz type 1 atrioventricular block, and tremor artifact), orthostatic hypotension, cardiac death, etc.

Radiologic Manifestations: (a) osteoporosis, osteomalacia, or rickets; (b) arthropathy, osteochondritis dissecans, subarticular cysts, para-articular calcific deposits, chondrocalcinosis, irregularity of vertebral body contour, "squaring" of vertebral bodies, Schmorl nodes, wedge-shaped vertebral bodies, juvenile kyphosis, disk space narrowing; (c) spontaneous fractures; (d) skeletal maturation retardation; (e) portal hypertension, increased computed tomographic (CT) density of the liver (case report), splenomegaly, pancreatic distortion due to splenomegaly; (f) renal stones; (g) cholelithiasis; (h)

CT: low attenuation in the basal ganglia (reversible under treatment); cavitation of the basal ganglia; selective dilatation of the frontal horn secondary to atrophic changes in the caudate and anterior lenticular nuclei; red nucleus, dentate nucleus, brain stem, and frontal cortex occasionally involved; (i) magnetic resonance imaging: increased signal in the brain stem and in the lenticular, thalamic, caudate, and dentate nuclei; (j) positron-emission tomography (PET): diffusely reduced glucose metabolism.

REFERENCES

Aisen AM, et al.: Wilson disease of the brain: MR imaging. *Radiology* 157:137, 1985.

Betend B, et al.: Les 13 desserts de Noël. Révélation inattendue d'une maladie de Wilson. *Arch. Fr. Pediatr.* 40:101, 1983.

Chen XR, et al.: Computed tomography in hepatolenticular degeneration (Wilson's disease). *Comput. Radiol.* 7:361, 1983.

Chu NS: Sensory evoked potentials in Wilson's disease. *Brain* 109:491, 1986.

Dixon AK, et al.: Computed tomography of the liver in Wilson Disease. *J. Comput. Assist. Tomogr.* 8:46, 1984.

Dixon AK, et al.: Pancreatic distortion due to splenomegaly in Wilson's disease. *Lancet* 2:47, 1983.

Gonin J, et al.: Association d'un syndrome des cheveux incoiffables et d'une maladie de Wilson. *Ann. Pediatr. (Paris)* 31:311, 1984.

Hawkins RA, et al.: Wilson's disease studied with FDG and positron emission tomography. *Neurology* 37:1707, 1987.

Heckmann J, et al.: Abnormal copper metabolism: Another "non-Wilson's" case. *Neurology* 38:1493, 1988.

Kuan P: Cardiac Wilson's disease. *Chest* 91:579, 1987.

Lingam S, et al.: Neurological abnormalities in Wilson's disease are reversible. *Neuropediatrics* 18:11, 1987.

Mayer DP, et al.: Asymptomatic carrier state in Wilson disease. *J. Comput. Assist. Tomogr.* 7:146, 1983.

Odievre M, et al.: Hypertransaminasémie persistante révélatrice d'une maladie de Wilson. A propos de trois observations. *Ann. Pediatr. (Paris)* 31:43, 1984.

Rosenfield N, et al.: Cholelithiasis and Wilson disease. *J. Pediatr.* 92:210, 1978.

Rubinstein SS, et al.: Clinical assessment of 31 patients with Wilson's disease. Correlations with structural changes on magnetic resonance imaging. *Arch. Neurol.* 44:365, 1987.

Saito T: Presenting symptoms and natural history of Wilson disease. *Eur. J. Pediatr.* 146:261, 1987.

Selekler K, et al.: Computed tomography in Wilson's disease. *Arch. Neurol.* 38:727, 1981.

Slovis TL, et al.: Varied manifestations of Wilson's disease. *J. Pediatr.* 78:578, 1971.

Weizman Z, et al.: Wilson's disease associated with pancreatitis. *J. Pediatr. Gastroenterol. Nutr.* 7:931, 1988.

Wiebers DO, et al.: Renal stones in Wilson's disease. *Am. J. Med.* 67:249, 1979.

Wilson SAK: Progressive lenticular degeneration: A familial nervous disease associated with cirrhosis of the liver. *Brain* 34:295, 1911–12.

Xie Yu-zhang (Hsieh Yu-chang), et al.: Radiologic study of 42 cases of Wilson disease. *Skeletal Radiol.* 13:114, 1985.

Yuzbasiyan-Gurkan V, et al.: Linkage of the Wilson disease gene to chromosome 13 in North-American pedigrees. *Am. J. Hum. Genet.* 42:825, 1988.

WINCHESTER SYNDROME

Mode of Inheritance: Autosomal recessive.

Clinical Manifestations: (a) short stature; (b) polyarthralgia, progressive joint deformities, flexion contractures of small and large joints; (c) coarse facial features; (d) skin thickening, hyperpigmentation, hypertrichosis, gum hypertrophy; (e) peripheral corneal opacities; (f) skin biopsy: fibroblastic hyperplasia, abnormal collagen bundles in the deep dermis, characteristic ultrastructural dilatation of mitochondria in fibroblasts (electron microscopy), excessive collagen turnover; (g) other reported abnormalities: intestinal lymphangiectasia and protein-losing enteropathy; excessive oligosaccharides in the urine (tentatively identified as a branched trisaccharide containing one fucose and two galactose units).

Radiological Manifestations: Extensive progressive skeletal disease: (a) *bone resorption, most marked in the carpals and metacarpal articular margin;* (b) osteoporosis; (c) thinning of long bones; (d) *resorption of the distal phalanges;* (e) subluxation of C_1 on C_2, kyphoscoliosis; (f) misshapen pelvis, destruction of the femoral heads; (g) expanded clavicle, wide and thin ribs; (h) delayed closure of the anterior fontanelle, widely open sutures and prominent frontal region, flat mandibular condyles, delayed tooth eruption; (i) other reported abnormalities: compression fracture of the vertebrae, protrusio acetabuli, ankylosis involving the small joints of the feet; radial and ulnar artery hypoplasia, hypervascularity in areas of apparent active bone resorption.

Differential Diagnosis: (a) coarse facial features and severe joint disease: Farber disease, Scheie syndrome; (b) bone and joint disease: juvenile rheumatoid arthritis (Fig ME–W–1).

REFERENCES

Bracq H, et al.: Ostéolyse progressive generalisée déformante. A propos d' une observation. *Chir. Pediatr.* 21:401, 1980.

Dunger DB, et al.: Two cases of Winchester syndrome: With increased urinary oligosaccharide excretion. *Eur. J. Pediatr.* 146:615, 1987.

Hollister DW, et al.: The Winchester syndrome: A nonlysosomal connective tissue disease. *J. Pediatr.* 84:701, 1974.

Stumpf DA, et al.: The Winchester syndrome and mucopolysaccharide metabolism. *J. Pediatr.* 86:646, 1975.

Winchester P, et al.: A new acid mucopolysaccharidosis with skeletal deformities simulating rheumatoid arthritis. *A.J.R.* 106:121, 1969.

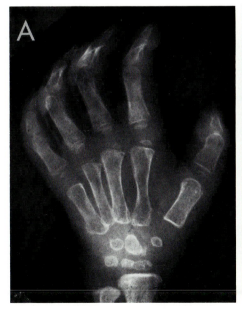 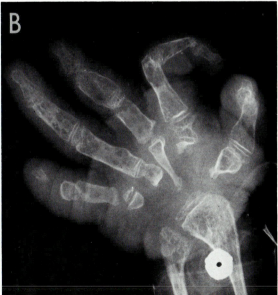

FIG ME–W–1.
Winchester syndrome. **A,** destruction of carpal ossification centers at 2½ years of age in one of two sisters with the syndrome. **B,** at 12 years of age, only small portions of metacarpals remain, and destruction of the phalanges of the fifth finger has occurred. (From Winchester P, Grossman H, Lim WN et al.: A new acid mucopolysaccharidosis with skeletal deformities simulating rheumatoid arthritis. *A.J.R.* 106:121, 1969. Used by permission.)

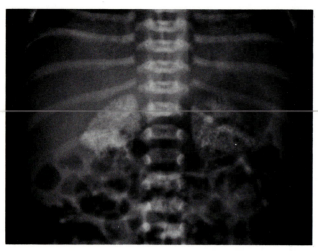

FIG ME–W–2.
Wolman disease in a 7½-month-old male with hepatosplenomegaly and regularly distributed calcification in the adrenal
glands. (From Queloz JM, Capitanio MA, Kirkpatrick JA: Wolman's
disease. *Radiology* 104:357, 1972. Used by permission.)

WOLMAN DISEASE

Synonyms: Lysosomal acid lipase deficiency; familial
xanthomatosis.

Mode of Inheritance: Autosomal recessive.

Frequency: Approximately 40 published cases (Foster et
al.).

Enzyme Deficiency: Lysosomal acid lipase (acid cholesteryl ester hydrolase).

Clinical Manifestations: Onset in early infancy: (a) failure to thrive; (b) diarrhea, steatorrhea; (c) protuberant abdomen; (d) hepatosplenomegaly; (e) anemia; (f) storage of cholesteryl esters and triglycerides in various tissues (liver,
spleen, intestine, kidneys, thymus, adrenal glands, blood
cells); (g) death in infancy.

Radiological Manifestations: (a) *punctate calcific foci
distributed throughout enlarged adrenal glands*, flattening of
the superior pole of the kidneys without displacement of the
kidneys or distortion of the pelvicaliceal system, marked
echodensity of the adrenals, cortical calcification and markedly enlarged adrenal glands (computed tomographic [CT]
examination); (b) *hepatosplenomegaly*, decreased attenuation
value (CT) of the liver, attenuation value that may be less
than that of the spleen; (c) paucity of subcutaneous fat; (d)
generalized osteoporosis; (e) multiple "growth lines" in
bones; (f) involution of the thymus.

Differential Diagnosis: Gaucher disease; Niemann-Pick
disease; multipolysaccharidoses; glycogen storage disease;
diseases associated with adrenal calcification ("physiological
neonatal involution", hemorrhage, neoplasma, granulomatous disease) (Figs ME–W–2 and ME–W–3).

Notes: (a) presumably Wolman disease is allelic to cholesteryl ester storage disease (CESD), with similar genetic and
enzymatic defects, but a distinctive clinical course and biochemical findings (enzyme activity reduced 200-fold in fibroblasts with Wolman disease as compared with 50- to 100-
fold in CESD cells; (b) Wolman disease with hypolipoproteinemia and acanthocytosis (Eto et al.): malabsorption of
lipid, growth failure, vomiting, and adrenal calcification.

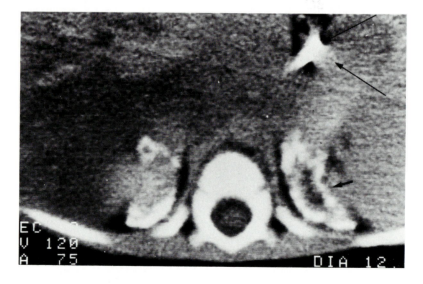

FIG ME–W–3.
Wolman disease. Abdominal CT of the adrenal level shows bilateral adrenal enlargement with distinctive cortical distribution of
calcifications *(short arrow)*. The liver and spleen are greatly enlarged, and there is diffuse fatty infiltration of the liver. A nasogas-
tric tube and a small amount of contrast is present in the stomach
(long arrows). (From Dutton RV: Wolman's disease. Ultrasound and
CT diagnosis. *Pediatr. Radiol.* 15:144, 1985. Used by permission.)

REFERENCES

Bretagne MC: La maladie de Wolman. *J. Radiol.* 62:197, 1981.

Dutton RV: Wolman's disease. Ultrasound and CT diagnosis. *Pediatr. Radiol.* 15:144, 1985.

Eto Y, et al.: Wolman's disease with hypolipoproteinemia and acanthocytosis: Clinical and biochemical observations. *J. Pediatr.* 77:862, 1970.

Foster D, et al.: Maladie de Wolman (cas radiologique du mois). *Arch. Fr. Pediatr.* 44:521, 1987.

Gross MS, et al.: Les lipases acides et les mutations responsables des maladies de Wolman et de surcharge a esters due cholestérol. *Ann. Genet. (Paris)* 26:10, 1983.

Harrison RB, et al.: Radiographic findings in Wolman's disease. *Radiology* 124:188, 1977.

Hill SC, et al.: CT findings in acid lipase deficiency: Wolman disease and cholesteryl ester storage disease. *J. Comput. Assist. Tomogr.* 7:815, 1983.

Kamalian N, et al.: Wolman disease with jaundice and subarachnoid hemorrhage. *Am. J. Dis. Child.* 126:671, 1973.

Neuhauser EBD, et al.: Wolman's disease: A new lipoidosis. *Ann. Radiol. (Paris)* 8:175, 1965.

Queloz JM, et al.: Wolman's disease. *Radiology* 104:357, 1972.

Schaub J, et al.: Wolman's disease: Clinical, biochemical and ultrastructural studies in an unusual case without striking adrenal calcification. *Eur. J. Pediatr.* 135:45, 1980.

Wolman M, et al.: Primary familial xanthomatosis with involvement and calcification of the adrenals. *Pediatrics* 28:742, 1961.

XANTHINURIA, HEREDITARY

Synonym: Xanthine oxidase deficiency.

Mode of Inheritance: Probably autosomal recessive.

Clinical Manifestations: (a) *deficiency of the enzyme xanthine-oxydase,* which catalyses the transformation of hypoxanthine to xanthine and xanthine to uric acid; enzyme deficiency demonstrable by evaluation of the liver or intestinal mucosa; (b) *xanthinuria;* hypouricemia; hypouric aciduria; increased urinary excretion of oxypurines, hypoxanthine, and xanthine; *xanthine stones;* (c) muscle cramp, myopathy, polyarthritis.

Radiologic Manifestations: *Nephrolithiasis.*

Notes: (a) the disease may present as the classic form (isolated xanthine oxidase deficiency) or a defect of a molybdenum-containing cofactor present in both xanthine oxidase and sulfite oxidase complexes; the second form is associated with severe neurological manifestations and early death in infancy; (b) a high incidence of the classic form in individuals of Lebanese extraction has been reported.

REFERENCES

Carpenter TO, et al.: Hereditary xanthinuria presenting in infancy with nephrolithiasis. *J. Pediatr.* 109:307, 1986.

Holmes EW, Wyngaarden JB: Hereditary xanthinuria, In Stanbury JB, et al. (eds.): *The Metabolic Basis of Inherited Disease,* ed 5. New York, McGraw-Hill International Book Co., 1983, p 1192–1201.

Maynard J, et al.: Hereditary xanthinuria in 2 Pakistani sisters: Asymptomatic in one with β-thalassemia but causing xanthine stone, obstructive uropathy and hypertension in the other. *J. Urol.* 139:338, 1988.

Ogier H, et al.: Double dèficit en sulfite et xanthine oxydase, cause d'encéphalopathie due à une anomalie héréditaire du métabolisme due molybdène. *Ann. Med. Interne (Paris)* 133:594, 1982.

ZELLWEGER SYNDROME

Synonym: Cerebrohepatorenal syndrome.

Mode of Inheritance: Autosomal recessive.

Frequency: More than 130 cases reported up to 1986; incidence of 1:25,000 to 1:100,000 newborns (Zellweger).

Pathology: (a) brain dysgenesis: microgyria, pachygyria, agenesis or hypoplasia of the corpus callosum, cerebral/cerebellar heterotopias, enlarged lateral ventricles, cerebellar hypoplasia, olivary hypoplasia, sudanophilic leukoencephalomyelopathy, gliosis, glycogen storage; (b) renal cortical microcysts, tubular ectasia, hydronephrosis; (c) cirrhosis, biliary dysgenesis, siderosis, absent peroxisomes, abnormal mitochondria, diminished smooth endoplasmic reticulum; (d) congenital heart disease: ventricular septal defect, patent ductus arteriosus; (e) other reported abnormalities: pancreatic islet cell hyperplasia, thymic hypoplasia.

Biochemical Abnormalities: absence of peroxisomes in hepatocytes and renal proximal tubule cells; marked deficiency of plasmalogens in the liver, kidney, brain, muscle, and heart; deficiency of peroxisomal enzyme dihydroxyacetone phosphate acyltransferase (DHAPAT); accumulation of very long chain fatty acids.

Laboratory Diagnostic Tests: (a) prenatal: demonstration of a deficiency of the enzyme DHAPAT in the amniotic fluid cells, absence of peroxisomes in cultured amniotic fluid cells; (b) postnatal: absence of peroxisome in the liver biopsy specimen, absence of DHAPAT activity, high levels of saturated very long chain fatty acids in cultured fibroblasts.

Clinical Manifestations: (a) *craniofacial dysmorphism*: macrocephaly, round flat face, high forehead, micrognathia, widely open suture and fontanelles, ocular hypertelorism, mongoloid slant of the orbital fissures, epicanthal folds, periorbital edema, external ear defect, high-arched palate; (b) *marked muscular hypotonia, decreased or absent reflexes, psychomotor retardation, seizures,* nystagmus, poor sucking, severe hearing impairment, marked abnormal neurophysiological study (electroencephalography, brain stem auditory evoked potentials, and somatosensory evoked potentials); (c) cataract, prominent Y-suture, glaucoma, corneal clouding, Brushfield spots, pigmentary retinopathy, optic nerve dysplasia/hypoplasia, blindness, extinguished electroretinogram; (d) *hepatomegaly,* proteinuria, hypoprothrombinemia, abnormal liver function values, elevated serum iron level and iron-binding capacity, hemosiderosis and iron deposition in macrophages of the bone marrow; (e) other reported abnormalities: jaundice of unusual degree and duration in newborn, congenital cardiovascular anomalies, camptodactyly, cubitus valgus, deep sacral dimple, hypospadias, cryptorchidism, hypertrophic pyloric stenosis, microdeletion of the proximal long arm of chromosome 7.

Radiologic Manifestations: (a) *chondral, articular, and periarticular soft-tissue calcifications,* especially in the patellae, acetabular regions, hyoid bone, and areas of the greater trochanters; (b) bell-shaped thorax; (c) limb anomalies: flexion deformities of the fingers, cubitus valgus, metatarsus adductus, talipes equinovarus, rocker-bottom feet, metatarsus varus; (d) retarded bone age; (e) dolichocephaly, wide-open sutures, large fontanelles, ventricular dilatation; (f) renal cortical cysts (computed tomography, ultrasonography) (Figs ME–Z–1 and ME–Z–2).

REFERENCES

Bartoletti S, et al.: The cerebro-hepato-renal (Zellweger's syndrome): Report of four cases. *Radiology* 127:741, 1978.

Bleeker-Wagemakers EM, et al.: Long term survival of a patient with cerebrohepato-renal (Zellweger) syndrome. *Clin. Genet.* 29:160, 1986.

Bowen P, Lee CSN, Zellweger H, et al.: A familial syndrome of multiple congenital defects. *Bull. Johns Hopkins Hosp.* 114:402, 1964.

Eyssen H, et al.: Bile acid abnormalities and the diagnosis of cerebro-hepato-renal syndrome (Zellweger Syndrome). *Acta Paediatr. Scand.* 74:539, 1985.

Goldfischer SL: More on Zellweger's syndrome, infantile Refsum's disease, and rhizomelic chondrodysplasia punctata. *N. Engl. J. Med.* 315:766, 1986.

Govaerts L, et al.: A neurophysiological study of children with the cerebro-hepato-renal syndrome of Zellweger. *Neuropediatrics* 16:185, 1985.

Govaerts L, et al.: Disturbed adrenocortical function in cerebro-hepato-renal syndrome of Zellweger. *Eur. J. Pediatr.* 143:10, 1984.

Hajra AK, et al.: Prenatal diagnosis of Zellweger cerebrohepatorenal syndrome. *N. Engl. J. Med.* 312:445, 1985.

Heymans HSA, et al.: Deficiency of plasmalogens in the cerebro-hepato-renal (Zellweger) syndrome. *Eur. J. Pediatr.* 142:10, 1984.

Kelley RI: The cerebrohepatorenal syndrome of Zellweger, morphologic and metabolic aspects. *Am. J. Med. Genet.* 16:503, 1983.

Luisiri A, et al.: Sonography of the Zellweger syndrome. *J. Ultrasound Med.* 7:169, 1988.

Moser AE, et al.: The cerebrohepatorenal (Zellweger) syndrome. Increased levels and impaired degradation of very-

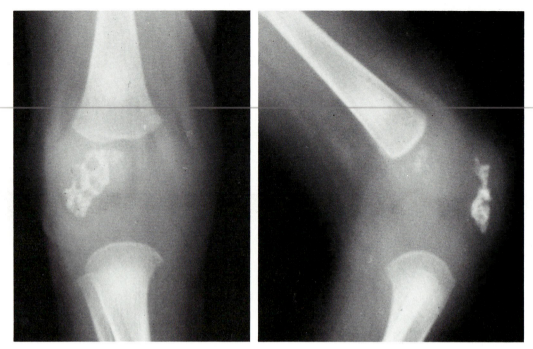

FIG ME–Z–1.
Zellweger syndrome in a 1-month-old female infant. Extensive irregular calcification of the patella is present. (From Poznanski AK, Nosan Chuk JS, Baublis J, et al.: The cerebro-hepato-renal syndrome (CHRS) (Zellweger's syndrome). *A.J.R.* 109:313, 1970. Used by permission.)

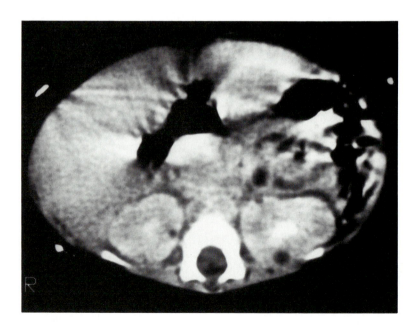

FIG ME–Z–2.
Zellweger syndrome: computer tomography of the kidneys with contrast. There are bilateral cortical cysts with additional cysts evident at other levels. (From Weese-Mayer DE, Smith KM, Reddy JK, Salafasky I, Poznanski AK: Computerized tomography and ultrasound in the diagnosis of cerebro-hepato-renal syndrome of Zellweger. *Pediatr. Radiol.* 17:170, 1987. Used by permission.)

low-chain fatty acids and their use in prenatal diagnosis. *N. Engl. J. Med.* 310:1141, 1984.

Naritomi K, et al.: Zellweger syndrome and a microdeletion of the proximal long arm of chromosome 7. *Hum. Genet.* 80:201, 1988.

Opitz JM: The Zellweger syndrome: Book review and bibliography. *Am. J. Med. Genet.* 22:419, 1985.

Poznanski AK, et al.: Cerebro-hepato-renal syndrome (CHRS) (Zellweger's syndrome). *A.J.R.* 109:313, 1970.

Schutgens RBH, et al.: Prenatal detection of Zellweger syndrome. *Lancet* 2:1339, 1984.

Suzuki Y, et al.: Zellweger-like syndrome with detectable hepatic peroxisomes: A variant form of peroxisomal disorder. *J. Pediatr.* 113:841, 1988.

Wanders RJA, et al.: A prenatal test for the cerebro-hepato-renal (Zellweger) syndrome by demonstration of the absence of catalase-containing particles (peroxisomes) in cultured amniotic fluid cells. *Eur. J. Pediatr.* 145:136, 1986.

Weese-Mayer DE, et al.: Computerized tomography and ultrasound in the diagnosis of cerebro-hepato-renal syndrome of Zellweger. *Pediatr. Radiol.* 17:170, 1987.

Zellweger H: The cerebro-hepato-renal (Zellweger) syndrome and other peroxisomal disorders. *Dev. Med. Child Neurol.* 29:821, 1987.

ZOLLINGER-ELLISON SYNDROME

Pathology: (a) *non—beta islet cell tumors of the pancreas* (adenocarcinoma, adenoma, or hyperplasia); (b) *peptic ulcer or ulcers;* (c) *ectopic gastrinoma.*

Clinical Manifestations: (a) *severe recurrent peptic ulcers;* (b) *watery diarrhea;* (c) *malabsorption syndrome;* (d) *gastric hypersecretion hyperchlorhydria;* (e) radioimmunoassay of circulating serum gastrin; (f) other associated abnormalities: endocrine abnormalities in about 30% of cases (pituitary tumor, hyperparathyroidism, insulinoma, multiple endocrine adenomatosis, duct adenocarcinoma of the pancreas, ovarian mucous cyst adenocarcinoma), osteoblastic bone metastasis, Cushing syndrome.

Radiologic Manifestations: (a) *peptic ulcer or ulcers of the stomach, duodenum, and jejunum in an atypical location; large mucosal folds of the stomach, duodenum, and jejunum; gastric hypersecretion; megaduodenum;* small-bowel edema; *increased intraluminal fluid; dilatation of the jejunum and ileum;* peptic esophagitis and esophageal ulceration; (b) ultrasonography of gastrinomas: homogeneous area of low echogenicity in the pancreas, tumor calcification; (c) computed tomography for localization and staging of islet cell tumors: calcification, tumor enhancement after contrast medium, hepatic metastases, secondary abnormalities (thickening of the gastric, duodenal, or jejunal wall; increased fluid in the duodenum or small bowel); (d) celiac arteriography: *tumor stain,* prominent gastric and intestinal venous opacification, transhepatic selective catheterization of the pancreatic veins for venous sampling and reliable localization of gastrin-secreting islet cell tumors; (e) other reported abnormalities: nephrocalcinosis, hypervascular liver metastases, bone metastases, Zollinger-Ellison syndrome as part of the

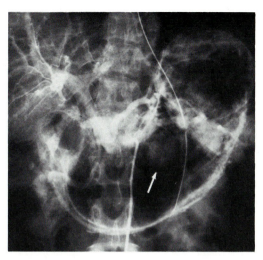

FIG ME—Z—3.
Zollinger-Ellison syndrome in a 29-year-old female. In the late arterial phase of selective angiography, a faint "blush" 2.5 cm in diameter is shown *(arrow)* at junction of the body and tail of the pancreas. This was the site of multiple pancreatic adenomas removed at surgery. Note the dense opacification of greater curvature in the region of the body of the stomach. (From Alfidi RJ, et al.: Arteriographic manifestations of the Zollinger-Ellison syndrome. *Cleve. Clin. Q.* 36:41, 1969. Used by permission.)

multiple endocrine neoplasm 1 (MEN-1) syndrome, kidney stones, esophageal involvement related to gastroesophageal reflux (esophagitis, stricture formation, Barrett esophagus).

Notes: (a) clinical manifestations suggestive of gastrinoma: peptic ulceration in unusual locations, multiple upper gastrointestinal ulcers, therapy-resistant ulcers, frequent and early recurrence of ulcers, postoperative recurrence of ulcers, familial history of duodenal ulcer disease, presence of basal hyperchlorhydria, diarrhea or steatorrhea of long duration, family history of endocrine tumors (pituitary, parathyroid, pancreas), symptoms related to hypercalcemia, enlarged gastric or duodenal folds associated with ulcer disease; (b) arteriography and computed tomography are complimentary examinations (Fig ME—Z—3).

REFERENCES

Agha FP: Esophageal involvement in Zollinger-Ellison syndrome. *A.J.R.* 144:721, 1985.

Alfidi RJ, et al.: Arteriographic manifestations of the Zollinger-Ellison syndrome. *Cleve. Clin. Q.* 36:41, 1969.

Bhagavan BS, et al.: Ectopic gastrinoma and Zillinger-Ellison syndrome. *Hum. Pathol.* 17:584, 1986.

Cocco AE, et al.: Zollinger-Ellison syndrome associated with ovarian mucinous cystadenocarcinoma. *N. Engl. J. Med.* 293:485, 1975.

Dodds WJ, et al.: MEN I syndrome and islet cell lesions of the pancreas. *Semin. Roentgenol.* 20:17, 1985.

Margolis RM, et al.: Zollinger-Ellison syndrome associated with pancreatic cystadenocarcinoma. *N. Engl. J. Med.* 311:1380, 1984.

Maton PN, et al.: Cushing's syndrome in patients with the Zollinger-Ellison syndrome. *N. Engl. J. Med.* 315:1, 1986.

Maton PN, et al.: Role of selective angiography in the management of patients with Zollinger-Ellison syndrome. *Gastroenterology* 92:913, 1987.

Mihas AA, et al.: Zollinger-Ellison syndrome associated with ductal adenocarcinoma of the pancreas. *N. Engl. J. Med.* 298:144, 1978.

Muhletaler CA: Radiology of the Zollinger-Ellison syndrome. *Rev. Interam. Radiol.* 7:87, 1982.

Nord KS, et al.: Zollinger-Ellison syndrome associated with a renal gastrinoma in a child. *J. Pediatr. Gastroenterol. Nutr.* 5:980, 1986.

Van den Abbeele AD, et al.: Bone metastases in Zollinger-Ellison syndrome demonstrated by scintigraphy. *Clin. Nucl. Med.* 12:954, 1987.

Wank SA, et al.: Prospective study of the ability of computed axial tomography to localize gastrinomas in patients with Zollinger Ellison syndrome. *Gastroenterology* 92:905, 1987.

Wolfe MM, et al.: Zollinger-Ellison syndrome. Current concepts in diagnosis and management. *N. Engl. J. Med.* 317:1200, 1987.

Zollinger RM: Islet cell tumors and the alimentary tract. *A.J.R.* 126:933, 1976.

Zollinger RM, Ellison EH: Primary peptic ulcerations of jejunum associated with islet cell tumors of pancreas. *Ann. Surg.* 142:709, 1955.

PART III

Skeletal Dysplasias
Ralph S. Lachman, M.D.

ACHONDROGENESIS TYPE I

Synonyms: Achondrogenesis type Parenti-Fraccaro, achondrogenesis type IA (Houston-Harris), achondrogenesis type IB (Fraccaro).

Frequency: Rare (46 cases reported to 1988; 0.23 per 10,000 live births).

Mode of Inheritance: Autosomal recessive.

Clinical Manifestations: (a) *marked micromelic dwarfism:* (b) *fetal hydrops;* (c) *barrel-shaped chest, distended abdomen, short neck and trunk;* (d) *lethal;* (e) *polyhydramnios;* (f) other reported abnormalities: patent ductus arteriosis, patent foramen ovale, undescended testes, inguinal hernia, blue sclera, urinary tract duplication and hydronephrosis, auditory canal atresia, cleft palate, corneal clouding, ear deformities, aplastic testes, anal atresia.

Radiologic Manifestations: (a) *poorly mineralized skull, multiple calvarial bone plaques;* (b) *absent or minimal ossification of vertebral bodies;* (c) *short and thin ribs with splayed ends, multiple fractures, beaded appearance;* (d) *deformed and short iliac wings, absent ossification of pubis and sacrum;* (e) *marked shortness, broadness, and bowing of tubular bones, concave ends of tubular bones associated with multiple lateral spurs, trapezoid, or wedged femurs;* (f) can be diagnosed in the second trimester by ultrasound (approximately eight cases to date) (Figs SK–A–1 and SK–A–2).

Chondro-osseous Morphology: (a) severe disturbance in endochondral ossification; (b) bulky epiphyseal cartilage; (c) *abundant cartilage matrix;* (d) *chondrocytes in enlarged lacunae (type IA);* (e) *ring around the chondrocytes (type IB).*

Differential Diagnosis, Significant: (a) Achondrogenesis type II; (b) hypochondrogenesis; (c) pycnoachondrogenesis (achondrogenesis I–like with *dense bones*). autosomal recessive (Camera, 1952).

Special Comments: Fraccaro's original case thought to actually represent achondrogenesis type II (Yang et al., 1975). More recently Rimoin's group has shown that Parenti's case is actually type II radiographically and histologically and that there are two distinct subgroups (Borochowitz et al.).

REFERENCES

Benacevraf B, et al.: Achondrogenesis type 1: Ultrasound diagnosis in utero. *J. Clin. Ultrasound* 12:357–359, 1984.

Bokesoy I, et al.: A case of achondrogenesis type 1. *Hum. Genet.* 67:349–350, 1984.

Borochowitz Z, et al.; Achondrogenesis type 1: Delineation of further heterogeneity and identification of two distinct sub-groups. *J. Pediatr.* 112:23–31, 1988.

Camera G: Pyknoachondrogenesis: An association of skeletal defects resembling achondrogenesis with generalized bone sclerosis. A new condition? *Clin. Genet.* 30:335–337, 1986.

Fraccaro M: Contributo allo studio dell malattie del mesenchima osteopoietico L'acondrogenesi. *Folia Hered. Pathol. (Milano)* 1:190, 1952.

Glenn LW, Teng SSK: In utero sonographic diagnosis of achondrogenesis. *J. Clin. Ultrasound* 13:195–198, 1985.

Golbus MS, et al.: Prenatal diagnosis of achondrogenesis. *J. Pediatr.* 91:464, 1977.

Graham D, et al.: Early second trimester sonographic diagnosis of achondrogenesis. *J. Clin. Ultrasound* 11:336–338, 1983.

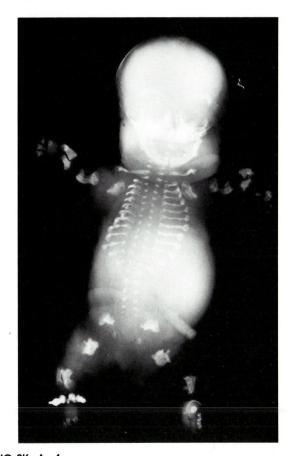

FIG SK–A–1.
Achondrogenesis type IA (Houston-Harris). Stillborn fetus. Note rib fractures, arched iliac wings, ossified ischia.

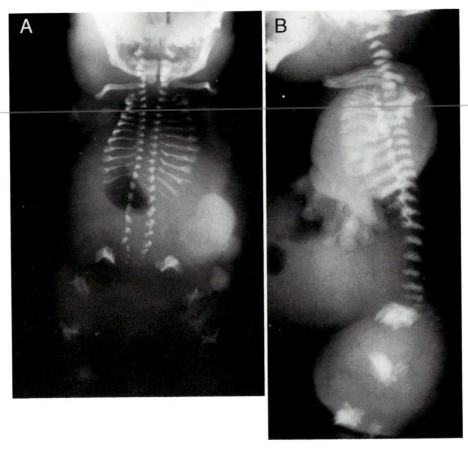

FIG SK–A–2.
Achondrogenesis type IB (Fraccaro). **A,** stillborn fetus. Note no rib fractures, crenated iliac wings, unossified ischium. **B,** stillborn fetus. No vertebral body ossification, very short ribs, trapezoid femurs.

Houston CS, et al.: Fatal neonatal dwarfism. *J. Can. Assoc. Radiol.* 23:45–61, 1972.

Molz G, et al.: Achondrogenesis type I: Light and electron microscopic studies. *Eur. J. Pediatr.* 134:69, 1980.

Schulte MJ, et al.: Letale Achondrogenesis: Eine Übersicht über 56 Fälle. *Klin. Paediatr.* 191:327, 1978.

Smith WL, et al.: In utero diagnosis of achondrogenesis, type I. *Clin. Genet.* 19:51, 1981.

Whitley CB, Gorlin RJ: Achondrogenesis: New nosology with evidence of genetic heterogeneity. *Radiology* 148:693–698, 1983.

Yang SS, et al.: Proposed readjustment of eponyms for achondrogenesis, (letter to the editor). *J. Pediatr.* 87:333–334, 1975.

Yang S-S, et al.: Two types of heritable lethal achondrogenesis. *J. Pediatr.* 85:796, 1974.

ACHONDROGENESIS TYPE II

Synonyms: Achondrogenesis type Langer-Saldino; achondrogenesis types III and IV; thanatophoric dysplasia type II.

Frequency: Uncommon (0.2 per 100,000 births).

Mode of Inheritance: Autosomal recessive.

Clinical Manifestations: (a) *marked micromelic dwarfism;* (b) fetal hydrops; (c) *distended abdomen, barrel-shaped thorax;* (d) *short trunk;* (e) enlarged cranium in some; (f) often lethal; (g) cleft palate.

Radiologic Manifestations: (a) *lack of mineralization of all or many vertebral bodies;* (b) *nonossified sacrum, ischium, pubis, talus and calcaneus;* (c) *marked shortness of long bones and tubular bones of hands and feet;* (d) concave metaphyses; (e) enlarged calvaria with *normal ossification;* (f) *small iliac wings with concave inferior and medial margins;* (g) *variable shortening of ribs;* (h) can be diagnosed in the second trimester by ultrasound (Fig SK–A–3).

Chondro-osseous Morphology and Biochemistry: (a) *increased vascularity in reserve and proliferative zones;* (b) enlarged lucanae with normal sized cells; (c) irregular columns, abnormal trabeculae with bone spurs; (d) *reduced cartilage matrix* (e) electron microscopy: dilated rough endoplasmic reticulum and decreased glycogen; (f) molecular defect of type II collagen.

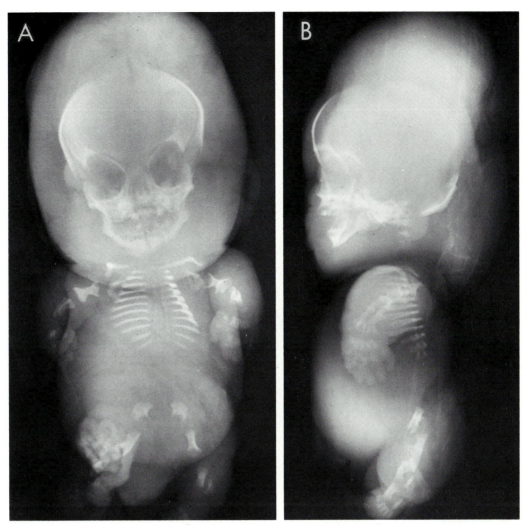

FIG SK–A–3.
Achondrogenesis type II. Anteroposterior **(A)** and lateral **(B)** radiographs of stillborn infant with achondrogenesis showing edematous soft tissue, especially around the head. The "detached" or "floating" appearance of the skull is the result of virtually total absence of ossification throughout the vertebral column. The skull is well mineralized, and the clavicles are of normal length. Note that in the lateral view the arm does not reach beyond the chest, a finding that exemplifies extreme micromelia. There is also outward bowing of the distal ends of the femora. (From Saldino RM: Radiographic diagnosis of neonatal short-limbed dwarfism. *Med. Radiogr. Photogr.* [Kodak] 49:61, 1973. Reproduced with permission.)

Differential Diagnosis, Significant: (a) achondrogenesis type 1; (b) hypochondrogenesis; (c) spondyloepiphyseal dysplasia congenita.

Special Comments: It appears that achondrogenesis type II and hypochondrogenesis represents a spectrum with marked phenotypic variability on radiographic and morphologic grounds (Borochowitz et al.).

REFERENCES

Anderson PE, Jr: Achondrogenesis type II in twins. *Br. J. Radiol.* 54:61, 1981.

Borochowitz Z, et al.: Achondrogenesis II—hypochondrogenesis: Variability vs. heterogeneity. *Am. J. Med. Genet.* 24:273–288, 1986.

Chen H, et al.: Achondrogenesis: A review with special consideration of achondrogenesis type II (Langer-Saldino). *Am. J. Med. Genet.* 10:379–394, 1981.

Dorfman HD, et al.: Case report 122: Lethal short-limbed dwarfism: Achondrogenesis type 2 (Fraccaro-Langer-Saldino). *Skel. Radiol.* 5:189, 1980.

Eyre DR, et al.: Nonexpression of cartilage type II collagen in a case of Langer-Saldino achondrogenesis. *Am. J. Hum. Genet.* 39:52–67, 1986.

Mahoney BS, et al.: Antenatal sonographic diagnosis of achondrogenesis. *J. Ultrasound Med.* 3:333–335, 1984.

Saldino RM: Lethal short-limbed dwarfism: Achondrogenesis and thanatophoric dwarfism. *Am. J. Roentgenol.* 112:185, 1971.

Whitley CB, Gorlin RJ: Achondrogenesis: New nosology
with evidence of genetic heterogeneity. *Radiology*
148:693–698, 1983.
Yang SS, et al.: Two types of heritable lethal achondrogenesis. *J. Pediatr.* 85:796, 1974.
Yang SS, et al: Proposed readjustment of eponyms for
achondrogenesis (letter to the editor). *J. Pediatr.* 87:333,
1975.

ACHONDROPLASIA

Synonyms: Chondrodystrophia fetalis.

Mode of Inheritance: Autosomal dominant trait; spontaneous mutation in four of five cases; three rare familial cases
(Optiz; Dodinual).

Frequency: Most common nonlethal skeletal dysplasia
(approximately 1 per 26,000 live births).

Clinical Manifestations: (a) *short-limbed, short trunked
dwarfism* with relatively long trunk; (b) *large head with prominent forehead*, saddle nose; (c) gibbus in thoracolumbar region in infants; swayback with prominent buttocks in children and adults; (d) flat thorax; (e) bowed legs; (f) *trident
hands* with fingers of equal length; (g) robust individual with
normal mentality; (h) *neurologic complications; hydrocephalus* (infrequent, communicating), megaloencephaly; compression at various levels, spinal cord, and nerve roots (paresthesias, deep tendon reflex changes, intermittent neurogenic
claudication, progressive paraparesis and quadriparesis);
brain stem compression by tight foramen magnum (sleep apnea and sudden infant death) (Reid); (i) other reported abnormalities: conductive and/or sensorineural deafness, choanal
atresia, poor respiratory reserve, reduced zinc and increased
copper values in the hair in children with achondroplasia and

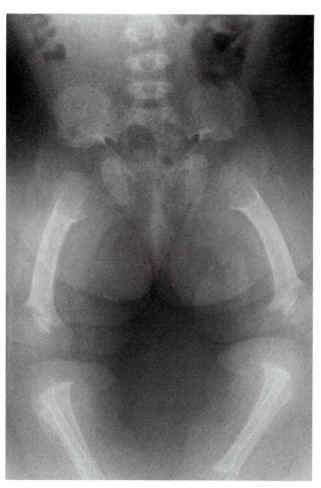

FIG SK–A–4.
Achondroplasia in a 3-month-old girl. Diminution in the interpediculate distance, squared-off iliac wings, narrow sciatic notches, flat
and irregular acetabular roofs, short thick tubular bones, V-shaped
notches in the growth plate regions, and flared metaphyses.

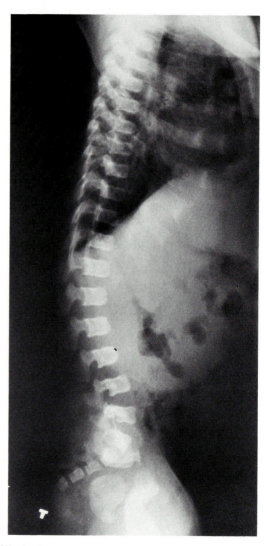

FIG SK–A–5.
Achondroplasia in a 5-month-old girl. Mild thoracolumbar kyphosis, posterior tilt of the sacrum, short pedicles, narrow spinal canal,
and concavities in the posterior borders of the lumbar vertebral
bodies.

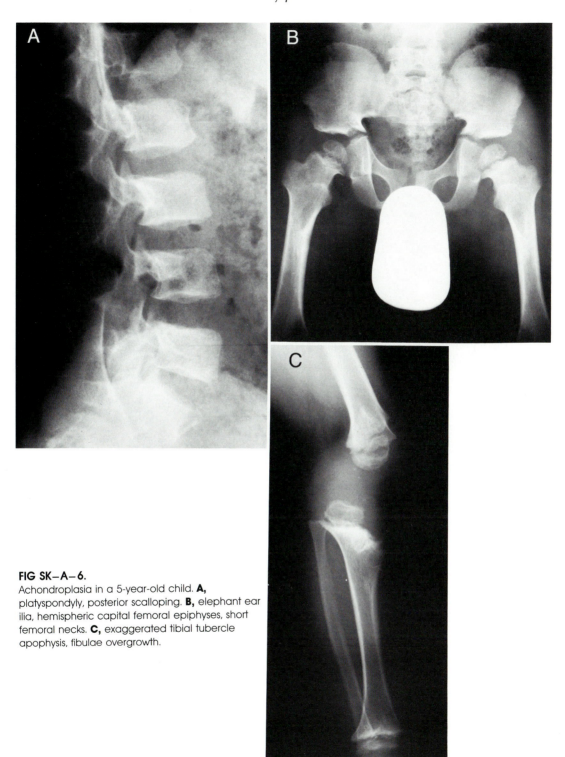

FIG SK–A–6.
Achondroplasia in a 5-year-old child. **A,** platyspondyly, posterior scalloping. **B,** elephant ear ilia, hemispheric capital femoral epiphyses, short femoral necks. **C,** exaggerated tibial tubercle apophysis, fibulae overgrowth.

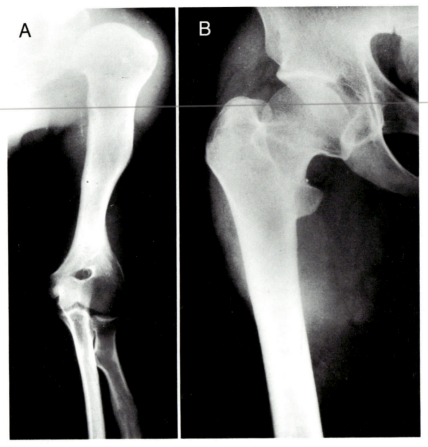

FIG SK—A—7.
Achondroplasia in an adult. **A,** rhizomelia, enlarged deltoid insertion area. **B,** short femoral neck, hemispheric femoral head, enlarged greater and lesser trochanters.

FIG SK—A—8.
Achondroplasia in a 2½-year-old child. CT scan shows moderate ventricular enlargement, prominent subarachnoid space.

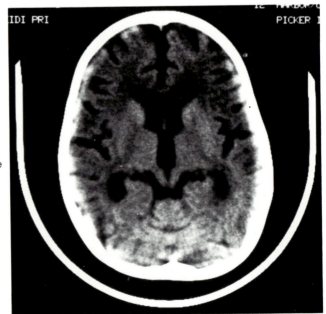

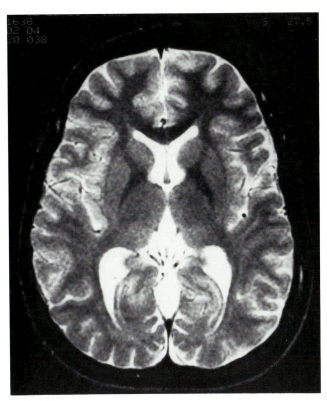

FIG SK–A–9.
Achondroplasia in a 17-year-old patient. MRI shows no significant ventricular dilitation.

in their parents; ankylosing spondylitis (Randolph); (j) complications: serious obesity (Hecht).

Radiologic Manifestations: (a) *large skull with relatively small base, narrow foramen magnum,* upward tilt of petrous pyramid, low position of mastoid process, small posterior fossa due to craniosynostosis at base of skull, small angle of base of skull (85 to 120 degrees compared with the normal 110 to 145 degrees), *megaloencephaly, dilatation of lateral ventricles,* communicating hydrocephalus (uncommon); CT, cochlea rotation (Cobb); MRI, brain stem evaluation: tight foramen (Wassman 1988); (b) *short flat vertebral bodies; bullet shaped (in early life); lack of normal increase in interpedicular distance from upper lumbar vertebrae caudally;* short pedicles with *narrow vertebral canal;* disk herniation, anterior wedging of one or more vertebral bodies, degenerative spondylosis and arthrosis; (c) champagne glass appearance of pelvis, *squared iliac wings (elephant ear), short narrow sciatic notch,* flat acetabular roof; (d) *micromelia, short and thick tubular bones,* notched growth plates (V-shaped), ball-in-a-socket epiphyseal-metaphyseal junctions, flared metaphyses, broad and relatively short metacarpals and phalanges; *fibular overgrowth* (e) thick stubby sternum, *short ribs* with deep concave rib ends; (f) ultrasound diagnosis can be made in the second trimester (Figs SK–A–4 to SK–A–11).

Therapeutic Modalities: Leg lengthening.

Chondro-osseous Morphology: (a) *regular, well-organized endochondral ossification;* (b) *short columns* with wide septae; suggests quantitative decrease in rate of endochondral ossification.

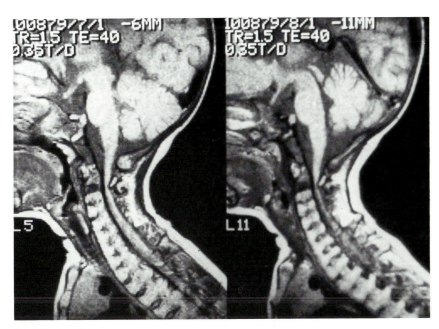

FIG SK–A–10.
Achondroplasia in an adult (21 years old). MRI shows significant hypoplasia of the cervical cord at C2, narrow foramen magnum.

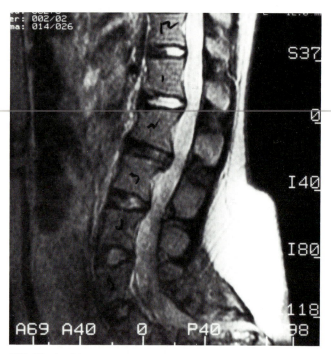

FIG SK—A—11.
Achondroplasia in a 17-year-old patient. MRI shows posterior scalloping of vertebral bodies with indentation by subarachnoid (dural) structures of lumbar spine, and severe lordosis.

Differential Diagnosis, Significant: Hypochondroplasia.

Special Comments: Achondroplasia was and is incorrectly overdiagnosed in many newborn infants with a skeletal dysplasia. The radiologic features of homozygous achondroplasia lie between those of heterozygous achondroplasia and thanatophoric dysplasia.

REFERENCES

Aldegheri R, et al.: Lengthening of the lower limbs in achondroplastic patients. *J. Bone Joint Surg. Br.* 70B:69–73, 1988.

Beighton P, et al.: Gibbal achondroplasia. *J. Bone Joint Surg. Br.* 63-B:328, 1981.

Blondeau, M. et al.: Compression de la moelle cervicale dans l' achondroplasie. *Sem. Hop. (Paris)* 60:771–775, 1984.

Caffey J: Achondroplasia of pelvis and lumbosacral spine: Some roentgenographic features. *Am. J. Roentgenol.* 80:449, 1958.

Cobb SR, et al.: CT of the temporal bone in achondroplasia. *AJNR* 9:1195–1199, 1988.

Depresseux JC, et al.: CSF scanning in achondroplastic children with cranial enlargement. *Dev. Med. Child Neurol.* 17:224, 1975.

Dodinual P, LeMarec B: Genetic counseling in unexpected familial recurrences of achondroplasia. *Am. J. Med. Genet.* 28:949–954, 1987.

Elejalde BR, et al.: Prenatal diagnosis in two pregnancies of an achondroplastic woman. *Am. J. Med. Genet.* 15:437–439, 1983.

Galanski M., et al.: Neurological complications and myelographic features of achondroplasia. *Neuroradiology* 17:59–63, 1978.

Ganal A, et al.: Leg lengthening in achondroplastic children. *Clin. Orthop.* 144:194, 1979.

Hecht JT, et al.: Obesity in achondroplasia. *Am. J. Med. Genet.* 31:597–602, 1988.

Hecht JT, et al.: Computerized tomography of the foramen magnum: Achondroplastic, values compared to normal standards. *Am. J. Med. Genet.* 20:355–360, 1985.

Kahanovitz N, et al.: The clinical spectrum of lumbar spine disease in achondroplasia. *Spine* 7:137–140, 1982.

Kaitila I, et al.: Achondroplastic dwarfism with generalized periosteal elevation in infancy. *Birth Defects* 11(6):356, 1975.

Katz J, Mayhew JF: Air embolism in the achondroplastic dwarf. *Anesthesiology* 63:205–207, 1985.

Kurtz AB. et al.: In utero analysis of heterozygous achondroplasia. *J. Ultrasound Med.* 5:137–140, 1986.

Langer LO, Jr, et al.: Achondroplasia. *Am. J. Roentgenol.* 100:12, 1967.

McArdle DQ, et al.: Brain tumor and achondroplasia: A case report and review of the literature. *Neurosurgery* 15:111–113, 1984.

Maynard JA, et al.: Histochemistry and ultrastructure of the growth plate in achondroplasia. *J. Bone Joint Surg. Am.* 63-A:969, 1981.

Morgan DF, Young RF: Spinal neurological complications of achondroplasia. *J. Neurosurg.* 52:463–472, 1980.

Nehme A-ME, et al.: Skeletal growth and development of the achondroplastic dwarf. *Clin. Orthop.* 116:8, 1976.

Oestreich AE: Choanal atresia with achondroplasia. *J. Pediatr.* 96:343, 1980.

Opitz JM: "Unstable premutation" in achondroplasia: Penetrance vs. phenotrance (editorial comment). *Am. J. Med. Genet.* 19:251–254, 1984.

Parrot J: Les malformations achondroplastiques. *Soc. Antrhop. Paris,* 1878.

Pauli RM, et al.: Homozygous achondroplasia with survival beyond infancy. *Am. J. Med. Genet.* 16:459–473, 1983.

Pauli RM, et al.: Apnea and sudden unexpected death in infants with achondroplasia. *J. Pediatr.* 104:342–348, 1984.

Randolph LM, et al.: Achondroplasia with ankylosing spondylitis. *Am. J. Med. Genet.* 31:117–121, 1988.

Reid CS, et al.: Cervicomedullary compression in young patients with achondroplasia. *J. Pediatr.* 110:522–530, 1987.

Rimoin DL: Endochondral ossification in achondroplastic dwarfism. *N. Engl. J. Med.* 283:728, 1970.

Rosenfeld RG, Hintz RL: Normal somatomedin and somatomedin receptors in achondroplastic dwarfism. *Horm. Metab. Res.* 12:76–79, 1980.

Silverman FN: Achondroplasia, in Kaufmann HJ (ed.): *Progress in Pediatric Radiology,* vol. 4. Basel, S. Karger, 1973, p. 94.

Stokes DC, et al.: Respiratory complications of achondroplasia. *J. Pediatr.* 102:534–541, 1983.

Wassman ER Jr, et al.: Achondroplasia and zinc deficiency. *J. Pediatr.* 97:503, 1980.

Wassman ER, Rimoin DL: Cervicomedullary compression with achondroplasia (letter). *J. Pediatr.* 113:411, 1988.

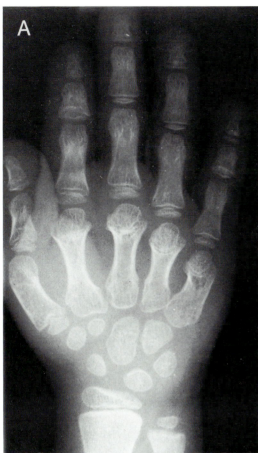
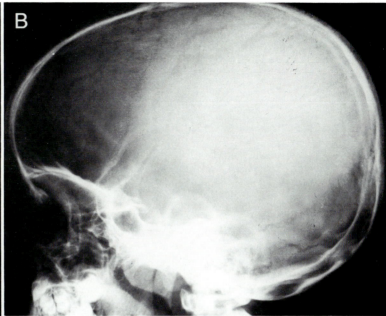

FIG SK–A–12.
Acrodysostosis in a 7-year-old child. **A,** cone epiphyses, brachydactyly (especially brachymetacarpia). **B,** normal cranium with midface hypoplasia.

Yamada H, et al.: Neurological manifestations of pediatric achondroplasia. *J. Neurosurg.* 54:49, 1981.

ACRODYSOSTOSIS

Synonyms: Peripheral dysostosis, PNM syndrome (peripheral dysostosis with pug nose and mental retardation), peripheral dysostosis (Brailsford).

Mode of Inheritance: Probably autosomal dominant (most cases nonfamilial, but older paternal age).

Frequency: Rare (about 40 cases to 1987; Frey).

Clinical Manifestations: (a) *growth failure;* (b) *short stature;* (c) *brachymelic dwarfism with shortening more marked in upper limbs;* (d) optic atrophy, strabismus, hypertelorism; *blue eyes* (Japanese); (e) *short and saddle nose;* (f) *hypogonadism;* (g) *psychomotor retardation,* seizures, choreoathetosis; pontine glioma (one case); (h) impaired hearing; (i) pigmented nevi; broad, very short, oval fingernails.

Radiologic Manifestations: (a) *brachycephaly, hypoplastic nasal bones, large mandibular angle and prognathism, thick calvaria,* delayed dental formation, internal hydrocephalus; CT, absence of nasal bones and nasal spine; (b) *peripheral dysostosis (short metacarpals, metatarsals, and phalanges, cone-shaped epiphyses,* premature skeletal maturation, in particular in the hands and feet), long bones less involved (thick and undertubulated); (c) other reported manifestations: irregularity of the end plates of thoracic and lumbar vertebrae; dorsal kyphosis; narrow interpedicular distances; small vertebrae; collapse of vertebrae; wide external auditory meatus; protrusio accetabuli (Fig SK–A–12).

Differential Diagnosis, Significant: (a) peripheral dysostosis without pug nose or mental retardation; (b) pseudohypoparathyroidism, pseudopseudohypoparathyroidism; (c) brachydactyly E; (d) acromesomelic dysplasia.

Special Comments: Pseudohypoparathyroidism, pseudopseudohypoparathyroidism, and brachydactyly type E (with or without type D) may all be variable expressions of the same trait.

REFERENCES

Frey VG, et al.: Die acrodysostose eine autosomal-dominant vererbte periphere dysplasia. *Kinderarztl. Prax.* 50:149–153, 1982.
Giedion A: Acrodysplasias. *Prog. Pediatr. Radiol.* 4:325–345, 1973.

Graudal N, et al.; Coexistent pseudohypoparathyroidism and D brachydactyly in a family. *Clin. Genet.* 30:449–455, 1986.

Joshi RM, et al.: Acrodysostosis syndrome. *Indian J. Pediatr.* 54:271–273, 1987.

MacNicol MF, Makris D: Acrodysostosis and protrusio acetabuli. *J. Bone Joint Surg. Br.* 70B:38–39, 1988.

Maroteaux P, Malmut G: L'acrodysostose. *Presse Med.* 76:2189, 1968.

Niikawa N, et al.: Acrodysostosis and blue eyes. *Hum. Genet.* 53:285, 1980.

Reiter S: Acrodysostosis. *Pediatr. Radiol.* 7:53, 1978.

Robinow M, et al.: Acrodysostosis: A syndrome of peripheral dysostosis, nasal hypoplasia, and mental retardation. *Am. J. Dis. Child.* 121:195, 1971.

Undereiner F, et al.: L'acrodysostose: A propos d'un cas avec étude tomodensimétrique crâniocérébrale. *Ann. Pediatr.* 28:429, 1981.

ACRODYSPLASIA WITH RETINITIS PIGMENTOSA AND NEPHROPATHY

Synonyms: Saldino-Mainzer syndrome; cone-shaped epiphyses–nephropathy–retinitis pigmentosa.

Mode of Inheritance: Autosomal recessive.

Frequency: Rare (13 reported cases to 1988).

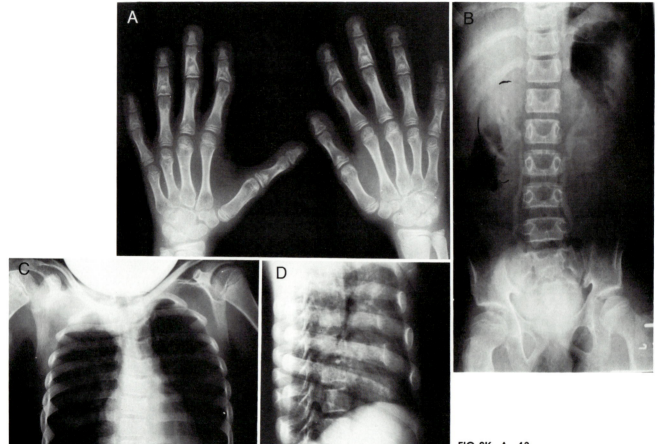

FIG SK–A–13.
Acrodysplasia with retinitis pigmentosa and nephropathy (Saldino-Mainzer syndrome) in a 14-year-old girl. **A,** cone epiphyses in middle phalanges. **B,** excretory urography shows poor concentration, loss of renal cortex; small capital femoral epiphyses. **C** and **D,** short ribs and narrow chest.

Clinical Manifestations: Onset of symptoms in childhood: (a) *nephronophthisis,* chronic renal failure, elevated blood pressure; polydypsia, polyuria; (b) *short middle phalanges of hands and feet;* (c) retinitis pigmentosa, *tapetoretinal degeneration;* (d) cerebellar ataxia; (e) hepatic fibrosis; (f) pigmented midline nevi.

Radiologic Manifestations: (a) *Cone-shaped epiphyses of hands and feet* (Giedion type 28 or 28A, also associated with types 38, 38A, 37, etc.), relative shortening of middle phalanges 2–4 in variable intensity (profile method of Poznanski); (b) flattened capital femoral epiphyses, widened femoral neck, irregular areas of sclerosis in metaphyseal region; (c) excretory urography demonstrating *poor concentration of excreted contrast medium and diminution of renal size;* (d) other reported abnormalities: hypoplastic iliac wings; small proximal humeral epiphyses; widening of ribs, quadrangular vertebral bodies, and short spinous process (Fig SK–A–13).

Morphological Changes: Kidneys and eyes: diffuse tubular atrophy, interstitual fibrosis and thickened basement membranes; Leber congenital amaurosis (tapetoretinal degeneration with focal depigmented retinal pigment epithelial lesions).

Differential Diagnosis, Significant: The conorenal syndromes: (a) asphyxiating thoracic dystrophy; (b) acrodysplasias.

Special Comments: Senior-Loken syndrome (nephronopthisis and tapetoretinal degeneration) may represent part of the spectrum of Saldino-Mainzer syndrome (Ellis).

REFERENCES

Bodaghi E, et al.: Familial nephropathy with congenital liver fibrosis, degenerative retinitis and cone-shaped epiphysis. *Int. J. Pediatr. Nephrol.* 1:153–156, 1980.

Chakera TMH: Peripheral dysostosis associated with juvenile nephronophthisis. *Br. J. Radiol.* 48:765, 1975.

Diekmann L, et al.: Familiäre Nephropathie mit Retinitis pigmentosa und peripherer Dysostose. *Helv. Paediatr. Acta* 32:375, 1977.

Ellis DS, et al.: Leber's congenital amaurosis associated with familial juvenile nephronopthisis and cone-shaped epiphyses of the hands (Saldino-Mainzer syndrome). *Am. J. Ophthalmol.* 97:233–239, 1984.

Giedion A: Phalangeal cone-shaped epiphysis of the hands (PhCSEH) and chronic renal disease—The conorenal syndrome. *Pediatr. Radiol.* 8:32, 1979.

Kleinknecht C, et al.: Nephronophtise juvenile. *Rev. Pediatr.* 13:441, 1977.

Popović-Rolovic M, et al.: Juvenile nephronophthisis associated with retinal pigmentary dystrophy, cerebellar ataxia, and skeletal abnormalities. *Arch. Dis. Child.* 51:801, 1976.

Saldino RM, Mainzer F: Cone-shaped epiphyses (CSE) in siblings with hereditary renal disease and retinitis pigmentosa. *Radiology* 98:39, 1971.

Silengo MC: A Saldino-Mainzer—like syndrome: Retinitis pigmentosa, interstitial nephropathy, Madelung-mesomelia, brachydactyly. *Pediatr Radiol.* 17:238–241, 1987.

ACROMESOMELIC DYSPLASIA

Synonyms: Le nanisme acromésomélique; Achromesomeler Zwergwuchs.

Mode of Inheritance: Autosomal recessive.

Frequency: rare; 31 cases to 1988.

Clinical Manifestations: Abnormalities may be detectable at birth but usually become more obvious in first year of life: (a) *dwarfism;* (b) head size within normal range but prominent relative to patient's size; slight flatness of midface; short nose; (c) *shortness of forearms, hands, legs, and feet; stubby fingers;* large great toes; limitation of elbow motion; ligamentous laxity; (d) low thoracic kyphosis; increased lumbar lordosis; (e) normal intelligence; delayed head control; (f) growth hormone studies normal; longitudinal growth studies reveal early slowdown of growth velocity.

Radiologic Manifestations: By 2 years can be diagnosed radiographically; (a) scaphocephalic skull, basal angles of 135 to 140 degrees; (b) oval vertebral bodies in infancy, progressive development of relative shortness of dorsal margin of vertebral bodies, anterior beaking of vertebral bodies in the first 2 years of life, anterior vertebral wedging in adults, diminished interpedicular distances of lower vertebrae; (c) shortness of all tubular bones, *in particular those of forearms;* bowed radial shaft, dislocated radial head; hypoplasia of the distal end of ulna; *very short tubular bones of hands and feet; cone-shaped epiphyses of metacarpals and phalanges;* metaphyseal flaring of the long tubular bones; *premature fusion of the epiphyses in hands and feet;* characteristic *large great toes* with enlarged proximal and distal phalanges (d) other reported abnormalities: superiorly curved clavicles, hypoplasia of basilar segment of ilia, irregularity and delay in ossification of lateral margins of acetabulae; (e) has not been diagnosed prenatally. (Figs SK–A–14 and SK–A–15).

Differential Diagnosis, Significant: Pseudohyperparathyroidism, brachydactyly type E, acrodysostosis, pseudoachondroplasia, acro-*coxo*-mesomelic dwarfism, geleophysic dysplasia, Osebold-Remondini dysplasia.

Special Comments: New form (two sibs) with hypoplastic and dysplastic tubular bones of hands (delta phalanges) and hypoplastic fibula (Brahimi).

REFERENCES

Borrelli P, et al.: Acromesomelic dwarfism in a child with an interesting family history. *Pediatr. Radiol.* 13:165–168, 1983.

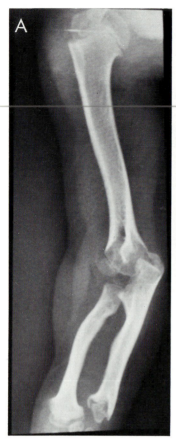
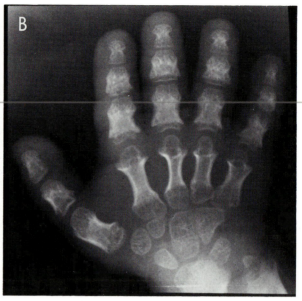

FIG SK—A—14.
Acromesomelic dysplasia. Upper limb of an 8-year-old child.
A, Shortness of forearm; abnormal configuration of humerus, radius, and ulna; bowing of radius and metaphyseal flaring. **B,** very short and stubby metacarpals and phalanges, cone-shaped epiphyses of metacarpals and phalanges. (From Langer LO, Garret RT: Acromesomelic dysplasia. *Radiology* 137:349, 1980. Reproduced with permission.)

Brahimi L, et al.: Acro-mesomelic dysplasia—a new type: Report of two siblings. *Pediatr Radiol* 18:67—69, 1988.

Frayer DW, et al.: Italian late upper paleolithic fossil with acromegalic dysplasia. *Nature* 330:60—62, 1987.

Hall CM, et al.; Acromesomelic dwarfism. *Br. J. Radiol.* 53:999, 1980.

Langer LO, et al.: Acromesomelic dysplasia. *Radiology* 137:349, 1980.

Langer LO, et al.: Acromesomelic dwarfism: Manifestations in childhood. *Am. J. Med. Genet.* 1:87—100, 1977.

Maroteaux P, et al.: Le nanisme acromésomélique. *Presse Med.* 79:1839, 1971.

Pfeiffer RA: Akromesomeler Zwergwuchs. *Fortsch. Roentgenstr.* 125:171, 1976.

Raes M, et al.: A boy with acromesomelic dysplasia. Growth course and hormone release. *Helv. Paediatr. Acta* 40:415—420, 1985.

Stichelbout P, et al.: La dysplasie acromesomelique. A propos d'une nouvelle observation. *Arch. Fr. Pediatr.* 41:487—489, 1984.

ACROMICRIC DYSPLASIA

Mode of Inheritance: Autosomal dominant.

Frequency: Very rare (six cases, one report, ?underreported).

Clinical Manifestations: Growth delay after 2 years: (a) *unusual facies,* narrow palpebral fissures, short nose, anteverted nostrils; (b) *small hands and feet;* limited finger flexion.

Radiologic Manifestations: (a) *short metacarpals and phalanges; mild proximal pointing* (2—5); pseudoepiphysis of first metacarpal; notch, base of second metacarpal; cone-shaped epiphyses of phalanges; (b) short long bones; laterally flat capital femoral epiphyses.

Differential Diagnosis, Significant: (a) brachydactyly syndromes, including pseudohypoparathyroidism; (b) geleophysic dysplasia.

REFERENCE

Maroteaux P, et al.: Acromicric dysplasia. *Am. J. Med. Genet.* 24:447—459, 1986.

ADENOSINE DEAMINASE DEFICIENCY WITH SEVERE COMBINED IMMUNODEFICIENCY AND CHONDRO-OSSEOUS DYSPLASIA

Synonyms: ADA deficiency with or without SCID; achondroplasia and Swiss-type agammaglobulinemia.

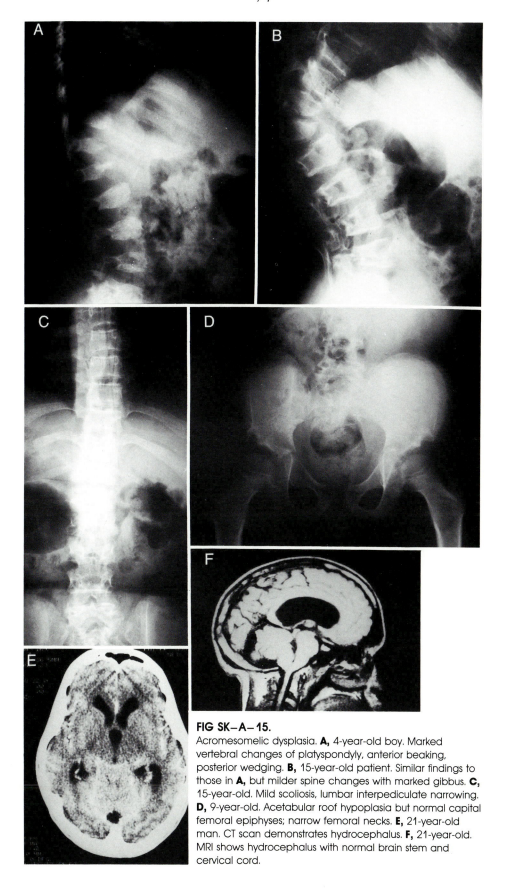

FIG SK–A–15.
Acromesomelic dysplasia. **A,** 4-year-old boy. Marked vertebral changes of platyspondyly, anterior beaking, posterior wedging. **B,** 15-year-old patient. Similar findings to those in **A,** but milder spine changes with marked gibbus. **C,** 15-year-old. Mild scoliosis, lumbar interpediculate narrowing. **D,** 9-year-old. Acetabular roof hypoplasia but normal capital femoral epiphyses; narrow femoral necks. **E,** 21-year-old man. CT scan demonstrates hydrocephalus. **F,** 21-year-old. MRI shows hydrocephalus with normal brain stem and cervical cord.

Mode of Inheritance: Autosomal recessive.

Frequency: Uncommon (about 35 families to 1984). About 50% of non-X-linked SCID, and 20% of all SCID (Hirshhorn).

Clinical Manifestations: (a) *recurrenct infections* (viral, bacterial, fungal); failure to thrive, *often fatal by 2 years;* diarrhea; rachitic rosary; (b) *absence of both cellular and humoral immunity;* (c) *very low level of ADA activity in peripheral blood mononuclear cells, erythrocytes, lymphocytes, and fibroblasts;* (d) other reported abnormalities: neurological; lymphoma, no increased cancer risk (Morrell); renal abnormalities (mesangial sclerosis 75%); cortical adrenal fibrosis; (e) prenatal diagnosis: ADA activity—amnionic cells, chorionic villus biopsy analysis (Dooley); fetal blood—fetoscopy (Cinch); (f) treatment: polyethylene glycol–modified ADA; bone marrow transplantation.

Radiologic Manifestations: (a) Long bones: irregularity of metaphyseal ends of long bones, splayed metaphyses, metaphyseal spurs perpendicular to long axis of bones; (b) ribs: short, wide, and cup-shaped at costochondral junctions; (c) vertebrae: "bone within bone" appearance, central breaking of lower thoracic vertebrae, mild platyspondyly; (d) pelvis; square-shaped iliac wings, flat acetabular roofs, irregular iliac crest, narrow sciatic notches; (e) resolution of bone lesions after enzyme replacement therapy; (f) absence of thymic shadow on chest roentgenograms.

Chondro-osseous Morphology: Ribs: absence of zone of proliferating cells, absent column formation, irregular calcified cartilage with poor trabecular formation (Cedarbaum, Kaitila).

Differential Diagnosis, Significant: (a) rickets; (b) metaphyseal chondrodysplasia, especially cartilage hair hypoplasia; (c) other SCID disease; (d) Menke syndrome, copper deficiency; (e) battered child syndrome.

Special Comments: Partial ADA deficiency has been associated with at least seven different alleles. Defects are located on chromosome 20.

REFERENCES

Cederbaum SD, et al.: The chondro-osseous dysplasia of ADA deficiency with severe combined immunodeficiency. *J. Pediatr.* 89:737–742, 1976.
Dooley T, et al.: First trimester diagnosis of ADA deficiency. *Prenatal Diagn.* 7:561–565, 1987.
Herman TE, et al.: Radiology of immunodeficiency syndromes. *Postgrad. Radiol.* 1:99, 1981.
Hershfield MS, et al.: Treatment of ADA deficiency with polyethylene glycol–modified ADA. *N. Engl. J. Med.* 316:589–598, 1987.
Hirschhorn R: Inherited enzyme deficiencies and immunodeficiency. *Clin. Immunol. Immunopathol.* 40:157–165, 1986.
Kaitila I, et al.: Chondroosseous histopathology in adenosine deaminase deficient combined immunodeficiency disease. *Birth Defects* 12:115–121, 1976.
Kapoor N, et al.: Lymphoma in a patient with SCID with ADA deficiency, following unsustained engraftment of histoincompatible T cell–depleted bone marrow. *J. Pediatr.* 108:435–437, 1986.
Lallemand D, et al.: Anomalies osseuses constitutionelles dans les déficits immunitaires congénitaux. *Ann. Radiol.* 22:108, 1979.
Linch DE, et al.: Prenatal diagnosis of three cases of severe combined immunodeficiency. *Clin. Exp. Immunol.* 56:223–232, 1984.
Morrell D, et al.: Cancer in families with severe combined immune deficiency. *JNCL* 78:455–458, 1987.
Silber GM, et al.: Reconstitution of T and B cell function after T lymphocyte depleted haploidentical bone marrow transplantation in SCID due to ADA deficiency. *Clin. Immunol. Immunopathol.* 44:317–320, 1987.
Wolfson JJ, Cross VF, in Meuwissen HJ, et al. (eds.): *Combined Immunodeficiency: A Molecular Defect.* New York, Academic Press, 1975, p. 255–277.
Yulish BS, et al.: Partial resolution of bone lesions: A child with severe combined immunodeficiency disease and adenosine deaminase deficiency after enzyme-replacement therapy. *Am. J. Dis. Child.* 134:61, 1980.

ANTLEY-BIXLER SYNDROME

Synonyms: Multisynostotic osteodysgenesis; campomelic dysplasia, short-limbed craniosynostotic form; trapezoidocephaly, midface hypoplasia, and cartilage abnormalities with multiple synostoses and skeletal fractures; trapezoidocephaly–multiple synostosis syndrome (TMS); acrocephalosynankia.

Mode of Inheritance: Autosomal recessive.

Frequency: Rare (11 cases reported to 1988).

Clinical Manifestations: (a) craniosynostosis *(trapezoidocephaly);* midface hypoplasia; low-set ears with abnormal helix; (b) narrow chest; (c) *fixed flexion at elbows; bowed femora;* clubfoot; camptodactyly; (d) respiratory death, usually within 8 months; (e) other reported abnormalities: cloverleaf skull (Kleeblattschadel), proptosis, choanal atresia, joint contractures, femoral fractures, external auditory canal atresia, cardiac and urogenital malformations, skin dimple.

Radiologic Manifestations: *Craniosynostosis (lambdoid and coronal sutures);* antegonial notching of mandible; gracile ribs; narrow vertical ilia, *humeroradial synostosis, bowed femurs;* sclerosis at end-plates of vertebral bodies; other less common features: clubfoot; carpal-tarsal synostosis; arachnodactyly; bowed ulna; long bone fractures; prenatal diagnosis (ultrasound) one case (Figs SK–A–16 and SK–A–17).

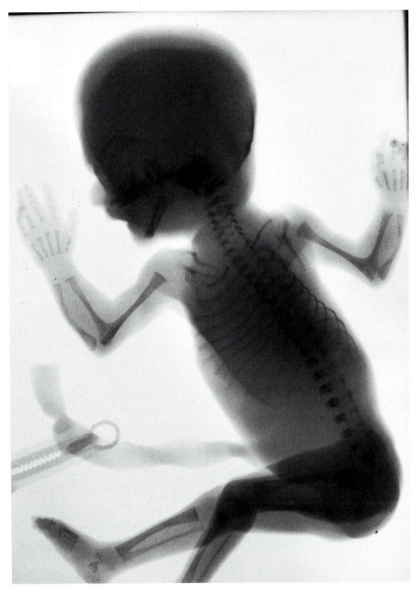

FIG SK–A–16.
Antley-Bixler syndrome in a stillborn infant. Radiohumeral synostosis, craniostenosis, antegonial notch (mandible), gracile ribs. (Courtesy of A. Schinzel, M.D., Zurich, Switzerland.)

Differential Diagnosis, Significant: Campomelic dysplasia, cloverleaf skull—limb anomalies, acrocephalosyndactyly (Pfeiffer, Apert).

Special Comments: The two patients with campomelic syndrome, short-boned craniostenotic form, appear to represent two cases of Antley-Bixler (Khajavi); this syndrome may have been described as early as 1926, as "acrocephalo-synankia" (Walbaum 1984).

REFERENCES

Antley RM, Bixler D: Trapezoidocephaly: Midfacial hypoplasia and cartilage abnormalities with multiple synostoses and skeletal fractures in Amsterdam. *Birth Defects* 11(2):397–401, 1975.

Antley RM, Bixler D: Developments in the trapezoidocephaly–multiple synostosis syndrome (invited editorial comments). *Am. J. Med. Genet.* 14:149–150, 1983.

Delozier CD, et al.: The syndrome of multisynostotic osteodysgenesis with long bone fractures. *Am. J. Med. Genet.* 7:391–403, 1980.

Delozier CD, Engel E: Multisynostotic osteodysgenesis and the problem of genetic counseling in newly-identified syndromes. *J. Génét. Hum.* 29:365–377, 1981.

Herva R, Seppanen U: Multisynostotic osteodysgenesis. *Pediatr. Radiol.* 15:63–64, 1985.

Khajavi A, et al.: Heterogeneity in the campomelic syndromes. Long and short bone varieties. *Radiology* 120:641–647, 1976.

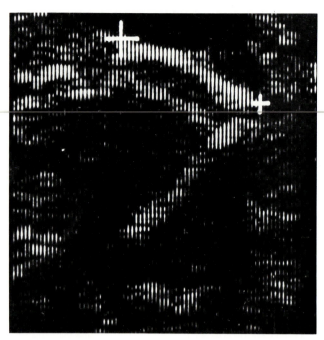

FIG SK—A—17.
Antley-Bixler syndrome in a 20-week fetus. Ultrasound study shows bowed forearms, humeroradial synostosis. (From Schinzel A, et al.: *Am. J. Med. Genet.* 14:139–147, 1983. Reproduced with permission.)

Robert E, et al.: Le syndrome d'Antley-Bixler. *J. Genet. Hum.* 32:291–298, 1984.

Robinson LK, et al.: The Antley-Bixler syndrome. *J. Pediatr.* 101:201–205, 1982.

Savoldelli G, Schinzel A: Prenatal ultrasound detection of humero-radial synostosis in a case of Antley-Bixler syndrome. *Prenatal Diagn* 2:219–223, 1982.

Schinzel A, et al.: Antley-Bixler syndrome in sisters. *Am. J. Med. Genet.* 14:139–147, 1983.

Walbaum R: Antley-Bixler syndrome (letter). *J. Pediatr.* 104:799, 1984.

Yasui Y, et al.: The first case of the Antley-Bixler syndrome with consanguinity in Japan. *Jinrui Idengaku Zasshi* 28:215–220, 1983.

ASPHYXIATING THORACIC DYSPLASIA

Synonyms: Jeune syndrome, thoracopelviphalangeal dysplasia, ATD.

Mode of Inheritance: Autosomal recessive.

Frequency: Uncommon (1 per 100,000 to 130,000 live births).

Clinical Manifestations: Wide spectrum of clinical manifestations ranging from lethal to latent forms without respiratory symptoms; (a) *respiratory distress* of varying severity in neonatal period; (b) *small, long, narrow thoracic cage;* (c) *short-limb dwarfism;* (d) *progressive nephropathy;* renal insuf-

ficiency, albuminuria, hypertension, chronic pyelonephritis, glomerular and tubular cysts, glomerular sclerosis; (e) hepatic fibrosis, proliferation of bile ducts, polycystic liver disease; (f) other reported abnormalities: recurrent respiratory infections, situs inversus, cystic disease of pancreas, impaired zymogen secretion, abdominal muscle dysplasia, reduced visual acuity, tapetoretinal degeneration, abnormalities of retinal pigmentation, neutropenia, epididymal cysts, abnormal phospholipids in lungs.

Radiologic Manifestations: (a) *Small, bell-shaped thoracic cage, handlebar clavicles, horizontally directed ribs, bulbous and irregular rib ends;* (b) *small pelvis, short flared iliac bones, trident appearance of acetabular margin, inferolateral spur of sciatic notch;* (c) *presence of proximal femoral ossification center at birth* in about two thirds of cases; (d) *cone-shaped epiphyses of hands* and premature fusions, short phalanges; (e) renal abnormalities: cystic disease, clubbing of calices, medullary smudging on excretory urography; (f) other reported abnormalities: carniosynostosis (sagittal suture), hydrocephalus (one case), absent twelfth rib, short fifth metatarsal, osteoporosis; (g) prenatally diagnosed by ultrasound (four cases) (Fig SK—A—18).

Chondro-osseous Morphology and General Pathology: (a) Ribs most severely affected; failure of enchondral ossification and markedly deficient and irregular chondrocyte columns at growth plates; ultrastructure: intracytoplasmic lipid droplets within chondrocytes; (b) pulmonary hypoplasia; normal lung growth; alveolar number and complexity normal; (c) renal-hepatic-pancreatic dysplasia; (d) nephronophthisis with medullary cystic changes; (e) retinal dystrophy, pigmentary retinopathy.

Differential Diagnosis, Significant: (a) chondroectodermal dysplasia (Ellis—van Creveld syndrome); (b) thoracolaryngopelvic dysplasia (Barnes syndrome); (c) short rib polydactyly syndrome, types 1 and 2; (d) metaphyseal chondrodysplasia with exocrine pancreatic insufficiency and cyclic neutropenia (Shwachman-Diamond syndrome).

Special Comments: ATD must be differentiated from autosomal dominant thoracolaryngopelvic dysplasia (Barnes syndrome).

REFERENCES

Borland LM: Anesthesia for children with Jeune's syndrome (asphyxiating thoracic dystrophy). *Anesthesiology* 66:86–88, 1987.

Burn J, et al.: Autosomal dominant thoracolaryngopelvic dysplasia: Barnes syndrome. *J. Med. Genet.* 23:345–349, 1986.

Elejalde BR, et al.: Prenatal diagnosis of Jeune syndrome. *Am. J. Med. Genet.* 21:433–438, 1985.

Forrest P, et al.: Hypoplastic lungs and abnormal phospholipids in asphyxiating thoracic dystrophy. *Aust. Paediatr.* 23:47–51, 1987.

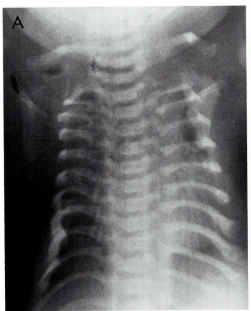
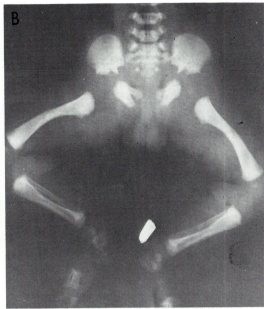

FIG SK—A—18.
Asphyxiating thoracic dysplasia in a newborn girl with respiratory distress. **A,** small, bell-shaped thoracic cage, horizontally directed ribs, and bulbous rib ends. **B,** small pelvis, short flared iliac bones, trident appearance of acetabular margins, inferolateral spur of sciatic notch, and short lower limbs. (Courtesy of Ronald A. Weintraub, M.D., Concord, Calif.)

Friedman JM, et al.: The Jeune syndrome (asphyxiating thoracic dystrophy) in an adult. *Am. J. Med.* 59:857, 1975.

Jeune M, et al.: Polychondrodystrophie avec blocage thoracique d'evolution fatale. *Pediatrie* 9:390, 1954.

Jequier JC, et al.: Asphyxiating thoracic dysplasia, in Kaufmann HJ (ed.): *Progress in Pediatric Radiology*, vol 4, Basel, S. Karger, 1973, p. 184.

Kozlowski K, et al.: Asphyxiating thoracic dystrophy without respiratory disease: Report of two cases of the latent form. *Pediatr. Radiol.* 5:30, 1976.

Langer LO: Thoracic-pelvic-phalangeal dystrophy: Asphyxiating thoracic dystrophy of the newborn, infantile thoracic dystrophy. *Radiology* 91:447, 1968.

Lipson M, et al.: Prenatal diagnosis of asphyxiating thoracic dysplasia. *Am. J. Med. Genet.* 18:273–277, 1984.

Oberklaid F, et al.: Asphyxiating thoracic dysplasia. *Arch. Dis. Child.* 52:758, 1977.

Pirnar T, Neuhauser EBD: Asphyxiating thoracic dystrophy of the newborn. *AJR* 98:358–364, 1966.

Schinzel A, et al.: Prenatal sonographic diagnosis of Jeune syndrome. *Radiology* 154:777–778, 1985.

Shah KJ: Renal lesion in Jeune's syndrome. *Br. J. Radiol.* 53:432, 1980.

Singh M, et al.: Hydrocephalus in asphyxiating thoracic dystrophy. *Am. J. Med. Genet.* 29:391–395, 1988.

Skiptunas SM, Weiner S: Early prenatal diagnosis of asphyxiating thoracic dysplasia (Jeune's syndrome): Value of fetal thoracic measurement. *J. Ultrasound Med.* 6:41–43, 1987.

Todd DW, et al.: A thoracic expansion technique for Jeune's asphyxiating thoracic dystrophy. *J. Pediatr. Surg.* 21:161–163, 1986.

Turkel SB, et al.: Necropsy findings in neonatal asphyxiating, thoracic dystrophy. *J. Med. Genet.* 22:112–118, 1985.

Williams AJ, et al.: Lung structure in asphyxiating thoracic dystrophy. *Arch. Pathol. Lab. Med.* 108:658–661, 1984.

Wilson DJ, et al.: Retinal dystrophy in Jeune's syndrome. *Arch Ophthalmol.* 105:651–657, 1987.

ATELOSTEOGENESIS

Synonyms: Spondylo-humero-femoral hypoplasia; giant cell chondroplasia, AO.

Classification: AO-1, AO-2, AO-3.

Mode of Inheritance: AO-1, sporadic; AO-2, autosomal recessive; AO-3, sporadic (possible new dominant mutation).

Frequency: Very rare (AO-1, 10 cases to 1988; AO-2, 7 cases to 1988; AO-3, 5 cases to 1988).

Clinical Manifestations: *AO-1 and AO-2 neonatally lethal; AO-3 usually lethal in infancy; all types: (a) flat nasal root; midface hypoplasia; cleft palate; micrognathia; (b) generalized limb shortening, especially rhizomelic; radial or ulnar deviation of fingers; large joint dislocations; equinovarus; (c) narrow chest; (d) other reported abnormalities: encephalocele (AO-1, one case; Chervenak).*

Radiologic Manifestations: AO-1: *(a) coronal and sagittal clefts; vertebral hypoplasia (thoracic), platyspondyly, scoliosis; (b) absent, short, globular, or clubbed (distally tapered) humeri; shortened femora with round metaphyses and proximal flaring; shortened, bowed radius and ulna; shortened, bowed tibia; absent fibulae; (c) short-wide well-ossified distal*

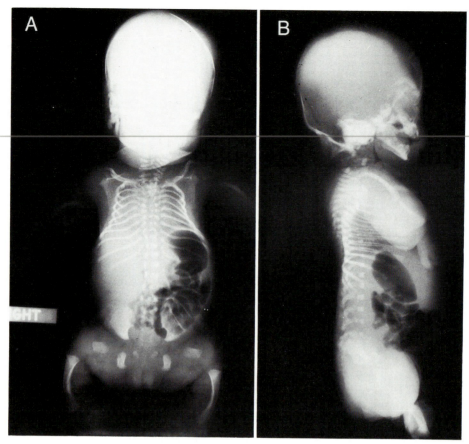

FIG SK–A– 19.
Atelosteogenesis type 1 in a newborn infant. **A,** marked aplasia-hypoplasia of humeri and femora, short bowed tibiae, absent fib-ulae, sagittal vertebral clefts. **B,** coronal clefts, thoracic vertebral hypoplasia.

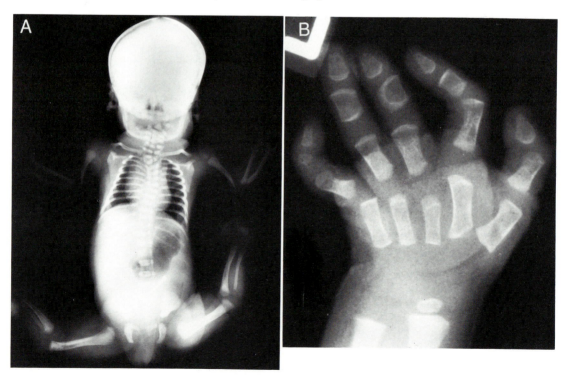

FIG SK–A– 20.
Atelosteogenesis type 3. **A,** newborn infant. Scoliosis, distal ta-pered humeri and femura, knee and elbow dislocations. **B,** 2-year-old child. "Tombstone"-shaped proximal phalanges, wide dis-tal phalanges.

phalanges; dysharmonic ossification of short tubular bones of *hands* (and feet); *short metacarpals* (and metatarsals); triangular first metacarpal; (d) abnormal pelvis, 11 shortened ribs; elongated clavicles; antenatal diagnosis (ultrasound; one case; Chervenak) (Fig SK–A–19).

AO-2: *infrequent coronal and sagittal clefting;* scoliosis; normal sacrosciatic notch; *short, dumbbell humeri (bifid distally); short dumbbell femurs; gap between first and second digits; enlarged second and third metacarpals; rounded hypoplastic middle phalanges; hypoplastic, formed fibula.*

AO-3: *hypoplastic maxilla and mandible,* prominant occiput; segmentation defects of *cervical spine with double curve (S) configuration;* almost normal ribs (12); *vertical blocklike ischia; club or globular humeri with precocious proximal epiphyseal ossification; tombstone-shaped proximal phalanges; widened distal phalanges;* harmonious ossification of tubular hand bones; *bifid digits;* absent fibula (two of five cases) (Fig SK–A–20).

Chondro-osseous Morphology: AO-1, acellularity with or without giant cells in resting zone; AO-2, cystic areas and threadlike radiations in resting zone; AO-3, mild hypocellularity; otherwise normal.

Differential Diagnosis, Significant: AO-1: (a) Boomerang syndrome; AO-2: (a) diastrophic dysplasia-like syndromes; (b) de la Chapelle dysplasia; AO-3: (a) otopalatodigital type 2 (Stern).

Special Comments: (?)Another atelosteogenesis type (different chondro-osseous morphology; fetal diagnosis) (ultrasound) (Herzberg). de la Chapelle and Boomerang dysplasia may not represent separate disorders from atelosteogenesis types 2 or 1 (family of similar disorders).

REFERENCES

AO-1

Chervenak FA, et al.: Antenatal diagnosis of frontal cephalocele in a fetus with atelosteogenesis. *J. Ultrasound Med.* 5:111–113, 1986.

Maroteaux P, et al.: Atelosteogenesis. *Am. J. Med. Genet.* 13:15–25, 1982.

Sillence DO, et al.: Spondylo-humero-femoral hypoplasia (giant cell chondroplasia). *Am. J. Med. Genet.* 13:7–14, 1982.

Yang, et al.: Two lethal chondrodysplasias with giant chondrocytes. *Am. J. Med. Genet.* 15:615–625, 1983.

AO-2

McAlister W, et al.: A new neonatal short limbed dwarfism. *Skeletal Radiol.* 13:271–275, 1985.

Sillence DO, et al.: Atelosteogenesis: Evidence for heterogeneity. *Pediatr. Radiol.* 17:112–118, 1987.

Herzberg AJ, et al: Variant of atelosteogenesis? Report of a 20-week fetus. *Am. J. Med. Genet.* 29:883–890, 1988.

AO-3

Stern HJ, et al.: Atelosteogenesis type 3: A distinct skeletal dysplasia with features overlapping atelosteogenesis and oto-palato-digital syndrome type 2. *Am. J. Med. Genet.* in press.

BOOMERANG DYSPLASIA

Mode of Inheritance: Not known; sporadic.

Frequency: Very rare (three cases, 1988).

Clinical Manifestations: *Lethal* severe *neonatal dwarfism;* polyhydramnios; edema; omphalocele.

Radiologic Manifestations: (a) lower extremities: *boomerang tibiae;* other bones absent; upper extremities: absent humerus and radius (or ulna); (b) absent thoracolumbar vertebral body ossification; (c) bell-shaped thorax; large iliac wings, small iliac bodies; absent pubic bone ossification.

Chondro-osseous Morphology: Similar to atelosteogenesis type 1 (giant cells).

Differential Diagnosis, Significant: Atelosteogenesis.

Special Comments: This might be the same disorder as ateleosteogenesis type 1.

REFERENCES

Kozlowski K, et al.: Case report: Boomerang dysplasia. *Br. J. Radiol.* 58:369–371, 1985.
Tenconi R, et al.: Boomerang dysplasia. *Fortschr. Roentgenstr.* 138:378–380, 1983.

BRACHYOLMIA

Synonyms: Spondylodysplasia, brachyrachia.

Mode of Inheritance: Type 1 (Hobaek and Toledo), autosomal dominant; type 2 (Maroteaux), autosomal recessive; type 3, autosomal dominant (very severe).

Frequency: Uncommon. (52 cases, all types); Hobaek type most common form (21 cases to 1988).

Clinical Manifestations: All types: (a) Normal birth length, *later markedly short-trunked,* early childhood presen-

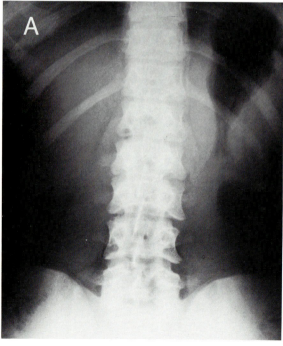
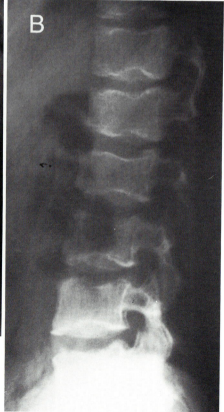

FIG SK–B–1.
Brachyolmia type 1 in a 13-year-old patient. **A,** close-set pedicles, platyspondyly. **B,** platyspondyly, end plate indentations and irregularity.

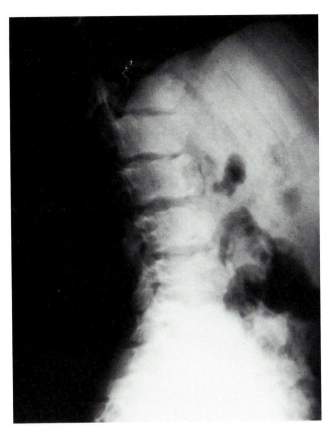

FIG SK–B–2.
Brachyolmia type 3 in an 8-year-old patient. Rounded anterior vertebral bodies, platyspondyly, moderate end-plate irregularity.

tation; (b) corneal opacities (only Toledo type); (c) scoliosis; (d) "subclinical" extremity shortening.

Radiologic Manifestations: Type 1 (Hobaek and Toledo): (a) *Squared-off platyspondyly, narrow intervertebral spaces, marked end plate irregularity, close-set pedicles* in anteroposterior (AP) view; (b) precocious anterior rib calcification (Toledo type) (Fig SK–B–1). Type 2 (Maroteaux): Same as type 1 but (a) *rounded vertebral edges,* mild end plate irregularity, normal intervertebral disk spaces; (b) precocious falx calcification. Type 3: Same as type 2 but *more severe involvement* without precocious calcification; (c) *severe cervical platyspondyly* (Fig SK–B–2).

Chondro-osseous Morphology: Nonspecific; regular growth plate with somewhat short columns and wide septae.

Differential Diagnosis, Significant: Spondylometaphyseal dysplasia (mild forms).

Special Comments: Three distinct radiographic and four distinct clinical types occur (Shohat). *Brachyolmia is platyspondyly without* significant *tubular bone* (epiphyseal, metaphyseal, diaphyseal) *involvement.*

REFERENCES

Fontaine G, et al.: La dysplasie spondyloaire pure ou brachyolmie. *Arch. Franc. Pediatr.* 32:695–708, 1975.
Horton WA, et al.: Brachyolmia, recessive type (Hobaek): A clinical, radiographic, and histochemical study. *Am. J. Med. Genet.* 16:201–211, 1983.
Shohat M, et al.: Brachyolmia (?spondylodysplasia): Clinical, radiographic and genetic evidence of heterogeneity. *Am. J. Med. Genet.,* 33:209, 1988.

C

CAMPOMELIC DYSPLASIA

Synonyms: Camptomelic dysplasia; classic or long-limbed campomelic syndrome.

Mode of Inheritance: Autosomal recessive; often sex-reversed XY females (H-Y antigen deficiency).

Frequency: Common (approximately 124 cases reported to 1988; 0.5 per 100,000 births).

Clinical Manifestations: *(a) dwarfism; (b) respiratory distress in neonatal period* due to maldevelopment of trachea; *(c) peculiar small facies* with macrocephaly, micrognathia, and malformed ears; *(d) cleft palate; (e) prenatal bowing of lower limbs; (f) pretibial skin dimpling;* (g) generalized hypotonia; (h) CNS anomalies; (i) commonly death in infancy; (j) polyhydramnios; (k) other reported abnormalities: hydronephrosis (38%); congenital heart defects (21%); malformed inner ear; *(l) complications:* air embolism; recurrent aspiration; apnea; scoliosis, dislocated hips.

Radiologic Manifestations: *(a) Enlarged and elongated skull* with high flat forehead and bulging occiput and relatively narrow base; antegonal notching of mandible; *(b) hypoplasia and poor ossification of cervical vertebrae* (63%); (c) bell-shaped thorax, *11 pairs of ribs,* absence of ossification of sternum, narrow tracheal air column; *(d) hypoplastic scapula; some shortness and angulation of upper limbs,* radial head dislocation, stubbiness of tubular bones of hands, squared-off appearance of distal phalanges, clinodactyly of fifth digits; (e) contracted pelvis, *narrow and tall iliac wings, poor or absent ossification of pubis and ala of sacrum, squat vertical ischia,* hip dislocation; *(f) angulation of proximal femoral shaft with apex located anteriorly and laterally, hypoplasia and angulation of tibia and hypoplastic fibula; (g) lack of ossification of talus,* talipes equinovarus; *(h) prenatal diagnosis (ultrasound)* Figs SK–C–1 to SK–C–3).

Differential Diagnosis, Significant: (a) Congenital bowing of the long bones (bent femurs); (b) "short bone varieties" of campomelic dysplasia (kyphomelic dysplasia; Antley-Bixler syndrome); (c) Larsen syndrome; (d) diastrophic dysplasia.

Special Comments: Several patients with campomelic dysplasia but without campomelia (bent limbs) have been identified; the "short bone varieties" of campomelic dysplasia (Khajavi 1976) represent two distinct syndromes: the normocephalic form is now known as *kyphomelic dysplasia,* and the craniostenotic type appears to be identical to *Antley-Bixler syndrome (see Kyphomelic dysplasia and Antley-Bixler syndrome).*

REFERENCES

Balcar I, Bieber FR: Sonographic and radiologic findings in campomelic dysplasia. *AJR* 141:481–482, 1983.

Beluffi G, Fraccaro M: Genetical and clinical aspects of campomelic dysplasia. *Prog. Clin. Biol. Res.* 104:53–65, 1982.

Bricarelli FD, et al.: Sex-reversed XY females with campomelic dysplasia are H-Y negative. *Hum. Genet.* 57:15, 1981.

Fryns JP, et al.: Prenatal diagnosis of campomelic dwarfism. *Clin. Genet.* 19:199, 1981.

Furman W, et al: Campomelic-like syndrome (AR): Abnormal hands and feet (missing digits). *Prog. Clin. Biol. Res.* 104:519–524, 1982.

Hall BD, et al.: Campomelic dysplasia: Further elucidation of a distinct entity. *Am. J. Dis. Child.* 134:285, 1980.

Hoefnagel D, et al.: Campomelic dwarfism associated with gonadal dysgenesis and chromosome anomalies. *Clin. Genet.* 13:489, 1978.

Houston CS, et al.: The campomelic syndrome: Review, report of 17 cases and follow-up of the currently 17-year-old boy first reported by Maroteaux et al. in 1971. *Am. J. Med. Genet.* 15:3–28, 1983.

Khajavi A, et al.: Heterogeneity in the campomelic syndromes: Long and short bone varieties. *Radiology* 120:641–647, 1976.

Lazjuk GI, et al.: Campomelic syndrome: Concepts of the bowing and shortening in the lower limbs. *Teratology* 35:1–8, 1987.

Maroteaux P, et al.: Le syndrome campomelique. *Presse Med.* 79:1157, 1971.

Mellows HJ, et al.: The campomelic syndrome in two female siblings. *Clin. Genet.* 18:137, 1980.

Moedjono SJ, et al.: The campomelic syndrome in a singleton and monozygotic twins. *Clin. Genet.* 18:397, 1981.

Nobuhiro T, et al.: The campomelic syndrome: Temporal bone histopathologic features and otolaryngologic manifestations. *Arch. Otolaryngol.* 105:449, 1979.

Nogami H, et al.: Congenital bowing of long bones: Clinical and experimental study. *Teratology* 33:1–7, 1986.

Pazzaglia UE, Beluffi G: Radiology and histopathology of the bent limbs in campomelic dysplasia: Implications in the aetiology of the disease and review of theories. *Pediatr. Radiol.* 17:50–55, 1987.

Pretorius DH, et al.: Specific skeletal dysplasias in utero: Sonographic diagnosis. *Radiology* 159:237–242, 1986.

Puck SM, et al.: Absence of H-Y antigen in an XY female with campomelic dysplasia. *Hum. Genet.* 57:23, 1981.

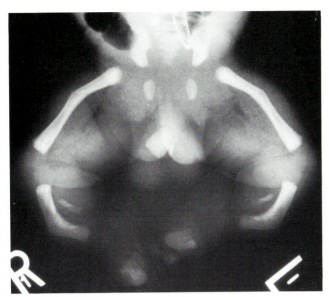

FIG SK–C–1.
Campomelic dysplasia, classic; newborn. Long femurs, hypoplastic ilia, bent long bones, hypoplastic fibulae.

Redon JY, et al.: Un diagnostic antenatal de dysplasie campomelique. *J. Gynecol. Obstet. Biol. Reprod.* 13:437–441, 1984.
Shafai T, et al.: Campomelic syndrome in siblings. *J. Pediatr.* 89:512, 1976.

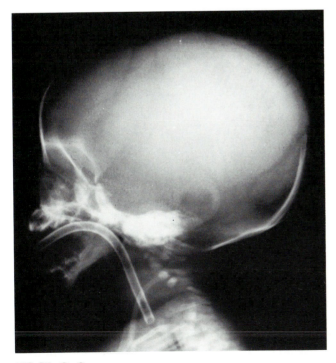

FIG SK–C–2.
Campomelic dysplasia, classic newborn. Cervical spine hypoplasia and kyphosis; large head, small face.

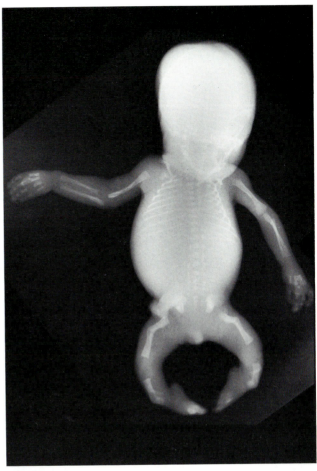

FIG SK–C–3.
Campomelic dysplasia, classic, fetus at 21 weeks' gestation.

Slater P, et al.: The campomelic syndrome: Prenatal ultrasound investigations. *S. Afr. Med. J.* 67:863–866, 1985.

CHERUBISM

Synonyms: Familial fibrous dysplasia of the jaw; familial benign giant cell tumor of the jaw; familial multilocular cystic disease of the jaw.

Mode of Inheritance: Autosomal dominant.

Frequency: Common (about 165 reported cases); 3% of tumoral jaw lesions.

Clinical Manifestations: Onset 18 months to 4 years, subsidence after puberty; (a) *hard, painless, and often symmetric swelling of jaws;* (b) everted thickened lips; upturned eyes; (c) lymphadenopathy (in some); (d) abnormal dentition; (e) complications: difficult intubation; proliferation of tissue from tooth extraction sites; progressive exophthalmos; speech, swallowing, and chewing problems.

Radiologic Manifestations: 1. Children: (a) *expansion of mandible, symmetric* or unilateral; (b) *well-defined multilocular soap bubble appearing radiolucency extending from molar region to notch; maxilla less often involved;* anterior rib and proximal femoral involvement rare; (c) miscellaneous dental manifestations: incomplete development or resorption of roots, noneruption, displacement of teeth, dental agenesis (Figs SK–C–4 and SK–C–5).

2. Adult: granular and sclerotic changes remaining at site of previous disease activity.

Chondro-osseous Morphology and Electron Microscopy: Three stages: *osteolytic stage,* groups of well-vascularized round and giant cells rich in acid phosphatases; *connective tissue rebuilding stage,* fibroblastic cells; *bone-forming stage* (Chomette).

Differential Diagnosis, Significant: (a) Giant cell reparative granuloma; (b) polyostotic fibrous dysplasia; (c) histiocytosis X; (d) aneurysmal bone cyst; (e) Caffey disease; (f) malignant hemangiopericytoma; (g) leukemia; (h) odontogenic cysts and tumors; (i) other tumors (Kozlowski).

Special Comments: Separate autosomal recessive syndrome of *cherubism, gingival fibromatosis,* epilepsy, and mental retardation *(Ramon syndrome)* with juvenile rheumatoid arthritis.

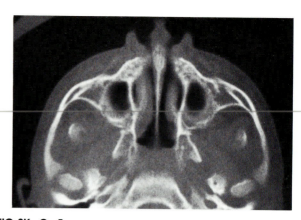

FIG SK–C–5.
Cherubism. CT revealing maxillary involvement. (From Bianchi SD, Boccardi A, Mela F, et al.: The computed tomographic appearance of cherubism. *Skeletal Radiol.* 16:6–10, 1987. Reproduced with permission.)

REFERENCES

Bianchi SD, et al.: The computed tomographic appearances of cherubism. *Skeletal Radiol.* 16:6–10, 1987.

Bixler D, et al.: Cherubism: A familial study to delineate gene action on mandibular growth and development. *Birth Defects* 7:222, 1971.

Cavezian R, et al.: Contribution à l'étude radiologique du cherubinisme. A propos de 2 observations, apport de la tomodensitométrie. *J. Radiol.* 62:373, 1981.

Chomette B, et al.: A peculiar form of osteodysplasia: Cherubism. *Arch. Anat. Cytol. Pathol.* 35:69–75, 1987.

Cornelius EA, et al.: Cherubism—Hereditary fibrous dysplasia of the jaw: Roentgenographic features. *Am. J. Roentgenol.* 106:136, 1969.

Hille JJ, et al.: Cherubism: Two case reports and a review of the literature. *J. Dent. Assoc. S. Afr.* 41:461–466, 1986.

Ireland AJ, Eveson JW: Cherubism—A report of a case with unusual post-extraction complication. *Br. Dent. J.* 164:116–117, 1988.

Jones WA: Familial multilocular cystic disease of jaws. *Am. J. Cancer* 17:946, 1933.

Kozlowski K, et al.: Mandibular and para-mandibular tumors in children. Report of 16 cases. *Pediatr. Radiol.* 11:183–192, 1981.

Maydew RP, Berry RA: Cherubism with difficult laryngoscopy and tracheal intubation. *Anesthesiology* 62:810–812, 1985.

Wackerle B, et al.: Radiologic findings in cherubism: Orthopantomography, CT, MRI. *Röntgenpraxis* 40:104–107, 1987.

CHONDRODYSPLASIA PUNCTATA

Classification: See Table SK–C–1.

CHONDRODYSPLASIA PUNCTATA, CONRADI-HÜNERMANN–TYPE

Synonyms: Dysplasia epiphysealis congenita; stippled epiphyses; chondrodysplasia punctata, dominant type; chon-

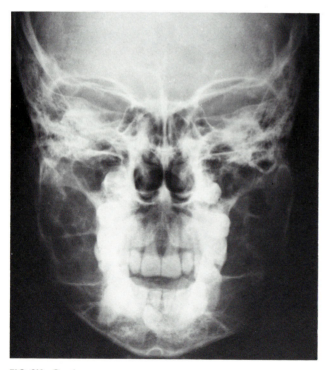

FIG SK–C–4.
Cherubism in a 12-year-old boy. Mandible is markedly widened and teeth are displaced medially; cystic appearance of lesions is striking. (From Shuler RK, Silverman FN: *Ann. Radiol.* 8:45, 1965. Reproduced with permission.)

drodysplasia epiphysealis punctata; chondrodystrophia calcificans congenita; Conradi-Hünermann disease.

Mode of Inheritance: Autosomal dominant.

Frequency: Common; one of most frequently seen types of chondrodysplasia punctata; most are new mutations (only 11 families reported).

Clinical Manifestations: (a) *craniofacial dysmorphism:* asymmetric head, frontal bossing, *flat nasal bridge,* dysplastic auricles, mongoloid palpebral fissures; hypertelorism, *high-arched palate;* (b) *ocular abnormalities: cataract* (17%), corneal opacity, nystagmus, microphthalmos, microcornea, glaucoma, dislocated lens; (c) *cutaneous abnormalities: linear and blotchy pattern of skin lesions* consisting of congenital ichthyosiform erythroderma and hyperkeratosis, atrophoderma; circumscribed alopecia, sparse eyebrows and lashes; layered or split nails; (d) *asymmetric shortening of limbs;* (e) other reported abnormalities: dysfunction of joints (flexion contracture, lateral dislocation of patellae), clubfoot or valgus deformity, hexadactyly; scoliosis, vertebral clefting or wedging; short necks; pulmonary artery stenosis.

Radiologic Manifestations: (a) *asymmetric* (less often, symmetric) mild *shortening of all long bones;* (b) *punctate calcific deposits* in infantile cartilaginous skeleton (spinal col-

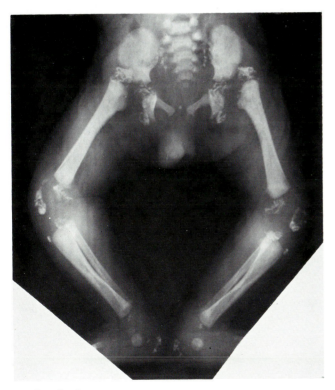

FIG SK−C−6.
Chondrodysplasia punctata Conradi-Hunermann type, newborn. Stippled calcifications in pubic, sacral, hip, knee, and ankle regions. (Courtesy of Children's Hospital of San Francisco.)

TABLE SK−C−1.

Chondrodysplasia punctata

Conradi-Hünermann, autosomal dominant type
Rhizomelic, autosomal recessive type
X-linked dominant type
Sheffield, mild type
X-linked recessive type
Other variants
   Lethal, (?)autosomal recessive, subgroup A of Conradi-Hünermann type (Spranger 1974)
   Variable expression, autosomal or X-linked dominant type (Rattel)
   Mesomelic dysplasia with punctate epiphyseal calcificatype (Burck)
   Noonan-like varient of chondrodysplasia punctata (Saul)

umn, sternum, rib ends, coracoid processes, and glenoid fossae of scapulae, carpal and tarsal bones, ischium, pubis, Y cartilage of iliac bone and hyoid), in *soft tissue surrounding joints, epiphyseal centers,* and in cartilage of trachea and larynx; (c) *multiple dense calcifications of vertebrae in infancy; vertebral body deformities, scoliosis in childhood;* (d) other reported abnormalities: peripheral pulmonary artery stenosis at angiography; os odontodeum and C1−C2 instability; tracheal stenosis; (e) ultrasound diagnosis of fetal ascites (Straub) (Fig SK−C−6).

Chondro-osseous Morphology: (a) pathological calcification foci in areas of chondrocyte clusters; (b) numerous vascular channels in epiphyseal cartilage areas; (c) some scattered growth plate disruption (Gaulier).

Differential Diagnosis, Significant: (a) Other forms of chondrodysplasia punctata *(see Table* SK−C−1); (b) warfarin embryopathy; (c) alcohol embryopathy; (d) Zellweger syndrome; (e) multiple epiphyseal dysplasias; (f) other: see Gamut "stippled calcifications."

Special Comments: (a) Chondrodysplasia punctata, Conradi-Hünermann type, as well as the rhizomelic type, appears to represent a peroxisomal enzyme deficiency disease (Holmes); may be X-linked case; (b) chondrodysplasia punctata, Conradi-Hünermann type, is rarely lethal, but then called subgroup A; surviving early infancy, severe and asymmetric called subgroup B; mild with symmetric changes called subgroup C (Spranger 1974).

REFERENCES

Anderson PE, Justesen P: Chondrodysplasia punctata. *Skeletal Radiol.* 16:223−226, 1987.
Bethem D: Os odontoideum in chondrodystrophia calcificans congenita. *J. Bone Joint Surg. [Am.]* 64A:1385−1386, 1982.
Burck U: Mesomelic dysplasia with punctate epiphyseal calcifications. *Eur. J. Pediatr.* 138:67−72, 1982.
Camera G, et al: Condrodisplasia punctata autosomica dom-

inante con calcificazioni laringo-tracheali. _Pathologia_ 77:693–698, 1985.

Comings DE, et al.: Conradi's disease. _J. Pediatr._ 72:63–69, 1968.

Conradi E: Vorzeitiges Auftreten von Knochenund eigenartigen Verkalkungskermen bei Chondrodystrophia foetalis hypoplastica: Histologische und Roentgenuntersuchungen. _J. Kinderheilkd._ 80:86, 1914.

Curless RG: Dominant chondrodysplasia punctata with neurologic symptoms. _Neurology_ 33:1095–1097, 1983.

Galluzzi F, et al.: Deficit della chemiotassi cellulare in un caso di condrodistrofia punctata tipo Conradi-Hünermann. _Minerva Pediatr._ 32:555–562, 1980.

Gaulier A, et al.: Lethal chondrodysplasia punctata, Conradi-Hünermann subtype A: One case. _Pathol. Res. Pract._ 182:72–79, 1987.

Holmes RD, et al.: Peroxisomal enzyme deficiency in the Conradi-Hunermann form of chondrodysplasia punctata (letter). _N. Engl. J. Med._ 316:1608, 1987.

Hünermann C: Chondrodystrophia calcificans congenita als abortive Form der Chondrodystrophie. _Ztschr. Kinderheilkd._ 51:1, 1931.

Kozlowski S: Chondrodysplasia punctata in a nine-year-old girl presenting as "unclassified multiple malformation syndrome." _Pediatr. Radiol._ 9:236, 1980.

Paltzik RL, et al.: Conradi-Hunermann disease. _Cutis_ 29:174–180, 1982.

Saul RA, Stevenson RE: Chondrodysplasia punctata: Another variant. _Proc Greenwood Genetic Center_ 1:58–62, 1982.

Silengo MC, et al.: Clinical and genetic aspects of Conradi-Hünermann disease. _J. Pediatr._ 97:911, 1980.

Spranger J, et al.: Chondrodysplasia punctata (chondrodystrophia calcificans). I: Typ. Conradi-Hünermann. _Fortschr. Roentgenstr._ 113:717, 1970.

Spranger JW, et al.: Heterogeneity of chondrodysplasia punctata. _Humangenetik_ 11:190–212, 1974.

Straub W, et al.: Fetal ascites associated with Conradi's disease. _J. Clin. Ultrasound_ 11:234–236, 1983.

Theander G, et al.: Calcification in chondrodysplasia punctata: Relation to ossification and skeletal growth. _Acta Radiol. [Diagn.]_ 19:205, 1978.

Trowitzsch E, et al.: Severe pulmonary arterial stenosis in Conradi-Hunermann disease. _Eur. J. Pediatr._ 145:116–118, 1986.

CHONDRODYSPLASIA PUNCTATA, RHIZOMELIC TYPE

Synonyms: Chondrodysplasia punctata, recessive type; dysplasia epiphysealis congenita, stippled epiphyses; chondrodysplasia epiphysealis punctata; chondrodystrophia calcificans.

Mode of Inheritance: Autosomal recessive.

Frequency: Common; one of most frequently seen types of chondrodysplasia punctata (1 per 84,000 live births).

Clinical Manifestations: (a) _symmetric rhizomelic short-limb dwarfism;_ (b) _craniofacial dysmorphism:_ flat face, upward slanting palpebral fissures, microcephaly, lymphedema of cheeks, micrognathia; (c) _cataracts_ (72%); (d) _ichthyosi-_ _form skin lesions, alopecia;_ (e) _joint contractures;_ (f) other reported abnormalities: foot deformities; cleft palate; congenital heart disease; optic atrophy; facial paralysis; mental retardation; spastic quadriplegia; umbilical cord hernia; pulmonary hypoplasia; (g) usually fatal within first year of life; survival to age 10½ years, 1 case (Saul).

Radiologic Manifestations: (a) _symmetric shortening of proximal and other long bones,_ (b) _punctate calcific deposits in infantile cartilaginous skeleton and periarticular regions, mild or absent stippling of axial skeleton,_ laryngeal and tracheal calcification less common; (c) gradual diminution or disappearance of stippling in first year of life; (d) _coronal clefts of vertebrae;_ (e) prenatal diagnosis, ultrasound (Figs SK–C–7 and SK–C–8).

Chondro-osseous Morphology: (a) severe disturbance of enchondral bone formation; (b) lack of columnar arrangement; (c) cancellous bone formed directly on resting cartilage, especially in necrotic areas.

Differential Diagnosis, Significant: (a) other forms of chondrodysplasia punctata (Table SK–C–1); (b) warfarin embryopathy; (c) alcohol embryopathy; (d) Zellweger syndrome; (e) chromosome 18 and 21 syndromes; (f) other: _see Gamut_ "stippled calcifications."

Special Comments: Chondrodysplasia punctata, rhizomelic type, is a peroxisomal disorder without an abnormality in bile acid synthesis (Clayton).

REFERENCES

Chandavasa O, Desposito F: Umbilical cord hernia in a child with autosomal recessive chondrodysplasia punctata. _J. Med. Genet._ 23:84–86, 1985.

Clayton PT, et al.: Plasma bile acids in patients with peroxisomal dysfunction syndromes. _Eur. J. Pediatr._ 146:166–173, 1987.

Connor JM, et al.: Lethal neonatal chondrodysplasias in the west of Scotland 1970–1983. _Am. J. Med. Genet._ 22:243–253, 1985.

Gilbert EF, et al.: Chondrodysplasia punctata—rhizomelic form. _Eur. J. Pediatr._ 123:89, 1976.

Harrod ME, et al.: Prenatal diagnosis of rhizomelic chondrodysplasia punctata. _Proc. Greenwood Genetic Center._ 4:148, 1985.

Heselson NG, et al.: Lethal chondrodysplasia punctata. _Clin. Radiol._ 29:679, 1978.

Moser HW: Peroxisomal disorders. _J. Pediatr._ 108:89–91, 1986.

Saul RA, Stevenson RE: Prolonged survival in chondrodysplasia punctata, rhizomelic type. _Proc. Greenwood Genetic Center_ 1:63–65, 1982.

Spranger JW, et al.: Chondrodysplasia punctata (chondrodystrophia calcificans). II: Der rhizomele Typ. _Fortschr. Roentgenstr._ 114:327, 1971.

Theander G, et al.: Calcification in chondrodysplasia punctata: Relation to ossification and skeletal growth. _Acta Radiol [Diagn.]_ 19:205, 1978.

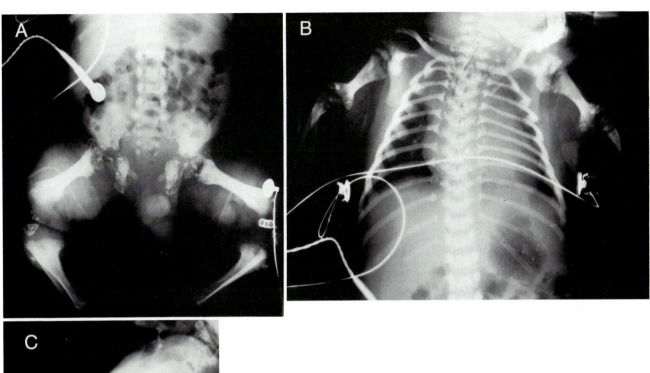

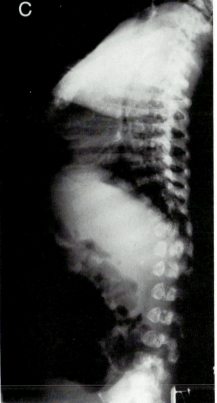

FIG SK−C−7.
Chondrodysplasia punctata, rhizomelic type. **A,** newborn: stippling, rhizomelia (short femurs). **B,** newborn: stippling (also of spine), rhizomelia (short humeri). **C,** 10-week-old infant: coronal clefting of vertebrae, posterior tracheal calcification.

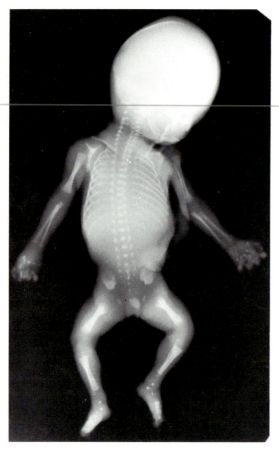

FIG SK—C—8.
Chondroplasia punctata, rhizomelic type; 19-week fetus: rhizomelia; stippling, especially in ankles.

CHONDRODYSPLASIA PUNCTATA, SHEFFIELD TYPE

Synonym: Chondrodysplasia punctata, mild form.

Mode of Inheritance: Not known.

Frequency: Uncommon but underdiagnosed; about 25 reported cases.

Clinical Manifestations: (a) *Failure to thrive;* (b) *mental retardation,* mild; (c) *abnormal, typical facies; flattened tip of nose;* depressed nasal bridge; (d) older parental age; 2:1 male-female ratio.

Radiologic Manifestations: (a) *stippling* (paint-splattered) replacing ossification of *calcaneus* in infancy; hypoplastic and/or multicentered calcaneus in later life; (b) sacral and coccygeal stippling; rarely, stippling in other areas (greater trochanter of femur, lateral masses of vertebrae, proximal humerus); (c) coronal and sagittal clefts of vertebrae (Fig SK—C—9).

Differential Diagnosis, Significant: (a) other forms of chondrodysplasia punctata (*see Table* SK—C—1); (b) warfarin

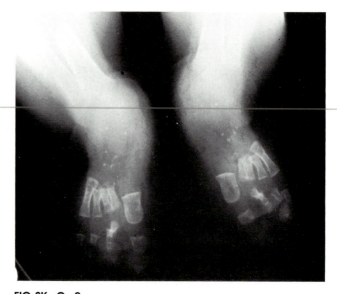

FIG SK—C—9.
Chondrodysplasia punctata, Sheffield type; 6-month-old infant: punctate calcifications in talocalcaneal area.

embryopathy; (c) alcohol embryopathy; (d) Zellweger syndrome; (e) chromosome 18 and 21 syndromes; (f) Osebold-Remondini syndrome; (g) other: *see Gamut* "stippled calcification."

REFERENCES

Sheffield LJ, et al.: Chondrodysplasia punctata: 23 cases of a mild and relatively common variety. *J. Pediatr.* 89:916–923, 1976.

CHONDRODYSPLASIA PUNCTATA, X-LINKED DOMINANT TYPE

Synonyms: Chondrodysplasia punctata, Conradi-Hünermann type subgroup B.

Mode of Inheritance: X-linked dominant; lethal in males.

Frequency: Uncommon; 43 reported cases.

Clinical Manifestations: (a) *skin lesions in a linear or blotchy pattern;* congenital ichthyosiform erythroderma, atrophoderma (especially hair follicles); circumscribed alopecia (sparse eyebrows and lashes); flattened, split nails; (b) flat nasal bridge; frontal bossing; high arched palate; (c) *asymmetric shortening of limbs;* (d) flexion contractures; foot deformities; polydactyly (three cases); (e) *scoliosis;* neck shortening; (f) *cataracts* (65%).

Radiological Manifestations: (a) *identical to Conradi-Hünermann type;* (b) *stippling of epiphyseal center regions and vertebral column;* asymmetric shortening of long bones (especially femurs and humeri); dislocated patellae; clefting or wedging of vertebrae; (c) *gradual disappearance of stippling in later life.*

Differential Diagnosis, Significant: (a) other forms of chondrodysplasia punctata, especially Conradi-Hünermann type *(Table* SK – C – 1); (b) incontinenti pigmenti; (c) warfarin embryopathy; (d) alcohol embryopathy; (e) Zellweger syndrome; (f) multiple epiphyseal dysplasias; (g) other: see Gamut "stippled calcification."

Special Comments: This X-linked disorder has an interesting clinical and radiographic genetic homologue in the mouse (Happle). This disorder may have mild affectation in female family members (Mueller). X-linked affectation may be difficult to substantiate, because the manifestations are so similar to the autosomal dominant disorder (Conradi-Hünermann) and rest primarily on the typical skin changes.

REFERENCES

Happle R, et al.: Sex-linked chondrodysplasia punctata? *Clin. Genet.* 11:73 – 76, 1977.
Happle R: X-linked dominant chondrodysplasia punctata. *Hum. Genet.* 53:65 – 73, 1979.
Happle R, et al.: Homologous genes for X-linked chondrodysplasia punctata in man and mouse. *Hum. Genet.* 63:24 – 27, 1983.
Kolde G, Happle R: Histologic and ultrastructural features of the ichthyotic skin in X-linked dominant chondrodysplasia punctata. *Acta Venereol.* 64:389 – 394, 1984.
Manzke H, et al.: Dominant sex-linked inherited chondrodysplasia punctata: A distinct type of chondrodysplasia punctata. *Clin. Genet.* 17:97 – 107, 1980.
Mueller RF, et al.: X-linked dominant chondrodysplasia punctata: *Am. J. Med. Genet.* 20:137 – 144, 1985.
Norwood C, et al.: Further delineation of X-linked dominant chondrodysplasia punctata. *Proc Greenwood Genetic Center* 4:130 – 131, 1985.
Scheibenreiter S, Melzer E: Chondrodystrophia calcificans congenita observed over 6 years. *Padiatr. Padol.* 17:521 – 528, 1982.

CHONDRODYSPLASIA PUNCTATA, X-LINKED RECESSIVE TYPE

Mode of Inheritance: X-linked recessive; deletion of portion of short arm of X chromosome.

Frequency: Very rare; two families, four patients.

Clinical Manifestations: (a) *nasal hypoplasia;* hearing loss, cataract; (b) *ichthyosis;* sparse hair; (c) *mental retardation;* mild short stature; (d) *no steroid sulfatase enzyme activity.*

Radiologic Manifestations: (a) *resembles Conradi-Hünermann type;* (b) *diffuse stippling* of epiphyseal, paravertebral, laryngeal, and tracheal areas; rapid disappearance of stippling; (c) hypoplasia of distal phalanges; (d) fetal postmor-

tem radiographs 14-22 weeks: distal phalangeal hypoplasia and abnormal metaphyseal cupping of long bones; (e) *normal length of long bones.*

Differential Diagnosis, Significant: (a) other forms of chondrodysplasia punctata, especially Conradi-Hünermann type *(see Table* SK – C – 1); (b) warfarin and alcohol embryopathy; (c) Zellweger syndrome; (d) other forms of ichthyosis; (e) other: *see Gamut* "stippled calcification."

Special Comments: Only males affected; female carriers have mildly short stature.

REFERENCES

Curry CJR, et al.: Inherited chondrodysplasia punctata due to a deletion of the terminal short arm of an X chromosome. *N. Engl. J. Med.* 311:1010 – 1015, 1984.

CHONDROECTODERMAL DYSPLASIA

Synonyms: Ellis – van Creveld syndrome; chondrodysplasia ectodermica; chondrodysplasia tridermica; mesoectodermal dysplasia.

Mode of Inheritance: Autosomal recessive.

Frequency: Common; about 170 cases reported to 1988 (0.9 per 100,000 births); high incidence in Amish, 89 cases (McKusick).

Clinical Manifestations: Present at birth: (a) *disproportionate short-limbed dwarfism (centrifugal shortening);* (b) *polydactyly hands* (almost 100%), *feet* (about 25%); (c) *hidrotic ectodermal dysplasia: koilonychia and hypoplasia of nails, hypoplasia and dysplasia of teeth* (natal teeth, retarded eruption of teeth, irregularity and incompleteness of teeth, dentine defect, dental caries), *sparse hair;* (d) *congenital heart disease* (60%); atrial septal defect and single atrium most common anomalies; (e) *fusion between upper lip and gum;* (f) other reported associated abnormalities: strabismus, cleft palate, lobar emphysema, situs inversus, nephrocalcinosis, neonatal gallstones, various genital anomalies, mental retardation; renal tubular dysplasia and dysgenesis; Dandy-Walker malformation; homozygosity for 9qh+; retinal dystrophy; cerebral heterotopias; respiratory tract infections (infancy); (g) prenatal diagnosis: fetoscopy.

Radiologic Manifestations: (a) *shortness of ribs;* (b) *short and heavy tubular bones;* (c) *bowed femur; premature ossification of capital femoral epiphysis; hypoplasia of proximal tibial ossification center;* short medial and long lateral slope of metaphysis; genu valgum; *exostosis of medial aspect of proximal tibial shaft;* marked shortening of fibula; (d) *flared hypoplastic iliac wing (trident);* small sciatic notch; (e) bowed humerus; *bony spike in medial side of distal metaphysis of humerus in newborn; enlarged proximal end of ulna and distal end of radius;* synmetacarpalism; fusion of capitate and

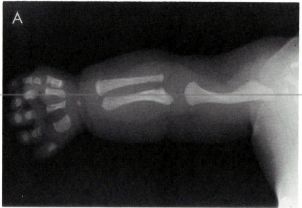

FIG SK–C–10.
Chondroectodermal dysplasia (Ellis–van Creveld syndrome).
One-day-old term infant boy with dwarfism, polydactyly, hypoplastic nails, two erupted teeth, multiple frenula, bitemporal alopecia, and congenital heart disease (common atrium, preductal coarctation of aorta, patent ductus arteriosus, and persistent left superior vena cava). **A,** tubular bones are short, heavy, and mildly bowed; carpal ossification and polydactyly are present. **B,** flared hypoplastic iliac wings, trident deformity of acetabular roofs, premature ossification of femoral capital epiphyses, lack of ossification of epiphyses in knee region, marked shortening of fibulae and three ossification centers in each tarsal region.

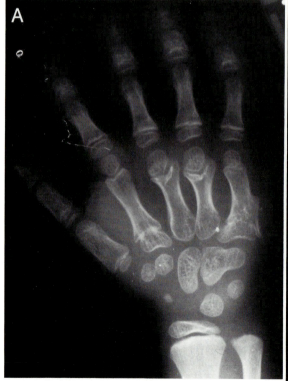

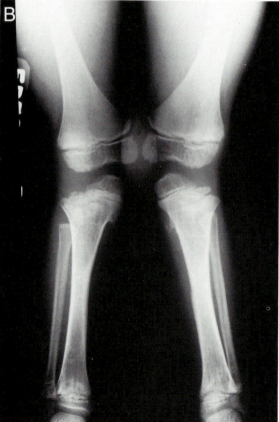

FIG SK–C–11.
Chondroectodermal dysplasia (Ellis–van Creveld syndrome) in a 7-year-old child. . **A,** residua of polydactyly, cone-shaped epiphyses, beginning carpal fusion. **B,** severe hypoplasia of lateral portions of proximal tibial epiphyses.

hamate (7%); *ninth carpal bone* (after 5 years, all cases; other carpal fusions (71%); delay in maturation of carpal bones and accelerated maturation of phalanges; *cone-shaped epiphyses of middle phalanges 2–5; polydactyly of hands and feet*; synmetatarsalism; missing tarsal bone; (f) skull and spine usually normal; (g) prenatal diagnosis (ultrasound): limb shortening (may not be present); *polydactyly; short ribs* four cases, confirmed. (Figs SK–C–10 and SK–C–11)

Differential Diagnosis, Significant: (a) asphyxiating thoracic dysplasia; (b) short-rib polydactyly syndromes.

REFERENCES

Berardi JC, et al.: Syndrome d'Ellis van Creveld. Apport de l'echographie dans le diagnostic prenatal. *J. Gynecol. Obstet. Biol. Reprod.* 14:43–47, 1985.

Blackburn MG, et al.: Ellis–van Creveld syndrome: A report of previously undescribed anomalies in two siblings. *Am. J. Dis. Child.* 122:267, 1971.

Bui TH, et al.: Prenatal diagnosis of chondroectodermal dysplasia with fetoscopy. *Prenat. Diagn.* 4:155–159, 1984.

Caffey J: Chondroectodermal dysplasia (Ellis–van Creveld syndrome): Report of three cases. *Am. J. Roentgenol.* 68:875, 1952.

Calver D, et al.: The extra digit. A pointer to the eye? *Trans. Ophthal. Soc. UK* 101:35–38, 1981.

Christian JC, et al.: A family with three recessive traits and homozygosity for a long 9qh+ chromosome segment. *Am. J. Med. Genet.* 6:301–308, 1980.

Ellis RWB, van Creveld S: A syndrome characterized by ectodermal dysplasia, polydactyly, chondrodystrophia and congenital morbus cordis. *Arch. Dis. Child.* 15:65, 1940.

Jéquier S, et al.: The Ellis–van Creveld syndrome, in Kaufmann HJ (ed.): *Progress in Pediatric Radiology*, vol. 4. Basel, Karger, 1973, p. 167.

Kunze VP: Ellis–van Creveld syndrome. *Kinderarztl. Prax.* 48:193–198, 1980.

Lynch JI, et al.: Congenital heart disease and chondroectodermal dysplasia. *Am. J. Dis. Child.* 115:80, 1968.

McKusick VA: The Amish. *Endeavor* 4:52–57, 1980.

Mahoney MJ, Hobbins JC: Prenatal diagnosis of chondroectodermal dysplasia (Ellis–van Creveld syndrome) with fetoscopy and ultrasound. *N. Engl. J. Med.* 297:258–260, 1977.

Muller LM, Cremin BJ: Ultrasonic demonstration of fetal skeletal dysplasia. *S. Afr. Med. J.* 67:222–226, 1985.

Rosenberg S, et al.: Brief clinical report: Chondroectodermal dysplasia (Ellis–van Creveld) with anomalies of CNS and urinary tract. *Am. J. Med. Genet.* 15:291–295, 1983.

Suguna Bai NS, et al.: Ellis–van Creveld syndrome. *Indian J. Pediatr.* 50:227–229, 1983.

Taylor GA, et al.: Polycarpaly and other abnormalities of the wrist in chondroectodermal dysplasia: The Ellis–van Creveld syndrome. *Radiology* 151:393–396, 1984.

Verschaerer V, et al.: The radiological diagnosis of the Ellis–van Creveld syndrome in the newborn. Report of one case. *J. Belge. Radiol.* 69:267–270, 1986.

Zangwill KM, et al: Dandy-Walker malformation in Ellis–van Creveld syndrome. *Am. J. Med. Genet.* 31:123–129, 1988.

CLEIDOCRANIAL DYSPLASIA

Synonyms: Scheuthauer-Marie-Sainton syndrome; cleidocranial dysostosis; mutational dysostosis; osteodental dysplasia; generalized dysostosis; pelvicocleidocranial dysplasia; cleidocranial-pubic dysostosis.

Historical Note: First mentioned in Homer's *Iliad* (Carter).

Mode of Inheritance: Autosomal dominant; spontaneous mutation in one third of cases; rare autosomal recessive in two families (Goodman).

Frequency: Very common; more than 800 patients reported to 1988 (0.5 per 100,000 live births).

Clinical Manifestations: (a) respiratory distress in newborn due to thoracic cage deformity; (b) *large brachycephalic head; large fontanelles and wide sutures in infancy, with delay in closure*; small face, saddle nose; (c) *delay in dental eruption; dental impaction; supernumerary teeth*; (d) *marked mobility of droopy shoulders*; (e) narrow chest; (f) abnormal gait; (g) mild shortness of stature; (h) other reported abnormalities: cleft palate; deafness; fragile bones; bilateral macrodactyly of second toes; β-thalassemia (one family); schwannoma (one case); syringomyelia (three cases); progressive scoliosis; Raynaud phenomenon; telangiectasia and epilepsy; diabetes.

Radiologic Manifestations: (a) *brachycephalic skull* with increased biparietal diameter, frontal bossing, *wide-spaced sutures, multiple sutural* (wormian) *bones*; absent parietal bone ossification; *anterior fontanelle remains open in adults*; posterior occipital synchondrosis persisting until 4 or 5 years of life; prominent notch in posterior border of foramen magnum; hypoplasia of body of sphenoid; hypoplasia of facial bones; *broad mandible, prognathism*; delayed closure of mental suture; high-arched palate; underdeveloped sinuses and mastoids; structural ossicular chain abnormalities; curved abnormal clivus; (b) persistence of synchondrosis between vertebral bodies and neural arches; spina bifida; scoliosis, kyphosis, *posterior wedging of thoracic vertebrae*, high incidence of spondylolysis of lumbar vertebrae; (c) short ribs with prominent downward slope, 11 ribs; lack of normal ossification of sternum; (d) *total aplasia (10%) or partial aplasia of clavicles; small scapulae*; broad appearance of tubular bones, various anomalies of bones of hands (*relatively long second and fifth metacarpals, short middle phalanges, tapering terminal phalanges, pseudepiphyses of metacarpals; cone-shaped epiphyses*; delay in skeletal maturation, supernumerary ossicles at different sites); (e) *absence or delayed ossification of pubic bones*, wide pubic symphysis in adults; *underdeveloped vertical, hypoplastic iliac wings*; cephalopelvic disproportion causing severe dystocia; (f) coxa vara or coxa valga; *undermodeling of long bones*; deformed femoral head and neck; congenital pseudoarthrosis of femur and tibia (three cases); shortness or absence of fibulae; deformity of ankle

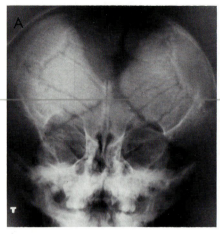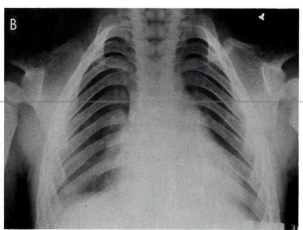

FIG SK–C–12.
Cleidocranial dysplasia in a 5-year-old boy with "soft shoulders" large head, prominent anterior fontanelle open down through forehead, and poor teeth. **A,** widely open sutures and fontanelle, and wormian bones. **B,** partial aplasia of clavicles, droopy shoulders, small scapulae, spina bifida, wide ribs.

joints, cone-shaped epiphyses of phalanges of toes; supernumerary epiphyseal centers of metatarsals; (g) delay in deciduous dentition; *very slow appearance of permanent teeth, some remaining unerupted, teeth irregularly placed; dental caries due to defective enamel, dentine, and cementum;* absent or supernumerary teeth; dentigerous cysts; early loss of "permanent" teeth. (Fig SK–C–12)

Differential Diagnosis, Significant: (a) pycnodysostosis; (b) congenital clavicular hypoplasia (including pseudoarthrosis of the clavicle-neurofibromatosis); (c) mandibuloacral dysplasia; (d) craniomandibular dermatodysostosis; (e) osteogenesis imperfecta; (f) hypophosphatasia; (g) parietal foraminal–cleidocranial dysplasia; (h) Yunis-Varon syndrome; (i) spondylomegaepiphyseal–metaphyseal dysplasia (SMMD); (j) partial trisomy 11q8, 11q/22q9, 20p trisomy; (k) scapuloiliac dysostosis.

Special Comments: (a) animal model, mouse (Sillence); ultrasound nomogram for evaluation of fetal clavicular size (Yarkoni); (b) recessively inherited cleidocranial dysplasia with imperforate anus, urogenital abnormalities, and psoriatic skin lesions has been reported in sibs (Fukuda).

REFERENCES

Alexander WN, Ferguson RL: Beta thalassemia minor and cleidocranial dysplasia: *Oral Surg.* 49:413–418, 1980.

Carter CO: Cleidocranial dysostosis in the *Iliad. Lancet* 2:323, 1973.

Fauré C, et al.: Cleidocranial dysplasia, in Kaufmann HJ (ed.): *Progress in Pediatric Radiology,* Basel, Karger, 1973, vol. 4, p. 211.

Dore DD, et al.: Cleidocranial dysostosis and syringomyelia. *Clin. Orthop.* 214:229–234, 1987.

Fukuda K, et al.: Two siblings with cleidocranial dysplasia associated with atresia ani and psoriasis-like lesions: A new syndrome? *Eur. J. Pediatr.* 136:109–111, 1981.

Goodman RM, et al.: Evidence for an autosomal recessive form of cleidocranial dysostosis. *Clin. Genet.* 8:20–29, 1975.

Hawkins HB, et al.: The association of cleidocranial dysostosis with hearing loss. *Am. J. Roentgenol.* 125:944, 1975.

Jarvis JL, et al.: Cleidocranial dysostosis: A review of 40 new cases. *Am. J. Roentgenol.* 121:5, 1974.

Keats TE: Cleidocranial dysostosis: Some atypical roentgen manifestations: *AJR* 100:71–74, 1967.

Kreiborg S, et al.: Abnormalities of the cranial base in cleidocranial dysostosis. *Am. J. Orthod.* 79:549–557, 1981.

Marie P, Sainton P: Observation d'hydrocéphalie héréditaire (pére et fils) par vice de dévelopment du crâne et du cerveau. *Bull. Mem. Soc. Med. Hop. Paris* 14:706, 1897.

Scheuthauer G: Kombination rudimentarer Schlüsselbeine mit Anomalien des Schädels beim erwachsenen Menschen. *Allg. Wien. Med. Ztg.* 16:293, 1871.

Sillence DO, et al: Animal models: Skeletal anomalies in mice with cleidocranial dysplasia. *Am. J. Med. Genet.* 27:75–85, 1987.

Tan KL, Tan LKA: Cleidocranial dysostosis in infancy. *Pediatr. Radiol.* 11:114–116, 1981.

Yarkoni S, et al. Clavicular measurement: A new biometric parameter for fetal evaluation. *J. Ultrasound Med.* 4:467, 1985.

CRANIODIAPHYSEAL DYSPLASIA

Synonym: Leontiasis ossea.

Mode of Inheritance: Usually autosomal recessive; autosomal dominant, one family (Schaefer).

Frequency: Rare; about 19 cases to 1988.

Clinical Manifestations: (a) *progressive facial and cranial thickening;* (b) *mental and growth retardation* in many cases; (c) nasal obstruction; (d) increasing deafness; (e) loss of vision; (f) seizures secondary to vascular occlusion; sudden death.

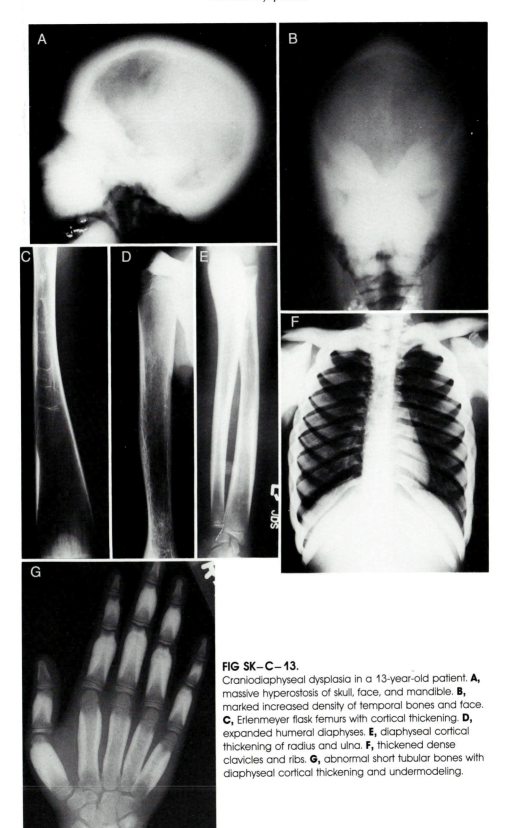

FIG SK–C–13.
Craniodiaphyseal dysplasia in a 13-year-old patient. **A,** massive hyperostosis of skull, face, and mandible. **B,** marked increased density of temporal bones and face. **C,** Erlenmeyer flask femurs with cortical thickening. **D,** expanded humeral diaphyses. **E,** diaphyseal cortical thickening of radius and ulna. **F,** thickened dense clavicles and ribs. **G,** abnormal short tubular bones with diaphyseal cortical thickening and undermodeling.

Radiologic Manifestations: (a) *marked thickening* and sclerosis of calvaria and facial bones *(leontiasis ossea);* hydrocephalus; cranial foraminal obliteration; (b) obliteration of paranasal sinuses; (c) *moderate widening and sclerosis of ribs;* (d) *extensive thickening and sclerosis of clavicles;* (e) *straight and cylindrical long bone diaphyses; hyperostotic diaphyseal widening, with increased cortex of other tubular bones* (hands and feet); (f) increased density of neural arches of vertebrae. (Fig SK−C−13)

Differential Diagnosis, Significant: Craniotubular dysplasia, especially: (a) craniometaphyseal dysplasia; (b) sclerosteosis; (c) Van Buchem syndrome.

Special Comments: The movie "Mask" (Universal Studios, 1985) accurately depicts a patient with craniodiaphyseal dysplasia (Kaitila; Kirkpatrick).

REFERENCES

Bonucci E, et al.: Histologic, microradiographic and electron-microscopic investigations of bone tissue in a case of craniodiaphyseal dysplasia. Virchows Arch. [A] 373:167−175, 1977.

Briani S, Cuvaliere R: Un caso di osteopatia petrofizzante poliostoficá con monstrusá et abnorme localizzazione craniofacciole. *Clin. Orthop.* 12:351−366, 1960.

de Souza O: Leontiasis ossea: Porto Alegre (Brazil). *Faculdade Med. Rev. Cursos* 13:47, 1927.

Gemmel JH: Leontiasis ossea: A clinical and roentgenological entity. *Radiology* 25:723, 1935.

Gorlin R, et al.: Genetic craniotubular bone dysplasias and hyperostosis: A critical analysis. *Birth Defects* 5(4):79−95, 1969.

Halliday J: A rare case of bone dysplasia. *Br. J. Surg.* 37:52, 1949.

Joseph R, et al.: Dysplasie cranio-diaphysaire progressive: Ses relation avec la dysplasie diaphysaire progressive de Camurti-Engelmann. *Ann. Radiol.* 1:477, 1958.

Kaitila I, et al.: Craniodiaphyseal dysplasia. *Birth Defects* 11(6):359−362, 1975.

Kirkpatrick D, et al.: The craniotubular bone modeling disorders: A neurosurgical introduction to rare skeletal dysplasias with cranial nerve compression. *Surg. Neurol.* 7:221−232, 1977.

Levy MH, Kozlowski K: Cranial-diaphyseal dysplasia: Report of a case. *Australas. Radiol.* 31:431−435, 1987.

Macpherson RI: Craniodiaphyseal dysplasia: A disease or group of diseases? *J. Can. Assoc. Radiol.* 25:22, 1974.

Scarfo GB, et al.: Idrocefalo associato à displasia craniodiafisaria. *Radiol. Med.* 65:249, 1979.

Schaefer B, et al.: Dominantly inherited craniodiaphyseal dysplasia: A new craniotubular dysplasia. *Clin. Genet.* 30:381−391, 1986.

Stransky E, et al.: On Paget's disease with leontiasis ossea and hyperthreosis starting in early childhood. *Ann. Paediatr.* 199:393−408, 1962.

Tucker AS, et al.: Craniodiaphyseal dysplasia: Evolution over a five-year period. *Skeletal Radiol.* 1:47, 1976.

CRANIOMETAPHYSEAL DYSPLASIA

Synonym: Pyle disease, separated out as *distinct* (Gorlin).

Mode of Inheritance: Autosomal recessive more severe, 15 patients in 9 sibships (Penchaszadeh); autosomal dominant milder and more common.

Frequency: Uncommon; approximately 66 cases to 1988.

Clinical Manifestations: (a) *Abnormal craniofacial features:* large and broad head; frontal bossing; hypertelorism; flat nasal root; large mandible; open mouth due to nasal obstruction; (b) neurologic manifestations: cranial nerve involvement (optic atrophy, progressive deafness, facial nerve paralysis); hemiplegia, quadriplegia, medullary compression; (c) defective dentition; (d) mental and motor retardation; (e) vascular occlusion.

Radiologic Manifestations: (a) *progressive diffuse hyperostosis of cranial vault, base, and facial bones; cranial foraminal narrowing;* accentuated bands of ossification along cranial sutures; (b) *obliteration of paranasal sinuses and mastoids;* (c) *hypertelorism;* (d) *flaring and widening of metaphyses of tubular bones;* (e) ground glass alveolar bone (mandible) with loss of lamina dura; (f) other reported abnormalities: cervical spine deformity (two cases); hydrocephalus. (Fig SK−C−14)

Differential Diagnosis, Significant: Craniotubular dysplasia especially: (a) craniodiaphyseal dysplasia; (b) Pyle dysplasia; (c) sclerosteosis; (d) frontometaphyseal dysplasia.

Special Comments: Although the clinical and radiographic findings are more severe in autosomal recessive disease, the genetics may be unclear in an isolated case because of clinical and familial heterogeneity and overlap. Reciprocal translocation 46,XX,t(12;18)(q13q12) in a single case (Yamada).

REFERENCES

Allen HA, et al.: Vascular involvement in cranial hyperostosis. *AJNR* 3:193−195, 1982.

Beighton P, et al.: Craniometaphyseal dysplasia—Variability of expression within a large family. *Clin Genet.* 15:252, 1979.

Bricker SL, et al.: Dominant craniometaphyseal dysplasia. *Dentomaxillofac. Radiol.* 12:95−100, 1983.

Carlson DH, et al.: Craniometaphyseal dysplasia: A family with three documented cases. *Radiology* 103:147, 1972.

Carnevale A, et al.: Autosomal dominant craniometaphyseal dysplasia. Clinical variability. *Clin. Genet.* 23:17−22, 1983.

Gorlin RJ, et al.: Pyle's disease (familial metaphyseal dysplasia): A presentation of two cases and argument for its sep-

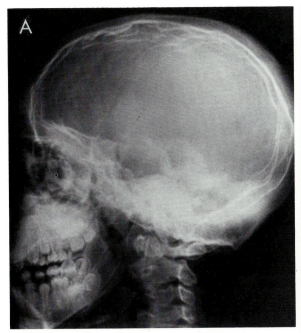

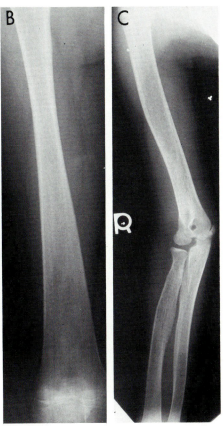

FIG SK–C–14.
Craniometaphyseal dysplasia in a 10-year-old girl with a history of right-sided facial weakness at 3 years of age and gradual bilateral hearing loss. **A,** diffuse hyperostosis of cranial vault, base, and facial bones. **B** and **C,** flaring and widening of metaphyses of tubular bones.

aration from craniometaphyseal dysplasia. *J. Bone Joint Surg. [Am.]* 52–A:347, 1970.

Halal F, et al: (Cranial)-metaphyseal dysplasia with maxillary hypoplasia and brachydactyly (characteristic facies). *Am. J. Med. Genet.* 13:71–79, 1982.

Holt JF: The evolution of cranio-metaphyseal dysplasia. *Ann. Radiol.* 9:209, 1966.

Hudgins RJ, Edwards MDB: Craniometaphyseal dysplasia associated with hydrocephalus: Case report. *Neurosurgery* 29:617–618, 1987.

Jend H: Cranial-metaphyseal-striatiform dysplasia (linen striata). *Eur. J. Radiol.* 1:261–265, 1981.

Penchaszadeh VB, et al.: Autosomal recessive craniometa-physeal dysplasia. *Am. J. Med. Genet.* 5:43–55, 1980.

Rimoin DL, et al.: Craniometaphyseal dysplasia (Pyle's disease): Autosomal dominant inheritance in a large kindred. *Birth Defects* 5(4):96–104, 1969.

Saper JR, et al.: Cranial metaphyseal dysplasia: A cause of recurrent bilateral facial palsy. *Arch. Neurol.* 31:204, 1974.

Shea J, et al.: Craniometaphyseal dysplasia: The first successful surgical treatment for associated hearing loss. *Laryngoscope* 91:1369–1374, 1981.

Yamada H, et al.: Cervical spinal deformity in craniometa-physeal dysplasia. *Surg. Neurol.* 27:284–290, 1987.

D

de la CHAPELLE DYSPLASIA

Synonyms: "Ring around the chondrocyte" dysplasia; neonatal osseous dysplasia type I.

Mode of Inheritance: Autosomal recessive.

Frequency: Very rare; four cases to 1988.

Clinical Manifestations: *Neonatally lethal;* (a) *cleft palate, small thorax; equinovarus with wide-spaced first and second toes;* (b) tracheomalacia, malformed stenotic larynx; pulmonary hypoplasia (c) genitourinary system anomalies; (d) polyhydramnios.

Radiologic Manifestations: (a) short slender ribs, small vertebrae, *platyspondyly; "tongue" anterior projection;* (b) *clubbed humerus* with proximal metaphyseal widening; irregular short curved radius; absent ulna (or triangular remnant); short bent femurs; short bent tibia; absent fibula *(or triangular remnant)* (c) small irregular ileum; flat horizontal acetabular roofs.

Chondro-osseous Morphology: Distinctive; resting cartilage contains "ring" around the chondrocytes (lacunar halo).

Differential Diagnosis, Significant: (a) atelosteogenesis; (b) boomerang dysplasia.

Special Comments: de la Chapelle dysplasia may be the same condition as atelosteogenesis type 2.

REFERENCES

de la Chapelle A, et al.: Une rare dysplasie osseuse lethale de transmission recessive autosomique. *Arch. Fr. Pediatr.* 29:759–770, 1972.
Salonen R.: Neonatal osseous dysplasia: *Prog. Clin. Biol. Res.* 104:171–172, 1982.
Whitley CB, et al.: de la Chapelle dysplasia. *Am. J. Med. Genet.* 25:29–39, 1986.

DIAPHYSEAL DYSPLASIA (ENGELMANN DISEASE)

Synonyms: Camurati-Engelmann disease; progressive diaphyseal dysplasia; osteopathica hyperostotica (sclerotisans) multiplex infantilis.

Mode of Inheritance: Autosomal dominant.

Frequency: Common; approximately 138 cases to 1988.

Clinical Manifestations: Usual onset in childhood: (a) *waddling gait; muscular weakness; extremity pain;* asthenic habitus; decreased muscle mass; genu valgum; shiny tightly stretched skin over tibia and maxilla; (b) other clinical abnormalities: diverse ocular manifestations including diplopia, cataract, vision loss, *exopthalmos* (50%), optic atrophy, tortuosity of retinal veins; progressive hearing loss; delayed puberty; increased intracranial pressure; Raynaud phenonemon; splenomegaly; facial palsy; vestibular dysfunction; recurrent bone marrow hypoplasia; elevated ESR; (c) clinical response to steroid therapy (Low; Naveh); (d) other reported abnormalities: neurofibromatosis (three patients, one family, Weickert); tumoral calcinosis (Thurman); *muscular dystrophy type of presentation* (Low); low muscle carnitine (Bye).

Radiologic Manifestations: (a) frontal and occipital bossing; *sclerotic changes at base of skull,* which may involve the cranial vault, and facial bones; narrowing of cranial nerve passages; dental caries; increased intracranial pressure (rare); (b) sclerosis of cervical vertebrae; (c) progressive *cortical sclerosis (internal and external) of diaphysis of long and short tubular bones,* rare metaphyseal involvement, asymmetric or unilateral sclerosis in some; *narrowing of medullary cavity;* (d) rare involvement of clavicles (medial two thirds), scapulae, and pelvic bones; (e) bone scintigraphy: increased bone activity, which may be discordant compared with radiographic manifestations; (f) other reported abnormalities: compression of vessels entering and leaving cranial vault); (g) CT findings: endosteal involvement greater than periosteal thickening; posterior vertebral involvement (body and arches)(Figs SK–D–1 to SK–D–3.

Chondro-osseous and Muscular Morphology: Rapid new bone formation (periosteal and endosteal; woven osteod; lack of haversian system development (Wirth); myopathic and vascular changes; atrophic muscle fibers; collagen accumulation; perivascular basement membrane thickening (Naveh) predomination of fast twitch fibers (Bosselmann).

Differential Diagnosis, Significant: (a) Ribbing disease (see Special Comments); (b) craniotubular dysplasias especially, van Buchem syndrome, craniodiaphyseal dysplasia; (c) Paget disease; (d) hyperphosphatasemia; (e) hyperostosis generalisata with striations of the bones; (f) diaphyseal medullary stenosis with *bone malignancy* (Hardcastle); (g) diaphyseal dysplasia, bowing, fractures, and *ichthyosis* (Koller).

Special Comments: Ribbing disease (hereditary multiple diaphyseal sclerosis) is thought to represent a milder form of diaphyseal dysplasia, with the same autosomal dominant inheritance. A porcine model for diaphyseal dysplasia is called

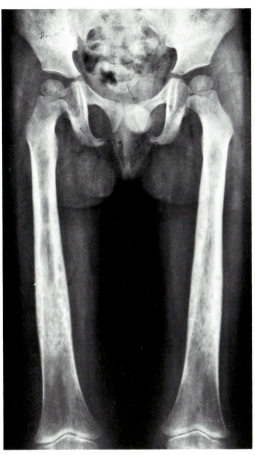

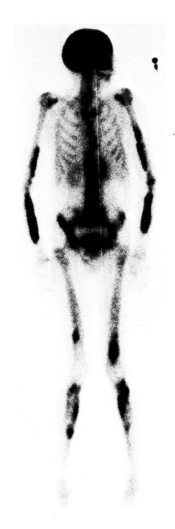

FIG SK–D–1.
Diaphyseal dysplasia (Engelmann disease) in a 3½-year-old boy who tired easily, had a peculiar wobbling gait, and complained of muscle pain on exertion. Internal and external cortical thickening of femoral shafts; metaphyses are normal. (From Girdany BR, Sane S, Graham CB: Engelmann's disease, in Kaufmann HJ (ed.): *Progress in Pediatric Radiology,* vol. 4. Basel, Karger, 1973, p. 414. Reproduced with permission.)

FIG SK–D–2.
Diaphyseal dysplasia (Engelmann disease) in a 47-year-old man. Bone scintigraphy shows diffusely increased activity. (From Kumar B, Murphy WA, Whyte MP: *Radiology* 140:87, 1981. Reproduced with permission.)

congenital porcine hyperostosis (Gibson). There is significant clinical variability within this syndrome.

REFERENCES

Bosselmann E, et al.: Myopathische Veranderangen bei der Diaphysaren Dysplasie: Camurati-Engelmann. *Beitr. Orthop. Tramatol.* 34:316–321, 1987.

Brodrick JD: Luxation of the globe in Engelmann's disease. *Am. J. Ophthalmol.* 83:870, 1977.

Bye AME: Progressive diaphyseal dysplasia and a low muscle carnitine. *Pediatr. Radiol.* 18:340, 1988.

Camurati M: Di un raro caso di osteite simmetrica ereditaria degli arti inferiori. *Chir. Organi Mov.* 6:662, 1922.

Crisp AJ, Brenton DP: Engelmann's disease of bone: A systemic disorder? *Ann. Rheum. Dis.* 41:183–188, 1982.

Engelmann G: Ein Fall von Osteopathia hyperostica (sclerotisans) multiplex infantalis. *Fortschr. Roentgenstr.* 39:1011, 1929.

Fallon MD, et al.: Progressive diaphyseal dysplasia (Engelmann's disease). *J. Bone Joint Surg. [Am.]* 62A:465, 1980.

Gibson JA, Rogers RJ: Congenital porcine hyperostosis (letter). *Austr. Veterin. J.* 56:254–255, 1980.

Hundley JD, Wilson FC: Progressive diaphyseal dysplasia. *J. Bone Joint Surg. [Am.]* 55A:461–474, 1973.

Kaftori JK, et al.: Progressive diaphyseal dysplasia (Camurati-Engelmann): Radiographic followup and CT findings. *Radiology* 164:777–782, 1987.

Koller ME: A familial syndrome of diaphyseal cortical thickening of the long bones, bowed legs, tendency to fracture and icthyosis. *Pediatr. Radiol.* 8:179–182, 1979.

Kumar B, et al.: Progressive diaphyseal dysplasia (Engelmann disease): Scintigraphic-radiographic-clinical correlations. *Radiology* 140:87–92, 1981.

Low LCK, et al.: Progressive diaphyseal dysplasia mimicking childhood myopathy. *Aust. Paediatr. J.* 21:193–196, 1985.

Lundy MM, et al.: Scintigraphic findings in progressive diaphyseal dysplasia. *J. Nucl. Med.* 23:324–325, 1982.

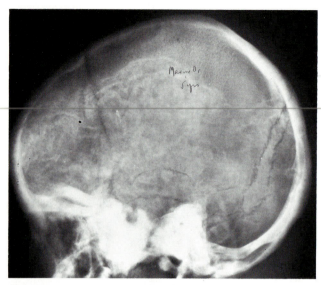

FIG SK–D–3.
Diaphyseal dysplasia (Engelmann disease) in a 5-year-old girl. Lateral film of skull shows marked sclerosis that affects base of skull and orbits. There are wavy bands of increased density in bones of cranial vault. (From Girdany BR, Sane S, Graham CB: Engelmann's disease, in Kaufmann HJ (ed.): *Progress in Pediatric Radiology*, vol. 4. Basel, Karger, 1973, p. 414. Reproduced with permission.)

Minford AMB, et al.: Engelmann's disease and the effect of corticosteroids: A case report. *J. Bone Joint Surg. [Br.]* 63B:597–600, 1981.
Naveh Y, et al.: Muscle involvement in progressive diaphyseal dysplasia. *Pediatrics* 76:944–949, 1985.
Naveh Y, et al: Progressive diaphyseal dysplasia: Evaluation of corticosteroid therapy. *Pediatrics* 75:321–323, 1985.
Naveh Y, et al.: Progressive diaphyseal dysplasia: Genetics and clinical and radiologic manifestations. *Pediatrics* 74:399–405, 1984.
Shier CK, et al.: Ribbing's disease: Radiographic-scintigraphic correlation and comparative analysis with Engelmann's disease. *J. Nucl. Med.* 28:244–248, 1987.
Thurman TF, et al.: Tumoral calcinosis and Engelmann disease. *Birth Defects* 12(5):136, 1976.
Van Dalsem VF, et al.: Progressive diaphyseal dysplasia. *J. Bone Joint Surg. [Am.]* 61A:596–598, 1979.
Verbruggen LA, et al.: Clinical and scintigraphic evaluation of corticosteroid treatment in a case of progressive diaphyseal dysplasia: *J. Rheumatol.* 12:809–813, 1985.
Weickert H, et al.: Diaphysäre dysplasie (Camurati-Engelmann). *Z. Orthop.* 121:744–748, 1983.
Wirth CR et al.: Diaphyseal dysplasia (Englemann's syndrome). *Clin. Orthop.* 171:186–195, 1982.
Yoshioka H, et al.: Muscular changes in Engelmann's disease. *Arch. Dis. Child.* 55:716, 1980.

DIAPHYSEAL MEDULLARY STENOSIS WITH BONE MALIGNANCY (HARDCASTLE)

Synonym: Hereditary bone dysplasia with malignant change.

Mode of Inheritance: Autosomal dominant.

Frequency: Very rare; 21 cases in three families.

Clinical Manifestations: *Fractures,* minimal trauma presentation; *cataract; osseous malignant fibrous histiocytoma (fibrosarcoma)* in 9 of 23 affected (second to fifth decades).

Radiologic Manifestations: *Diaphyseal cortical thickening; metaphyseal striations* and cystic changes.

Differential Diagnosis, Significant: (a) Kenny-Caffey disease; (b) Engelmann disease; (c) Paget disease.

REFERENCES

Hardcastle P, et al.: Hereditary bone dysplasia with malignant change. *J. Bone Joint Surg.* 68A:1079–1089, 1986.

DIASTROPHIC DYSPLASIA

Synonyms: Atypical achondroplasia; achondroplasia with clubbed hands and feet; cherub dwarf; diastrophic variant; epiphyseal dysostosis without dwarfism.

Mode of Inheritance: Autosomal recessive.

Frequency: Common; more than 300 cases reported to 1988 (0.2 per 100,000 births); high incidence in Finland (150 patients; Kaitila, personal communication).

Clinical Manifestations: Present at birth; (a) *variable micromelic dwarfism;* (b) *clubfoot, symphangilism of feet;* deformed great toes; (c) *ulnar deviation of hand;* irregular length of fingers; abduction of hypermobile and proximally inserted thumb *(hitchhiker thumb);* (d) *flexion contracture* and limitation of motion of peripheral joints; progressive postnatal joint dislocation; (e) progressive postnatal dorsal *lordosis* and *scoliosis;* (f) *deformed earlobes;* cystic masses in anthelix, which may rupture, with prominent scar formation *(cauliflower ear);* (g) *cleft or high-arched palate;* (h) other reported abnormalities: inguinal hernia; thick pectinate strands at root of iris; micrognathia; hyperelasticity of skin; cryptorchidism; abnormal glucose metabolism, lethal in neonatal period (12 cases; Gustavson); quadriplegia, cardiac malformations; mental retardation in some; trisomy 18 (trisomy E) mosaicism; death.

Radiologic Manifestations: (a) *short, thick, and clubbed tubular bones,* with delay in appearance of epiphyses, fragmentation of ossifying epiphyseal centers, epiphyseal invagination; (b) irregular length and form of metacarpals, metatarsals, and phalanges; *short, often ovoid first metacarpal with proximally located thumb;* longitudinal bracketed epiphysis; (c) *severe talipes equinovarus* with metatarsal fusions; (d) *deformed tarsal and carpal bones; accessory irregular carpal centers;* accelerated carpal center development; (e) delta wrist deformity; radial head dislocation; (f) abnormal pelvis; hypoplastic acetabulum and glenoid; (g) *multiple subluxations or dislocations;* (h) *progressive scoliosis and kyphosis;* platyspondyly and hypoplasia of cervical vertebrae; hyperplasia or hypoplasia of odontoid process; subluxation of atlas over axis; narrow interpediculate distances in lumbar region; *cervical kyphosis,* which may be progressive, causing neurologic changes; cord compression (MRI); significant cervical and sacral *posterior process clefting;* (i) *collapsible trachea due to abnormal cartilage tissue;* (j) *ossification of pinnae;*

premature costochondral and laryngeal cartilage calcification; intracranial calcification; (k) dislocated, multiple ossification centers or hypoplastic patellae; (l) prenatal diagnosis (ultrasound), (Fig SK–D–4).

Chondro-osseous Morphology and General Pathology:
(a) cystic areas in cartilage matrix with degenerating cells and fibrotic appearance; secondary fibro-ossification (dystrophic bone formation); (b) probably same process in ear and trachea; (c) electron microscopy; thick collagen fibers with ab-

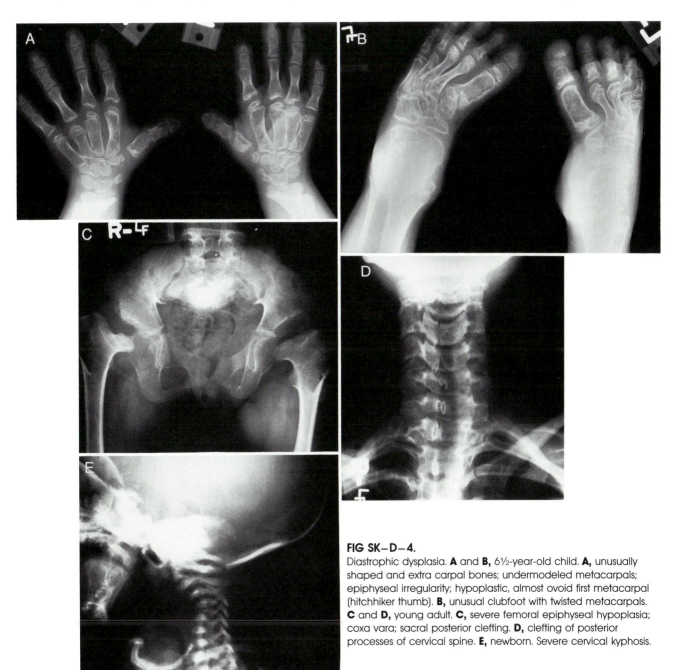

FIG SK–D–4.
Diastrophic dysplasia. **A** and **B,** 6½-year-old child. **A,** unusually shaped and extra carpal bones; undermodeled metacarpals; epiphyseal irregularity; hypoplastic, almost ovoid first metacarpal (hitchhiker thumb). **B,** unusual clubfoot with twisted metacarpals. **C** and **D,** young adult. **C,** severe femoral epiphyseal hypoplasia; coxa vara; sacral posterior clefting. **D,** clefting of posterior processes of cervical spine. **E,** newborn. Severe cervical kyphosis.

normal periodicity; (d) defect appears to represent abnormal collagen organization in cartilage.

Differential Diagnosis, Significant: (a) anthrogryposis; (b) spondyloepiphyseal dysplasia; (c) pseudodiatrophic dysplasia; (d) multiple epiphyseal dysplasia with clubbed feet.

Special Comments: (a) diastrophic variant cases with milder manifestations and classic diastrophic dysplasia are the same disorder (Lachman); (b) pseudodiastrophic dysplasia is entirely different; (c) short-limbed skeletal dysplasia with *congenital macular colobomas;* dumbbell long bones; generalized epiphyseal delay; histologic findings similar to diastrophic dysplasia (Smith).

REFERENCES

Bethem D, et al.: Disorders of the spine in diastrophic dwarfism. *J. Bone Joint Surg. [Am.]* 62A:529, 1980.
Eteson DJ, et al.: Pseudodiastrophic dysplasia: A distinct newborn skeletal dysplasia. *J. Pediatr.* 109:635–641, 1986.
Gollop TR, Eisler A: Prenatal ultrasound diagnosis of diastrophic dysplasia at 16 weeks. *Am. J. Med. Genet.* 27:321–324, 1987.
Gustavson KH, et al.: Lethal and non-lethal diastrophic dysplasia. *Clin. Genet.* 28:321–334, 1985.
Hall JG: Diastrophic dwarfism with ossicle malformation. *Birth Defects* 7(4):125, 1971.
Herring JA: The spinal disorders in diastrophic dwarfism. *J. Bone Joint Surg. [Am.]* 60A:177, 1978.
Holmgren G, et al.: A pair of siblings with diastrophic dysplasia and E trisomy mosaicism. *Hum. Hered.* 34:266–268, 1984.
Horton WA, et al.: Diastrophic dwarfism: A histochemical and ultrastructural study of the endochondral growth plate. *Pediatr. Res.* 13:904, 1979.
Horton WA, et al.: The phenotypic variability of diastrophic dysplasia. *J. Pediatr.* 93:609, 1978.
Kaitila J, et al.: Detection of diastrophic dysplasia in early pregnancy. *Duodecim* 99:861–868, 1983.
Krecak J, Starshak RJ: Cervical kyphosis in diastrophic dwarfism: CT and MR findings. *Pediatr. Radiol.* 17:321–322, 1987.
Lachman R, et al.: Diastrophic dysplasia: The death of a variant. *Radiology* 140:79, 1981.
Lamy M, Maroteaux P: Le nanisme diastrophique. *Presse Med.* 52:1977, 1960.
Langer LO: Diastrophic dwarfism in early infancy. *Am. J. Roentgenol.* 93:399, 1965.
Mantagos S, et al.: Prenatal diagnosis of diastrophic dysplasia. *Am. J. Obstet. Gynecol.* 139:111–113, 1981.
O'Brian GD, et al.: Early prenatal diagnosis of diastrophic dwarfism by ultrasound. *Br. Med. J.* 280:1300, 1980.
Queenan JT, et al.: Ultrasound measurement of fetal limb bones. *Am. J. Obstet. Gynecol.* 138:297–302, 1980.
Rintala A, et al.: Cleft palate in diastrophic dysplasia. *Scand. J. Plast. Reconstr. Surg. Hand Surg.* 20:45–49, 1986.
Smith RD, et al.: Brief clinical report: Congenital macular colobomas and short limb skeletal dysplasia. *Am. J. Med. Genet.* 5:365–371, 1980.
Stanescu V, et al.: Abnormal pattern of segment long spacing (SLS) cartilage collagen in diastrophic dysplasia. *Coll. Relat. Res.* 2:111–116, 1982.
Taybi H: Diastrophic dwarfism. *Radiology* 80:1, 1963.
Walker BA, et al.: Diastrophic dwarfism. *Medicine* 51:41–59, 1972.

DISTAL OSTEOSCLEROSIS

Mode of Inheritance: Autosomal dominant.

Frequency: Very rare; one report; five affected in two generations, one family; female affliction milder.

Clinical Manifestations: Clinically silent.

Radiologic Manifestations: (a) *mild calvarial hyperostosis and sclerosis at base;* (b) *expanded clavicles;* (c) mesomelic involvement; *radius, ulna, tibia, and fibula bowed, with cortical widening and sclerosis* ; (d) mild ilial sclerosis and striations of femoral neck; (e) vertebral pedicle sclerosis.

Differential Diagnosis, Significant: (a) craniotubular dysplasias; (b) osteopetrosis; (c) endosteal hyperostoses (van Buchem and Worth); (d) Weismann-Netter syndrome.

REFERENCES

Beighton P, et al.: Distal osteosclerosis. *Clin. Genet.* 18:298–304, 1980.

DOLICHOSPONDYLIC DYSPLASIA

Synonym: High vertebral body dwarfism.

Mode of Inheritance: Autosomal dominant (variable expressivity).

Frequency: Very rare; about eight cases to 1988.

Clinical Manifestations: *Short stature;* low IQ; unusual facies (in some).

Radiologic Manifestations: (a) *tall vertebral bodies;* (b) *gracile hand bones;* (c) steep ribs; (d) coxa vara.

Differential Diagnosis: 3-M syndrome (facies).

Special Comment: High vertebrae are often *secondary* to severe hypotonia with or without weight bearing.

REFERENCES

Barber et al.: Case report. *Birth Defects* 15(5B):355, 1979.
Flannery DB: Dolichospondylic dysplasia: Syndromic short stature with tall vertebral bodies. *Proc. Greenwood Genet. Center.* 3:96–97, 1984.

Fuhrmann W, et al.: Dwarfism with disproportionate high vertebral bodies. *Humangenetik* 16:271–282, 1972.
Rochiccioli P, Malpuech G: Dwarfism with high vertebral bodies. *Ann. Pediatr.* 30:709–712, 1983.

DYGGVE-MELCHIOR-CLAUSEN DYSPLASIA

Synonyms: Smith-McCort syndrome; modified hyaluronic acid mucopolysaccharidosis; pseudo-Morquio syndrome, type A.

Mode of Inheritance: Autosomal recessive.

Frequency: Uncommon; 47 cases to 1988 (includes Smith-McCort syndrome).

Clinical Manifestations: Usually diagnosed within the first year; (a) *small at birth; short stature;* (b) *microcephaly; psychomotor retardation* often severe (80%); feeding problems in infancy; (c) *short trunk, sternal protrusion;* scoliosis; *thoracic kyphosis* and *lumbar lordosis;* (d) *restricted joint mobility, waddling gait.*

Radiologic Manifestations: (a) microcephaly; (b) *spine: platyspondyly, anterior beaking of vertebral bodies, double vertebral hump with notch-like ossification defect of end plates,* posterior scalloping of vertebral bodies, elongation of vertebral laminae, *hypoplastic odontoid process; C1-C2 dislocation;* normal interpediculate distances; (c) thorax: broad chest, prominent anterior convexity of sternum, wide costochondral junctions; (d) *pelvis:* small iliac wings, irregular and *lacy iliac crests;* wide sacroiliac joint, small sacrosciatic notch; wide pubic ramus and ischiopubic synchondrosis; flat acetabular roof with irregular ossification; lateral displacement of femoral head; wide pubic symphysis; (e) shoulder: small scapula with irregularly ossified concave inferior angle, flat glenoid fossa, flaring of acromion; (f) *long bones:* shortening of long bones to varying degree, *irregular metaphyses (especially hips); multicentric ossification and deformities of proximal humeral and femoral epiphyses;* flat epiphyses in older children; (g) *hands and feet:* small carpal bones; short metacarpal and metatarsal bones; cone-shaped epiphyses, accessory epiphyses. (Figs SK–D–5 and SK–D–6)

Chondro-osseous Morphology and Biochemical Findings: Resting chondrocytes excessively vacuolated with cytoplasmic inclusions; at growth plate, degenerating cells replace columns with dystrophic calcification (lacy pelvis); EM: widened cysternae of rough endoplasmic reticulum; increased amounts of glucosaminoglycans in cartilage; elevated abnormal serum α_2-macroglobulin; normal proteoglycan degradation.

Differential Diagnosis, Significant: (a) Morquio disease (MPS IV); (b) spondyloepiphyseal dysplasia tarda.

Special Comments: *Morquio-like phenotype without mucopolysacchariduria, lacy pelvis,* and *double-humped*

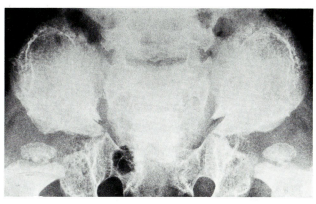

FIG SK–D–5.
Dyggve-Melchior-Clausen syndrome. Pelvis and hip joints of a patient at age 6 years. Characteristic lacy appearance of iliac crest, small iliac wing, wide sacroiliac joint, small sacroiliac notch, wide pubic ramus and ischiopubic synchondrosis, flat acetabular roof, lateral displacement of femoral head, and wide pubic symphysis. (From Schorr S, Legum C, Ochshorn M, et al.: *Am. J. Roentgenol.* 128:107, 1977. Reproduced with permission.)

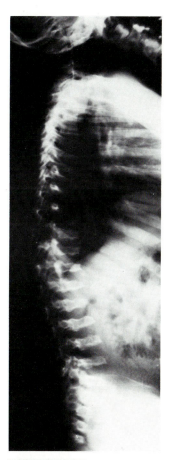

FIG SK–D–6.
Dyggve-Melchior-Clausen syndrome in a 4-year-old child. Flattened irregular vertebral bodies with a pointed end directed forward. Changes are most marked in lumbar part. (From Dyggve HV, Melchior JC, Clausen J: *Arch. Dis. Child.* 37:525, 1962. Reproduced with permission.)

centrally indented vertebral bodies are characteristic and diagnostic; some cases with the above described skeletal manifestations and normal intelligence have been reported as Smith-McCort syndrome (Kappers; Spranger); one family, X-linked recessive (Yunis); probably spondyloepiphyseal dysplasia tarda (Spranger).

REFERENCES

Beck M, et al.: Dyggve-Melchior-Clausen syndrome: Normal degradation of proteodermatan sulfate proteokeratan sulphate and heparin sulfate. *Clin. Chim. Acta* 141:7–15, 1984.

Dyggve HV, Melchior JC, Clausen J: Morquio-Ulrich's disease. *Arch. Dis. Child.* 37:525, 1962.

Engfeldt B, et al.: Dyggve-Melchior-Clausen dysplasia. Morphological and biochemical findings in cartilage growth zones. *Acta Paediatr. Scand.* 72:259–274, 1983.

Hall-Craggs MA, Chapman M: Case report 431. *Skeletal Radiol.* 16:422–424, 1987.

Horten WA, Scott CI: Dyggve-Melchior-Clausen syndrome: A histochemical study of the growth plate. *J. Bone Joint Surg.* 64A:408–415, 1982.

Kappers B: Smith-McCort syndrome. *Fortschr. Roentgenstr.* 130:213, 1979.

Rastogi SC, et al.: Abnormal serum alpha-2 macroglobulin in Dyggve-Melchior-Clausen syndrome. *J. Clin. Chem. Clin. Biochem.* 18:67–68, 1980.

Schorr S, et al.: The Dyggve-Melchior-Clausen syndrome.

Smith R, McCort J: Osteochondrodystrophy (Morquio-Brailsford type). *Calif. Med.* 88:55, 1958.

Spranger J: X-linked Dyggve-Melchior-Clausen syndrome (letter). *Clin. Genet.* 19:304, 1981.

Spranger J, et al.: Heterogeneity of Dyggve-Melchior-Clausen dwarfism. *Hum. Genet.* 33:279, 1976.

Spranger J, et al.: The Dyggve-Melchior-Clausen syndrome. *Radiology* 114:415, 1975.

Yunis E, et al.: X-linked Dyggve-Melchior Clausen syndrome. *Clin. Genet.* 18:284–290, 1980.

DYSCHONDROSTEOSIS

Synonym: Léri-Weill disease.

Mode of Inheritance: Autosomal dominant, more severe and apparently more common in females.

Frequency: Very common; most common form of mesomelic dysplasia.

Paleopathologic Note: Observed in a sixth century skeleton.

Clinical Manifestations: (a) *mild to moderate mesomelic dwarfism with shortness of forearms and lower legs;* (b) *Madelung deformity with dorsal and external bowing deformity of forearms, dorsal subluxation of ulna,* limitation of motion of elbow and wrist; (c) other reported abnormalities:ligamental laxity, Yq to Yp translocation 2:8(q32:p.13) balanced translocation, mental retardation.

Radiologic Manifestations: (a) *shortening and bowing of radius and triangulation of distal radial epiphysis;* widening of distance between radius and ulna; *wedging of carpal bones between distal radius and ulna;* (b) *subluxation or dislocation of distal ulna;* (c) elbow dislocation, cubitus valgus; (d) *shortening and mild curvature of tibia;* (e) other reported abnormalities: shortness of metacarpals and metatarsals; genu valgum; coxa valga; beaking of medial tibial metaphysis; lumbar spine stenosis; degenerative joint changes.

Differential Diagnosis, Significant: (a) posttraumatic Madelung deformity; (b) multiple exostosis with Madelung deformity; (c) Turner syndrome; (d) acromesomelic dysplasia and other forms of mesomelic dysplasia.

Special Comments: (a) mesomelic dysplasia, type Langer appears to represent the homozygous state for dyschondrosteosis (six families); (b) dyschondrosteosis with hereditary nephritis (one family; Funderburk); (c) dyschondrosteosis-like bone dysplasia with brachydactyly and cone epiphyses, autosomal recessive (Fasanelli).

REFERENCES

Beals RK, et al.: Dyschondrosteosis and Madelung's deformity. Report of three kindreds and review of the literature. *Clin. Orthop.* 116:24, 1976.

Carter AR, et al.: Dyschondrosteosis (mesomelic dwarfism)—A family study. *Br. J. Radiol.* 47:634, 1974.

Dawe C, et al.: Clinical variation in dyschondrosteosis. *J. Bone Joint Surg. [Br.]* 64B:377–381, 1982.

Fasanelli S, et al.: A possibly new form of familial bone dysplasia resembling dyschondrosteosis. *Pediatr. Radiol.* 13:25–31, 1983.

Felman AH, et al.: Dyschondrosteose. *Am. J. Dis. Child.* 120:329, 1970.

Funderburk S, et al.: A family with concurrent mesomelic shortening and hereditary nephritis. *Birth Defects* 12(6):47–61, 1976.

Galliard L, et al.: Micromélie avec malformation symétrique du radius. *Bull. Mem. Soc. Med. Hop. (Paris)* 21:1103, 1904. (Quoted from Goldberg et al.)

Goldberg EE, et al.: Dyschondrosteosis. *Am. J. Dis. Child.* 132:1038, 1978.

Lagier R, et al.: Dyschondrosteosis (Leri-Weill syndrome) observed in a VIth century skeleton. *Skeletal Radiol.* 3:102–104, 1978.

Léri A, Weill J: Une affection congénitale et symétrique du developpement osseux: La dyschondrosteose. *Bull. Mém. Soc. Med. Hop. (Paris)* 53:1491, 1929.

Youlton R, et al.: Translocation on XY chromosomes in a woman with dyschondrosteosis and sterility. *Rev. Med. Chil.* 113:228–230, 1985.

DYSOSTEOSCLEROSIS

Mode of Inheritance: Probably autosomal recessive.

Frequency: Rare; 12 well-documented cases to 1988, 11 males.

Clinical Manifestations: (a) *short stature, unusual facies* (narrow midface, narrow beaklike nose, micrognathia); (b) *progressive mental and motor retardation;* (c) *cranial nerve involvement;* reduced visual acuity, optic atrophy, blindness; facial palsy; (d) *depressed skin plaques;* (e) abnormal teeth: lack of eruption of permanent teeth, yellowish color, enamel hypoplasia, premature loss of teeth; (f) *bone fragility.*

Radiologic Manifestations: (a) *sclerosis of vault and base of skull;* sclerosis of mastoids; failure of pneumatization of paranasal sinuses; flattening of mandibular angle; narrow optic canal and other foramina; (b) *punctate sclerosis of vertebral bodies; progressive platyspondyly;* (c) *short, thick, sclerotic ribs;* short thick sternum; sclerosis of clavicles and scapulae; (d) *club-shaped tubular bones;* Erlenmeyer flask config-

uration of widened distal femoral shaft and metaphysis; *metaphyseal dense lines* adjacent to relatively transparent diaphysis; thin cortex of tubular bones; *phalangeal tuft resorption;* (e) multiple fractures. (Fig SK–D–7)

Chondro-osseous Morphology: Abnormalities in transition of cartilage to bone; defect in resorption of calcified cartilage with absence of subsequent bone formation.

Differential Diagnosis, Significant: (a) Osteopetrosis; (b) craniometaphyseal dysplasia; (c) pycnodysostosis; (d) frontometaphyseal dysplasia.

Special Comments: Vertebral body changes *(flattening with punctate densities)* are a helpful diagnostic feature.

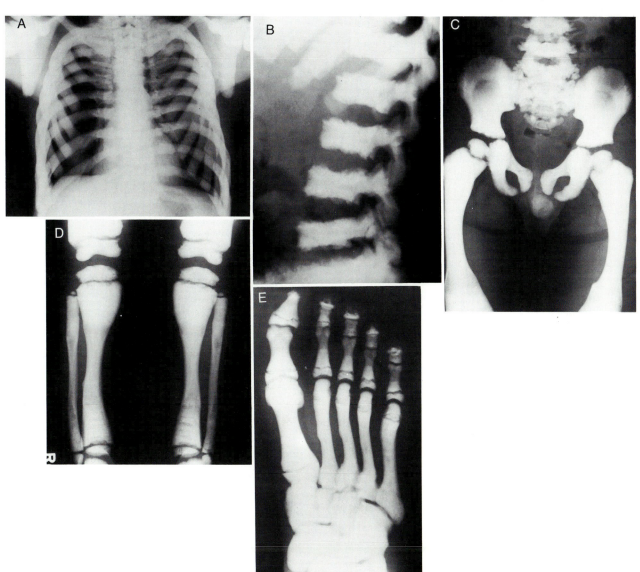

FIG SK–D–7.
Dysosteosclerosis. **A** and **B,** 10-year-old child. **A,** dense bones; wide ribs. **B,** dense platyspondyly with end plate irregularity. **C** and **D,** 5-year-old child. **C,** dense bones; distal clubbed femurs. **D,** proximal and distal modeling defects and striations with dense bones. **E,** 16-year-old patient. Acro-osteolysis; healed metatarsal fractures; distal phalangeal resorption.

REFERENCES

Ellis RWB: Osteopetrosis. *Proc. R. Soc. Med.* 27:1563, 1934.

Field CE: Albers-Schonberg disease: An atypical case. *Proc. R. Soc. Med.* 32:320–324, 1938.

Fryns JP, et al.: Dysosteosclerosis in a mentally retarded boy. *Acta Paediatr. Belg.* 33:53–56, 1980.

Houston CS, et al.: Dysosteosclerosis. *Am. J. Roentgenol.* 130:988, 1978.

Kaitila I, Rimoin DL: Histologic heterogeneity in the hyperostotic bone dysplasias. *Birth Defects* 12(6)71–79, 1976.

Leisti J, et al.: Dysosteosclerosis (case report). *Birth Defects* 11(6):349–351, 1975.

Pascual-Castroviejo I, et al.: X-linked dysosteosclerosis: Four familial cases. *Eur. J. Pediatr.* 126:127, 1977.

Roy C, et al.: Un nouveau syndrome osseaux avec anomalies cutanées et troubles neurologiques. *Arch. Fr. Pediatr.* 25:893, 1968.

Spranger J, et al.: Die Dysosteosklerose. *Fortschr. Roentgenstr.* 109:504–512, 1968.

Stehr L: Pathogeneses und Klinik der Osteoskerosen. *Arch Orthop. Trauma Surg.* 41:156–182, 1941.

Utz VW: Manifestations der Dysosteoskerlose im Kieferbereich. *Dtsch. Zahnaerztl* 25:48–50, 1970.

DYSPLASIA EPIPHYSEALIS HEMIMELICA

Synonyms: Trevor disease; Fairbank disease; tarsomegaly; epiphyseal osteochondroma; epiphyseal exostosis; unilateral epiphyseal dysplasia; tarsoepiphyseal aclasis; fragmentation osseuse hypertrophiante.

Mode of Inheritance: No known hereditary factor, male-female ratio 3:1.

Frequency: Common; 136 cases reported to 1988.

Clinical Manifestations: (a) *unilateral asymmetric hard swelling of knee and/or ankle* with or without pain or restriction of motion; (b) varus or valgus according to site of involvement; painful flat foot; (c) sites of involvement: *talus (most common); distal femoral epiphysis; distal tibial epiphysis;* carpal bones (eight cases); scapula; *upper extremity less commonly affected than lower* extremity; (d) quiescent following epiphyseal plate fusion; (e) no association with malignancy.

Radiologic Manifestations: (a) *overgrowth of one side of epiphysis with irregular contour and ossification;* (b) overgrowth of adjacent bones; advanced bone age in unaffected epiphyses; (c) adjacent (probably secondary) metaphyseal and growth plate involvement; (d) less common findings: loose bodies in affected joints; osteochondral fractures; (e) arthrography, CT, and MRI helpful Fig SK–D–8).

Chondro-osseous Morphology: Exostosis (with cartilaginous cap) arising from an *epiphysis, apophysis, or round bone* (Oates).

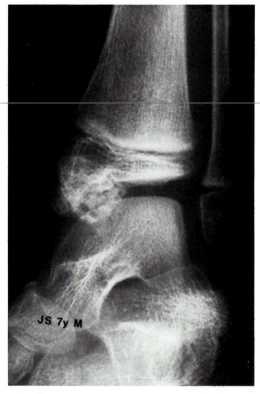

FIB SK–D–8.
Dysplasia epiphysealis hemimelica in a 7-year-old boy. External oblique view of left ankle shows irregularly calcified mass extending from medial malleolus. (From Carlson DH, Wilkinson RH: *Radiology* 133:369, 1979. Reproduced with permission.)

Differential Diagnosis, Significant: (a) solitary or multiple exostosis; (b) multiple enchondromatosis; (c) metachondromatosis; (d) synovial chondromatosis.

Special Comments: (a) familial dysplasia epiphysealis hemimelica associated with chondromas and osteochondromas has been reported; (b) case of mixed sclerosing bone dysplasia (melorheostosis and osteopathia striata lesions) with dysplasia epiphysealis hemimelica; (c) severe case manifested at birth (Wiedemann); *usual presentation 2 to 14 years;* seven cases diagnosed before 1 year.

REFERENCES

Azouz EM, et al.: The variable manifestations of dysplasia epiphysealis hemimelica. *Pediatr. Radiol.* 15:44–49, 1985.

Buckwalter JA, et al.: Dysplasia epiphysealis hemimelica of the ulna. *Clin. Orthop.* 135:36, 1978.

Bugliani LU, et al.: Dysplasia epiphysealis hemimelica of the scapula. *J. Bone Joint Surg. [Am.]* 62A:292, 1980.

Calderoni P, et al.: Dysplasia epiphysealis hemimelica (a review of 19 cases). *Ital. J. Orthop. Traumatol* 10:243–249, 1984.

Carlson DH, Wilkinson RH: Variability of unilateral epiphyseal dysplasia (dysplasia epiphysealis hemimelica). *Radiology* 133:369, 1979.

Enriquez J, et al.: A unique case of dysplasia epiphysealis hemimelica of the patella. *Clin. Orthop.* 160:168, 1981.

Fairbank TJ: Dysplasia epiphysealis hemimelica (tarso-epiphyseal aclasis). *J. Bone Joint Surg. [Br.]* 38B:237, 1956.

Gillier P, et al.: Dysplasie epiphysaire hemimelique: Un cas inhabituel. *Rev. Chir. Orthop.* 71:595–597, 1985.

Greenspan A, et al.: Mixed sclerosing bone dysplasia coexisting with dysplasia epiphysealis hemimelica (Trevor-Fairbank disease). *Skeletal Radiol.* 15:452–454, 1986.

Hensinger RN, et al.: Familial dysplasia epiphysealis hemimelica, associated with chondromas and osteochondromas: Report of a kindred with variable presentation. *J. Bone Joint Surg. [Am.]* 56A:1513, 1974.

Ho AMW, et al.: The role of arthrography in the management of dysplasia epiphysealis hemimelica. *Skeletal Radiol.* 15:224–227, 1986.

Kettelkamp DB, et al.: Dysplasia epiphysealis hemimelica. A report of fifteen cases and a review of the literature. *J. Bone Joint Surg.* 48A:746, 1966.

Lamesch AJ: Dysplasia epiphysealis hemimelica of the carpal bones. *J. Bone Joint Surg. [Am.]* 65A:308–400, 1983.

Mouchet A, Belot J: La tarso-megalie. *J. Radiol.* 10:289–293, 1926.

Oates E, et al.: Case report 305. *Skeletal Radiol.* 13:174–178, 1985.

Sherlock DA, Benson MKD: Dysplasia epiphysealis hemimelica of the hip. *Acta Orthop. Scand.* 57:173–175, 1986.

Trevor D: Tarso-epiphyseal aclasis: A congenital error of epiphyseal development. *J. Bone Joint Surg. [Br.]* 32B:204, 1950.

Wiedemann HR, et al.: Dysplasia epiphysealis hemimelica: Trevor disease. Severe manifestations in a child. *Eur. J. Pediatr.* 136:311–316, 1981.

DYSSEGMENTAL DYSPLASIA

Synonyms: Rolland-Desbuquois syndrome; chondrodysplastic dwarfism–cleft palate–micrognathia syndrome; lethal anisospondylic camptomicromelic dwarfism; nanisme dyssegmentaire (dysplasie dyssegmentaire); micromelic chondrodysplasia.

Mode of Inheritance: Autosomal recessive.

Classification: *Two distinct types:* (a) *type Rolland-Desbuquois (R-D), mild* (Fig SK–D–10); (b) *type Silverman-Handmaker (S-H), severe, lethal* (Fig SK–D–9).

Frequency: Uncommon; 34 cases (R-D 12, S-H 22) to 1988.

Type: R-D (Rolland-Desbuquois type).

Clinical Manifestations: (a) *survival beyond the newborn period* until 3 years; (b) encephalocele (one case); *micrognathia, cleft palate; orbital hypoplasia; flat face;* (c) *short neck; narrow chest;* (d) decreased joint mobility; (e) other re-

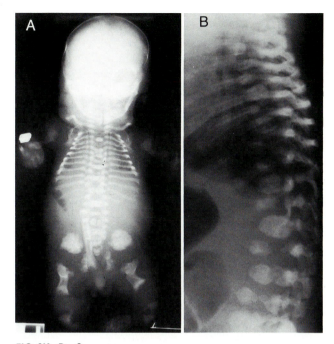

FIG SK–D–9.
Dyssegmental dysplasia, Silverman-Handmaker type, newborn. **A,** small thorax, anisospondyly, small round dense ilia. **B,** severe anisospondyly (segmentation defects; absent, oversized, and clefted vertebral bodies).

ported abnormalities: congenital heart disease (one case); hirsutism; hydrocephalus; ear abnormality; *French ethnic background.*

Radiologic Manifestations: (a) shallow orbits; *midface hypoplasia; mild micrognathia;* (b) *moderately short, flared ribs;* (c) spine: *coronal clefts and oversized vertebrae* (lateral view); *sagittal clefting* (AP view); coronal clefts and lack of ossification of cervical spine; (d) *short, broad long tubular bones; dumbbell femurs;* bowed long bones; (e) short, broad tubular bones (hands and feet); enlarged first metatarsal; accelerated ossification in newborn; (f) pelvis: *wide flared ilia* with small sacrosciatic notches; broad pubis and ischia.

Chondro-osseous Morphology: Relatively normal growth plate; extensive patches of broad collagen fibers in resting cartilage.

Type: S-H (Silverman-Handmaker type).

Clinical Manifestations: (a) stillborn or death within 48 hours; (b) *encephalocele or occipital defect* (50% of cases); micrognathia; ear abnormalities; *orbital hypoplasia; flat face;* (c) *short neck; very narrow chest;* (d) *severe microcamptomelia; decreased joint mobility;* (e) other reported abnormalities: cleft palate (rare); congenital heart disease (including patent ductus arteriosus); genitourinary abnormalities; Dandy-Walker malformation and cerebellar hypoplasia; (f) *Hispanic ethnic background.*

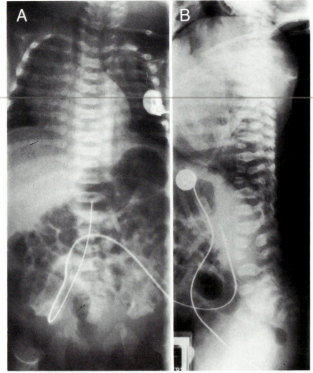

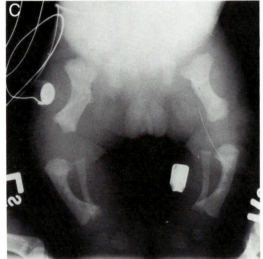

FIG SK–D–10.
Dyssegmental dysplasia, Rolland-Desbuquois type, newborn. **A,** platyspondyly but almost no anisospondyly (AP); wide, flared ilia. **B,** moderate anisospondyly (lateral). **C,** short broad dumbbell femura and tibiae.

Radiologic Manifestations: (a) shallow orbits; *severe midface hypoplasia; micrognathia;* (b) *very short, flared ribs;* small asphyxiated appearing thorax; (c) spine: *anisospondyly (severe segmentation defects;* absent, oversized, or clefted vertebral bodies) of entire spine; (d) *extremely short, broad tu-* bular bones, with angulation of long bones; (e) hypoplastic first metacarpal; (f) pelvis: *characteristic small round ilia with very dense ossification;* small sacrosciatic notches; broad pubis and ischia; (g) malformed scapula with prominent acromion; (h) prenatal diagnosis (ultrasound) at 18 and 20 weeks gestation.

Chondro-osseous Morphology and Biochemical Abnormalities: (a) disorganized growth plate; failure of aggregation of calcospherites; disarranged collagen fibers of bone; mucoid degeneration and absence of patches of broad collagen fibers in resting cartilage; puddlelike intercellular aggregates; (b) abnormal gel electrophoretic patterns of collagen peptides suggest deficiency in α_1 chains.

Differential Diagnosis, Significant: (a) Kniest dysplasia; (b) Weissenbacher-Zweymüller syndrome (OSMED); (c) micrognathic dwarfism (Maroteaux); (d) Kniest-like dysplasia (Sconyers); (e) Kniest-like dysplasia: whistling face (Burton).

Special Comments: (a) differentiation between the two types of dyssegmental dysplasia can be made radiographically by the *AP spine* and *iliac wing changes,* as well as severity; (b) first description of dyssegmental dysplasia in 1900 (Gorlin).

REFERENCES

Aleck KA, et al.: Dyssegmental dysplasias. *Am. J. Med. Genet.* 27:295–312, 1987.

Anderson PE, et al.: Dyssegmental dysplasia in siblings: Prenatal ultrasonic diagnosis. *Skeletal Radiol.* 17:29–31, 1988.

Burton BK, et al.: A new skeletal dysplasia. *J. Pediatr.* 109:642–648, 1986.

Gorlin RJ: Letter to Editor. *Am. J. Med. Genet.* 28:1015–1016, 1987.

Handmaker SD, et al.: Dyssegmental dwarfism: A new syndrome of lethal dwarfism. *Birth Defects* 13(3D):79, 1977.

Kim HJ, et al: Prenatal diagnosis of dyssegmental dwarfism. *Prenatal Diagn.* 6:143–150, 1986.

Maroteaux P, et al.: Le nanisme micrognathe. *La Presse Med.* 78:2371–2374, 1970.

Rolland JC, Laugier J, Grenier B, Desbuquois G: Nanisme chondrodystrophique et division palatine chez un nouveau-ne. *Ann. Pediatr.* 19:139–143, 1972.

Sconyers SM, et al.: A distinct chondrodysplasia resembling Kniest dysplasia: *J. Pediatr.* 103:898, 1983.

Silverman FN: Forms of dysostotic dwarfism of uncertain classification. *Ann. Radiol.* 12:1005, 1969.

Stoss H: Dyssegmentale dysplasie. *Pathologe* 6:88–95, 1985.

Svejcar J: Biochemical abnormalities in connective tissue of osteodysplasty of Melnick-Needles and dyssegmental dwarfism. *Clin. Genet.* 23:369–375, 1983.

ENCHONDROMATOSES

Classification: See Table SK−E−1.

ENCHONDROMATOSIS (OLLIER)

Synonyms: Multiple enchondromata; dyschondroplasia; internal chondromatosis; Ollier disease.

Mode of inheritance: Sporadic; rare (5) familial cases.

Frequency: Very common; probably underreported.

Clinical Manifestations: Presents at all ages, usually in infancy: (a) *asymmetry in length and shape of involved limbs, enlargement of metaphyseal regions, lumps and bumps on hands* and feet; (b) *kyphoscoliosis (rare); pathological fracture;* gait disturbance; (c) *granulosa cell tumor of ovary;* parasellar chondrosarcoma; astrocytoma; *malignant transformation (about 30%); chondrosarcomas.*

Radiologic Manifestations: Unilateral or bilateral abnormalities: (a) *irregular, elongated, or oval tumorous radiolu-* cent defects in metaphyses of tubular bones with extension in direction of diaphysis, irregular calcification within enchondromatous lesions; (b) *long bones, short tubular bones of hands and feet, pelvic bones and ribs commonly involved;* (c) carpal, tarsal, base of skull, and spine rarely involved.

Chondro-osseous Morphology and Pathophysiology: Enchondroma (cartilaginous rests) surrounded by lamellar bone; resting cartilage displaced into the metaphysis (Langenskiöld) (Fig SK−E−1).

Differential Diagnosis, Significant: (a) metaphyseal chondrodysplasias, (b) spondylometaphyseal dysplasias, (c) other endochromatoses (Table SK−E−1).

REFERENCES

Cannon SR, Sweetnam DR: Multiple chondrosarcomas in dyschondroplasia. *Cancer* 55:836−840, 1985.
Goodman SB, et al.: Ollier's disease with multiple sarcomatous transformations. *Hum. Pathol.* 15:91−93, 1984.

TABLE SK−E−1.
Enchondromatoses (Classification)*

Condition	Major Radiographic Features	Etiology	State of Delineation
I Ollier disease	Multiple enchondromas of tubular and flat bones, unevenly distributed, in various stages of development, sparing calvaria and vertebrae	Sporadic	Definitive
II Maffucci syndrome	Same as Ollier disease, with multiple cutaneous hemangiomas	Sporadic	Definitive
III Metachondromatosis	Multiple enchondromas with prominent marginal or solid calcifications, exostoses, rapid progression and regression, affecting preferably short tubular bones	Autosomal dominant	Definitive
IV Spondyloenchondrodysplasia	Irregularly distributed, mostly discrete enchondromas of long tubular bones; generalized severe platyspondyly	? Autosomal recessive	Probable
V Enchondromatosis with irregular vertebral lesions	Multiple enchondromas of long tubular and flat bones, generalized and irregular dysplasia of vertebral bodies	No hereditary factor known	Tentative
VI Generalized enchondromatosis (with mild platyspondyly)	Generalized, evenly distributed enchondromas with severe involvement of hands and feet, mild platyspondyly, and skull deformity	No hereditary factor known	Tentative
VII Enchondromatosis with vertebral anomalies and irregularities	Generalized moderate enchondromatosis with hemivertebrae and end plate irregularity	Sporadic	Tentative

*Adapted and modified from Spranger J, et al.: Two peculiar types of enchondromatosis. *Pediatr. Radiol.* 7:215, 1978 Reproduced with permission.

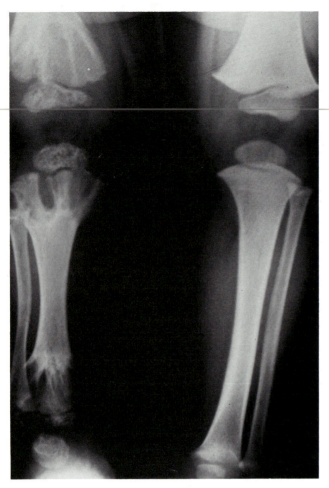

FIG SK–E–1.
Enchondromatosis (Ollier). At ends of long bones of right leg are masses of unossified cartilage. The adjacent epiphyses are irregular. (From Mainzer F, Minagi H, Steinbach HL: The variable manifestations of multiple enchondromatosis. *Radiology* 99:377, 1971. Reproduced with permission.)

Grenet P, et al.: Dyschondroplasie et tumeur de l'ovarie. *Ann. Pediatr.* 19:759, 1972.

Langenskiöld A: The stages of development of the cartilaginous foci in dyschondroplasia. *Acta Orthop. Scand.* 38:174–180, 1967.

Liu J, et al.: Bone sarcomas associated with Ollier's disease. *Cancer* 59:1376–1385, 1987.

Mainzer F, et al.: The variable manifestations of multiple enchondromatosis. *Radiology* 99:377, 1971.

Mitchell ML, Ackerman LV: Case report 405. *Skel. Radiol.* 16:61–66, 1987.

Ollier L: De la dyschondroplasie. *Bull. Soc. Chir. Lyon* 3:22, 1899.

Reuter K, Weber AL: Parasellar chondrosarcoma in a patient with Ollier's disease. *Neuroradiology* 22:151–154, 1981.

Saul RA: Hereditary enchondromatosis. *Proc. Greenwood Genet. Center* 6:48–50, 1987.

Schwartz HS, et al.: The malignant potential of enchondromatosis. *J. Bone Joint Surg. [Am.]* 69A:269–274, 1987

Shapiro F: Ollier's disease. *J. Bone Joint Surg. [Am.]* 64A:95–103, 1982.

Spranger J, et al.: Two peculiar types of echondromatosis. *Pediatr. Radiol.* 7:215, 1978.

Tamimi HK, Bolen JW: Enchondromatosis (Ollier's disease) and ovarian juvenile granulosa cell tumor. *Cancer* 53:1605–1608, 1984.

Vaz RM, Turner C: Ollier disease (enchondromatosis) associated with ovarian juvenile granulosa cell tumor and precocious pseudopuberty. *J. Pediatr.* 108:945–947, 1986.

ENDOSTEAL HYPEROSTOSIS (VAN BUCHEM TYPE)

Synonyms: Hyperostosis corticalis generalisata; van Buchem disease.

Mode of Inheritance: Autosomal recessive.

Historical Note: High incidence in families on the Isle of Urk. In 1637, 151 of 300 survived the plague. In 1971, entire population was composed of descendents of about 75 marriages in the 17th century (van Buchem, 1971).

Frequency: Rare; about 40 cases to 1988; high incidence among the Dutch.

Clinical Manifestations: Usually onset of symptoms at puberty: (a) *widened and thickened chin without acquired prognathism or malocclusion;* (b) normal head size; (c) mild exophthalmos; (d) *facial nerve palsy,* optic atrophy, deafness (e) *elevated alkaline phosphatase;* (f) increased intracranial pressure; (g) other reported abnormalities: aneurysmal bone cyst; spinal cord compression.

Radiologic Manifestations: (a) *endosteal diaphyseal hyperostosis of tubular bones and narrowing of medullary cavity, normal or widened diaphysis of long bones, periosteal excrescences;* (b) *endosteal sclerosis of neurocranium with loss of diploë, foraminal involvement of cranial nerves 2, 5, and 7;* (c) *osteosclerosis and hyperostosis of mandible;* (d) *osteosclerosis and endosteal sclerosis of ribs and clavicles;* (e) milder osteosclerosis of pelvis and vertebrae; (f) other reported abnormalities: empty sella, ventricular dilatation (Fig SK–E–2).

Differential Diagnosis: (a) sclerosteosis; (b) endosteal hyperostosis, Worth type; (c) osteopetrosis, pycnodysostosis, and dysosteosclerosis; (d) the craniotubular dysplasias, including craniometaphyseal, craniodiaphyseal, frontometaphyseal, and Melnick-Needles; (e) diaphyseal dysplasia; (f) osteoectasia with hyperphosphatasia; (g) polyostotic fibrous dysplasia.

Special Comments: The differentiation from sclerosteosis may be difficult; van Buchem disease is milder, and syndactyly does not occur (Beighton). van Buchem disease is distinguished from Worth disease (autosomal dominant) by its severity and periosteal excrescences.

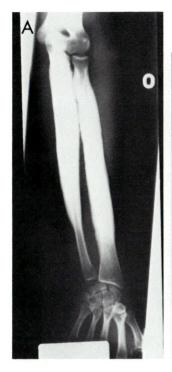 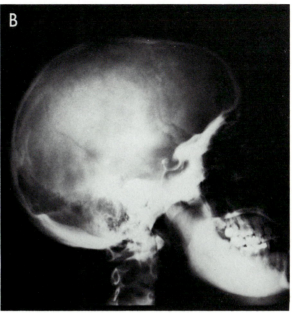

FIG SK–E–2.
Endosteal hyperostosis (van Buchem) in a 21-year-old female. **A,** cortical thickness of tubular bones and lack of involvement of distal radius. **B,** severe osteosclerosis and hyperostosis of mandible and lesser involvement of base of skull. (From Eastman JR, Bixler D: Generalized cortical hyperostosis [van Buchem disease]: Nosologic considerations. *Radiology* 125:297, 1977. Reproduced with permission.)

REFERENCES

Beighton P, et al.: The syndromic status of sclerosteosis and van Buchem disease. *Clin. Genet.* 25:175–181, 1984.

Dixon JM, et al.: Two cases of van Buchem's disease. *J. Neurol. Neurosurg. Psychiatry* 45:913–918, 1982.

Kitasawa Y, et al.: A case of van Buchem's disease with multiple cranial neuropathy. *Rinsho Shinkeigaku* 26:28–33, 1986.

Miguez AM, et al.: Partially empty sella turcica in van Buchem's disease. *Med. Clin. (Barc.)* 87:719–721, 1986.

van Buchem FSP, et al.: An uncommon familial systemic disease of the skeleton: Hyperostosis corticalis generalisata familiaris. *Acta Radiol.* 44:109, 1955.

van Buchem FSP, et al.: Hyperostosis corticalis generalisata: Report of seven cases. *Am. J. Med.* 33:387, 1962.

van Buchem FSP: Hyperostosis corticulis generalisata: Eight new cases. *Acta Med. Scand.* 189:257–267, 1971.

Veth RPH, et al.: van Buchem's disease and aneurysmal bone cyst. *Arch. Orthop. Trauma Surg.* 104:65–68, 1985.

ENDOSTEAL HYPEROSTOSIS (WORTH TYPE)

Synonyms: Hyperostosis corticalis generalisata "congenita"; autosomal dominant osteosclerosis; idiopathic osteosclerosis; endosteal hyperostosis, dominant type; Worth disease.

Mode of Inheritance: Autosomal dominant.

Frequency: Uncommon, approximately 50 cases to 1988.

Clinical Manifestations: Onset of disease in late childhood: (a) craniofacial features: prominent forehead, *progressive asymmetric enlargement of mandible* associated with increased gonial angle, widening of nasal root; (b) cranial nerve involvement uncommon (facial, optic, and auditory); coughing; headaches (uncommon); (c) usually normal alkaline phosphatase levels.

Radiologic Manifestations: (a) *endosteal sclerosis of neurocranium, loss of diploë, mandibular hyperostosis and sclerosis, increased mandibular angle;* (b) *endosteal sclerosis of diaphysis of tubular long bones, mild involvement of tubular bones of hands and feet; diminution of medullary cavity;* (c) mild distortion of contour and sclerotic changes of vertebrae, ribs, clavicles, and pelvis; (d) CT: reduction in size of posterior fossa and foramen magnum; (e) other reported abnormalities: mottled sclerosis of maxilla and mandible (sparing ramus) with embedded teeth and odontomas (Fig SK–E–3).

Chondro-osseous Morphology: Thickened but normal mature lamellar bone (Gelman).

Differential Diagnosis, Significant: (a) endosteal hyperostosis, van Buchem type; (b) craniometaphyseal dysplasia;

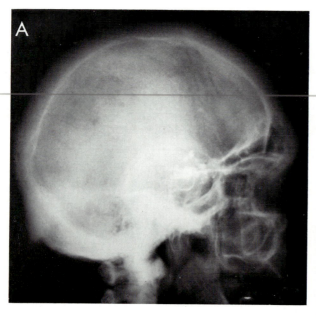
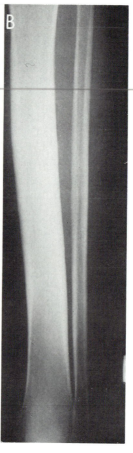

FIG SK−E−3.
Endosteal hyperostosis (Worth)—autosomal dominant osteosclerosis. **A,** in a 57-year-old man, thickening and sclerosis of calvaria and base of skull. **B,** 31-year-old daughter of previous patient. Diaphyseal cortical thickening of tibia and fibula. (From Gelman MI: Autosomal dominant osteosclerosis. *Radiology* 125:289, 1977. Reproduced with permission.)

(c) craniodiaphyseal dysplasia; (d) frontometaphyseal dysplasia; (e) Melnick-Needles syndrome; (f) polyostotic fibrous dysplasia; (g) Paget disease.

Special Comments: Endosteal hyperostosis, autosomal dominant type, described by Nakamura et al., with mottled sclerosis of the jaw and dental changes may represent a different entity. The Worth type of endosteal hyperostosis is distinguished from van Buchem by less severe involvement and lack of periosteal excrescences.

REFERENCES

Eastman JR, Bixler D: Generalized cortical hyperostosis (van Buchem disease). *Radiology* 125:297–304, 1977.

Gelman MI: Autosomal dominant osteosclerosis. *Radiology* 125:289, 1977.

Gorlin RJ, et al.: Autosomal dominant osteosclerosis. *Radiology* 125:547, 1977.

Jend-Rossmann I, et al.: Form veranderungen des Gesichtesskeletts bei Kraniotubulaeren Dysplasien und Hyperostosen. *Dtsch. Zahnartzl. Z.* 38:681–688, 1983.

Maroteaux P, et al.: L'hyperostose corticale generalisée à transmission dominante (type Worth). *Arch. Fr. Pediatr.* 28:685, 1971.

Moretti C, et al.: Endosteal hyperostosis, dominant type: Report on 8 cases in the same kindred. *Radiol. Med. (Torino)* 68:151–158, 1982.

Nakamura T, et al.: Autosomal dominant type of endosteal hyperostosis with unusual manifestations of sclerosis of the jaw bones. *Skel. Radiol.* 16:48–51, 1987.

Perez-Vincente JA, et al.: Autosomal dominant endosteal hyperostosis. *Clin. Genet.* 31:161–169, 1987.

Ruckert EW, et al.: Surgical treatment of van Buchem's disease. *J. Oral Maxillofac. Surg.* 43:801–805, 1985.

Vayssairat M, et al.: Nouveaux cas familiaux d'hyperostose corticale généralisée à transmission dominante (type Worth). *J. Radiol.* 57:719, 1976.

Worth HM, et al.: Hyperostosis corticalis generalisata congenita. *J. Can. Assoc. Radiol.* 17:67, 1966.

EXOSTOSIS (MULTIPLE CARTILAGINOUS)

Synonyms: Osteochondromatosis; diaphyseal aclasis.

Mode of Inheritance: Autosomal dominant: higher incidence and increased severity in males.

Frequency: Very common; especially high incidence in the Chamorros (Micronesians) in Guam (1/1,000) (Krooth).

Clinical Manifestations: Onset: infancy and early childhood; (a) *lumps and bumps,* usually nontender; inadvertent

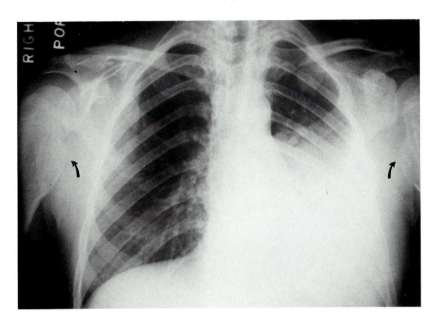

FIG SK—E—4.
Exostoses, multiple (and hemothorax) in a 12-year-old girl with a history of chest pain and shortness of breath of several hours' duration. Left pleural effusion is present. Blood was aspirated from left hemithorax. Note exostoses of proximal humeri and clavicles *(arrows).* In follow-up films of left hemithorax, an irregularity of the anterior end of the sixth rib was noted. (Courtesy of Donald Stern, M.D., and Philip M. Sapunor, M.D., Walnut Creek, Calif.)

radiographic diagnosis; *short stature;* (b) other clinical findings: genu valgum, coxa vara, *local pain;* weakness; pseudoaneurysm (26 cases); hemothorax (3 cases); spontaneous disappearance (Merle, Copeland); Madelung-like forearm deformities; (c) sites commonly affected in order of frequency: *shoulders, knees, ankles,* etc. (d) *malignant transformation:* usually chondrosarcoma; variable incidence figures (from *1% or 2% to 20%*).

Radiologic Manifestations: (a) *exostosis originating from metaphyses, apex directed away from epiphyses;* (b) abnormality of tubulation; (c) *disproportionate shortening of ulnae and fibulas resulting in deformity of forearms and legs;* (d) *any enchondral bone area may also be involved,* i.e., flat bones, short tubular bones, ribs, spine (7%), base of skull; (e) popliteal pseudoaneurysm of adjacent osteochondroma; (f) bone scintigraphy (^{99m}Tc diphosphate): abnormal uptake in actively growing osteochondroma and in chondrosarcoma; (g) overlying cystic bursa (ultrasonographic demonstration); (h) CT (and MRI) useful in spinal involvement and neural encroachment (Fig SK—E—4).

Chondro-osseous Morphology: Cartilaginous cap over normal, mature enchondral bone.

Differential Diagnosis, Significant: See gamut—Exostosis, especially: (a) Langer-Gideon syndrome (TRP 2); (b) metachondromatosis; (c) Turner syndrome.

Special Comments: (a) the gene for multiple exostosis may be located on the 8q region (Hall); (b) animal models (dog and horse); (c) exostoses-anetodermis brachydactyly E. Syndrome (Mollica).

REFERENCES

Bouvier JF, et al.: Radionuclide bone imaging in diaphyseal aclasis with malignant change. *Cancer* 57:2280–2284, 1986.

Copeland RL, et al.: Spontaneous regression of osteochondromas. *J. Bone Joint Surg. [Am.]* 67A:971–973, 1985.

Craig EV: Subacromial impingement syndrome in hereditary multiple exostosis. *Clin. Orthop. Rel. Res.* 209:182–184, 1986.

Doige CE: Multiple cartilaginous exostoses in dogs. *Vet. Pathol.* 24:276–278, 1987.

Epstein DA, et al.: Bone scintigraphy in hereditary multiple exostoses. *Am. J. Roentgenol.* 130:331, 1978.

Ferrari G, et al.: Paraparesis in hereditary multiple exostoses. *J. Neurosurg.* 29:973, 1979.

Greenway G, et al.: Popliteal pseudoaneurysm as a complication of an adjacent osteochondroma: Angiographic diagnosis. *Am. J. Roentgenol.* 132:294, 1979.

Hall JG, et al.: Familial multiple exostosis: No chromosome 8 deletion observed. *Am. J. Med. Genet.* 22:639–640, 1985.

Kraus RA, et al.: Popliteal vein compression by a fibular osteochondroma. *Podiatr. Radiol.* 6:173–174, 1986.

Krooth RS, et al.: Diaphyseal aclasis (multiple exostosis) on Guam. *Am. J. Hum. Genet.* 13:340–347, 1961.

Leone NC, et al.: Hereditary multiple exostosis. *J. Hered.* 78:171–177, 1987.

Merle P, et al.: Evanescent exostosis. *J. Radiol.* 61:291–292, 1980.

Mollica F, et al.: New syndrome: Exostoses, anetodermia, brachydactyly. *Am. J. Med. Genet.* 19:665, 1984.

Prichett JW: Lengthening of the ulna in patients with hereditary multiple exostosis. *J. Bone Joint Surg. [Br.]* 68B:561–565, 1986.

Propper RA, et al.: Hemothorax as a complication of costal cartilaginous exostoses. *Pediatr. Radiol.* 9:135, 1980.

Shapiro F, et al.: Hereditary multiple exostoses: Anthropometric, roentgenographic, and clinical aspects. *J. Bone Joint Surg. [Am.]* 61A:815, 1979.

Vallance R, et al.: Vascular complications of osteochondroma. *Clin. Radiol.* 36:539–642, 1985.

Vinstein AL, et al.: Hereditary multiple exostoses. *Am. J. Roentgenol.* 112:405, 1971.

Voegeli E, et al.: Case report 143: Multiple hereditary osteocartilaginous exostoses affecting right femur with an overlying giant cystic bursa (exostosis bursata). *Skeletal. Radiol.* 6:134, 1981.

Volpi N, et al.: Familial multiple exostosis syndrome: A phacomatosis of bone tissue. *Acta Neurol. (Napoli)* 8:516–527, 1987.

F

FIBROCHONDROGENESIS

Synonym: Fibrodischondrogenesis.

Mode of Inheritance: Autosomal recessive.

Frequency: Very rare; 6 cases described to 1988.

Clinical Manifestations: *Neonatally lethal short-limbed skeletal dysplasia*; (a) normal head size, frontal bossing, wide sutures, flat base of nose, small palpebral fissures, short neck; (b) *narrow bell-shaped thorax, protuberant abdomen*; (c) *short, bowed lower limbs,* hands and feet not affected; (d) other reported abnormalities: omphalocele, patent foramen ovale, cleft palate, microstomia, small abnormal ear pinnae.

Radiologic Manifestations: (a) undermineralized skull, collapsed, soft tissue edema; (b) long thin clavicles; *very short, cupped ribs,* small scapulae; (c) *platyspondyly, posterior vertebral body hypoplasia (pinched)*; (d) hypoplastic pelvic bones, squared iliac wings, medial acetabular spike (trident roof); (e) *very short long bones, dumbbell-shaped; metaphyseal flare; short fibulas;* ectopic ossification (spurs); (f) generalized brachydactyly, fragmented distal tufts (Fig SK−F−1).

Chondro-osseous Morphology: Disorganized growth plate; characteristic fibrous matrix around chondrocytes; defect probably abnormal organization of type 2 collagen.

Differential Diagnosis, Significant: Lethal neonatal skeletal dysplasias, especially (a) thanatophoric dysplasia, (b) spondyloepiphyseal dysplasia congenita, (c) Kniest dysplasia, (d) metatropic dysplasia.

REFERENCES

Colavita N, Kozlowski K: Neonatal death dwarfism: A new form. *Pediatr. Radiol.* 14:451−452, 1984.
Eteson DJ, et al.: Fibrochondrogenesis: Radiologic and histologic studies. *Am. J. Med. Genet.* 19:277−290, 1984.
Lazzaroni-Fossati F: La fibrodischondrogenesi. *Minerva Pediatr.* 31:1273, 1979.
Lazzaroni-Fossati F, et al.: La fibrochondrogenèse. *Arch. Fr. Pediatr.* 35:1096, 1978.
Stanescu V, et al.: Pathogenic mechanisms in osteochondrodysplasias. *J. Bone Joint Surg. [Am.]* 66A:817−835, 1984.
Whitley CB, et al.: Fibrochondrogenesis. *Am. J. Med. Genet.* 19:265−275, 1984.

FRONTOMETAPHYSEAL DYSPLASIA

Synonyms: Gorlin-Cohen syndrome; Gorlin-Holt syndrome.

Mode of Inheritance: X-linked; severe expression in males, variable in females.

Frequency: Rare; about 29 cases to 1988.

Clinical Manifestations: (a) *"Mephistophelean" facial appearance:* very prominent supraorbital ridge, wide nasal bridge, antimongoloid palpebral fissures, small and pointed chin, and *hirsutism* above eyebrows; (b) malocclusion, dental anomalies, renal abnormalities (including obstructive uropathy; congenital stridor and respiratory infections; (c) other reported abnormalities: poorly developed musculature,

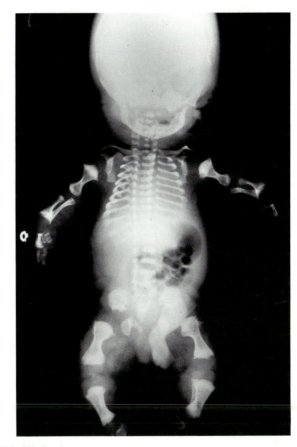

FIG SK−F−1.
Fibrochondrogenesis in a stillborn: long thin clavicles, short cupped ribs, short dumbbell long bones, small femoral spurs.

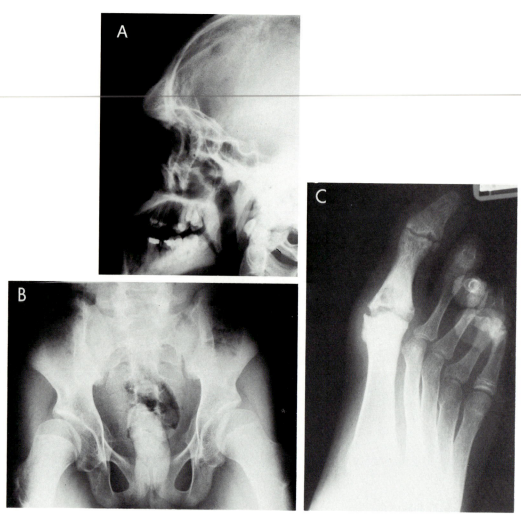

FIG SK−F−2.
A, frontometaphyseal dysplasia, young adult: frontal bone projection with no pneumatization of frontal sinus. **B** and **C**, 17-year-old boy. **B,** bilateral coxa valga and wide femoral neck. **C,** elongation of metatarsal bones and lack of normal tubulation, degenerative changes of first metatarsophalangeal and interphalangeal joints, and flexion deformity of toes.

pseudomarfanoid appearance, winged scapulae, joint contractures, restricted radioulnar or elbow movement, large hands and feet, finger anomalies, genu valgum and/or tibia recurvata, relatively short trunk, progressive hearing loss, (mixed conductive and sensorineural type), ocular disturbance (esotropia, anisotropia, amblyopia, hyperopia), mitral valve prolapse.

Radiologic Manifestations: (a) *thick-frontal ridge, often absence of pneumatization of frontal sinuses;* (b) antegonial notching of body of mandible, *marked hypoplasia of angle and condyloid process of mandible;* (c) defective dentition; (d) irregular rib contours, "coat hanger" deformity of lower ribs; (e) *increased density of diaphysis of long bones and Erlenmeyer flask deformity of metaphyses;* long bones may be mildly affected or unaffected (Levine); (f) dislocation of radial head; (g) fusion of carpal bones, subluxation at proximal interphalangeal joints of hands; elongation of metacarpals and phalanges, barrel-like widening of middle phalanges of fingers, increased carpal angle; (h) *marked flaring of iliac wings;* coxa valga, increased lumbar interpediculate distance; (i) other reported abnormalities: osteolytic changes of carpal bones, large foramen magnum, anterior location of odontoid process, fusion of cervical vertebrae, small metaphyseal exostoses, short and broad femoral neck, small femoral head, scoliosis, ossicular chain abnormalities including fixed malleus, mitral valve prolapse (ultrasound), subglottic stenosis (Fig SK−F−2).

Differential Diagnosis, Significant: (a) craniotubular dysplasias including: Pyle disease; Craniometaphyseal dysplasia; (b) Melnick-Needles syndrome.

REFERENCE

Arenberg IK, et al.: Otolaryngologic manifestations of frontometaphyseal dysplasia. *Arch. Otolaryngol.* 99:52–58, 1974.

Beighton P, Hamersma H: Fronto-metaphyseal dysplasia. *J. Med. Genet.* 17:53–56, 1980.

Danks DM, et al.: Frontometaphyseal dysplasia. *Am. J. Dis. Child.* 123:254–258, 1982.

Fitzsimmons JS, et al.: Fronto-metaphyseal dysplasia. Further delineation of the clinical syndrome. *Clin. Genet.* 22:195–205, 1982.

Gorlin RJ, et al.: Frontometaphyseal dysplasia: a new syndrome. *Am. J. Dis. Child.* 118:488, 1969.

Gorlin RJ, Winter RB: Frontometaphyseal dysplasia: Evidence for X-linked inheritance. *Am. J. Med. Genet.* 5:81–84, 1980.

Holt JF, et al: Frontometaphyseal dysplasia. *Radiol. Clin. North Am.* 10:225, 1972.

Kanemura T, et al.: Frontometaphyseal dysplasia with congenital urinary tract malformation. *Clin. Genet.* 16:399, 1979.

Kassner EG, et al.: Frontometaphyseal dysplasia: Evidence for autosomal dominant inheritance. *Am. J. Roentgenol.* 27:927, 1976.

Kleinsorge Von H, et al.: Das Gorlin-Cohen syndrome (fronto-metaphysäre Dysplasie). *Fortsch. Roentgenstr.* 127:451, 1977.

Levine M, et al.: Familial frontal dysplasia. *Birth Defects* 11(5):313–314, 1975.

Lischi G: Le torus supraorbitalis: Variation crânienne rare. *J. Radiol. Electr.* 48:463, 1967.

Medler RC, et al.: Frontometaphyseal dysplasia presenting as scoliosis. *J. Bone Joint Surg. [Am.]* 60A:392, 1978.

Park JM, et al.: Mitral valve prolapse in a patient with fronto-metaphyseal dysplasia. *Clin. Pediatr.* 25:469–471, 1986.

Sauvegrain J, et al.: Dysplasie fronto-métaphysaire. *Ann. Radiol.* 18:155, 1975.

Stern SD, et al.: The ocular and cosmetic problems in frontometaphyseal dysplasia. *J. Pediatr. Ophthalmol. Strabismus* 9:151–161, 1972.

Weiss L, et al.: Frontometaphyseal dysplasia. *Am. Dis. J. Child.* 130:259–261, 1976.

GELEOPHYSIC DYSPLASIA

Mode of Inheritance: Autosomal recessive.

Frequency: Very rare, about 12 cases to 1988.

Clinical Manifestations: *Nonlethal, "acrofacial dysplasia"*; (a) *happy-natured facies*; (b) *small hands and feet*, small nails, thick tight skin, high-pitched voice; (c) growth retardation, recurrent respiratory and middle ear infections, hepatosplenomegaly, (d) joint contractures; (e) *cardiac failure*, upper airway obstruction *(tracheal narrowing)* (Peters).

Radiologic Manifestations: (a) *short, plump tubular bones of hands and feet* (± metacarpal proximal pointing), broad proximal phalanges, short long tubular bones, *irregular small capital femoral epiphyses*; (b) osteopenia, broad ribs; (c) *J-shaped sella turcica* (personal experience) (Fig SK–G–1).

Cellular Morphology and Biochemistry: Lysosomal storage vacuoles in hepatocytes; primary disorder of glycoprotein metabolism with lysosomal storage (skin, *liver*, heart, trachea).

Differential Diagnosis, Significant: (a) acromicric dysplasia; (b) mucopolysacchridoses and mucolipidoses.

Special Comments: (a) acromicric dysplasia may represent a milder form of geleophysic dysplasia (Lipson); (b) terminology note: geleo = *happy,* physis = *nature.*

REFERENCES

Koiffmann CP: Familial recurrence of geleophysic dysplasia. *Am. J. Med. Genet.* 19:483–486, 1984.

Leroy JG, et al.: Acrofacial dysplasia and geleophysic dysplasia. *Proc. Greenwood Genet. Center* 4:113–114, 1985.

Lipson AH, et al.: Geleophysic dysplasia: Acromicric dysplasia with evidence of glycoprotein storage. *Am. J. Med. Genet.* 3(suppl.):181–189, 1987.

Peters M, et al.: Narrow trachea in mucopolysaccharidoses. *Pediatr. Radiol.* 15:225–228, 1985.

Spranger J, et al.: Geleophysic dysplasia. *Am. J. Med. Genet.* 19:487–499, 1984.

Spranger J, et al.: Acrofacial dysplasia resembling geleophysic dysplasia. *Am. J. Med. Genet.* 19:501–506, 1984.

GREBE CHONDRODYSPLASIA

Synonyms: Achondrogenesis, Brazilian type (Achondrogenesis type 2—"incorrect" term); nonlethal achondrogenesis; achondrogenesis, Grebe-Quelce-Salgado type; Grebe disease; Grebe syndrome.

Mode of Inheritance: Autosomal recessive.

Frequency: Rare; about 70 cases reported but 47 cases belong to one pedigree; 7 families with multiple affected individuals.

Clinical Manifestations: Very distinct clinical phenotype; (a) *short-limbed dwarfism with normal head and trunk* ; (b) severity of shortening progressively increased from proximal to distal segments; (c) *valgus deformity of forearms and hands, fingers resembling toes*; (d) *shortening of lower limbs more severe than upper limbs, broad feet with rudimentary toes, valgus foot deformity*, (e) normal intelligence; (f) polydactyly; (g) early death.

Radiologic Manifestations: (a) lower extremities: almost normal; *short,* or absent femurs; *very short* to absent *tibias* and *fibulas; hypoplastic* and dysplastic *tarsal bones;* absent or *very hypoplastic metatarsals; very hypoplastic* or absent *phalanges with distal phalanges always ossified;* (b) upper extremities: *short humeri, short radius* and ulna with *ulna even shorter and hypoplastic in its distal third,* hypoplastic or *absent carpals,* absent or very hypoplastic *metacarpals,* hypoplastic or *absent phalanges but distal phalanges always present* (Figs SK–G–2 SK–G–3).

Differential Diagnosis, Significant: None; distinctive phenotype (see Special comments).

Special Comments: (a) a clay figurine from central Mexico (preclassical period circa 1300–800 B.C.) appears to depict the characteristic features of Grebe chondrodysplasia. (Garcia-Castro); (b) several other forms of severe short-limbed (normal trunk and head) dwarfism mimic Grebe chondrodysplasia (Romeo 1977, Teebi, Plauchu); (c) two families have been reported with Grebe chondrodysplasia in which other family members have only mild skeletal anomalies of the hand (brachydactyly) (Kumar 1984).

REFERENCES

Bo F, et al.: A kindred of Miao nationality affected with Grebe-Quelco-Salgado achondrogenesis. *Acta Genet. Sinica* 12:378–386, 1985.

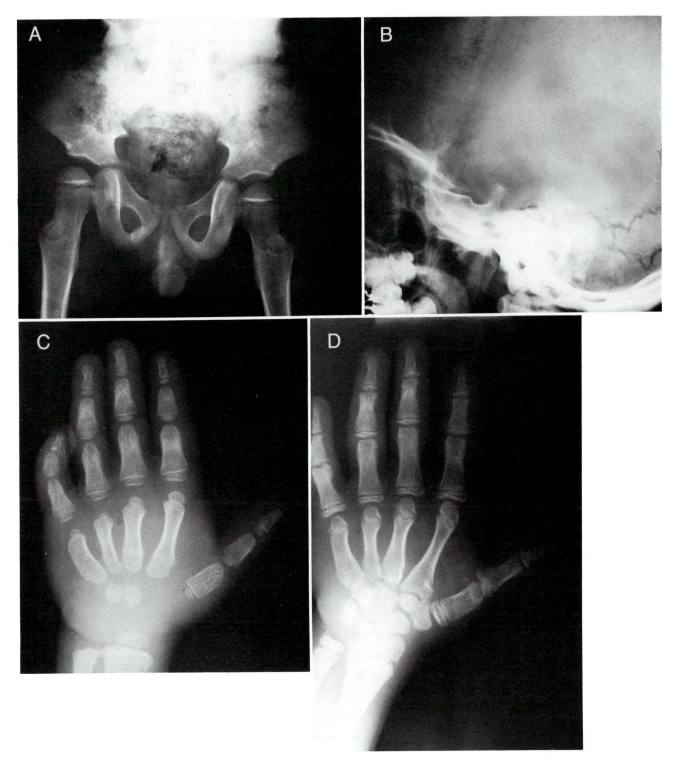

FIG SK–G–1.
Geleophysic dysplasia in **A,** a 5-year-old child: small capital femoral epiphyses, hip valgus, flared iliac wings; **B,** in a 10-year-old child: J-shaped sella; **C,** in a 7-year-old child: MPS-like hands: mild proximal pointing, brachydactyly; **D,** in an adolescent aged 15 years: less MPS-like hands: just brachydactyly (especially brachymetacarpalia).

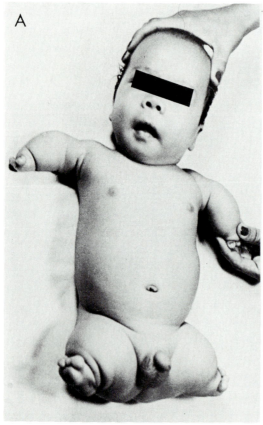

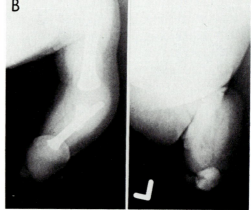

FIG SK–G–2.
Grebe chondrodysplasia. Marked shortening of upper and lower limbs. (From Garcia-Castro JM, Pérez-Comas A: Nonlethal achon-drogenesis (Grebe-Quelce-Salgado type) in two Puerto Rican sib-ships. *J. Pediatr.* 87:948, 1975. Reproduced with permission.)

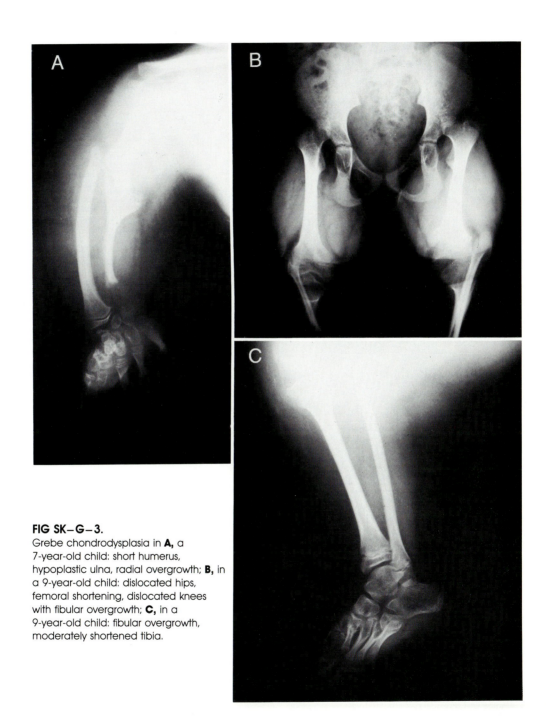

FIG SK–G–3.
Grebe chondrodysplasia in **A,** a
7-year-old child: short humerus,
hypoplastic ulna, radial overgrowth; **B,** in
a 9-year-old child: dislocated hips,
femoral shortening, dislocated knees
with fibular overgrowth; **C,** in a
9-year-old child: fibular overgrowth,
moderately shortened tibia.

Curtis D: Heterozygote expression in Grebe chondrodysplasia (letter). *Clin. Genet.* 29:455–456, 1986.

Freire-Maia N, Lenz MD: Case discussion. *Birth Defects* 5(4):14–16, 1969.

Garcia-Castro JM, et al.: Nonlethal achondrogenesis (Grebe-Quelce-Salgado type) in two Puerto Rican sibships. *J. Pediatr.* 87:948, 1975.

Grebe H: Die Achondrogenesis. Ein einfach rezessives Erbmerkmal. *Folia Hered. Pathol.* 2:23, 1952.

Khan PM, Khan A: Grebe chondrodysplasia in three generations of an Andhra family in India. *Prog. Clin. Biol. Res.* 104:69–80, 1982.

Kumar D, et al.: Grebe chondrodysplasia and brachydactyly in a family. *Clin. Genet.* 25:68–72, 1984.

Plauchu H, et al.: Acro-coxo-mesomelic dwarfism: A new variety of autosomal recessive dwarfism. *Ann. Genet.* 27:83–87, 1984.

Quelce-Salgado A: A new type of dwarfism with various bone aplasias and hypoplasias of the extremities. *Acta Genet.* 14:63, 1964.

Romeo G, et al.: Grebe chondrodysplasia and similar forms of severe short-limbed dwarfism. *Birth Defects* 13(30):109–115, 1977.

Romeo G, et al.: Heterogeneity of nonlethal severe short-limbed dwarfism. *J. Pediatr.* 91:918, 1977.

Teebi AS, et al.: Severe short-limbed dwarfism resembling Grebe chondrodysplasia. *Hum. Genet.* 74:386–390, 1986.

HYDROPS-ECTOPIC CALCIFICATION— MOTH-EATEN SKELETAL DYSPLASIA (HEM)

Mode of Inheritance: Autosomal recessive.

Frequency: Very rare, only two siblings reported.

Clinical Manifestations: (a) *lethal, severe hydrops;* (b) *large head,* narrow thorax, *short limbs* (rhizomelia).

Radiologic Manifestations: (a) deficient skull ossification, micrognathia, small maxilla, high orbits, *laryngeal and tracheal calcifications;* (b) platyspondyly with multiple extra ossification centers; (c) *extraneous calcification* in anterior ribs, sternum, iliac apophysis, pubis, ischium, epiphyseal areas; (d) *moth-eaten long bones,* brachydactyly.

Chondro-osseous Morphology: Bizarre, severely disordered; no column formation; calcification extends into metaphysis, deficient bone formation; mesenchyme-like tissue ingrowth; nodular deposits of calcification.

REFERENCE

Greenberg CR, et al.: A new autosomal recessive lethal chondrodystrophy with congenital hydrops. *Am. J. Med. Genet.* 29:623–632, 1988.

HYPEROSTOSIS GENERALISATA WITH STRIATIONS OF THE BONES

Synonym: Hyperostosis generalisata with pachydermia.

Mode of Inheritance: Autosomal dominant (or X-linked); reported only in males.

Frequency: Very rare; 12 cases to 1988 (seven in two related families).

Clinical Manifestations: Childhood or *adult* onset: (a) bone and muscle pain or *asymptomatic;* (b) normal calcium, phosphorus; slightly elevated alkaline phosphatase; (c) clubbing, and pachydermia.

Radiologic Manifestations: (a) *sclerosis of cranial base;* (b) *widened, sclerotic ribs;* (c) *long bones:* widened, *thickened cortex, densely thickly striated;* (d) similar involvement in pelvis, hands, and feet; (e) other reported abnormalities: bone islands, shaggy periosteal bone formation.

Differential Diagnosis, Significant: (a) diaphyseal dysplasia (Camurati-Engelmann); (b) osteopathia striata with cranial sclerosis; (c) mixed sclerosing-bone-dystrophy; (d) pachydermoperiostitis.

REFERENCES

Fairbank HAT: *An Atlas of General Affectations of the Skeleton.* London, E and S. Livingstone Ltd., 1951, p. 118,
Gonet LCL, Wright MJ: Hyperostosis generalisata with striations of bones. *Br. J. Radiol.* 32:818–821, 1959.
Jones DN: Hyperostosis generalisata with striations of the bones: A further report in two related families. *Clin. Radiol.* 30:87–94, 1979.
Rucher TN, Alfidi RJ: A rare familial affection of the skeleton. *Radiology* 82:63–66, 1964.
Uehlinger E: Hyperostosis generalisata mit pachydermie. *Virchows. Arch. Path. Anat. Physiol.* 308:396, 1941.

HYPOCHONDROGENESIS

Synonyms: Achondrogenesis 2–hypochondrogenesis; lethal spondyloepiphyseal dysplasia (SED) congenita; thanatophoric dysplasia type 2.

Mode of Inheritance: Sporadic, probably autosomal recessive (Borochowitz).

Frequency: Uncommon; about 70 cases to 1988.

Clinical Manifestations: *Live-born* but survive only for a few months *(respiratory death):* short-trunked, *short-limbed* dwarfism; *large head, pear shaped abdomen, flat face, small thorax, cleft palate* (8/11).

Radiologic Manifestations: *Like SED congenita but more severe:* (a) skull: ossification defect behind foramen magnum; (b) chest: *short ribs* with anterior and posterior flare; (c) pelvis: hypoplastic iliac wings, flat acetabular roofs, *unossified pubic bones,* vertical ischia; (d) spine: *ossified ovoid, flat vertebral bodies;* (e) *talus and calcaneus unossified,* no epiphyseal centers are ossified; (f) long bones: *short broad femora; moderate metaphyseal irregularity, generalized;* relatively long fibulas, generalized micromelia (Fig SK–H–1).

Chondro-osseous Morphology: Distinctive (same as achondrogenesis 2, but less severe); hypervascularity and hypercellularity of cartilage with dilatation of rough endoplasmic reticulum cysternae *"marble-like inclusions";* different from SED congenita (Borochowitz).

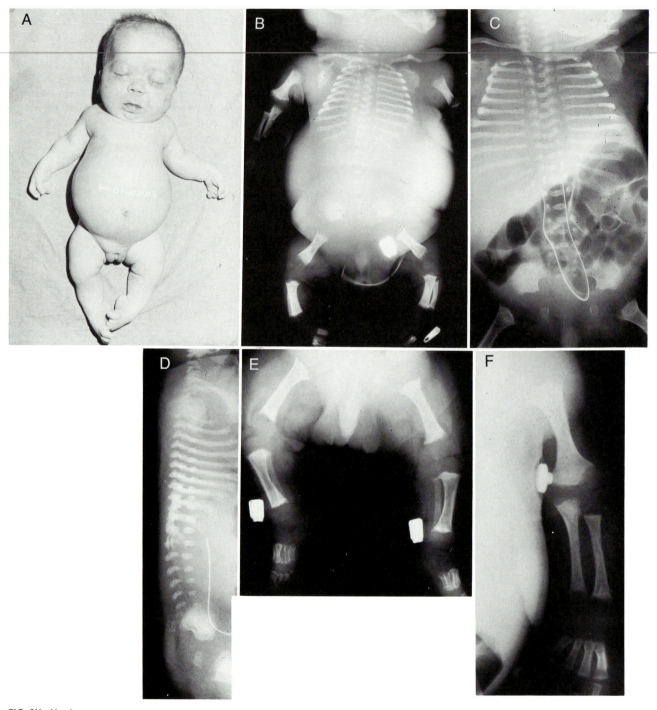

FIG SK–H–1.

Hypochondrogenesis in **A,** a 6-week-old infant postmortem; clinical appearance: narrow chest, protuberant abdomen, short limbs, large head; **B,** in a newborn: severe affectation; **C,** in a newborn, milder case: hypoplastic vertebrae, unossified cervical and sacral ends, vertical ischia, absent pubic ossification; **D,** in a newborn: hypoplastic flattened vertebrae; **E,** in a newborn: micromelia, mild metaphyseal irregularity; **F,** in a 3-week-old infant: severe metaphyseal irregularity and ossification defects.

Differential Diagnosis, Significant: (a) achondrogenesis type 2; (b) SED congenita; (c) spondyloepimetaphyseal dysplasia (SEMD)–Strudwick.

Historical Note and Special Comments: Maroteaux and Stanescu defined hypochondrogenesis as a form of neonatal skeletal dysplasia that clinically and *radiographically* mimicked *SED congenita* but exhibited the chondro-osseous morphology of achondrogenesis type 2 (Maroteaux 1981). It is now felt that hypochondrogenesis represents clinical variability within one disorder that is best termed *achondrogenesis 2–hypochondrogenesis* (Borochowitz). *SED congenita* can often be distinguished by its *lack of metaphyseal changes,* and its less lethal course.

REFERENCES

Borochowitz Z, et al.: Achondrogenesis 2–hypochondrogenesis: variability versus heterogeneity. *Am. J. Med. Genet.* 24:273–288, 1986.

Hendrickx G, et al.: Hypochondrogenesis: An additional case. *Eur. J. Pediatr.* 140:278–281, 1983.
Macpherson RI, Wood BP: Spondyloepiphyseal dysplasia congenita: A cause of lethal neonatal dwarfism. *Pediatr. Radiol.* 9:217–224, 1980.
Maroteaux P, et al.: Correspondence: Spondyloepiphyseal dysplasia congenita. *Pediatr. Radiol.* 10:250, 1981.
Maroteaux P, et al.: Hypochondrogenesis. *Eur. J. Pediatr.* 141:14–22, 1983.
Naumoff P: Thoracic dysplasia in spondyloepiphyseal dysplasia congenita. *Am. J. Dis. Child.* 131:653–654, 1977.
Stanescu V, et al.: Pathogenic mechanisms in osteochondrodysplasias. *J. Bone Joint Surg. [Am.]* 66A:817–835, 1984.

HYPOCHONDROPLASIA

Synonyms: Chondrohypoplasia; mild or incomplete achondroplasia.

Mode of Inheritance: Autosomal dominant.

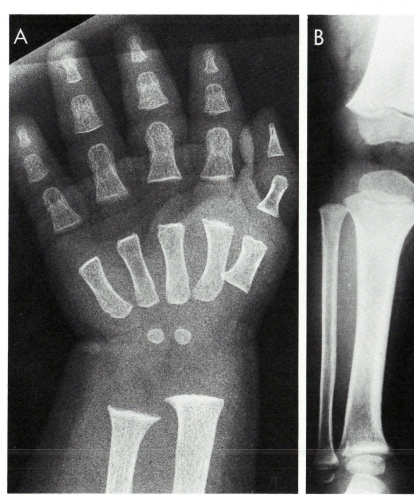

FIG SK–H–2.
Hypochondroplasia. **A,** 7-month-old infant. Metacarpals, proximal and middle phalanges, and less markedly distal phalanges are short and broad; **B,** 18-month-old child. Leg bones are short and plump with wide metaphyses. Fibula is disproportionately long.

(From Hall BD, Spranger J: Hypochondroplasia: Clinical and radiological aspects in 39 cases. *Radiology* 133:95, 1979. Reproduced with permission.)

Frequency: Very common, underdiagnosed; one of the 5 most frequent autosomal dominant disorders (Ginter).

Clinical Manifestations: (a) *mild, markedly variable short-limb dwarfism,* detectable in childhood, *thick body build;* (b) macrocephaly, *frontal bossing;* (c) *broad and stubby hands and feet;* (d) other reported abnormalities: scoliosis, lordosis, *bowlegs,* squint, cataract, ptosis, unusual facies, asymmetric face, frontal bossing, mild mental retardation, abdominal protrusion, mild generalized joint laxity, multiple exostosis.

Radiologic Manifestations: (a) *skull fairly normal,* except frontal bossing, *midface hypoplasia,* slight shortening of bases and narrowing of foramen magnum; (b) *decrease in interpediculate distance from first to fifth lumbar vertebrae,* posterior scalloping, platyspondyly; (c) short iliac bones, flat acetabular roof, small sacroiliac incisura, small posteriorly tilted sacrum and exaggerated lumbar lordosis; (d) *long bones:* short, with wide-appearing diaphysis, mild flaring of metaphyseal-epiphyseal junction, slight shortening of ulna relative to radius, elongation of ulnar styloid, short distal portion of ulna, elongation of distal fibula, short and broad femoral neck, rectangular proximal tibial epiphyses; (e) *mild to moderate brachydactyly,* characteristic pattern profile (Hall); (f) other reported abnormalities: delayed closure of fontanelles, increased depth of cranial vault, bone cysts, unilateral postaxial toe polydactyly; (g) prenatal diagnosis (ultrasound) at 22 weeks (Fig SK–H–2).

Chondro-osseous Morphology: Similar to but less severe than achondroplasia; short columns (growth plate); thick septae; periosteal overgrowth.

Differential Diagnosis, Significant: (a) achondroplasia; (b) normal; (c) cartilage hair hypoplasia.

Special Comments: Hypochondroplasia and achondroplasia are probably allelic diseases (McKusick, Sommer); successful leg lengthening; probable animal models: dachshund, basset hound, and Welsh corgi.

REFERENCES

De Bastiani G, et al.: Chondrodiastasis-controlled symmetrical distraction of the epiphyseal plate. *J. Bone Joint Surg. Br.* 68B:550–556, 1986.

Dominguez R, et al.: Multiple exostotic hypochondroplasia. *Pediatr. Radiol.* 14:356–359, 1984.

Ginter EK, et al.: Medical-genetic study of Kostroma district population. *Genetika* 21:1372–1379, 1985.

Hall BD, et al.: Hypochondroplasia: Clinical and radiological aspects in 39 cases. *Radiology* 133:95, 1979.

Léri A, et al.: Hypochondroplasie hereditaire. *Bull. Mem. Soc. Med. Hop.* (Paris) 48:1780, 1924.

McKusick V, et al.: Observations suggesting allelism of the achondroplasia and hypochondroplasia genes. *J. Med. Genet.* 10:11–16, 1973.

Newman DE, et al.: Hypochondroplasia. *J. Can. Assoc. Radiol.* 26:95, 1975.

Sommer A, et al.: Achondroplasia-hypochondroplasia complex. *Am. J. Med. Genet.* 26:949–957, 1987.

Stoll C, et al.: Prenatal diagnosis of hypochondroplasia. *Prenat. Diagn.* 5:423–426, 1985.

Verheijen J, Bouw J: Canine: Intervertebral disk disease. *Vet. Q.* 4:125–134, 1982.

Waynne-Davies R, et al.: Achondroplasia and hypochondroplasia: Clinical variation and spinal stenosis. *J. Bone Joint Surg. [Br.]* 63B:508, 1981.

KNIEST DYSPLASIA

Synonyms: Syndrome of bone dysplasia, retinal detachment and deafness; metatropic dwarfism type 2; pseudometatropic dysplasia; Swiss-cheese cartilage dysplasia.

Mode of Inheritance: Autosomal dominant.

Frequency: Uncommon, approximately 50 cases to 1988.

Clinical Manifestations: (a) *disproportionate dwarfism;* (b) *round face, prominent eyes, flat midface, cleft palate;* (c) *myopia; vitreoretinal degeneration,* retinal detachment, cataract, blindness, pseudoglioma, congenital glaucoma; (d) *progressive conduction deafness;* (e) *limited joint motion, large and painful joints,* hand arthropathy; (f) *kyphoscoliosis,* lordosis; (g) other reported abnormalities: short neck, hip dislocation, delay in sitting and walking, abnormal gait; (h) increased urinary secretion of keratan sulfate (intermittent) (7 cases).

Radiologic Manifestations: Progressive bone changes from infancy: (a) *shortness and dumbbell appearance of long bones due to splaying of metaphyses and epiphyses, irregular punctate epiphyses, fluffiness and irregularity of growth plate, cloud effect;* (b) loss of normal trabecular pattern, groundglass appearance of bones; (c) *flattened and squared-off epiphyses of tubular bones of hands, narrowing of joint spaces;* (d) trefoil-shaped pelvis; (e) marked coxa vara; (f) *platyspondyly,* with irregular end-plates, *coronal clefts of vertebral bodies in infancy,* narrow interpediculate distances of lumbar vertebrae; (g) other reported abnormalities: cephalometrics: increased neurocranium; flat cranial base; short (or tall), wide odontoid; C1–C2 fusion anteriorly *(no C1–C2 dislocations)* (Fig SK–K–1).

Chondro-osseous Morphology: (a) *Swiss-cheese cartilage* (resting), *distinctive* (Lachman); (b) electron microscopy intracytoplasmic accumulation of metachromatic material; dilated rough endoplasmic reticulum suggests abnormality of proteoglycan metabolism in cartilage (Stanescu).

Differential Diagnosis, Significant: (a) Morquio disease; (b) metatropic dysplasia; (c) spondyloepiphyseal dysplasia congenita; (d) juvenile rheumatoid arthritis and other arthropathies; (e) "Kniest-like dysplasias"; (f) OSMED (Weissenbacher-Zweymuller) dysplasia.

Special Comments: The dyssegmental dysplasias share some clinical, radiologic, and histologic features with Kniest dysplasia; several rare *Kniest-like dysplasias* have been described that must be differentiated from Kniest dysplasia. The type described by *Hunter* et al. has the following differentiating features: milder than Kniest; possibly AR; primarily hand and spine involvement. The type described by *Currarino* has more severe coronal clefts and milder long bone involvement. The chief differentiating feature of the dysplasia described by *Perri* is that it is milder than Kniest dysplasia. Burton's type has the following differentiating features: autosomal recessive, microstomia (pursed lips), ectopia lentis, no coronal clefts, no joint stiffness; brachydactyly. *Crowle's* patients had these differentiating features: autosomal recessive; early death; more vertebral body hypoplasia and platyspondyly; metaphyseal irregularities; markedly shortened diaphyses. *Farag's* family also had autosomal recessive inheritance, no cloud effect, and persistently anteriorly wedged vertebrae. The *Sconyers'* patients' differentiating features were as follows: growth plate and resting cartilage changes; autosomal recessive; markedly shortened diaphyses and metaphyseal changes; lethal.

REFERENCES

Burton BK, et al.: A new skeletal dysplasia. *J. Pediatr.* 109:642–648, 1986.

Crowle P, et al.: A form of metatropic dwarfism in two brothers. *Pediatr. Radiol.* 4:172–174, 1976.

Currarino G: Unusual bone dysplasia featuring severe platyspondyly and vertebral "coronal cleft in infancy, and changes of metaphyseal chondrodysplasia in childhood. *Pediatr. Radiol.* 16:433–436, 1986.

Douglas GR: The ocular findings in Kniest dysplasia, letter. *Am. J. Ophthalmol.* 100:860–861, 1985.

Farag TI, et al.: A family with spondyloepimetaphyseal dwarfism: A "new" dysplasia or Kniest disease with autosomal recessive inheritance. *J. Med. Genet.* 24:597–601, 1987.

Frayha RA, et al.: Hand arthropathy: A clue to the diagnosis of the Kniest dysplasia. *Rheumatol. Rehabil.* 19:167–169, 1980.

Friede H, et al.: Craniofacial and mucopolysaccharide abnormalities in Kniest dysplasia. *J. Craniofac. Genet. Dev. Biol.* 5:267–276, 1985.

Gnamey D, et al.: La maladie de Kniest: Une observation familiale. *Arch. Fr. Pediatr.* 33:143, 1976.

Hunter AGW, et al.: An unusual skeletal dysplasia with platyspondyly and marked digital involvement: A new entity? *Prog. Clin. Biol. Res.* 104:111–118, 1982.

Kniest W: Zur Abgrenzung der Dysostosis enchondralis von der Chondrodystrophie. *Z. Kinderheilkd.* 70:633, 1952.

Kniest W: Das Kniest-Syndrom und seine Differentialdiagnose. *Dtsch. Gesundh.-Wesen* 34:1317, 1979.

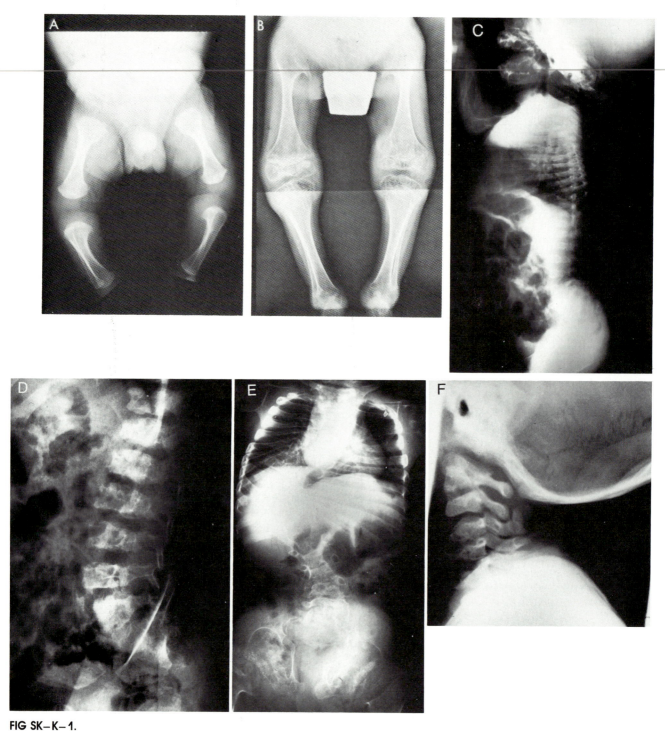

FIG SK–K–1.
Kniest dysplasia. **A,** at age 6 weeks; **B,** at age 5 years. Shortness and dumbbell appearance of long bones due to splaying of metaphyses and epiphyses, irregular ossification of epiphyses, flattened and squared-off epiphyses, narrowing of joint spaces, and coxa vara; **C,** Kniest dysplasia in a newborn: Lumbar coronal clefts, platyspondyly; **D,** in a 6-year-old child: platyspondyly, end-plate irregularity, no residual clefting; **E,** in an 8-year-old child: severe kyphoscoliosis, cloud-effect at femoral epiphyseal plate; **F,** in early infancy: cervical vertebral ossification defects and clefting.

Kozlowski K, et al.: Kniest syndrome: Report of two cases. *Australas. Radiol.* 21:60, 1977.

Lachman RS, et al.: The Kniest syndrome. *Am. J. Roentgenol.* 123:805, 1975.

Maumenee IH, Traboulsi EI: The ocular findings in Kniest dysplasia. *Am. J. Ophthalmol.* 100:155–160, 1985.

Perri G: The radiological features of a new bone dysplasia. *Pediatr. Radiol.* 11:109–113, 1981.

Sconyers SM et al.: A distinct chondrodysplasia resembling Kniest dysplasia. *J. Pediatr.* 103:898–904, 1983.

Siggers D, et al.: The Kniest syndrome. *Birth Defects* 10(9):193, 1974.

Stanescu V, et al.: Pathogenic mechanisms in osteochondro-dysplasias. *J. Bone Joint Surg. [Am.]* 66A:817–835, 1984.

KYPHOMELIC DYSPLASIA

Synonyms: Short-limbed campomelic dysplasia, normo-cephalic type; pseudocampomelia.

Mode of Inheritance: Autosomal recessive.

Frequency: Rare; approximately 14 cases reported to 1988.

Clinical Manifestations: Disproportionate short stature apparent at birth; mild truncal shortening; *severe rhizomelic/mesomelic limb shortening; bowed extremities, especially lower; skin dimples over bowing;* narrow chest; facial he-mangiomata; whistling face phenotype; joint restriction.

Radiologic Manifestations: (a) *short femurs with metaphyseal flare and irregularity; 11 moderately short ribs with flared ends;* short and broad tubular bones; other flared and irregular metaphyses; bowed humeri and other long bones; mild platyspondyly; camptodactyly; (b) prenatal diagnosis (ultrasound) reported twice (SK–K–2).

Differential Diagnosis, Significant: (a) classic campo-melic dysplasia; (b) congenital bowing of the long bones (bent femurs); (c) Antley-Bixler syndrome (short-limbed camptomelic syndrome, craniostenotic form); (d) Larsen syndrome; (e) diastrophic dysplasia; (f) femoral-facial syndrome.

REFERENCES

Angle CR: Congenital bowing and angulation of long bones. *Pediatrics* 13:257–268, 1954.

Fryns JP, et al.: Prenatal diagnosis of campomelic dwarfism. *Clin. Genet.* 19:199–201, 1981.

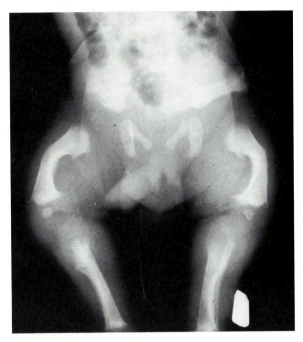

FIG SK–K–2.
Kyphomelic dysplasia in a newborn: shortened bent femurs with distal metaphyseal irregularity.

Fryns JP, et al.: Congenital bowing of the long bones. *Acta Paediatr. Scand.* 72:789–791, 1983.

Hall BD, Spranger JW: Familial congenital bowing with short bones. *Radiology* 132:611–614, 1979.

Hall BD, Spranger J: Congenital bowing of the long bones. *Eur. J. Pediatr.* 133:131–138, 1980.

Hall BD, Mier R: Kyphomelic dysplasia: Whistling face (Freeman-Sheldon) phenotype, limb bowing and metaphyseal dysplasia. Proceedings of the Greenwood Genetic Center, vol 4. 1985, p 172.

Khajavi A, et al.: Heterogeneity in the campomelic syndromes: Long- and short-bone varieties. *Radiology* 120:641–647, 1976.

Maclean RN, et al.: Skeletal dysplasia with short, angulated femora (kyphomelic dysplasia). *Am. J. Med. Genet.* 14:373–380, 1983.

Pavone L, et al.: Camptomelic dwarfism associated with camptodactyly in a new-born infant from consanguineous parents. *Acta Paediatr. Belg.* 33:129–132, 1980.

Rezza E, et al.: Familial congenital bowing with short thick bones and metaphyseal changes, a distinct entity. *Pediatr. Radiol.* 14:323–327, 1984.

Viljoen D, Beighten P: Kyphomelic dysplasia. *Dysmorph. Clin. Genet.* 1:136–141, 1988.

Winter, R. et al.: Prenatal diagnosis of campomelic dyspla-sia by ultrasonography. *Prenatal Diagn.* 5:1-8, 1985.

LENZ-MAJEWSKI HYPEROSTOTIC DWARFISM

Mode of Inheritance: Sporadic cases.

Frequency: Very rare: four cases to 1988.

Clinical Manifestations: (a) *intrauterine growth retardation;* (b) *mental retardation;* (c) *physical features: delayed closure of fontanelles, hypertelorism, nasal obstruction, dental enamel dysplasia, hyperextensible joints, proximal symphalangism, interdigital webbing, cryptorchidism, loose skin, prominent cutaneous veins, emaciation ("progeria").*

Radiologic Manifestations: (a) *progressive sclerosis of skull, facial bones, and vertebrae;* (b) *broad clavicles and ribs;* (c) *diaphyseal undermodeling and midshaft cortical thickening, metaphyseal and epiphyseal hypostosis, short middle phalanges;* (d) *retarded skeletal maturation* (Fig SK−L−1).

Chondro-osseous Morphology: Tetracycline kinetics reveal increased bone formation and defective coupling.

Differential Diagnosis, Significant: (a) progeria; (b) craniodiaphyseal dysplasia; (c) diaphyseal dysplasia (Camurati-Engelmann); (d) cutis laxa.

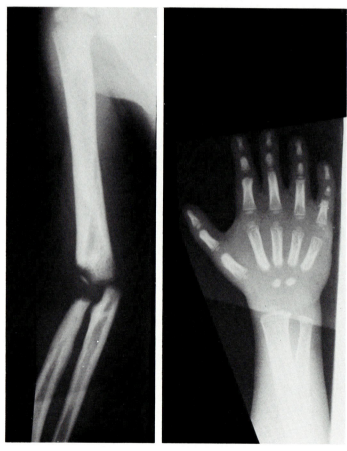

FIG SK−L−1.
Lenz-Majewski syndrome. Upper limb radiograms at 4 years of age show cortical thickening of tubular bones and early signs of proximal symphalangism in third and fourth digits. (From Robinow M, Johansen AJ, Smith TH: The Lenz-Majewski hyperostotic dwarfism. *J. Pediatr.* 91:417, 1977. Reproduced with permission.)

REFERENCES

Braham RL: Multiple congenital abnormalities with diaphyseal dysplasia (Camurati-Engelmann's syndrome). *Oral Surg.* 27:20, 1969.

Lenz WD, Majewski F: A generalized disorder of the connective tissues with progeria, choanal atresia, symphalangism, hypoplasia of dentine and craniodiaphyseal hypostosis. *Birth Defects* 10(12):133, 1974.

Robinow M, Johanson AJ, Smith TH: The Lenz-Majewski hyperostotic dwarfism. *J. Pediatr.* 91:417, 1977.

M

MAFFUCCI SYNDROME

Synonyms: Multiple enchondromatosis with hemangiomata; hemangiomatosis chondrodystrophica.

Mode of Inheritance: Sporadic

Frequency: Common, about 149 cases reported to 1988.

Clinical Manifestations: (a) *hemangiomatosis of skin,* often cavernous, often of limbs and other soft tissues; arteriovenous shunts; (b) *dwarfism with deformity of affected extremities;* (c) huge and hard nodules and masses (enchondromas); (d) head and neck manifestations: involvement of base skull, extension into pharynx, involvement of cranial nerves, dysphagia due to neck mass, airway compression and distortion, epistaxis due to nasopharyngeal involvement; (e) *associated with malignant tumors: chondrosarcoma, 18% incidence* (23/129 cases), usually after age 40, often multiple; intracranial chondrosarcoma, 3 cases; *angiosarcoma,* multifocal, 2 cases; other: pancreatic and biliary *adenocarcinoma; brain tumors* (glioma, astrocytoma), 3 cases; (f) other neoplasms: MEA type 1: parathyroid adenoma, 2 cases (nephrolithiasis); adenomatous goiter; thyroid adenoma; pituitary adenoma; mesothelioma; paraganglioma (chemodectoma) (Armstrong); fibroadenoma of breasts; (g) other reported abnormalities: vitiligo; gastrointestinal hemangiomas (uncommon); lymphangioma; aneurysms; inversion of chromosome 1; (h) complications: *pathologic fractures;* platelet trapping.

Radiologic Manifestations: (a) large expansile *enchondromas* of long bones and bones of hands and feet; (b) malignant degeneration of bone lesions; (c) soft tissue masses and *phleboliths;* (d) angiographic demonstration of *hemangiomas of soft tissues* and bones; *phlebectasia;* (e) bone scan does not differentiate benign from malignant; (f) CT and MRI helpful (Fig SK–M–1).

Chondro-osseous Morphology: Typical enchondromas and hemangiomas.

Differential Diagnosis, Significant: See Enchondromatoses Table SK–E–1; (1) Ollier's disease; (b) blue rubber bleb nevus syndrome; (c) Klippel-Trenaunay-Weber syndrome; (d) metaphyseal chondrodysplasia calcificans (van Crefeld); (e) fibrocartilaginous lesions with hemangiomata and lipomas.

Special Comments: (a) the syndrome of fibrocartilaginous lesions (parosteal) and lipomas as well as typical enchondromas and hemangiomas may represent a separate Maffucci-like syndrome (Bender). (b) a case of a Maffucci-like syndrome with exostoses resembles Maffucci syndrome and a chondrosarcoma developed (metachondromatosis with hemangiomata?) (Saha).

REFERENCES

Armstrong EA, et al.: Maffucci's syndrome complicated by an intracranial chondrosarcoma and a carotid body tumor. *J. Neurosurg.* 55:479–483, 1981.

Bender BL, Yunis E: Fibrocartilaginous lesions of bone and hemangiomas and lipomas of soft tissue resembling Maffucci's syndrome. *J. Bone Joint Surg. [Am.]* 61A:1104–1108, 1979.

Cheng FCY, et al.: Maffucci's syndrome with fibroadenomas of the breasts. *J. R. Coll. Surg. Edinb.* 26:181–183, 1981.

Davidson TI, et al.: Angiosarcoma arising in a patient with Maffucci syndrome. *Eur. J. Surg. Oncol.* 11:381–384, 1985.

Howie FMC, et al.: Case report 492. *Skel. Radiol.* 17:368–374, 1988.

Lewis RJ, et al.: Maffucci's syndrome: Functional and neoplastic significance. *J. Bone Joint Surg. [Am.]* 55A: 1465, 1973.

Lofferer O, et al.: Uber das Vorkommen von arteriovenosen Kurzschlussen bei der Haemangiomatosis Chondrodystrophica. *Wien. Klin. Wochenschr.* 24:698–707, 1986.

Lowell SH, et al.: Head and neck manifestations of Maffucci's syndrome. *Arch. Otolaryngol.* 105:427, 1979.

Maffucci A: Di un caso encondroma ed angioma multiplo. *Mov. Med. Chir.* 3:399, 1881.

Matsumoto N, et al.: Maffucci's syndrome with intracranial manifestation and chromosome abnormality. *No Shinkei Geka* 14:403–410, 1986.

Minami M, et al.: Bone scintigraphy in Maffucci syndrome. *Radiat. Med.* 2:49–55, 1984.

Nemoto Y, et al.: A case of Maffucci's syndrome associated with primary hyperparathyroidism. *Endocrinol. Jpn.* 28:363–367, 1981.

Saha MM, et al.: Coexistence of enchondromatosis: exostosis and hemangiomata. *Australas. Radiol.* 31:71–74, 1987.

Sarwar M, et al.: Intracranial chondromas. *Am. J. Roentgenol.* 127:973, 1976.

Schnall AM, et al.: Multiple endocrine adenomas in a patient with the Maffucci syndrome. *Am. J. Med.* 61:952, 1976.

Schwartz HE, et al.: The malignant potential of enchondromatosis. *J. Bone Joint Surg. [Am.]* 69A:269–274, 1987.

Simpson A, Singh SR: Aneurysm of the superior mesenteric artery: A case of Maffucci's syndrome. *Br. J. Surg.* 71:241–242, 1984.

Slaysman ML, et al.: Mesothelioma of the male genital tract in a patient with Maffucci's syndrome. *South. Med. J.* 75:1007–1010, 1982.

TABLE SK–M–1.
Mesomelic Dysplasia (Classification)*

	Dyschondrosteosis	Langer Type	Nievergelt type	Rheinhardt-Pfeiffer type	Werner Type	Robinow type	Ellis-van Creveld Type	Acromesomelia, Maroteaux Type	Acromesomelia, Campailla-Martinelli Type
Mode of inheritance	AD†	AR	AD	AD	AD	AD	AR	AR	AR
Age at onset	Late childhood	Birth	Birth	Birth	Birth	Birth	Birth	Birth	Birth
Extent of short stature	Mild	Dwarfed	Dwarfed	Mild	Dwarfed	Mild	Moderate	Dwarfed	Dwarfed
Degree of shortening‡ upper/lower extremities	++/+	+++/+++	++/+++	+/+	–/+++	++/+ –	++/++	++/++	++/+
Acromelia	–	–	–	–	–	–	++	+++	++
Radiologic changes in									
Ulnae	Madelung deformity	Distal hypoplasia	Rhomboid	Distal hypoplasia	–	Distal hypoplasia	Short	Distal hypoplasia	Distal hypoplasia
Radii	Short and curved	Short and deformed, proximal hypoplasia	Rhomboid, proximal dislocation	Flat and curved, proximal dislocation	–	Short, proximal dislocation	Short	Short and curved, proximal dislocation	Short and curved
Tibiae	Short	Short, proximal hypoplasia	Rhomboid	Short	Rudimentary	—	Short, proximal erosion	Short	Short
Fibulas	Short	Proximal hypoplasia, rudimentary	Rhomboid	Proximal hypoplasia, curved	Proximal dislocation	—	Short	Short	Short
Metacarpals/tarsals	?short	—	Tarsal synostosis	—	?fusion	—	Short	Short and stubby	Short IV and V metatarsals
Phalanges	?short	—	—	—	Poly (syn) dactyly, thumb aplasia	—	Short and stubby	Short and stubby	Short II and III phalanges
Other radiologic/ clinical changes	Cubitus valgus, coxa valga, ?exostoses, elbow contracture	Mandibular hypoplasia, ulnar deviation of hands	Radio-ulnar synostosis, elbow contracture, clubfoot	Bowing of forearm, ulnar deviation of hands, cutaneous dimple	Thick humerus, hypoplastic patella	Craniofacial dysmorphism, hypoplastic external genitalia, vertebral rib abnormalities	Acetabular changes, genu valgum, heart defect, narrow chest, ectodermal abnormalities	Scaphocephaly, short vertebrae?, elbow contracture	Scoliosis, vertebral anomalies

*From Kaitila II, et al.: Mesomelic skeletal dysplasias. *Clin. Orthop.* 114:94, 1976. Reproduced with permission.

†AD, autosomal dominant; AR, autosomal recessive.

‡(+++) signifies marked, (++) moderate, (+) slight shortening; (–) signifies proportionately normal size.

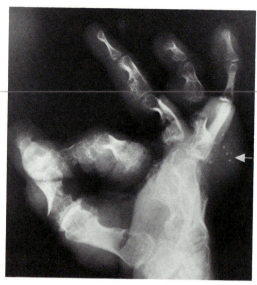

FIG SK—M—1.
Maffucci syndrome. Multiple enchondromas and vascular calcification of soft tissues *(arrow)*. (Courtesy of Robert S. Arkoff, M.D., San Francisco).

Stiegler H, Frey KW: Maffucci syndrom. *Munch. Med. Wschr.* 125:853–854, 1983.
Sun T, et al.: Chondrosarcoma in Maffucci's syndrome. *J. Bone Joint Surg. [Am.]* 67A:1214–1218, 1985.

MELORHEOSTOSIS

Synonyms: Léri disease; Léri type osteopetrosis; osteosis eburnisans monomelica; flowing hyperostosis.

Historical Note: Found in a 1,500-year-old prehistoric skeleton from Alaska; first described by Léri and Joanny in 1922.

Mode of Inheritance: Sporadic.

Frequency: Common, about 300 cases reported to 1988; incidence: 0.9 cases per million estimated.

Clinical Manifestations: (a) bone pain; (b) joint stiffness; (c) segmental or total *asymmetry* of limbs; (d) skin and soft tissue abnormalities: edematous infiltration, anomalous pigmentation, muscle wasting, muscle contracture, fibrotic changes in muscles and tendons, hypertrophy of fingers, band type of linear scleroderma overlying osseous lesions, vascular abnormalities (hemangiomas, vascular nevi), glomus tumors, lymphedema, neurofibromas, arterial and arteriovenous aneurysms (including Klippel-Trenaunay-Weber changes); (e) other reported abnormalities; lipoma of cord (Ruby, Garver); fibrolipomatous lesion, osteosarcoma, carpal tunnel syndrome (one case; Böstman); (f) symptomatic relief with vasodilator therapy.

Radiologic Manifestations: Monostotic or polyostotic involvement of *limbs,* shoulder girdles, pelvis, less commonly spine, ribs, and skull: (a) *linear dense cortical hyperostosis following long axis of bones resembling melted wax running down side of a candle;* (b) extension of hyperostosis into medullary cavity; (c) small bone deposit within soft tissues; (d) premature closure of epiphyseal growth line; (e) scintigraphy (^{99m}Tc-labeled pyrophosphate): increased activity and uptake (Fig SK—M—2).

Chondro-osseous Morphology: Irregularly arranged haversian systems with dense, thick trabeculae.

Differential Diagnosis, Significant: (a) Paget disease; (b) scleroderma; (c) osteopathia striata; (d) dysplasia epiphysealis hemimelica.

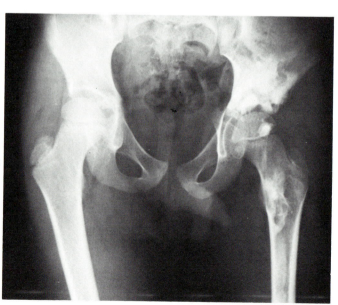

FIG SK—M—2.
Melorheostosis. Several dense areas present in left iliac wing above acetabulum. Left femur shows involvement, with cortical thickening and localized increased density in femoral head and lesser trochanter. (From Beauvais P, Fauré C, Montagne JP, et al.: Léri's melorheostosis: Three pediatric cases and a review of the literature. *Pediatr. Radiol.* 6:153, 1977. Reproduced with permission.)

Special Comments: (a) because the bony lesions follow sclerotomes, may represent an acquired postnatal neuropathy of sensory nerves; (b) may be associated with osteopoikilosis and osteopathia striata (see Mixed Sclerosing Bone Dysplasia).

REFERENCES

Applebaum RE, et al.: Synchronous left subclavian and axillary artery aneurysms associated with melorheostosis. *Surgery* 99:249–253, 1986.

Beauvais P, et al.: Leri's melorheostosis: Three pediatric cases and a review of the literature. *Pediatr. Radiol.* 6:153, 1977.

Bostman OM, Bakalim GE: Carpal tunnel syndrome in a melorheostotic limb. *J. Hand Surg.* 10B:101–102, 1985.

Bostman OM, et al.: Osteosarcoma arising in a melorheostotic femur. *J. Bone Joint Surg. [Am.]* 69A:1232–1237, 1987.

Drane WE, et al.: Detection of melorheostosis on bone scan. *Clin. Nucl. Med.* 12:548–551, 1987.

Garver P, et al.: Melorheostosis of the axial skeleton with associated fibrolipomatous lesions. *Skeletal Radiol.* 9:41–44, 1982.

Kumar B, et al.: Klippel-Trenaunay-Weber syndrome with melorheostosis. *J. Assoc. Physicians India* 31:313–316, 1983.

Leri A, Joanny J: Une affection non décrite des os: Hyperostose "en coulée" sur toute la longueur d'un membre ou "mélorheostose." *Bull. Soc. Med. Hop.* (Paris) 46:1141, 1922.

Morris JM, et al.: Melorheostosis. Review of the literature and report of an interesting case with nineteen-year follow-up. *J. Bone Joint Surg. [Am.]* 45A:1191, 1963.

Murray RO, et al.: Melorheostosis and sclerotome: A radiological correlation. *Skeletal Radiol.* 4:57, 1979.

Pascaud-Ged E, et al.: Melorheostosis, osteopoikilosis and linear sclerederma. *Ann. Radiol.* 24:643–646, 1981.

Ruby N, Vivian G: Case report 478. *Skeletal Radiol.* 17:216–219, 1988.

Semble EL, et al.: Successful symptomatic treatment of melorheostosis with nifedipine. *Clin. Exp. Rheumatol.* 4:277–280, 1986.

Soffa DJ, et al.: Melorheostosis with linear sclerodermatous skin changes. *Radiology* 114:577, 1975.

Young D, et al.: Melorheostosis in children: Clinical features and natural history. *J. Bone Joint Surg. [Br.]* 61B:415, 1979.

MESOMELIC DYSPLASIA (CLASSIFICATION)

Definition: A heterogeneous group of bone dysplasias with dysproportionate shortening of middle segment of limbs with or without hand and foot involvement (Table SK–M–1; Fig SK–M–3).

Special Comments: *Other forms of mesomelic dysplasia:* (a) AD, tibial and radial hypoplasia with *elongated fibulae* (Leroy); (b) AR, mesomelia, *midface hypoplasia,* congenital heart disease, hypertrichosis, *polydactyly,* hydronephrosis, narrow fingernails, and *clubfeet* (Shinzel); (c) mesomelia, *icthyosis,* and *claw-shaped hands* (D'Avanzo); (d) mesomelia (short ulnae, *long fibulae),* brachymetacarpal, micrognathia, *dislocated radial heads and patellae,* contractures and mild syndactyly (Burck; Sandomenico); (e)mesomelia (especially arms), *delayed skull ossification,* unusual facies, *pterygium colli,* hypospadias, *flexion deformities of fingers* (Lohr); (f) AR, mesomelia, unusual facies, *tongue hamartomas, polydactyly, club-feet* (OFD type IV) (Burn); (g) mesomelia (hypogenesis of radii) *thumb duplication, hypotrichosis,* hypoplastic dermal ridges and nails (Brunoni); (h) AR *lethal* mesomelia, micrognathia, microglossia, *tongue cysts, ambiguous genitalia,* web neck, clubfeet; heart, renal, and brain abnormalities (Rutledge); (i) AD, mesomelia, absence or hypoplasia of second phalanges, phalangeal synostosis, *carpal tarsal coalitions* (see Osebold-Remondini syndrome); (j) AD, mesomelia (confined to *forearms),* radial and ulnar shortening (Fryns); (k) see Carraro syndrome: hypoplasia of tibia with *clubbed feet* (Wendler).

REFERENCES

Beighton P: Autosomal recessive inheritance in the mesomelic dwarfism of Campailla and Martinelli. *Clin. Genet.* 5:363, 1974.

Brunoni D: Syndrome identification 114. Mesomelic dwarfism, skeletal abnormalities and ectodermal dysplasia. *J. Clin. Dysmorph.* 2:14, 1984.

Burck U et al: Mesomelic dysplasia with short ulna, long fibula, brachymetacarpy and micrognathia. *Pediatr. Radiol.* 9:161, 1980.

Burn J et al: Orofacial digital syndrome with mesomelic limb shortening. *J. Med. Genet.* 21:189, 1984.

D'Avanzo M, Colavita C: Su di un caso di nanismo melico. *Pediatria.* 87:427, 1979.

Fryns JP et al: Isolated mesomelic shortening of forearm in father and daughter. *Clin. Genet.* 33:57, 1988.

Kaitila II, et al.: Mesomelic skeletal dysplasias. *Clin. Orthop.* 114:94–106, 1976.

Leroy JG et al: Dominant mesomelic dwarfism of the hypoplastic tibia, radius type. *Clin. Genet.* 7:280, 1975.

Lohr H et al: Mesomelic dysplasia: Associated with other abnormalities. *Eur. J. Pediatr.* 137:313, 1981.

Maroteaux P, et al.: Essai de classification des chondrodysplasies à prédominance mésomelique. *Arch. Fr. Pediatr.* 34:945–958, 1977.

Rheinhardt K, Pfeiffer RA: Ulnofibulare dysplasie. *Fortschr. Rontgenstr.* 107:379–391, 1967.

Rutledge JC et al: A "new" lethal multiple congenital anomaly syndrome: *Am. J. Med. Genet.* 19:255, 1984.

Sandomenico C et al: Mesomelic dysplasia with "normal or relatively long fibula," slight micrognathia and brachymetarsals in a six-year-old girl. *Pediatr. Radiol.* 13:47, 1982.

Shinzel A Gideon A: A syndrome of severe midface retraction, multiple skull anomalies, clubfeet and cardiac and renal malformations in sibs. *Am. J. Med. Genet.* 1:361, 1978.

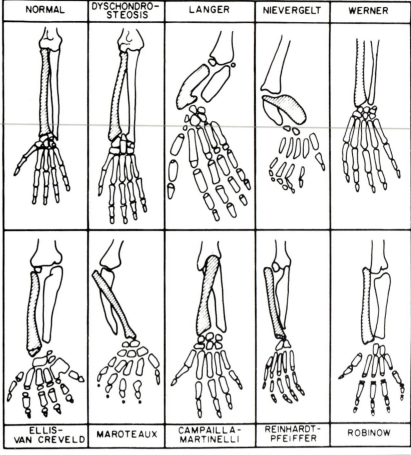

FIG SK—M—3.

A, mesomelic skeletal dysplasias. A schematic presentation of the characteristic radiographic features of various forms of mesomelic skeletal dysplasias. Drawings are from original case reports, which were of patients of different ages and therefore present different development stages for each dysplasia. Right forearm and hand, radius is shadowed. Normal, adult; dyschondrosteosis, adult; Langer type, 4 years; Nievergelt type, 2½ years; Werner type, adult; Ellis-van Creveld type, 6 years; Campailla-Martinelli type, adult; Reinhardt-Pfeiffer type, 9 years; Robinow type, 5½ years. (From Kaitila II, Leisti JT, Rimoin DL: Mesomelic skeletal dysplasias. *Clin. Orthop.* 114:94, 1976. Reproduced by permission.) **B,** mesomelic skeletal dysplasias. Right leg, fibula has been shadowed. Normal, adult; dyschondrosteosis, adult; Langer type, 2½ years (Courtesy of Dr. Ralph Lachman, Torrance, California); Nievergelt type, 2 years; Werner type, 10 months; Ellis-van Creveld type, 6 years; Maroteaux type, 13 years; Campailla-Martinelli type, adult; Reinhardt-Pfeiffer type, 14 years; Robinow type, 5½ years (Courtesy of Meinhard Robinow, M.D., and Frank Johnson, M.D., Dayton.) (From Kaitilia II, Leisti JT, Rimoin DL: Mesomelic skeletal dysplasias. *Clin. Orthop.* 114:94, 1976. Reproduced by permission.)

MESOMELIC DYSPLASIA, LANGER TYPE

Synonyms: Homozygous dyschondrosteosis; mesomelic dwarfism of the hypoplastic ulna, fibula, mandibular type.

Mode of Inheritance: Probably homozygosity for the autosomal dominant gene of dyschondrosteosis.

Frequency: Very rare; seven families to 1988 with parental involvement documented.

Clinical Manifestations: (a) *marked shortness of shanks and forearms;* (b) mild hypoplasia of mandible; (c) normal intelligence.

Radiologic Manifestations: (a) *shortness and broadness of long bones of limbs with bones of forearms and lower legs relatively shorter;* (b) varus deformity of humeral head, prominent deltoid tubercle; (c) marked angulation of shaft of radius, deformed radial head, short and broad ulna, some distortion of carpals; (d) short femoral neck, large trochanters and femoral condyles; (e) *marked shortening and thickening of tibia; lateral angulation of tibia, late appearance and early fusion of epiphyses of tibia;* (f) *hypoplasia or absence of ossification of proximal one half of fibula, absent or poor ossification of epiphyseal center of fibula;* (g) increased lumbar lordosis (see Fig SK–M–3).

Differential Diagnosis, Significant: All the mesomelic dysplasias, especially: (a) dyschondrosteosis, heterozygous; (b) Nievergelt; (c) Reinhardt-Pfeiffer.

Special Comments: The heterozygous-state parents may appear clinically normal and show only subtle radiographic findings of dyschondrosteosis.

REFERENCES

Blanckaert D, et al.: Le nanisme mésomelique de type Langer. *Arch. Fr. Pediatr.* 35:37, 1978.
Böök JA: A clinical genetical study of disturbed skeletal growth (chondrodysplasia). *Hereditas* 36:161, 1950.
Brailsford JF: Dystrophies of the skeleton. *Br. J. Radiol.* 8:533, 1935.
Espiritu C, et al.: Mesomelic dwarfism as the homozygous expression of dyschondrosteosis. *Am. J. Dis. Child.* 129:375–377, 1975.
Fryns JP, Van den Berghe H: Langer type of mesomelic dwarfism as the homozygous expression of dyschondrosteosis. *Hum. Genet.* 46:21–27, 1979.
Goldblatt J, et al.: Heterozygous manifestations of Langer mesomelic dysplasia. *Clin. Genet.* 31:19–24, 1987.
Jones MC, Pickney LE: Mesomelic dysplasia of Langer: Relationship to dyschondrosteosis. Proceedings of the Greenwood Genetic Center, vol 2. 1983, pp 89–90.
Kemperdick H, Majewski F: Mesomeler Zuergwnchs vom Type Langer als Homozygote Form der Dyschondrosteose. *Fortschr. Rontgenstr.* 136:583–587, 1982.
Kunze J, et al.: Mesomelic dysplasia, type Langer: A ho-

mozygous state for dyschondrosteosis. *Eur. J. Pediatr.* 134:269, 1980.
Langer LO, Jr.: Mesomelic dwarfism of hypoplastic ulna, fibula, mandible type. *Radiology* 89:654, 1967.

MESOMELIC DYSPLASIA, NIEVERGELT TYPE

Synonyms: Nievergelt syndrome; Nievergelt-Pearlman syndrome; multiple synostosis syndrome.

Mode of Inheritance: Autosomal dominant.

Frequency: Rare; 16 reports in the literature (including the Pearlman-like cases), about 28 cases (6 affected in the original family; Hess).

Clinical Manifestations: (a) short-limb mesomelic dwarfism; (b) deformed lower limbs, bony protuberances and cutaneous dimples at medial and lateral aspects of lower legs, genu valgum, abducted feet; (c) bony protuberance and cutaneous dimple of forearms, limitation of joint motion at elbow, fingers, and jaw; (d) other reported abnormalities: hearing loss.

Radiologic Manifestations: (a) *hypoplasia of radius and ulna,* elbow dysplasia with subluxation of radial head, radioulnar synostosis; (b) carpal coalition, brachydactyly, clinodactyly; (c) *hypoplasia of tibia and fibula, rhomboidal shape of tibia and fibula, relative overgrowth of fibula;* (d) tarsal synostosis; (e) clubfoot.

Differential Diagnosis, Significant: (a) other mesomelic dysplasias; (b) Grebe dysplasia.

Special Comments: Pearlman's cases appear to represent a *separate disorder,* although Maroteaux feels that this may be clinical variability in a single disorder and should be termed *multiple synostosis syndrome* (see Multiple Synostosis Syndrome).

REFERENCES

Dubois HS: Nievergelt-Pearlman syndrome. *J. Bone Joint Surg. [Br.]* 52B:325, 1970.
Guilbert F: Nievergelt's syndrome and bilateral tempomandibular ankylosis. *Rev. Stomatol. Chir. Maxillofac.* 77:381–382, 1976.
Hess OM, et al.: Familial mesomelic dysplasia (Nievergelt syndrome). *Schweiz. Med. Wochenschr.* 108:1202–1206, 1978.
Maroteaux P, et al.: La maladie des synostoses multiples. *Nouv. Presse Med.* 1:3041, 1972.
Murakami Y: Nievergelt-Pearlman syndrome with impairment of hearing. *J. Bone Joint Surg. [Br.]* 57B:367–372, 1975.
Nievergelt K: Positiver Vaterschaftsnachweis auf Grund erbli-

cher Missbildungen der Extremitäten. *Arch. Julius Klaus-Stift. Vererbungsforsch.* 19:157, 1944.

Nixon JR: The multiple synostoses syndrome. *Clin. Orthop. Rel. Res.* 135:48–51, 1978.

Pearlman HS et al.: Familial tarsal and carpal synostosis with radial head subluxation (Nievergelt's syndrome). *J. Bone Joint Surg. [Am.]* 46A:585, 1964.

Solonen KA, et al.: Nievergelt syndrome and its treatment. *Ann. Chir. Gynaecol. Fenn.* 47:142, 1958.

Wiedemann HR, Dibbern H: Nievergelt syndrome. *Med. Welt.* 31:374–375, 1980.

Young LW, Wood BP: Nievergelt syndrome. *Birth Defects* 10(5):81, 1974.

MESOMELIC DYSPLASIA, WERNER TYPE

Synonym: Werner mesomelic dysplasia.

Mode of Inheritance: Autosomal dominant (? more severe, lethal autosomal recessive form: Kozlowski).

Frequency: Rare; 6 families and about 15 cases.

Clinical and Radiologic Manifestations: (a) *mesomelia, bilateral tibial aplasia or hypoplasia;* (b) *preaxial polydactyly and syndactyly of hands and feet* (up to 9 digits), *absence of the thumbs;* (c) forearm (radial, ulnar) hypoplasia, infrequent; (d) fibular hypoplasia; (e) other reported abnormalities: congenital heart disease (ventricular septal defect), Hirschsprung disease. (Fig SK–M–3)

Differential Diagnosis, Significant: (a) other mesomelic dysplasias; (b) polydactyly syndromes; (c) acromesomelic dysplasia.

Special Comments: *Marked clinical and intrafamilial variability; lethal forms* including cleft palate, abnormal facies, microphthalmy, encephalocele, renal aplasia and bicornate uterus (Meckel or hydrolethalis-like) and upper extremity hypoplasia with elbow dislocation (Kozlowski).

REFERENCES

Eaton GO, McKusick VA: A seemingly unique polydactyly syndrome in 4 persons in 3 generations. *Birth Defects* 5:221–225, 1969.

Hall CM: Werner's mesomelic dysplasia with ventricular septal defect and Hirschsprung's disease. *Pediatr. Radiol.* 10:247–249, 1981.

Kozlowski K, Eklof O: Werner mesomelic dysplasia. *J. Belge Radiol.* 70:337–339, 1987.

Pashayan H, et al.: Bilateral aplasia of the tibia, polydactyly and absent thumbs in father and daughter. *J. Bone Joint Surg. [Br.]* 53B:495–499, 1971.

Pfeiffer RA, Roseskan M: Agenesis of the tibia, duplication of the fibulae and mirror image polydactyly in mother and child. *Z. Kinderheilkd* 111:38, 1971.

Werner P: Uber einen selten fall von Zwergwuchs. *Arch. Gynaekol.* 104:278, 1915.

Yajnovsky O, et al.: A syndrome of polydactyly-syndactyly and triphalangeal thumbs in 3 generations. *Clin. Genet.* 6:51–59, 1974.

METACHONDROMATOSIS

Mode of Inheritance: Autosomal dominant.

Frequency: Rare; 27 well-documented cases to 1988.

Clinical Manifestations: *Painless lumps and bumps.*

Radiologic Manifestations: (a) juxtametaphyseal *osteocartilaginous exostoses pointing toward growth plate and joint*, most common in tubular bones of hands and feet; (b) *enchondromatous lesions* of iliac crest and proximal femur; (c) tonguelike projections of ventral aspect of thoracic and lumbar vertebral bodies, irregularity of end plates of vertebrae (enchondromata); (d) *unpredictable evolution* with frequent spontaneous disappearance of lesions (Fig SK–M–4).

Chondro-osseous Morphology: Classic changes of osteocartilaginous exostoses and enchondromas at different sites (Lachman).

Differential Diagnosis, Significant: (a) multiple exostosis; (b) multiple enchondromatosis (Ollier's disease); (c) TRP II (Langer-Giedeon syndrome).

Special Comments: Metachondromatosis appears to represent the combination of exostoses and enchondromas in the same individual. The combination of metachondromatosis with hemangiomata (Maffucci syndrome with exostosis) has been reported. The patient had a chondrosarcoma.

REFERENCES

Bassett GS, Cowell HR: Metachondromatosis. *J. Bone Joint Surg. Am.* 67:811–814, 1985.

Beals RK: Metachondromatosis. *Clin. Orthop. Rel. Res.* 169:167–170, 1982.

Hinkel GK et al.: Beitrag zur. Metachondromatose. *Helv. Paediatr. Acta* 39:481–489, 1984.

Kennedy LA: Metachondromatosis. *Radiology* 148:117–118, 1983.

Kozlowski K, et al.: Metachondromatosis: Report of a case in a 6-year-old boy. *Australas. Paediatr. J.* 11:42, 1975.

Lachman RS, et al.: Metachondromatosis. *Birth Defects* 10(8):171–178, 1974.

Maroteaux P: La metachondromatose. *Z. Kinderheilkd.* 109:246, 1971.

Saha MM, et al: Coexistence of enchondromatosis, exostosis, and hemangiomata. *Australas. Radiol.* 31:71, 1987.

Vanek J: Metachondromatosis 3 Beobachtungen mit erblichem verkommen. *Beitr. Orthop. Traumatol.* 29:103–107, 1982.

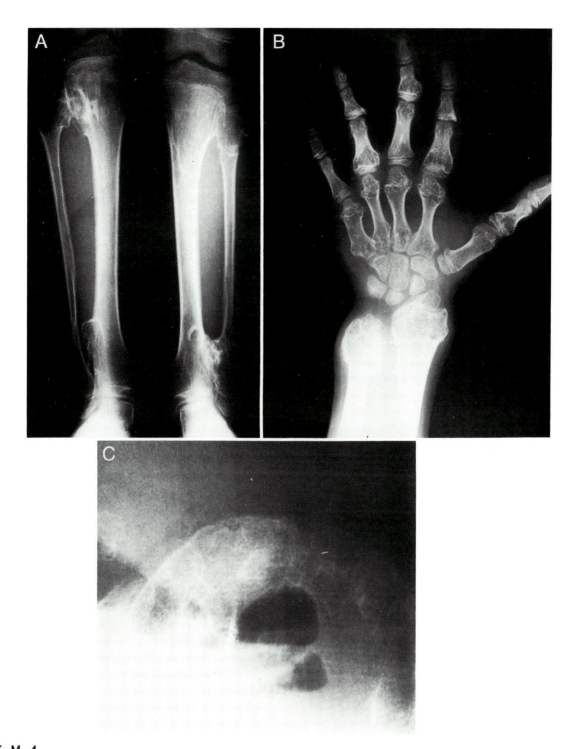

FIG SK−M−4.
Metachondromatosis in **A,** a 9-year-old male: multiple exostoses in the metaphyseal areas of tibia and fibula; **B,** a 9-year-old: exostosis in short tubular bones of hand pointing toward the growth plate; **C,** in a 9-year-old: iliac crest showing areas of uncalcified cartilage extending into ileum from the apophysis (enchondromata).

METAPHYSEAL CHONDRODYSPLASIA (CLASSIFICATION)*

Types:
Common and/or well known

1. Jansen, 1934
2. Schmid, 1949
3. McKusick (cartilage-hair hypoplasia), 1965
4. Metaphyseal chondrodysplasia (MChD) with pancreatic insufficiency and neutropenia (Shwachman-Diamond syndrome), 1964
5. Adenosine deaminase deficiency, 1975

Rare

1. Vaandrager, 1960
2. Spahr (small capital femoral epiphyses), 1961
3. Mixed (Kozlowski), 1962
4. Mild (Kozlowski), 1964
5. Pena, 1965
6. MChD with hereditary lymphopenic agammaglobulinemia (Gatti), 1969
7. Wiedemann-Spranger, 1970
8. MChD with cone epiphyses (Hoeffel, 1984; Bellini, 1987)
9. Congenital lethal MChD, Sedaghatian type (Opitz, 1987)
10. MChD with ectodermal dysplasia (Bellini; Jequier) and cone epiphyses
11. Others (see Lachman, 1988 [Table 4B])

*Adapted from Kozlowski K: Metaphyseal chondroplasias. *Clin. Orthop.* 114:83, 1976.

REFERENCES

Bellini F: Su un caso di disostosi peuiferica. *Minerva Pediatr.* 18:106–110, 1966.

Bellini F, et al.: Wedge-shaped epiphyses of the knees in two siblings. *Helv. Paediatr. Acta* 39:365–372, 1984.

Gatti RA, et al.: Hereditary lymphopenic agammaglobulinaemia associated with a distinctive form of a short-limbed dwarfism and ectodermal dysplasia. *J. Pediatr.* 75:675, 1969.

Hoeffel JC, et al.: Metaphyseal dyschondroplasia with cone-shaped epiphyses. *Br. J. Radiol.* 60:707–710, 1987.

Jequier S, et al.: Metaphyseal chondrodysplasia with ectodermal dysplasia. *Skeletal Radiol.* 7:107–112, 1981.

Kozlowski K: Metaphyseal dysostosis. Report of five familial and two sporadic cases of mild type. *Am. J. Roentgenol.* 91:602, 1964.

Kozlowski K, et al.: Metaphyseal dysostosis of mixed type in a female child. *Am. J. Roentgenol.* 88:443, 1962.

Lachman RS, et al.: Metaphyseal chondrodysplasia, Schmid type: Clinical and radiographic deliniation with a review of the literature. *Pediatr. Radiol.* 18:93–102, 1988.

Opitz JM, et al.: Sedaghatian congenital lethal metaphyseal chondrodysplasia. *Am. J. Med. Genet.* 26:583–590, 1987.

Pena J: Disostosis metafisaria. Una revision. Con aportacion de una observacion familiar. Una forma mieva de la enfermedael. *Radiologia* 47:3, 1965.

Vaandrager GJ: Metafysaire dysostosis. *Ned. Tijdschr. Geneeskd.* 104:547, 1960.

Wiedemann HR, et al.: Chondrodysplasia metaphysaria (dysostosis metaphysaria)—ein neuer Typ. *Z. Kinderheilkd.* 108:171, 1970.

METAPHYSEAL CHONDRODYSPLASIA, JANSEN TYPE

Mode of Inheritance: Autosomal dominant.

Frequency: Rare; 17 patients to 1988.

Clinical Manifestations: Symptoms present in infancy (rarely newborn), *significant variability:* (a) *marked short stature;* (b) typical facies: hypertelorism, exophthalmos, receding chin; (c) *waddling gait, contracture deformities* of joints, in particular flexion of hips and knees, *gradual swelling at joints, short clubbed fingers* (80%); (d) *bowing of legs* resulting in monkeylike squatting stance in childhood; (e) other reported abnormalities: hypercalcemia, hypophosphatemia, asphyxiating thorax; hearing loss.

Radiologic Manifestations: (a) underdeveloped base of skull, brachycephaly, platybasia, prominent supraorbital and zygomatic arches, underdevelopment of paranasal sinuses with sclerotic base (58%), hypoplasia and irregular mineralization of mandible; (b) *extensive irregularity in mineralization of markedly expanded and cupshaped metaphyses* (early), *radiolucent nonossified cartilage mixed with scattered islands of bone and calcification in metaphyseal region* (later); large epiphyses with relatively normal bone structure; (c) short and mildly broad diaphyses; (d) bowing of long bones, in particular in lower limbs, shortness of tubular bones; *hands in childhood: wide distance between epiphyses and metaphyses;* (e) irregular mineralization of anterior rib ends, acetabular and glenoid areas, sternal end of clavicles, pubic symphysis, ischiopubic junction, and sacroiliac joint borders; (f) persistence of dwarfism and skeletal deformities in adult life, *marked improvement in roentgenographic appearance of metaphyseal bone texture;* (g) other reported abnormalities: generalized osteopenia (70%), spindly ribs (56%), pathological fractures (45%), subperiosteal bone resorption (50%), choanal atresia (Fig SK–M–5).

FIG SK–M–5.

A, Metaphyseal chondrodysplasia, Jansen type, in a 1-year-old: moderate metaphyseal changes in long and short tubular bones of arm and hand. **B,** same patient, 7 years old: marked metaphyseal defects at wrists; increased distance between epiphyses and metaphyses with metaphyseal changes in hands. **C,** metaphyseal chondrodysplasia, Jansen type, in 1-year-old: moderate metaphyseal changes in knees and ankles. **D,** same patient, 7 years old: marked progression of metaphyseal changes with fragmentation.

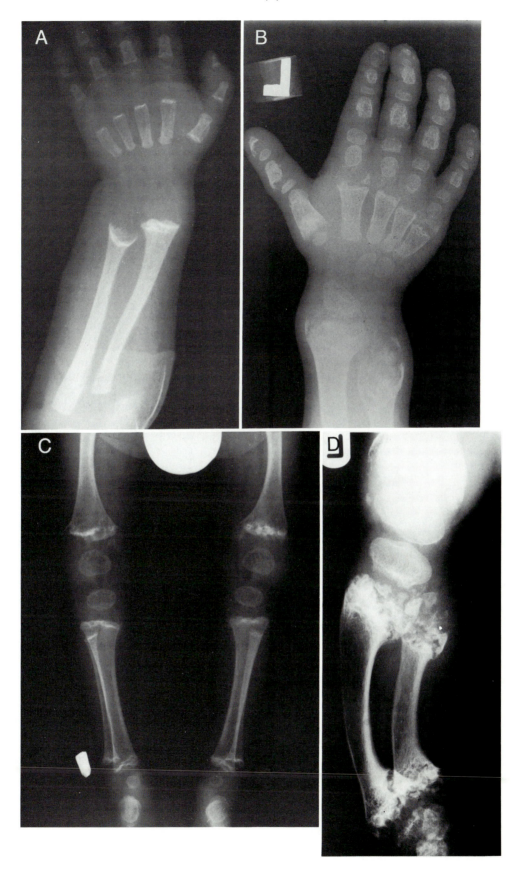

Chondro-osseous Morphology: Similar to other forms of metaphyseal chrondrodysplasia, but very severe. Clusters of proliferating and hypertrophic cells instead of columns, dense wide fibrous matrix, irregular vascular invasion, tongues of cartilage extend into metaphysis.

Differential Diagnosis, Significant: (a) hyperparathyroidism (infancy); (b) rickets (infancy); (c) other MChD; (d) multiple enchondromatosis (older child, adult); (e) battered child syndrome.

REFERENCES

Cameron JAP, et al.: Metaphyseal dysostosis. *J. Bone Joint Surg. [Br.]* 36B:622–629, 1954.

Charrow J, Poznanski AK: The Jansen type of metaphyseal chondrodysplasia. *Am. J. Med. Genet.* 18:321–327, 1984.

De Haas WHD, de Boer W: Metaphyseal dysostosis. *J. Bone Joint Surg. [Br.]* 51B:290–299, 1969.

Gordon SL, et al.: Jansen's metaphyseal dysostosis. *Pediatrics* 58:556, 1976.

Gram PB et al.: Metaphyseal chondrodysplasia of Jansen. *J. Bone Joint Surg. [Am.]* 41A:951–959, 1959.

Holthusen W, et al.: The skull in metaphyseal chondrodysplasia type Jansen. *Pediatr. Radiol.* 3:137, 1975.

Jansen M: Ueber atypische Chondrodystrophie Achondroplasia und ueber eine noch nicht beschriebene angeborene Wachstumsstörung des Knochensystems: Metaphysäre Dysostosis. *Z. Orthop. Chir.* 61:255, 1934.

Kikuchi S, et al.: Metaphyseal dysostosis (Jansen type). *J. Bone Joint Surg.* 58B:102, 1976.

Nazará Z, et al.: Further clinical and radiological features in metaphyseal chondrodysplasia Jansen type. *Radiology* 140:697, 1981.

Ozonoff MB: Metaphyseal dysostosis of Jansen. *Radiology* 93:1047, 1969.

Ozonoff MB: Asphyxiating thoracic dysplasia as a complication of metaphyseal chondrodysplasia (Jansen type). *Birth Defects* 10(12):72–77, 1974.

Scotoliff HA: Metaphyseal dysostosis, Jansen type. *J. Bone Joint Surg.* 55A:623–629, 1973.

Silverthorn KG, et al.: Mark Jansen's metaphyseal chondrodysplasia with long-term follow-up. *Pediatr. Radiol.* 17:119–123, 1987.

METAPHYSEAL CHONDRODYSPLASIA, McKUSICK TYPE

Synonyms: Cartilage hair hypoplasia (CHH); MChD, McKusick type.

Mode of Inheritance: Autosomal recessive.

Frequency: Common; especially in Amish (1.5 per 1,000) and in Finland (88 cases by 1988).

Historical Data: In the Amish 80% of affected individuals can trace their ancestry to Catherine or Jacob Hochstetler who emigrated to the United States in the mid-1700s.

Clinical Manifestations: (a) *sparse, thin, and light-colored hair*, microscopy: small caliber; (b) *short-limb dwarfism in early childhood*; (c) short and pudgy hands with short nails, *bowed legs*; (d) other reported abnormalities: intestinal absorptive defect, Hirschsprung disease, chronic neutropenia, anemia, combined deficient antibody-mediated immunity and deficient cell-mediated immunity, generalized cell defect with marked T cell impairment as well as deficient proliferation of B cells and fibroblasts, increased incidence of malignancies Hodgkin lymphoma, thrombocytopenic purpura, rotavirus infection, long menstrual cycles, *increased susceptibility to chickenpox*.

Radiologic Manifestations: (a) *chondrodysplasia manifested by flaring, cupping, marginal serration, fragmentation and scalloping of metaphyses of tubular bones, most prominent at knees*, irregular cystlike radiolucencies in metaphyses with extension into diaphyses, abnormal epiphyseal shape corresponding to deformed metaphyseal zones; (b) smallness and irregularity of contour of carpal and tarsal bones; (c) *marked shortening of metacarpals, metatarsals, and phalanges, metaphyseal cupping* and mildly cone-shaped epiphyses;

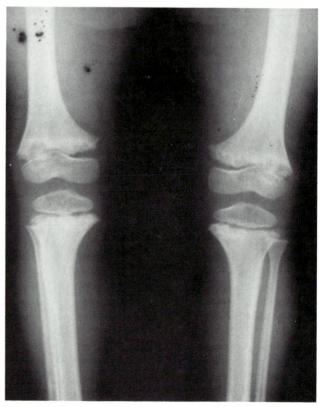

FIG SK–M–6.
Metaphyseal chondrodysplasia (McKusick)—cartilage-hair hypoplasia (CHH) in a 6-year-old male. Note irregularity of metaphyses, most marked in knee regions. Metaphyses have a sharp border. (From Irwin GAL: Cartilage-hair-hypoplasia [CHH] variant of familial metaphyseal dysostosis. *Radiology* 86:926, 1966. Reproduced with permission.)

(d) cupping and cystlike radiolucencies at costochondral junctions, mild flaring of lower rib cage, short sternum; (e) smallness of vertebrae and mild irregularity of their end-plates, prominent lumbar lordosis, mild scoliosis, moderate forward subluxation of C1 and C2 in flexion (several cases); (f) *small femoral heads, relative smallness of size of pelvis* with narrowness of ischium and pubic bones, shallow acetabular fossae and small inferior iliac spine (Fig SK–M–6).

Chondro-osseous Morphology: Nonspecific but similar to all the metaphyseal chondrodysplasias.

Differential Diagnosis, Significant: (a) other MChD; (b) ADA deficiency.

Special Comments: A single family—sib with CHH and other sibs with wrinkly skin syndrome. (Goodman et al.: *Prog. Clin. Biol. Res.* 104:205–214, 1982.)

REFERENCES

Allanson JE, Hall JG: Obstetric and obstet gynecologic problems in women with chondrodystrophies 67:74–78, 1986.

Ashby GH, Evans DIK: Cartilage hair hypoplasia with thrombocytopenic purpura, autoimmune hemolytic anemia and cell mediated immunodeficiency. *J. R. Soc. Med.* 19:113–114, 1986.

Harris RE, et al.: Cartilage hair hypoplasia, defective T cell reaction and Blackfan-Diamond anemia in an Amish child. *Am. J. Med. Genet.* 8:291–297, 1981.

Irwin GAL: Cartilage-hair-hypoplasia (CHH) variant of familial metaphyseal dysostosis. *Radiology* 86:926, 1966.

Lischka A, et al.: Radiologische Verandernngen bei metaphysurer Chondrodystrophie Typ McKusick. *Monatsschr Kinderheilkd* 132:550–553, 1984.

McKusick VA: Metaphyseal dysostosis and thin hair: A "new" recessively inherited syndrome? *Lancet* 1:832, 1964.

McKusick VA, et al.: Dwarfism in the Amish II cartilage hair hypoplasia. *Bull. Johns Hopkins Hosp.* 116:285–326, 1965.

Polmar SH, Pierce GF: Cartilage hair hypoplasia: Immunological aspects and their clinical implications. *Clin. Immunol. Immunopathol.* 40:87–93, 1986.

Ray HC, et al.: Cartilage-hair hypoplasia in Kaufmann HJ (ed.): *Progress in Pediatric Radiology*, vol. 4. Basel, Karger, 1973, p. 270.

Roberts MA, Arnold RM: Hodgkin's lymphoma in a child with cartilage hair hypoplasia: Case report. *Milit. Med.* 149:280–281, 1984.

Seige M: Metaphysäre chondrodysplasie vom typ McKusick (Knorpel-Haar-Hypoplasie). *Monatsschr. Kinderheilkd.* 128:157, 1980.

Wood DJ, et al.: Chronic enteric virus infection in two T-cell immunodeficient children. *J. Med. Virol.* 24:435–444, 1988.

METAPHYSEAL CHONDRODYSPLASIA, SCHMID TYPE

Synonym: MChD, Schmid type.

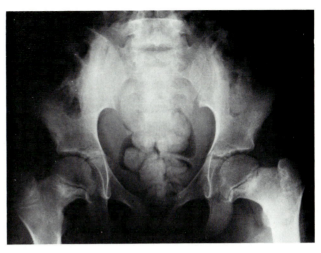

FIG SK–M–7.
Metaphyseal chondrodysplasia (Schmid). A 10-year-old female with bowing of legs noted soon after birth. Bilateral coxa vara, increase in density of provisional zone of calcification, and unevenness of ossification in metaphyseal regions are present. (From Taybi H, Mitchell AD, Friedman CD: Metaphyseal dysostosis and the associated syndrome of pancreatic insufficiency and blood disorders. *Radiology* 93:563, 1969. Reproduced with permission.)

Mode of Inheritance: Autosomal dominant.

Frequency: Uncommon, 53 cases to 1988.

Clinical Manifestations: (a) *short-limbed, short stature presenting in the second year;* (b) *bowed legs, waddling gait;* (c) increasing shortness with age.

Radiologic Manifestations: (a) *diffuse metaphyseal flaring, irregularity and growth plate widening, most severe at knees;* (b) *enlarged capital femoral epiphyses (75%), coxa vara (70%), femoral bowing (70%);* irregular acetabular roof (20%): (c) *ribs: anterior cupping, splaying and sclerosis (100%);* (d) *no hand and vertebral involvement* (Fig SK–M–7).

Chondro-osseous Morphology: Nonspecific, similar to other metaphyseal chondrodysplasias (MChD).

Differential Diagnosis, Significant: (a) other MChD, well defined; (b) non-Schmid, unspecified MChD; (c) autosomal recessive Spahr MChD; (d) Schmid +type, Spondylometaphyseal dysplasia.

REFERENCES

Lachman RS, et al.: Metaphyseal chondrodysplasia, Schmid type: Clinical and radiographic delineation with a review of the literature. *Pediatr. Radiol.* 18:93–102, 1988.

Schmid F: Beitrag zur Dysostosis enchondralis metaphysaria. *Monatsschr. Kinderheilkd.* 97:393, 1949.

METAPHYSEAL CHONDRODYSPLASIA WITH EXOCRINE PANCREATIC INSUFFICIENCY AND CYCLIC NEUTROPENIA

Synonyms: Shwachman-Diamond syndrome, Shwachman syndrome, Shwachman-Bodian syndrome; MChD, Shwachman-Diamond type.

Mode of Inheritance: Autosomal recessive.

Frequency: Very common.

Clinical Manifestations: Onset of symptoms in infancy: (a) growth retardation, low birth weight (30%); (b) *short-limbed dwarfism;* (c) *malabsorption syndrome resulting from exocrine pancreatic insufficiency;* (d) *recurrent infections* (85%); (e) *leukopenia and/or neutropenia* (95%), defective neutrophil chemotaxis corrected with thiamine, thrombocytopenia (70%); (f) respiratory distress in neonatal period; (g) other reported abnormalities: eczema, galactosuria, hepatic dysfunction, liver cirrhosis, dysgammaglobulinemia (often reduction of IgA, less often IgG or IgM), renal dysfunction, den-

tal abnormalities, septicemia, bronchopneumonia, disseminated visceral hemorrhages, anemia 50%, *leukemia,* central pontine myelinolysis, focal pontine leukencephaly, *increased spontaneous chromosome breakage*

Radiologic Manifestations: (a) *metaphyseal changes in particular in hip and knee regions* consisting of small lucent patches and sclerotic serrations at or adjacent to provisional zone of calcification (62%); (b) *irregularity in ossification at anterior rib ends* (90% by age 2½ years); (c) coxa vara, slipping of capital femoral epiphysis may develop; (d) other reported abnormalities: abnormal tubulation of long bones, clinodactyly, phalangeal hypoplasia, narrowing of sacrosciatic notches, skeletal maturation retardation, lipomatosis of the pancreas (computerized tomography and ultrasound. (Figs SK–M–8 and SK–M–9).

Differential Diagnosis, Significant: (a) other MChD; (b) adenosine deaminase deficiency; (c) Fanconi anemia; (d) cystic fibrosis; (e) chronic diarrhea and neutropenia not associated with pancreatic insufficiency.

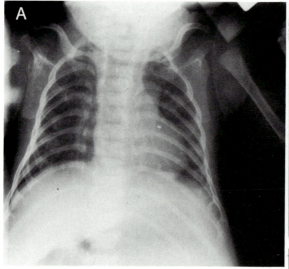
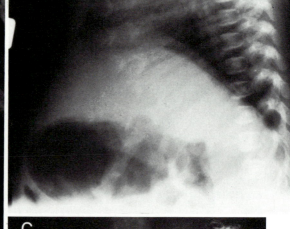
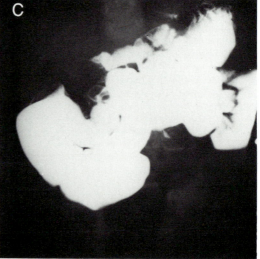

FIG SK–M–8.
A and **B,** metaphyseal chondrodysplasia (MChD) with exocrine pancreatic insufficiency and cyclic neutropenia (Shwachman type) in a 3-month-old: chest films, anteroposterior and lateral, showing anterior rib cupping and splaying. **C,** MChD (Shwachman type) in a 6-month-old: small bowel examination with dilatation of loops suggesting malabsorption.

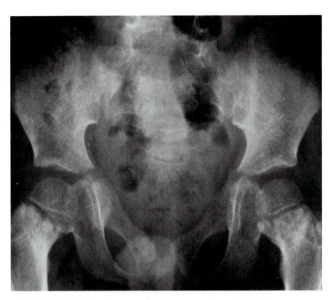

FIG SK—M—9.
Metaphyseal chondrodysplasia with exocrine pancreatic insufficiency and cyclic neutropenia, Shwachman type. An 8-year-old male with exocrine pancreatic insufficiency, nonpersistent neutropenia, and metaphyseal chondrodysplasia. Note dense and irregular bone formation in femoral neck. (From Taybi H, Mitchell AD, Friedman CD: Metaphyseal dysostosis and associated syndrome of pancreatic insufficiency and blood disorders. *Radiology* 93:563, 1969. Reproduced with permission.)

Special Comments: Scott Hamilton, the 1984 gold-medal-winning Olympic figure skater, has the Shwachman-Diamond syndrome.

REFERENCES

Aggett PJ, et al.: Shwachman's syndrome: A review of 21 cases. *Arch. Dis. Child.* 55:331, 1980.

Danks DM, et al.: Metaphyseal chondrodysplasia, neutropenia, and pancreatic insufficiency presenting with respiratory distress in the neonatal period. *Arch. Dis. Child.* 51:697, 1976.

Giedion A, et al.: Metaphysäre Dysostose und angeborene Pankreasinsuffizienz. *Fortschr. Roentgenstr.* 108:51, 1968.

Kuraziel JC, Dondelinger R: Fatty infiltration of the pancreas in Shwachman's syndrome: CT demonstration, *Eur. J. Radiol.* 4:202–204, 1984.

LaBrunne M, et al.: Syndrome de Shwachman. *Arch. Fr. Pediatr.* 41:561–563, 1984.

Liebman WM, et al.: Shwachman-Diamond syndrome and chronic liver disease. *Clin. Pediatr.* 18:695, 1979.

Mah V, et al.: Focal pontine leukoencephalopathy in a patient with Shwachman-Diamond syndrome. *Can. J. Neurol. Sci.* 14:608–610, 1987

Marino LR, et al: Chronic diarrhea and neutropenia associated with pancreatic insufficiency: A non Shwachman-Diamond entity. *J. Pediatr. Gastroenterol. Nutr.* 2:559, 1983.

Michels VV, Donovan GK: Shwachman syndrome: Unusual presentation as asphyxiating thoracic dystrophy. *Birth Defects* 18(3B):129–134, 1982.

McLennan TW, et al.: Shwachman's syndrome: The broad spectrum of bony abnormalities. *Radiology* 112:167, 1974.

Robberecht E, et al.: Pancreatic lipomatosis in the Shwachman-Diamond syndrome. *Pediatr. Radiol.* 15:348–349, 1985.

Shwachman H, et al.: The syndrome of pancreatic insufficiency and bone marrow dysfunction. *J. Pediatr.* 65:645, 1964.

Spycher MA, et al.: Electron microscopic examination of cartilage in the syndrome of exocrine pancreatic insufficiency, neutropenia, metaphyseal dysostosis and dwarfism. *Helv. Paediatr. Acta* 29:471, 1974.

Stanley P, et al.: Metaphyseal chondrodysplasia with dwarfism, pancreatic insufficiency and neutropenia. *Pediatr. Radiol.* 1:119, 1973.

Steinsapir KD, Vinters HV: Central pontine myelinolysis in a child with Shwachman-Diamond syndrome. *Hum. Pathol.* 16:741–743, 1985.

Stuts P, et al.: Letter to editor. *Lancet* 1:1072–1073, 1984.

Tada H, et al.: A case of Shwachman syndrome with increased spontaneous chromosome breakage. *Hum. Genet.* 77:289–291, 1987.

Taybi H, Mitchell AD, Friedman CD: Metaphyseal dysostosis and associated syndrome of pancreatic insufficiency and blood disorders. *Radiology* 93:563, 1969.

Woods WG, et al.: The occurrence of leukemia in patients with the Shwachman syndrome. *J. Pediatr.* 99:425, 1981.

METAPHYSEAL—SELLA TURCICA DYSPLASIA, ROSENBERG

Synonym: Ulna-metaphyseal dysplasia syndrome.

Mode of Inheritance: Autosomal dominant.

Frequency: Very rare; 3 cases in 1 family.

Clinical Manifestations: *Thickened wrists; wrist-pain.*

Radiologic Manifestations: (a) *metaphyseal irregularities;* widened epiphyseal plate; *wide metaphyses;* (b) *thickened dorsum sella;* (c) *wedged vertebrae, end plate sclerosis, mild platyspondyly, coxa valga.*

Differential Diagnosis, Significant: (a) Madelung deformity (dyschondrosteosis); (b) spondylometaphyseal dysplasia; (c) metaphyseal chondrodysplasias.

REFERENCE

Rosenberg E, Lohr H: A new hereditary bone dysplasia with characteristic bowing and thickening of the distal ulna. *Eur. J. Pediatr.* 145:40–45, 1986.

METATROPIC DYSPLASIA

Synonym: Hyperplastic achondroplasia.

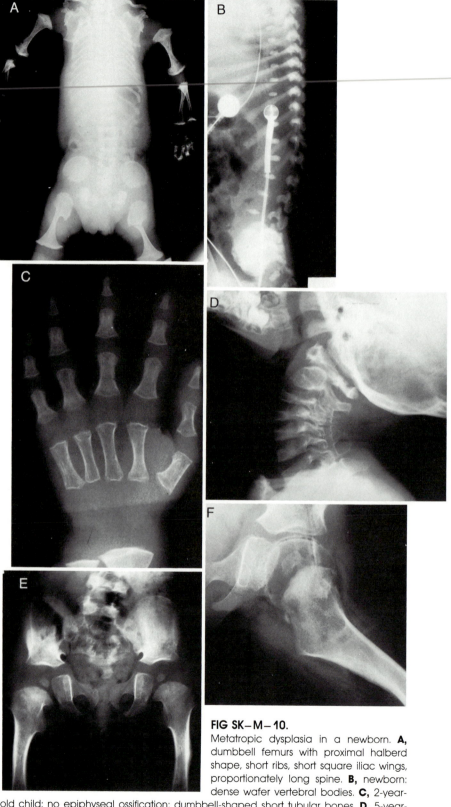

FIG SK—M—10.
Metatropic dysplasia in a newborn. **A,** dumbbell femurs with proximal halberd shape, short ribs, short square iliac wings, proportionately long spine. **B,** newborn: dense wafer vertebral bodies. **C,** 2-year-old child: no epiphyseal ossification; dumbbell-shaped short tubular bones. **D,** 5-year-old child: odontoid hypoplasia, platyspondy. **E,** 2-year-old child: short square iliac wings, halberd femurs with miniepiphyses. **F,** 2-year-old child, arthrogram of hip: capital femoral epiphyseal anlage is normal-appearing and smooth.

Mode of Inheritance: Nonlethal autosomal recessive type, nonlethal autosomal dominant type; lethal autosomal recessive type.

Frequency: Uncommon, about 43 cases reported to 1988.

Clinical Manifestations: (a) *short-limbed dwarfism wtih normal or slightly elongated trunk and narrow and cylindric thorax at birth;* (b) limitation of extension of some of joints (hips, knees), progressive joint enlargement; (c) *tail* (small caudal appendage or cutaneous fold in coccygeal region) *very severe progressive scoliosis or kyphoscoliosis;* (d) *relatively greater increase in length of limbs compared with trunk in childhood;* (e) other reported abnormalities: cyanosis, sleep apnea, neurologic deficits, cleft palate.

Radiologic Manifestations: (a) early micromelic period (perinatal): *dumbbell femurs and humeri, halberd proximal femurs,* generalized shortening of all tubular bones (including hands and feet), *dense, wafer vertebral bodies,* elongated clavicles, *short ribs with anterior and posterior flare,* increased distance between ribs and spine, short, square scapulae, *short square iliac wings, flat irregular acetabular roof,* narrow sacrosciatic notches; (b) later kyphoscoliotic period (childhood and adult): *trumpet-like metaphyses of long bones,* marked epiphyseal delay, *elongated fibula, dumbbell-shaped short tubular bones of hands and feet;* carpal ossification delay; *unusual sharply etched tarsal bones; increasingly severe scoliosis and kyphosis, hypoplastic odontoid, C1–C2 dislocation with flexion,* hydrocephalus; anteriorly wedged vertebrae; (c) other reported abnormalities: accessory ossification centers of ischia, dense metaphyseal lines (Fig SK–M–10).

Chondro-osseous Morphology: Absence of normal primary spongiosa, thin seal of bone at chondro-osseous junction, arrest of enchondral growth suggesting uncoupling of endochondral and perichondral growth (Boden); vacuolated resting cartilage with metachromatic staining.

Differential Diagnosis, Significant: (a) Kniest dysplasia; (b) metatropic variants; (c) fibrochondrogenesis; (d) Morquio disease; (e) spondyloepiphyseal-metaphyseal dysplasia, dominant "metatropic" type–Langer.

Special Comments: Metatropic dysplasia is the *"dwarf with a tail";* although heterogeneity exists in metatropic dysplasia, the various genetic forms are difficult to separate; several atypical forms of metatropic dysplasia have been described; Colavita and Kozlowski's case of neonatal death dwarfism actually represents a case of fibrochondrogenesis, not metatropic dysplasia (see fibrochondrogenesis).

REFERENCES

Beck M, et al.: Heterogeneity of metatropic dysplasia. *Eur. J. Pediatr.* 140:231–237, 1983.

Belik J, et al.: Respiratory complications of metatropic dysplasia. *Clin. Pediatr.* 24:504–511, 1985.

Boden SD, et al.: Metatropic dwarfism. *J. Bone Joint Surg.* 69A:174–183, 1987.

Colavita N, Kozlowski K: Neonatal death dwarfism: A new form. *Pediatr. Radiol.* 14:451, 1984.

Gefferth K: Metatropic dwarfism, in Kaufmann HJ (ed.): *Progress in Pediatric Radiology,* vol. 4. Basel, Karger, 1973, p. 137.

Johnston CE: Scoliosis in metatropic dysplasia. *Orthopedics* 6:491–498, 1983.

Maroteaux P, et al.: Der metatropische Zwergwuchs. *Arch. Kinderheilkd.* 173:211, 1966.

Perri G: A severe form of metatropic dwarfism. *Pediatr. Radiol.* 7:183, 1978.

Shohat M, et al.: Odontoid hypoplasia, cervical spine subluxation and hydrocephalus in metatropic dysplasia. *J. Pediatr.,* in press.

MIXED SCLEROSING BONE DYSPLASIA

Synonyms: Combined melorheostosis, osteopoikilosis, osteopathia striata and generalized sclerosis; MSBD.

Mode of Inheritance: Sporadic.

Frequency: Very rare; 8 cases to 1988.

Clinical Manifestations: *Asymptomatic,* elevated creatine phosphokinase, mild anemia, hypophosphatemia, hypocalcemia, markedly increased alkaline phosphatase, increased parathormone, subcutaneous nodules, lymphedema, hemangiomata.

Radiologic Manifestations: Combinations of *melorheostotic* (dense, dripping wax), *dense linear striations, bone islands* and often generalized sclerosis involving the entire skeleton (including sclerosis of skull and mandible at times), asymmetric; (a) MRI changes (Pacifici); (b) bone scans: increased uptake in all types of lesions.

Differential Diagnosis, Significant: (a) osteopathia striata with cranial sclerosis; (b) osteopetrosis.

Special Comments: MSBD probably should be confined to the combination of melorheostosis (MO), osteopoikilosis (OP) and osteopathia striata (OS) with or without focal sclerosis. Whyte however has alluded to 3 other types: type 2: OS with cranial sclerosis; type 3: OS with cortical hyperostosis and metadiaphyseal changes; type 4: OP with diaphyseal dysplasia. Another type: MO, OP, and scleroderma (Pascaud-Ged).

REFERENCES

Abrahamson MN: Disseminated asymptomatic osteosclerosis with features resembling melorheostosis, osteopoikilosis, and osteopathia striata. *J. Bone Joint Surg. [Am.]* 50A: 991–996, 1968.

Elkeles A: Mixed sclerosing bone dystrophy with regression of melorheostosis, letter. *Br. J. Radiol. [Am.]* 49:97, 1976.

Ewald FC: Unilateral mixed sclerosing bone dystrophy associated with unilateral lymphangiectasia and capillary hemangioma. *J. Bone Joint Surg.* 54A:878–880, 1972.

Kanis JA, Thomson JG: Mixed sclerosing bone dystrophy with regression of melorheostosis. *Br. J. Radiol.* 48:400–403, 1975.

Pacific R, et al.: Mixed-sclerosing bone dystrophy. *Calcif. Tissue Int.* 38:175–185, 1986.

Pascaud-Ged E, et al.: Melorheostosis osteopoikilosis and linear scleroderma. *Ann. Radiol.* 24:643–646, 1981.

Walker GF: Mixed sclerosing bone dystrophies. *J. Bone Joint Surg. [Br.]* 46B:546–552, 1964.

Whyte MP, et al.: Mixed-sclerosing bone dystrophy. *Skeletal Radiol.* 6:95–102, 1981.

MULTIPLE EPIPHYSEAL DYSPLASIA

Synonyms: Fairbank disease; Ribbing disease; dysplasia epiphysealis multiplex.

Mode of Inheritance: Autosomal dominant.

Frequency: Very common.

Historical Note: First described by Barrington Ward in 1912 (*Lancet 1:157, 1912*).

Clinical Manifestations: Clinical presentation and diagnosis often in late childhood or adolescence: (a) *limp, pain, and stiffness in hips, knees, and ankles*; (b) *early onset large joint arthrosis*, first decade on; limitation of joint motion; (c) *mild short-limbed dwarfism*; (d) slightly stubby hands and feet; (e) other reported abnormalities: os trigonum syndrome.

Radiologic Manifestations: (a) *delay in appearance of secondary ossification centers of tubular bones and ossification centers of hands and wrists*; (b) *small, irregular, fragmented, and in some cases flattened epiphyses of tubular bones, most pronounced in hips* and lower limbs; (c) relatively long fibula with external malleolus in low position, shallow acetabulum; (d) subsidiary ossification centers; (e) irregularity in shape and ossification of cuboid bones of wrists, ankles; (f) shortness of tubular bones of hands and feet with irregular epiphyses; (g) mild irregularity of end-plates of vertebrae, anterior wedging and Schmorl nodes in second and third decades; (h) MRI (1 case) normal epiphyseal imaging-decreased size, irregularity (Toby); (i) measurement standards of distal femoral epiphysis: measured 2 or more SD below the mean in 19 cases (Schlesinger); hip arthrography shows normal anlage for capital femoral epiphyses with decrease in joint space size (Lachman); (j) other reported abnormalities: subluxated radial head, slipped capital femoral epiphysis, dislocated patella, double-layered patella, genu valgum or varum, osteochondritis dessicans of knee (Versteylen) (Fig SK–M–11).

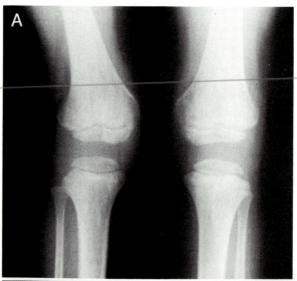

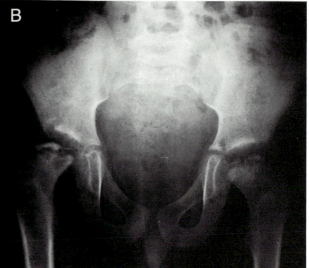

FIG SK–M–11.
Multiple epiphyseal dysplasia, Fairbanks type, in a 6-year-old child. **A,** marked epiphyseal ossification delay and dysplasia at the knees. **B,** small dense fragmented epiphyseal centers of proximal femurs, and acetabular hypoplasia.

Differential Diagnosis, Significant: (a) Meyer dysplasia; (b) Legg-Perthes disease; (c) spondyloepiphyseal dysplasias; (d) varying juvenile arthropathies; (e) chondrodysplasia punctata (C–H type); (f) Mseleni joint disease (Solomon L, et al.: *South. Med. Assoc. J.* 69:15–17, 1986); (g) Wolcott-Rallison syndrome.

Special Comments: Some separate a very *mild*, common *Ribbing* type from the more *severe Fairbank* type. Ribbing MED may have involvement only of the hips; both are autosomal dominant.

Other MED Syndromes: *MED* with *myopia* and *deafness* (Beighton, MacDermot), epiphyseal dysplasias with *mi-*

crocephaly and *immune deficiency* (Aylsworth) with *microcephaly, mental retardation* and *nystagmus (Lowry-Wood syndrome)*, autosomal recessive.

REFERENCES

Aylsworth AS, et al: Proceedings of the Greenwood Genetics Center, vol 7. 1988, p 198.

Beighton P, et al: Dominant inheritance of multiple epiphyseal dysplasia, myopia and deafness. *Clin. Genet.* 14:173, 1978.

Dahners LE, et al.: Findings at arthrotomy in a case of double layered patellae associated with multiple epiphyseal dysplasia. *J. Pediatr. Orthop.* 2:67–70, 1982.

Fairbank HAT: Generalized disease of skeleton. *Proc. R. Soc. Med.* 28:1611, 1935.

Herring JA: Legg-Perthes disease versus multiple epiphyseal dysplasia: Instructional case. *J. Pediatr. Orthop.* 7:341–343, 1987.

Hulvey JT, Keats T: Multiple epiphyseal dysplasia. *A.J.R.* 106:170–177, 1969.

Lachman RS, et al.: Arthrography of the hip: A clue to the pathogenesis of the epiphyseal dysplasias. *Radiology* 108:317–322, 1973.

Lowry RB, Wood BJ: Syndrome of epiphyseal dysplasia, short stature, microcephaly, and nystagmus. *Clin. Genet.* 8:269, 1975.

MacDermot KD, et al: Epiphyseal dysplasia of the femoral head, mild vertebral abnormality, myopia, and sensorineural deafness. *J. Med. Genet.* 24:602, 1987.

Mena HR, et al.: Multiple epiphyseal dysplasia: A family case report. *J.A.M.A.* 236:2629, 1976.

Molay M, et al.: Os trigonum syndrome in a patient with multiple epiphyseal dysplasia. *J. Foot Surg.* 21:265–268, 1982.

Murphy MC, et al.: Multiple epiphyseal dysplasia. *J. Bone Joint Surg. [Am.]* 55A:814, 1973.

Nevin NC, et al: Syndrome of short stature microcephaly, mental retardation, and multiple epiphyseal dysplasia--Lowry-Wood syndrome. *Am. J. Med. Genet.* 24:33, 1986.

Patrone NA, Kredich DW: Arthritis in children with multiple epiphyseal dysplasia. J. Rheumatol. 12:145–149, 1985.

Ribbing S: Studien ueber hereditäre, multiple Epiphysenstörungen. *Acta Radiol.* Suppl. 34, 1937.

Schlesinger AE, et al.: Distal femoral epiphysis with normal standards for thickness and application to bone dysplasias. *Radiology* 159:515–519, 1986.

Toby EB, et al.: Magnetic resonance imaging of pediatric hip disease. *J. Pediatr. Orthop.* 5:665–671, 1985.

Versteylen RJ, et al.: Multiple epiphyseal dysplasia complicated by severe osteochondritis dessicans of the knee. *Skeletal Radiol.* 17:407–412, 1988.

Radiologic Manifestations: (a) *sclerosis of base of skull* and mastoids, *delay in closure of anterior fontanelle, micrognathia,* hypoplasia of coronoid process of mandible with wide angle between horizontal and vertical rami, loculation of unknown nature in mandibular rami, impacted molar teeth, underdeveloped paranasal sinuses; (b) *tall vertebrae* (especially those of axis, atlas, and occipital condyles), anterior concavity of the body of thoracic vertebrae, decreased lumbar disk space; (c) *cortical irregularity and ribbon appearance of ribs;* (d) cortical irregularity and flaring of clavicles, delayed sternal ossification centers; (e) flared iliac wings, flat acetabular roofs, *tapered ischia;* (f) *metaphyseal flaring of short and long bones, long femoral necks; subtrochanteric narrowing,* bowed radius and tibia (**S**-shaped), coxa valga; (g) delay in general ossification; (h) other reported abnormalities: sigmoid configuration of clavicles, pectus excavatum, hourglass vertebrae, delayed closure of anterior fontanelle, ureterovesical obstruction; (i) prenatal diagnosis with ultrasound in 16-week fetus; Donnenfeld; (j) *lethal male cases: absent digits, cervical lordosis; dystrophic calcification* (soft tissue and long bones) (Fig SK–O–2).

Biochemical Abnormalities: Increased collagen synthesis and content.

Differential Diagnosis, Significant: (a) precocious osteodysplasty; (b) frontometaphyseal dysplasia; (c) Hajdu-Cheney syndrome.

Special Comments: Precocious osteo-dysplasty (autosomal recessive) appears to be a separate disorder (Donnenfeld).

REFERENCES

Bartolozzi P, et al.: Melnick-Needles syndrome: Osteodysplasty with kyphoscoliosis. *J. Pediatr. Orthop.* 3:387–391, 1983.

Donnenfeld AE, et al.: Melnick-Needles syndrome in males. *Am. J. Med. Genet.* 27:159–173, 1987.

Fryns JP, et al.: Osteodysplasty: A rare skeletal dysplasia. *Acta Paediatr. Belg.* 32:65, 1979.

Gorlin RJ, et al.: Melnick-Needles syndrome: Radiographic alterations in the mandible. *Radiology* 128:351, 1978.

Klint RB, et al.: Melnick-Needles osteodysplasia associated with pulmonary hypertension, obstructive uropathy and marrow hypoplasia. *Pediatr. Radiol.* 6:49, 1977.

Krajewska-Walasek M, et al.: Melnick-Needles syndrome in males. *Am. J. Med. Genet.* 27:153–158, 1987.

Maroteaux P, et al.: L'ostéodysplastie (syndrome de Melnick et de Needles). *Presse Med.* 76:715, 1968.

Melnick JC, Needles CF: An undiagnosed bone dysplasia: A 2 family study of 4 generations and 3 generations. *Am. J. Roentgenol.* 97:39, 1966.

Moadel E, et al.: Osteodysplastia (Melnick-Needles syndrome). *Radiology* 123:154, 1977.

Švejcar J: Biochemical abnormalities in connective tissue of osteodysplasty of Melnick-Needles and dyssegmental dwarfism. *Clin. Genet.* 23:369–375, 1983.

OSTEODYSPLASTY, PRECOCIOUS

Mode of Inheritance: Autosomal recessive.

Frequency: Very rare; 10 cases (5 male).

Clinical Manifestations: (a) *low birth weight;* (b) *hypertelorism, exophthalmos; micrognathia, round face, dental malalignment;* (c) *severely short bowed limbs;* genu valga; *small hands and feet;* (d) scoliosis, narrow chest; (e) frequent urinary and respiratory infections; *frequent death in childhood.*

Radiologic Manifestations: *Same as Melnick-Needles* plus (a) *hypoplasia of distal phalanges* (fingers and toes); (b) *markedly shortened long bones.*

Differential Diagnosis, Significant: (a) osteodysplasty, Melnick-Needles; (b) pycnodysostosis; Hajdu-Cheney syndrome.

REFERENCES

de Toni T, et al.: La sindrome di Melnick-Needles. *Minerva Pediatr.* 35:447–454, 1983.

Donnenfeld AE: Melnick-Needles syndrome in males. *Am. J. Med. Genet.* 27:159–173, 1987.

Grosse KP, Bowing B: Osteodysplastie, in Spranger J, Tolksdorf B (eds): *Klinische Genetik in der Padiatrie.* Stuttgart, Thieme Verlag, 1979, p. 80–86.

Kozlowski K, et al.: Precocious type of osteodysplasia. *Acta Radiol. Diagn.* 14:171–176, 1973.

ter Haar B, et al.: Melnick-Needles syndrome: Indication for an autosomal recessive form. *Am. J. Med. Genet.* 13:469–477, 1982.

Theodorou SD, et al.: Osteodysplasty (Melnick-Needles syndrome in a male). *Prog. Clin. Biol. Res.* 104:139–142, 1982.

OSTEOGENESIS IMPERFECTA

Synonyms: Approximately forty, including Lobstein disease, Ekman syndrome, osteopsathyrosis, van der Hoeve syndrome, Vrolik disease; OI.

Historical Data: First good description, Ekman 1788; first in-depth description, Lobstein 1833; mythical Danish prince (Ivar Benlos) carried into battle on a shield (unable to walk on his soft legs); Egyptian mummy dated 1,000 B.C. (Gray); high gene frequency in Africa (Zimbabwe): 2 major tribal groups, mutation occurred about 2,000 years ago (Viljoen).

Frequency: Very common; 4 per 100,000 births; most common second trimester ultrasound diagnosis of short bent limbs.

Classification: *Type I: Autosomal dominant; group A, normal teeth; group B, dentinogenesis imperfecta (DI)*

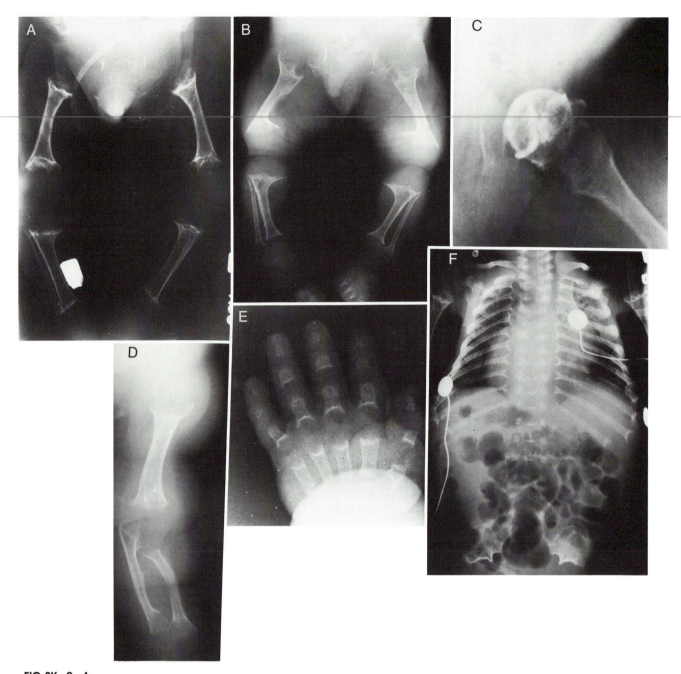

FIG SK–0–1.
Opsismodysplasia in **A,** a full-term newborn: short bones; metaphyseal flare, no epiphyseal centers, slit ischial ossification; **B,** a child aged 5½ years: still unossified epiphyses; **C,** an infant aged 1½ years: hip arthrogram—normal capital femoral epiphyseal cartilaginous anlage; **D,** an infant aged 1 year: upper extremity— flared metaphyses; no epiphyseal ossification; **E,** an infant aged 6 months: brachydactyly with marked metaphyseal flare; **F,** a newborn: anterior and posterior rib flaring and cupping; dense hypoplastic vertebral body ossification; hypoplastic cupped acetabula. *(Continued.)*

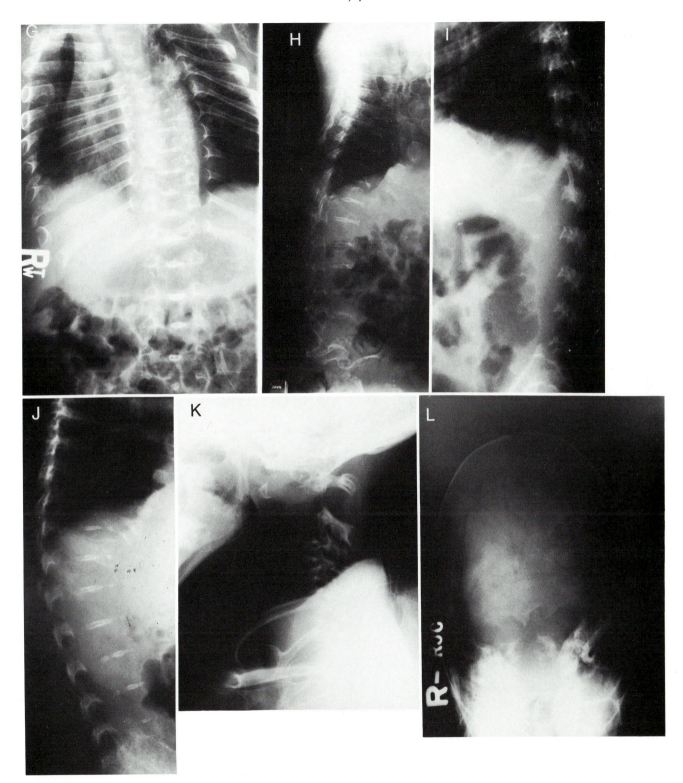

FIG SK–O–1 (cont).
G, and **H,** a child aged 5½ years: very little increase in vertebral body ossification (anteroposterior and lateral); **I,** a newborn: minimal vertebral body ossification with almost normally ossified posterior elements; **J,** an infant aged 1½ years: tiny wafer vertebral ossification with maintenance of apparent disk space distances; **K,** an infant aged 6 months: severe cervical vertebral body ossification defects with C1–C2 dislocation; **L,** a newborn: ossification defect of skull around and posterior to foramen magnum; remaining skull density is normal.

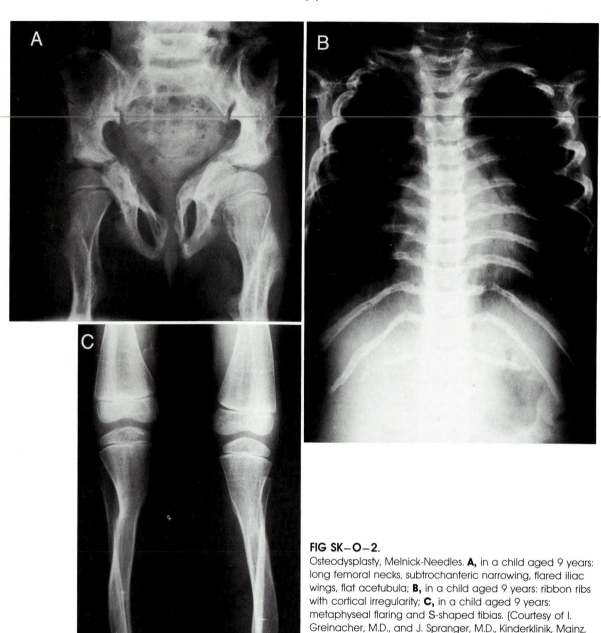

FIG SK–O–2.
Osteodysplasty, Melnick-Needles. **A,** in a child aged 9 years: long femoral necks, subtrochanteric narrowing, flared iliac wings, flat acetubula; **B,** in a child aged 9 years: ribbon ribs with cortical irregularity; **C,** in a child aged 9 years: metaphyseal flaring and S-shaped tibias. (Courtesy of I. Greinacher, M.D., and J. Spranger, M.D., Kinderklinik, Mainz, West Germany.)

Clinical Manifestations: (a) *osseous fragility* (none to moderately severe); (b) *blue sclerae* (all ages); (c) *hearing loss* (50% by age 40); (d) other reported abnormalities: joint hypermobility; postfracture deformities; *easy bruisability*, premature arcus senilis; joint dislocations; asymptomatic mitral valve prolapse and aortic root dilatation (rare); (e) other important features: marked reduction in fracture frequency after puberty, long bone deformity less severe than in other types, hyperextensibility joint changes.

Radiologic Manifestations: (a) *osteoporosis*; (b) *fractures* (none to multiple); (c) large or normal calvarium; *wormian bones*; (d) *radiographic DI* (group B) hypoplastic dentine, short roots, late eruption, caries; (e) kyphoscoliosis.

Classification: *Type II: New dominant mutations (majority); recurrences due to gonadal mosaicism; less than 5% autosomal recessive (especially group C); perinatally lethal; group A: broad crumpled long bones (accordion-like), beaded ribs; group B: broad crumpled long bones, no beading (usually), rib fractures, survival possible; group C: thin fractured long bones, thin mildly beaded ribs (possibly autosomal recessive), very rare type.*

Clinical Manifestations: Connective tissue fragility, blue sclera, nonimmune hydrops (about 15%, group A), microscopic calcification of aorta and endocardium (group A), respiratory distress, micrognathia, small nose.

Radiologic Manifestations: (a) *almost no ossification of skull or wormian bones* with severe demineralization; (b) *beaded ribs, shortened crumpled long bones* (especially femurs and humeri), multiple fractures, *diffuse osteoporosis with thin cortices*, angulated tibiae, short tubular bones just osteoporotic; (c) flattened acetabulae and iliac wings (Fig SK–O–3).

Classification: *Type III: Autosomal recessive, rare disorder.*

Clinical Manifestations: *Nonlethal, severely affected, limb deformities at birth,* poor growth, kyphoscoliosis, pulmonary hypertension, *fractures often at birth and numerous fractures by 2 years of age;* "triangular facies" with frontal bossing, *blue sclerae at birth but change to white later;* DI may be present.

Radiologic Manifestations: *Osteoporosis, severe, generalized;* (a) *skull:* face and basiocciput reasonably well ossified; *membranous skull severely deossified; wormian bones;* (b) *long bones:* mild shortening, *marked angulations; overmodeling;* later metaphyseal and diaphyseal widening; "popcorn" calcification; (c) *codfish vertebrae.*

Classification: *Type IV: Autosomal dominant; normal sclera; group A: normal teeth; group B: DI.*

Clinical Manifestations: *Osseous fragility (mild to moderate);* (a) *newborn:* fractures (25%); (b) *childhood: fractures (maximal);* (c) *similar to type I but no bleeding diathesis, less deafness, greater long bone deformity and kyphoscoliosis, normal sclera.*

Radiologic Manifestations: See Type I.

Complications: Nonunion of fractures; flail chest; cardiomyopathy; atrial rupture; aortic root stiffness; central retinal artery occlusion; bleeding diathesis; aortic root dilatation (12%); apareunia; upper cervical cord compression (Pauli) metabolic acidosis; coarctation of the aorta; decreased skin strength (type 1) pulmonary emboli with rod fixation; brittle hair; retinoblastoma family; diaphragmatic hernia; malignant hyperpyrexia (4 cases); ulnar artery aneurysm; mitral valve prolapse; *osteosarcoma;* hangman's fracture.

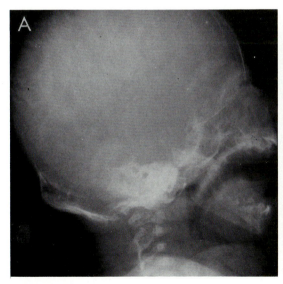
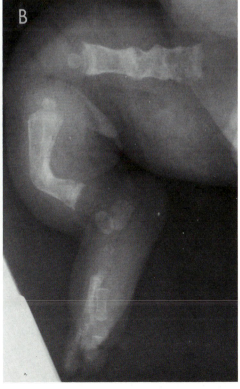

FIG SK–O–3.
Osteogenesis imperfecta type II. **A,** newborn with poorly ossified skull and wormian bones. **B,** bones of lower limb are markedly deformed (accordion-shaped femora); healing or healed fractures are present. (From Taybi H: Osteogenesis imperfecta congenita. *Semin. Roentgenol.* 8:184, 1973. Reproduced with permission.)

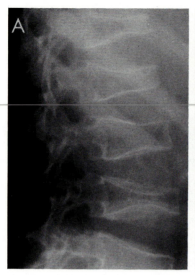
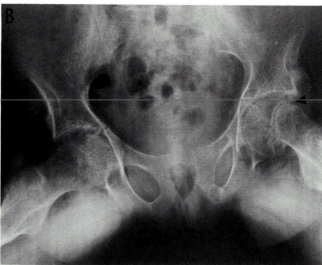

FIG SK—O—4.
Osteogenesis imperfecta type I or IV in an 8-year-old female. **A,** osteoporosis and flat biconcave vertebral bodies. **B,** same patient at 11 years of age. Slipped capital femoral epiphysis and osteoporosis.

General Radiologic Manifestations: (a) "popcorn" calcifications; (b) epiphyseal involvement (cone epiphyses); (c) *basilar impression* (d) *hyperplastic callus formation;* (e) bone scanning assessment; (f) CT for bone mineral content analysis; CT of petrous bone (narrow middle ear cavity with proliferation of dysplastic bone); CT—macrocephaly; cortical atrophy; (g) biphosphonate treatment produces dense metaphyseal lines; (h) prenatal diagnosis, ultrasound second trimester (3 cases, type 1; 12 cases, type 2; 2 cases, type 3; 5 cases, unspecified); *limb shortening* and bowing, fetal fractures; decreased skull echoes (may be misleading); rib fractures and beading (Fig SK—O—4).

Chondro-osseous and Biochemical Defects: *Molecular defects of type 1 collagen;* patients with severe radiographic changes have molecules that are overmodified over a longer extent; point mutations with amino acid substitutions; smaller apatite crystal size; decreased trabecular bone volume, thin cortices and reduced calcification rate.

Differential Diagnosis, Significant: (a) steroid-induced osteoporosis, including Cushing disease; (b) postmenopausal osteoporosis and multiple myeloma; (c) scurvy; (d) battered child syndrome; (e) juvenile osteoporosis; (f) malignant osteoporosis; (g) campomelic and kyphomelic dysplasia; (h) dentinogenesis imperfecta (without bone involvement; Gage); (i) osteoporosis—pseudoglioma syndrome; copper deficiency.

Other OI-like Syndromes: (a) *Grant syndrome;* (b) *hyperimmunoglobulinemia E syndrome* with osteoporosis and recurrent fractures; (c) *OI, microcephaly, cataracts* (Buyse); (d) *arthropathic form of OI* (Penttinen); (e) *OI,* macrocephaly, wormian bones, *brachytelephalangy,* hyperextensible joint; *congenital blindness,* oligophrenia (Heide); (f) *OI, total alopecia, hoarseness, skin aging* (Kääriäinen); (g) OI, *cranio-* synostosis, ocular proptosis, hydrocephalus (Cole); (h) *OI, maxillary* and *mandibular lesions, coarse trabecular bone structure* (Levin).

Special Comments: (a) osteogenesis imperfecta appears to be a "family" of similar disorders with many different point mutations not only within specific types but even among subgroups; the concept of OI congenita and tarda are no longer valid; (b) linkage analysis has been used effectively for prenatal diagnosis (Tsipouras 1987).

REFERENCES

Buyse M, et al.: A syndrome of osteogenesis imperfecta microcephaly, and cataracts. *Birth Defects* 14(6B):95, 1978.

Byers PH, et al.: Perinatal lethal osteogenesis imperfecta (OI type 2). *Am. J. Hum. Genet.* 42:237–248, 1988.

Cardemas N, et al.: Flail chest in the newborn. *Clin. Pediatr.* 27:161–162, 1988.

Cole DC, et al.: Bone fragility, craniosynostosis, ocular proptosis, hydrocephalus, and distinctive facial features: A newly recognized type of osteogenesis imperfecta. *J. Pediatr.* 110:76, 1987.

deGuembecker C, et al: Radiologic features of the epiphyseal abnormality in osteogenesis imperfecta. *J. Radiol.* 64:249–253, 1983.

Devogelaer JP, et al.: Radiological manifestations of biphosphonate treatment with APD in a child suffering from osteogenesis imperfecta. *Skeletal Radiol.* 16:360–363, 1987.

Fisher LW, et al.: Two bovine models of osteogenesis imperfecta exhibit decreased apatite crystal size. *Calcif. Tissue Int.* 40:282–285, 1987.

Forslund BO, et al.: Brittle hair in osteogenesis imperfecta. *Acta Dermatol. Venereol.* 64:418–420, 1984.

Gage JP: Dentinogenesis imperfecta: A new prospective. *Aust. Dent. J.* 30:285–290, 1985.

Gamble JG, et al.: Nonunion of fractures in children who have osteogenesis imperfecta. *J. Bone Joint Surg. [Am.]* 70A:439–443, 1988.

Gray PHK: A case of osteogenesis imperfecta associated with dentinogenesis imperfecta dating from antiquity. *Clin. Radiol.* 21:106–108, 1970.

Heide T: Ein Syndrom bestehend aus Osteogenesis imperfecta, Makrozephalus mit Schaltknochen und prominenten Stirnhöckern, Brachytelephalangie, Gelenküberstreckbarkeit, kongenitaler Amaurose und Oligophrenie bei drei Geschwistern. *Klin. Padiatr.* 193;334, 1981.

Hollister DW: Molecular basis of osteogenesis imperfecta. *Curr. Probl. Dermatol.* 17:76–94, 1987.

Hortop J, et al.: Cardiovascular involvement in osteogenesis imperfecta. *Circulation* 73:54–61, 1986.

Jardin C, et al.: Tomographic and CT features of the petrous bone in Lobstein's disease. *J. Neuroradiol.* 12:317–326, 1985.

Kääriainen H, et al.: A dominant syndrome resembling osteogenesis imperfecta with total alopecia, hoarseness, and premature aging of the skin. *Prog. Clin. Biol. Res.* 104:167, 1982.

Kalath S, et al.: Increased aortic root stiffness associated with osteogenesis imperfecta. *Ann Biomed. Eng.* 15:91–99, 1987.

Kramer EL: Bone scan appearance of osteogenesis imperfecta in an adult. *Clin. Nucl. Med.* 11:331–333, 1986.

Kurtz D, et al.: Vertebral bone mineral content in osteogenesis imperfecta. *Calcif. Tissue Int.* 37:14–18, 1985.

Levin LS, et al.: Osteogenesis imperfecta with unusual skeletal lesions: Report of three families. *Am. J. Med. Genet.* 21:257, 1985.

McCall RE, Bax JA: Hyperplastic callus formation in osteogenesis imperfecta following Intramedullary rodding. *J. Pediatr. Orthop.* 4:361–364, 1984.

Moore JB, et al.: Ulnar artery aneurysm in osteogenesis imperfecta. *Hand* 15:91–95, 1983.

Morton ME: Excessive bleeding after surgery in osteogenesis imperfecta. *Br. J. Oral Maxillofacial Surg.* 25:507–511, 1987.

Oxlund H, et al.: Reduced strength of skin in osteogenesis imperfecta. *Eur. J. Clin. Invest.* 15:408–411, 1985.

Paterson CR, et al.: Clinical and radiological features of osteogenesis imperfecta type 4A. *Acta Paediatr. Scand.* 76:548–552, 1987.

Pauli RM, Gilbert EF: Upper cervical cord compression as cause of death in osteogenesis imperfecta type 2. *J. Pediatr.* 108:579–581, 1986.

Pentinnen R, et al.: An arthropathic form of osteogenesis imperfecta, *Acta Paediatr. Scand.* 69:263, 1980.

Pozo JL, et al.: Basilar impression in osteogenesis imperfecta. *J. Bone Joint Surg. [Br.]* 66B:233–238, 1984.

Rampton AJ, et al.: Occurrence of malignant hyperpyrexia in a patient with osteogenesis imperfecta. *Br. J. Anaesth.* 56:1443–1446, 1984.

Reid BS, et al.: Osteosarcoma arising in osteogenesis imperfecta. *Pediatr. Radiol.* 8:110, 1979.

Robinson LP, et al.: Prenatal diagnosis of osteogenesis imperfecta type 3. *Prenat. Diagn.* 7:7–15, 1987.

Rodriguez RP, et al.: Apareunia as a complication of osteogenesis imperfecta. *Orthopedics* 9:1233–1234, 1986.

Romero R, et al.: *Prenatal Diagnosis of Congenital Anomalies.* Appleton and Lange, 1987, pp. 354–357.

Rush GA, et al.: Hangman's fracture in a patient with osteogenesis imperfecta. *J. Bone Joint Surg. [Am.]* 66A:778–779, 1984.

Rutkowski R, et al.: Osteosarcoma in osteogenesis imperfecta. *J Bone Joint Surg. [Am.]* 61A:606–608, 1979.

Sadat-Ali M, et al.: Metabolic acidosis in osteogenesis imperfecta. *Eur. J. Pediatr.* 145:582–583, 1986.

Ste-Marie LG, et al.: Iliac bone histomorphometry in adults and children with osteogenesis imperfecta. *J. Clin. Pathol.* 37:1081–1089, 1984.

Schwarz T, Gotsman WS: Mitral valve prolapse in osteogenesis imperfecta. *Isr. J. Med. Sci.* 17:1087–1088, 1981.

Sigmund J, et al.: Aortic coarctation and osteogenesis imperfecta. *Pediatr. Padol.* 21:343–349, 1986.

Sillence DO, et al.: Osteogenesis imperfecta type II: Delineation of the phenotype with reference to genetic heterogeneity. *Am. J. Med. Genet.* 17:407, 1984.

Sillence DO: Personal communication, 1988.

Spranger J: Invited editorial comment. *Am. J. Med. Genet.* 17:425–428, 1984.

Tsipouras P, et al.: Neurologic correlates of osteogenesis imperfecta. *Arch. Neurol.* 43:150–152, 1986.

Tsipouras P, et al.: Prenatal prediction of osteogenesis imperfecta (OI type 4). *J. Med. Genet.* 24:406–409, 1987.

Viljoen D, Beighton P: Osteogenesis imperfecta type 3: An ancient mutation in Africa? *Am. J. Med. Genet.* 27:907–912, 1987.

Weil NH: Osteogenesis Imperfecta.: Historical background. *Clin. Orthop. Rel. Res.* 159:6, 1981.

Wisser J, et al.: Osteogenesis imperfecta in prenatal ultrasound diagnosis. *Pädiatr. Praxis* 35:115–123, 1987.

OSTEOGLOPHONIC DYSPLASIA

Synonym: Craniofacial dysostosis with fibrous metaphyseal defects.

Mode of Inheritance: Autosomal dominant.

Frequency: Very rare; nine patients to 1988.

Clinical Manifestations: (a) *dwarfism with short stubby extremities;* (b) *craniofacial features: acrocephaly, cloverleaf deformity, frontal bossing,* hypertelorism, marked mandibular prognathism, unerupted teeth, high-arched palate, anteverted nares; (c) short neck; (d) lumbar lordosis; (e) other reported abnormalities: inflammatory arthritis and hypophosphatemic osteomalacia; mental retardation.

Radiologic Manifestations: (a) *craniosynostosis,* midface hypoplasia, prognathism, cystic changes in mandibular ramus; (b) *unerupted teeth;* (c) *platyspondyly with anterior projection,* narrow spinal canal, posterior scalloping of lumbar vertebral bodies; (d) *gross dysplastic changes in metaphyses and epiphyses of long bones (neonatal; one case), irregular areas of radiolucency (fibrous defects),* loss of cortical bone adjacent to radiolucent lesions; (e) *shortening and broadening of metacarpals, metatarsals, and phalanges, wide medullary cavities, pointed proximal end of metacarpals,* slight irregularity of carpal bones; (f) distorted pelvis with radiolucent areas present in ilia (Fig SK–O–5).

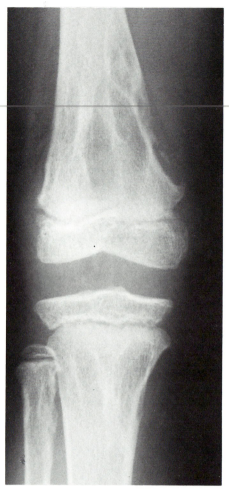

FIG SK—O—5.
Osteoglophonic dwarfism. Knee roentgenogram shows large eccentric areas of radiolucency in metaphyses with absence of cortical bone. (From Keats TE, Smith TH, Sweet DE: Craniofacial dysostosis with fibrous metaphyseal defects. *Am. J. Roentgenol.* 124:271, 1975. Reproduced with permission.)

Chondro-oseous Morphology: Metaphyseal lesions are benign whorls of fibrous tissue (Keats).

Differential Diagnosis, Significant: (a) mucopolysaccharidoses, (b) spondyloenchondromatosis.

Special Comment: The term *osteoglophonic* (of Greek origin) refers to "hollowed out" appearance of the bony structures in this disease.

REFERENCES

Beighton P, et al.: Osteoglophonic dwarfism. *Pediatr. Radiol.* 10:46, 1980.
Keats TE, Smith TH, Sweet DE: Craniofacial dysostosis with fibrous metaphyseal defects. *Am. J. Roentgenol.* 124:271, 1975.
Kelley RI, et al.: Osteoglophonic dwarfism in two generations. *J. Med. Genet.* 20:436—440, 1983.
Reynolds JF, et al.: Osteoglophonic dysplasia: Natural history and confirmation of autosomal dominant inheritance. *Proc. Greenwood Genet. Center* 7:167—168, 1988.

OSTEOMESOPYKNOSIS

Mode of Inheritance: Autosomal dominant.

Frequency: Very rare; 10 cases to 1988.

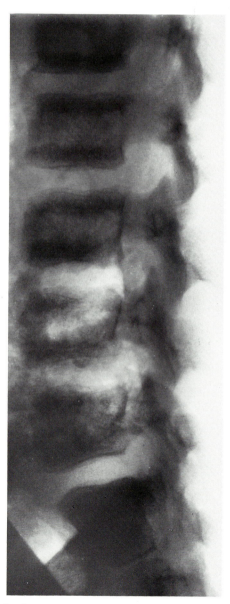

FIG SK—O—6.
Osteomesopyknosis. Dense vertebral plates in 10-year-old boy. (From Maroteaux P: L'ostéomesopycnose. *Arch. Fr. Pediatr.* 37:153, 1980. Reproduced with permission.)

Clinical Manifestations: Most cases symptomatic in the adolescent and young adult: *back pain.*

Radiologic Manifestations: (a) *sclerosis of vertebral bodies along end-plates, pelvis,* and in some cases in proximal segment of femora; (b) CT: patchy sclerotic lesions (Fig SK–O–6).

Differential Diagnosis, Significant: (a) osteopetrosis; (b) dysosteosclerosis; (c) fibrous dysplasia.

REFERENCES

Maroteaux P: L'osteomésopycnose: Une nouvelle affection condensante de transmission dominante autosomique. *Arch. Fr. Pediatr.* 37:153–157, 1980.
Proschek R, et al.: Osteomesopyknosis. *J. Bone Joint Surg. [Am.]* 67A:652–653, 1985.
Stoll CG, et al.: Brief clinical report: Osteomesopyknosis. *Am. J. Med. Genet.* 8:349–353, 1981.

OSTEOPATHIA STRIATA

Synonyms: Voorhoeve disease; OS.

Mode of Inheritance: Sporadic, isolated case reports.

Frequency: Probably uncommon; underreported; about 12 cases to 1988.

Clinical Manifestations: Asymptomatic.

Radiologic Manifestations: (a) *vertical fine dense linear striations especially at the ends of long tubular bones,* all bones reported affected except skull and clavicle; (b) normal uptake of ^{99m}Tc pyrophosphate (bone imaging).

Differential Diagnosis, Significant: (a) osteopathia striata (OS) with cranial sclerosis; (b) Goltz syndrome; (c) OS with familial dermopathy and white forelock (X-linked or autosomal dominant) (Whyte); (d) sponastrime dysplasia; (e) mixed sclerosing bone dysplasia.

REFERENCES

Bernard C, et al.: A propos d'an cas d'Osteopathie striee. *Sem. Hop. Paris* 60:573–576, 1984.
Carlson DH: Osteopathia striata revisited. *J. Assoc. Can. Radiol.* 28:190, 1977.
Gehweiler JA, et al.: Osteopathia striata: Voorhoeve's disease. *Am. J. Roentgenol.* 118:450, 1973.
Paling MR, et al.: Osteopathia striata with sclerosis and thickening of the skull. *Br. J. Radiol.* 54:427, 1981.
Voorhoeve N: L'image radiologique non encore décrite d'une anomalie du squelette: Ses rapports avec la dyschondroplasie et l'osteopathia condensans disseminata. *Acta Radiol.* 3:407, 1924.
Whyte MP, et al.: ^{99m}TC-pyrophosphate bone imaging in

osteopoikilosis, osteopathia striata, and melorheostosis. *Radiology* 127:439, 1978.
Whyte MP, et al.: Osteopathia striata associated with familial dermopathy and white forelock. *Am. J. Med. Genet.* 5:227, 1980.

OSTEOPATHIA STRIATA (OS) WITH CRANIAL SCLEROSIS

Synonym: Cranial sclerosis with striated bone disease.

Mode of inheritance: Autosomal dominant.

Frequency: Rare; 22 cases reported to 1988.

Clinical Manifestations: (a) *often asymptomatic* (50%); (b) vague recurrent joint pain; (c) hearing difficulties including deafness; (d) facial disfigurement, macrocephaly, and cranial nerve dysfunction resulting from cranial deformity; facial nerve palsy; cleft and high arched palate (50%); (e) other reported abnormalities: mental retardation, premature cortical cataracts, frequent respiratory infections.

Radiologic Manifestations: (a) *vertical linear fine striations* especially in long bones; (b) *increased bone density in other bones,* i.e., ribs, vertebrae, pelvis, carpal and tarsal bones; (c) *increased skull density, especially basal* (60%); also frontal, facial (including mandible), and calvarial; hypoplastic paranasal sinuses (45%) (Fig SK–O–7).

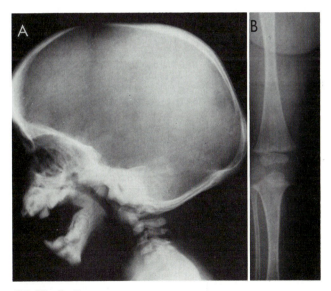

FIG SK–O–7.
Osteopathia striata with cranial sclerosis. Female child with frontal bossing, depressed nasal bridge, apparent hypertelorism, and some weakness and underdevelopment of musculature. **A,** skull of patient at 2 years and 5 months showing thick calvaria, also thick and dense basilar region. **B,** striation of long bones in particular in distal shaft and metaphysis of femur in same patient at 2 years and 3 months of age. (From Taybi H, et al.: Osteopathia striata. *Birth Defects* 5[4]:105, 1969. Reproduced with permission.)

Differential Diagnosis, Significant: (a) OS; (b) Goltz syndrome, (c) OS with familial dermopathy and white forelock, (d) sponsastrime dysplasia; (e) mixed sclerosing bone dysplasia; (f) other craniotubular dysplasias.

Special Comments: OS with cranial sclerosis appears to represent an entity different from isolated OS. A case of OS with cranial sclerosis in the mother had other multiple anomalies in her son (short fibulas; cervical kyphosis; hand anomalies: delta phalanx (Cuarrino).

REFERENCES

Cortina H, et al.: Familial osteopathia striata with cranial condensation. *Pediatr. Radiol.* 11:87, 1981.

Currarino G, et al.: Severe craniofacial sclerosis with multiple anomalies in a boy and his mother. *Pediatr. Radiol.* 16:441, 1986.

De Keyser J, et al.: Osteopathia striata with cranial sclerosis. *Clin. Neurol. Neurosurg.* 85:41–48, 1983.

Horan FT, et al.: Osteopathia striata with cranial sclerosis. An autosomal dominant entity. *Clin. Genet.* 13:201, 1978.

Kornreich L, et al.: Osteopathia striata, cranial sclerosis with cleft palate and facial nerve palsy. *Eur. J. Pediatr.* 147:101–103, 1988.

Nakamura T, et al.: Osteopathia with cranial sclerosis affecting three family members. *Skeletal Radiol.* 14:267–269, 1985.

Paling MR, et al.: Osteopathia striata with sclerosis and thickening of the skull. *Br. J. Radiol.* 54:344, 1981.

Piechowiak H, et al.: Cranial sclerosis with striated bone disease. *Klin. Padiatr.* 198:418–424, 1986.

Robinow M, Unger F: Syndrome of osteopathia striata, macrocephaly and cranial sclerosis. *Am. J. Dis. Child.* 138:821–823, 1984.

Schnyder PA: Osseous changes of osteopathia striata associated with cranial sclerosis. *Skeletal Radiol.* 5:19, 1980.

Taybi H, et al.: Osteopathia striata. *Birth Defects* 5(4):105, 1969.

Winter RM, et al.: Osteopathia striata with cranial sclerosis: Highly variable expression within a family including cleft palate in two neonatal cases. *Clin. Genet.* 18:462, 1980.

OSTEOPETROSIS

Synonyms: Albers-Schönberg disease; marble bone disease; congenital osteosclerosis; osteosclerosis fragalis generalisata.

Types and Modes of Inheritance: (a) *precocious* (malignant, congenital, infantile)—*autosomal recessive;* (b) *delayed* (benign, adult, tarda)—*autosomal dominant;* (c) *intermediate form* (mild recessive)—*autosomal recessive;* (d) *carbonic anhydrase 2 deficiency syndrome* (osteopetrosis with renal tubular acidosis)—*autosomal recessive.*

Frequency: Very common; more than 600 cases to 1988; from 1:500,000 to 5.5 per 100,000 births; delayed form is most common (intermediate form, 22 cases; 11 families to 1988; carbonic anhydrase 2 deficiency, 30 cases).

Clinical Manifestations: (a) newborn and infancy: *anemia* or pancytopenia, jaundice, *hepatosplenomegaly,* infections, early death, nonimmune hydrops; phagocytic abnormalities (neutrophil defect); obstructive sleep apnea; (b) childhood: physical retardation, cranial nerve palsies, progressive deafness and blindness, *fractures* (50%) including vertebral arch, macrocephaly, anemia, *osteomyelitis,* choanal atresia; (c) *adult: may be asymptomatic,* bone pain (25%), dental abscesses, carpal tunnel syndrome; (d) other reported abnormalities: nasal obstruction and adenoidal facies, hypertelorism, flattened nose, nystagmus, diffuse retinal degeneration (electroretinography), renal tubular acidosis (familial, associated with cerebral calcification, marble brain disease), vitamin D-resistant rickets (rare in United States); hypophosphatemia (7%), tetany, elevated acid phosphatase (39%), delayed and impaired teeth production, periodontal disease, hypogonadotropic hypogonadism, postsplenectomy sepsis, cerebrovascular thrombosis and hemorrhage, cervical spine compression myelopathy; tumors: non-Hodgkin lymphoma, bronchogenic CA; (e) prenatal diagnosis—ultrasound (fractures, macrocephaly, hydrocephalus, "increased bone echoes"—14 to 24 weeks).

Radiologic Manifestations: (a) *thick and dense skull,* most marked at base, *narrowness of neural and vascular foramina,* arterial and venous angiograms—severe stenosis, underdevelopment or lack of development of paranasal sinuses; (b) *uniformly dense skeleton* or generalized increased density with alternate radiolucent bands in metaphyses and diaphyses of long bones, bone scan—increased uptake, diffuse—especially bone ends; (c) *splaying of metaphyses* and rib ends; (d) *"bone-within-bone" appearance;* (e) pathologic fractures; (f) osteomyelitis; (g) "sandwich" appearance of vertebral bodies; (h) CT—hydrocephalus with calvarial thickening, foraminal narrowing; MRI—lack of marrow signal, carpal bones—uneven signal; (i) other reported abnormalities: delayed skeletal maturation, sunburst appearance of calvaria, intracranial calcification (basal ganglia especially), rickets, bone remodeling and new nonsclerotic bone formation following successful bone marrow transplantation for infantile malignant osteopetrosis, bone scan—cold spots, pseudoavascular necrosis of hips; sternum—multiple rudimentary centers persist; mandible—short body, wide ramus (Fig SK–O–8).

Treatment: (a) steroids (with low calcium, high phosphate diet; Dorantes)—questionable results; (b) calcitriol therapy (Key; Blazar)—good results in some; (c) bone marrow transplantation (about 14 patients; Kaplan; Nisbet; Orchard)—excellent results with bone marrow take.

Chondro-osseous Morphology: Osteosclerosis (50% to 60% increase of mineral content), narrowing and fibrosis of medullary spaces, abundant osteoid, osteomalacic appearance (Silvestrini), abnormal osteoclasts (not responsive to PTH, cell membrane abnormality; van Tran), ankylosis of cementum to bone (mandible; Younai).

Differential Diagnosis, Significant: (a) dysosteosclerosis; (b) pycnodysostosis; (c) axial osteomalacia; (d) Paget disease;

76:423–426, 1983; (4) Tien RD, et al.: An irregularly generalized osteosclerosis. *Skeletal Radiol.* 17:281–284, 1988; (5) Osteosclerosis *with empty sella* (Merle).

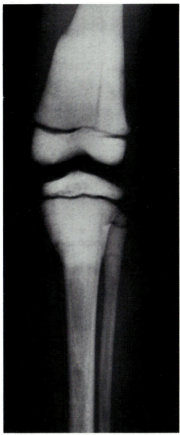

FIG SK–O–8.
Osteopetrosis. A 6½-year-old male who had a bone survey after discovery of osteopetrosis in his sister. Metaphyseal flaring and sclerotic bone changes are present. Alternate horizontal radiolucent bands of femur, tibia, and fibula and longitudinal radiolucent striation are seen.

(e) osteoblastic metastases; (f) chronic renal failure; (g) sclerosteosis and other sclerosing bone dysplasias; (h) osteosclerosis and mental retardation.

Special Comments: (a) the *intermediate form* has significant interfamilial variability; consists of short stature, increased upper and lower segments and decreased span, radiologically between delayed and precocious types (Kahler; Kaibara; Horton); (b) *carbonic anhydrase 2 deficiency type* consists of severe osteopetrosis, *renal tubular acidosis*, characteristic facies, abnormal teeth, *diffuse dense cerebral calcifications* (Ohlsson; Cumming); *mouse model*: mutation at Car-2 locus of chromosome 3 (Lewis); (c) *autosomal dominant osteopetrosis*-heterogeneity: 2 "distinct" types (type 1: pronounced sclerosis of skull and thickened cranial vault with almost normal spine; type 2: skull, only dense base with rugger jersey spine; Anderson); (d) *other osteopetrotic syndromes*: (1) Jagadha, V, et al.: Infantile osteopetrosis and neuronal storage disease (AR). *Acta Neuropathol* 75:233–240, 1988. (2) Lerman-Sagie T, et al.: Osteopetrosis, *COFS* and *myopathy. Am. J. Med. Genet.* 28:137–142, 1987; (3) Dowd PJ: Osteopetrosis and *icthyosis. R. Soc. Med.*

REFERENCES

Albers-Schónberg H: Eine bisher nicht beschriebene Allgemeinekrankung des Skelettes im Roentgenbilde. *Fortschr. Roentgenstr.* 11:261, 1907.
Al-Mefty O, et al.: Optic nerve decompression in osteopetrosis. *J. Neurosurg.* 68:80–84, 1988.
Anderson PE, Bollerslev J: Heterogeneity of autosomal dominant osteopetrosis. *Radiology* 164:223–225, 1987.
Beard CJ, et al.: Neutrophil defect associated with malignant infantile osteopetrosis. *J. Lab. Clin. Med.* 108:498–505, 1986.
Blazar BR, et al.: Letter to editor. *N. Engl. J. Med.* 311:55, 1984.
Bollerslev J: Osteopetrosis: Agenetic and epidemiological study. *Clin. Genet.* 31:86–90, 1987.
Carter M, et al.: Severe sleep apnea in a child with osteopetrosis. *Clin. Pediatr.* 27:108–110, 1988.
Dorantes LM, et al.: Juvenile osteopetrosis: Effects on blood and bone of prednisone and a low calcium, high phosphate diet. *Arch. Dis. Child.* 61:666–670, 1986.
Dumont M, et al.: Osteopetrosis appearance on bone scan. *Clin. Nucl. Med.* 8:446, 1983.
El Khazen N, et al.: Lethal osteopetrosis with multiple fractures in utero. *Am. J. Med. Genet.* 23:811–819, 1986.
Grabbe E, et al.: Manifestation of osteopetrosis of the sternum. *Fortschr. Roentgenstr.* 141:356–357, 1984.
Graham CB, et al.: Osteopetrosis, in Kaufmann HJ (ed.): *Progress in Pediatric Radiology,* vol. 4. Basel, Karger, 1973, p. 375.
Gupta DS, et al.: Osteomyelitis of the mandible in marble bone disease. *Int. J. Oral Maxillofacial Surg.* 15:201–205, 1986.
Kaplan FS, et al.: Successful treatment of infantile malignant osteopetrosis by bone-marrow transplantation. *J. Bone Joint Surg.* 70A:617–623, 1988.
Key L, et al.: Treatment of congenital osteopetrosis with high dose calcitriol. *N. Engl. J. Med.* 310:409–414, 1984.
Makin GJV, et al.: Major cerebral arterial and venous disease in osteopetrosis. *Stroke* 17:106–110, 1986.
Manolios N, et al.: Pseudo-avascular necrosis of the hips in a sporadic case of osteopetrosis. *Clin. Rheumatol.* 6:408–411, 1987.
Mathur BP, Karan S: Non immune hydrops fetalis due to osteopetrosis congenita. *Indian Pediatr.* 21:651–653, 1984.
Mazur J, Wortsman J: Hypogonadotropic hypogonadism from osteopetrosis. *Clin. Orthop. Rel. Res.* 162:202–206, 1982.
McCleary L, et al.: Case report: Myelopathy secondary to congenital osteopetrosis of the cervical spine. *Neurosurgery* 20:487–489, 1987.
Merle P, et al.: Primary empty sella turcica in children: Report of two familial cases. *Pediatr. Radiol.* 8:209–212, 1979.
Nagele M, et al.: Osteopetrosis: MRI findings. *ROFO* 147:687–689, 1987.
Nisbet NW: Bone marrow transplantation in precocious osteopetrosis. *Br. Med. J.* 294:463–464, 1987.
Orchard PJ, et al.: Haploidentical bone marrow transplantation for osteopetrosis. *Am. J. Pediatr. Hematol. Oncol.* 9:335–340, 1987.

Rakic M, et al.: Adult-type osteopetrosis presenting as carpal tunnel syndrome. *Arthritis Rheum.* 29:926–928, 1986.

Rao VM, et al.: Osteopetrosis: M.R. characteristics at 1.5 T. *Radiology* 161:217–220, 1986.

Sand JJ, et al.: Non-bacterial thrombotic endocarditis and nondisseminated malignancy with osteopetrosis. *Eur. Neurol.* 27:167–172, 1987.

Shibuya H, et al.: Non Hodgkin's lymphoma in a patient with osteopetrosis. *Lymphology* 19:90–92, 1986.

Silvestrini G, et al.: Adult osteopetrosis. *Appl. Pathol.* 5:184–189, 1987.

Van Tran P, et al.: Osteoclast abnormalities in idiopathic osteopetrosis. *Virchows Arch. [A]* 408:269–280, 1985.

Younai F, et al.: Osteopetrosis. *Oral Surg. Oral Med. Oral Pathol.* 65:214-221, 1988.

Zamboni G, et al.: Association of osteopetrosis and vitamin D-resistant rickets. *Helv. Paediatr. Acta* 32:363, 1977.

Carbonic Anhydrase 2 Deficiency

Cochat P, et al.: Carbonic anhydrase 2 deficiency. *Pediatrie* 42:121–128, 1987.

Cumming WA, Ohlsson A: Intracranial calcification in children with osteopetrosis caused by carbonic anhydrase 2 deficiency. *Radiology* 157:325–327, 1985.

Lewis SE, et al.: Null mutation at the mouse Car-2 locus: An animal model for human carbonic anhydrase 2 deficiency syndrome. *Proc. Natl. Acad. Sci.* 85:1962–1966, 1988.

Ohlsson A, et al.: Carbonic anhydrase 2 deficiency. *Pediatrics* 77:371–380, 1986.

Intermediate Form

Horton WA, et al.: Osteopetrosis: Further heterogeneity. *J. Pediatr.* 97:580–585, 1980.

Kahler SG, et al.: A mild recessive form of osteopetrosis. *Am. J. Med. Genet.* 17:451–464, 1984.

Kaibura N, et al.: Intermediate form of osteopetrosis with recessive inheritance. *Skeletal Radiol.* 9:47–51, 1982.

OSTEOPOIKILOSIS

Synonyms: Osteopathia condensans disseminata, disseminated dermatofibrosis with osteopoikilosis (Bushke-Ollendorff syndrome); dermato-osteopoikilosis; juvenile elastoma and osteopoikilosis.

Mode of Inheritance: Autosomal dominant.

Frequency: Very common; 6 per 100,000 films; underreported; more than 200 cases to 1988.

Clinical Manifestations: (a) often asymptomatic; (b) *association with cutaneous* and *subcutaneous fibrous pea-sized nodules* (bone and skin lesions may be present separately in members of same family); (c) other reported abnormalities: giant cell tumor, osteosarcoma, lumbar spine stenosis.

Radiologic Manifestations: (a) *small foci of bone sclerosis of different sizes and shapes* (round, oval, or lenticular) located in spongiosa of skeleton, particularly in pelvis, metaphyses and epiphyses of long bones, tarsals, and carpals; (b) normal uptake of ^{99m}Tc pyrophosphate on bone imaging (Fig SK–O–9).

Chondro-osseous and Skin Morphology: Bone lesions—specific foci of compact bone; skin lesions—excessive amounts of elastic or pre-elastic fibers in dermis; electron microscopy—clumps of elastin coated with free fibrils (Verbou).

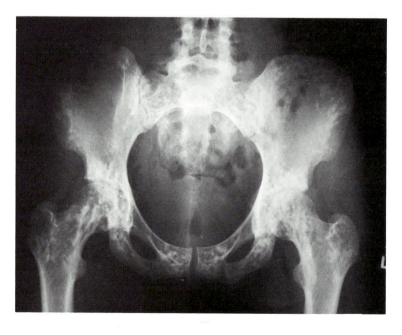

FIG SK–O–9.
Osteopoikilosis in a 38-year-old woman. Foci of bone sclerosis of different sizes in pelvic bones and femora. (From Whyte MP, Murphy WA, Siegel BA: ^{99m}Tc pyrophosphate bone imaging in osteopoikilosis, osteopathia striata, and melorheostosis. *Radiology* 127:439, 1978. Reproduced with permission.)

Differential Diagnosis, Significant: (a) bone metastases; (b) melorheostosis; (c) osteopathia striata; (d) enostoses (bone islands).

Special Comments: Unclear whether Bushke-Ollendorff syndrome is a separate entity from just osteopoikilosis; separate syndrome of *osteopoikilosis, melorheostosis,* and *scleroderma;* association of *osteosclerosis* and *osteopoikilosis* in one family (Strossberg et al.).

REFERENCES

Albers-Schönberg HE: Eine seltene, bisher nicht bekannte Strukturanomalie de Skelettes. *Fortschr. Roentgenstr.* 23:174, 1915.

Ayling RM, Evans PEL: Giant cell tumor in a patient with osteopoikilosis. *Acta Orthop. Scand.* 59:74–76, 1988.

Gershman I, et al.: Osteopoikilosis: Familial documentation. *Am. J. Dis. Child.* 134:416, 1980.

Grassberger A, et al.: Knochenszintigramm bei Osteopoikilosis familiaris. *Radiol. Clin.* 44:372, 1975.

Langier R et al.: Osteopoikilosis: A radiological and pathological study. *Skeletal Radiol.* 11:161–168, 1984.

Mindell ER, et al.: Osteosarcoma associated with osteopoikilosis. *J. Bone Joint Surg. [Am.]* 60A:406, 1978.

Onitsuka H: Roentgenologic aspects of bone islands. *Radiology* 123:607, 1977.

Pascaud-Ged E, et al.: Mélorhéostose, osteopoecilie et sclérodermie en bandes. *Ann. Radiol.* 24:643, 1981.

Strossberg JM, et al.: Osteosclerosis associated with osteopoikilosis. *J.A.M.A.* 246:2030, 1981.

Verbou J, Graham R: Review article: Buschke-Ollendorff syndrome. *Clin. Exp. Dermatol.* 11:17–26, 1986.

Weisz GM: Lumbar spinal canal stenosis in osteopoikilosis. *Clin. Orthop.* 166:89–92, 1982.

Whyte MP, Murphy WA, et al.: ^{99m}Tc-pyrophosphate bone imaging in osteopoikilosis, osteopathia striata, and melorheostasis. *Radiology* 127:439, 1978.

OSTEOPOROSIS-PSEUDOGLIOMA SYNDROME

Synonyms: Ocular form of osteogenesis imperfecta; pseudoglioma with bone fragility.

Mode of Inheritance: Autosomal recessive.

Frequency: Rare, about 32 cases to 1988 (13 families).

Clinical Manifestations: Onset in infancy: (a) *very poor vision; microphthalmos; iris, lens* and *anterior chamber abnormalities; vitrioretinal abnormalities; cataracts;* (b) *short stature,* mental retardation, microcephaly, discolored teeth; (c) *muscular hypotonia, hyperextensible joints,* elbow limitation of motion; (d) short spine, barrel chest, kyphoscoliosis, *spontaneous fractures;* (e) other reported abnormalities: congenital heart disease (ventricular septal defect); thin, sparse hair; seizures; obesity.

Radiologic Manifestations: (a) *osteoporosis,* wormian bones, *platyspondyly,* craniosynostosis, *fractures, long bone deformities;* (b) CT—ocular calcification, eye-structural abnormalities.

Differential Diagnosis, Significant: (a) osteogenesis imperfecta (OI); (b) other osteoporosis syndromes, i.e., malignant osteoporosis; (c) OI, macrocephaly; wormian bones, *brachydactyly,* hyperextensible joints, and *Leber's retinal dystrophy* (Heide).

Special Comments: Osteoporosis-pseudoglioma syndrome may just be another form of OI (Beighton, 1985, Frontali, 1986; Superti-Furga; Somer); awaiting biochemical confirmation.

REFERENCES

Bartsocas CS, et al.: Syndrome of osteoporosis with pseudoglioma. *Ann. Genet.* 25:61–62, 1982.

Beighton P, et al.: The ocular form of osteogenesis imperfecta. *Clin. Genet.* 28:69–75, 1985.

Beighton P: Letter to editor. *Clin. Genet.* 29:263, 1986.

Frontali M, et al.: Osteoporosis-pseudoglioma syndrome. *Am. J. Med. Genet.* 22:35–47, 1985.

Frontali M, Dalla Piccola B: Letter to editor. *Clin. Genet.* 29:262, 1986.

Heide T: Ein Syndrom bestehend aus Osteogenesis imperfecta, Makrozephalus mit Schaltknochen und prominenten Stirnhöckern, Brachytelephalangie, Gelenküberstreckbarkeit, kongenitaler Amaurose und Oligophrenie bei drei Geschwisten. *Klin. Padiatr.* 193:334, 1981.

Somer H, et al.: Osteoporosis-pseudoglioma syndrome: Clinical, morphological and biochemical studies. *J. Med. Genet.* 25:543–549, 1988.

Superti-Furga A, et al.: Letter to editor. *Clin. Genet.* 29:184-185, 1986.

Teebi AS, et al.: Osteoporosis-pseudoglioma syndrome with congenital heart disease: *J. Med. Genet.* 25:32–36, 1988.

OSTEOSCLEROSIS—DOMINANT TYPE, STANESCU

Synonyms: Stanescu dysostosis; dominant osteosclerosis—Stanescu type.

Mode of Inheritance: Autosomal dominant.

Frequency: Very rare; 14 cases to 1988; 3 reports; 11 in one family (Stanescu).

Clinical Manifestations: (a) short stature, (b) *craniofacial malformation (brachycephaly, small face;* proptosis, beaked nose), (c) short neck, (d) *brachydactyly,* rhizomelia, (e) dental decay and malocclusion, (f) abnormal dermatoglyphics (Dipierri).

Radiologic Manifestations: *(a) brachy-turrencephaly;* decreased sinuses and mastoid air cells; *obtuse mandibular angle; (b) dense, thickened cortices of long bones; generalized brachydactyly* with normal distal phalanges.

Differential Diagnosis, Significant: (a) pycnodysostosis; (b) frontometaphyseal dysplasia.

Special Comments: Hall's isolated case may represent another entity. Her patient did not have the cortical thickening and increased density; a normal mandibular angle as well as scoliosis and platyspondyly (Hall).

REFERENCES

Dipierri JE, Guzman JD: A second family with autosomal dominant osteosclerosis—type Stanescu. *Am. J. Med. Genet.* 18:13–18, 1984.
Hall JG: Craniofacial dysostosis: Either Stanescu dysostosis or a new entity. *Birth Defects* 10(12):521–523, 1974.
Stanescu V, et al.: Syndrome hereditaire dominant, reunissant une dysostose craniofaciale de type particulier une insuffisance de croissance d'aspect chondrodystrophique, et un epaississement massif de la corticale des os longs. *Rev. Fr. Endocrinol. Clin.* 4:219–231, 1963.

OTO-PALATO-DIGITAL SYNDROME—TYPE 2

Synonyms: Cranio-oro-digital syndrome; facio-palato-osseous syndrome (FPO); OPD–2.

Mode of Inheritance: X-linked, minor to no manifestations in the female.

Frequency: Very rare; 7 well described cases to 1988 (all male).

Clinical Manifestations: Newborn presentation with *facial* and *limb anomalies*: (a) large anterior fontanelle and wide sutures, low set ears, *"pugilist" face*, prominent forehead, hypertelorism, antimongoloid slant and flat nasal bridge, *microstomia* and *micrognathia, cleft palate*; (b) *"tree frog" hands and feet, flexed overlapping fingers*; syndactyly; *short, broad first digits*; undescended testes; (c) other reported abnormalities: respiratory failure.

Radiologic Manifestations: (a) skull: mildly reduced ossification; *midface hypoplasia*; vertical clivus; *small mandible* with obtuse angle; (b) long bones: increased density; *bowing; hypoplastic or absent fibula; elbow dislocations*; (c) hands and feet: *markedly hypoplastic metacarpals and metatarsals* (some fail to ossify); *hypoplasia of phalanges; very short proximal first digits*; camptodactyly, peg-shaped epiphyses; (d) wavy, shortened ribs; precocious sternal fusion; sloping clavicles; flat acetabular roof; flared ilia.

Chondro-osseous Morphology: Normal (Brewster).

Differential Diagnosis, Significant: (a) oto-palato-digital syndrome 1 (milder); (b) atelosteogenesis, type 3 (more severe); (c) trisomy 18; (d) oro-facio-digital syndrome 2.

Special Comments: Separation from OPD-1 is suggested by severity and certain salient features (fibula, clavicle, and rib changes, etc.; Fitch 1983). Separation from atelosteogenesis type 3 depends on *less severe phenotype* (down-slanting palpebral fissures, abnormal ears, microstomia, cleft palate, no club feet; *increased survival; different hand changes* (triangular first metacarpal, bifid fingers); usually *normal length long bones* with fibular aplasia or hypoplasia (see AO–3).

REFERENCES

Andre M, et al.: Abnormal facies, cleft palate, and generalized dysostosis. *J. Pediatr.* 98:747–752, 1981.
Brewster TG, et al.: Oto-palato-digital syndrome type 2. *Am. J. Med. Genet.* 20:249–254, 1985.
Fitch N, et al.: A familial syndrome of cranial, facial, oral and limb anomalies. *Clin. Genet.* 10:226–231, 1976.
Fitch N, et al.: The oto-palato-digital syndrome, proposed type 2. *Am. J. Med. Genet.* 15:655–664, 1983.
Kozlowski K, et al.: Oto-palato-digital syndrome with severe x-ray changes in two half brothers. *Pediatr. Radiol.* 6:97–102, 1977.

OTO-SPONDYLO-MEGAEPIPHYSEAL DYSPLASIA

Synonyms: Bone dysplasia with deafness; Weissenbacher-Zweymuller syndrome phenotype (some cases); otospondylofacial dysplasia; OSMED.

Mode of Inheritance: Autosomal recessive.

Frequency: Very rare; six cases to 1988.

Clinical Manifestations: (a) birth: *characteristic facies, short limbed dwarfism*, small jaw, *cleft palate* (67%); (b) later-life: *deafness*, joint pains, recurrent pulmonary infections, *enlarged joints*.

Radiologic Manifestations: (a) newborn—*coronal clefts of spine, dumbbell femurs*, square iliac wings, short long bones, mandibular hypoplasia; (b) infancy and early childhood—*absent or small capital femoral epiphyses*; (c) later life—enlarged odontoid, *platyspondyly*, anterior wedging, narrow rib cage, *square iliac wings*, generalized mild long bone shortening, *megaepiphyses*, normal to advanced bone age, abnormal pattern profile, large epiphyses of hands and feet.

Differential Diagnosis: (a) Kniest dysplasia; (b) metatropic dysplasia; (c) megaepiphyseal dysplasias; (d); spondyloepiphyseal dysplasia; (e) Weissenbacher-Zweymuller syndrome; (f) micrognathic dwarfism; (g) megaepiphyseal dysplasia with osteoporosis, wrinkled skin, and aging (McAlister).

Special Comments: Patients with OSMED have the Weissenbacher-Zweymuller phenotype in infancy but develop large epiphyses, unlike other patients with that phenotype, and have epiphyseal ossification delay. It may be that OSMED belongs to a spectrum of disease that includes Stickler and Marshall syndromes as well as micrognathic dwarfism.

REFERENCES

Giedon A, et al.: Oto-spondylo-megaepiphyseal dysplasia (OSMED). *Helv Paediatr. Acta* 37:361–380, 1982.

Haller JO, et al.: The Weissenbacher-Zweymuller syndrome of micrognathia and rhizomelic chondrodysplasia at birth with subsequent normal growth. *AJR* 125:936–943, 1975.

Insley J, Astley R: A bone dysplasia with deafness. *Br. J. Radiol.* 47:244–251, 1974.

McAlister W, et al.: Macroepiphyseal dysplasia with symptomatic osteoporosis, wrinkled skin, and aged appearance. *Skeletal Radiol* 15:47, 1986.

Scribanu N, et al.: The Weissenbacher-Zweymüller phenotype in the neonatal period as an expression in the continuum of manifestations of the hereditary arthroophthalmopathies. *Ophthalmol. Paediatr. Genet.* 8:159, 1987.

Winter RM, et al.: The Weissenbacher-Zweymüller, Stickler, and Marshall syndromes. Further incidence of their identity. *Am. J. Med. Genet.* 16:189, 1983.

PARASTREMMATIC DYSPLASIA

Mode of Inheritance: Probably autosomal dominant.

Frequency: Very rare; eight patients reported to 1988.

Clinical Manifestations: (a) stiff babies in first year of life, full clinical picture by age 10; (b) delay in walking, abnormal gait; (c) *contracture of large joints and progressive skeletal deformities* (twisted dwarfism); (d) *severe dwarfism*.

Radiologic Manifestations: (a) decreased bone density; (b) cranial vault deformities secondary to osteoporosis (occipital flattening, etc.); (c) *bowing of long bones;* (d) *"flocky" or "woolly" appearance of zones of enchondral bone formation, calcific stippling of metaphyses, epiphyses, and apophyses;* (e) *genu valgum;* (f) *kyphoscoliosis, platyspondyly* (Fig SK–P–1).

Differential Diagnosis, Significant: (a) Morquio disease (MPS IV); (b) Dyggve-Melchior-Clausen syndrome; (c) metatropic dysplasia; (d) Kniest dysplasia; (e) a new familial chondrodystrophy simulating parastremmatic dwarfism (Golden et al.) also called SMD Richmond type-X linked.

REFERENCES

Ajuria-Gottwald ML, Morla BE: Parastremmatic dwarfism. *Bol. Med. Hosp. Infant. Mex.* 39:748–752, 1982.
Golden WL, et al.: A new familial chondrodystrophy simulating parastremmatic dwarfism. *MCV Quarterly* 13:189, 1977.
Horan F, et al.: Parastremmatic dwarfism. *J. Bone Joint Surg.* 58B:343, 1976.
Langer LO, et al.: An unusual bone dysplasia: Parastremmatic dwarfism. *Am. J. Roentgenol.* 110:550, 1970.

PROGRESSIVE PSEUDORHEUMATOID CHONDRODYSPLASIA

Synonyms: Spondyloepiphyseal dysplasia tarda with progressive arthropathy; progressive pseudorheumatoid arthritis (arthropathy); progressive pseudorheumatoid arthritis of childhood; PPAC.

Mode of Inheritance: Autosomal recessive.

Frequency: Rare; about 30 cases reported to 1988; increased incidence in Arab populations (five families).

Clinical Manifestations: Onset, 3 to 8 years: (a) *walking difficulties, easy fatigability, muscular weakness;* (b) *joint stiffness and prominence;* large-joint contractures; (c) normal sed rate, negative rheumatoid factor; (d) decreased cervical spine mobility, kyphoscoliosis; (e) other reported abnormalities: pseudogout; flexion deformities of fingers.

Radiologic Manifestations: (a) *platyspondyly, anterior end plate erosions* and gouge defects (Scheuermann-like); (b) *hands: narrowed joint spaces, widened metaphyses, flattened epiphyses;* (c) *hips: enlarged femoral heads, joint space narrowing,* acetabular irregularity; (d) similar changes in other joint space—epiphyseal areas; (e) chondrocalcinosis (Fig SK–P–2).

Chondro-osseous and Synovial Morphology: Abnormal clustering of chondrocytes with pycnotic nucleus and defective column formation—nonspecific; normal synovium at biopsy; calcium pyrophosphate dihydrate crystals in synovial fluid.

Differential Diagnosis, Significant: (a) rheumatoid arthritis (seronegative); (b) polymyositis; (c) muscular dystrophy; (d) collagen diseases; (e) ankylosing spondylitis (HLA-B27 negative); (f) Kniest dysplasia; (g) multiple epiphyseal dysplasia; (h) spondyloepiphyseal dysplasias; (i) Scheuermann disease.

Special Comments: Spondyloepiphyseal dysplasia tarda with progressive arthropathy appears to represent the same disorder (Wynne-Davies).

REFERENCES

Bradley JD: Pseudoseptic pseudogout in progressive pseudorheumatoid arthropathy of childhood. *Ann. Rheum. Dis.* 46:709–712, 1987.
Kozlowski K, et al.: Radiographic features of progressive pseudorheumatoid arthritis. *Australas. Radiol.* 30:244–250, 1986.
Spranger J, et al.: Progressive pseudorheumatoid arthropathy of childhood (PPAC), letter. *Am. J. Med. Genet.* 14:399–401, 1983.
Spranger J, et al.: Progressive pseudorheumatoid arthritis of childhood (PPAC). *Eur. J. Pediatr.* 140:34–40, 1983.
Wynne-Davies R, et al.: Spondyloepiphyseal dysplasia tarda with progressive arthropathy. *J. Bone Joint Surg. [Br.]* 64:442–445, 1982.

PSEUDOACHONDROPLASIA

Synonym: Pseudoachondroplastic spondyloepiphyseal dysplasia.

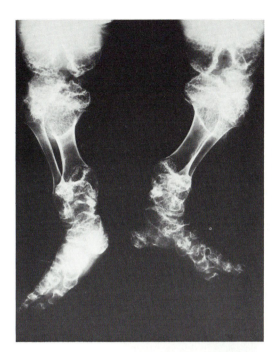

FIG SK—P—1.
Parastremmatic dysplasia. Anteroposterior views of lower limbs at age 9 years. Metaphyses and epiphyses are greatly enlarged and show "flocky" appearance of bone. (From Horan F, Beighton P: Parastremmatic dwarfism. *J. Bone Joint Surg.* 58B:343, 1976. Reproduced with permission.)

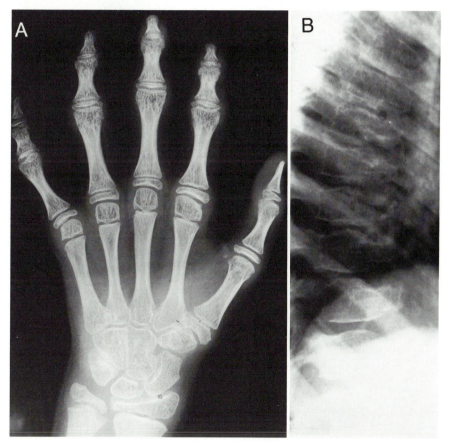

FIG SK—P—2.
Progressive pseudorheumatoid chondrodysplasia, late childhood. **A,** narrowed joint spaces, widened metaphyses, flat epiphyses. **B,** platyspondyly, anterior end plate erosions. (From Kozlowski K, Kennedy J, Lewis IC: Radiographic features of progressive pseudorheumatoid arthritis. *Australas. Radiol.* 30:244–250, 1986. (Reproduced with permission.)

Mode of Inheritance: Most autosomal dominant; rarely gonadal mosaicism rather than autosomal recessive (Hall 1987).

Frequency: Common; about 150 cases to 1988; under-reported.

Clinical Manifestations: (a) *short-limbed, short trunked dwarfism,* usually detectable in second to fourth years of life; (b) *marked shortness of hands and feet;* (c) *normal attractive facial appearance;* (d) hyperlordosis, scoliosis, kyphosis; (e) waddling gait, valgus deformity of legs, knock-knee (in some), bowing of long bones, ulnar deviation of wrists, flexion contractures of hips, knees, and elbows (late), tibiotarsal joint varus or valgus deformities, *marked ligamentous laxity* (especially at knees); (f) normal intelligence; (g) immune deficiency (h) growth curves available.

Radiologic Manifestations: *spinal, metaphyseal, and epiphyseal changes;* (a) *normal craniofacial bones;* (b) *shortness of tubular bones;* (c) *irregular mushroomed metaphyses;* (d) *fragmentation and irregularities of developing epiphyses; miniepiphyses* (hips and phalanges); (e) *characteristic platyspondyly,* irregularity and exaggeration of epiphyseal grooves of vertebral end plates; biconcave appearance of vertebral bodies (late); *atlantoaxial dislocation* (Finidori), abnormal spinal curvature in later childhood; (f) spatulate appearance of ribs; (g) irregularity of acetabulum, large ilium, short pubis and ischium, coxa vara; (h) *rounded proximal ends of metacarpals;* hypoplastic abnormally formed carpals (Fig SK—P—3).

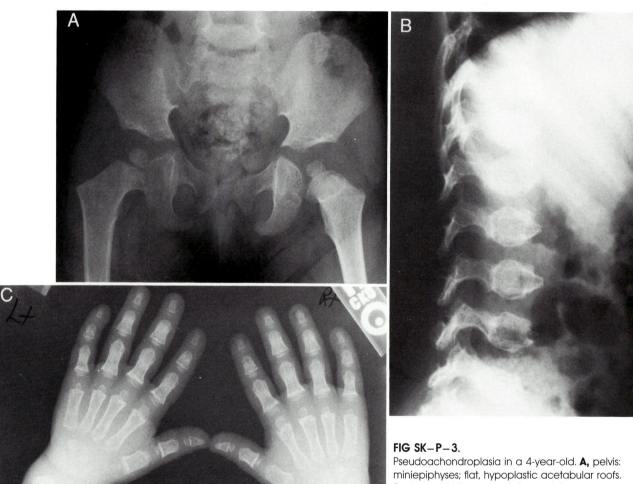

FIG SK—P—3.
Pseudoachondroplasia in a 4-year-old. **A,** pelvis: miniepiphyses; flat, hypoplastic acetabular roofs. **B,** characteristic spine; platyspondyly; exaggeration of epiphyseal grooves of end plates; superior and inferior humps. **C,** hands: small epiphyses, metaphyseal irregularities; proximal metacarpal irregularities.

Chondro-osseous Morphology: Disorganized growth plate; nests and clustered cells in proliferating zone, poor column formation; inclusions in cartilage cells; electron microscopy—large lamellar dilatations of rough endoplasmic reticulum; studies suggest packaging and transport defect of proteoglycans to golgi apparatus (Stanescu 1984).

Differential Diagnosis, Significant: (a) achondroplasia; (b) spondyloepiphyseal and spondyloepimetaphyseal dysplasias; (c) Morquio disease (MPS type IVA).

Special Comments: First described in 1959 by Marateaux and Lamy. "Achondroplast with a normal face"; delineation into 4 types no longer felt to be warranted; animal model—miniature poodle; cartilage contains undersulfated chondroitin sulfate proteoglycan (type 2 collagen).

REFERENCES

Bingel SA, et al: Undersulfated chondroitin sulfate in cartilage from a miniature poodle with SED. *Connect. Tissue Res.* 15:283–302, 1986.
Dennis NR, et al.: The severe recessive form of pseudoachondroplastic dysplasia. *Pediatr. Radiol.* 3:169, 1975.
Finidori G, et al.: Les déformations osteo-articulaires dans la dysplasie pseudo-achondroplastique. *Chir. Pediatr.* 21:191, 1980.
Hall JG: Pseudoachondroplasia. *Am. J. Dis. Child.* 128:834, 1974.
Hall JG, et al.: Gonadal mosaicism in pseudachondroplasia. *Am. J. Med. Genet.* 28:143–151, 1987.
Heselson NG, et al.: Pseudoachondroplasia: A report of 13 cases. *Br. J. Radiol.* 50:473, 1977.
Horten WA, et al.: Growth curves for height for diastrophic dysplasia, spondyloepiphyseal dysplasia congenita, and pseudachondroplasia. *Am. J. Dis. Child.* 136:316–319, 1982.
Kultursay N, et al.: Pseudachondroplasia with immune deficiency. *Pediatr. Radiol.* 18:505–508, 1988.
Riser WH, et al.: Pseudoachondroplastic dysplasia in miniature poodles. *J. Am. Vet. Med. Assoc.* 15:335–341, 1980.
Stanescu V, et al.: The biochemical defect of pseudoachondroplasia. *Pediatrics* 138:221–225, 1982.
Stanescu V, et al.: Pathogenic mechanisms in osteochondrodysplasias. *J. Bone Joint Surg. [Am.]* 66A:817–835, 1984.
Wynne-Davies R, et al.: Pseudachondroplasia. *J. Med. Genet.* 23:425–434, 1986.

PSEUDODIASTROPHIC DYSPLASIA

Synonym: Nanisme pseudodiastrophique.

Mode of Inheritance: Autosomal recessive.

Frequency: Very rare, 7 cases reported to 1988.

Clinical Manifestations: (a) often fatal in the first year; *short at birth*; (b) blue-gray sclera, *hypertelorism, flat nasal bridge, large malformed ears* (folded superior helix), *cleft palate*; (c) *rhizomelia*, elbow dislocations, *interphalangeal dislocations* (hands), *clubfeet*, contractures; (d) *scoliosis* (early onset), C-1, C-2 dislocation.

Radiologic Manifestations: (a) *mild to moderate platyspondyly; ovoid vertebral bodies;* (b) *elbow dislocations;* short metacarpals, *interphalangeal joint dislocations;* proximal fibular overgrowth; (c) long clavicles (newborn), mildly short ribs with anterior flare, horizontal acetabular roof (Fig SK–P–4).

Chondro-osseous Morphology: Almost normal (unlike diastrophic dysplasia).

Differential Diagnosis, Significant: (a) diastrophic dysplasia; (b) distal arthrogryposis.

REFERENCES

Burgio GR: Nanisme pseudodiastrophique. *Arch. Fr. Pediatr.* 31:681–696, 1974.
Canki N, et al.: Le nanisme pseudodiastrophique. *J. Genet. Hum.* 27:247–252, 1979.
Eteson DJ, et al.: Pseudodiastrophic dysplasia: A distinct newborn skeletal dysplasia. *J. Pediatr.* 109:635–641, 1986.

PYCNODYSOSTOSIS

Synonym: Pyknodysostosis.

Mode of Inheritance: Autosomal recessive.

Frequency: Uncommon; approximately 125 cases to 1988.

Clinical Manifestations: (a) *short-limbed dwarfism;* (b) prominent calvaria with *smallness of facial structures;* (c) prominent nose; (d) micrognathia; (e) dental abnormalities: delayed eruption, persistent deciduous teeth, irregular permanent teeth, partial anodontia, dental infections; (f) *fractures, shortness of fingers;* (g) flattened nails, cyst-like deficits in ungual tufts of fingers; (h) other reported abnormalities: varying degrees of respiratory distress, tendency to vomit, aspiration pneumonia, long uvula with obstructive effect on nasopharynx and oropharynx, hypoventilation during sleep related to position of uvula, rickets.

Radiologic Manifestations: (a) craniofacial abnormalities: frontal and occipital bossing, wormian bones, *delayed closure of fontanelles and sutures,* obtuse or absense of angle of mandible, *dense skull,* in particular the orbital rims (harlequin appearance), mastoid cells and sinuses underdeveloped or absent; (b) *generalized osteosclerosis;* (c) *hypoplasia or re-*

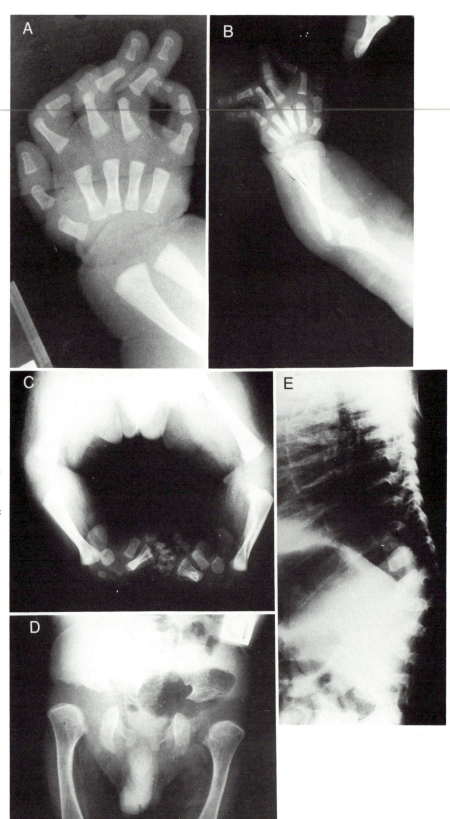

FIG SK—P—4.
Pseudodiastrophic dysplasia in **A,** a
newborn: multiple interphalangeal
dislocations; **B,** an infant aged 7 months:
elbow dislocation and finger dislocations;
C, an infant aged 2 months: very severe
clubbed feet; no proximal tibial
epiphyseal ossification and tiny distal
femoral epiphyses; **D,** an infant aged 5
months: broad, rounded proximal femoral
metaphyses without epiphyseal
ossification; flat acetabular roofs; **E,** an
infant aged 5 months: gibbus; hypoplastic
lumbar vertebrae with platyspondyly.

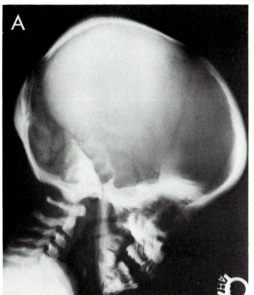

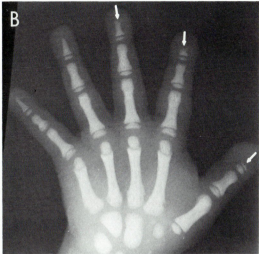

FIG SK–P–5.
Pycnodysostosis in a 5-year-old girl. **A,** dense bones, widely open cranial sutures, prognathism, obtuse angle of mandible, lack of normal development of mastoids and paranasal sinuses. **B,** gen-eralized osteosclerosis, partial absence of ossification of distal phalanx of thumb and middle and index fingers *(arrows)*.

sorption of acromial end of clavicle; (d) mild narrowing of thorax; (e) *partial or total aplasia or resorption of distal pha-langes, often with fragmentation;* (f) *brittle bones, pathologic fractures,* fractures of vertebral arches, spondylolisthesis; (g) partial disappearance of hyoid bone and other bones, cranio-synostosis, rickets (Fig SK–P–5).

Chondro-osseous Morphology: Narrow small islands of cells instead of columns; short thick primary trabeculae; in-clusions in chondrocytes; possible phospholipid disorder (Stanescu).

Differential Diagnosis, Significant: (a) cleidocranial dys-plasia; (b) osteopetrosis and other dense bone disorders; (c) acro-osteolysis syndromes.

Special Comments: Identified as a separate syndrome by Maroteaux and Lamy in 1962; "malady of Toulouse-Lautrec," the impressionist painter (Maroteaux 1965).

REFERENCES

Bennani-Smires C, et al.: La pycnodysostose. *J. Radiol.* 65:689–695, 1984.
Benz G, Schmid-Rüter E: Pycñodysostosis with heterozygous beta-thalassemia. *Pediatr. Radiol.* 5:164–171, 1977.
Bernard R, et al.: Pycnodysostose et crânioosténose. *Ann. Pediatr.* 27:383, 1980.
Grunebaum M, Landdau B: Pycñodysostosis. *Br. J. Radiol.* 41:359–361, 1968.
Maroteaux P, Lamy M: La pycnodysostose. *Presse Med.* 70:999, 1962.
Maroteaux P, Lamy M: The malady of Toulouse-Lautrec. *JAMA* 191:111–113, 1965.
Srivastava KK, et al.: Pycnodysostosis (report of four cases). *Australas. Radiol.* 22:70, 1978.
Stanescu V, et al.: Pathogenic mechanisms in osteochondro-dysplasias. *J. Bone Joint Surg. [Am.]* 66A:817–835, 1984.
Theander G: Partial disappearance of the hyoid bone in pyk-nodysostosis. Report of a case. *Acta Radiol. [Diagn]* 19:237, 1978.
Yousefzadeh DK, et al.: Radiographic studies of upper air-way obstruction with cor pulmonale in a patient with pyc-nodysostosis. *Pediatr. Radiol.* 8:45, 1979.
Zachariades N, Koundouris I: Maxillofacial symptoms in 2 patients with pyknodysostosis. *J. Oral Maxillofacial Surg.* 42:819–823, 1984.

PYLE DYSPLASIA

Synonym: Familial metaphyseal dysplasia.

Archeological Note: A skeleton from the Mochica cul-ture of Peru (200–800 A.D.) had Pyle disease.

Frequency: Rare; approximately 30 cases to 1988.

Clinical Manifestations: *Often asymptomatic* or *only few clinical findings:* (a) muscle weakness; (b) joint pain; (c) *genu valgum* with onset early in life; (d) scoliosis; (e) limitation of extension of elbows.

Radiologic Manifestations: (a) *mild skull involvement:* prominent supraorbital ridge, mild hyperostosis of vault, mild prognathism; (b) thickening of clavicles, ribs, and ischiopubic

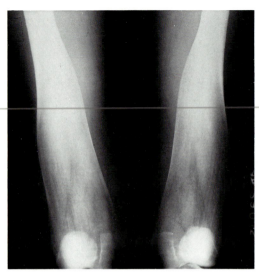

FIG SK–P–6.
Pyle dysplasia. Femora show marked Erlenmeyer-flasklike flare,
which extends far up diaphysis. (From Gorlin RJ, Koszalka A,
Spranger J.: Pyle's disease (familial metaphyseal dysplasia). *J.
Bone Joint Surg. [Am.]* 52A:347, 1970. Reproduced with permis-
sion.)

bones; (c) *marked undertubulation of long bones,* in particular femora distally *(Erlenmeyer flask deformity);* (d) *flaring of
metacarpals distally and phalanges proximally;* (e) mild platyspondyly (infrequent); (f) bone fragility (infrequent) (Fig
SK–P–6).

Differential Diagnosis, Significant: The craniotubular
dysplasias, especially: (a) craniometaphyseal dysplasia; (b)
craniodiaphyseal dysplasia; (c) sclerosteosis; as well as (d)
Gaucher disease; (e) Niemann Pick disease.

Special Comments: Several Pyle-like entities have been
described: (a) metaphyseal dysplasia with maxillary hypoplasia and brachydactyly–autosomal dominant (Halal); (b) a familial metaphyseal dysplasia with characteristic radial
deformity–autosomal dominant (Hohle; Fried); (c) isolated
case of metaphyseal dysplasia with defective tooth enamel,
blue sclera, high palate and no cranial sclerosis (Taneli); (d)
metaphyseal dysplasia with a hemimelic distribution (Polivka).

REFERENCES

Backwin H, et al.: Familial metaphyseal dysplasia. *Am. J.
Dis. Child.* 53:1521, 1937.
Cohn M: Konstitutionelle Hyperspongiosierung des skeletts
mit partiellem Riesenwuchs. *Fortschr. Roentgenstr.*
47:293, 1933.
Fried K, Krause J: Die Metaphysare Dysplasie-Morbus Pyle.
Fortschr. Roentgenstr. 116:224–228, 1972.
Gorlin RJ, et al.: Pyle's disease (familial metaphyseal dysplasia): The presentation of two cases and argument for its
separation from craniometaphyseal dysplasia. *J. Bone Joint
Surg. [Am.]* 52A:347, 1970.
Halal F, et al.: Metaphyseal dysplasia with maxillary hypoplasia and brachydactyly. *Am. J. Med. Genet.* 13:71–
79, 1982.
Heselson NG, et al.: The radiological manifestations of
metaphyseal dysplasia (Pyle disease). *Br. J. Radiol.*
52:431, 1979.
Hohle B, St Braun H: Eine Neue Form der Familiaren Meta-
physaren Dysplasie. *Helv. Paediatr. Acta* 37:151–160,
1982.
Polivka D: Metaphyseal dysplasia with hemimelic distribution. *Acta Chir. Orthop. Traumatol. Cech.* 39:98–104,
1972.
Pyle E: A case of unusual bone development. *J. Bone Joint
Surg.* 13:874, 1931.
Raad MS, et al.: Autosomal recessive inheritance of metaphyseal dysplasia (Pyle disease). *Clin. Genet.* 14:251,
1978.
Shibuya H, et al.: The radiological appearances of familial
metaphyseal dysplasia. *Clin. Radiol.* 33:439–444, 1982.
Taneli B: A type of Pyle's metaphyseal dysplasia (or simula-
tion?): A case report. Abstract 72. European Society of
Pediatric Radiology, Paris, May 1983.
Taybi H: Generalized skeletal dysplasia with multiple anom-
alies: A note on Pyle's disease. *Am. J. Roentgenol.*
88:450, 1962.
Urteaga BO, et al.: Craniometaphyseal dysplasia (Pyle's disease) in an ancient skeleton from the Mochica culture of
Peru. *Am. J. Roentgenol.* 99:712, 1967.
Vohra V: Pyles disease: Familial metaphyseal dysplasia. A
case report. *Australas. Radiol.* 31:75–78, 1987.

R

ROBINOW SYNDROME

Synonyms: Mesomelic dysplasia, type Robinow; fetal face syndrome; Robinow-Silverman-Smith syndrome; mesomelic dwarfism with hemivertebrae and small genitalia; Covesdem syndrome.

Mode of Inheritance: Genetic heterogeneity; autosomal dominant and autosomal recessive forms; 25% recurrence risk (Butler et al., 1987).

Frequency: Rare, 40 cases reported to 1988.

Clinical Manifestations: *Marked phenotypic variability* (especially in females): (a) *characteristic facies:* large head, macrocephaly, prominent forehead, facial nevus (23%), flat nasal bridge, short and upturned nose, mandibular hydpoplasia, apparent ocular hypertelorism, S-shaped lower eyelids, triangular mouth with downturned angles, micrognathia; (b) *oral abnormalities:* dental malalignment, crowded teeth, delayed exfoliation of deciduous teeth, retained molar teeth, notching of teeth, macroglossia, hyperplastic gingivae, absent or rudimentary uvula (18%), cleft lip, cleft palate (9%); (c) *mesomelic shortening of limbs with disproportionate shortening of forearms, small hands (89%), and feet; nail dysplasia;* (d) *hypoplastic external genitalia;* primary hypogonadism (Lee); (e) *growth delay;* (f) other reported abnormalities: scoliosis (50%), ankyloglossia, hepatosplenomegaly, digital anomalies, stenotic orifice of eustachian tubes, low-set ears with an overhanging helix (53%), abnormal palmar creases and single flexion creases of fingers, developmental or mental retardation (5 of 27), inguinal and/or umbilical hernia (20%), Hodgkin disease, abnormal umbilicus, thrombocytopenia.

Radiologic Manifestations: (a) *mesomelic brachymelia with disproportionate shortening of forearms,* ulna shorter than radius, luxation of radius; (b) brachymesophalangism V, clinodactyly V, shortening of other phalanges, short metacarpals, *bifid terminal phalanges of hands and feet,* distinctive pattern profile; (c) *multiple rib anomalies (40%), fusions;* (d) *hemivertebrae (70%), vertebral fusions, narrow interpediculate distances (66%);* (e) urinary system anomalies (29%), renal duplication, hydronephrosis (Fig SK–R–1).

Differential Diagnosis, Significant: Hurler syndrome; other mesomelic dysplasias; Aarskog syndrome.

Special Comments: Robinow syndrome without mesomelia has been reported in 5 patients. Mesomelia may be more severe in the autosomal recessive patients. The *"fetal face"* term is used because of the resemblance of the face to

that of the fetus at 8 weeks. The recessive form has been referred to as *Covesdem syndrome.*

REFERENCES

Bain MD, et al.: Robinow syndrome without mesomelic "brachymelia": a report of five cases. *J. Med. Genet.* 23:350–354, 1986.

Butler MG, Wadlington WB: Robinow syndrome: Report of two patients and review of literature. *Clin. Genet.* 31:77–85, 1987.

Butler MG, et al.: Metacarpophalangeal pattern profile analysis in Robinow syndrome. *Am. J. Med. Genet.* 27:219–223, 1987.

Friedman JM: Umbilical dysmorphology. *Clin. Genet.* 28:343–347, 1985.

Khayat D, et al.: Robinow syndrome: A case with thrombocytopenia. *Arch. Fr. Pediatr.* 40:327–330, 1983.

Lee PA, et al.: Micropenis. III. Primary hypogonadism, partial androgen insensitivity syndrome and idiopathic disorders. *Johns Hopkins Med. J.* 147:175–181, 1980.

Robinow M, Silverman FN, Smith HD: A newly recognized dwarfing syndrome. *Am. J. Dis. Child.* 117:645, 1969.

Wadia RJ: Covesdem syndrome. *J. Med. Genet.* 16:162, 1979.

"ROUND DISTAL FEMORAL EPIPHYSEAL" MICROMELIC DYSPLASIA—MAROTEAUX

Synonyms: Recessive lethal chondrodysplasia "round femoral inferior epiphysis type"; thanatophoric-like dysplasia—Glasgow variant.

Mode of Inheritance: Autosomal recessive.

Frequency: Very rare; 9 cases to 1988.

Clinical Manifestations: *Lethal* (newborn of shortly after); relatively large head, short limbs; normal trunk; narrow thorax.

Radiologic Manifestations: *Short long bones with incurving (especially femurs); large round distal femoral precocious ossification;* metaphyseal enlargement and irregularity; slightly short ribs; hypoplastic iliac wings; normal skull, spine, hands, and feet; prenatal diagnosis (ultrasound), 18 weeks.

Chondro-osseous Morphology: *Nonspecific;* normal resting zone; irregular columns; reduced proliferative zone. Short trabeculae and bony bridging.

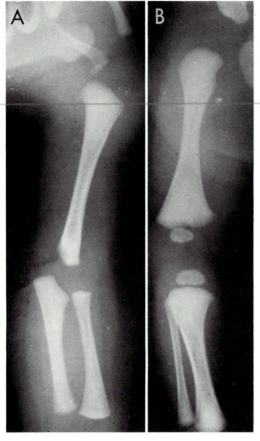

FIG SK–R–1.
Robinow syndrome. Newborn male with moderate mesomelic brachymelia. (From Robinow M, Silverman FN, Smith HD: A newly recognized dwarfing syndrome. *Am. J. Dis. Child.* 117:645, 1969. Reproduced with permission.)

Differential Diagnosis: (a) thanatophoric variants and dysplasia; (b) micromelic dysplasia.

REFERENCES

Conner JM, et al.: Lethal neonatal chondrodysplasias in the west of Scotland. *Am. J. Med. Genet.* 22:243–253, 1985.
Holmgren G, et al.: Semi lethal bone dysplasia in 3 sibs. *Clin. Genet.* 26:249–251, 1984.
Maroteaux P, et al.: Recessive lethal chondrodysplasia, "round femoral inferior epiphysis type. *Eur. J. Pediatr.* 147:408–411, 1988.

RUVALCABA SYNDROME

Synonyms: Tricho-rhino-phalangeal syndrome, type 3; Hunter syndrome; Sugio-Kajii syndrome.

Mode of Inheritance: Autosomal dominant.

Frequency: Rare; 23 patients to 1988.

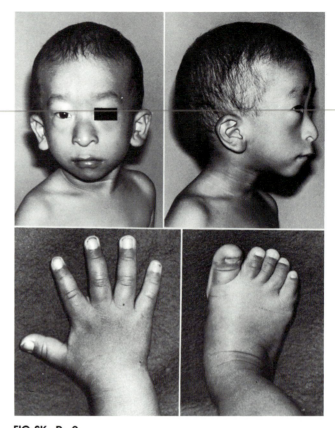

FIG SK–R–2.
Ruvalcaba syndrome, early childhood. clinical appearance: narrow beaked nose; small hands and feet. (From Sugio Y, Kajii T: Ruvalcaba syndrome. *Am. J. Med. Genet.* 19:741–753, 1984. Reproduced with permission.)

Clinical Manifestations: *Mental retardation, short stature, microcephaly; characteristic facial appearance with narrow beaked nose,* narrow thorax with pectus carinatum, hypoplastic genitalia, small hands and feet; other reported manifestations: sparse hair, posterior and low-set ears, scoliosis, large areolae, hypoplastic skin, hyperchromic skin areas, white forelock, tapetoretinal dystrophy.

Radiologic Manifestations: *Short metacarpals and phalanges, short metatarsals, cone epiphyses (55%),* bulbous metacarpal and metatarsal ends with narrow diaphyses, lunate-scaphoid fusion; craniostenosis; osteochondrosis of spine (Fig SK–R–2).

Differential Diagnosis, Significant: Tricho-rhino-phalangeal syndrome type 1.

Special Comment: Not to be confused with Ruvalcaba-Myhre-Smith syndrome (macrocephaly, GI polyposis, and penile macules); Hunter patients and the Sugio-Kajii cases may represent separate (and allelic) disorders (Niikawa).

REFERENCES

Bianchi E, et al.: Ruvalcaba syndrome: *Eur. J. Pediatr.* 142:301–303, 1984.

Hunter A, et al.: A new syndrome of mental retardation with characteristic facies and brachyphalangy. *J. Med. Genet.* 14:430–437, 1977.

Hunter A: Ruvalcaba syndrome (letter). *Am. J. Med. Genet.* 21:785–786, 1985.

Niikawa N, Kamei T: The Sugio-Kajii syndrome: Proposed tricho-rhino-phalangeal syndrome, type III (letter). *Am. J. Med. Genet.* 24:759–760, 1986.

Revalcaba RHA et. al.: A new familial syndrome with osseous dysplasia and mental deficiency. J. Pediatr. 79; 450–455, 1971.

Sugio, Y. and Kajii, T.: Ruvalcaba Syndrome: Amer. J. Med. Genet. 19; 741–753, 1984.

S

SCHNECKENBECKEN DYSPLASIA

Synonyms: Snail-pelvis dysplasia; cochlea pelvis dysplasia.

Mode of Inheritance: Autosomal recessive.

Frequency: Very rare; 10 cases to 1988.

Clinical Manifestations: (a) *consanguinity, polyhydramnios; lethal neonatal;* (b) *large head,* short neck, flat midface, cleft palate (1/9), edema.

Radiologic Manifestations: (a) *dumbbell very short long bones,* metaphyseal irregularity; *wide fibula;* (b) *round vertebral bodies,* posterior vertebral body absence; normal posterior elements; (c) short splayed ribs, handle-bar clavicles, hypoplastic scapulae; (d) *snail-shaped ilia,* flat acetabular roofs, sacral stenosis, precociously ossified ischium; (e) brachydactyly, precociously ossified carpal and tarsal bones; (f) intrauterine diagnosis (18-week fetus)—ultrasound (Fig SK–S–1).

Chondro-osseous Morphology: Characteristic resting cartilage; increased cellular density; hypervascularity; normal-sized chondrocytes with central nucleus; no lacunar space.

Differential Diagnosis, Significant: (a) thanatophoric dysplasia and variants; (b) achondrogenesis-hypochondrogenesis; (c) Kniest-like dysplasia.

Special Comment: I have called this skeletal dysplasia "Schneckenbecken dysplasia" because of the diagnostic iliac wing configuration.

REFERENCES

Borochowitz Z, Jones KL, Silbey R, Adomian R, Lachman R, Rimoin DL: A distinct lethal neonatal chondrodysplasia with snail-like pelvis: Schneckenbecken dysplasia. *Am. J. Med. Genet.* 25:47–59, 1986.
Knowles S, Winter R, Rimoin D: A new category of lethal short-limbed dwarfism. *Am. J. Med. Genet.* 25:41–46, 1986.

SCLEROSTEOSIS

Synonyms: Osteopetrosis with syndactyly; sklerosteose; endosteal hyperostosis, type sclerosteosis.

Mode of Inheritance: Autosomal recessive.

Frequency: Uncommon; about 60 cases to 1988; high incidence among Afrikaner population of South Africa.

Clinical Manifestations: Progressive skeletal deformity with onset in early childhood: (a) *acquired craniofacial dysmorphism:* prominent frontal bone, *mandibular prognathism,* relative midfacial hypoplasia, proptosis, hypertelorism, *dental malocclusion;* (b) *gigantism;* (c) *cranial nerve palsy,* especially *seventh nerve,* sensorineural hearing loss; (d) *characteristic syndactyly,* usually of second and third fingers; (e) dysplastic nails; (f) increased intracranial pressure, headaches; (g) elevated serum alkaline phosphatase level; (h) other reported abnormalities: divergent strabismus; excess lacrimation; anesthetic management problems.

Radiologic Manifestations: (a) *cranial sclerosis* (infancy onset); obliteration of cranial nerve foramina; (b) *dense massive mandible;* dental malocclusion; (c) *sclerotic vertebral end plates* and pedicles; (d) *wide dense clavicles and ribs;* dense pelvis and scapulae; (e) cortically dense, expanded later massive long tubular bones; (f) expanded, dense short tubular bones (hands and feet); *bony and soft tissue syndactyly* (especially 2 and 3); (g) CT demonstration of cranial abnormalities (Fig SK–S–2).

Chondro-osseous Morphology: Craniotomy specimens—increased bone and osteoid volume; increased osteoblast activity suggesting osteoblast function disorder.

Differential Diagnosis, Significant: (a) osteopetrosis; (b) van Buchem disease and other sclerosing bone dysplasias.

REFERENCES

Beighton P, et al.: The syndromic states of sclerosteosis and van Buchem disease. *Clin. Genet.* 25:175–181, 1984.
Beighton P: Sclerosteosis. *J. Med. Genet.* 25:200–203, 1988.
Cremin BJ: Sclerosteosis in children. *Pediatr. Radiol.* 8:173, 1979.
Geyser PG, et al.: Anesthetic management in sclerosteosis. *S. Afr. Med. J.* 61:488, 1982.
Hansen HG: Sklerosteose, in Opitz H, Schmidt F (eds.): *Handbuch der Kinderheilkunde,* vol. 6. Berlin, Springer, 1967, p. 351.
Hill SC, et al.: Cranial CT findings in sclerosteosis. *AJNR* 7:505–511, 1986.
Nager GT, Hamersma H: Sclerosteosis involving the temporal bone: Histopathiologic aspects. *Am. J. Otolaryngol.* 7:1–16, 1986.
Stein SA, et al.: Sclerosteosis. *Neurology* 33:267–277, 1983.

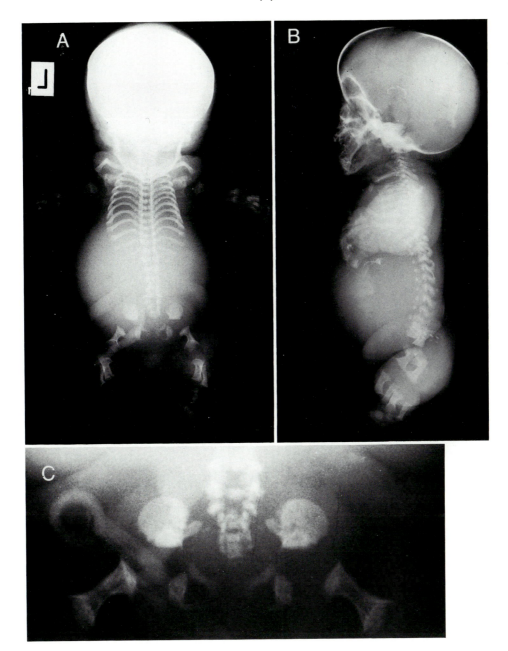

FIG SK–S–1.
Schneckenbecken dysplasia in a stillborn. **A,** large skull; narrow chest; short ribs, micromelia. **B,** large skull; midface hypoplasia, anterior vertebral body ossification, short ribs. **C,** iliac wings in the shape of a snail.

Sugiura Y, et al.: Sclerosteosis. *J. Bone Joint Surg.* 57A:273–276, 1975.
Truswell AS: Osteopetrosis with syndactyly. A morphological variant of Albers-Schönberg disease. *J. Bone Joint Surg.* 40:208, 1958.

Note:: SRP without polydactyly has been seen in type 3 and type Beemer. Types 1 and 3 may be variability within the same disorder (Sillence). Type 2 and type Beemer may also represent the same disorder with some variability.

SHORT RIB–POLYDACTYLY SYNDROMES (SRP)

Classification: *type 1*: Saldino-Noonan, AR; *type 2*: Majewski, AR; *type 3*: Verma-Naumoff, AR; *type*: Beemer, AR.

SHORT RIB-POLYDACTYLY SYNDROME, TYPE 1 (SALDINO-NOONAN)

Synonyms: Lethal form of chondroectodermal dysplasia—le Marec; Saldino-Noonan syndrome; SRP–1.

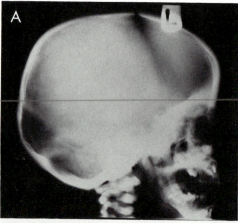

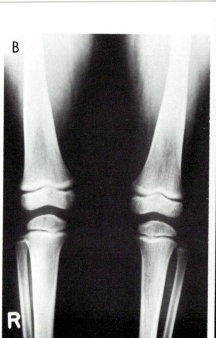

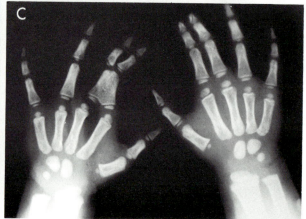

FIG SK–S–2.
Sclerosteosis. A 3-year-old female with a history of intermittent transient facial palsies. **A,** lateral skull showing increased density at base of the skull. **B,** knees with increased metaphyseal density. **C,** hands showing bony and soft tissue syndactyly. (From Cremin BJ: Sclerosteosis in children. *Pediatr. Radiol.* 8:173, 1979. Reproduced with permission.)

Mode of Inheritance: Autosomal recessive.

Frequency: Uncommon; 63 cases to 1988 (including type 3).

Clinical Manifestations: (a) *primarily female (9/13); hydropic appearance at birth;* (b) *dolichocephaly, natal teeth micrognathia;* (c) *extremely short and narrow thorax, protuberant abdomen;* (d) *marked micromelia (flipper-like extremities), postaxial and occasionally preaxial polydactyly, severe brachydactyly;* (e) *other reported abnormalities: renal anomalies, genital anomalies (sex reversal), cardiovascular anomalies: gastrointestinal anomalies, imperforate anus, hypoplastic lungs;* (f) *death in perinatal period;* (g) *prenatal diagnosis— fetoscopy.*

Radiologic Manifestations: (a) *dolichocephaly, poor mineralization of frontal bones, mandibular hypoplasia;* (b) *severely shortened horizontally oriented ribs,* small scapulae, superiorly located deformed clavicles, misshapen and square vertebral bodies, coronal cleft of vertebral bodies, small iliac bones, flattened acetabular roofs; (c) *hypoplasia and grossly misshapen ragged-ended tubular bones—in particular distally; metaphyseal spurs, pointed femora on both ends, absent fibulas deficiency in ossification of metacarpals, metatarsals, and phalanges;* (d) *prenatal diagnosis—4 cases (ultrasound) (Fig SK–S–3).*

Chondro-osseous Morphology: Shortened or absent zone of proliferation, loss of columnization, irregularly dispersed hypertrophic cells, *does not separate type 1 from 3 (Sillence).*

Differential Diagnosis, Significant: (a) SRP other types especially; (b) asphyxiating thoracic dysplasia; (c) Ellis–van Creveld.

Special Comment: *Distinguishing features from type 3; more genitourinary and cardiovascular anomalies, female sex preponderance, pointed femoral ends; absent fibulas.*

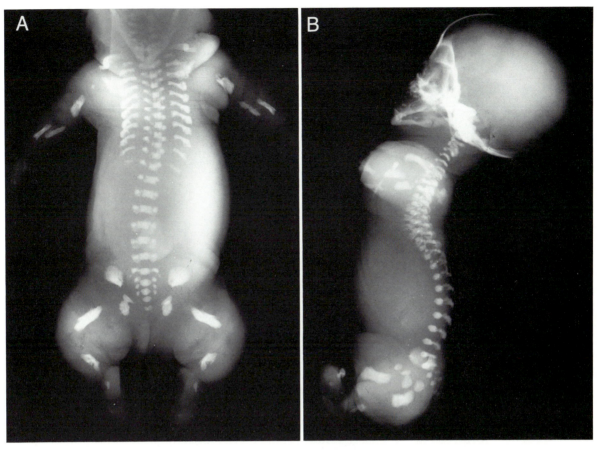

FIG SK–S–3.

A, and **B,** short rib–polydactyly syndrome, type 1 (Saldino-Noonan) in a stillborn: tiny ribs; hypoplastic scapulae; metaphy-seal spurs; micromelia; pointed femoral ends; hypoplastic ilia, absent fibulas.

REFERENCES

Cherstvoy ED, et al.: Difficulties in classification of the short rib-polydactyly syndromes. *Eur. J. Pediatr.* 133:57, 1980.

Grote W, et al.: Prenatal diagnosis of a short-rib-polydactyly syndrome type Saldino-Noonan at 17 weeks gestation. *Eur. J. Pediatr.* 140:63–66, 1983.

Johnson VP, et al.: Midtrimester prenatal diagnosis. Short limb dwarfism (Saldino-Noonan syndrome). *Birth Defect Conference,* San Diego, June 14–19, 1981.

LeMarec B, et al.: Lethal neonatal form of chondroectodermal dysplasia. *Ann. Radiol.* 16:19–26, 1973.

Richardson MM, et al.: Prenatal diagnosis of recurrence of Saldino-Noonan dwarfism. *J. Pediatr.* 91:467–471, 1977.

Saldino RM, Noonan CD: Severe thoracic dystrophy with striking micromelia, abnormal osseous development, including the spine and multiple visceral abnormalities. *Am. J. Roentgenol.* 114:257, 1972.

Sillence D, et al.: Perinatally lethal short rib-polydactyly syndrome. *Pediatr. Radiol.* 17:474–480, 1987.

Stromme Koppang H, et al.: Oral abnormalities in the Saldino-Noonan syndrome. *Virhows Arch.* 398:247–262, 1983.

Toftager-Larsen K, Benzie RJ: Fetoscopy in prenatal diagnosis of the Majewski and Saldino Noonan types of short rib polydactyly syndrome. *Clin. Genet.* 26:56–60, 1984.

SHORT RIB–POLYDACTYLY SYNDROME, TYPE 2 (MAJEWSKI)

Synonyms: Majewski syndrome; SRP–2.

Mode of Inheritance: Autosomal recessive.

Frequency: Rare; about 23 well-documented cases to 1988.

Clinical Manifestations: (a) *hydropic appearance at birth;* (b) *facial features:* prominent forehead, low-set and malformed ears, *lobulated tongue,* tight frenulum, micrognathia, *cleft lip/palate,* short and flat nose; (c) *extremely short and narrow thorax, protuberant abdomen;* (d) *marked micromelia, in particular distally,* preaxial and/or postaxial *polysyndactyly, brachydactyly, hypoplasia,* or *aplasia of nails;* (e) other reported abnormalities: dry skin, *cystic kid-*

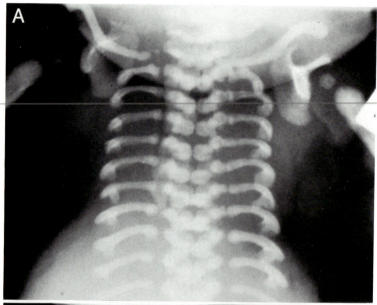

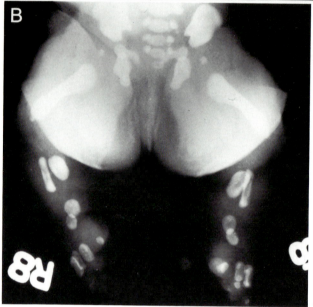

FIG SK—S—4.
Short rib-polydactyly syndrome, type 2 (Majewski) in a neonate. **A,** short ribs, precocious humeral ossification; sagittal vertebral clefts. **B,** precocious femoral ossification; round femoral ends; round hypoplastic tibias, short fibula.

neys, genital anomalies, pancreatic fibrosis, *gastrointestinal anomalies,* brain anomalies (arhinencephaly, cerebral dysgenesis), *hypoplastic epiglottis and larynx,* cardiovascular anomalies (atrial septal defect); (f) *death in perinatal period;* (g) prenatal diagnosis (fetoscopy).

Radiologic Manifestations: (a) *underdeveloped mandible, irregular teeth;* (b) *extremely short and horizontally located ribs;* (c) *mesomelia, marked shortening of tubular bones, in particular extreme shortness of tibiae (ovoid configuration), rounded metaphyseal ends of long tubular bones, precocious ossification of proximal femoral epiphysis, poly-* dactyly, distal phalangeal hypoplasia, symphalangism; (d) almost *normal pelvis;* (g) prenatal diagnosis (ultrasound) (Figs SK—S—4 and Sk—S—5).

Chondro-osseous Morphology and Chromosomal Findings: Mildly abnormal growth plate similar to other SRP types; *additional chromosome material* at 17p11 on high-resolution prometaphase analysis (Pauli).

Differential Diagnosis, Significant: (a) OFD-2 (Mohr); (b) other SRP, especially type Beemer; (c) asphyxiating thoracic dysplasia.

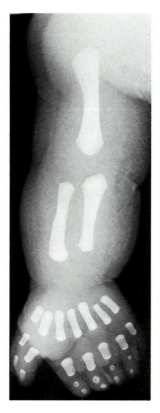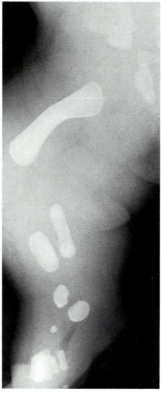

FIG SK—S—5.
Short rib—polydactyly syndrome, type 2 (Majewski). Short tubular bones, polydactyly with seven fingers, marked disproportion between distal and proximal bones. (From Bergström K, Gustafson K-H, Jorulf H, et al.: *Skeletal Radiol.* 4:134, 1979. Reproduced with permission.)

Special Comment: OFD type 2 (Mohr) and SRP-2 may be mild and severe expressions of the same disorder (Silengo).

REFERENCES

Bergström K, et al.: A case of Majewski syndrome with pathoanatomic examination. *Skeletal Radiol.* 4:134, 1979.

Black IL, et al.: Parental consanguinity and Majewski syndrome. *J. Med. Genet.* 19:141–157, 1982.

Chen H, et al.: Short rib-polydactyly syndrome Majewski type. *Am. J. Med. Genet.* 7:215–222, 1980.

Gembruch U, et al.: Early prenatal diagnosis of SRP type 1 (Majewski). *Prenat. Diagn.* 5:357, 1985.

Majewski F, et al.: Polysyndaktylie verkürzte Gliemassen und Genitalfehlbildungen. Kennzeichen eines selbatändigen Syndroms? *Z. Kinderheilkd.* 111:118, 1971.

McCormac RM, et al.: Short rib-polydactyly syndrome type 2 (Majewski syndrome). *Pediatr. Pathol.* 2:457–467, 1984.

Meizner I, et al.: Prenatal ultrasound diagnosis of fetal thoracic and intrathoracic abnormalities. *Isr. J. Med. Sci.* 22:350–354, 1986.

Pauli RM, et al.: Short rib polydactyly type Majewski. *Proc. Greenwood Genet. Center* 7:168–169, 1988.

Silengo MC, et al.: Oro-facio-digital syndrome II: Transitional type between the Mohr and the Majewski syndrome: Report of two new cases. *Clin. Genet.* 31:331, 1987.

Spranger J, et al.: Short-rib-polydactyly (SRP) syndromes, types Majewski and Saldino-Noonan. *Z. Kinderheilkd.* 116:73, 1974.

Thomson GSM, et al.: Antenatal detection of recurrence of Majewski dwarf. *Clin. Radiol.* 33:509–517, 1982.

Toftager-Larsen K, Benzie RJ: Fetoscopy in prenatal diagnosis of Majewski and Saldino-Noonan types of short rib-polydactyly syndrome. *Clin. Genet.* 26:56–60, 1984.

Walley VM, et al.: Brief clinical report: SRP, Majewski type. *Am. J. Med. Genet.* 14:445–452, 1983.

SHORT RIB—POLYDACTYLY SYNDROME, TYPE 3 (VERMA-NAUMOFF)

Synonyms: Verma-Naumoff syndrome; SRP–3.

Mode of Inheritance: Autosomal recessive.

Frequency: Uncommon (including type 1); 63 cases to 1988, *more frequent than type 1.*

Clinical Manifestations: *similar to but milder than type 1:* (a) *micromelic dwarfism, polydactyly of hands and feet (often no polydactyly);* (b) *narrow thorax, hypoplastic lung;* (c) *cleft lip/palate;* (d) other reported abnormalities: congenital anomalies (renal, genital [sex reversal 3/20], gastrointestinal, cardiovascular).*

Radiologic Manifestations: (a) *short cranial base, bulging forehead, flattened occiput, sunken root of nose;* (b) *short ribs, hypoplastic thin vertebrae with irregular margins of vertebral bodies,* increased intervertebral disk spaces; (c) *severely shortened tubular bones, round metaphyseal ends with*

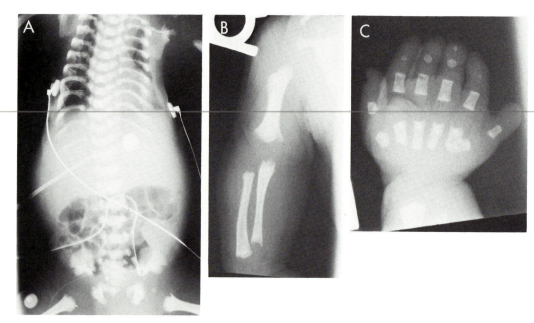

FIG SK–S–6.
Short rib–polydactyly syndrome type 3 (Verma-Naumoff). **A,** narrow thorax, short ribs, deformed scapulae and pelvic bones. **B,** right upper limb—marked shortness of tubular bones and spurs at

ends of tubular bones. **C,** polydactyly, fusion of fifth and sixth metacarpals, absence of ossification of several phalanges, and shortness of digits.

lateral spikes (3-pronged ball in V groove) *of long bones—especially femora* and *tibias; shortening of all short tubular bones* (hands and feet); *progressive distally;* (d) prenatal diagnosis (ultrasound)—2 cases: 31 weeks—polyhydramnios, etc., 30 weeks (Fig SK–S–6).

Chondro-osseous Morphology: Same as SRP 1, cases with PAS-stained inclusions.

Differential Diagnosis, Significant: Other SRP especially type 1; Ellis van Creveld syndrome; asphyxiating thoracic dysplasia.

Special Comment: *Distinguishing features from type 1:* 50% male, often no polydactyly; ball in cone (V-groove) end of bones; normal to hypoplastic fibulas; trident acetabulae, less severe radiographic involvement.

REFERENCES

Belloni C, et al.: Short rib-polydactyly syndrome, type Verma-Naumoff. *Fortschr. Roentgenstr.* 134:431, 1981.
Bernstein R, et al.: Short rib polydactyly syndrome: *J. Med. Genet.* 22:46–53, 1985.
Meizner I, Bar-Ziv J: Prenatal ultrasonic diagnosis of SRPS type 3. *J. Clin. Ultrasound* 13:284–287, 1985.
Naumoff P, et al.: Short rib-polydactyly syndrome type 3. *Radiology* 122:443, 1977.
Sillence D, et al.: Perinatally lethal short rib polydactyly syndromes. *Pediatr. Radiol.* 17:474–480, 1987.
Steffelaar JW, et al.: Prenatal diagnosis in a prima gravida of the short rib polydactyly syndrome. *Ned. Tijdschr. Geneeskd.* 132:405–407, 1988.

Verma IC, et al.: Autosomal recessive form of lethal chondrodystrophy with severe thoracic narrowing, rhizoacromelic micromelia, polydactyly and genital anomalies. *Birth Defects* 11:167–174, 1975.
Yang SS, et al.: Short rib polydactyly syndrome, type 3 with chondrocyte inclusion: *Am. J. Med. Genet.* 7:205–213, 1980.
Yang SS, et al.: Three conditions in neonatal asphyxiating thoracic dysplasia (Jeune) and short rib polydactyly syndrome spectrum. *Am. J. Med. Genet. (suppl.)* 3:191–207, 1987.

SHORT RIB SYNDROME TYPE–BEEMER

Synonyms: SRP without polydactyly type Beemer; Beemer syndrome; SRP–Beemer.

Mode of Inheritance: Autosomal recessive.

Frequency: Very rare; 6 cases reported to 1988.

Clinical Manifestations: Same as SRP type 2 (Majewski) *except no polydactyly;* normal tongue.

Radiologic Manifestations: Same as SRP 2 *except more normally developed tibia;* (a) prenatal diagnosis (ultrasound).

Differential Diagnosis, Significant: (a) other SRP especially type 2; (b) asphyxiating thoracic dysplasia.

Special Comment: SRP-Beemer may represent clinical variability in SRP type 2 (Majewski): *without polydactyly,* rather than a separate disorder.

REFERENCES

Beemer FA, et al.: A new short rib syndrome: *Am. J. Med. Genet.* 14:115–123, 1982.

Passarge E: Letter to editor. *Am. J. Med. Genet.* 14:403–405, 1983.

Winter RM: A lethal short rib syndrome without polydactyly. *J. Med. Genet.* 25:349–357, 1988.

Wladimiroff JW, et al.: Early diagnosis of skeletal dysplasia by real time ultrasound. *Lancet* 1:661, 1981.

SPONASTRIME DYSPLASIA

Mode of Inheritance: Autosomal recessive.

Frequency: Very rare; 6 cases, 2 families.

Clinical Manifestations: *Nonlethal; short stature;* late infancy more severe in the male; (a) *"oriental look"*—midface hypoplasia, saddle nose; (b) kyphoscoliosis, lumbar lordosis.

Radiologic Manifestations: (a) *striations in metaphyses;* (b) spine: osteoporosis; *pear-shaped vertebrae; cod-fish vertebrae;* (c) typical pattern profile (Fig SK–S–7).

Chondro-osseous Morphology: *Characteristic:* pseudocystic transformation; reduction and abnormal arrangement of collagen fibrils—defect in collagen synthesis and proteoglycans.

Differential Diagnosis, Significant: Osteopathia striata.

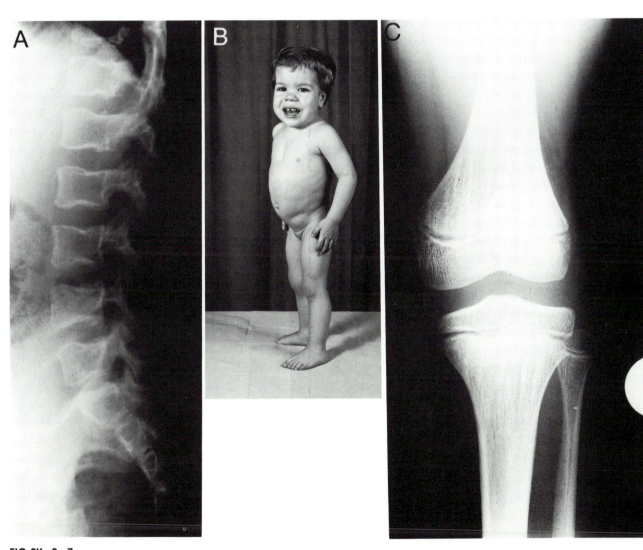

FIG SK–S–7.
Sponastrime dysplasia in **A,** a female aged 6½ years: superior and inferior indentations of vertebral bodies; osteoporosis; **B,** a child aged 2½ years: characteristic facies with midface hypoplasia and saddle nose; **C,** a female aged 11½ years: well established linea striata; slightly small epiphyseal ossification.

Special Comment: Terminology: Spon = *spondylo;* Nas = *nasal;* Stri Me = *striated metaphyses.*

REFERENCES

Fanconi S, et al.: The sponastrime dysplasia. *Helv. Paediatr. Acta* 38:267–280, 1983.
Lachman RS, et al.: Sponastrime dysplasia: A radiologic-pathologic correlation. *Pediatr. Radiol.,* 19:417, 1989.

SPONDYLOENCHONDRODYSPLASIA

Synonym: Enchondromatosis with severe platyspondyly.

Mode of Inheritance: Probably autosomal recessive.

Frequency: Very rare, 5 well-documented cases reported to 1988.

Clinical Manifestations: (a) *short stature;* rhizomelia; genu valgum; increased anteroposterior diameter of chest; thoracic kyphosis; lumbar lordosis; (b) *prominent joints and ends of long bones* and ribs.

Radiologic Manifestations: (a) *enchondromatous involvement of long bones, flat bones* but sparing of hands and feet; (b) *severe platyspondyly with marked end plate irregularity* (enchondroma) (Fig SK–S–8).

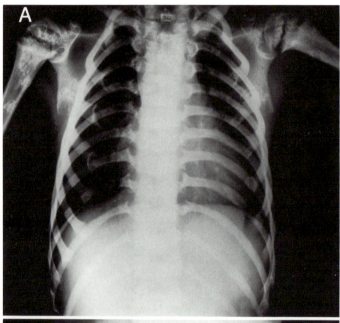
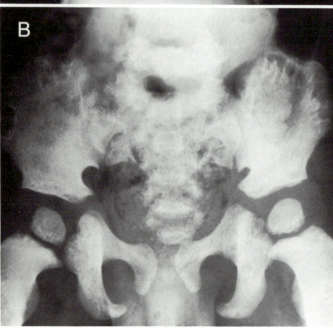
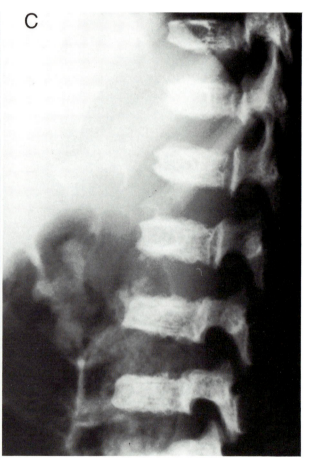

FIG SK–S–8.
Spondyloenchondrodysplasia in a child aged 6 years.
A, multiple enchondromata in humeri, ribs, scapulae.
B, enchondromatous changes in ilia. **C,** characteristic spine; platyspondyly with end plate (enchondromatous) irregularity. (Courtesy of I. Greinacher, M.D., and J. Spranger, M.D., Kinderklinic, Mainz, West Germany).

Differential Diagnosis, Significant: (a) Ollier disease; (b) enchondromatosis with vertebral involvement, including: Spranger type 1, with irregular vertebral lesions; Spranger type 2, with mild platyspondyly; Azouz type, with vertebral anomalies and platyspondyly; (c) metachondromatosis; (d) spondylometaphyseal dysplasia, unclassified forms.

Special Comments: This probably autosomal recessive disorder can be differentiated from Spranger type 1, which has *normal height vertebral bodies* with *irregular end plates,* and from Spranger type 2, which has *mild platyspondyly* and *severe hand involvement.* The Azouz type has *hemivertebrae,* end plate irregularity and moderate hand involvement. The three aforementioned disorders are all sporadic. (Table SK–E–1)

REFERENCES

Spondyloenchondrodysplasia

Chagnon S, et al.: Spondylo-enchondrodysplasie. *J. Radiol.* 66:75–79, 1985.
Mainzer F, et al.: The variable osc enchondromatosis. *Radiology* 99:377, 1971.
Sauvegrain J, et al.: Chondromes multiples avec atteinte rachidienne. Spondylo-enchondroplasie et autres formes. *J. Radiol.* 61:495–501, 1980.
Schorr S, et al.: Spondyloenchondro-dysplasia. *Radiology* 118:133–139, 1976.

Enchondromatosis with Spinal Involvement

Azouz EM: Case report 418. *Skeletal Radiol.* 16:236–239, 1987.
Spranger J, et al.: Two peculiar types of enchondromatosis. *Pediatr. Radiol.* 7:215–219, 1978.

SPONDYLO-EPI-METAPHYSEAL DYSPLASIAS (SEMD) (CLASSIFICATION)

Common Forms:

1. SEMD Strudwick type (AR).
2. SEMD with joint laxity (AR).
3. SEMD, dominant "metatropic" type. (AD).
4. SEMD, Irapa type (AR).

Rare Forms:

1. SEMD with cone epiphyses (Perri 1987).
2. SEMD with micromelia (Kozlowski 1974).
3. SEMD with severe platyspondyly (Tehranzadeh 1978).

AR = autosomal recessive; AD = autosomal dominant.

REFERENCES

Benson KT, et al.: Anesthesia for cesarean section in patient with spondylometaepiphyseal dysplasia. *Anaesthesia* 63:548–550, 1985.

Kozlowski K: Micromelic type of spondylo-metaepiphyseal dysplasia. *Pediatr. Radiol.* 2:61, 1974.
Langer L, et al.: SEMD dominant "metatropic" type. Birth Defects meeting, Baltimore, Md, 1988.
Perri G, et al.: Unusual cone shaped epiphyses in spondyloepiphyseal dysplasia. *Pediatr. Radiol.* 17:223–225, 1987.
Tehranzadeh J, et al.: Complex spondylo-epi-metaphyseal dysplasia with severe platyspondyly in two brothers. *Australas. Radiol.* 22:173, 1978.

SPONDYLO-EPI-METAPHYSEAL DYSPLASIA, IRAPA TYPE

Synonym: SEMD-IRAPA.

Mode of Inheritance: Autosomal recessive.

Frequency: Rare; 16 cases to 1988; first reported in Irapa tribe of Venezuelan Indians.

Clinical Manifestations: Onset during childhood, with *joint pains* and *walking difficulty; short stature,* proportionate; *joint limitation; wide costochondral junctions; generalized joint enlargement; brachydactyly with long second digit.*

Radiologic Manifestations: (a) *generalized platyspondyly with end plate irregularity;* (b) *epiphyseal ossification delay; wide irregular metaphyses* (especially proximal femoral and distal humeral); *short long bones;* (c) *hypoplastic ilia; hypoplastic acetabular roof; symphysis pubis irregularity; coxa vara;* (d) *small irregular carpals;* capitate-hamate fusion; *short, distally widened metacarpals* (3,4,5); (e) *anterior rib flaring;* (f) early-onset severe *osteoarthritis,* all joints; osteopenia.

Differential Diagnosis, Significant: (a) other SEMD; (b) SED; (c) Morquio disease.

REFERENCES

Arias S, et al.: L'osteochondrodysplasie spondylo-epiphyso-metaphysaire type Irapa. *Nouv. Presse Med.* 5:319–323, 1976.
Arias S: Letter to editor. *Am. J. Med. Genet.* 8:251–253, 1981.
Cantu JM: Reply, letter to editor. *Am. J. Med. Genet.* 8:253–256, 1981.
Hernandez A, et al.: Autosomal recessive Spondylo-epi-metaphyseal dysplasia (Irapa type) in a Mexican family. *Am. J. Med. Genet.* 5:179–188, 1980.

SPONDYLO-EPI-METAPHYSEAL DYSPLASIA, STRUDWICK TYPE

Synonyms: Spondylo-meta-epiphyseal dysplasia—Strudwick; SEMD-Strudwick; SED congenita with metaphyseal involvement.

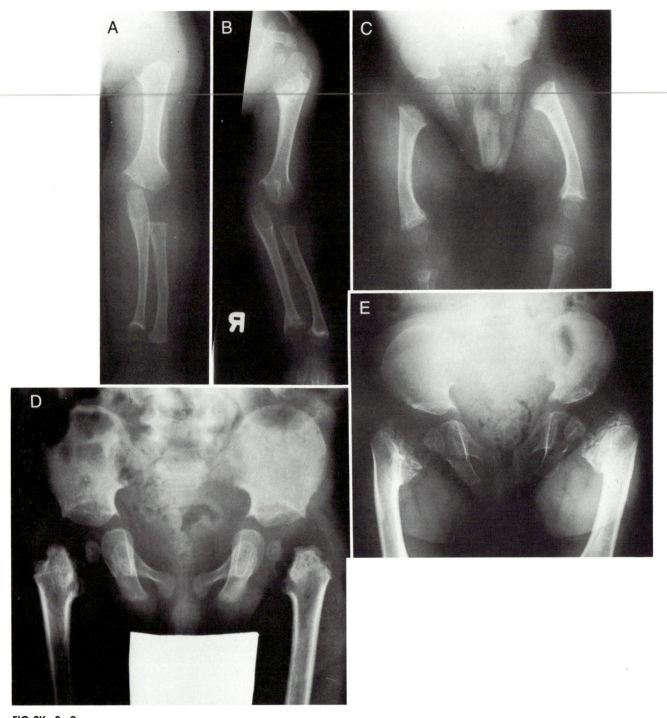

FIG SK–S–9.
Spondylo-epi-metaphyseal dysplasia (SMED) Strudwick in **A,** an infant aged 1 year: metaphyseal changes, proximal humerus, distal ulna; no epiphyseal ossification; **B,** a child aged 3 years: dappled metaphyses, proximal humerus, distal ulna and radius; hypoplastic epiphyseal ossification; **C,** an infant aged 1 year: rounded proximal femoral metaphyses, hypoplastic acetabulae; absent pubic ossification; distal femoral metaphyseal changes; **D,** a 2½ year old male: stick-proximal femora, dappling; hypoplastic epiphyses; **E,** in a child aged 3 years: dappling (fragmentation) of metaphyses *(Continued.)*

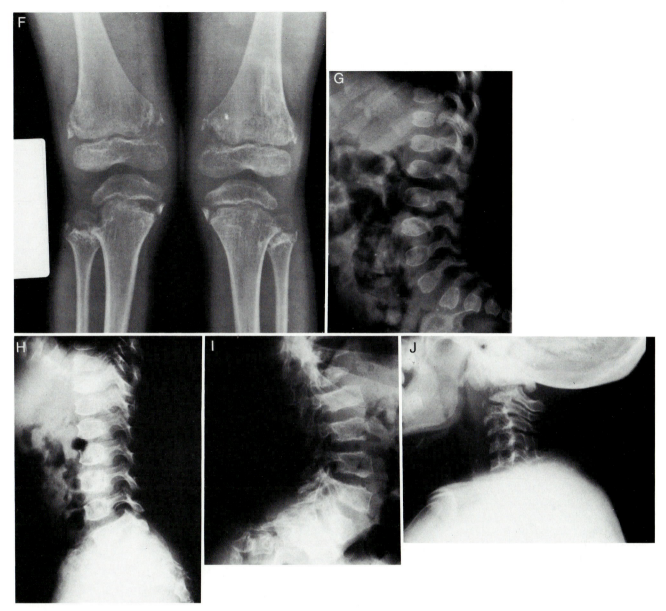

FIG SK–S–9 (cont).

F, a 7½ year old male: metaphyseal infractions at knees with metaphyseal irregularity—more severe in fibula than tibia; epiphyseal hypoplasia; **G,** an infant aged 9 months: platyspondylic, hypoplastic vertebral bodies; **H,** a child aged 3 years: mild platyspondyly with superior and inferior rounding; **I,** a 6-year-old female: severe platyspondyly; **J,** a child aged 5 years: severe cervical hypoplasia with C1-C2 subluxation.

Mode of Inheritance: Probably autosomal recessive.

Frequency: Rare; about 19 cases reported to 1988; probably underreported.

Clinical Manifestations: (a) *short-trunked, short-limbed dwarfism* at birth; (b) *cleft palate;* (c) *pectus carinatum,* protruberant abdomen, lordosis; (d) *myopia,* (e) normal intelligence; (f) *genu valga* (later).

Radiologic Manifestations: 1. Newborn and infancy: identical to SED congenita; (a) *marked generalized epiphyseal delay, "club-shaped" proximal temora,* generalized brachymelia; (b) platyspondyly. 2. Early childhood (3–5 years): (a) *metaphyseal irregularity and sclerosis (dappling-alternating sclerosis and lucency); more severe distal ulna* than radius, *fibula* than tibia; (b) pelvis, normal iliac wings, narrow sciatic notches; *delayed pubic bone ossification; coxa vara;* (c) *platyspondyly,* sometimes pear-shaping of vertebrae; scoliosis; *odontoid hypoplasia;* (d) ribs, *bulbous or splayed anteriorly* (Fig SK–S–9).

Chondro-osseous Morphology: Chondrocyte clustering in proliferative and hypertrophic zones; broad trabeculae and spicules; *inclusion bodies in chondrocytes;* electron microscopy—dilated rough endoplasmic reticulum filled with granular material.

Differential Diagnosis, Significant: (a) *SED congenita;* (b) other SEMDs.

REFERENCES

Anderson CE, et al.: Spondylometaepiphyseal dysplasia, Strudwick type. *Am. J. Med. Genet.* 13:243–256, 1982.

Bartsocas CS, et al.: A variant of spondyloepiphyseal dysplasia congenita. *Prog. Clin. Biol. Res.* 104:163–166, 1982.

Kousseff BG, Nichols P: Letter to editor. Autosomal recessive spondylometaepiphyseal dysplasia, type Strudwick. *Am. J. Med. Genet.* 17:547–550, 1984.

Spranger JW, Maroteaux P: Editorial comment: Genetic heterogeneity of spondyloepiphyseal dysplasia congenita. *Am. J. Med. Genet.* 13:241–242, 1982.

SPONDYLO-EPI-METAPHYSEAL DYSPLASIA WITH JOINT LAXITY

Synonym: SEMD-joint laxity.

Mode of Inheritance: Autosomal recessive (Afrikaner-German origin).

Frequency: Rare; 19 cases reported to 1988.

Clinical Manifestations: (a) *neonatal dwarfism; articular hypermobility; newborn kyphoscoliosis* (especially thoracic); *elbow deformities; club feet;* (b) characteristic facies (oval face, long upper lip, protruberant eyes); (c) spatulate terminal phalanges, ulnar deviation of fingers; (d) *soft doughy* stretchy *skin;* (e) cleft or high palate (43%), congenital heart disease (28%); dislocated hips (27%); (f) other reported abnormalities: mental retardation, myopia and lens dislocation; Hirschsprung disease; congenital megaureter; (g) complications: often early death (mid-childhood); paraplegia; *cardiorespiratory failure.*

Radiologic Manifestations: *Kyphoscoliosis; platyspondyly* (oval vertebrae); *end plate irregularity;* flared iliac wings; narrow sacrosciatic notch; *coxa valga; late ossification of capital femoral epiphyses; generalized epiphyseal delay; widened distal radius and ulna; radial head dislocation;* widened metaphyses; abnormal coarse trabecular structure (cyst-like lucencies); exostosis-like projections; shortened tubular bones of hands and feet; *metaphyseal irregularity.*

Differential Diagnosis, Significant: (a) *diastrophic dysplasia;* (b) pseudodiastrophic dysplasia; (c) spondyloepiphyseal dysplasia congenita; (d) other SEMD; (e) mucopolysaccharidoses; (f) Larsen syndrome; (g) metatropic dysplasia.

REFERENCES

Beighton P, Kozlowski K: Spondylo-epi-metaphyseal dysplasia with joint laxity and severe progressive kyphoscoliosis. *Skeletal Radiol.* 5:205–212, 1980.

Beighton P, et al.: The manifestations and natural history of spondylo-epi-metaphyseal dysplasia with joint laxity. *Clin. Genet.* 26:308–317, 1984.

Kozlowski K, Beighton P: Radiographic features of spondylo-epi-metaphyseal dysplasia with joint laxity and kyphoscoliosis. *Fortschr. Rontgenstr.* 141:337–341, 1984.

SPONDYLOEPIPHYSEAL DYSPLASIA CONGENITA

Synonyms: SED, Spranger-Wiedemann; SED-congenita.

Mode of Inheritance: Autosomal dominant (rarely autosomal recessive, possibly gonadal mosaicism).

Frequency: Common: about 162 well-documented cases to 1988.

Clinical Manifestations: (a) *small stature with short trunk at birth;* (b) flat face, hypertelorism, cleft palate; (c) *myopia, vitreoretinal degeneration, retinal detachment;* (d) short neck, cervical myopathy *(C1-C2 instability);* (e) *barrel-shaped thorax, pectus carinatum;* (f) *increase in thoracic kyphosis and marked lumbar lordosis, short spine;* (g) shortness of limbs; (h) *muscular hypotonia, waddling gait;* (i) relatively normal hands and feet, genu valgum or varum; (j) other reported abnormalities: restrictive lung disease (pulmonary function tests); laryngeal hypoplasia; height growth curves available (Horten); degenerative arthrosis of hips.

Radiologic Manifestations: (a) neonate and infancy: *ovoid or "pear-shaped" vertebrae;* generalized long bone shortening with normal modeling; *absent pubic* (and hypoplastic ischial) *ossification; no ossification of epiphyses at knees; no talus or calcaneal ossification; no metaphyseal changes;* (b) childhood and later life: *platyspondyly,* severe with irregularity; *odontoid hypoplasia, C1-C2 dislocation; marked epiphyseal delay and irregularity;* short normal appearing long bones; unusual high located greater trochanter; coxa vara; (c) prenatal diagnosis (ultrasound)—femoral length measurements (Fig SK–S–10).

Chondro-osseous Morphology and Biochemical Defect: Mild growth plate disorganization; PAS-positive cytoplasmic inclusions in chondrocytes; fine granular material in rough endoplasmic reticulum; small retinal type 2 collagen fibers; mutation in the CO L2A1 locus on *chromosome 12 (type 2 collagen gene).*

Differential Diagnosis, Significant: (a) Morquio disease; (b) hypochondrogenesis; (c) spondylo-epi-metaphyseal dysplasias (Strudwick type and others); (d) other forms of SED; (e) Stickler syndrome.

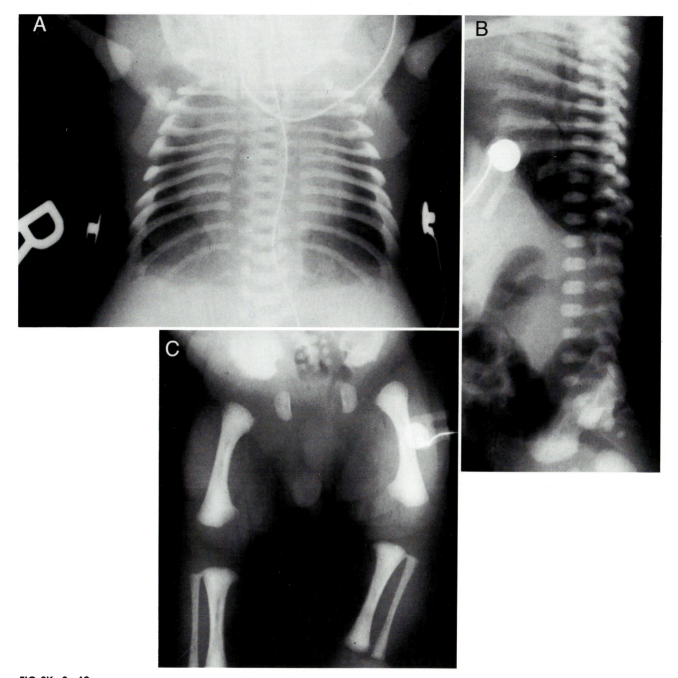

FIG SK–S–10.
Spondyloepiphyseal dysplasia (SED) congenita in a full-term newborn. **A,** short ribs, small thorax. **B,** platyspondyly; some round, ovoid vertebral bodies; short ribs. **C,** absent pubic ossification; absent epiphyseal center (at knees, etc.); no talus (or calcaneal) ossification.

Special Comments: The term *SED congenita* has been used for a variety of disorders, and may even represent a part of a family (Spranger, 1985) but should be thought of as a specific condition as it can be quite specifically diagnosed outside the newborn period and then separated from other conditions (i.e., SEMD Strudwick); this is important for genetic counseling as well as clinical management (i.e., C1-C2 dislocation). A lethal form (termed hypochondrogen-esis) is best thought of as a separate condition as there is a gradation of radiologic and clinical defects from achondro-genesis type 2 on the one end through hypochondrogenesis and into SED congenita. The chondro-osseous morphology of SED congenita is characteristic and different. Intrafamilial variability is not a problem in these disorders as a general rule.

REFERENCES

Borochowitz Z, et al.: Achondrogenesis 2-hypochondrogenesis: Variability versus heterogeneity. *Am. J. Med. Genet.* 24:273–288, 1986

Francomano CA, et al.: Type 2 collagen gene analysis in the epiphyseal dysplasias. Birth Defects meeting, Baltimore, Md, 1988.

Hamidi-Toosi S, et al.: Vitreoretinal degeneration in spondyloepiphyseal dysplasia congenita. *Arch. Ophthalmol.* 100:1104–1107, 1982.

Harrod MJE, et al.: Genetic heterogeneity in spondyloepiphyseal dysplasia congenita. *Am. J. Med. Genet.* 18:311–320, 1984.

Horten WA, et al.: Growth curves for height for spondyloepiphyseal dysplasia *Am. J. Dis. Child.* 136:316–319, 1982.

Murray T, et al.: Spondyloepiphyseal dysplasia congenita: Light and electron microscopic studies of the eye. *Arch. Ophthalmol.* 103:407–411, 1985.

Spranger J: Pattern recognition in bone dysplasias. *Prog. Clin. Biol. Res.* 200:315–342, 1985.

Spranger JW, et al.: Dysplasia spondyloepiphysaria congenita. *Helv. Paediatr. Acta* 21:598, 1966.

Spranger JW, et al.: Spondyloepiphyseal dysplasias. *Birth Defects* 10(9):19, 1974.

Spranger JW, Langer LO: Spondyloepiphyseal dysplasia congenita. *Radiology* 94:313–322, 1970.

Yagi Y, et al.: Anesthesia for patients with spondyloepiphyseal dysplasia congenita. *Masui* 36:793–796, 1987.

Yang SS, et al.: Spondyloepiphyseal dysplasia congenita. *Arch. Pathol. Lab. Med.* 104:208–211, 1980.

SPONDYLOEPIPHYSEAL DYSPLASIA TARDA

Synonym: SED tarda.

Mode of Inheritance: X-linked recessive; also autosomal dominant form; and autosomal recessive with arthropathy form.

Frequency: Common, about 85 cases of X-linked recessive form; about 16 cases of the autosomal dominant form; 33 cases of the autosomal recessive form with progressive arthropathy (to 1988).

Clinical Manifestations: Usually diagnosed in *adolescence or adult life:* (a) *short stature; in particular, short trunk;* (b) back and hip pain; (c) limitation of joint motion; (d) dorsal kyphosis, lumbar hyperlordosis; (e) short neck; (f) other reported abnormalities; congenital megaloblastic anemia and proteinuria; osteosarcoma; poikiloderma and cutaneous lymphoma.

Radiologic Manifestations: (a) *platyspondyly, hump-shaped mound of bone in central and posterior portions of superior and inferior endplates* of lumbar vertebrae with absence of ring epiphyses, platyspondyly of thoracic and cervical segments of lesser severity, *narrow disk spaces,* scoliosis, hypoplastic cone-shaped odontoid process; (b) *mild to moderate epiphyseal dysplasia,* (small, irregular epiphyses); (c)

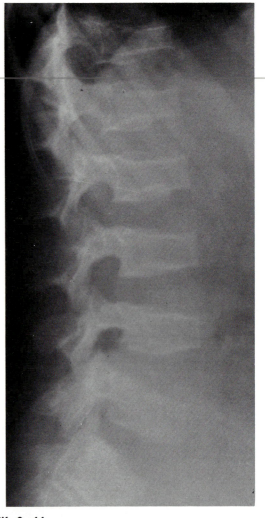

FIG SK—S—11.
Spondyloepiphyseal dysplasia (tarda) in a 13-year-old male. Platyvertebrae, hump-shaped mound of bone in central and posterior portions of superior and inferior end plates. Patient also had mild epiphyseal dysplasia.

small bony pelvis, short femoral neck, coxa vara; (d) *premature osteoarthritic changes in young adults, spondyloarthrosis* (thinning of intervertebral disk spaces, disk calcification and vacuum phenomenon) (Fig SK—S—11).

Differential Diagnosis, Significant: (a) Morquio disease; (b) multiple epiphyseal dysplasia; (c) Scheuermann disease; (d) spondyloperipheral dysplasia; (e) Wolcott-Rallison syndrome (SED with diabetes mellitus); (f) Stickler syndrome.

Special Comment: The radiological characteristics of all types of SED tarda are the same. The commonest type is *X-linked recessive;* some cases of an *autosomal dominant type* have been described (Conner; de Pino Neto; Barber); a more recently described form *with progressive arthopathy* especially common in Arab families appears to be autosomal recessive. It may be the same as *progressive pseudorheumatoid arthropathy of childhood-Spranger;* (Wynne-Davies; Kaibrara; Al-Amadi; Teebi; Miladi); another *autosomal recessive form with mental retardation* (Kohn).

REFERENCES

Al-Amadi SA, et al.: Spondyloepiphyseal dysplasia tarda with progressive arthropathy. *J. Med. Genet.* 21:193–196, 1984.

Barber KE, et al.: A family with multiple musculoskeletal abnormalities. 43:275–284, 1984.

Branford WA, et al.: Two first cousins with SED tarda (X-linked recessive form), one also with poikiloderma atrophicans vasculare progressing to lymphocytic lymphoma. *J. Med. Genet.* 19:210–213, 1982.

Conner JM, et al.: An adult female with spondyloepiphyseal dysplasia tarda. *J. Med. Genet.* 19:234–236, 1982.

Iceton, JA, Horne G: Spondyloepiphyseal dysplasia tarda. *J. Bone Joint Surg. [Br.]* 68B;616–619, 1986.

Kaibara N, et al.: Spondyloepiphyseal dysplasia tarda with progressive arthropathy. *Skeletal Radiol.* 10:13–16, 1983.

Kohn G, et al.: Spondyloepiphyseal dysplasia: A new autosomal recessive variant with mental retardation. *J. Med. Genet.* 24:366–377, 1987.

Langer LO: Spondyloepiphyseal dysplasia tarda, hereditary chondrodysplasia with characteristic vertebral configuration in the adult. *Radiology* 82:833, 1964.

Marandian MH, et al.: Coexistence d'une dysplasie spondylo-epiphysaire tardive et d'ne anemie megaloblastique congenitale avec proteinurie. *Pediatrie* 40:49–53, 1985.

Maroteaux P, et al.: La dysplasie spondyloepiphysaire tardive: Description clinique et radiologique. *Presse Med.* 65:1205, 1957.

Matsumoto T, et al.: A case of spondyloepiphyseal dysplasia tarda associated with osteosarcome. *Jpn. J. Human Genet.* 29:39–43, 1984.

Miladi M, et al.: Spondyloepiphyseal dysplasia tarda with progressive arthropathy. A report of 3 cases. *Int. Orthop.* 11:271–275, 1987.

Monteiro de Pino Neto J, et al.: Classic X-linked spondyloepiphyseal dysplasia tarda in a woman with normal karyotype. *Prog. Clin. Biol. Res.* 104:127–132, 1982.

Poker N, et al.: Spondyloepiphyseal dysplasia tarda. *Radiology* 85:474, 1965.

Teebi AS, Al-Awadi SA: SED tarda with progressive arthropathy. Letter to editor. *J. Med. Genet.* 23:188–191, 1986.

Wynne Davies R, et al.: Spondyloepiphyseal dysplasia tarda with progressive arthropathy *J. Bone Joint Surg. [Br.]* 64B:442–445, 1982.

SPONDYLO-MEGAEPIPHYSEAL-METAPHYSEAL DYSPLASIA

Synonyms: Spondylopubosternal achondrogenesis with dental-epiphyseal acceleration; SMMD.

Mode of Inheritance: Autosomal recessive.

Frequency: Very rare; approximately 8 cases to 1988.

Clinical Manifestations: *Short-trunked;* mildly short-limbed; short stature.

Radiologic Manifestations: (a) *absent* (or only anterior) *vertebral body ossification;* (b) long bones: *metaphyseal irregularities, widened epiphyseal plate; megaepiphyses;* hands: *metaphyseal cupping and irregularity;* carpal ossification retardation, large epiphyses; (c) *absent to hypoplastic pubis; intact clavicles;* vertical high ilia.

Differential Diagnosis: (a) cleidocranial dysplasia; (b) spondylometaphyseal dysplasias.

REFERENCE

Silverman FN, Reiley MA: Spondylo-megaepiphyseal-metaphyseal dysplasia: *Radiology* 156:365–371, 1985.

SPONDYLOMETAPHYSEAL DYSPLASIA (SMD) (CLASSIFICATION)

Types:

1. Kozlowski (only well-described form, most common)—AD.
2. Schmidt (Schmidt; Sutcliffe; case 1, 1965).
3. Algerian (Kozlowski, 1988)—AD.
4. Murdock (Di Stefano).
5. Richmond (Golden)—X-linked.
6. Others, less common (Felman—SEMD; Gustavson); Leone—testicular dysgenesis; Kozlowski 1979, 1982; Garcia-Castro; Lerman-Sagie—mucopolysachariduria; Ouadfel Meziane—AR; Borochowitz—AD; Sutcliffe—case 2; Hunter—interphalangeal changes).

AR-autosomal recessive; AD-autosomal dominant.

REFERENCES

Borochowitz Z, et al.: Spondylometaphyseal dysplasia: Further heterogeneity. *Skeletal Radiol.* 17:181–186, 1988.

Di Stefano A, et al.: Murdock-type spondylo-metaphyseal dysostosis. *Minerva Pediatr.* 34:303–308, 1982.

Felman AH, et al.: Spondylometaphyseal dysplasia. A variant form. *Radiology* 113:409, 1974.

Garcia-Castro JM, et al.: A new variant of spondylometaphyseal dysplasia with autosomal dominant mode of inheritance. *J. Med. Genet.* 19:104–109, 1982.

Golden WL, et al.: A new familial chondrodystrophy simulating parastremmatic dwarfism. *MCV Quarterly* 13:189–191, 1977.

Gustavson KH, et al.: Spondylometaphyseal dysplasia in two sibs of normal parents. *Padiatr. Radiol.* 7:90–96, 1978.

Hunter AGW, et al.: An unusual skeletal dysplasia with platyspondyly and marked digital metaphyseal involvement: A new entity? *Prog. Clin. Biol. Res.* 104:111–118, 1982.

Kozlowski K, et al.: Spondylo-metaphyseal dysplasia (report of a case of common type and three cases of "new varieties"). *Fortschr. Roentgenstr.* 130;222, 1979.

Kozlowski, K, et al.: Spondylometaphyseal dysplasia. *Prog. Clin. Biol. Res.* 104:89–101, 1982.

Kozlowski K, et al.: A new type of spondylometaphyseal dysplasia—Algerian type. *Pediatr. Radiol.* 18:221–226, 1988.

Lachman R, et al.: The spondylometaphyseal dysplasias. Clinical Radiologic and pathologic correlation. *Ann. Radiol.* 22:125–135, 1979.

Leone C; Metaphyseal chondrodysplasia with atypical vertebral changes in a case of anorchia. *Radiol. Med.* 65:799–805, 1979.

Lerman-Sagie T, et al.: Case report 416. *Skeletal Radiol.* 16:175–178, 1987.

Ouadfel Meziane A, et al.: Spondylometaphyseal dysplasia, autosomal recessive. *Ann. Genet.* 30:216–220, 1987.

Schmidt BJ, et al.: Metaphyseal dysostosis. *J. Pediatr.* 63:106, 1963.

Sutcliffe J: Metaphyseal dysostosis. *Ann. Radiol.* 9:215, 1965.

SPONDYLOMETAPHYSEAL DYSPLASIA, KOZLOWSKI TYPE

Synonym: SMD–Kozlowski type.

Mode of Inheritance: Autosomal dominant.

Frequency: Uncommon; underreported; about 45 cases to 1988.

Clinical Manifestations: *Abnormalities noted in early childhood:* (a) *moderate dwarfism,* most marked in trunk region, short neck; (b) scoliosis or kyphoscoliosis; (c) mildly curved (varus) limbs, short and stubby hands and feet; (d) normal craniofacial appearance; (e) *limitation of joint motion with gait disturbances.*

Radiologic Manifestations: (a) *generalized severe platyspondyly* with an increase in height of intervertebral disk spaces, *open staircase vertebral bodies, medially placed pedicles,* kyphosis or kyphoscoliosis, early osteoarthritic spine changes; (b) *widening, sclerosis, and irregularity of metaphyses of tubular bones, irregularity of physeal surface(s) of femoral epiphyseal ossification centers, coxa vara;* (c) shortness of iliac bones and flaring of iliac wings; (d) *skeletal maturation retardation especially carpals* (i.e., no carpal centers by 5 or 6 years of age); (e) hypoplasia of sphenoids and basiocciput bones (Fig SK–S–12).

Chondro-osseous Morphology: Short irregular columns, wide septae; metachromatic inclusions; electron microscopy

suggests lysosomal disorder involving proteoglycans in chondrocytes (Stanescu).

Differential Diagnosis, Significant: (a) other SMD types; (b) spondyloenchondromatosis; (c) SEMD Strudwick and others; (d) brachyolmia.

REFERENCES

Kozlowski K: Spondylo-metaphyseal dysplasia, in Kaufmann HJ (ed.): *Progress in Pediatric Radiology,* vol. 4. Basel, Karger, 1973, p. 299.

Kozlowski K, Maroteaux P, Spranger JW: La dysostose spondylo-métaphysaire. *Presse Med.* 75:2769, 1967.

Lachman R, et al.: The spondylometaphyseal dysplasias: Clinical, radiologic and pathologic correlation. *Ann. Radiol.* 22:125, 1979.

Pettersson H, et al.: Spondylometaphyseal dysplasia in a mother and her child. *Acta Radiol.* (Diagn) 20:241, 1979.

Stanescu V, et al.: Pathogenic mechanisms in osteochondrodysplasia. *J. Bone Joint Surg.* [Am.] 66A:817–835, 1984.

SPONDYLOPERIPHERAL DYSPLASIA

Mode of Inheritance: Autosomal dominant.

Frequency: Rare; 14 cases to 1988.

Clinical Manifestations: (a) short stature, normal facies; (b) back pain, small hands and feet.

Radiologic Manifestations: (a) *brachydactyly* (E—especially metacarpals and distal phalanges); (b) *mild platyspondyly;* wedging, biconcave deformity; (c) *mild epiphyseal hypoplasia* (especially hips—in young); (d) metaphyseal modeling defect tibia; severe elbow epiphyseal abnormalities (Kelly), shortened ulna.

Differential Diagnosis, Significant: (a) spondyloepiphyseal dysplasias; (b) brachydactyly E and pseudohypoparathyroidism; (c) unique skeletal dysplasia with absence of distal ulnae (Goldblatt), but no hand, foot, hip, and joint manifestations.

FIG SK–S–12.
Spondylometaphyseal dysplasia (SMD), Kozlowski type, in **A,** a father and son: truncal shortening; short neck; normal facies; in a child aged 5 years: **B,** severe scoliosis; open staircase vertebral bodies; medially placed pedicles; **C,** severe generalized platyspondyly; and **D,** severe carpal ossification delay; metaphyseal changes (cupping) of short tubular bones of the hand, radius and ulna.

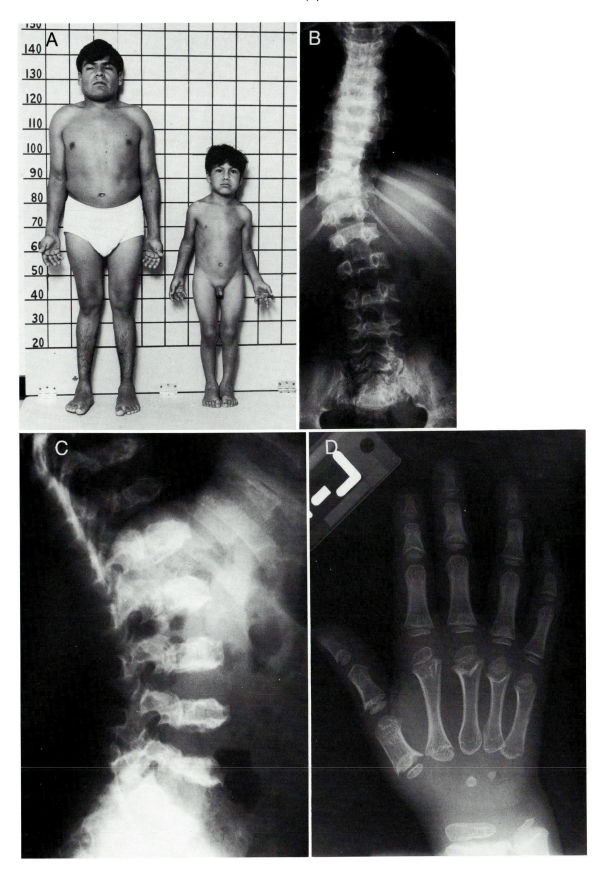

REFERENCES

Goldblatt J, et al.: Unique skeletal dysplasia with absence of the distal ulnae. *Am. J. Med. Genet.* 28:625, 1987.

Kelly TE, et al.: An unusual familial spondyloepiphyseal dysplasia spondyloperipheral dysplasia. *Birth Defects* 13;149−165, 1977.

Sybert VP, et al.: Variable expression in a dominantly inherited skeletal dysplasia with similarities to brachydactyly E and spondyloepiphyseal/spondloperipheral dysplasia. *Clin. Genet.* 15:160−166, 1979.

Vanek J: Spondyloperipheral dysplasia. *J. Med. Genet.* 20:117−121, 1983.

T

THANATOPHORIC DYSPLASIA

Synonym: TD.

Mode of Inheritance: Sporadic; probably lethal new autosomal dominant mutation.

Frequency: Very common; 1.7 per 100,000 births; by far the *most common form of lethal neonatal skeletal dysplasia.*

Clinical Manifestations: (a) *marked short-limb dwarfism;* (b) *marked curvature of limbs;* (c) *relatively large head and near normal length of trunk;* (d) *small thoracic cage,* respiratory distress, respiratory acidosis; (e) *death often soon after birth;* (212-day survivor: Tonoki; more than 14 months (Mac-Donald); respirator, tracheostomy; (f) polyhydramnios during pregnancy.

Radiologic Manifestations: (a) *small face, short and narrow skull base,* relatively large calvaria, frontal bossing *Kleeblattschadel (cloverleaf skull);* (b) *long narrow trunk, very short ribs, wide-cupped costochondral junctions, posterior rib scalloping, small abnormally formed scapulae;* (c) *severe platyspondyly, anterior rounded vertebral bodies,* anterior spike (infrequent), apparent wide disk spaces, diffuse interpediculate narrowing; *U-* or *H-shaped appearance* on AP projection; (d) *characteristic short and small iliac bones, horizontal acetabular roofs, small sacroiliac notches; medial and lateral spikes;* (e) *marked shortness and bowing of long bones of limbs,* "French telephone receiver femora," *irregularity and flaring of metaphyses;* (f) *extreme shortness, broadness, and deformity of tubular bones of hands and feet;* (g) increased subcutaneous tissues; (h) prenatal diagnosis, ultrasound (short curved femora, large or cloverleaf skull, etc.), 9 cases diagnosed in second trimester, many in third; term *intrauterine radiograph* helpful for obstetrical management (Romero) (Figs SK–T–1 and SK–T–2).

Chondro-osseous and Neuropathologic Morphology: Variable growth plate changes from almost normal areas to poorly organized regions without columns or clusters; tufts of fibrous tissue, ossifying and disrupting growth plate (Ornoy); type 1 collagen suggesting foci of membranous ossification (Horton). Abnormal sulci with polymicrogyria and neuronal heterotopia; marked hypoplasia of middle and posterior cranial fossae (Shigematsu).

Differential Diagnosis, Significant: (a) *thanatophoric variants;* (b) *homozygous achondroplasia;* (c) *achondrogenesis I and II;* (d) *asphyxiating thoracic dysplasia;* (e) *short rib-polydactyly syndromes;* (f) *new neonatal short-limbed dwarf(s): hypoplastic humeri* (McAlister).

Special Comment: Thanatophoric dysplasia (TD) with Kleeblatt-Schadel (KB) may or may not represent a separate entity, the TD with KB usually have straight femora; histology appears to be the same, only less severe, in KB cases (Langer 1986, 1987; Horten; Rimoin; *interesting perspective:* a parent's point of view (Stabosz).

REFERENCES

Horton WA, et al.: Abnormal ossification in thanatophoric dysplasia. *Bone* 9:53–61, 1988.
Langer LO: Thanatophoric dwarfism. *Radiology* 92:285, 1969.
Langer L, et al.: The relationship of thanatophoric dysplasia and Kleeblattschadel. *Proc. Greenwood Genet. Center* 5:154, 1986.
Langer LO, et al.: Thanatophoric dysplasia and cloverleaf skull. *Am. J. Med. Genet.* 3:167–179, 1987.
MacDonald IM, et al.: Prolonged survival in two cases of thanatophoric dysplasia. *Proc. Greenwood Genet. Center* 5:151–152, 1986.
Maroteaux P, et al.: Le nanisme thanatophore. *Presse Med.* 75:2519, 1967.
McAlister W, et al.: New neonatal short limb dwarfism. *Skeletal Radiol.* 13:271, 1985.
Ornoy A, et al.: The role of mesenchyme-like tissue in the pathogenesis of thanatophoric dysplasia. *Am. J. Med. Genet.* 21:613–630, 1985.
Rimoin DL: Prenatal abnormal bone growth: A perspective. *Prog. Clin. Biol. Res.* 187:131–140, 1985.
Romero R, et al.: Thanatophoric Dysplasia in Prenatal Diagnosis of Congenital Anomalies. Norwalk, Conn, Appleton and Lange, 1986, pp. 335–339.
Shigematsu H, et al.: Neuropathological and Golgi study on a case of thantophoric dysplasia. *Brain Dev.* 7:628–632, 1985.
Stabosz RD: Thanatophoric dwarfism: A parent's point of view. *Deleware Med. J.* 57:221–225, 1985.
Tonoki H: A boy with thanatophoric dysplasia surviving 212 days. *Clin. Genet.* 32:415–416, 1987.
Young RS, et al.: Thanatophoric dwarfism and cloverleaf skull ("Kleeblattschadel"). *Radiology* 106:401–406, 1973.

THANATOPHORIC VARIANTS

Synonyms: Atypical thanatophorics; platyspondylic lethal neonatal short-limbed dwarfism.

Classification: *Torrance type; San Diego type; Luton type (Middlesex type).*

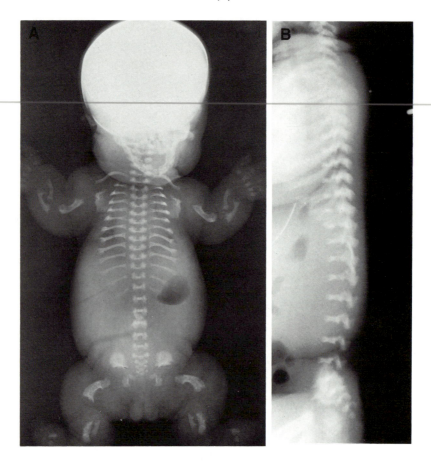

FIG SK–T–1.
Thanatophoric dysplasia in a newborn. **A,** marked short-limb dwarfism, marked flattening of vertebral bodies, short ribs with wide-cupped costochondral junctions, short and small iliac bones, horizontal acetabular roofs, marked shortness and bowing of long bones of limbs, irregularity and flaring of metaphyses, and "French telephone receiver" femora. **B,** severe platyspondyly with characteristic anteriorly rounded vertebral bodies.

Mode of Inheritance: Not known; isolated cases.

Frequency: Very rare; 6 cases (personal experience with about 6 more cases).

Clinical Manifestations: All types; *lethal;* large head; short neck; coarse facies; tiny chest; protuberant abdomen; very short arms and legs.

Radiologic Manifestations: *All types; decreased ossification of cranial base;* short thin ribs; *disk (wafer) platyspondyly;* hypoplastic ilia, ischia, pubic bones; *wide sacrosciatic notches;* flat acetabular roofs; *short relatively straight long bones (femora), sometimes widened; metaphyseal cupping (or rounding)* (Figs SK–T–3 and SK–T–4).

Chondro-osseous Morphology: *Torrance type*—hypercellular resting cartilage, large cells; normal growth plate; *San Diego type*—normal resting cartilage, large cells, poor column formation; *Luton type*—hypercellular resting cartilage, normal and large cells, normal column formation, focal degenerating chondrocyte incorporation and focal disorganization; probably a type 2 collagen abnormality.

Differential Diagnosis, Significant: (a) thanatophoric dysplasia; (b) round distal femoral epiphyseal micromelic dysplasia—Maroteaux.

Special Comment: Difficult to impossible to differentiate these three types on radiographic grounds. *Chondro-osseous morphology is specific.* They are called thanatophoric variants because clinically they look just like classic thanatophoric dysplasia but are easily diagnosed as *separate entities* by their radiologic findings.

REFERENCES

Horten WA, et al.: Further heterogeneity within lethal neonatal short-limbed dwarfism: The platyspondylic types. *J. Pediatr.* 94:736–742, 1979.

Kaibara N, et al.: Torrance type of lethal neonatal short-limbed platyspondylic dwarfism. *Skeletal Radiol.* 10:17–19, 1983.

Winter RM, Thompson EM: Lethal, neonatal, short-limbed platyspondylic dwarfism. *Hum. Genet.* 61:269–272, 1982.

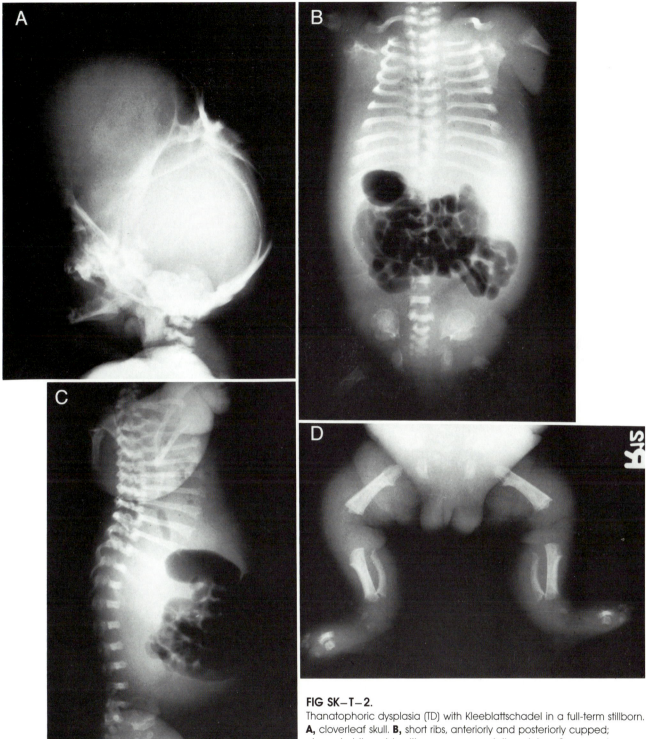

FIG SK–T–2.
Thanatophoric dysplasia (TD) with Kleeblattschadel in a full-term stillborn. **A,** cloverleaf skull. **B,** short ribs, anteriorly and posteriorly cupped; characteristic pelvis with narrow sacrosciatic notches, 3-pronged acetabulae. **C,** more mature appearing platyspondyly with rounded anterior edges. **D,** "French telephone receiver" femora without the curve; more mature appearing long bones.

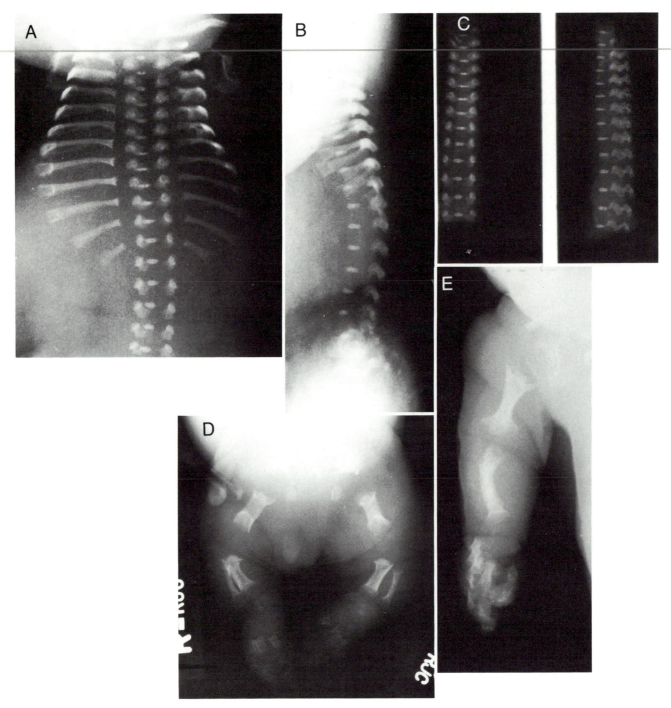

FIG SK–T–3.
Thanatophoric variant, Torrance type in a stillborn. **A,** dense platy-spondyly; short ribs. **B,** dense wafer platyspondyly. **C,** (postmortem radiographs): characteristic dense platyspondyly. **D,** micromelia, metaphyseal cupping; ischiopubic hypoplasia. **E,** upper extremity micromelia and metaphyseal cupping.

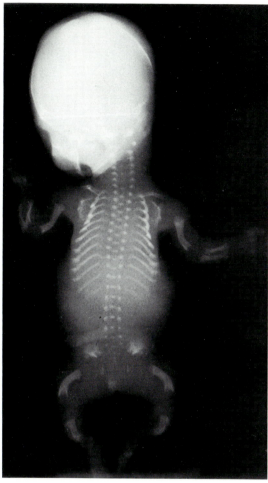

FIG SK–T–4.
Thanatophoric variant, San Diego type in a fetus of 16–19 weeks' gestation: large head, small body; micromelia; metaphyseal cupping.

TRICHO-RHINO-PHALANGEAL DYSPLASIA, TYPE I

Synonyms: Giedion syndrome; TRP type 1.

Mode of Inheritance: Autosomal dominant; chromosome 8 abnormality.

Frequency: Common; about 135 cases to 1988.

Clinical Manifestations: (a) *sparse and slowly growing scalp hair,* medially thick and laterally thin eyebrows; (b) *brachyphalangy,* thin nails; (c) peculiar, somewhat *pear-shaped or "hose" nose; thin upper lip; long philtrum; large ears;* mandibular micrognathia; *recurrent respiratory infections;* progressive hip symptoms; (d) other reported abnormalities: poor alignment and delayed eruption of teeth, mother-of-pearl-like discoloration of fingernails, renal disease, congenital heart disease, idiopathic hypoglycemia, mental retardation (unusual), seizures; winged scapula; scoliosis and lordosis; exczematoid skin rash; ulcerative colitis (Tuzovic);

(e) short stature below third percentile; (f) osteoarthrosis (adults) of hips.

Radiologc Manifestations: (a) *type 12 cone-shaped epiphyses of phalanges;* (b) ivory epiphyses; (c) *Perthes-like changes of hips* (18 cases); degenerative hip changes in adults; (d) *brachymetacarpalism,* brachymetatarsalism; *specific pattern profile;* (e) other reported abnormalities: flattened distal femoral epiphyses; midface hypoplasia; micrognathia; kyphoscoliosis; delayed bone age; radial head hypoplasia-dislocation; acetabular roof hypoplasia; pes planus; absense of patellae (Fig SK–T–5).

Hair Electron-Microscopic Morphology: Extremely reduced hair shaft diameter, dimples and surface pattern abnormalities, abnormal cuticle cells, and spacing exposing cortex.

Differential Diagnosis, Significant: (a) TRP type 2 (Langer-Gideon); (b) Ruvalcaba syndrome; (c) peripheral dysostosis; (d) the conorenal syndromes and other cone-shaped epiphyses syndromes.

Special Comments: The *Ruvalcaba syndrome* has many features of TRP type 1; differences include hair abnormalities, and Perthes-like changes in TRP; with somewhat different face and nose and bulbous epiphyses and narrow diaphyses in Ruvalcaba syndrome; a single case of TRP type 1 with female phenotype and X chromosome analysis has been reported (Resentini 1986); a case of deletion of 1q21 to 1q25 clinically has some features of TRP type 1 (Schinzel); distinguishing features from TRP type 2 (Langer-Gideon) include *lack of:* microcephaly; *mental retardation; multiple exostoses;* redundant loose skin, lax joints; skin nevi.

REFERENCES

Balza OR, et al.: Neurological changes in TRP type 1. *An. Esp. Pediatr.* 22:143–148, 1985.
Beals RK: Tricho-rhino-phalangeal dysplasia. *J. Bone Joint Surg. [Am.]* 55A:821, 1973.
Bennett CG, et al.: Facial and oral findings in TRPS 1. *Pediatr. Dent.* 3:348–352, 1984.
Cope R, et al.: The trichorhinophalangeal dysplasia syndrome. *J. Pediatr. Orthop.* 6:133–138, 1986.
Felman AH, et al.: The trichorhinophalangeal syndrome: Study of 16 patients in one family. *Am. J. Roentgenol.* 129:631, 1977.
Ferrández A, et al.: The trichorhinophalangeal syndrome, report of 4 familial cases belonging to 4 generations. *Helv. Paediatr. Acta* 35:559, 1980.
Fryns JP, Van den Berghe H: 8q24-12 Interstitial deletion in trichorhinophalangeal syndrome type 1. *Hum. Genet.* 74:188–189, 1986.
Gaarsted C, et al.: A Danish kindred with tricho-rhino-phalangeal syndrome type 1. *Eur. J. Pediatr.* 139:84–87, 1982.
Giedion A: Das tricho-rhino-phalangeale syndrome. *Helv. Paediatr. Acta* 21:475, 1966.
Goodman RM, et al.: New observations in the trichorhino-

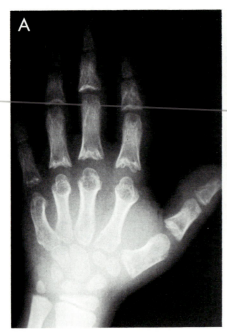

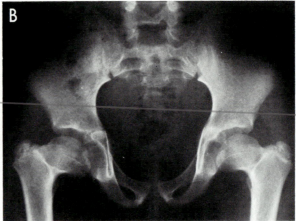

FIG SK−T−5.
Trichorhinophalangeal dysplasia type 1, in a 9-year-old girl. **A,** cone-shaped epiphyses, premature fusion of epiphyses and short metacarpals and phalanges. **B,** bilateral coxa vara, coxa plana, and premature closure of growth plates.

phalangeal syndrome. *J. Craniofac. Genet. Dev. Biol.* 1:15−29, 1981.

Jorgenson RJ, et al.: Heterogeneity in the trichorhinophalangeal syndromes. *Birth Defects* 19:167−179, 1983.

King GJ, et al.: A cephalometric study of the craniofacial skeleton in trichorhinophalangeal syndrome. *Am. J. Orthod.* 75:70, 1979.

Klingmüller G: Ueber eigenteumliche Konstitutionsanomalien der zwei Schwestern und ihre Beziehungen zu neueren entwicklungspathologischen befunden. *Hautarzt* 7:105−113, 1956.

Kozlowski K, et al.: Tricho-rhino-phalangeal syndrome. *Australas. Radiol.* 16:411, 1972.

Noltorp S, et al.: TRP type 1: Symptoms and signs, radiology and genetics. *Ann. Rheum Dis.* 45:31−36, 1986.

Parizel PM, et al.: The tricho-rhino-phalangeal syndrome revisited. *Eur. J. Radiol.* 7:154−156, 1987.

Preus EP, et al.: Clinical and scanning electron microscopic findings in a solitary case of trichorhino-phalangeal syndrome type 1. *Acta Derm. Venereol.* 64:249−253, 1984.

Resentini M, et al.: Gideon syndrome with a 46XY karyotype in a female subject. *Pathologica* 78:657−660, 1986.

Sanchez JM, et al.: Complex translocation in a boy with trichorhinophalangeal syndrome. *J. Med. Genet.* 22:314−318, 1985.

Say B, et al.: Pattern profile analysis of the hand in trichorhinophalangeal syndrome. *Pediatrics* 59:123, 1977.

Schinzel A, et al.: Interstitial deletion of long arm of chromosome 1, del (1) (q21−q25) in a profoundly retarded 8-year-old girl with multiple anomalies. *Clin. Genet.* 18:305, 1980.

Schlesinger AE, Poznanski AK: Flattening of the distal femoral epiphyses in the trichorhinophalangeal syndrome. *Pediatr. Radiol.* 16:498−500, 1986.

Tuzovic S, et al.: Das trichorhinophalangeal syndrome. *Rontgenblatter* 35:391−397, 1982.

TRICHO-RHINO-PHALANGEAL DYSPLASIA, TYPE 2 (LANGER-GIEDION)

Synonyms: Alè-Calò syndrome; multiple exostoses-mental retardation syndrome (MEMR syndrome); acrodysplasia with exostoses (Giedion-Langer); Giedon-Langer syndrome; TRP type 2.

Mode of Inheritance: Sporadic; many but not all cases have deletion of the long arm of chromosome 8 (22 cases); one familial case described.

Frequency: Uncommon; approximately 41 cases reported.

Clinical Manifestations: (a) *characteristic facies with pear-shaped or bulbous nose, prominent ears,* prominent elongated philtrum, thin upper lip; (b) *sparse scalp hair;* (c) *microcephaly;* (d) *short stature;* (e) *mental retardation* (very common); (f) other reported abnormalities: micrognathia, exotropia, winged scapula, joint laxity, loose skin, skin nevi, absent or delayed speech, frequent respiratory infections, hearing loss, delayed pubertal development, syndactyly, polydactyly, limb hypoplasia, clinobrachydactyly, cryptorchidism, coloboma, deep voice, umbilical hernia (Naselli).

Radiologic Manifestations: (a) *type 12 cone-shaped epiphyses of phalanges;* shortened metacarpals; (b) *multiple cartilaginous exostoses;* (c) *Perthes-like femoral head changes;* (d) other radiologic manifestations: cerebral atrophy (CT); multiple fractures (Fig SK−T−6).

Differential Diagnosis, Significant: (a) TRP type 1; (b) Ruvalcaba syndrome; (c) hereditary multiple exostoses; (d)

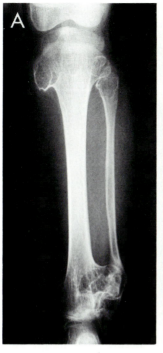
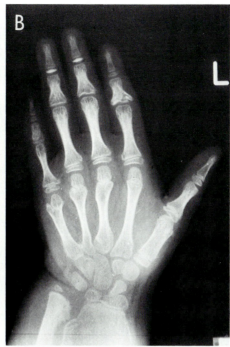

FIG SK–T–6.
Trichorhinophalangeal dysplasia, type 2 (Langer-Giedion) in a 12-year-old girl. **A,** multiple exostoses of tibia and fibula. **B,** cone-shaped epiphyses of middle phalanges of left hand. (From Mura-

syndrome of exostoses, anetodermia, brachydactyly (Mollica).

Special Comments: Distinguishing features from TRP type 1 include: microcephaly; *mental retardation; multiple exostoses;* redundant loose skin, lax joints; skin nevi.

REFERENCES

Alè G, Calò S: Su di un caso di disostosi periferica associata con esostosi osteogeniche multiple ed iposomia disuniforme e disarmonica. *Ann. Radiol.* [Diagn] 34:376, 1961.

Bühler EM, et al.: Chromosome deletion and multiple cartilaginous exostoses. *Eur. J. Pediatr.* 133:163, 1980.

Fryns JP, et al.: Langer-Giedion syndrome and deletion of the long arm of chromosome 8. *Hum. Genet.* 58:231, 1981.

Giedion A: Die periphere Dysostose (PD)-ein Sammelbegriff. *Fortschr. Roentgenstr.* 110:507, 1969.

Giedion A, et al.: The widened spectrum of multiple cartilaginous exostosis (MCE). *Pediatr. Radiol.* 3:93, 1975.

Langer LO: The thoracic-pelvic-phalangeal dystrophy. *Birth Defects* 4(4):55, 1969.

Mirovsky Y, et al.: Multiple exostoses-mental retardation syndrome. *Clin. Orthop.* 185:72–76, 1984.

Mollica F, et al.: New syndrome: Exostoses, anetodermia, brachydactyly. *Am. J. Med. Genet.* 19:665, 1984.

Murachi S, et al.: Familial tricho-rhino-phalangeal syndrome type II. *Clin. Genet.* 19:149, 1981.

Naselli A, et al.: La sindrome tricorinofalagea con esostosi. *Minerva Pediatr.* 39:25–31, 1987.

chi S, Nogami H, Oki T, et al.: Familial tricho-rhino-phalangeal syndrome type II. *Clin. Genet.* 19:149, 1981. Reproduced with permission.)

Okuno T, et al.: Langer-Giedeon syndrome with del. 8(q24.13-q24.22). *Clin. Genet.* 32:40–45, 1987.

Rogers RC, et al.: Tricho-rhino-phalangeal syndrome with exostoses (Langer-Giedion syndrome). *Proc. Greenwood Genet. Center* 6:44–47, 1987.

Stolzfus E, et al.: Langer-Giedion syndrome: Type II tricho-rhino-phalangeal dysplasia. *J. Pediatr.* 91:277, 1977.

Turlean C, et al.: Langer-Giedion syndrome with and without del. 8q (q24.13-q24.22). *Hum. Genet.* 62:183–187, 1982.

Zaletaev DV et al.: Langer-Giedion syndrome and a deletion in the long arm of chromosome 8. *Genetika* 13:907–912, 1987.

TUBULAR STENOSIS DYSPLASIA (KENNY-CAFFEY)

Synonyms: Kenny syndrome; diaphyseal tubular stenosis; dwarfism and congenital medullary stenosis; Kenny-Caffey syndrome.

Mode of Inheritance: Autosomal dominant (or X-linked).

Frequency: Rare; 21 cases to 1988 (12 cases in 5 families).

Clinical Manifestations: (a) prenatal growth retardation; low birth weight; *proportionate short stature* (18/20); (b) delayed anterior fontanelle closure; *hyperopia or myopia; microphthalmia;* macrocephaly; (c) *symptomatic hypocalcemia;* anemia; (d) normal intelligence (11/13); (e) other reported ab-

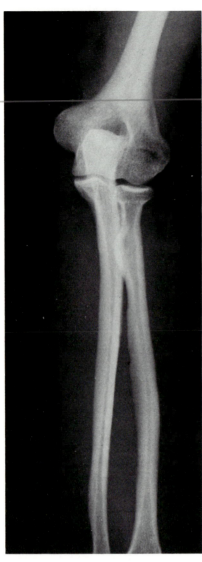

normalities: prominent metopic suture; papilledema; tetany; idiopathic hypoparathyroidism (Fanconi).

Radiologic Manifestations: (a) *lack of differentiation of calvaria into diploic space and inner and outer tables* or thin calvarial tables; (b) *symmetric internal thickening of cortex and narrowing of medullary cavity of tubular bones*; (c) delayed bone age (Fig SK–T–7).

Differential Diagnosis, Significant: (a) hypocalcemic states; (b) hypoparathyroidism including pseudohypoparathyroidism; (c) diaphyseal medullary stenosis with bone malignancy–Hardcastle.

REFERENCES

Caffey J: Congenital stenosis of medullary spaces in tubular bones and calvaria in two proportionate dwarfs—mother and son; coupled with transitory hypocalcemic tetany. *Am. J. Roentgenol.* 100:1, 1967.

Fanconi S, et al.: Kenny syndrome. *J. Pediatr.* 109:469–475, 1986.

Frech RS, et al.: Medullary stenosis of the tubular bones associated with hypocalcemic convulsions and short stature. *Radiology* 91:457, 1968.

Kenny FM, Linarelli L: Dwarfism and cortical thickening of tubular bones: Transient hypocalcemia in a mother and son. *Am. J. Dis. Child.* 111:201, 1966.

Larsen JL, et al.: Unusual cause of short stature. *Am. J. Med.* 78:1025–1032, 1985.

Lee WK, et al.: The Kenny-Caffey syndrome. *Am. J. Med. Genet.* 14:773–782, 1983.

Majewski F, et al.: The Kenny syndrome, a rare type of growth deficiency with tubular stenosis, transient hypoparathyroidism and anomalies of the refraction. *Eur. J. Pediatr.* 136:21–30, 1981.

Sarria A, et al.: Estonosis tubular diafisaria (sindrome de Kenny-Caffey), Presentacion de cuatro observaciones. *An. Esp. Pediatr.* 13:373, 1980.

Wilson MG, et al.: Dwarfism and congenital medullary stenosis (Kenny syndrome). *Birth Defects* 10(12):128–132, 1974.

FIG SK–T–7.
Tubular stenosis (Kenny-Caffey) dysplasia. Medullary stenosis limited to more central segments of shafts in 41-year-old female. (From Caffey J: Congenital stenosis of medullary spaces in tubular bones and calvaria in two proportionate dwarfs—mother and son; coupled with transitory hypocalcemic tetany. *Am. J. Roentgenol.* 100:1, 1967. Reproduced with permission.)

WEISSENBACHER-ZWEYMULLER PHENOTYPE (SYNDROME)

Frequency: Rare.

Clinical Manifestations: (a) *micrognathia*; (b) *rhizomelic shortening* of limbs in infancy.

Radiologic Manifestations: (a) *dumbbell widening of metaphyses* of long bones, in particular femora and humeri, prominent trochanters; (b) *bulbous deformity of ischial and pubic bones, broad iliac wings*; (c) *vertebral coronal clefts*; (d) improvement in configuration of bones in childhood (Fig SK–W–1).

Special Comment: The original case developed into otospondylo-megaepiphyseal dysplasia (OSMED); this phenotype may be part of a continuum that includes Stickler, Marshall, OSMED, and micrognathic dwarfism.

REFERENCES

Cortina H, et al.: The Weissenbacher-Zweymüller syndrome. *Pediatr. Radiol.* 6:109, 1977.
Kelly TE, et al.: The Weissenbacher-Zweymuller syndrome. *Am. J. Med. Genet.* 11:113–119, 1982.
Scribanu N, et al.: The Weissenbacher-Zweymuller phenotype in the neonatal period. *Ophthalmol. Paediatr. Genet.* 8:159–163, 1987.
Weissenbacher G, Zweymüller E: Coincidental occurrence of Pierre Robin and fetal chondrodysplasia. *Monatsschr. Kinderheilkd.* 112:315, 1964.
Winter RM, et al.: The Weissenbacher-Zweymuller, Sticker and Marshall syndromes. *Am. J. Med. Genet.* 16:189–199, 1983.

WOLCOTT-RALLISON SYNDROME

Synonyms: Epiphyseal dysplasia with diabetes mellitus; ED–diabetes mellitus.

Mode of Inheritance: Autosomal recessive.

Frequency: Very rare; seven cases to 1988.

Clinical Manifestations: (a) *infancy-onset diabetes mellitus*; (b) *small stature and walking difficulties* (second year),

joint pain; (c) other reported abnormalities: renal insufficiency, chronic neutropenia (1 patient), seizure disorder.

Radiologic Manifestations: (a) *generalized epiphyseal ossification delay, small, fragmented epiphyses*; (b) *resorption of capital femoral epiphyses with dislocation*; (c) *generalized platyspondyly* (Fig SK–W–2).

Chondro-osseous Morphology: Nonspecific; paucity of chondrocytes, lack of columnization, poorly vascularized resorptions zones—like in MED; dilated rough endoplasmic reticulum on electron microscopy; thick collagen fibers.

Differential Diagnosis, Significant: (a) SED, other types; (b) Morquio disease; (c) Dyggve-Melchior-Clausen syndrome; (d) *MED, juvenile cataracts, insulin resistance, and early ma-*

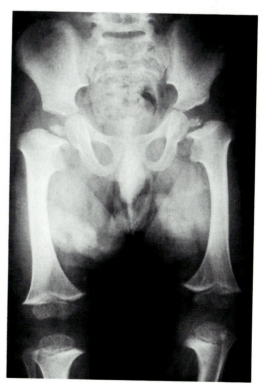

FIG SK–W–1.
Weissenbacher-Zweymüller phenotype in a 2-year-old male. Widening of metaphyses, in particular in femoral neck region. (From Cortina H, Aparici R, Beltran J, et al.: The Weissenbacher-Zweymüller syndrome. *Pediatr. Radiol.* 6:109, 1977. Reproduced with permission.)

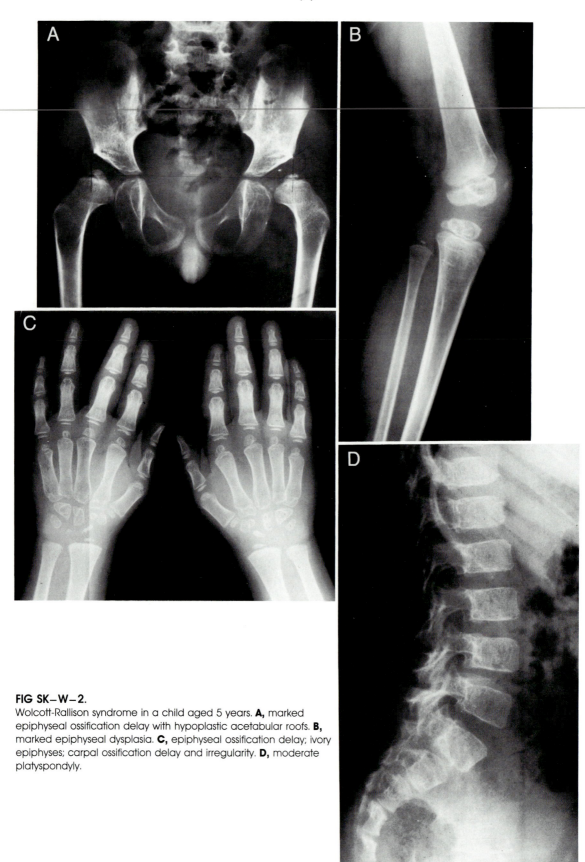

FIG SK—W—2.
Wolcott-Rallison syndrome in a child aged 5 years. **A,** marked
epiphyseal ossification delay with hypoplastic acetabular roofs. **B,**
marked epiphyseal dysplasia. **C,** epiphyseal ossification delay; ivory
epiphyses; carpal ossification delay and irregularity. **D,** moderate
platyspondyly.

lignancy (hepatocellular carcinoma, breast carcinoma (Streeten).

REFERENCES

Stoss H, et al.: Wolcott-Rallison syndrome: Diabetes mellitus and spondyloepiphyseal dysplasia. *Eur. J. Pediatr.* 138:120–129, 1982.

Streeten EA, et al.: Poster—Birth Defect Meeting. Baltimore, Md, 1988.

Wolcott CD, Rallison ML: Infancy-onset diabetes mellitus and multiple epiphyseal dysplasia. *J. Pediatr.* 80:292, 1972.

YUNIS-VARÓN SYNDROME

Synonym: Cleidocranial dysostosis with micrognathism, bilateral absence of thumbs and first metatarsal with distal aphalangia.

Mode of Inheritance: Autosomal recessive.

Frequency: Very rare (7 patients in 4 families).

Clinical Manifestations: (a) dolichocephalic skull; wide fontanelles; facial hypoplasia, micrognathia; narrow arched palate; low-set malformed ears; (b) *clavicular agenesis;* (c) *absent thumbs; distal aphalangia;* (d) *sparse peach fuzz hair;* (e) progressive growth retardation or death in infancy; (f) cardiomyopathy (arrhythmia).

Radiologic Manifestations: (a) separated sutures; *hypoplastic facial bones; micrognathia;* (b) *hypoplasia or agenesis of clavicles,* thin clavicles; (c) iliac hypoplasia; (d) *agenesis of thumbs;* distal aphalangia of hands and feet; other phalangeal hypoplasia; hypoplasia-agenesis of phalanges of first toe; *hypoplasia of first metatarsal;* (e) cardiomegaly.

Differential Diagnosis, Significant: Cleidocranial dysplasia.

REFERENCES

Hughes HE, Partington MW: Brief clinical report: The syndrome of Yunis and Varon—Report of a further case. *Am. J. Med. Genet.* 14:539–544, 1983.

Partington MW: Cardiomyopathy added to the Yunis-Varon syndrome. *Proc. Greenwood Genet. Center* 7:224–225, 1988.

Yunis, E. and Varon, H.: Cleidocranial dysostosis, severe micrognathism, bilateral absense of thumbs and first metacarpal bone and distal aphalangia. *Am. J. Dis. Child.* 134:649-653, 1980.

SELECTED REFERENCES

Felson B, Reeder MM: *Gamuts in Radiology.* Cincinnati, Audiovisual Radiology of Cincinnati, Inc, 1987.

Jones KL: *Smith's Recognizable Patterns of Human Malformation.* Philadelphia, WB Saunders, 1988.

Kozlowski K, Beighton P: *Gamut Index of Skeletal Dysplasias: An Aid to Radiodiagnosis.* Berlin, Springer-Verlag, 1984.

McKusick VA: *Mendelian Inheritance in Man,* ed 8. Baltimore, The Johns Hopkins University Press, 1988.

Poznanski AK: *The Hand in Radiologic Diagnosis With Gamuts and Pattern Profiles,* Philadelphia. WB Saunders, 1984.

Appendix A

List of Subjects in Gamuts

Gamuts

ABDOMEN

Ascites
Alpha-1-antitrypsin deficiency
Budd-Chiari syndrome
Chromosome XO syndrome
Fetal cytomegalovirus infection
Fetal toxoplasmosis infection
Galactosialidosis
Gaucher disease
GM$_1$ gangliosidosis
Hepatic fibrosis–renal cystic disease
Hypothyroidism
Mediterranean fever
Meigs syndrome
Ménétrier disease
Nephrotic syndrome
Ovarian hyperstimulation syndrome
Pancreatic disease, subcutaneous fat necrosis, and polyserositis
Pancreatitis, hereditary
POEMS syndrome
Tyrosinosis, type I
Vitamin A intoxication
Wilson disease

Diaphragmatic hernia
Chromosome 9p− syndrome
Chromosome 13 trisomy syndrome
Chromosome 18 trisomy syndrome
de Lange syndrome
DiGeorge syndrome
Ehlers-Danlos syndrome
Fetal hydantoin syndrome
Fryns syndrome
Marfan syndrome

Hepatomegaly
Aase syndrome
Alagille syndrome
Alpha1-antitrypsin deficiency
Amyloidosis
Beckwith-Wiedemann syndrome
Budd-Chiari syndrome
Chédiak-Higashi syndrome
Cholesterol ester storage disease
Chronic granulomatous disease of childhood
Cystic fibrosis
Cystinosis
Diabetes mellitus (infants born to diabetic mothers)
Ethanolaminosis
Farber syndrome
Felty syndrome
Fetal cytomegalovirus infection
Fetal herpes simplex infection
Fetal rubella syndrome
Galactosemia
Galactosialidosis
Gaucher disease
Geleophysic dysplasia
Geophagia-dwarfism-hypogonadism syndrome
Glycogenosis, type I
Glycogenosis, type III
GM$_1$ gangliosidosis
Hepatic fibrosis–renal cystic disease
Histiocytosis X
Homocystinuria

Hyperlipoproteinemia
Infantile multisystem inflammatory disease
Iron deficiency anemia
Juvenile xanthogranuloma
Kasabach-Merritt syndrome
Lipoatrophic diabetes
Mauriac syndrome
Moore-Federman syndrome
Mucolipidosis II
Mucopolysaccharidosis I-H/S
Mucopolysaccharidosis I-H
Mucopolysaccharidosis II
Mucopolysaccharidosis III
Mucopolysaccharidosis VI
Mulibrey nanism
Nephrogenic hepatic dysfunction syndrome
Niemann-Pick disease
Osteopetrosis
POEMS syndrome
Polycystic disease
Pyruvate kinase deficiency
Reye syndrome
Sarcoidosis
Sea-blue histiocyte syndrome
Sickle cell anemia
Thalassemia
Tyrosinosis, type I
Vaquez-Osler syndrome
Waldenström syndrome
Weber-Christian syndrome
Wilson disease
Wolman disease
Zellweger syndrome

Hernia
Aarskog syndrome
Achondrogenesis, type I
Acrocephalopolysyndactyly, Carpenter type
Acrocephalopolysyndactyly, Sakati type
Amniotic band syndrome
Aniridia-Wilms tumor association
Beckwith-Wiedemann syndrome
Cantrell syndrome
CHARGE association
Chondrodysplasia punctata
Chromosomal abnormalities
Coffin-Lowry syndrome
Coffin-Siris syndrome
Cutis laxa
de Lange syndrome
Diastrophic dysplasia
Ehlers-Danlos syndrome
Femoral-facial syndrome
Fetal alcohol syndrome
Fetal hydantoin syndrome
Fetal trimethadione syndrome
Fetal valproate syndrome
Fibrochondrogenesis
Fibrodysplasia ossificans progressiva
Freeman-Sheldon syndrome
Gastrocutaneous syndrome
Gerodermia osteodysplastica hereditaria
Goltz syndrome
Hajdu-Cheney syndrome

Homocystinuria
Hypothyroidism
Marshall-Smith syndrome
Meckel syndrome
Mucolipidosis II
Mucopolysaccharidosis I-H
Mucopolysaccharidosis II
Mucopolysaccharidosis VI
Myotonic dystrophy
Opitz syndrome
Osteogenesis imperfecta
Persistent Müllerian duct syndrome
Pterygium syndrome (popliteal)
Pterygium syndrome
Rieger syndrome
Robinow syndrome
Ruvalcaba syndrome
Sandifer syndrome
Shprintzen-Goldberg syndrome
Smith-Lemli-Opitz syndrome
Splenogonadal fusion-limb deformity
Testicular feminization
Tricho-rhino-phalangeal syndrome, type 2
Weaver syndrome
Williams syndrome

Liver, calcification[235]
Abscess
Cholelithiasis
Chronic granulomatous disease of childhood
Fetal herpes simplex infection
Fetal toxoplasmosis infection
Fetal varicella infection
Hemangioma
Ischemic hepatic necrosis (neonate)
Neoplasms
Visceral larva migrans

Liver, cirrhosis
Alpha$_1$-antitrypsin deficiency
Caroli syndrome
Cruveilhier-Baumgarten syndrome
Cystic fibrosis
Galactosemia
Glycogenosis, type III
Glycogenosis, type IV
Hemochromatosis
Hemophilia
Hypothyroidism (adult)
Lipodystrophy (lipodystrophic diabetes)
Odontomas-esophageal stenosis-liver cirrhosis syndrome
Sarcoidosis
Sea-blue histiocyte syndrome
Thalassemia
Tyrosinosis, type I
Weber-Christian syndrome
Wilson disease

Liver, fatty infiltration
Cushing syndrome
Cystic fibrosis
Diabetes mellitus
Fructose intolerance
Glycogenosis, type I
Hyperalimentation
Hyperlipemia, familial

Kwashiorkor
Lipodystrophy
Lipoproteinemia
Malnutrition
Reye syndrome
Steroid therapy

Liver, fibrosis
Acrodysplasia with retinitis pigmentosa and nephropathy (Saldino-Mainzer)
Asphyxiating thoracic dysplasia
Caroli syndrome
Fetal alcohol syndrome
Hemochromatosis
Hepatic fibrosis-renal cystic disease
Meckel syndrome
Mucopolysaccharidosis I-H
Rendu-Osler-Weber syndrome

Splenomegaly
Aase syndrome
Alpha$_1$-antitrypsin deficiency
Amyloidosis
Banti syndrome
Chédiak-Higashi syndrome
Cholesterol ester storage disease
Chronic granulomatous disease of childhood
Cogan syndrome
Cruveilhier-Baumgarten syndrome
Cystinosis
Diabetes mellitus (infant born to diabetic mother)
Dysgammaglobulinemia
Ethanolaminosis
Farber syndrome
Felty syndrome
Fetal cytomegalovirus infection
Fetal herpes simplex infection
Galactosialidosis
Gaucher disease
Geophagia-dwarfism-hypogonadism syndrome
Glycogenosis, type I
Glycogenosis, type III
GM$_1$ gangliosidosis
Hemochromatosis
Hepatic fibrosis-renal cystic disease
Histiocytosis X
Hyperlipoproteinemia
Hypersplenism syndrome
Hyperthyroidism
Infantile multisystem inflammatary disease
Iron deficiency anemia
Juvenile xanthogranuloma
Lipoatrophic diabetes
Mucolipidoses
Mucopolysaccharidoses
Niemann-Pick disease
Osteopetrosis
POEMS syndrome
Pyruvate kinase deficiency
Sarcoidosis
Sea-blue histiocyte syndrome
Vaquez-Osler syndrome
Waldenström syndrome
Wilson disease

ALIMENTARY SYSTEM

Achalasia, esophagus
Achalasia-adrenal-alacrima syndrome
Achalasia-deafness-vitiligo[208]
Amyloidosis
Familial achalasia
Scleroderma

Anorectal anomaly
Achondrogenesis, type I
Acrocephalosyndactyly, Apert type
Baller-Gelord syndrome
Cat-eye syndrome
Caudal dysplasia syndrome
CHARGE association
Chromosome 21 trisomy and other chromosomal abnormalities
Currarino triad
DiGeorge syndrome
Dyskeratosis congenita
Familial anorectal malformation[28]
Femoral-facial syndrome
Fetal hydantoin syndrome
FG syndrome
Fraser syndrome
G syndrome (239)
Imperforate anus—radial defects
IVIC syndrome
Jarco-Levin syndrome
Johanson-Blizzard syndrome
Kaufman-McKusick syndrome
Meckel syndrome
Mermaid syndrome
Opitz syndrome
Pallister-Hall syndrome
Persisting mesonephric duct syndrome
Polydactyly-imperforate anus—vertebral anomalies
Potter syndrome
Prune-belly syndrome
Rieger syndrome
Schinzel syndrome
Short rib—polydactyly syndrome (Saldino-Noonan)
Smith-Lemli-Opitz syndrome
Splenogonadal fusion/limb malformation
Thanatophoric dysplasia
Townes-Brocks syndrome
VATER association

Biliary tract, abnormal
Alagille syndrome
Asplenia syndrome
Bardet-Biedl syndrome
Caroli syndrome
Hepatic fibrosis-renal cystic disease
Polysplenia syndrome

Calcification, alimentary system[235]
Appendolith
Hereditary multiple bowel atresias
Hirschsprung disease
Imperforate anus
Intestinal atresia
Intestinal duplication
Intestinal stenosis
Meckel diverticulum stone
Meconium peritonitis
Mesenteric cyst
Mummified pieces of small bowel
Neoplasm
Omental cyst

Colitis
Acquired immune deficiency syndrome
Behçet syndrome
Chronic granulomatous disease of childhood
Hemolytic uremic syndrome
Hermansky-Pudlak syndrome
Kawasaki syndrome

Diverticulum, alimentary system
Cutis laxa
Diverticulosis of jejunum—macrocytic anemia—steatorrhea syndrome
Ehlers-Danlos syndrome
Groll-Hirschowitz syndrome
Jadassohn-Lewandowsky syndrome
Multiple endocrine neoplasia, type 2a
Multiple endocrine neoplasia, type 2b
Noonan syndrome
Oculogastrointestinal muscular dystrophy
Scleroderma
Williams syndrome

Esophagus, dysfunction
Amyloidosis
Behçet syndrome
Chronic granulomatous disease of childhood
Chromosome 21 trisomy syndrome
CREST syndrome
Cutis laxa
Dermatomyositis
Diabetes mellitus
Ehlers-Danlos syndrome
Ethanolaminosis
G syndrome
Hyperthyroidism
Hypothyroidism
Intestinal pseudo-obstruction (idiopathic)
Kugelberg-Welander syndrome
Mixed connective tissue disease
Myasthenia gravis
Myotonic dystrophy
Nemaline myopathy
Paraneoplastic syndrome
Riley-Day syndrome
Scleroderma

Esophagus, narrowing
Dyskeratosis congenita
Epidermolysis bullosa dystrophica
Jadassohn-Lewandowsky syndrome
Odontomas—esophageal stenosis—liver cirrhosis syndrome
Plummer-Vinson syndrome
Stevens-Johnson syndrome

Esophagus, rupture
Behçet syndrome
Boerhaave syndrome
Epidermolysis bullosa dystrophica
Mallory-Weiss syndrome

Esophagus, varices
Banti syndrome
Budd-Chiari syndrome
Cruveilhier-Baumgarten syndrome
Cystic fibrosis
Gaucher disease
Hepatic fibrosis-renal cystic disease
Superior vena cava syndrome
Wilson disease

Functional disorders (gastrointestinal)[4]
Amyloidosis
Celiac disease
Chronic granulomatous disease of childhood
Deficiency of argyrophil neurones in the myenteric plexus[233]
Deprivation dwarfism
Dermatomyositis
Diabetes mellitus
Fabry disease
Groll-Hirschowitz syndrome
Hypoparathyroidism
Hypothyroidism
Intestinal pseudo-obstruction (idiopathic)
Kugelberg-Welander syndrome
Mediterranean fever
Megacystitis-microcolon-intestinal hypoperistalsis syndrome
Multiple endocrine neoplasia syndrome, 2b
Muscular dystrophies
Oculogastrointestinal muscular dystrophy
Systemic lupus erythematosus

Gallstone
Bouvert syndrome
Caroli syndrome
Chondroectodermal dysplasia
Cystic fibrosis
Hemophilia
Hyperlipoproteinemias
Hyperparathyroidism (primary)
Immunoglobulin A deficiency[57]
Mirizzi syndrome
Paroxysmal nocturnal hemoglobulinuria
Pyruvate kinase deficiency
Sickle cell anemia
Somatostatinoma syndrome
Spherocytosis
Thalassemia
Wilson disease

Hemorrhage
Banti syndrome
Blue rubber bleb nevus syndrome
Budd-Chiari syndrome
Carcinoid syndrome
Ehlers-Danlos syndrome
Hemolytic uremic syndrome
Hemophilia
Henoch-Schönlein syndrome
Malabsorption syndrome
Mallory-Weiss syndrome
Neurofibromatosis
Peutz-Jeghers syndrome
Postcoarctectomy syndrome
Pseudoxanthoma elasticum
Rendu-Osler-Weber syndrome
Wiskott-Aldrich syndrome

Intestinal obstruction
Apple peel syndrome
Cast syndrome
Chronic granulomatous disease of childhood
Henoch-Schönlein syndrome
Intestinal atresia, familial
Meconium plug syndrome
Mediterranean fever
Neurofibromatosis
Small left colon syndrome
Splenogonadal fusion—limb deformity
Superior mesenteric artery syndrome

Intestinal pseudo-obstruction[4]
Amyloidosis
Celiac disease
Diabetes mellitus
Fetal cytomegalovirus infection
Hypokalemia
Hypoparathyroidism
Hypothyroidism
Intestinal pseudo-obstruction (idiopathic)
Kawasaki syndrome
Myotonic dystrophy
Oculogastrointestinal muscular dystrophy[114]
Porphyria
Rickets
Scleroderma
Sprue

Malabsorption
Abetalipoproteinemia
Acrodermatitis enteropathica
Addison disease
Agammaglobulinemia, X-linked
Alpha-chain disease
Amyloidosis
Anorexia nervosa
Blind loop syndrome
Carcinoid syndrome
Celiac compression syndrome
Celiac syndrome
Chronic granulomatous disease of childhood
Cronkhite-Canada syndrome
Cystic fibrosis
Dermatomyositis
Diabetes mellitus
Disaccharidosis
Diverticulosis of jejunum—macrocytic anemia—steatorrhea syndrome
Ehlers-Danlos syndrome
Henoch-Schönlein syndrome
Histiocytosis X
Hyperthyroidism
Hypoparathyroidism
Hypopituitarism
Immune disorders and lymphoid hyperplasia
Islet cell tumor
Johanson-Blizzard syndrome
Kwashiorkor syndrome
Lymphangiectasia
Malabsorption syndrome
Metaphyseal chondrodysplasia (McKusick)
Multiple endocrine neoplasia, type 2b
Nephrotic syndrome
Pancreatitis
POEMS syndrome
Postgastrectomy syndrome
Protein-losing enteropathy
Shwachman syndrome
Scleroderma
Short bowel syndrome
Sprue
Stagnant small intestine syndrome
Steatorrhea, idiopathic
WDHA syndrome
Whipple disease
Zollinger-Ellison syndrome

Malrotation, intestinal
Apple peel syndrome
Asplenia syndrome
Cantrell syndrome

Cat-eye syndrome
Chromosomal abnormalities (13, 18, 21, etc.)
Coffin-Siris syndrome
de Lange syndrome
FG syndrome
Marfan syndrome
Meckel syndrome
Mobile cecum syndrome
Osteodysplasty, Melnick-Needles
Polysplenia syndrome
Prune-belly syndrome
Thoracoabdominal wall defect syndrome
Zellweger syndrome

Meconium plug
Cystic fibrosis
Hirschsprung disease
Meconium plug syndrome
Small left colon syndrome

Megacolon
Amyloidosis
Celiac disease
Cystic fibrosis
Dermatomyositis
Diabetes mellitus
Fetal cytomegalovirus infection
Functional constipation
Hinman syndrome
Hirschsprung disease
Hypothyroidism
Metachromatic leukodystrophy
Metaphyseal chondrodysplasia (McKusick)
Multiple endocrine neoplasia, type 2b
Muscular dystrophies
Neurofibromatosis
Neurogenic megacolon
Ogilvie syndrome
Piebaldism-Waardenburg syndrome[118]
Riley-Day syndrome
Scleroderma
Sotos syndrome
Sprue

Microcolon
Apple peel syndrome
Hirschsprung disease

Inspissated milk syndrome
Intestinal atresia, familial
Meconium ileus
Small left colon syndrome

Polyps, alimentary tract
Bannayan syndrome
Behçet syndrome
Cowden syndrome
Cronkhite-Canada syndrome
Familial juvenile type polyposis coli
Familial polyposis of colon
Familial polyposis of entire gastrointestinal tract
Gardner syndrome
Generalized juvenile polyposis with pulmonary arteriovenous malformation
Peutz-Jeghers syndrome
Polyposis with exostoses
Ruvalcaba-Myhre-Smith syndrome
Tumor of neural crest origin and intestinal polyposis[249]
Turcot syndrome

Steatorrhea
Abetalipoproteinemia
Diverticulosis of jejunum–macrocytic anemia–steatorrhea syndrome
Hypoparathyroidism
Immune disorder and lymphoid hyperplasia
Intestinal pseudo-obstruction (idiopathic)
Short bowel syndrome
Somatostatinoma syndrome
Waldenström syndrome
Wolman disease

Ulcer, gastrointestinal
Cutis laxa
Degos syndrome
Gastrocutaneous syndrome
Hyperparathyroidism (primary)
Ménétrier disease
Multiple endocrine neoplasia
Paroxysmal nocturnal hemoglobinuria
Sarcoidosis
Zollinger-Ellison syndrome

BLOOD

Alkaline phosphatase, high
Axial osteomalacia
Caffey disease
Endosteal hyperostosis (van Buchem)
Fibrogenesis imperfecta ossium
Hyperostosis-hyperphosphatemia syndrome
Hyperphosphatasemia
Rickets
Sclerosteosis

Anemia
Aarskog syndrome
Aase syndrome
Aluminum intoxication
Banti syndrome
Celiac disease
Chédiak-Higashi syndrome
Congenital dyserythropoietic anemia[24]
Copper deficiency
Cronkhite-Canada syndrome

Diamond-Blackfan syndrome
Diaphyseal dysplasia-anemia[83]
Diverticulosis of jejunum–macrocytic anemia–steatorrhea syndrome
Dubowitz syndrome
Dyskeratosis congenita
Fabry syndrome
Fanconi anemia
Felty syndrome
Geophagia-dwarfism-hypogonadism syndrome
Glucagonoma syndrome
Goodpasture syndrome
Hemolytic uremic syndrome
Hemosiderosis (idiopathic pulmonary)
Histiocytosis X
Holt-Oram syndrome
Hypereosinophilia syndrome
Hyperostosis-hyperphosphatemia
Hyperthyroidism
Hypothyroidism

Hypophosphatasia
Infantile multisystem inflammatory disease
Iron-deficiency anemia
Jervell and Lange-Nielsen syndrome
Kenny-Caffey syndrome
Kwashiorkor syndrome
Lead intoxication
Lowe syndrome
Ménétrier syndrome
Metaphyseal chondrodysplasia (McKusick)
Mixed connective tissue disease
Nephronophthisis of Fanconi
Niemann-Pick disease
Osteopetrosis
Paraneoplastic syndromes
Paroxysmal nocturnal hemoglobulinuria
Peutz-Jeghers syndrome
Plummer-Vinson syndrome
Polyglandular autoimmune disease
Porphyria
Pyruvate kinase deficiency
Sea-blue histiocyte syndrome
Shwachman syndrome
Sickle cell anemia
Somatostatinoma syndrome
Spherocytosis
Stagnant small intestine syndrome
TAR syndrome
Thalassemia
Tricho-rhino-phalangeal dysplasia, type 2
Tyrosinosis, type I
Vitamin A deficiency
Vitamin B_{12} deficiency
Waldenström syndrome
Wegener granulomatosis
Weismann-Netter syndrome
Wilson disease
Wiskott-Aldrich syndrome

Hemorrhage
Afibrinogenemia (congenital)
Amyloidosis
Cogan syndrome
Hemophilia
Hermansky-Pudlack syndrome
Osteogenesis imperfecta, type I
Scurvy
Wiskott-Aldrich syndrome

Hypercalcemia
Adrenal insufficiency
Aluminum intoxication
Blue diaper syndrome
Cancer
Familial hypercalcemia[139]
Hyperparathyroidism (neonatal)
Hyperparathyroidism (primary)
Hyperthyroidism
Hypophosphatasia
Hypothyroidism
Infantile hypercalcemia[6, 159]
Liver disease, chronic
Metaphyseal chondrodysplasia (Jansen)
Milk-alkali syndrome
Multiple endocrine neoplasia, type I
Oxalosis
Paraneoplastic syndromes
Sarcoidosis
Vitamin D intoxication
Williams syndrome

Hyperphosphatemia
Acromegaly
Glomerular failure
Hyperostosis-hyperphosphatemia syndrome
Hyperparathyroidism (secondary)
Kenny-Caffey syndrome
Osteodysplasty, Melnick-Needles
Osteopetrosis
Pseudohypoparathyroidism
Transient hyperphosphatemia of infancy[177]
Tumoral calcinosis
Vitamin D intoxication

Hypocalcemia
Acidosis
DiGeorge syndrome
Hyperparathyroidism (secondary)
Hypoalbuminic states
Hypoparathyroidism
Kenny-Caffey syndrome
Malabsorption syndromes
Nephronophthisis (Fanconi)
Normal neonate
Osteopetrosis
Paraneoplastic syndromes
Pseudohypoparathyroidism
Renal tubular acidosis
Rickets
Uremia

Hypoglycemia
Beckwith-Wiedemann syndrome
Glycogenoses
Hyperinsulinism
Hypopituitarism (anterior lobe)
Islet cell dysplasia
Laron dwarfism
Neurofibromatosis
Paraneoplastic syndromes
Silver-Russell syndrome

Hypokalemia
Cystinosis
Fanconi syndrome
Kwashiorkor syndrome
Renal tubular acidosis
WDHA syndrome

Hypophosphatemia
Bone metastases
Fanconi syndrome
Hyperparathyroidism (neonatal)
Hyperparathyroidism (primary)
Increased carbohydrate metabolism
Malabsorption syndrome
Nutritional deficiency
Paraneoplastic syndromes
Pregnancy
Rickets, vitamin D-resistant

Immune disorders
Acquired immune deficiency syndrome (AIDS)
Addison-hypoparathyroidism-moniliasis[173]
Agammaglobulinemia, X-linked
Alpha-chain disease
Ataxia-telangiectasia
Beckwith-Wiedemann syndrome
Bloom syndrome
Celiac disease
Chromosome 21 trisomy syndrome
Chromosome XO syndrome
Cockayne syndrome

DiGeorge syndrome
Dubowitz syndrome
Dyskeratosis congenita
Ehlers-Danlos syndrome
Fanconi anemia
Felty syndrome
Hallermann-Streiff syndrome
Henoch-Schönlein syndrome
Histiocytosis X
Hypergammaglobulinemia E syndrome
Hyperostosis-hyperphosphatemia syndrome
Hypopituitarism (Fleischer syndrome)
Immotile cilia syndrome
Immune deficiency and dwarfism
Immune disorders and lymphoid hyperplasia
Incontinentia pigmenti
Infantile multisystem inflammatory disease
Lichtenstein syndrome
Lymphoproliferative syndrome (X-linked)
Mannosidosis
Metaphyseal chondrodysplasia (McKusick)
Myotonic dystrophy
POEMS syndrome
Polyglandular autoimmune disease
Sarcoidosis
Schwartz-Jampel syndrome
Shwachman syndrome
Sjögren syndrome
Thymic tumor syndromes
Tropical splenomegaly syndrome
Waldenström macroglobulinemia
Wiskott-Aldrich syndrome

Pancytopenia
Aase syndrome
Diamond-Blackfan syndrome
Dyskeratosis congenita
Fanconi anemia
Hypothyroidism (infants)
Pancytopenia and multiple dysmorphic features[209]
Paroxysmal nocturnal hemoglobinuria

Polycythemia
Asplenia syndrome
Beckwith-Wiedemann syndrome
Diabetes mellitus (infant born to diabetic mother)
Paraneoplastic syndromes
Pickwickian syndrome
Rendu-Osler-Weber syndrome
von Hippel-Lindau syndrome

Thrombocythemia
Caffey disease
Henoch-Schönlein syndrome
Kawasaki syndrome
Paraneoplastic syndromes

Thrombocytopenia
Banti syndrome
Chédiak-Higashi syndrome
Chromosome 13 trisomy syndrome
Chromosome 18 trisomy syndrome
Congenital thrombocytopenia with multiple malformation and neurologic dysfunction[79]
Dyskeratosis congenita
Fanconi syndrome
Fetal cytomegalovirus infection
Fetal herpes simplex infection
Fetal rubella syndrome
Hemolytic uremic syndrome
Hyperthyroidism
Kasabach-Merritt syndrome
Klippel-Trenaunay syndrome
Mixed connective tissue disease
Osteopetrosis
Roberts syndrome
Sea-blue histiocyte syndrome
Shwachman syndrome
TAR syndrome
Wiskott-Aldrich syndrome

CARDIOVASCULAR SYSTEM

ARTERIES (SYSTEMIC)

Aneurysm
Behçet syndrome
Chromosome XO syndrome
Contractural arachnodactyly
Ehlers-Danlos syndrome
Exostoses (multiple cartilaginous)
Familial intracranial aneurysm(s)
Hughes-Stovin syndrome
Hypothenar hammer syndrome
Kawasaki syndrome[25]
Maffucci syndrome
Marfan syndrome
Neurofibromatosis
Progeria
Relapsing polychondritis[29]
Rendu-Osler-Weber syndrome
Takayasu arteritis
Tuberous sclerosis

Aortic valvular disease
Alkaptonuria
Chromosome XO syndrome
Chronic granulomatous disease of childhood
Cogan syndrome
Ehlers-Danlos syndrome
Floppy valve syndrome
Hyperlipoproteinemia
Manosidosis
Marfanoid hypermobility syndrome
Marfan syndrome
Mucolipidosis III
Mucopolysaccharidoses
Osteogenesis imperfecta, types I, II, and IV
Reiter syndrome
Relapsing polychondritis
Subaortic stenosis—short stature
Supravalvular aortic stenosis, autosomal dominant[17]
Takayasu syndrome
Williams syndrome

Arteriosclerosis/atherosclerosis
Alkaptonuria
Arterial calcification of infancy
Cholesterol storage disease
Homocystinuria
Mucolipidosis II
Mucopolysaccharidoses (IH, IH/S, II, VI)
Osteogenesis imperfecta, 2
Prader-Willi syndrome

Progeria
Pseudoxanthoma elasticum
Takayasu arteritis
Werner syndrome

Arteriovenous fistula
Ehlers-Danlos syndrome
Fibrous dysplasia (polyostotic)
Pseudoxanthoma elasticum
Red-eyed shunt syndrome
Rendu-Osler-Weber syndrome

Calcification of arteries
Alkaptonuria
Arterial calcification of infancy
Burger disease
Chondrodysplasia punctata
Cushing syndrome
Degos syndrome
Diabetes mellitus
Eisenmenger syndrome
Glycogenosis, type I
Gout
Homocystinuria
Hypercalcemia, idiopathic
Hyperlipoproteinemia
Hyperparathyroidism
Hypoparathyroidism
Hypothyroidism
Leriche syndrome
Lipodystrophy (lipodystrophic diabetes)
Milk-alkali syndrome
Nephrotic syndrome
Osteogenesis imperfecta, type II
Oxalosis
Progeria
Pseudoxanthoma elasticum
Raynaud disease
Sarcoidosis
Singleton-Merten syndrome
Takayasu arteritis
Tumoral calcinosis
Vitamin D intoxication
Werner syndrome

Claudication
Popliteal artery entrapment syndrome
Pseudoxanthoma elasticum
Subclavian steal syndrome
Takayasu arteritis
Thoracic outlet syndrome
Vaquez-Osler syndrome

Coarctation of aorta
Chromosome XO syndrome
Cutis laxa
Familial coarctation of aorta–ptosis–deafness[49]
Marfan syndrome
Marfanoid hypermobility syndrome
Neurofibromatosis
Postcoarctectomy syndrome
Sturge-Weber syndrome
Tuberous sclerosis

Coronary artery, abnormality
Arterial calcification of infancy
Hyperlipoproteinemias
Hyperthyroidism
Kawasaki syndrome
Marfan syndrome
Pseudoxanthoma elasticum

Takayasu arteritis
Werner syndrome

Dilatation of arteries
Acromegaly
Chromosome X, fragile[227]
Chromosome XO syndrome
Contractural arachnodactyly
Cutis laxa
Ehlers-Danlos syndrome
Homocystinuria
Larsen syndrome
Marfan syndrome
Marfanoid hypermotility syndrome
Menkes syndrome
Neurofibromatosis
Osteogenesis imperfecta, types I, IV
Pseudoxanthoma elasticum
Rendu-Osler-Weber syndrome

Dissection of arteries
Chromosome XO syndrome
Ehlers-Danlos syndrome
Marfan syndrome
Marfanoid hypermobility syndrome

Hypertension, systemic
Adrenal hyperplasia, congenital
Aldosteronism (primary)
Alkaptonuria
Alport syndrome
Carcinoid syndrome
Chromosome XO syndrome
Degos syndrome
Fabry syndrome
Hemolytic uremic syndrome
Hyperphosphatasemia
Hyperthyroidism
Mucopolysaccharidosis, IH
Nephronophthisis (Fanconi)
Neurofibromatosis
Osteolysis with nephropathy
Paraneoplastic syndromes
Postcoarctectomy syndrome
Progeria
Pseudoxanthoma elasticum
Riley-Day syndrome
Sleep apnea syndrome
Takayasu arteritis
Tuberous sclerosis
Williams syndrome

Hypotension, systemic
Addison syndrome
Cyclical edema syndrome
Hypopituitarism (anterior lobe)
Neurofibromatosis
Riley-Day syndrome
Sheehan syndrome
Subclavian steal syndrome

Obstruction (partial or total)
Anterior tibial syndrome
Blue digit syndrome
Celiac axis compression syndrome
Chronic granulomatous disease of childhood
Cogan syndrome
Compartment syndromes
Degos syndrome
Ehlers-Danlos syndrome
Homocystinuria
Hypothenar hammer syndrome

Kawasaki syndrome
Leriche syndrome
Menkes syndrome
Moyamoya
Mucopolysaccharidosis, IH
Neurofibromatosis
Popliteal artery entrapment syndrome
Pseudoxanthoma elasticum
Quadrilateral space syndrome
Raynaud syndrome
Tuberous sclerosis

Raynaud phenomenon
CREST syndrome
Raynaud syndrome
Scleroderma

Rupture, arterial
Ehlers-Danlos syndrome
Marfan syndrome
Neurofibromatosis

Steal, arterial
Steal syndromes (vascular)
Subclavian steal syndrome

Tortuosity, elongation, arterial
Cutis laxa
Ehlers-Danlos syndrome
Menkes syndrome
Pseudoxanthoma elasticum

Vasculitides
Behçet syndrome
Buerger disease
Churg-Strauss syndrome
Cogan syndrome
Cryoglobulinemia
Henoch-Schönlein syndrome
Kawasaki syndrome
Lymphomatoid granulomatosis
Reiter syndrome
Relapsing polychondritis
Sweet syndrome
Takayasu arteritis
Wegener granulomatosis

Vasomotor symptoms
Carcinoid syndrome
Dumping syndrome
Reflex sympathetic dystrophy syndrome
Riley-Day syndrome
Thevenard syndrome

HEART

Calcification, heart[235]
Alkaptonuria
Arterial calcification of infancy
Hyperparathyroidism
Marfan syndrome
Mucopolysaccharidoses
Singleton-Merten syndrome

Cardiac failure
Abetalipoproteinemia
Addison disease
Adrenal hyperplasia, congenital
Alkaptonuria
Alport syndrome
Amyloidosis
Arterial calcification of infancy
Carcinoid syndrome
Cardiomyopathies

Carnitine deficiency
Cogan syndrome
Diabetes mellitus (infants born to diabetic mothers)
Duchenne muscular dystrophy
Fabry syndrome
Floppy valve syndrome
Geleophysic dysplasia
Glycogenosis, type II
Hamman-Rich syndrome
Hemochromatosis
Hemolytic uremic syndrome
Henoch-Schönlein syndrome
Hypereosinophilic syndrome (idiopathic)
Hyperthyroidism
Hypoparathyroidism
Hypoplastic left heart syndrome
Hypoplastic right heart syndrome
Iron deficiency anemia
Kasabach-Merritt syndrome
Kawasaki syndrome
McCune-Albright syndrome
Mucolipidosis II
Mucopolysaccharidoses
Mulibrey nanism
Myotubular myopathy
Pickwickian syndrome
Progeria
Sickle cell anemia
Takayasu arteritis
Thalassemia
Twin-to-twin transfusion syndrome
Werner syndrome

Cardiomegaly
Adrenal hyperplasia (congenital)
Alpha$_1$-antitrypsin deficiency syndrome
Amyloidosis
Arterial calcification of infancy
Beckwith-Wiedemann syndrome
Carcinoid syndrome
Cardiomyopathies
Cardiovocal syndrome
Carnitine deficiency
Diabetes mellitus (infants born to diabetic mothers)
Duchenne muscular dystrophy
Erdheim-Chester disease
Ethanolaminosis
Fabry syndrome
Floppy valve syndrome
Friedreich ataxia
Gaucher disease
Glycogenosis, type II
Hemochromatosis
Hemolytic uremic syndrome
Hypereosinophilic syndrome, idiopathic
Hyperthyroidism
Hypoparathyroidism
Hypoplastic left heart syndrome
Hypoplastic right heart syndrome
Hypothyroidism
Iron deficiency anemia
Kasabach-Merritt syndrome
Kawasaki syndrome
Kugelberg-Welander syndrome
Lutembacher syndrome
Mitral valve prolapse syndrome
Mucolipidosis II
Mucopolysaccharidosis I-H
Mucopolysaccharidosis I-H/S
Mucopolysaccharidosis I-S
Myotubular myopathy

Pickwickian syndrome
Postcardiotomy syndrome
Postmyocardial infarction syndrome
Pseudoxanthoma elasticum
Pyruvate kinase deficiency
Relapsing polychondritis
Rendu-Osler-Weber syndrome
Sarcoidosis
Scleroderma
Sialidosis
Sickle cell anemia
Singleton-Merten syndrome
Takayasu arteritis
Thalassemia
Twin-to-twin transfusion syndrome
Vaquez-Osler syndrome
Vitamin B_1 deficiency
Werner syndrome

Cardiomyopathy
Acanthocytosis-neurologic disease
African myocardiopathy
Amyloidosis
Aspartyglycosaminuria
Becker muscular dystrophy
Carnitine deficiency syndrome
Catalase deficiency-aniridia-del[11] (p15.1 p12)–cardiomyopathy[84]
Degos syndrome
Duchenne muscular dystrophy
Emery-Dreifuss muscular dystrophy
Fabry disease
Facioscapulohumeral muscular dystrophy
Farber disease
Fetal rubella syndrome
Friedreich ataxia
Fucosidosis, type I
Gaucher disease
Glycogenosis, type II
Glycogenosis, type III
GM_1 gangliosidosis
Hemochromatosis
Hemolytic uremic syndrome
Hyperphosphatasemia
Hyperthyroidism
Hypothyroidism
Idiopathic hypertrophic subaortic stenosis
Kearns-Sayre syndrome
Keshan disease[81]
Kugelberg-Welander syndrome
Leigh disease
LEOPARD syndrome
Limb-girdle muscular dystrophy
Mannosidosis type I
Mitochondrial diseases
Mucolipidosis, type II, type III
Mucopolysaccharidoses
Myotubular myopathy
Nemaline myopathy
Niemann-Pick disease
Noonan syndrome
Palmoplantar keratosis[193]
Polymyositis-dermatomyositis
Polyneuropathy of Roussy-Lévy[150]
Pseudoxanthoma elasticum
Refsum syndrome
Sarcoidosis
Scleroderma
Uremia
Vitamin B deficiency (Beriberi)
Werdnig-Hoffmann disease

Congenital heart disease
Asplenia syndrome
Cantrell syndrome
Cardioauditory syndromes
Cardiofacial syndrome (Cayler)
Cardiomelic syndrome (ulnar agenesis)[230]
Cardiovocal syndrome
CHARGE association
Chondroectodermal dysplasia
DiGeorge syndrome
Eisenmenger syndrome
Fetal rubella syndrome
Holt-Oram syndrome
Koussef syndrome
LEOPARD syndrome
Lutembacher syndrome
Noonan syndrome
Polysplenia syndrome
Scimitar syndrome
Shone syndrome
Sternal-cardiac malformation association
VATER association
Velocardiofacial syndrome (Shprintzen)
Williams syndrome

Microcardia
Addison syndrome
Adrenal hyperplasia
Kwashiorkor
Malnutrition (severe)

Mitral valve disease
Alkaptonuria
Chromosome X, fragile[227]
Contractural arachnodactyly
Cutis laxa
Ehlers-Danlos syndrome
Floppy valve syndrome
Mannosidosis
Marfan syndrome
Marfanoid hypermobility syndrome
Mitral valve insufficiency-deafness-skeletal malformations
Mitral valve prolapse syndromes
Mucolipidoses (II, III)
Mucopolysaccharidoses (IH, IH/S, II, VII)
Osteogenesis imperfecta (I, III, IV)
Pseudoxanthoma elasticum
Relapsing polychondritis
Takayasu arteritis

Myocardial infarction
Alkaptonuria
Arterial calcification of infancy
Degos syndrome
Fabry disease
Homocystinuria
Kawasaki syndrome
Mucopolysaccharidoses (IH, II, VI)
Pseudoxanthoma elasticum
Takayasu arteritis

Pericardial effusion
Amyloidosis
Anorexia nervosa
Behçet syndrome
Chromosome XO syndrome
Degos syndrome
Erdheim-Chester syndrome
Gout
Hypothyroidism
Kawasaki syndrome
Mediterranean fever

Mixed connective tissue disease
Nephrotic syndrome
Pancreatic disease, subcutaneous fat necrosis, polyserositis
Pericarditis-arthritis-camptodactyly
Polyserositis
Postcardiotomy syndrome
Postmyocardial infarction syndrome
Reiter syndrome
Sarcoidosis
Scleroderma
Stevens-Johnson syndrome
Superior vena cava syndrome
Thalassemia
Uremia
Vitamin B deficiency (beriberi)
Waldenström syndrome
Wegener granulomatosis
Wissler syndrome
Yellow nail syndrome

Valve thickening
Alkaptonuria
Aspartylglycosaminuria
Mannosidosis
Mucolipidoses (II, III)
Mucopolysaccharidoses

LYMPHATICS
Lymphangiectasia, intestinal[34]
Aplasia cutis[34]
Chromosome XO syndrome
Colonic polyps
Cystic fibrosis
DiGeorge syndrome
Hypobetalipoproteinemia
IgA deficiency
Noonan syndrome

Lymphatic abnormalities
Acquired lymphedema
Cyclical edema syndrome
G syndrome
Hereditary lymphedema syndromes
Klippel-Trenaunay syndrome
Lymphedema-hypoparathyroidism syndrome
Neurofibromatosis
Primary lymphatic dysplasia
Waldenström syndrome

PULMONARY ARTERY
Embolism, thrombosis
Behçet syndrome
Nephrotic syndrome
Vaquez-Osler syndrome

Hypertension, cor pulmonale
Alpha$_1$-antitrypsin deficiency syndrome
Crouzon syndrome
Cutis laxa
Cystic fibrosis
Ehlers-Danlos syndrome
Eisenmenger syndrome
Familial primary pulmonary hypertension[105]
Idiopathic pulmonary hemosiderosis
Marfan syndrome
Mucopolysaccharidoses (IH, IH/S, II, VI)
Osteodysplasty, Melnick-Needles
Pulmonary hypertension-cerebrovascular malformation-lymphedema[8]
Robin syndrome
Sarcoidosis

Scleroderma
Sleep apnea syndrome
Takayasu arteritis
Tuberous sclerosis

Pulmonary artery stenosis
Alagille syndrome
Carcinoid syndrome
Cardioauditory syndrome (pulmonary stenosis and deaf-mutism)
Chondrodysplasia punctata (Conradi-Hünermann)
Chromosome XO syndrome
Cutis laxa
Fetal rubella syndrome
Keutel syndrome
LEOPARD syndrome
Noonan syndrome
Pulmonary valve dysplasia syndrome
Takayasu syndrome
Williams syndrome

Pulmonary artery aneurysm
Behçet syndrome
Ehlers-Danlos syndrome
Hughes-Stovin syndrome
Marfan syndrome
Polyarteritis nodosa
Takayasu arteritis

Pulmonary artery rupture
Cutis laxa
Ehlers-Danlos syndrome (IV, VI)
Marfan syndrome

VEINS
Anomalies
Aplasia cutis congenita
Asplenia syndrome
Chromosome XO syndrome
Cruveilhier-Baumgarten syndrome
Hepatic fibrosis-renal cystic disease
Obui-Himo syndrome
Polysplenia syndrome
Scimitar syndrome
Wiedemann-Rautenstrauch syndrome
Wrinkly skin syndrome

Obstruction
Achondroplasia
Budd-Chiari syndrome
Iliocaval compression syndrome[234]
May-Thurmer syndrome
Obui-Himo syndrome
Pseudotumor cerebri
Superior vena cava syndrome
Thoracic outlet syndrome

Portal vein hypertension
Alagille syndrome
Alpha$_1$-antitrypsin deficiency
Banti syndrome
Budd-Chiari syndrome
Cholesterol ester storage disease
Cruveilhier-Baumgarten syndrome
Cystic fibrosis
Gaucher disease
Glycogenosis III
Glycogenosis IV
Hepatic fibrosis—renal cystic disease
Rendu-Osler-Weber syndrome
Tropical splenomegaly syndrome
Wilson disease

Thrombosis
Aplasia cutis congenita
Behçet syndrome
Budd-Chiari syndrome
Carpal tunnel syndrome
Diabetes mellitus (infants born to diabetic mothers)
Glucagonoma syndrome
Homocystinuria
Hughes-Stovin syndrome
Iliocaval compression syndrome[234]
Inferior vena cava syndrome[101]
Nephrotic syndrome
Paget-Schrotter syndrome
Pancreatitis, hereditary
Paraneoplastic syndromes
Paroxysmal nocturnal hemoglobulinuria

Superior vena cava syndrome
Tolsa-Hunt syndrome
Trousseau syndrome
Vaquez-Osler syndrome

Varices (peripheral)
Ehlers-Danlos syndrome
Fabry syndrome
Inferior vena cava syndrome[101]
Klippel-Trenaunay syndrome
Maffucci syndrome
Marfan syndrome
Occipital horn syndrome
Rendu-Osler-Weber syndrome
Superior vena cava syndrome

ENDOCRINE SYSTEM

ADRENAL

Adrenal calcification
Addison disease
Amyloidosis
Beckwith-Wiedemann syndrome
Cholesterol ester storage disease
Cushing syndrome
Fetal herpes simplex infection
Hemorrhage
Niemann-Pick disease
Wolman disease

Adrenal insufficiency
Achalasia-adrenal-alacrima syndrome
Addison disease
Addison-hypoparathyroidism-moniliasis[173]
Adrenal hypoplasia, congenital[254]
Adrenogenital syndrome
Adrenoleukodystrophy
Amyloidosis
Autoimmune disease
Deprivation dwarfism
Glucocorticol deficiency, familial
Hemochromatosis
Histiocytosis X
Iatrogenic: steroid withdrawal
Inflammatory diseases
Micropenis–congenital adrenal hypoplasia[30]
Neoplasms
Pituitary diseases
POEMS syndrome
Polyglandular autoimmune disease
Sheehan syndrome
Waterhouse-Friderichsen syndrome

Large adrenal gland
Addison disease
Adrenogenital syndrome
Amyloidosis
Multiple endocrine neoplasia (pheochromocytoma)
Normal (newborn)

GONADS
Hypogenitalism, hypogonadism[10, 42]
Achondrogenesis, type I
Acrocephalopolysyndactyly, Carpenter type
Acrocephalosyndactyly, Summit type
Acrodysostosis
Alstrom syndrome[42]

Bardet-Biedl syndrome
Biemond syndrome II
Bloom syndrome
Börjeson-Forssman-Lehmann syndrome
Cerebellar ataxia-hypogonadism, familial
Chromosome 21 trisomy syndrome
Chromosome XO syndrome
Chromosome XXXXY syndrome
Chromosome XXY syndrome
Cockayne syndrome
Cushing syndrome
de Lange syndrome
De Sanctis-Cacchione syndrome
Ectodermal dysplasia (hypohidrotic)
Fibrodysplasia ossificans congenita
Fröhlich syndrome
Genital anomaly with cardiomyopathy
Geophagia-dwarfism-hypogonadism syndrome
Goltz syndrome
Hallermann-Streiff syndrome
Hemochromatosis
Histiocytosis X
Hypopituitarism (anterior lobe)
Hypothyroidism
Jaffe-Campanacci syndrome
Kallmann syndrome
Laron dwarfism
Laurence-Moon syndrome
LEOPARD syndrome
Marfan syndrome
Martsolf syndrome
Mauriac syndrome
Mental retardation, male hypogonadism–skeletal anomalies
Mental retardation–growth retardation–deafness–microgenitalism
Myotonic dystrophy
Nevoid basal cell carcinoma syndrome (Gorlin)
Odontotrichomelic hypohidrotic dysplasia
Osteopetrosis
Prader-Willi syndrome
Pseudohypoparathyroidism
Reifenstein syndrome
Robinow syndrome
Rothmund-Thomson syndrome
Seckel syndrome
Thalassemia
Werner syndrome

Ovarian tumor or cyst
Cystic fibrosis
Enchondromatosis

Hypothyroidism (juvenile)
Lipodystrophy (lipoatrophic diabetes)
McCune-Albright syndrome
Meigs syndrome
Nevoid basal cell carcinoma syndrome (Gorlin)
Ovarian hyperstimulation syndrome
Peutz-Jeghers syndrome
Polycystic ovary syndrome
Polysplenia syndrome

Puberty, precocious
Adrenal enzyme deficiencies
Adrenal tumor
Constitutional
Enchondromatosis
Gonadal lesions
Hypothalamic lesions
Hypothyroidism
Idiopathic
McCune-Albright syndrome
Paraneoplastic syndromes
Shapiro syndrome
Tuberous sclerosis

PANCREAS

Diabetes mellitus
Achondroplasia
Chromosome XO syndrome
Chromosome XXY syndrome
Cystinosis
Femoral-facial syndrome
Fetal rubella syndrome
Glucagonoma syndrome
Hemochromatosis
Lipodystrophy (lipoid diabetes)
Mauriac syndrome
McCune-Albright syndrome
Myotonic dystrophy
Patterson syndrome
Polyglandular autoimmune disease
Prader-Willi syndrome
Renal-hepatic-pancreatic dysplasia
Ruvalcaba-Myhr-Smith syndrome
Somatostatinoma syndrome
Sotos syndrome
Thalassemia
Troell-Junet syndrome
Werner syndrome
Wolcott-Rallison syndrome

PARATHYROID

Hyperparathyroidism
Bartter syndrome
Cystinosis
Fibrous dysplasia (polyostotic)
McCune-Albright syndrome
Neurofibromatosis
Oxalosis

Hypoparathyroidism
Addison-hypoparathyroidism-moniliasis[173]
Endocrine-moniliasis syndrome
Hallermann-Streiff syndrome
Paraneoplastic syndromes
Polyglandular autoimmune disease
Thalassemia

PITUITARY

Diabetes insipidus
Bardet-Biedl syndrome
Histiocytosis X
Paraneoplastic syndromes

Hyperpituitarism
Acromegaly
Fibrous dysplasia (polyostotic)
Gigantism
Histiocytosis X
Prolactin-secreting pituitary adenoma

Hypopituitarism
Caudal dysplasia sequence
de Morsier syndrome
Deprivation dwarfism
Diamond-Blackfan syndrome
Diencephalic syndrome
Fanconi syndrome
Pallister-Hall syndrome
Shapiro syndrome
Thalassemia

THYROID

Goiter
Cowden syndrome
Deaf-mutism-goiter-euthyroidism syndrome
Familial multinodular goiter (autosomal dominant)[50]
Hyperthyroidism
McCune-Albright syndrome
Multinodular goiter, cystic renal lesions, and digital anomalies[56]
Multiple endocrine neoplasia, type 2b
Pendred syndrome
Troell-Junet syndrome
Weismann-Netter syndrome

Thyroid dysfunction
Alagille syndrome
Anorexia nervosa
Chromosome 21 trisomy syndrome
Chromosome XO syndrome
Cowden syndrome
Cystinosis
de Morsier syndrome
Deaf-mutism—goiter—euthyroidism syndrome
Deprivation syndrome
DiGeorge syndrome
Fetal rubella syndrome
Fibrous dysplasia (polyostotic)
Johanson-Blizzard syndrome
Kocher-Debré-Sémélaigne syndrome
McCune-Albright syndrome
Paraneoplastic syndromes
POEMS syndrome
Polyglandular autoimmune disease
Pseudohypoparathyroidism
Thalassemia
Troell-Junet syndrome
Tuberous sclerosis

GENITOURINARY SYSTEM

Ambiguous genitalia[10]
Adrenal hyperplasia, congenital (female)
Aniridia-Wilms tumor
Anorchia, familial (embryonic testicular regression)
Chromosome 13 ring syndrome
Chromosome 13q− syndrome
Johanson-Blizzard syndrome
Male pseudohermaphrotidism
Meckel syndrome
Pterygium syndrome (popliteal web)

Anorchia
Anorchia and cone-shaped epiphyses[210]
Chromosome 18q− syndrome
Familial anorchia (embryonic testicular regression)

Bladder, absent or small
Cerebro-oculo-facio-skeletal syndrome
Mermaid syndrome
Neurogenic bladder
Polycystic kidney disease (infantile)
Potter syndrome

Bladder diverticulum
Cutis laxa
Ehlers-Danlos syndrome
Fetal alcohol syndrome
Menkes syndrome
Williams syndrome

Bladder dysfunction
Caudal dysplasia syndrome
Cutis laxa
Diabetes mellitus
Ehlers-Danlos syndrome
Hinman syndrome
Hypothyroidism (adult)
Megacystis-microcolon-intestinal hypoperistalsis syndrome
Myotonic dystrophy
Neurofibromatosis
Prune-belly syndrome
Shy-Drager syndrome
Tethered conus syndrome
Urofacial syndrome

Bladder, large
Bartter syndrome
Diabetes insipidus
Diabetes mellitus
Hinman syndrome
Intestinal pseudo-obstruction (idiopathic)
Kaufman-McKusic syndrome
Megacystis-megaureter syndrome
Megacystis-microcolon-intestinal hypoperistalsis syndrome
Neurogenic bladder
Prune-belly syndrome
Psychogenic retention syndrome

Bladder wall calcification
Hypercalcemia, idiopathic
Hyperparathyroidism
Hyperuricemia
Neurogenic bladder
Oxalosis
Prune-belly syndrome
Stevens-Johnson syndrome
Urachal cyst

Calculus[191]
Abetalipoproteinemia
Alkaptonuria
Calcinosis universalis
Cushing syndrome
Cystinosis
Cystinuria
Enteric hyperoxaluria
Glycogenosis, type I
Gout
Hemophilia
Hypercalcemia
Hypercalciuria, idiopathic
Hypercortisonism
Hyperparathyroidism (primary)
Hyperthyroidism
Hyperuricosuria
Malabsorption
Medullary sponge kidney
Milk-alkali syndrome
Myeloproliferative disorders
Osteomalacia
Osteoporosis
Oxalosis
Pyridoxine deficiency
Renal tubular acidosis
Sarcoidosis
Vaquez-Osler syndrome
Vitamin D intoxication
Williams syndrome
Wilson disease
Xanthine oxidase deficiency

Clitoromegaly
Adrenal hyperplasia, congenital
Chromosome 5p− syndrome
Chromosome 18 trisomy syndrome
Fraser syndrome
Johanson-Blizzard syndrome
Roberts syndrome

Cryptorchidism[10]
Aarskog syndrome
Acrocephalopolysyndactyly, Carpenter type
Acrocephalopolysyndactyly, Sakati type
Acrocephalosyndactyly, Hermann-Opitz type
Acrocephalosyndactyly, Saethre-Chotzen type
Aniridia-Wilms tumor association
Arthrogryposis multiplex congenita
Beckwith-Wiedemann syndrome
Biedl-Bardet syndrome
Cerebro-oculo-facio-skeletal syndrome
Chromosomal abnormalities
Cockayne syndrome
de Lange syndrome
Diastrophic dysplasia
Dubowitz syndrome
Fanconi anemia
Fetal rubella syndrome
Frazer syndrome
Gordon syndrome
Hallermann-Streiff syndrome
Hypopituitarism
Kallmann syndrome
Lenz microphthalmia syndrome
LEOPARD syndrome
Lissencephaly (Miller-Dieker syndrome)
Lowe syndrome
Marfan syndrome
Meckel syndrome
Myotonic dystrophy
N syndrome

Nevoid basal-cell carcinoma syndrome (Gorlin)
Noonan syndrome
Opitz syndrome
Pena-Shokeir syndrome
Persistent Müllerian duct syndrome
Prader-Willi syndrome
Prune-belly syndrome
Pterygium syndromes
Roberts syndrome
Robinow syndrome
Rothmund-Thomson syndrome
Rubinstein-Taybi syndrome
Seckel syndrome
Senter syndrome (erythroderma-sensory deafness)[220]
Silver-Russell syndrome
Smith-Lemli-Opitz syndrome
Splenogonadal fusion-limb deformity
Testicular feminization
Treacher Collins syndrome
Urofacial syndrome (Ochoa)
Velocardiofacial syndrome
Zellweger syndrome

Genital anomalies

Aarskog syndrome
Adrenogenital syndrome
Amniotic band syndrome
Bardet-Biedl syndrome
Chondroectodermal dysplasia
Chromosome 13 trisomy syndrome
Chromosome 18 trisomy syndrome
Chromosome 21 trisomy syndrome
Chromosome 4p− syndrome
Chromosome XO syndrome
Chromosome XXXXY syndrome
Chromosome XXY syndrome
Drash syndrome
Fetal alcohol syndrome
Fetal trimethadione syndrome
Fraser syndrome
Fryns syndrome
Gardner-Silengo-Wachtel syndrome
Hand-foot-genital syndrome
Jarcho-Levin syndrome
Johanson-Blizzard syndrome
Kaufman-McKusick syndrome
LEOPARD syndrome
Mayer-Rokitansky-Küster syndrome
Nager syndrome
Noonan syndrome
Persistent Müllerian duct syndrome
Prune-belly syndrome
Pterygium syndrome, popliteal
Renal, genital, and middle ear anomalies
Roberts syndrome
Robinow syndrome
Rüdiger syndrome
Seckel syndrome
Smith-Lemli-Opitz syndrome
Splenogonadal fusion/limb deformity
Testicular feminization
Urogenital dysplasia (hereditary)
Young syndrome

Hypospadias

Aniridia-Wilms tumor association
Biemond syndrome II
Branchiogenitoskeletal syndrome
Chromosomal abnormalities
Dubowitz syndrome
Familial hypospadias

Fanconi anemia
Fetal primidone syndrome
Fraser syndrome
G syndrome
Gardner-Silengo-Wachtel syndrome
Hand-foot-genital syndrome
Lenz microphthalmia
LEOPARD syndrome
Male pseudohermaphroditism
N syndrome
Opitz syndrome
Polycystic kidney disease (infantile)
Potter syndrome
Radial hypoplasia−triphalangeal thumbs−hypospadias−maxillary
   diastema
Reifenstein syndrome
Rieger syndrome
Schinzel-Giedion syndrome
Sensorineural deafness−hypospadias−metacarpal and metatarsal
   synostoses[190]
Silver-Russell syndrome
Smith-Lemli-Opitz syndrome
Splenogonadal fusion−limb deformity
VATER association
Zellweger syndrome

Kidney, anomalies

Acro-renal-ocular syndrome[94]
Acrorenal syndrome (Dieker-Opitz)
Adrenal hyperplasia (congenital)
Aminopterin fetopathy
Anorectal malformation, hereditary
Asplenia syndrome
Baller-Gerold syndrome
Beckwith-Wiedemann syndrome
Branchio-oto-ureteral syndrome
Brancho-oto-renal dysplasia
Chromosome 13 trisomy syndrome
Chromosome 18 trisomy syndrome
Chromosome XO syndrome (Turner)
de Lange syndrome
Dietl syndrome
EEC syndrome
Fanconi anemia
Femoral-facial syndrome
Fetal alcohol syndrome
Fetal rubella syndrome
Fetal trimethadione syndrome
Fraser syndrome
Freeman-Sheldon syndrome
Fryns syndrome
Hemihypertrophy
Johanson-Blizzard syndrome
Klippel-Feil syndrome
Kousseff syndrome
Lenz microphthalmia syndrome
Limb duplication-renal agenesis
Mayer-Rokitansky-Küster syndrome
Mermaid syndrome
Noonan syndrome
Perlman syndrome[171]
Persisting mesonephric duct syndrome
Poland syndrome
Polysplenia syndrome
Potter syndrome
Radial ray aplasia-renal anomalies
Renal, genital, and middle ear anomalies
Renal-digital-ear anomalies
Roberts syndrome
TAR syndrome

Urogenital adysplasia (hereditary)
VATER association

Kidney, cyst

Acrocephalosyndactyly, Apert type
Aplasia cutis congenita
Asphyxiating thoracic dysplasia
Asplenia syndrome
Axial osteomalacia
Bardet-Biedl syndrome
Beckwith-Wiedemann syndrome
Brancho-oto-renal dysplasia
C syndrome
Chromosomal abnormalities
Cystic hamartoma of kidney and lung
Dandy-Walker syndrome
Darier disease
DiGeorge syndrome
Ehlers-Danlos syndrome
Femoral-facial syndrome
Fetal alcohol syndrome
Fetal hydantoin syndrome
Fryns syndrome
Glutaric aciduria, type II
Goldenhar syndrome
Hemihypertrophy
Hepatic fibrosis-renal cystic disease
Joubert syndrome
Kaufman-McKusick syndrome
Lissencephaly
Marden-Walker syndrome
Meckel syndrome
Medullary sponge kidney
Neophronophthisis (Fanconi)
Orofaciodigital syndrome I
Pallister-Hall syndrome
Polycystic kidney disease
Polysplenia syndrome
Potter syndrome
Prune-belly syndrome
Renal-hepatic-pancreatic dysplasia
Retinal-renal dysplasia syndrome
Roberts syndrome
Serpentine fibula-polycystic kidney syndrome[71]
Short rib-polydactyly syndrome (types 1, 2, and 3)
Smith-Lemli-Opitz syndrome
Tuberous sclerosis
VATER association
von Hippel-Lindau syndrome
Williams syndrome
Zellweger syndrome

Kidney, large[33]

Acromegaly
Amyloidosis
Bartter syndrome
Beckwith-Wiedemann syndrome
Cystic kidney disease
Diabetes insipidus
Diabetes mellitus
Gaucher disease
Glomerulonephritis, familial and hereditary
Glomerulonephritis, idiopathic
Glycogenosis, type I
Goodpasture syndrome
Hemihypertrophy
Hemolytic uremic syndrome
Hemophilia (hemorrhage)
Henoch-Schönlein syndrome
Histiocytosis X
IgA glomerulonephritis

Lipodystrophy (lipoatrophic diabetes)
Lipoid nephrosis
Lupus nephritis
Mucopolysaccharidoses
Neonatal transient nephromegaly
Nephrotic syndrome
Nephrocalcinosis
Nieman-Pick disease
POEMS syndrome
Sarcoidosis
Senior syndrome
Sickle cell disease
Steroid therapy
Tuberous sclerosis
Tyrosinemia
Uric acid nephropathy
Venous thrombosis
Wegener granulomatosis
Weinberg-Zumwalt syndrome[251]
Wolman disease

Kidney, small

Acrodysplasia with retinitis pigmentosa and nephropathy (Saldino-Mainzer)
Alport syndrome
Bardet-Biedl syndrome
Bartter syndrome
Collagen diseases
Diabetes mellitus
Fibromuscular arterial dysplasia
Glomerulonephritis, chronic
Gout
Hyperparathyroidism
Lead nephropathy
Medullary cystic disease
Nephronophthisis (Fanconi)
Tuberous sclerosis

Labia major, aplasia or hypoplasia

Chromosomal abnormalities
de Lange syndrome
Femoral-facial syndrome
Fetal alcohol syndrome
Pterygium syndromes
Robinow syndrome

Nephrocalcinosis

Alkaptonuria
Alport syndrome
Amelogenesis imperfecta—nephrocalcinosis syndrome
Aminoaciduria
Bartter syndrome
Blue diaper syndrome
Chondroectodermal dysplasia
Cushing syndrome
Ehlers-Danlos syndrome
Glycogenosis, type I
Gout
Hemolytic uremic syndrome
Hepatic fibrosis-renal cystic disease
Hypercalcemia, idiopathic
Hyperchloremic acidosis
Hyperparathyroidism
Hyperphosphatasia
Hyperthyroidism
Hyperuricemia
Hypophosphatasia
Hypothyroidism (juvenile)
Medullary sponge kidney
Milk-alkali syndrome
Nail-patella syndrome

Osteoporosis
Oxalosis
Paraneoplastic syndromes
Parenchymal necrosis
Pseudohypoparathyroidism
Renal tubular acidosis
Rickets, vitamin D resistant
Sarcoidosis
Shwachman syndrome
Sickle cell anemia
Sjögren syndrome
Vitamin D intoxication
Wilson disease
Xanthin oxidase deficiency
Zollinger-Ellison syndrome

Nephropathy

Acrodysplasia with retinitis pigmentosa and nephropathy (Saldino-Mainzer)
Alagille syndrome
Alkaptonuria
Alport syndrome
Amelogenesis imperfecta—nephrocalcinosis syndrome
Amyloidosis
Asphyxiating thoracic dysplasia
Bardet-Biedl syndrome
Bartter syndrome
Behçet syndrome
Carbonic anhydrase II deficiency
Cockayne syndrome
Cystinosis
Cystinuria
Diabetes mellitus
Drash syndrome
Fabry disease
Fanconi syndrome
Gaucher disease
Glycogenosis, type I
Glycogenosis, type V
Goodpasture syndrome
Gout
Hemolytic uremic syndrome
Hemophilia
Henoch-Schönlein syndrome
Hepatic fibrosis-renal cystic disease
Hereditary renal disease and preauricular pits[134]
Hyperparathyroidism
Juvenile megaloblastic anemia
Lesch-Nyhan syndrome
Lowe syndrome
Mediterranean fever
Milk-alkali syndrome
Nail-patella syndrome
Nephronophthisis-encephalopathy[157]
Nephronophthisis (Fanconi)
Nephrotic syndrome
Optic nerve coloboma-renal interstitial fibrosis[250]
Osteolysis with nephropathy
Oxalosis
Paraneoplastic syndromes
Pulmonary-renal syndromes
Renal tubular acidosis
Riley-Day syndrome
Senior-Loken syndrome[219]
Sickle cell disease
Tyrosinemia
Vitamin D intoxication
Waldenström syndrome
Wegener granulomatosis
Wilson disease

Wiskott-Aldrich syndrome
Zellweger syndrome

Penis, large

Adrenal hyperplasia, congenital
Cerebro-oculo-facio-skeletal syndrome
Klippel-Trenaunay-Weber syndrome
Lipoatrophic diabetes
Neurofibromatosis
Roberts syndrome

Penis, small[10]

Aarskog syndrome
Acrocephalopolysyndactyly, Sakati type
Aniridia-Wilms tumor association
Arthrogryposis multiplex congenita
Bardet-Biedl syndrome
CHARGE association
Chromosomal abnormalities
Hypopituitarism (anterior lobe)
Laron dwarfism
Micropenis-congenital adrenal hypoplasia[30]
Rudiger syndrome
Ruvalcaba syndrome
Short rib-polydactyly syndromes
Silver-Russell syndrome
Smith-Lemli-Opitz syndrome

Scrotum, bifid

Aarskog syndrome
Bardet-Biedl syndrome
Chromosome 18 ring
Chromosome XXXXY
Cranio-fronto-nasal dysplasia—like syndrome
Pterygium syndrome (popliteal)
Triploidy

Testes, small/hypoplastic[10]

Chromosome 18p− syndrome
Chromosome XXXY syndrome
Chromosome XXY syndrome
Chromosome XXYY syndrome
Chromosome XY gonadal dysgenesis
De Sanctis-Cacchione syndrome
Drash syndrome
Dyskeratosis congenita syndrome
Myotonic dystrophy
Rudimentary testes with Leydig cell deficiency[1]
Schwartz-Jampel syndrome

Testes, large

Chromosome X: fragile
Hemihypertrophy
Proteus syndrome

Uterus, bicornuate and/or vaginal duplication

Acrocephalosyndactyly, Apert type
Beckwith-Wiedemann syndrome
Chromosome 13 trisomy syndrome
Chromosome 18 trisomy syndrome
Fraser syndrome
Jarcho-Levin syndrome
Johanson-Blizzard syndrome
Mayer-Rokitansky-Küster syndrome
Roberts syndrome
Schinzel-Giedion syndrome

Vaginal anomaly

Chromosomal abnormalities
Fraser syndrome
Johanson-Blizzard syndrome
Male pseudohermaphroditism

Mayer-Rokitansky-Küster syndrome
MURCS association (Müllerian duct, renal, and cervical vertebral defects)[67]
Renal-genital-middle ear syndrome[243]
Roberts syndrome
VATER association

Vaginal atresia
Antley-Bixler syndrome
Dyskeratosis congenita syndrome

EEC syndrome
Fraser syndrome
Mayer-Rokitansky-Küster syndrome
Mermaid syndrome
MURCS association (Müllerian duct, renal, and cervical vertebral defects)[67]
Renal, genital, and ear anomalies

HEAD

EAR
Deafness (partial or total)
Acrocephalopolysyndactyly, Carpenter type
Acrocephalosyndactyly, Apert type
Acrocephalosyndactyly, Saethre-Chotzen type
Acrodysostosis
Alport syndrome
Baller-Gerold syndrome
Bardet-Biedl syndrome
Behçet syndrome
Branchio-oto-renal dysplasia syndrome
Branchio-oto-ureteral syndrome
Camptodactyly-sensorineural hearing loss syndrome
Cardioauditory syndromes
Carraro syndrome
Cerebro-costo-mandibular syndrome
Charcot-Marie-Tooth syndrome
CHARGE association
CHILD syndrome
Chromosomal abnormalities (13, XO, etc.)
Cleidocranial dysplasia
Cockayne syndrome
Craniodiaphyseal dysplasia
Craniometaphyseal dysplasia
Cruzon syndrome
de Lange syndrome
Deaf-mutism—goiter—euthyroidism syndrome
Deafness and metaphyseal dysostosis
Deafness, hypospadias, and synostosis of metacarpals and metatarsals[190]
Diaphyseal dysplasia (Engelmann)
Diastrophic dysplasia
Door syndrome
DR (Duane-radial dysplasia) syndrome
Dyskeratosis congenita syndrome
EEC syndrome
Facio-audio-symphalangism syndrome
Facio-auriculo-radial dysplasia
Fanconi anemia
Fetal cytomegalovirus infection
Fetal herpes simplex infection
Fetal rubella syndrome
Fetal trimethadione syndrome
FG syndrome
Fibrodysplasia ossificans progressiva
Flynn-Aird syndrome
Fountain syndrome
Frontometaphyseal dysplasia
Frontonasal dysplasia
Goldenhar syndrome
Goltz syndrome
Groll-Hirschowitz syndrome
Hajdu-Cheney syndrome
Hay-Wells syndrome of ectodermal dysplasia[102]
Hyperphosphatasemia

Hypopituitarism (anterior lobe)
Hypothyroidism (juvenile)
Infantile multisystem inflammatory disease
Jervell and Lange-Nielsen syndrome
Johanson-Blizzard syndrome
Kartagener syndrome
Keratoderma hereditaria mutilans
Keutel syndrome
Klein-Waardenburg syndrome
Klippel-Feil syndrome
Kniest syndrome
Lacrimo-auriculo-dento-digital syndrome
Larsen syndrome
LEOPARD syndrome
Levy-Hollister syndrome
Mannosidosis
Marshall syndrome
McCune-Albright syndrome
Mesomelic dysplasia, Nievergelt
Metaphyseal chondrodysplasia (Jansen)
Microangiopathic syndrome of encephalopathy—hearing loss—retinal arteriolar occlusion
Microtia
Mitral valve insufficiency—deafness—skeletal malformations
Mondini malformation[156]
Mucolipidosis I
Mucopolysaccharidosis I-H
Mucopolysaccharidosis II
Mucopolysaccharidosis VI
Multiple synostosis syndrome
MURCS association (Müllerian duct, renal, cervical spine)[67]
N syndrome
Nager anomaly
Naso-digito-acoustic syndrome
Noonan syndrome
Oculo-dento-osseous dysplasia
Oculo-palato-skeletal syndrome
Oro-facio-digital syndrome II (Mohr)
Osteodysplasty, Melnick-needles
Osteogenesis imperfecta, types I, IV
Osteolysis, familial expansile
Osteopetrosis
Osteopathia striata
Otodental dysplasia
Oto-spondylo-megaepiphyseal dysplasia
Oto-palato-digital syndrome I
Oto-palato-digital syndrome II
Otosclerosis in twins[64]
Pallister-Killian syndrome
Pendred syndrome
Perrault syndrome (ovarian dysgenesis—sensorineural deafness)[175]
Pigmentary-hearing loss (oculocutaneous albinism)
Postaxial acrofacial dysostosis (Miller)
Progeria
Refsum syndrome

Relapsing polychondritis
Renal, genital, and ear anomalies
Renal, genital, and middle ear anomalies
Renal tubular acidosis
Rieger syndrome
Robin sequence
Sclerosteosis
Senter syndrome[220]
Stewart-Bergstrom syndrome
Stickler syndrome
Townes-Brock syndrome
Treacher Collins syndrome
Tricho-rhino-phalangeal dysplasia, type 2
Triphalangeal thumb—onychodystrophy—deafness
Trotter syndrome
Usher syndrome
Velocardiofacial syndrome (Shprintzen)
Waardenburg syndrome
Weill-Marchesani syndrome
Wildervanck syndrome

External ear calcification

Acromegaly
Addison syndrome
Alkaptonuria
Calcium pyrophosphate dihyrate deposition disease
Cushing syndrome
Diabetes mellitus
Diastrophic dysplasia
Familial cold hypersensitivity
Gout
Hypercalcemia
Hyperparathyroidism
Hyperthyroidism
Hypoparathyroidism
Hypopituitarism (anterior lobe)
Idiopathic
Keutel syndrome
Odonto-tricho-melic hypohidrotic dysplasia
Relapsing polychondritis
Systemic chondromalacia (von Meyenberg disease)

External ear, malformation

Aarskog syndrome
Achondrogenesis, type I
Acrocephalopolysyndactyly, Sakati type
Acrocephalosyndactyly, Saethre-Chotzen type
Aminopterin-like syndrome without aminopterin
Aminopterin fetopathy
Amniotic band syndrome
Anderson syndrome
Aniridia-Wilms tumor association
Antley-Bixler syndrome
Aural atresia—mental retardation—multiple anomalies[48]
Auriculo-osteodysplasia syndrome (Beals)
Baller-Gerold syndrome
Beckwith-Wiedemann syndrome
Blepharophimosis syndrome
Bloom syndrome
Börjeson-Forssman-Lehmann syndrome
Branchio-oto-renal dysplasia
C syndrome
Campomelic dysplasia
Cat-eye syndrome
Cerebro-costo-mandibular syndrome
CHARGE association
Chromosomal abnormalities (13, 18, 21, XO, etc.)
Cleidocranial dysplasia
Coffin-Lowry syndrome
Cohen syndrome
Contractural arachnodactyly

Craniometaphyseal dysplasia
DiGeorge syndrome
Diastrophic dysplasia
Dubowitz syndrome
Dyschondrosteosis
Dyssegmental dysplasia
EEC syndrome
Ehlers-Danlos syndrome
Facio-auriculo-radial dysplasia
Fanconi anemia
Fetal alcohol syndrome
Fetal hydantoin syndrome
Fetal isotretinoin syndrome
Fetal primidone syndrome
Fetal rubella syndrome
Fetal trimethadione syndrome
FG syndrome
Fibrochondrogenesis
Fraser syndrome
Fryns syndrome
G syndrome
GM$_1$ gangliosidosis
Goldenhar syndrome
Greig cephalopolysyndactyly syndrome
Hay-Wells syndrome of ectodermal dysplasia[102]
Hydrolethalus syndrome
Hyperphosphatasia
Hypertelorism, microtia, facial clefting syndrome
Klippel-Feil syndrome
Kousseff syndrome
Lacrimo-auriculo-dento-digital syndrome
Langer-Giedion syndrome
Lenz-Majewski hyperostosis syndrome
Lenz microphthalmia syndrome
LEOPARD syndrome
Levy-Hollister syndrome
Lissencephaly syndrome
Mandibulofacial dysostosis
Marfan syndrome
Meckel syndrome
Möbius syndrome
MURCS association (Müllerian duct, renal, cervical spine defects)[67]
Nager syndrome
Neu-Laxova syndrome
Noonan syndrome
Opitz syndrome
Opsismodysplasia
Oro-facio-digital syndrome II
Osteodysplasty, Melnick-Needles
Osteogenesis imperfecta
Osteopetrosis
Oto-onycho-peroneal syndrome
Oto-palato-digital syndrome I
Pallister-Killian syndrome
Pena-Shokeir syndrome
Pallister-Hall syndrome
Postaxial acrofacial dysostosis (Miller)
Potter syndrome
Prader-Willi syndrome
Pseudodiastrophic dysplasia
Relapsing polychondritis
Renal-genital and ear anomalies
Roberts syndrome
Robinow syndrome
Rubinstein-Taybi syndrome
Schinzel-Giedion syndrome
Seckel syndrome
Short rib-polydactyly syndrome, type I
Short rib-polydactyly syndrome, type 2 (Majewski)

Shprintzen-Goldberg syndrome
Smith-Lemli-Opitz syndrome
Sturge-Weber syndrome
Thalidomide embryopathy
Townes-Brocks syndrome
Treacher Collins syndrome
Tricho-rhino-phalangeal syndrome (types 1 and 2)
VATER association
Velo-cardio-facial syndrome
Warfarin embryopathy
Wildervanck syndrome
Yunis-Varón syndrome
Zellweger syndrome
Zimmermann-Laband syndrome

Inner ear anomaly

Achondroplasia
Acrocephalosyndactyly, Apert type
Branchio-oto-renal dysplasia
Chromosome 21 trisomy
Cleidocranial dysplasia
DiGeorge syndrome
Fetal rubella syndrome
Fountain syndrome
Goldenhar syndrome
Hypertelorism, microtia, facial clefting syndrome
Klippel-Feil syndrome
Multiple synostosis syndrome
Neurofibromatosis
Osteogenesis imperfecta
Osteopetrosis
Pendred syndrome
Treacher Collins syndrome
Waardenburg syndrome
Wildervanck syndrome

Low-set ears

Acrocephalopolysyndactyly, Carpenter type
Aminopterin fetopathy
Campomelic dysplasia
Cat-eye syndrome
Chromosomal abnormalities
de Lange syndrome
DiGeorge syndrome
Fetal hydantoin syndrome
Fibrochondrogenesis
Frontonasal dysplasia sequence
Gardner-Silengo-Wachtel syndrome
German syndrome
Goldenhar syndrome
Hajdu-Cheney syndrome
Hallermann-Streiff syndrome
Joubert syndrome
Lissencephaly syndrome
Noonan syndrome
Oto-palato-digital syndrome I
Pena-Shokeir syndrome
Potter syndrome
Rubinstein-Taybi syndrome
Schinzel-Giedion syndrome
Schwartz-Jampel syndrome
Seckel syndrome
Short rib-polydactyly syndrome, type 2 (Majewski)
Shprintzen-Goldberg syndrome
Smith-Lemli-Opitz syndrome
Treacher Collins syndrome
Yunis-Varón syndrome

Mastoid, advance pneumatization

Acromegaly
Dyke-Davidoff-Masson syndrome
Lipodystrophy (lipoatrophic diabetes)

Mastoid, underdeveloped

Cleidocranial dysplasia
Cockayne syndrome
Craniodiaphyseal dysplasia
Craniometaphyseal dysplasia
Diaphyseal dysplasia (Engelmann disease)
Endosteal hyperostosis (van Buchem)
Frontometaphyseal dysplasia
Hypothyroidism
Mucopolysaccharidoses
Osteopathia striata
Osteopetrosis
Otopalatodigital syndrome I
Pycnodysostosis
Treacher Collins syndrome

Mastoiditis

Gradenigo syndrome
Histiocytosis X
Immotile cilia syndrome
Immune disorders
Wiskott-Aldrich syndrome

Middle ear anomaly

Achondroplasia
Acrocraniofacial dysostosis
Acrocephalosyndactyly, Apert type
Branchio-oto-renal dysplasia
Chromosome 13 trisomy syndrome
Chromosome 18 trisomy syndrome
Chromosome XO syndrome
Cleidocranial dysplasia
Craniometaphyseal dysplasia
DiGeorge syndrome
Duane syndrome
Dyschondrosteosis
EEC syndrome
Endosteal hyperostosis (van Buchem)
Facio-audio-symphalangism syndrome
Fanconi anemia
Fetal rubella syndrome
Frontometaphyseal dysplasia
Hypertelorism, microtia, facial clefting syndrome
Hypothyroidism
Klippel-Feil syndrome
Mucopolysaccharidoses
Oro-facio-digital syndrome II
Osteodysplasty, Melnick-Needles
Osteogenesis imperfecta
Osteopetrosis
Oto-palato-digital syndrome I
Renal, genital, and ear anomalies
Robin sequence
Treacher Collins syndrome
Wildervanck syndrome

Preauricular tags or pits

Acrocallosal syndrome
Acrocephalopolysyndactyly, Carpenter type
Antley-Bixler syndrome
Beckwith-Wiedemann syndrome
Branchio-oto-ureteral syndrome
Branchio-oto-renal syndrome
Cat-eye syndrome
Chromosomal abnormalities
Coffin-Siris syndrome
Frontonasal dysplasia sequence
Goldenhar syndrome
Langer-Giedion syndrome
Lenz microphthalmia syndrome
Nager syndrome

Oculo-cerebro-cutaneous syndrome (postauricular)
Townes-Brocks syndrome
Treacher Collins syndrome

EYE

Anophthalmia
Chromosome 13 trisomy syndrome
Goldenhar syndrome
Lenz microphthalmia syndrome
Microphthalmia and digital anomalies
Waardenburg anophthalmia syndrome

Blepharophimosis
Blepharophimosis, ptosis, epicanthus inversus syndrome[180]
Blepharophimosis syndrome, familial
Dubowitz syndrome
Freeman-Sheldon syndrome
Klein-Waardenburg syndrome
Oculo-palato-skeletal syndrome
Schwartz-Jampel syndrome
Smith-Lemli-Opitz syndrome

Blue sclerae
Aarskog syndrome
Achondrogenesis, type I
Chromosome 18 trisomy syndrome
Chromosome XO syndrome
Ehlers-Danlos syndrome
Grant syndrome
Hallermann-Streiff syndrome
Hyperphosphatasia
Hypophosphatasia
Incontinentia pigmenti
Iron deficiency anemia
Marfan syndrome
Marshall-Smith syndrome
Osteogenesis imperfecta
Roberts syndrome
Silver-Russell syndrome

Calcification, intraorbital
Cataract
Dermoid
Fetal cytomegalovirus infection
Fetal toxoplasmosis infection
Fraser syndrome
Glaucoma
Hypercalcemia
Hyperparathyroidism (primary)
Milk-alkali syndrome
Neurofibromatosis
Oculo-dento-osseous dysplasia
Retinoblastoma
Retrolental fibrodysplasia[236]
Vitamin D intoxication
von Hippel-Lindau syndrome

Cataract
Alport syndrome
Angelman syndrome
Aniridia-Wilms tumor association
Bardet-Biedl syndrome
Cataract—cerebellar atrophy—mental retardation—myopathy
Cerebro-oculo-facio-skeletal syndrome
Chondrodysplasia punctata
Chromosomal abnormalities
Clouston syndrome
Cockayne syndrome
Cutis verticis gyrata
Diabetes mellitus
Diaphyseal dysplasia (Engelmann)
Diaphyseal medullary stenosis with malignancy—Hardcastle

Fetal rubella syndrome
Fetal varicella syndrome
Flynn-Aird syndrome
Fronto-facio-nasal dysplasia
Galactosemia
Goldenhar syndrome
Goltz syndrome
Hallermann—Streiff syndrome
Homocystinuria
Hypochondroplasia
Hypoparathyroidism
Incontinentia pigmenti
Jadassohn-Lewandowsky syndrome
Klippel-Trenaunay-Weber syndrome
Kniest syndrome
Lowe syndrome
Mannosidosis
Marinesco-Sjögren syndrome
Marshall syndrome
Martsoff syndrome
Median cleft face syndrome
Menkes syndrome
Mevalonic aciduria
Moore-Federman syndrome
Morning glory syndrome
Myotonic dystrophy
Nail-patella syndrome
Nance-Horan syndrome
Neu-Laxova syndrome
Nevoid basal cell carcinoma syndrome (Gorlin)
Oculo-dento-osseous syndrome
Osteogenesis imperfecta
Osteopathia striata
Progeria
Proteus syndrome
Pseudohypoparathyroidism
Rieger syndrome
Roberts syndrome
Rothmund-Thomson syndrome
Rubinstein-Taybi syndrome
Schwartz-Jampel syndrome
Sclerosteosis
Smith-Lemli-Opitz syndrome
Stickler syndrome
Velo-cardio-facial syndrome
Warburg syndrome
Warfarin embryopathy
Werner syndrome
Zellweger syndrome

Cherry-red spots
Farber syndrome
Galactosialidosis
GM_1 gangliosidosis
GM_2 gangliosidosis, type 2
Leber congenital amaurosis
Metachromatic leukodystrophy
Niemann-Pick disease

Coloboma
Acro-renal-ocular syndrome[94]
Aniridia-Wilms tumor association
Beimond syndrome II
Cat-eye syndrome
CHARGE Association
Chromosomal abnormalities
Cohen syndrome
Contractural arachnodactyly
Crouzon syndrome
de Lange syndrome
Epidermal nevus syndrome

Fetal hydantoin syndrome
Fronto-facio-nasal dysplasia
Goldenhar syndrome
Goltz syndrome
Holoprosencephaly
Joubert syndrome
Marfan syndrome
Meckel syndrome
Median cleft face syndrome
Morning glory syndrome
Nager syndrome
Nasopalpebral lipoma-coloboma syndrome
Nevoid basal cell carcinoma syndrome (Gorlin)
Oculo-cerebro-cutaneous syndrome
Optic nerve coloboma-renal disease[250]
Pallister-Hall syndrome
Phillips-Griffith syndrome
Rieger syndrome
Rubinstein-Taybi syndrome
Scapuloiliac dysostosis
Sorsby syndrome
Sturge-Weber syndrome
Treacher Collins syndrome
Tricho-rhino-phalangeal dysplasia, type 2

Conjunctivitis
Acrodermatitis enteropathica
Granulomatous disease of childhood
Kawasaki syndrome
Reiter syndrome
Relapsing polychondritis[29]
Stevens-Johnson syndrome

Corneal opacity, dystrophy
Achondrogenesis, type I
Acrocephalopolysyndactyly, Carpenter type
Acrodermatitis enteropathica
Acromesomelic dysplasia
Chédiak-Higashi syndrome
Chromosomal abnormalities
Cockayne syndrome
Cutis laxa
Dermo-chondro-corneal dystrophy of François
Fabry syndrome
Fanconi syndrome
Fetal rubella syndrome
Fryns syndrome
Galactosialidosis
Indifference to pain
Jadassohn-Lewandowsky syndrome
Kearns-Sayre syndrome
Linear sebaceous nevus sequence
Lipodystrophy (Bernardinelli)
Lowe syndrome
Mannosidosis
Mietens syndrome
Mucolipidoses
Mucopolysaccharidoses
Nasopalpebral lipoma-coloboma syndrome
Neurofibromatosis
Ophthalmo-mandibulo-melic dysplasia
Osteogenosis imperfecta, type I
Rieger syndrome
Roberts syndrome
Rutherfurd syndrome
Scapuloiliac dysostosis
Senter syndrome[220]
Tangier disease[192]
Warfarin embryopathy
Winchester syndrome

Exophthalmos
Acrocephalosyndactyly
Caffey disease
Cloverleaf skull
Craniosynostosis
Crouzon syndrome
Cystic fibrosis
de Lange syndrome
Diaphyseal dysplasia (Engelmann)
Endosteal hyperostosis (van Buchem)
Erdheim-Chester disease
Fibrous dysplasia
Geoderma osteodysplastica hereditaria
Histiocytosis X
Hyperthyroidism
Infantile multisystem inflammatory disease
Metaphyseal chondrodysplasia (Jansen)
Neu-Laxova syndrome
Neurofibromatosis
Noonan syndrome
Osteodysplasty, Melnick-Needles
Osteodysplasty, precocious
Osteopetrosis
Osteosclerosis, dominant-type Stanescu
Red-eyed shunt syndrome
Relapsing polychondritis
Roberts syndrome
Sclerosteosis
Shprintzen-Goldberg syndrome

Eyelashes, abnormal, or unusual
Chondrodysplasia punctata
Chromosome 18 trisomy syndrome
de Lange syndrome
Distichiasis-lymphedema syndrome
Fronto-facio-nasal dysplasia
Hypothyroidism (infants)
Nasopalpebral lipoma-coloboma syndrome
Rothmund-Thomson syndrome
Treacher Collins syndrome

Eyelid, abnormal
Distichiasis-lymphedema syndrome
Fraser syndrome
N syndrome
Nasopalpebral lipoma-coloboma syndrome
Treacher Collins syndrome

Glaucoma
Aniridia-Wilms tumor association
Ehlers-Danlos syndrome
Fetal rubella syndrome
Goldenhar syndrome
Hallermann-Streiff syndrome
Homocystinuria
Kenny-Caffey syndrome
Klippel-Trenaunay-Weber syndrome
Lowe syndrome
Marfan syndrome
Marshall syndrome
Moore-Federman syndrome
Mucopolysaccharidoses
Nevoid basal cell carcinoma syndrome (Gorlin)
Neurofibromatosis
Oculo-dento-osseous syndrome
Rieger syndrome
Stickler syndrome
Sturge-Weber syndrome
Treacher Collins syndrome
von Hippel-Lindau syndrome
Weill-Marchesani syndrome
Zellweger syndrome

Hypertelorism (ocular, orbital)
Aarskog syndrome
Acrocallosal syndrome
Acrocephalosyndactyly, Apert type
Acrocephalosyndactyly, Pfeiffer type
Acrocephalosyndactyly, Saethre-Chotzen type
Acrodysostosis
Aminopterin fetopathy
Aminopterin-like syndrome without aminopterin
Beckwith-Wiedemann syndrome
Campomelic dysplasia
Cat-eye syndrome
CHARGE association
Chondrodysplasia punctata
Chromosomal abnormalities
Cleft lip sequence
Cleidocranial dysplasia
Cloverleaf skull
Coffin-Lowry syndrome
Cranio-fronto-nasal dysplasia
Cranio-fronto-nasal dysplasia-like syndrome
Craniometaphyseal dysplasia
Craniosynostosis (coronal)
Crouzon syndrome
de Lange syndrome
DiGeorge syndrome
Diamond-Blackfan syndrome
Dubowitz syndrome
Dyssegmental dwarfism
Ehlers-Danlos syndrome
Familial, normal variant
Fetal hydantoin syndrome
Fetal isotretinoin syndrome
FG syndrome
Fraser syndrome
Freeman-Sheldon syndrome
Frontometaphyseal dysplasia
Frontonasal dysplasia
G syndrome
German syndrome
Greig cephalopolysyndactyly syndrome
Holt-Oram syndrome
Hypertelorism, microtia, facial clefting syndrome
Larsen syndrome
Lenz-Majewski hyperostotic dwarfism
LEOPARD syndrome
Lissencephaly syndrome
Marden-Walker syndrome
Meckel syndrome
Median cleft face syndrome
Metaphyseal chondrodysplasia (Jansen)
Mucopolysaccharidosis, IH
Neu-Laxova syndrome
Nevoid basal cell carcinoma syndrome (Gorlin)
Noonan syndrome
Oculo-dento-osseous dysplasia
Opitz syndrome
Oro-facio-digital syndrome I
Oromandibular-limb hypogenesis syndromes
Osteodysplasty, precocious
Osteoglophonic dwarfism
Osteopetrosis
Oto-palato-digital syndrome I
Oto-palato-digital syndrome II
Pallister-Killian syndrome
Pena-Shokeir syndrome
Potter syndrome
Pterygium syndromes
Roberts syndrome
Robinow syndrome
Rubinstein-Taybi syndrome
Schinzel-Giedion syndrome
Sclerosteosis
Seckel syndrome
Simpson-Golabi-Behmel syndrome
Sjögren-Larsson syndrome
Sotos syndrome
Spondyloepiphyseal dysplasia congenita
Thalassemia
Treacher Collins syndrome
Unusual facies—arthrogryposis—advanced skeletal maturation syndrome[116]
W syndrome
Waardenburg syndrome
Warfarin embryopathy
Weaver syndrome

Hypotelorism (ocular, orbital)
Acro-fronto-nasal dysostosis
Chromosome 13 trisomy syndrome
Chromosome 20 syndrome
Chromosome 21 trisomy syndrome
Craniosynostosis (sagittal)
Craniotelencephalic dysplasia
DiGeorge syndrome
Fetal hydantoin syndrome
Holoprosencephaly
Meckel syndrome
Myotonic dystrophy
Oculo-dento-osseous syndrome
Phenylketonuria
Postaxial acrofacial dysostosis (Miller)
Tricho-rhino-phalangeal dysplasia, type 2
Trigonocephaly
Williams syndrome

Iris, abnormal
Aniridia-Wilms tumor association
Behçet syndrome
Goltz syndrome
Klein-Waardenburg syndrome
Reiger syndrome
Relapsing polychondritis
Shah-Waardenburg syndrome
Waardenburg syndrome

Lacrimal system, abnormal
Branchio-oto-renal dysplasia
Ectodermal dysplasia
EEC syndrome
Epidermal nevus syndrome
Fraser syndrome
Hay-Wells syndrome[102]
Hypomelanosis of Ito
Johanson-Blizzard syndrome
Lacrimo-auriculo-dento-digital syndrome
Lenz-Majewski hyperostotic dwarfism
Levy-Hollister syndrome
Mikulicz syndrome
Nasopalpebral lipoma-coloboma syndrome
Riley-Day syndrome
Sarcoidosis
Smith-Lemli-Opitz syndrome

Lens dislocation
Ehlers-Danlos syndrome
Homocystinuria
Marfan syndrome
Rieger syndrome
Stickler syndrome
Weill-Marchesani syndrome

Lens, opacity
Alport syndrome
Brachiolemia
Lowe syndrome
Stickler syndrome
Osteoporosis-pseudoglioma syndrome
Tuomaala syndrome

Microphthalmia
Amniotic band syndrome
Aplasia cutis congenita (Adams-Oliver)
Bardet-Biedl syndrome
Cat-eye syndrome
Cerebro-oculo-facio-skeletal syndrome
CHARGE association
Chromosomal abnormalities
Cohen syndrome
Fanconi anemia
Fetal alcohol syndrome
Fetal herpes simplex infection
Fetal isotretinoin syndrome
Fetal rubella syndrome
Fetal toxoplasmosis infection
Fetal varicella syndrome
Goldenhar syndrome
Goltz syndrome
Hallermann-Streiff syndrome
Holoprosencephaly
Hydrolethalus syndrome
Hypopituitarism (anterior lobe)
Incontinentia pigmenti
Kenny-Caffey syndrome
Lenz microphthalmia syndrome
Meckel syndrome
Median cleft syndrome
Neu-Laxova syndrome
Oculo-dento-osseous dysplasia
Oculo-cerebro-cutaneous syndrome
Osteoporosis-pseudoglioma syndrome
Pallister-Hall syndrome
Phenylketonuria
Proteus syndrome
Pseudohypoparathyroidism
Roberts syndrome
Scapuloiliac dysostosis
Thalidomide embryopathy
Treacher Collins syndrome
Warfarin embryopathy

Myopia
Alagille syndrome
Alport syndrome
Aminopterin fetopathy
Branchio-oto-renal dysplasia
Chomosomal abnormalities
Cohen syndrome
Cranioectodermal dysplasia
de Lange syndrome
Ehlers-Danlos syndrome
Fetal alcohol syndrome
Fetal trimethadione syndrome
Flynn-Aird syndrome
Gastrocutaneous syndrome
Hajdu-Cheney syndrome
Homocystinuria
Incontinentia pigmenti
Kenny-Caffey syndrome
Kniest syndrome
Marfan syndrome
Marshall syndrome
Marshall-Smith syndrome

Mucopolysaccharidosis I-S
Noonan syndrome
Postaxial polydactyly-myopia syndrome[55]
Proteus syndrome
Rubinstein-Taybi syndrome
Schwartz-Jampel syndrome
Spondylo-epimetaphyseal dysplasia, Strudwick type
Spondyloepiphyseal dysplasia congenita
Stickler syndrome
Tuomaala syndrome
Weill-Marchesani syndrome

Nystagmus
Aniridia-Wilms tumor association
Ataxia-telangiectasia syndrome
Bardet-Biedl syndrome
Biemond syndrome I
Börjeson-Frossman-Lehmann syndrome
Cerebro-oculo-facio-skeletal syndrome
Chédiak-Higashi syndrome
Chromosome X, fragile
Cockayne syndrome
Cranioectodermal dysplasia
de Morsier syndrome
Epidermal nevus syndrome
Fanconi anemia
Hajdu-Cheney syndrome
Hallermann-Streiff syndrome
Karsch-Neugenbauer syndrome
Marinesco-Sjögren syndrome
Mietens syndrome
Noonan syndrome
Parinaud syndrome
Proteus syndrome
Pseudohypoparathyroidism
Sorsby syndrome
Wallenberg syndrome
Zellweger syndrome

Optic atrophy
Acrodysostosis
Berk-Tabatznik syndrome
Bobble-head doll syndrome
Chondrodysplasia punctata
Cohen syndrome
Craniometaphyseal dysplasia
de Lange syndrome
de Morsier syndrome
Diaphyseal dysplasia (Engelmann)
Fetal alcohol syndrome
Fetal varicella syndrome
Foster Kennedy syndrome
GAPO syndrome
GM_2 gangliosidosis, type I
Hajdu-Cheney syndrome
Homocystinuria
Hyperphosphatasemia
Incontinentia pigmenti
Optic atrophy-spastic paraplegia syndrome
Refsum syndrome
Rieger syndrome
Sclerosteosis
Vitamin B_1 deficiency

Orbit, large
Craniosynostosis (coronal)
Glaucoma (congenital)
Histiocytosis X
Hyperthyroidism
Neurofibromatosis
Pseudotumor

Orbit, shallow
Cloverleaf skull
Crouzon syndrome
Larsen syndrome
Marshall-Smith syndrome
Mucopolysaccharidosis I-H
Weill-Marchesani syndrome

Orbit, small
Anophthalmos
Chromosome 13 trisomy syndrome
Fibrous dysplasia (polyostotic)
Hallermann-Streiff syndrome
Oculo-dento-osseous dysplasia
Microphthalmia

Papilledema
Diaphyseal dysplasia (Engelmann)
Foster Kennedy syndrome
Hughes-Stovin syndrome
Parinaud syndrome
POEMS syndrome
Pseudotumor cerebri
Riley-Smith syndrome

Ptosis (eyelid)
Aarskog syndrome
Aniridia-Wilms tumor association
Arthrogryposis syndrome
Börjeson-Forssman-Lehmann syndrome
Cerebro-oculo-facio-skeletal syndrome
CHARGE association
Chromosomal abnormalities (XO, etc.)
Coffin-Siris syndrome
Congenital ptosis-congenital heart disease[138]
EEC syndrome
Fetal alcohol syndrome
Fetal hydantoin syndrome
Fetal trimethadione syndrome
Freeman-Sheldon syndrome
Groll-Hirschowitz syndrome
Horner syndrome
Hypochondroplasia
Lymphedema-ptosis
Mannosidosis
Myesthenic syndromes
Myotonic dystrophy
Nail-patella syndrome
Neurofibromatosis
Noonan syndrome
Oculogastrointestinal muscular dystrophy
Pachydermoperiostosis syndrome
Pallister-Killian syndrome
Parinaud syndrome
Proteus syndrome
Raeder syndrome
Rubinstein-Taybi syndrome
Tricho-rhino-phalangeal syndrome, type 2

Retinopathy
Aase syndrome
Abetalipoproteinemia
Acrodysplasia with retinitis pigmentosa and nephropathy (Saldino-Mainzer)
Aicardi syndrome
Alagille syndrome
Alport syndrome
Bardet-Biedl syndrome
Behçet syndrome
Cockayne syndrome
Cohen syndrome
Diabetes mellitus

EEM syndrome (ectodermal dysplasia, ectodactyly, macular dystrophy)[178]
Fetal alcohol syndrome
Fetal herpes simplex infection
Fetal toxoplasmosis infection
Fetal varicella syndrome
Flynn-Aird syndrome
Holoprosencephaly
Hyperlipoproteinemia
Hypomelanosis of Ito
Incontinentia pigmenti
Kearns-Sayre syndrome
Kniest dysplasia
Lipoid proteinosis
Marshall syndrome
Microangiopathic syndrome of encephalopath–hearing loss–retinal arteriolar occlusion
Morning glory syndrome
Mucolipidosis IV
Neurofibromatosis
Nevoid basal cell carcinoma syndrome (Gorlin)
Osteopetrosis
Proteus syndrome
Refsum syndrome
Ruvalcaba syndrome
Sotos syndrome
Takayasu arteritis
Usher syndrome
Velo-cardio-facial syndrome
von Hippel-Lindau syndrome
Walker-Warburg syndrome
Wrinkly skin syndrome

Strabismus
Aarskog syndrome
Acrocephalosyndactyly, Apert type
Acrocephalosyndactyly, Pfeiffer type
Acrocephalosyndactyly, Saethre-Chotzen syndrome
Aplasia cutis congenita (Adams-Oliver syndrome)
Baller-Gerold syndrome
Bardet-Biedl syndrome
Biemond syndrome I
Blepharophimosis syndrome, familial
Chondroectodermal dysplasia
Chromosomal abnormalities (XO, etc.)
Clouston syndrome
Cohen syndrome
Crouzon syndrome
de Lange syndrome
Duane-radial dysplasia syndrome
Femoral-facial syndrome
Fetal alcohol syndrome
Fetal hydantoin syndrome
Fetal primidone syndrome
Fetal rubella syndrome
Fetal trimethadione syndrome
Freeman-Sheldon syndrome
Goldenhar syndrome
Goltz syndrome
Hallermann-Streiff syndrome
Hypomelanosis of Ito
Incontinentia pigmenti
Johanson-Blizzard syndrome
Langer-Giedion syndrome
Marden-Walker syndrome
Marinesco-Sjögren syndrome
Marshall syndrome
Mietens-Weber syndrome
Möbius syndrome
Mulibrey nanism
Multiple synostosis syndrome

Nevoid basal cell carcinoma syndrome (Gorlin)
Noonan syndrome
Opitz syndrome
Oromandibular-limb hypogenesis
Osteodysplasty, Melnick-Needles
Pallister-Killian syndrome
Prader-Willi syndrome
Rieger syndrome
Rubinstein-Taybi syndrome
Ruvalcaba-Myhr-Smith syndrome
Seckel syndrome
Smith-Lemli-Opitz syndrome
Sotos syndrome
TAR syndrome
W syndrome
Williams syndrome

EYEBROW

Eyebrow abnormalities[19]
Alopecia areata, totalis and universalis (absent)
Chromosome 10q+ (fine, arched)
Chromosome 12p+ (lateral extension)
Chromosome 18 trisomy (discontinuous)
Chromosome 3q+ (synophrys)
de Lange syndrome (synophrys)
Fucosidosis (heavy)
Hypertrichosis universalis congenita (double)
Ichthyosis-cheek-eyebrow syndrome (ICE syndrome) (absence of outer half)
KBG syndrome (redundant)
Klein-Waardenburg syndrome (heavy)
Metaphyseal chondrodysplasia, type McKusick (sparse)
Monilethrix (sparse)
Mucopolysaccharidosis I-H (heavy)
Mucopolysaccharidosis VI (heavy)
Oto-palato-digital syndrome I (lateral extension)
Partial eyebrow duplication-multiple malformation syndrome[19]
Progeria (absent)
Romberg syndrome (loss of median portion)
Rothmund-Thomson syndrome (sparse)
Waardenburg syndrome (premature graying)
Williams syndrome (medial flare)

Synophrys
Aarskog syndrome
Chromosomal abnormalities (13 trisomy, etc.)
de Lange syndrome
Fetal trimethadione syndrome
Mucopolysaccharidosis III
Nevoid basal cell carcinoma syndrome (Gorlin)
Unusual facies-arthrogryposis-advanced skeletal maturation syndrome[116]
Waardenburg syndrome

FACE

Facial asymmetry
Acrocephalosyndactyly, Saethre-Chotzen type
Aminopterin-like syndrome without aminopterin
Bencze syndrome
Cardiofacial syndrome (Cayler)
Dyke-Davidoff-Masson syndrome
Epidermal nevus syndrome
Fibrous dysplasia
Goltz syndrome
Hypochondroplasia
Klippel-Feil syndrome
Romberg syndrome[122]
Sturge-Weber syndrome
Velo-cardio-facial syndrome
Wildervanck syndrome

Facial hypoplasia
Aarskog syndrome
Anderson syndrome
Antley-Bixler syndrome
Atelosteogenesis
Binder syndrome
Bloom syndrome
Chromosome 18 trisomy syndrome
Chromosome 21 trisomy syndrome
Cleidocranial dysplasia
Cowden syndrome
Cranio-fronto-nasal dysplasia
Crouzon syndrome
Dyssegmental dysplasia
Fetal valproate syndrome
Freeman-Sheldon syndrome
Fronto-facio-nasal dysplasia[86]
GAPO syndrome
Geroderma osteodysplastica hereditaria
Goldenhar syndrome
Goltz syndrome
Hajdu-Cheney syndrome
Hallermann-Streiff syndrome
Holoprosencephaly
Keutel syndrome
Larsen syndrome
Mandibuloacral dysplasia
Maxillofacial dysostosis
Maxillonasal dysplasia
Nager anomaly
Progeria
Pycnodysostosis
Rieger syndrome
Riley-Day syndrome
Schinzel-Giedion syndrome
Schneckenbecken dysplasia
Seckel syndrome
Shprintzen-Goldberg syndrome
Stickler syndrome
The 3-M syndrome
Treacher Collins syndrome
Tuomaala syndrome
Weill-Marchesani syndrome
Wiedemann-Rautenstrauch syndrome
Wildervanck syndrome
Wrinkly skin syndrome
Yunis-Varón syndrome

MANDIBLE

Antegonial notching
Acro-cranio-facial dysostosis
Acrogeria
Antley-Bixler syndrome
Campomelic dysplasia
de Lange syndrome
Frontometaphyseal dysplasia
Goldenhar syndrome
Infantile multisystem inflammatory disease
Mandibuloacral dysplasia
Mandibulofacial dysostosis
Möbius syndrome
Neurofibromatosis
Oculo-dento-osseous dysplasia
Robin syndrome
Treacher Collins syndrome

Micrognathia
Achard syndrome
Achondrogenesis
Acrogeria
Aminopterin fetopathy

Aminopterin-like syndrome without aminopterin
Aniridia-Wilms tumor association
Arthrogryposis
Atelosteogenesis
Bloom syndrome
C syndrome
Campomelic dysplasia
Cat-eye syndrome
Catel-Manzke syndrome
Cerebro-costo-mandibular syndrome
Cerebro-oculo-facio-skeletal syndrome
CHARGE association
Charlie M syndrome
Chondrodysplasia punctata
Chromosome 13 trisomy syndrome
Chromosome 18 trisomy syndrome
Chromosome 22 trisomy syndrome
Chromosome 4p− syndrome
Chromosome 5 partial short arm deletion
Chromosome XO syndrome
Cockayne syndrome
Cohen syndrome
Contractural arachnodactyly
Cowden syndrome
de Lange syndrome
DiGeorge syndrome
Diastrophic dysplasia
Dubowitz syndrome
Dyssegmental dwarfism
Ehlers-Danlos syndrome
Femoral-facial syndrome
Fetal alcohol syndrome
Fetal isotretinoin syndrome
Fetal trimethadione syndrome
Fetal valproate syndrome
Fountain syndrome
Freeman-Sheldon syndrome
Frontometaphyseal dysplasia
GAPO syndrome
Gardener-Silengo-Wachtel syndrome
German syndrome
Glossopalatine ankylosis syndrome
Goldenhar syndrome
Grant syndrome
Hajdu-Cheney syndrome
Hallermann-Streiff syndrome
Hydrolethalus syndrome
Hypoglossia-hypodactylia syndrome
Johanson-Blizzard syndrome
Klippel-Feil syndrome
Larsen syndrome
Lenz-Majewski hyperostosis syndrome
Lissencephaly (Miller-Dieker syndrome)
Mandibuloacral dysplasia
Marden-Walker syndrome
Marshall-Smith syndrome
Meckel syndrome
Mesomelic dysplasia (Langer)
Metaphyseal chondrodysplasia, Jansen type
Midline cervical webbing/cleft-micrognathia-symphyseal spur
Möbius syndrome
MURCS association (Müllerian duct, renal, and cervical spine defects)[67]
Nager syndrome
Neu-Laxova syndrome
Noonan syndrome
Ophthalmo-mandibulo-melic dysplasia
Oro-facio-digital syndrome I
Oro-facio-digital syndrome II
Oromandibular-limb hypogenesis syndromes
Osteodysplasty, Melnick-Needles

Osteolysis with nephropathy
Oto-palato-digital syndrome, type 2
Pallister-Hall syndrome
Pallister-Killian syndrome
Pena-Shokeir syndrome
Postaxial acrofacial dysostosis syndrome (Miller)
Potter syndrome
Progeria
Pterygium syndromes
Pycnodysostosis
Roberts syndrome
Robin syndrome
Robinow syndrome
Rubinstein-Taybi syndrome
Rutledge lethal multiple congenital anomaly syndrome
Schwartz-Jampel syndrome
Seckel syndrome
Short rib-polydactyly syndrome, type 1
Short rib-polydactyly syndrome, type 2
Silver-Russell syndrome
Smith-Lemli-Opitz syndrome
Splenogonadal fusion/limb deformity
Stickler syndrome
TAR Syndrome
Treacher Collins syndrome
Tricho-rhino-phalangeal syndrome, types 1 and 2
Triploidy syndrome
Velo-cardio-facial syndrome
Weaver syndrome
Williams syndrome
Yunis-Varón syndrome
Zellweger syndrome

Prognathism

Achondroplasia
Acrocephalosyndactyly, Apert type
Acrodysostosis
Acromegaly
Anderson syndrome
Angelman syndrome
Ankylosed teeth-clinodactyly
Beckwith-Wiedemann syndrome
Binder syndrome
Chromosomal abnormalities (21, XO, fragile X, etc.)
Cleidocranial dysplasia
Cloverleaf skull
Cockayne syndrome
Crouzon syndrome
Diaphyseal dyspalsia (Engelmann)
Endosteal hyperostosis (van Buchem)
Endosteal hyperostosis (Worth)
Epidermolysis bullosa dystrophica
Fetal alcohol syndrome
Geodermia osteodysplastica hereditaria
Hajdu-Cheney syndrome
Hemihypertrophy (unilateral prognathism)
Hypothyroidism (juvenile)
LEOPARD syndrome
Mucolipidosis III
Mucopolysaccharidosis, IS
Multiple endocrine neoplasia, type 2b
Myotonic dystrophy
Nevoid basal cell carcinoma syndrome (Gorlin)
Normal variant
Oculo-dento-osseous dysplasia
Opitz syndrome
Osteoglophonic dwarfism
Pyle disease
Rieger syndrome
Sclerosteosis
Sotos syndrome
Williams syndrome

MOUTH
Abnormal tongue (miscellaneous)
Beckwith-Wiedemann syndrome
Cerebrocostomandibular syndrome
Chromosome 13 trisomy syndrome
Chromosome 21 trisomy syndrome
Glossopalatine ankylosis syndrome
Goldenhar syndrome
Hypoglossia-hypodactylia syndrome
Kocher-Debré-Sémélaigne syndrome
Meckel syndrome
Mucopolysaccharidosis I-H
Multiple endocrine neoplasia syndrome, type 2b
Oro-facio-digital syndrome I
Oro-facio-digital syndrome II
Oro-facio-digital syndrome III (Sugarman)
Oro-facio-digital syndrome IV (Temtamy-McKusick)
Pachynochia congenita syndrome
Robinow syndrome
Rutledge lethal multiple congenital anomaly syndrome

Cleft lip/palate
Aarskog syndrome
Aase syndrome
Aase-Smith syndrome
Achondrogenesis, type I
Achondrogenesis, type II
Acro-fronto-facio-nasal dysostosis syndrome
Acrocallosal syndrome
Acrocephalosyndactyly, Apert type
Adducted thumb syndrome
Aicardi syndrome
Aminopterin fetopathy
Amniotic band syndrome
Aplasia cutis congenita (Adams-Oliver syndrome)
Arthrogryposis
Ateleostogenesis
Bardet-Biedl syndrome
Bencze syndrome
Campomelic dysplasia
Catel-Manzke syndrome
Caudal dysplasia sequence
CHARGE association
CHILD syndrome
Chondroectodermal dysplasia
Chromosomal abnormalities
Cleft lip sequence
Cleidocranial dysplasia
Cranio-fronto-nasal dysplasia
Craniosynostosis-radial/fibular aplasia-cleft lip/palate syndrome
Crouzon syndrome
de la Chapelle dysplasia
de Lange syndrome
Diastrophic dysplasia
Dubowitz syndrome
Dyssegmental dwarfism
EEC syndrome
Femoral-facial syndrome
Fetal alcohol syndrome
Fetal hydantoin syndrome
Fetal valproate syndrome
Fetal trimethadione syndrome
Fronto-facio-nasal dysplasia
Gardner-Silengo-Wachtel syndrome
Goldenhar syndrome
Goltz syndrome
Gordon syndrome
Hay-Wells syndrome[102]
Holoprosencephaly
Hydrolethalus syndrome
Hypochondrogenesis
Hypoglossia-hypodactylia syndrome

Juberg-Hayward syndrome
Kniest dysplasia
Larsen syndrome
Marden-Walker syndrome
Marfan syndrome
Meckel syndrome
Median cleft face syndrome
MURCS association (Müllerian duct, renal, cervical spine defects)[67]
Neu-Laxova syndrome
Nevoid basal cell carcinoma syndrome (Gorlin)
Oculo-dento-osseous syndrome
Oculo-palato-skeletal dysplasia
Odontotrichomelic hypohidrotic dysplasia
Opitz syndrome
Oro-facio-digital syndrome I
Oro-facio-digital syndrome II
Oromandibular-limb hypogenesis syndrome
Osteopathia striata with cranial sclerosis
Oto-spondylo-megaepiphyseal dysplasia
Oto-palato-digital syndrome I
Oto-palato-digital syndrome II
Pallister-Hall syndrome
Phillips-Griffiths syndrome
Postaxial acrofacial dysostosis (Miller)
Pseudodiastrophic dysplasia
Pterygium syndromes
Roberts syndrome
Robin sequence
Robinow syndrome
Rosselli-Gulienetti syndrome
Seckel syndrome
Short rib-polydactyly syndrome, type 2 (Majewski)
Short rib-polydactyly syndrome, type 3 (Verma-Naumoff)
Simpson-Golabi-Behmel syndrome
Smith-Lemli-Opitz syndrome
Spondyloepimetaphyseal dysplasia, Strudwick type
Spondyloepimetaphyseal dysplasia with joint laxity
Spondyloepiphyseal dysplasia congenita
Stickler syndrome
Treacher Collins syndrome
Triploidy syndrome
Van der Woude syndrome[133, 217]
Velo-cardio-facial syndrome
Waardenburg syndrome

Lip defect (fistula or pit)
Acrocephalosyndactyly, Saethre-Choltzen type
Hypoglossia-hypodactylia syndrome
Oro-facio-digital syndrome
Pterygium syndrome
Van der Woude syndrome (lip pit-cleft lip syndrome)[133, 217]

Macroglossia
Acromegaly
Amyloidosis
Ateleostogenesis
Beckwith-Wiedemann syndrome
Chromosome 21 trisomy syndrome
Chromosome 4p trisomy syndrome
Familial macroglossia[201]
Glycogenosis, type II
GM_1 gangliosidosis
Hypothyroidism
Infant of diabetic mother
Kocher-Debré-Sémélaigne syndrome
Lethal congenital dwarfism with accelerated maturation[26]
Mucopolysaccharidosis I-H
Mucopolysaccharidosis, IS
Mucopolysaccharidosis, VI
Muscular dystrophy
Myotonia congenita

Neurofibromatosis
Robinow syndrome
Triploidy syndrome

Macrostomia
Angelman syndrome
Beckwith-Wiedemann syndrome
C syndrome
Chromosome 18p− syndrome
Chromosome 18q− syndrome
Goldenhar syndrome
Mucopolysaccharidosis, IS
Mucopolysaccharidosis IV
Neu-Laxova syndrome
Pallister-Killian syndrome
Simpson-Golabi-Behmel syndrome
Treacher Collins syndrome
Williams syndrome

Microglossia
Distal arthrogryposis
Freeman-Sheldon syndrome
Lenz-Majewski hyperostosis syndrome
Möbius syndrome
Oromandibular-limb hypogenesis syndrome
Pallister-Hall syndrome
Rutledge lethal multiple congenital anomaly syndrome
Short rib-polydactyly, type 2 (Majewski)

Microstomia
Bardet-Biedl syndrome
Cerebro-costo-mandibular syndrome
Chromosome 18 trisomy syndrome
Chromosome 21 trisomy syndrome
Cowden syndrome
Freeman-Sheldon syndrome
Hallermann-Streiff syndrome
Hypertelorism, microtia, facial clefting syndrome
Marden-Walker syndrome
Oromandibular-limb hypogenesis syndromes
Oto-palato-digital syndrome, type I
Oto-palato-digital syndrome, type II
Pena-Shokeir syndrome
Rapp-Hodgkin ectodermal dysplasia syndrome
Robinow syndrome
Ruvalcaba syndrome
Schwartz-Jampel syndrome
Skeletal dysplasia, "pursed" lips-ectopia lentis[35]
Treacher Collins syndrome
Trismus pseudocamptodactyly syndrome (Hecht syndrome)

Salivary duct ectasia
Mikulicz syndrome
Sarcoidosis
Sjögren syndrome

Salivary gland abnormality
Amyloidosis
Cystic fibrosis
Goldenhar syndrome
Hyperparathyroidism (primary)
Hypoglossia-hypodactylia syndrome
Lacrimo-auriculo-dento-digital syndrome
Levy-Hollister syndrome
Mikulicz syndrome
Treacher Collins syndrome

Stomatitis
Behçet syndrome
Chronic granulomatous disease of childhood
Fetal herpes simplex infection
Glucagonoma syndrome

Histiocytosis X
Iron deficiency anemia
Polyglandular autoimmune disease
Stevens-Johnson syndrome

NOSE

Bifid nose (partial or total)
Acro-fronto-facio-nasal dysostosis syndrome
Craniofrontonasal dysplasia
Frontofacionasal dysplasia
Hypertelorism, microtia, facial clefting syndrome
Median cleft face syndrome
Median cleft nose[120]
Orofaciodigital syndrome II

Choanal atresia[125]
Acrocephalosyndactyly, Apert type
Acrocephalosyndactyly, Pfeiffer type
Acrocephalosyndactyly, Saethre-Chotzen type
Amniotic band syndrome
Antley-Bixler syndrome
CHARGE association[125]
Chromosomal abnormalities (18, 21, XO)[125]
Crouzon syndrome
de Lange syndrome
DiGeorge syndrome
Familial choanal atresia[194]
Lenz-Majewski hyperostosis syndrome
Marshall-Smith syndrome
Schinzel-Giedion syndrome (stenosis)
Thalidomide embryopathy
Treacher Collins syndrome
Triploidy syndrome

Depressed or flat nasal bridge
Achondrogenesis, type II
Achondroplasia
Acrocephalopolysyndactyly, Carpenter type
Acrocephalosyndactyly, Pfeiffer type
Acrodysostosis
Aminopterin fetopathy
Anderson syndrome
Antley-Bixler syndrome
Atelosteogenesis
Binder syndrome
C syndrome
Campomelic dysplasia
Cephaloskeletal dysplasia (Taybi-Linder)
Chondrodysplasia punctata
Chromosomal abnormalities (21, XXXXY, XXXXX, etc.)
Cleidocranial dysplasia
Cloverleaf skull
Cranio-fronto-nasal dysplasia-like syndrome
Craniometaphyseal dysplasia
Ectodermal dysplasia (hypohidrotic)
Ehlers-Danlos syndrome
Fetal hydantoin syndrome
Fetal trimethadione syndrome
Fetal valproate syndrome
Fibrochondrogenesis
Fraser syndrome
Gardner-Silengo-Wachtel syndrome
GM_1 gangliosidosis
Hyperphosphatasia
Keutel syndrome
Kniest syndrome
Laron dwarfism
Larsen syndrome
Marshall syndrome
Marshall-Smith syndrome
Mietens-Weber syndrome
Mucolipidosis II

Mucopolysaccharidosis, I-H
Mucopolysaccharidosis, I-S
Mucopolysaccharidosis, VI
Neu-Laxova syndrome
Oro-facio-digital syndrome
Osteogenesis imperfecta, types I, II
Oto-palato-digital syndrome, type 2
Pallister-Killian syndrome
Proteus syndrome
Pseudohypoparathyroidism
Relapsing polychondritis
Robinow syndrome
Rothmund-Thomson syndrome
Rüdiger syndrome
Schinzel-Giedion syndrome
Stickler syndrome
Thanatophoric dysplasia
Triploidy syndrome
Warfarin embryopathy
Weill-Marchesani syndrome
Williams syndrome

Prominent nose, bulbous nose

Alagille syndrome
Coffin-Lowry syndrome
Facio-audio-symphalangism syndrome
Pycnodysostosis
Rubinstein-Taybi syndrome
Seckel syndrome
Smith-Lemli-Opitz syndrome
Tricho-rhino-phalangeal dysplasia, types 1 and 2
Velo-cardio-facial syndrome

Polyp

Azospermia-nasal polyposis[216]
Cystic fibrosis
Immotile cilia syndrome
Kartagener syndrome
Peutz-Jeghers syndrome

Small nose

Aarskog syndrome
Achondrodysplasia
Achondrogenesis, type II
Acrocephalosyndactyly, Apert type
Acrocephalosyndactyly, Pfeiffer type
Acrodysostosis
Acromesomelic dysplasia
C syndrome
Chromosomal abnormalities (13, 18, 21, XXXXY, etc.)
Craniometaphyseal dysplasia
de Lange syndrome
Femoral-facial syndrome
Fetal alcohol syndrome
Fetal hydantoin syndrome
Fetal trimethadione syndrome
Fetal valproate syndrome
Geleophysic dysplasia
Hallermann-Streiff syndrome
Lissencephaly (Miller-Dieker syndrome)
Marshall syndrome
Marshall-Smith syndrome
Mucolipidosis II
Mucopolysaccharidosis IV
Oculo-dento-osseous dysplasia
Osteogenesis imperfecta, II
Oto-palato-digital syndrome, type 1
Pallister-Hall syndrome
Pallister-Killiam syndrome
Pena-Shokeir syndrome
Robinow syndrome
Rothmund-Thomson syndrome

Treacher Collins syndrome
Waardenburg syndrome
Warfarin syndrome
Williams syndrome

SINUSES

Advanced pneumatization of sinuses

Acromegaly
Chromosome XO syndrome
Dyke-Davidoff-Masson syndrome
Homocystinuria
Lipodystrophy (lipoatrophic diabetes)
Marfan syndrome
Myotonic dystrophy
Normal variant

Sinusitis

Ataxia-telangiectasia
Cystic fibrosis
Immotile cilia syndrome
Immune deficiency diseases
Kartagener syndrome
Wiskott-Aldrich syndrome
Yellow nail syndrome
Young syndrome

Underdeveloped sinuses

Binder syndrome
Chromosome 21 trisomy syndrome
Cleidocranial dysplasia
Cockayne syndrome
Craniodiaphyseal dysplasia
Craniometaphyseal dysplasia
Fibrous dysplasia
Frontometaphyseal dysplasia
Fucosidosis
Hypopituitarism
Hypothyroidism
Median cleft face syndrome
Metaphyseal chondrodysplasia (Jansen)
Osteodysplasty, Melnick-Needles
Osteopathia striata with cranial sclerosis
Osteopetrosis
Oto-palato-digital syndrome, type 1
Prader-Willi syndrome
Pycnodysostosis
Schwarz-Lélek syndrome
Thalassemia
Treacher Collins syndrome

SKULL

Asymmetry

Acrocephalosyndactyly, Saethre-Chotzen type
Acrocephalosyndactyly, Waardenburg type
Dyke-Davidoff-Masson syndrome
Epidermal nevus syndrome
Fibrous dysplasia
Hemicerebral arterial ectasia[5]
Opitz syndrome (BBB syndrome)
Sturge-Weber syndrome
Wildervanck syndrome

Basilar invagination[237]

Achondroplasia
Ankylosing spondylitis
Arnold-Chiari malformation
Chromosome 21 trisomy
Cleidocranial dysplasia
Congenital craniovertebral junction anomalies[237]
Crouzon syndrome
Fibrous dysplasia
Hajdu-Cheney syndrome

Histiocytosis X
Hypoparathyroidism
Hypophosphatasia
Klippel-Feil syndrome
Mucopolysaccharidoses
Osteogenesis imperfecta
Osteomalacia
Osteopetrosis
Osteoporosis
Pycnodysostosis
Rickets

Cloverleaf skull malformation
Achondroplasia
Acrocephalopolysyndactyly, Carpenter type
Acrocephalosyndactyly, Apert type
Acrocephalosyndactyly, Pfeiffer type
Amniotic band syndrome
Antley-Bixler syndrome
Chromosome 13 partial trisomy
Cloverleaf skull-limb anomalies
Crouzon disease
Hypopituitarism
Osteoglophonic dysplasia
Thanatophoric dysplasia

Craniosynostosis[47]
Acrocraniofacial dysostosis
Acrocephalopolysyndactyly, Carpenter type
Acrocephalopolysyndactyly, Goodman type
Acrocephalopolysyndactyly, Sakati type
Acrocephalosyndactyly, Apert type
Acrocephalosyndactyly, Hermann-Opitz type
Acrocephalosyndactyly, Pfeiffer type
Acrocephalosyndactyly, Robinow-Sorauf type
Acrocephalosyndactyly, Saethre-Chotzen type
Acrocephalosyndactyly, Summit type
Acrocephalosyndactyly, Waardenburg type
Adducted thumb syndrome
Aminopterin fetopathy
Andersen-Pindborg syndrome
Antley-Bixler syndrome
Armendares syndrome (1974)
Asphyxiating thoracic dysplasia
Aural-cephalosyndactyly[132]
Baller-Gerold syndrome
Bardet-Biedl syndrome
Berant syndrome (1973)
C syndrome
Chondrodysplasia punctata
Chromosomal syndromes
Cloverleaf skull
Craniofacial dyssynostosis
Cranio-fronto-nasal dysplasia
Craniosynostosis-fibular aplasia[151]
Craniosynostosis-radial/fibular aplasia-cleft lip/palate syndrome
  (Hermann syndrome, 1969)
Craniosynostosis-ulnar aplasia[37]
Craniotelencephalic dysplasia
Crouzon syndrome
De Sanctis-Cacchione syndrome
Elejalde syndrome (1977)
Exobar-Bixler syndrome (1977)
Fairbank syndrome
Familial craniosynostosis[39, 189]
Fetal hydantoin syndrome
Fetal rubella syndrome
FG syndrome
Fucosidosis
Gorlin-Chaudhry-Moss syndrome
Hall syndrome
Hallermann-Streiff syndrome

Hootnick-Holmes syndrome (1972)
Hunter-McAlpine syndrome (1977)
Hypercalcemia, idiopathic
Hyperthyroidism
Hypophosphatasia
Hypothyrodism (juvenile)
Idaho syndrome I (Cohen, 1977)
Idaho syndrome II (Cohen, 1977)
Ives-Houston syndrome[115]
Jackson-Weiss syndrome
Lacheretz-Allain syndrome (craniosynostosis-radiohumeral fusion)
  (1974)
Lowe syndrome
Meckel syndrome
Median cleft face syndrome
Michels syndrome (1978)
Mucolipidosis III
Mucopolysaccharidosis I-H
Mucopolysaccharidosis VI
Osteoglophonic dwarfism
Osteopetrosis
Pycnodysostosis
Rickets
Seckel syndrome
Sickle cell anemia
Thalassemia
Thanatophoric dysplasia
Trigonocephaly, familial (Say-Meyer)
Ventruto syndrome (1976)
Vitamin D intoxication
Williams syndrome

Cranium bifidum
Aminopterin fetopathy
Familial cranium bifidum occultum[238]
Fronto-facio-nasal dysplasia
Median cleft face syndrome

Defect, acquired
Caffey disease
Histiocytosis X
Hyperparathyroidism
Sarcoidosis

Defective ossification/congenital defect
Aase syndrome
Aminopterin fetopathy
Aminopterin-like syndrome without aminopterin
Amniotic band sequence
Aplasia cutis congenita
Bardet-Biedl syndrome
Chromosomal abnormalities (13, 18, and 21 chromosomes)
Cleidocranial dysplasia
Cranium bifidum occultum
Dermal sinus
Ehlers-Danlos syndrome
Encephalocele
Fetal rubella syndrome
Fibromatosis, congenital
Frontonasal dysplasia
Goldenhar syndrome
Hallermann-Streiff syndrome
Hydrocephalus
Hydrops—ectopic calcification—moth-eaten skeletal dysplasia
Hyperparathyroidism
Hypochondrogenesis
Hypophosphatasia
Hypothyroidism
Lacunar skull
Median cleft face syndrome
Neurofibromatosis
Noonan syndrome

Occipital foramina
Oculo-cerebro-cutaneous syndrome
Osteogenesis imperfecta
Parietal foramina[143]
Parietal "foramina"-clavicular hypoplasia
Parietal thinning
Progeria
Rickets
Rubinstein-Taybi syndrome

Fontanelle, delayed closure, large

Aase syndrome
Aminopterin fetopathy
Aplasia cutis (scalp)
Chondrodysplasia punctata
Chromosome 13 trisomy syndrome
Chromosome 18 trisomy syndrome
Chromosome 21 trisomy syndrome
Cleidocranial dysplasia
Coffin-Lowry syndrome
Cranium bifidum
Cutis laxa
Familial idiopathic osteoarthropathy
Fetal hydantoin syndrome
Fetal primidone syndrome
Fetal rubella syndrome
G syndrome
GAPO syndrome
Goldenhar syndrome
Greig cephalopolysyndactyly syndrome
Hallermann-Streiff syndrome
Hypochondroplasia
Hypophosphatasia
Hypothyroidism
Infantile multisystem inflammatory disease
lenz-Majewski hyperostotic dwarfism
Osteodysplasty, Melnick-Needles
Osteogenesis imperfecta
Oto-palato-digital syndrome, type 1
Progeria
Pycnodysostosis
Rickets
Rubinstein-Taybi syndrome
Schinzel-Giedion syndrome
Silver-Russell syndrome
Wiedemann-Rautenstrauch syndrome
Winchester syndrome
Zellweger syndrome

Foramen magnum, large

Arnold-Chiari malformation
Dandy-Walker syndrome
Encelphalocele/meningocele
Frontometaphyseal dysplasia
Hydrolethalus
Rubinstein-Taybi syndrome

Foramen magnum, small

Achondrogenesis
Achondroplasia
Diastrophic dysplasia
Hypochondroplasia
Metatrophic dysplasia
Thanatophoric dysplasia

Frontal bossing

Achondrogenesis
Achondroplasia
Acrocallosal syndrome
Cleidocranial dysplasia
Cranio-fronto-nasal dysplasia
Craniometaphyseal dysplasia

Craniotelencephalic dysplasia
Diaphyseal dysplasia (Engelmann)
Diastrophic dysplasia
Frontometaphyseal dysplasia
GAPO syndrome
GM$_1$ gangliosidosis
Goldenhar syndrome
Greig cephalopolysyndactyly syndrome
Hallermann-Streiff syndrome
Hydrocephalus
Hypochondroplasia
Infantile multisystem inflammatory disease
Iron deficiency anemia
Larsen syndrome
Lissencephaly syndrome
Lowe syndrome
Marshall-Smith syndrome
Metatrophic dysplasia
Mucolipidosis II
Mucopolysaccharidoses
Nevoid basal cell carcinoma syndrome (Gorlin)
Osteoglophonic dwarfism
Osteopetrosis
Oto-palato-digital syndrome, type 1
Parietal "foramina"-clavicular hypoplasia
Progeria
Pycnodysostosis
Rickets, healed
Riley-Smith syndrome
Robinow syndrome
Schwarz-Lélek syndrome
Sclerosteosis
Sickle cell anemia
Silver-Russell syndrome
Sotos syndrome
Thalassemia
Thanatophoric dysplasia
The 3-M syndrome

Macrocephaly/macrocrania[60]

3-Hydroxy-3-methylglutaryl-CoA lyase deficiency[146]
Achondroplasia
Achondrogenesis
Acrocallosal syndrome
Agenesis of corpus callosum-macrocephaly[257]
Alexander disease
Bannayan syndrome
Beckwith-Wiedemann syndrome
Benign macrocephaly of infancy[186]
Canavan syndrome
Chromosome 8 trisomy syndrome
Cleidocranial dysplasia
Cowden syndrome
Cranioectodermal dysplasia
Cronkhite-Canada syndrome
Dandy-Walker syndrome
Duchenne muscular dystrophy
Familial megalencephaly[58]
GM$_1$ gangliosidosis
GM$_2$ gangliosidosis (Tay-Sachs disease)
Greig cephalopolysyndactyly syndrome
Growth hormone deficiency
Hemicerebral arterial ectasia[5]
Hydroanencephaly
Hydrocephalus
Hydrolethalus
Hypochondrogenesis
Hypochondroplasia
Hypomelanosis of Ito
Hypothyroidism
Infantile multisystem inflammatory disease

Kniest dysplasia
Laron syndrome
Macrocephaly and mesodermal hamartomas
Marfan syndrome
Metachromatic leukodystrophy
Mucolipidoses
Mucopolysaccharidoses
Multiple hemangiomatosis syndrome
Neurofibromatosis
Noonan syndrome
Osteogenesis imperfecta
Parietal "foramina"—clavicular hypoplasia
Pituitary dwarfism
Pituitary gigantism
Porencephaly
Proteus syndrome
Pycnodysostosis
Riley-Smith syndrome
Robinow syndrome
Ruvalcaba-Myhre-Smith syndrome
Schwarz-Lélek syndrome
Silver-Russell syndrome
Spondyloepiphyseal dysplasia congenita
Thanatophoric dysplasia
Thick skull
Tuberous sclerosis
Zellweger syndrome

Microcephaly
Adducted thumb syndromes
Anencephaly
Angelman syndrome
Aspartylglucosaminuria
Autosomal dominant microcephaly[206]
Beckwith-Wiedemann syndrome
Börjeson-Forssman-Lehman syndrome
C syndrome
Cephaloskeletal dysplasia (Taybi-Linder)
Cerebro-oculo-facio skeletal syndrome
Chondrodysplasia punctata
Chromosomal abnormalities (13, 18, 21, etc.)
Cockayne syndrome
Coffin-Siris syndrome
Craniosynostosis
Cutis verticis gyrata
de Lange syndrome
De Sanctis-Cacchione syndrome
Deprivation dwarfism
Dubowitz syndrome
Dyggve-Melchior-Clausen syndrome
Fanconi syndrome
Fetal alcohol syndrome
Fetal cytomegalovirus infection
Fetal herpes simplex infection
Fetal hydantoin syndrome
Fetal rubella syndrome
Fetal toxoplasmosis infection
Fetal trimethadione syndrome
Fraser syndrome
Goltz syndrome
Holoprosencephaly
Homocystinuria
Incontinentia pigmenti
Johanson-Blizzard syndrome
Juberg-Hayward syndrome
Kearns-Sayre syndrome
Lenz microphthalmia syndrome
Lesch-Nyhan syndrome
Lissencephaly syndrome
Marinesco-Sjögren syndrome
Martsolf syndrome

Meckel syndrome
Menkes syndrome
Myotonic dystrophy
Noonan syndrome
Prader-Willi syndrome
Progressive familial encephalopathy—basal ganglia calcification
Pyruvate dehydrogenase complex deficiencies
Riley-Day syndrome
Rubinstein-Taybi syndrome
Ruvalcaba syndrome
Seckel syndrome
Smith-Lemli-Opitz syndrome
Tuberous sclerosis
Wrinkly skin syndrome

Sella turcica, enlarged
Acromegaly and gigantism
Cushing syndrome
Empty sella syndrome
Hydrocephalus
Hydrolethalus syndrome
Hypogonadism
Hypopituitarism (empty sella)
Hypothyroidism (juvenile)
Mucolipidoses
Mucopolysaccharidoses
Nelson syndrome

Sella turcica, small
Cockayne syndrome
Chromosome 21 trisomy syndrome
Deprivation dwarfism
Fibrous dysplasia
Growth hormone deficiency
Hypopituitarism
Microcephaly
Myotonic dystrophy
Prader-Willi syndrome
Sheehan syndrome

Sutures, delayed closure and/or wide
Acrogeria
Aminopterin fetopathy
Chondrodysplasia punctata
Chromosomal abnormalities (13, 18, 21)
Cleidocranial dysplasia
Craniometaphyseal dysplasia
Cranium bifidum
Dandy-Walker syndrome
Deprivation dwarfism
Diencephalic syndrome
Fetal primidone syndrome
Fetal rubella syndrome
Growth hormone deficiency
Hajdu-Cheney syndrome
Hallermann-Streiff syndrome
Hydrocephalus
Hydrolethalus
Hyperparathyroidism
Hypoparathyroidism
Hypophosphatasia
Hypothyroidism
Laron syndrome
Lead intoxication
Mandibuloacral dysplasia
Osteogenesis imperfecta
Osteopathy, familial idiopathic (Currarino)
Osteoporosis
Pachydermoperiostosis
Progeria
Pseudotumor cerebri
Pycnodysostosis

Rickets
Rubinstein-Taybi syndrome
Schinzel-Giedion syndrome
Silver-Russell syndrome
Vitamin A deficiency
Vitamin A intoxication
Wiedemann-Rautenstrauch syndrome
Winchester syndrome
Zellweger syndrome

Thick skull

Aase-Smith syndrome
Achard syndrome
Acrodysostosis
Acromegaly
Aspartylglucosaminuria
Calvarial doughnut lesions–osteoporosis–dentinogenesis imperfecta
Calvarial hyperostosis, familial
Cerebral atrophy
Chromosome XXXXY syndrome
Clouston syndrome
Cockayne syndrome
Coffin-Lowry syndrome
Craniodiaphyseal dysplasia
Craniofacial sclerosis–multiple anomalies[53]
Craniometaphyseal dysplasia
Diaphyseal dysplasia (Engelmann)
Distal osteosclerosis
Dyke-Davidoff-Masson syndrome
Endosteal hyperostosis (van Buchem)
Endosteal hyperostosis (Worth)
Fanconi anemia
Fibrous dysplasia (polyostotic)
Fluorosis
Fountain syndrome
Frontometaphyseal dysplasia
Fucosidosis
Geophagia-dwarfism-hypogonadism syndrome
Homocystinuria
Hypercalcemia, idiopathic
Hyperostosis generalisata with striations of the bones
Hyperphosphatasemia
Hypoparathyroidism
Hypothyroidism
Infantile multisystem inflammatory disease
Iron deficiency anemia
Lenz-Majewski hyperostosis dwarfism
Lipodystrophy (lipoatrophic diabetes)
Mannosidosis
Marfan syndrome
Marshall syndrome
Microcephaly
Morgagni-Stewart-Morel syndrome[176]
Mucolipidosis I
Mucolipidosis II
Mucopolysaccharidosis I-H
Mucopolysaccharidosis II
Mucopolysaccharidosis III
Mucopolysaccharidosis VI
Myhre syndrome
Myotonic dystrophy
Neu-Laxova syndrome
Oculo-dento-osseous dysplasia
Osteogenesis imperfecta
Osteopathia striata
Osteopetrosis
Oto-palato-digital syndrome, type 1
POEMS syndrome
Polycythemia
Proteus syndrome

Pseudohypoparathyroidism
Pycnodysostosis
Pyle disease
Pyruvate kinase deficiency
Renal osteodystrophy
Rickets, treated
Riley-Smith syndrome
Sala syndrome
Schwarz-Lélek syndrome
Sickle cell anemia
Sjögren-Larsson syndrome
Spherocytosis
Thalassemia
Tricho-dento-osseous syndrome
Troell-Junet syndrome
Tuberous sclerosis
Vitamin D intoxication
Weill-Marchesani syndrome

Trigonocephaly

C syndrome (Opitz)
Chromosomal abnormalities
Familial trigonocephaly
Familial trigonocephaly–short stature–developmental delay (215)
Holoprosencephaly
Sporadic trigonocephaly

Wormian bones (sutural bones)[52]

Acrogeria
Aminopterin embryopathy
Aplasia cutis congenita
Chondrodysplasia punctata (Conradi-Hünermann)
Chromosome 21 trisomy syndrome
Cleidocranial dysplasia
Copper deficiency
Grant syndrome
Hajdu-Cheney syndrome
Hallermann-Streiff syndrome
Hydrocephalus
Hypophosphatasia
Hypothyroidism (cretinism)
Infantile multisystem inflammatory disease
Mandibuloacral dysplasia
Menkes syndrome
Metaphyseal chondrodysplasia, Jansen type
Normal variant
Osteoarthropathy, familial idiopathic (Currarino)
Osteogenesis imperfecta
Osteopetrosis, infantile type
Prader-Willi syndrome
Progeria
Pycnodysostosis
Rickets
Schinzel-Giedion syndrome
Zellweger syndrome

TEETH

Adontia or hypodontia

Aarskog syndrome
Acrofacial dysostosis
Bloom syndrome
Böök syndrome
Charlie M syndrome
Cherubism
Chondroectodermal dysplasia
Chromosome 21 trisomy
Chromosome XXXXY syndrome
Cleft lip sequence
Cleidocranial dysplasia
Coffin-Lowry syndrome
Crouzon syndrome

Ectodermal dysplasia (hypohidrotic)
EEC syndrome
Ehlers-Danlos syndrome
Epidermal nevus syndrome
Familial hypodontia—nail dysgenesis[111]
Frontometaphyseal dysplasia
GAPO syndrome (pseudoadontia)
Glossopalatine ankylosis syndrome
Goltz syndrome
Hallermann-Streiff syndrome
Hanhart syndrome
Hay-Wells syndrome (ankyloblepharon—ectodermal
  dysplasia—cleft lip-palate)[102]
Hypoglossia-hypodactylia syndrome
Hypophosphatasia
Incontinentia pigmenti
Johanson-Blizzard syndrome
Kirghizian dermato-osteolysis
Levy-Hollister syndrome
Oculo-dento-osseous syndrome
Odonto-tricho-melic hypohidrotic dysplasia
Oro-facio-digital syndrome I
Oro-facio-digital syndrome II
Osteogenesis imperfecta
Oto-palato-digital syndrome, type 1
Pseudohypoparathyroidism
Pycnodysostosis
Rapp-Hodgkin ectodermal dysplasia
Rieger syndrome
Rothmund-Thomson syndrome
Seckel syndrome
Sjögren-Larsson syndrome
Tricho-dento-osseous syndrome
Tricho-odonto-onychial dysplasia
Tuomaala syndrome
Van der Woude syndrome (lip pit, cleft lip)
Weill-Marshesani syndrome
Williams syndrome

Delayed eruption of teeth
Aarskog syndrome
Acrocephalosyndactyly, Apert type
Branchio-genito-skeletal syndrome
Charlie M syndrome
Chondroectodermal dysplasia
Chromosome 21 trisomy syndrome
Cleidocranial dysplasia
de Lang syndrome
Dubowitz syndrome
Fetal rubella syndrome
GAPO syndrome
Gardner syndrome
Goltz syndrome
Hallermann-Streiff syndrome
Hanhart syndrome
Hypoparathyroidism
Hypopituitarism (anterior lobe)
Hypothyroidism
Incontinentia pigmenti
Kocher-Debré-Sémélaigne syndrome
Levy-Hollister syndrome
Lissencephaly (Miller-Dieker syndrome)
Mucopolysaccharidoses
Nonerupting teeth-maxillo-zygomatic hypoplasia
Osteogenesis imperfecta
Osteoglophonic dwarfism
Pallister-Killian syndrome
Progeria
Pseudohypoparathyroidism
Pycnodysostosis
Rickets
Romberg syndrome

Tricho-dento-osseous syndrome
Wiedemann-Rautenstrauch syndrome
Williams syndrome
Winchester syndrome

Dental caries
Addison disease
Chondroectodermal dysplasia
Cleidocranial dysplasia
Cockayne syndrome
Diaphyseal dysplasia
Dubowitz syndrome
Dyskeratosis congenita
EEC syndrome
Epidermal nevus syndrome
Epidermolysis bullosa dystrophica
Flynn-Aird syndrome
Groll-Hirschowitz syndrome
Hallermann-Streiff syndrome
Hypoparathyroidism
Hypophosphatasia
Hypothyroidism
Jadassohn-Lewandowsky syndrome
Mucopolysaccharidoses
Nevoid basal cell carcinoma syndrome (Gorlin)
Oro-facio-digital syndrome I, II
Osteogenesis imperfecta
Osteopetrosis
Prader-Willi syndrome
Pyle disease
Rothmund-Thomson syndrome
Sjögren syndrome

Dental cyst
Branchio-genito-skeletal syndrome
Cleidocranial dysplasia
Gardner syndrome
Lowe syndrome
Mucopolysaccharidosis I-H
Mucopolysaccharidosis I-H/S
Nevoid basal cell carcinoma syndrome (Gorlin)
Opitz syndrome (BBB syndrome)
Rutherford syndrome

Dental defects
Aarskog syndrome
Acrocephalosyndactyly, Apert type
Amelogenesis imperfecta—nephrocalcinosis syndrome
Anderson syndrome
Angelman syndrome
Ankylosed teeth-clinodactyly
Bardet-Biedl syndrome
Branchio-genito-skeletal dysplasia
Calvarial doughnut lesions—osteoporosis—dentinogenesis imper-
  fecta
Cerebro-costo-mandibular syndrome
Cherubism
Chondroectodermal dysplasia
Chromosome 21 trisomy syndrome
Chromosome XXXXY syndrome
Chromosome XXY syndrome
Cleidocranial dysplasia
Coffin-Lowry syndrome
Cohen syndrome
Cranioectodermal dysplasia
Craniometaphyseal dysplasia
Crouzon syndrome
de Lange syndrome
Dentino-osseous dysplasia
DOOR syndrome
Dysosteosclerosis
Ectodermal dysplasia (hypohidrotic)
Ehlers-Danlos syndrome

Epidermal nevus syndrome
Fibrodysplasia ossificans progressiva
Fluorosis
Frontometaphyseal dysplasia
Gardner syndrome
Gerodermia osteodysplastica hereditaria
Goldenhar syndrome
Goltz syndrome
Gorlin-Chaudhry-Moss syndrome
Hajdu-Cheney syndrome
Hallermann-Streiff syndrome
Hay-Wells syndrome (ankyloblepharon—ectodermal
    dysplasia—cleft lip-palate)[102]
Homocystinuria
Hyperphosphatasemia
Hypoglossia-hypodactylia syndrome
Hypomelanosis of Ito
Hypoparathyroidism
Hypophosphatasia
Hypopituitarism (anterior lobe)
Hypothyroidism
Incontinentia pigmenti
Johanson-Blizzard syndrome
KBG syndrome
Lacrimo-auriculo-dento-digital syndrome
Lenz microphthalmia syndrome
Lenz-Majewski hyperostotic dwarfism
Levy-Hollister syndrome
Lowe syndrome
Marinesco-Sjögren syndrome
Marshall syndrome
Marshall-Smith syndrome
Mucopolysaccharidoses
Nance-Horan syndrome
Nevoid basal cell carcinoma syndrome (Gorlin)
Oculo-dento-osseous dysplasia
Oro-facio-digital syndrome I
Oro-facio-digital syndrome II
Osteogenesis imperfecta
Osteolysis, familial expansile
Osteopetrosis
Otodental dysplasia
Oto-palato-digital syndrome, type 1
Oto-palato-digital syndrome, type 2
Papillon-Lefèvre syndrome
Prader-Willi syndrome
Progeria
Proteus syndrome
Pseudohypoparathyroidism
Pyle syndrome
Rickets
Rieger syndrome
Robinow syndrome
Rothmund-Thomson syndrome
Rubinstein-Taybi syndrome
Rutherford syndrome
Scleroderma
Sclerosteosis
Seckel syndrome
Short rib-polydactyly syndrome, type I
Singleton-Merten syndrome
Sjögren-Larsson syndrome
Stickler syndrome

Thalidomide embryopathy
Treacher Collins syndrome
Tricho-dento-osseous syndrome
Tricho-odonto-onychial dysplasia
Weill-Marchesani syndrome
Werner syndrome
Weyer acrodental dysostosis
Wildervanck syndrome
Williams syndrome

Floating teeth

Familial dysgammaglobulinemia
Fibrous dysplasia
Gaucher disease
Histiocytosis X
Hyperparathyroidism
Hypophosphatasia
Papillon-Lefèvre syndrome

Malocclusion

Aarskog syndrome
Beckwith-Wiedemann syndrome
Binder syndrome
Cleidocranial dysplasia
FG syndrome
Fibrous dysplasia
Goldenhar syndrome
Mandibuloacral dysplasia
Martsolf syndrome
Mucopolysaccharidoses
Noonan syndrome
Osteodysplasty, Melnick-Needles
Osteodysplasty, precocious
Rieger syndrome
Robinow syndrome
Treacher Collins syndrome
Tricho-rhino-phalangeal syndrome, types 1 and 2
Williams syndrome

Natal teeth[144]

Adrenal hyperplasia, congenital
Chondroectodermal dysplasia
Hallermann-Streiff syndrome
Hypoglossia-hypodactylia syndrome
Jadassohn-Lewandowsky syndrome
Pena-Shokeir syndrome
Robin sequence
Sotos syndrome
Steatocystoma multiplex
Wiedemann-Rautenstrauch syndrome

Premature loss of teeth

Cleidocranial dysplasia
Groll-Hirschowitz syndrome
Hajdu-Cheney syndrome
Hyperphosphatasemia
Hypophosphatasia
Indifference to pain
Jadassohn-Lewandowsky syndrome
Mandibuloacral dysplasia
Papillon-Lefèvre syndrome
Tricho-dento-osseous syndrome
Werner syndrome

MUSCLES

Absent or deficient muscles

Familiar muscular aplasia[165]
Goodman camptodactyly syndrome A
Möbius syndrome
Poland syndrome

Potter syndrome
Prune-belly syndrome

Atrophy of muscles

Arthrogryposis
Camptodactyly-sensorineural hearing loss syndrome

Charcot-Marie-Tooth disease
Duchenne muscular dystrophy
Flynn-Aird syndrome
Freeman-Sheldon syndrome
Glycogen storage disease, type V
Kugelberg-Welander syndrome
Kuskokwim syndrome
Madelung disease
Multiple endocrine neoplasia syndrome, 2b
Myotonic dystrophy
Pancoast syndrome
Progeria
Rieger syndrome
Schwartz-Jampel syndrome
Spinal muscular atrophy
Tethered canus syndrome[197]
Werner syndrome

Diaphragm, abnormal
Beckwith-Wiedemann syndrome
Cantrell syndrome
Ehlers-Danlos syndrome
Familial congenital diaphragmatic defect[54,82]
Fetal hydantoin syndrome
Scimitar syndrome

Hypertonicity
Azorean neurologic disease
Canavan disease
Chromosome 13 trisomy syndrome
Chromosome 18 trisomy syndrome
de Lange syndrome
Fahr syndrome
Freeman-Sheldon syndrome
Fucosidosis
Hypothyroidism (Hoffmann syndrome)
Melorheostosis
Menkes syndrome
Schwartz-Jampel syndrome
Sjögren-Larsson syndrome
Stewart-Bergstrom syndrome
Stiff-man syndrome
Vitamin A intoxication
Weaver-Smith syndrome

Hypotonicity
Achondroplasia
Adducted thumb syndrome
Aluminum intoxication
Börjeson-Forssman-Lehmann syndrome
Canavan syndrome
Cerebro-oculo-facio-skeletal syndrome
Chromosome 13 trisomy syndrome
Chromosome 21 trisomy syndrome
Chromosome 5 partial short-arm deletion
Chromosome XXXXY syndrome
Cohen syndrome
Copper deficiency

Cutis verticis gyrata
Diaphyseal dysplasia (Engelmann)
Fetal alcohol syndrome
FG syndrome
Fukuyama-type muscular dystrophy
Galactosemia
German syndrome
Gerodermia osteodysplastica hereditaria
Glycogenosis, type II
GM_1 gangliosidosis
Hyperparathyroidism (neonatal)
Hypomelanosis of Ito
Hypothyroidism (infant)
Johanson-Blizzard syndrome
Lissencephaly syndrome
Lowe syndrome
Mannosidosis
Marfan syndrome
Marinesco-Sjögren syndrome
Mulibrey nanism
Multiple endocrine neoplasia, type 2b
Myotonic dystrophy
Nemaline myopathy
Osteoporosis-pseudoglioma syndrome
Pallister-Killian syndrome
Prader-Willi syndrome
Rieger syndrome
Smith-Lemli-Opitz syndrome
Spondyloepiphyseal dysplasia congenita
Werdnig-Hoffmann disease
Wrinkly skin syndrome
Zellweger syndrome

Large muscles
Hypothyroidism, adult (Hoffmann syndrome)
Kocher-Debré-Sémélaigne syndrome
Lipodystrophy (lipoatrophic diabetes)
Myhre syndrome

Myopathy
Aluminum intoxication
Carnitine deficiency
Cataract-cerebellar atrophy-mental retardation-myopathy
Glycogenesis, type II, III, V
GM_1 gangliosidosis
Hypothyroidism
MELAS syndrome
Myotubular myopathy
Nemaline myopathy
Rigid spine syndrome
Xanthine oxidase deficiency

Pectoral muscle deficiency
Holt-Oram syndrome
Isolated anomaly
Möbius syndrome
Poland syndrome

NECK

Branchial arch anomalies[46]
Auriculo-osteodysplasty (Beals)
Branchial cleft fistulas
Branchial pits
Branchio-oto-renal syndrome
DiGeorge syndrome
Goldenhar syndrome
Hemangiomatous branchial cleft syndrome
Hypertelorism-microtia-facial clefting (Bixler)
Levy-Hollister syndrome

Microtia-meatal atresia syndrome
Nager syndrome
Oto-facio-cervical syndrome
Postaxial acrofacial dysostosis syndrome (Miller)
Townes-Brocks syndrome

Lymphoid tissue, absence/hypoplasia
Ataxia-telangiectasia
DiGeorge syndrome
Immune disorders

Steroid therapy
Wiskott-Aldrich syndrome

Nuchal cyst[69]

Chromosome 13 trisomy
Chromosome 21 trisomy
Chromosome XO syndrome
Nuchal cyst—edema—cleft palate—short limb[69]
Nuchal cystic hygroma—cleft palate[51]
Pterygium syndrome
Roberts syndrome

Short neck

Aarskog syndrome
Achondrogenesis, type I
Achondrogenesis, type II
Atelosteogenesis
CHARGE association
Chondrodysplasia punctata
Chromosome 18 trisomy syndrome
Chromosome 21 trisomy syndrome
Chromosome XO syndrome
Chromosome XXXXY syndrome
Contractural arachnodactyly
Diamond-Blackfan syndrome
Dyssegmental dwarfism
Fetal alcohol syndrome
Fetal hydantoin syndrome
Fibrochondrogenesis
Freeman-Sheldon syndrome
Fryns syndrome
Hajdu-Cheney syndrome
Hyperphosphatasemia
Jarcho-Levin syndrome
Joubert syndrome
Klippel-Feil syndrome
Kniest syndrome
Kousseff syndrome
Meckel syndrome

Neu-Laxova syndrome
Noonan syndrome
Osteoglophonic dwarfism
Pallister-Killian syndrome
Schwartz-Jampel syndrome
Smith-Lemli-Opitz syndrome
Spondylocostal dysostosis
Spondyloepiphyseal dysplasia congenita
Spondyloepiphyseal dysplasia tarda
Spondylometaphyseal dysplasia (Kozlowski)
The 3-M syndrome
Warfarin embryopathy

Web Neck

Aase syndrome
Acrocephalosyndactyly, Hermann-Opitz type
Bardet-Biedl syndrome
Cerebro-costo-mandibular syndrome
Chromosomal abnormalities (13, 18, XO, XXXX, XXXXY, etc.)
DiGeorge syndrome
Diamond-Blackfan syndrome
Distichiasis-lymphedema syndrome
Fetal alcohol syndrome
Fetal hydantoin syndrome
Fetal primidone syndrome
Fetal trimethadione syndrome
Freeman-Sheldon syndrome
Golden-Lakim syndrome
Hypothyroidism, congenital
Klippel-Feil syndrome
Lenz microphthalmos syndrome
LEOPARD syndrome
Meckel syndrome
Midline cervical webbing/cleft—micrognathia—symphyseal spur
Noonan syndrome
Pterygium syndromes
Rutledge lethal multiple congenital anomaly syndrome

NERVOUS SYSTEM

Brain atrophy

Acanthocytosis-neurologic disease
Acrodermatitis enteropathica
Adrenoleukodystrophy
Angelman syndrome
Aplasia cutis congenita
Ataxia-telangiectasia
Azorean neurologic disease
Biotinidase deficiency
Börjesan-Forssman-Lehmann syndrome
Canavan disease
Cataract—cerebellar atrophy—mental retardation—myopathy
Ceroid lipofuscinosis (neuronal)
Chondrodysplasia punctata
Cushing syndrome
Cystinosis
De Sanctis-Cacchione syndrome
Deprivation dwarfism
Dyke-Davidoff-Masson syndrome
Encephalo-cranio-cutaneous lipomatosis
Epidermal nevus syndrome
Fetal isotretinoin syndrome
Fucosidosis
Galactosemia
Glutaric acidemia
GM$_1$ gangliosidosis

Hallervorden-Spatz disease
HHHH syndrome
Huntington chorea
Hyperammonemia (congenital)
Hypomelanosis of Ito
Incontinentia pigmenti
Krabbe disease
Leigh disease
Lesch-Nyhan syndrome
Lissencephaly
Maple syrup urine disease
Membranous lipodystrophy
Menkes syndrome
Metachromatic leukodystrophy
Mevalonic aciduria
Minamata disease
Ornithine transaminase deficiency
Pick disease
Proteus syndrome
Pyruvate dehydrogenase complex deficiency
Rett syndrome
Reye syndrome
Stiff-man syndrome
Sturge-Weber syndrome
Usher syndrome
Zellweger syndrome

Brain dysgenesis
Achondroplasia
Acrocephalosyndactyly, Apert type
Acrocephalosyndactyly, Pfeiffer type
Acrocephalosyndactyly, Saethre-Chotzen type
Aicardi syndrome
Aminopterin fetopathy
Aplasia cutis congenita
Bobble-head doll syndrome
Cephaloskeletal dysplasia (Taybi-Linder)
Cerebellar hypoplasia and dense bones[229]
Craniotelencephalic dysplasia
de Morsier syndrome
DiGeorge syndrome
Dyssegmental dwarfism
Encephalo-cranio-cutaneous lipomatosis
Epidermal nevus syndrome
Fetal alcohol syndrome
FG syndrome
Fryns syndrome
Fukuyama-type muscular dystrophy
Goldenhar syndrome
Holoprosencephaly
Hydrolethalus syndrome
Hypomelanosis of Ito
Incontinentia pigmenti
Iniencephaly
Jarcho-Levin syndrome
Joubert syndrome
Kallmann syndrome
Kearns-Sayre syndrome
Lissencephaly
Meckel syndrome
Median cleft face syndrome
Miller-Dieker syndrome
Mulibrey nanism
Nephronophthisis-encephalopathy[157]
Neu-Laxova syndrome
Nevoid basal cell carcinoma syndrome (Gorlin)
Oro-facio-digital syndrome I
Oro-facio-digital syndrome II
Porencephaly (familial)
Smith-Lemli-Opitz syndrome
Thanatophoric dysplasia
Walker-Warburg syndrome

Calcification, intracranial
Calcinosis (metastatic calcification)
Carbonic anhydrase II deficiency
Cerebro-oculo-facio-skeletal syndrome
Cockayne syndrome
Diastrophic dysplasia
Encephalo-cranio-cutaneous lipomatosis
Endocrine-moniliasis syndrome
Epidermal nevus syndrome
Fahr syndrome
Familial idiopathic basal ganglia calcification
Fetal cytomegalovirus infection
Fetal herpes simplex infection
Fetal rubella syndrome
Fetal toxoplasmosis infection
Goldenhar syndrome
Hallermann-Streiff syndrome
Homocystinuria
Hypercalcemia, idiopathic
Hyperlipoproteinemia
Hyperparathyroidism
Hypoparathyroidism
Hypopituitarism (anterior lobe)
Hypothyroidism (adult)
Idiopathic lenticular calcification

Infantile familial encephalopathy[199]
Kallmann syndrome
Kearns-Sayre syndrome
Lead intoxication
Lipoid proteinosis
Lipodystrophy (lipotrophic diabetes)
Lissencephaly
Marshall syndrome
Membranous lipodystrophy
Neurocutaneous melanosis sequence
Neurofibromatosis
Nevoid basal cell carcinoma syndrome (Gorlin)
Oculo-dento-osseous dysplasia
Osteopetrosis
Papillon-Lefèvre syndrome
Pelizaeus-Mezbacher disease
Polyglandular autoimmune disease
Porphyria
Progressive familial encephalopathy—basal ganglia calcification
Pseudohypoparathyroidism
Pseudoxanthoma elasticum
Romberg syndrome
Sturge-Weber syndrome
Tuberous sclerosis
Vitamin D intoxication
von Hippel-Lindau syndrome
Weismann-Netter syndrome
Wilson disease

Cerebrovascular malformations[170]
Bannayan-Zonana syndrome
Familial cavernous angioma syndrome
Familial intracranial aneurysm
Hemangiomas
Hereditary arteriovenous malformations
Polycystic kidney disease (autosomal dominant)
Rednu-Osler-Weber syndrome
Telangiectasias
von Hippel-Lindau syndrome

Corpus callosum, agenesis[221]
Acrocallosal syndrome
Acrocephalosyndactyly, Apert type
Aicardi syndrome
Andermann syndrome[3]
Chromosome 18 trisomy syndrome
Chromosome 8 trisomy syndrome
Cogan syndrome
Combined immunodeficiency, bilateral cataract, and hypopigmentation[61]
Dandy-Walker syndrome
de Morsier syndrome
Duplication of hands and feet, multiple joint dislocation, and hypsarrhythmia[211]
Facial anomalies, Robin sequence, and other anomalies[240]
Familial agenesis of the corpus callosum and macrocephaly[257]
Fetal alcohol syndrome
FG syndrome
Joubert syndrome
Lennox Gastaut syndrome
Median cleft face syndrome
Mucolipidosis IV
Neu-Laxova syndrome
Nevoid basal cell carcinoma syndrome (Gorlin)
Oculo-cerebro-cutaneous syndrome
Oro-facio-digital syndrome[20]
Rubinstein-Taybi syndrome
Shapiro syndrome

Cranial nerve paresis or paralysis
Amyloidosis
Behçet syndrome

Cardiofacial syndrome
Claude syndrome
Craniodiaphyseal dysplasia
Craniometaphyseal dysplasia
Dejerine-Sottas syndrome
Diaphyseal dysplasia (Engelmann)
Dysosteosclerosis
Endosteal hyperostosis (van Buchem)
Epidermal nevus syndrome
Garcin syndrome
Gradenigo syndrome
Hajdu-Cheney syndrome
Henoch-Schönlein syndrome
Hyperthyroidism
Jugular foramen syndrome
Kawasaki syndrome
Kearns-Sayre syndrome
Möbius syndrome
Neurocutaneous melanosis sequence
Nevoid basal cell carcinoma syndrome (Gorlin)
Oromandibular-limb hypogenesis syndromes
Osteopathia striata
Osteopetrosis
Paraneoplastic syndromes
Parinaud syndrome
Poland syndrome
Sclerosteosis
Trotter syndrome
Wallenberg syndrome
Wildervanck syndrome

Encephalopathy
Adrenoleukodystrophy
Aluminum intoxication (dialysis dementia)
Behçet syndrome
Binswanger disease[252]
Hemolytic uremic syndrome
Hemophilia
Hyperammonemia
Hypereosinophilic syndrome
Kawasaki syndrome
Lead intoxication
Lennox-Gastaut syndrome
Maple syrup urine disease
MELAS syndrome
Menkes syndrome
Metachondromatic leukodystrophies
Microangiopathic encephalopathy—hearing loss—retinal ateriolar occlusion
Oculo-cerebello-myoclonic syndrome
Progressive familial encephalopathy—basal ganglia calcification
Reye syndrome
Sarcoidosis
Sickle cell anemia
Vitamin B_{12} deficiency
Wilson disease

Hydrocephalus
Aase-Smith syndrome
Achondroplasia
Acrocallosal syndrome
Acrocephalosyndactyly, Apert type
Acrocephalosyndactyly, Pfeiffer type
Acrodysostosis
Aicardi syndrome
Aminopterin fetopathy
Amniopterin-like syndrome without aminopterin
Amniotic band sequence
Aplasia cutis congenita
Arnold-Chiari malformation
Bardet-Biedl syndrome

Biemond syndrome, II
Bobble-head doll syndrome
Caudal dysplasia sequence
Cloverleaf skull
Cockayne syndrome
Craniodiaphyseal dysplasia
Crouzon syndrome
Cystinosis
Dandy-Walker syndrome
Diabetes mellitus (infant born to diabetic mother)
Diencephalic syndrome
Epidermal nevus syndrome
Ethanolaminosis
Farber disease
Fetal alcohol syndrome
Fetal isotretinoin syndrome
Fetal toxoplasmosis infection
Fetal varicella syndrome
Fukuyama-type muscular dystrophy
Huntington chorea
Hydrocephalus (X-linked)
Hydrolethalus syndrome
Incontinentia pigmenti
Kasabach-Merritt syndrome
Klüver-Bucy syndrome
Lissencephaly syndrome
Mannosidosis
Meckel syndrome
Metachromatic leukodystrophies
Mucolipidosis IV
Mucopolysaccharidosis I-H
Mucopolysaccharidosis VI
Mulibrey manism
Neurocutaneous melanosis syndrome
Nevoid basal cell carcinoma syndrome (Gorlin)
Oro-digito-facial syndrome I (Papillon-Leage)
Osteopetrosis
Rieger syndrome
Riley-Day syndrome
Sarcoidosis
Sjögren-Larsson syndrome
Smith-Lemli-Opitz syndrome
Sotos syndrome
Thanatophoric dysplasia
Triploidy
Tuberous sclerosis
Vitamin A intoxication
Zellweger syndrome

Myelopathy, acquired
Adrenomyeloneuropathy
Burning hand syndrome
Calcium phosphate dihydrate deposition disease
Central cord syndrome
Dejerine-Sottas syndrome
Fluorosis
Guillain-Barré syndrome
Kugelberg-Welander syndrome
Mucopolysaccharidosis I-H
Mucopolysaccharidosis I-H/S
Mucopolysaccharidosis VI
Paraneoplastic syndromes
Schwartz-Jampel syndrome

Neuropathy, peripheral
Adrenoleukodystrophy-adrenomyeloneuropathy
Charcot-Marie-Tooth disease
Fetal varicella syndrome
Flynn-Aird syndrome
Fucosidosis
GM_1 gangliosidosis

Groll-Hirschowitz syndrome
Hajdu-Cheney syndrome
Lead intoxication
Oculogastrointestinal muscular dystrophy
POEMS syndrome
Refsum syndrome
Thevenard syndrome
Thyrotoxic periodic paralysis[129]
Vitamin B$_1$ deficiency
Wernicke-Korsakoff syndrome

Paralysis
Adrenoleukodystrophy
Aplasia cutis congenita
Berk-Tabatznik syndrome
Brown-Séquard syndrome
Craniometaphyseal dysplasia
Cross syndrome[76]
Cutis verticis gyrata
Dejerine-Sottas syndrome
Diastrophic dysplasia
Dyke-Davidoff-Masson syndrome
Epidermal nevus syndrome
Goldenhar syndrome
Groll-Hirschowitz syndrome
Hemophilia
Ichthyosis syndromes
Kawasaki syndrome
Kugelberg-Welander syndrome
Mucopolysaccharidosis IV A
Nevoid basal cell carcinoma syndrome (Gorlin)
Steele-Richardson-Olszewski syndrome[142]
Sturge-Weber syndrome
Takayasu arteritis
Tethered conus syndrome[197]

Septum pellucidum, absent[11]
Agenesis of the corpus callosum
Basilar encephalocele
de Morsier syndrome
Holoprosencephaly
Hydrocephalus (chronic, severe)

Porencephaly/hydroanencephaly
Schizencephaly

Stroke[170]
Adrenal mineralcorticoid excess (hypertension)
Amyloidosis
Atrial myxoma (familial)
Behçet syndrome
Cardiac conductive diseases (hereditary)
Cardiomyopathies
Cerebrovascular malformations
Coagulopathies
Defective release of plasminogen activator
Ehlers-Danlos syndrome
Fabry disease
Familial hemiplegic migraine
Familial porencephaly
Factor XII deficiency
Fibromuscular dysplasia (autosomal dominant)
Heparin cofactor II deficiency
Homocystinuria
Kearns-Sayre syndrome
Leigh disease
Lipoprotein metabolic disorders
Man-in-the-barrel syndrome
MELAS syndrome
Mitral valve prolapse
Moyamoya
Neurofibromatosis
Operculum syndrome
Organic acidemia
Platelet disorders
Polycythemia, hereditary
Prekallikrein deficiency
Protein C deficiency
Pseudoxanthoma elasticum
Sickle cell disease, hemoglobin SC disease
Spherocytosis
Sulfate oxidase deficiency
Tuberous sclerosis

RESPIRATORY SYSTEM

Bronchiectasis
Cystic fibrosis
Immotile cilia syndrome
Immune deficiency diseases
Kartagener syndrome
Young syndrome

Larynx, anomaly
Atelosteogenesis
Cardiovocal syndrome
Cerebro-costo-mandibular syndrome
Chondrodysplasia punctata
de la Chapelle syndrome
Diastrophic dysplasia
Epidermolysis bullosa
Fraser syndrome (atresia)
Frontometaphyseal dysplasia
G syndrome
Geleophysic dysplasia
Goldenhar syndrome
Jadassohn-Lewandowsky syndrome
Larsen syndrome
Lipoid proteinosis
Marshall-Smith syndrome
Multiple endocrine neoplasia syndrome, type 2b

Opitz syndrome
Pallister-Hall syndrome
Relapsing polychondritis
Short rib-polydactyly syndrome, type 2 (Majewski)
Thoraco-laryngo-pelvic dysplasia
Velo-cardio-facial syndrome (web)

Larynx, calcification
Adrenogenital syndrome
Chondrodysplasia punctata
Diastrophic dysplasia
Hydrops—ectopic calcification—moth-eaten skeletal dysplasia
Isolated, congenital
Keutel syndrome
Warfarin embryopathy

Pneumothorax, pneumomediastinum
Adult respiratory distress syndrome
Anorexia nervosa
Boerhave syndrome
Cystic fibrosis
Hamman-Rich syndrome
Hemosiderosis, idiopathic pulmonary
Histiocytosis X

Marfan syndrome
Respiratory distress syndrome

Trachea/bronchi calcification
Chondrodysplasia punctata
Isolated, idiopathic
Keutel syndrome
Relapsing polychondritis
Postoperative prosthetic mitral valve replacement[235]
Warfarin embryopathy

Trachea, short[137]
Brevicolis
Congenital heart disease (some)

DiGeorge syndrome
Skeletal dysplasias (some)

Tracheomegaly[256]
Bronchopulmonary dysplasia
Chronic bronchitis
Chronic cigarette smoking
Cystic fibrosis
Ehlers-Danlos syndrome
Emphysema
Immune deficiency diseases
Mourier-Kuhn syndrome[63]
Pulmonary fibrosis, diffuse

SKELETAL SYSTEM

LIMBS
Acro-osteolysis, distal phalangeal erosion
Acrodystrophic neuropathy
Acrogeria
Cleidocranial dysplasia
Dermatomyositis
Diabetes mellitus
Disseminated lipogranulomatosis
Dysosteosclerosis
Ectodermal dysplasia
Ehlers-Danlos syndrome
Epidermolysis bullosa
Familial
Gout
Hajdu-Cheney syndrome
Hyperparathyroidism
Hypertrophic osteoarthropathy
Ichthyosiform erythroderma
Indifference to pain
Lesch-Nyhan syndrome
Lipoid dermatoarthritis
Malabsorption syndrome
Mandibuloacral dysplasia
Mixed connective tissue disease
Neurotropic diseases
Osteomalacia
Osteopetrosis
Osteopoikilosis
Pachydermoperiostosis
Pityriasis rubra[66]
Polymyositis
Porphyria
Progeria
Pseudoxanthoma elasticum
Psoriasis
Pycnodysostosis
Rheumatoid arthritis
Rothmund-Thomson syndrome
Raynaud disease
Reiter syndrome
Sarcoidosis
Scleroderma
Sézary syndrome
Singleton-Merten syndrome
Sjögren syndrome
Syringomyelia
Theverand syndrome
Werner syndrome
Winchester sydrome

Adactyly, digital defects
Acrorenal syndrome (Dieker-Opitz)
Amniotic band sequence

Aplasia cutis congenita
Baller-Gerold syndrome
C syndrome
CHILD syndrome
Chromosome 18 trisomy
Chromosome 21 trisomy syndrome
Chromosome 45 monosomy (XXC−)
Cleft lip and palate, lower lip pits, and limb deficiency defects[133]
de Lange syndrome
EEC syndrome
Fetal hydantoin syndrome
Fetal phenitoin toxicity[117]
Grebe chondrodystrophy
Hypoglossia-hypodactylia syndrome
Keratoderma palmaris et plantaris familiaris (tylosis)
Möbius syndrome
Oculo-dento-osseous dysplasia
Onychonychia and absence and/or hypoplasia of distal phalanges
Oro-facio-digital syndrome I
Oromandibular-limb hypogenesis syndromes
Osteodysplasty, Melnick-Needles (lethal male)
Poland syndrome
Pterygium syndrome
Roberts syndrome
Splenogonadal fusion syndrome
Thalidomide embryopathy
Yunis-Varón syndrome
Zimmerman-Laband syndrome

Amputation (congenital, acquired)
Ainhum
Amniotic band syndrome
Diabetes mellitus
Indifference to pain
Intravascular coagulation (meningococcemia)
Keratoderma palmaris et plantaris familiaris (tylosis)
Lesch-Nyhan syndrome
Scleroderma

Anomalies of limbs, miscellaneous
Amniotic band sequence
C syndrome
CHILD syndrome
Cloverleaf skull, limb anomalies
Cranioectodermal dysplasia
de Lange syndrome
Duane syndrome–upper limb anomalies[179]
Duane/radial dysplasia syndrome
Dupan syndrome
Epidermoid nevus syndrome
Fetal hydantoin syndrome
Fetal trimethadione syndrome
Fetal varicella syndrome

Golden-Lakim syndrome
Goltz syndrome
Hallermann-Streiff syndrome
Holt-Oram syndrome
Humerospinal dysostosis
Hypoglossia-hypodactylia syndrome
Limb duplication—renal agenesis
Mermaid syndrome
Nager syndrome
Nevoid basal cell carcinoma syndrome (Gorlin)
Odontotrichomelic hypohidrotic dysplasia
Ophthalmomandibulomelic dysplasia
Oromandibular-limb hypogenesis syndromes
Potter syndrome
Prune-belly syndrome
Pterygium syndromes
Roberts syndrome
Robin syndrome
Splenogonadal fusion/limb deformity
Tabatznik syndrome
TAR syndrome
Thalidomide embryopathy
Treacher Collins syndrome
Upper limb-cardiovascular syndrome[147]
VATER association
Yunis-Varón syndrome

Arachnodactyly
Antley-Bixler syndrome
Chromosome XYY syndrome
Contractural arachnodactyly
Ehlers-Danlos syndrome
Frontometaphyseal dysplasia
Goodman camptodactyly syndrome B
Homocystinuria
Ichthyosis syndromes
Marden-Walker syndrome
Marfan syndrome
Multiple endocrine neoplasia, type 2b
Myotonic dystrophy
Nevoid basal cell carcinoma syndrome (Gorlin)
Rieger syndrome
Shprintzen-Goldberg syndrome
Sotos syndrome

Bowed tubular bones
Absent tibiae—triphalangeal thumbs—polydactyly
Achondrogenesis, type I
Achondrogenesis, type II
Achondroplasia
Acromesomelic dwarfism
Antley-Bixler syndrome
Blount disease
Boomerang dysplasia
Calvarial doughnut lesions—osteoporosis—dentinogenesis imperfecta
Campomelic dysplasia
Chondroectodermal dysplasia
Cloverleaf skull
Contractural arachnodactyly
de la Chapelle dysplasia
de Lange syndrome
Diabetes (infant born to diabetic mother)
Diastrophic dysplasia
Dyschondrosteosis
Dyssegmental dwarfism
Enchondromatosis
Epidermal nevus syndrome
Familial congenital bowing[95]
Fibrochondrogenesis
Fibrous dysplasia

GM$_1$ gangliosidosis
Grant syndrome
Hemihypertrophy
Homocystinuria
Hydrolethalus syndrome
Hyperparathyroidism
Hyperphosphatasemia
Hypochondroplasia
Hypophosphatasia
Infantile multisystem inflammatory disease
Intrauterine positional deformity
Isolated anomaly
Klippel-Trenaunay syndrome
Koller syndrome
Kyphomelic dysplasia
Larsen syndrome
Maffucci syndrome
Mesomelic dysplasia
Metaphyseal chondrodysplasia (Jansen)
Metaphyseal chondrodysplasia (McKusick)
Metaphyseal chondrodysplasia (Schmid)
Mucolipidoses
Mucopolysaccharidoses
Neurofibromatosis
Occipital horn syndrome
Oligohydramnios
Osteodysplasty, Melnick-Needles
Osteodysplasty, precocious
Osteogenesis imperfecta, all types
Osteolysis with nephropathy
Osteomalacia
Oto-palato-digital syndrome, type 1
Oto-palato-digital syndrome, type 2
Parastremmatic dwarfism
Physiologic bowing of infancy
Pseudoachondroplasia
Pseudoarthrosis
Pseudohypoparathyroidism
Rickets
Schwarz-Lélek syndrome
Serpentine fibula—polycystic kidney[71]
Short rib-polydactyly syndromes
Skeletal dysplasia—"pursed lips"—ectopia lentis[35]
Spondylometaphyseal dysplasia, type Kozlowski
Thanatophoric dysplasia
Weismann-Netter syndrome

Brachydactyly
Aarskog syndrome
Achondrogenesis
Achondroplasia
Acrocallosal syndrome
Acrocephalopolysyndactyly, Carpenter type
Acrocephalopolysyndactyly, Goodman type
Acrocephalopolysyndactyly, Sakati type
Acrocephalosyndactyly, Hermann-Opitz type
Acrocephalosyndactyly, Waardenburg type
Acro-cranio-facial dysostosis
Acrodysostosis
Acrodysostosis and protrusio acetabuli[155]
Acro-fronto-facio-nasal dysostosis
Acromesomelic dysplasia
Acrorenal syndrome (Dieker-Opitz)
Asphyxiating thoracic dysplasia
Atelosteogenesis
Biemond syndrome I
Brachydactyly syndrome, type E
Brachydactyly—ectrodactyly—onchodystrophy[130]
Brachymesophalangy nail dysplasia
C syndrome
Campomelic dysplasia

Cheirolumbar dysostosis[98, 248]
Chondroectodermal dysplasia
Chromosome 13 trisomy syndrome
Chromosome 18 trisomy syndrome
Chromosome 21 trisomy syndrome
Chromosome XXXXX syndrome
Chromosome XXXXY syndrome
Cleidocranial dysplasia
Deafness and metaphyseal dysostosis
Diastrophic dysplasia
DOOR syndrome
Dupan syndrome
Dyssegmental dwarfism
Facioaudiosymphalangism
Fanconi anemia
Fetal alcohol syndrome
Fibrodysplasia ossificans progressiva
Fountain syndrome
Geleophysic dysplasia
Goltz syndrome
Grebe chondrodysplasia
Hand-foot-genital syndrome
Hanhart syndrome
Hirschsprung disease—brachydactyly[200]
Holt-Oram syndrome
Hydrops—ectopic calcification—moth-eaten skeletal dysplsia
Hyperparathyroidism (secondary)
Hyperthyroidism
Hypochondroplasia
Hypoparathyroidism
Hypophosphatasia
Hypothyroidism
Indifference to pain (congenital)
Juberg-Hayward syndrome
Kabuki makeup syndrome
KBG syndrome
Keutel syndrome
Larsen syndrome
Lesch-Nyhan syndrome
Martsoff syndrome
Metaphyseal chondrodysplasia (McKusick)
Metatropic dysplasia
Mitral valve insufficiency—deafness—skeletal malformation
Möbius syndrome
Moore-Federman syndrome
Mucolipidosis II
Mucopolysaccharidoses
Neu-Laxova syndrome
Noonan syndrome
Oculo-dento-osseous dysplasia
Onchonychia and absence and/or hypoplasia of distal phalanges
Opsismodysplasia
Oro-facio-digital syndromes I and II
Osteoglophonic dwarfism
Osteosclerosis, dominant type
Oto-palato-digital syndrome, types 1 and 2
Pallister-Hall syndrome
Patterson syndrome
Peripheral dysostosis (Brailsford)
Poland syndrome
Progeria
Pseudoachondroplasia
Pseudohypoparathyrodism
Pterygium syndrome
Pycnodysostosis
Refsum syndrome
Rieger syndrome
Rothmund-Thomson syndrome
Rubinstein-Taybi syndrome
Rüdiger syndrome
Schneckenbecken

Short rib-polydactyly syndrome, type 1
Short rib-polydactyly syndrome, type 2
Short rib-polydactyly syndrome, type 3
Silver-Russell syndrome
Smith-Lemli-Opitz syndrome
Sorsby syndrome
Spondyloperipheral dysplasia
Spondyloepimetaphyseal dysplasia, Irapa type
Tabatznik syndrome
TAR syndrome
Thanatophoric dysplasia
Tricho-rhino-phalangeal syndrome, types 1 and 2
Tuomaala syndrome
Weill-Marchesani syndrome

Brachymetacarpalia

Acrodysostosis
Acromesomelic dysplasia
Aplasia cutis congenita
Atelosteogenesis
Beckwith-Wiedemann syndrome
Biemond syndrome I
Bilginturan brachydactyly[22]
Brachydactyly A-1[15]
Brachydactyly C[15]
Brachydactyly E[15]
C syndrome
Camptobrachydactyly[68]
Cephaloskeletal dysplasia (Taybi-Linder)
Cheirolumbar dysostosis[98, 248]
Chondrodysplasia punctata
Chromosome 18 trisomy syndrome
Chromosome 5, partial short arm deletion
Chromosome XO syndrome
Cockayne syndrome
Cohen syndrome
Cryptodontic metacarpalia[88]
de Lange syndrome
Deafness and metaphyseal dysostosis
Diastrophic dysplasia
Dyggve-Melchior-Clausen syndrome
Dyschondrosteosis
Dyssegmental dwarfism
Exostoses
Fanconi anemia
Fetal alcohol syndrome
Fibrodysplasia ossificans progressiva
Gorman syndrome[90]
Grebe chondrodysplasia
Hand-foot-genital syndrome
Holt-Oram syndrome
Hypoparathyroidism
Hypothyroidism
Larsen syndrome
Mucolipidosis II
Mucopolysaccharidosis I-H
Mucopolysaccharidosis II
Multiple epiphyseal dysplasia
Myotonic dystrophy
Nevoid basal cell carcinoma syndrome (Gorlin)
Osteoglophonic dwarfism
Otopalatodigital syndrome, type 2
Pallister-Hall syndrome
Pfeiffer-Weber syndrome[188]
Poland syndrome
Pseudohypoparathyroidism
Refsum syndrome
Rothmund-Thomson syndrome
Ruvalcaba syndrome
Short rib-polydactyly syndrome, type 1
Short rib-polydactyly syndrome, type 2

Short rib-polydactyly syndrome, type 3
Silver-Russell syndrome
Sjögren-Larsson syndrome
Sybert syndrome[231]
Tabatznik syndrome
Tricho-rhino-phalangeal syndrome, types 1 and 2
Tuomaala syndrome
Weill-Marchesani syndrome

Brachymetacarpalia, first metacarpal

Acrocraniofacial dysostosis
Cephaloskeletal dysplasia (Taybi-Linder)
de Lange syndrome
Diastrophic dysplasia
Dyssegmental dwarfism
Facio-audio-symphalangism syndrome
Fanconi syndrome
Fibrodysplasia ossificans progressiva
Hand-foot-genital syndrome
IVIC syndrome
Juberg-Hayward syndrome
Oto-palato-digital syndrome, type 2
Radial hypoplasia
Schinzel-Giedion syndrome

Broad metaphyses

Cockayne syndrome
Craniometaphyseal dysplasia
Diastrophic dysplasia
Dysosteosclerosis
Dyssegmental dysplasia
Fibrochondrogenesis
Frontometaphyseal dysplasia
Infantile multisystem inflammatory disease
Kniest dysplasia
Metatropic dysplasia
Oculo-dento-osseous dysplasia
Osteopetrosis
Oto-spondylo-megaepiphyseal dysplasia
Pseudoachondroplasia
Pyle disease
Schwarz-Lélek syndrome
Skeletal dysplasia—"pursed lips"—ectopia lentis[35]
Spondylomegaepiphyseal-metaphyseal dysplasia

Broad tubular bones

Achondrogenesis, type 1
Achondrogenesis, type 2
Chromosome 8 trisomy syndrome
Cleidocranial dysplasia
Craniodiaphyseal dysplasia
Diaphyseal dysplasia—anemia[83]
Diaphyseal dysplasia—proximal myopathy[36]
Diaphyseal dysplasia (Engelmann)
Dyschondrosclerosis
Dyssegmental dwarfism
Endosteal hyperostosis (van Buchem)
Endosteal hyperostosis (Worth)
Fibrogensis imperfecta ossium
Fibrous dysplasia
Gaucher disease
GM$_1$ gangliosidosis
Hyperphosphatasemia
Hypochondrogenesis
Infantile mutlisystem inflammatory disease
Iron deficiency anemia
Kyphomelic dysplasia
Mesomelic dysplasia (Langer)
Mucolipidoses
Mucopolysaccharidoses
Neu-Laxova syndrome
Niemann-Pick disease

Oculo-dento-osseous dysplasia
Opsismodysplasia
Osteogenesis imperfecta, type II
Osteopetrosis
Oto-palato-digital syndrome, type 1
Pachydermoperiostosis
Pleonosteosis
Pyle disease
Schwarz-Lélek syndrome
Singleton-Merten syndrome
Thalassemia
Thanatophoric dysplasia
Weissenbacher-Zweymüller syndrome

Calcaneus: multiple ossification centers, stippled calcification

Chondrodysplasia punctata, Sheffield type
Chromosome 21 trisomy syndrome
GM$_1$ gangliosidosis
Larsen syndrome
Mucolipidosis II

Camptodactyly[207]

Aarskog syndrome
Acro-fronto-facio-nasal dysostosis syndrome
Acrocephalopolysyndactyly, Goodman type
Adducted thumb syndrome (Christian)
Antley-Bixler syndrome
Camptobrachydactyly[68]
Camptodactyly—ichthyosis syndrome (Windmill vane camptodactyly)
Camptodactyly—joint contracture—facial anomalies—skeletal defects[207]
Camptodactyly—sensorineural hearing loss
Cerebro-oculo-facio-skeletal syndrome
Chromosomal abnormalities (8, 13, 18, 21, etc.)
Contractural arachnodactyly
Craniofrontal dysplasia
Distal arthrogryposis[97]
Distal symphalangism with camptodactyly
Familial camptodactyly-scoliosis[9]
Fetal alcohol syndrome
Freeman-Sheldon syndrome
Fryns syndrome
Golden-Lakim syndrome
Goltz syndrome
Goodman camptodactyly syndrome A
Goodman camptodactyly syndrome B
Gordon syndrome
Grebe chondrodysplasia
Greig cephalopolysyndactyly syndrome
Guadalajara camptodactyly
Holt-Oram syndrome
Jarcho-Levin syndrome
Klein-Waardenberg syndrome
Kuskokwim syndrome
Lenz microphthalmia syndrome
Marden-Walker syndrome
Marfan syndrome
Meckel syndrome
Nail-patella syndrome
Neu-Laxova syndrome
Oculo-dento-osseous dysplasia
Ophthalmomandibulomelic dysplasia
Oro-facio-digital syndrome I
Pena-Shokeir syndrome I, II
Pericarditis-arthritis-camptodactyly
Poland syndrome
Pterygium syndrome
Roberts syndrome
Tel-Hashomer camptodactyly

Triploidy
Trismus-pseudocamptodactyly (Hecht,, 1968)
W syndrome
Weaver-Smith syndrome
Williams syndrome
Zellweger syndrome

Carpal fusion
Acro-fronto-facio-nasal dysostosis
Acrocallosal syndrome
Acrocephalosyndactyly, Apert type
Acromegaly
Arthrogryposis
Baller-Gerold syndrome
Chondroectodermal dysplasia
Chromosome XO syndrome
Diastrophic dysplasia
Dyschondrosteosis
EEC syndrome
F syndrome
Facio-audio-symphalangism syndrome
Fetal alcohol syndrome
Frontometaphyseal dysplasia
Hand-foot-genital syndrome
Holt-Oram syndrome
IVIC syndrome
Keratoderma palmaris et plantaris familiaris (tylosis)
Klein-Waardenberg syndrome
Kniest dysplasia
LEOPARD syndrome
Liebenberg syndrome[148]
"Long-thumb" brachydactyly syndrome[109]
Mesomelic dysplasia, Nievergelt
Mitral valve insufficiency—deafness—skeletal malformation
Multiple synostosis syndrome
Occipital horn syndrome
Oto-palato-digital syndrome, type 1
Reflex sympathetic dystrophy
Rothmund-Thomson syndrome
Scleroderma
Spondyloepimetaphyseal dysplasia, Irapa
Stickler syndrome
Thalidomide embryopathy
Townes-Brocks syndrome

Clinodactyly
Aarskog syndrome
Acrocephalopolysyndactyly, Carpenter type
Acrocephalopolysyndactyly, Goodman type
Acrocephalosyndactyly, Saethre-Chotzen type
Aminopterin embryopathy
Ankylosed teeth-clinodactyly
Bardet-Biedl syndrome
Bloom syndrome
Brachydactyly A-1, A-2, A-3, C
Camptomelic dysplasia
Cephaloskeletal dysplasia (Taybi-Linder)
Cerebro-costo-mandibular syndrome
Chromsomal abnormalities (13, 18, 21, etc.)
Cohen syndrome
Cranio-fronto-nasal dysplasia
Cranio-fronto-nasal dysplasia-like syndrome
de Lange syndrome
DOOR syndrome
Dubowitz syndrome
EEC syndrome
Ehlers-Danlos syndrome
Fanconi anemia
Fetal alcohol syndrome
Fibrochondrogenesis
Fibrodysplasia ossificans progressiva

Fillippi syndrome
Goltz syndrome
Hand-foot-genital syndrome
Holt-Oram syndrome
Hypomelanosis of Ito
Kabuki make-up syndrome
Lenz microphthalmia syndrome
Lissencephaly (Miller-Dieker syndrome)
"Long thumb" brachydactyly syndrome[109]
Marfan syndrome
Meckel syndrome
Mesomelic dysplasia, Nievergelt
Myotonic dystrophy
Nail-patella syndrome
Naso-digito-acoustic syndrome
Noonan syndrome
Oculo-dento-osseous dysplasia
Oro-facio-digital syndrome I
Oro-facio-digital syndrome II
Osteo-onychodysplasia
Oto-palato-digital syndrome, type I
Poland syndrome
Prader-Willi syndrome
Pterygium syndrome
Rieger syndrome
Roberts syndrome
Robinow syndrome
Rubinstein-Taybi syndrome
Ruvalcaba syndrome
Seckel syndrome
Sensenbrenner syndrome
Shwachman syndrome
Silver-Russell syndrome
TAR syndrome
Treacher Collins syndrome
Tricho-rhino-phalangeal dysplasia, types 1 and 2
Triploidy
Weill-Marchesani syndrome
Williams syndrome
Zellweger syndrome

Club foot, metatarsus adductus
Aarskog syndrome
Aminopterin fetopathy
Amniotic band sequence
Arthrogryposis
Bloom syndrome
Campomelic dysplasia
Caudal regression syndrome
Cephaloskeletal dysplasia (Taybi-Linder)
Chondrodysplasia punctata
Chromosomal abnormalities
de Lange syndrome
Diastrophic dysplasia
Dubowitz syndrome
Ehlers-Danlos syndrome
Femoral-facial syndrome
Fetal valproate syndrome
Freeman-Sheldon syndrome
Gardner-Silengo-Wachtel syndrome
Hecht syndrome (trismus pseudocamptodactyly)
Homocystinuria
Humerospinal dysostosis
Kuskokwim syndrome
Larsen syndrome
Marinesco-Sjögren syndrome
Meckel syndrome
Mietens-Weber syndrome
Möbius syndrome
Mucopolysaccharidoses
Myotonic dystrophy

Nager syndrome
Nail-patella syndrome
Noonan syndrome
Pena-Shokeir syndrome
Potter syndrome
Pterygium syndrome
Roberts syndrome
Schinzel-Giedion syndrome
Schwartz-Jampel syndrome
Seckel syndrome
Smith-Lemli-Opitz syndrome
Waardenburg anophthalmia syndrome
Zellweger syndrome

Clubbing of digits
Acromegaly
Aplasia cutis congenita
Cronkhite-Canada syndrome
Cystic fibrosis
Hajdu-Cheney syndrome
Hamman-Rich syndrome
Hyperthyroidism
Hypertrophic osteoarthropathy
Hypothyroidism (myxedema)
Immotile cilia syndrome
Larsen syndrome
Osteoarthropathy, familial idiopathic (Currarino)
Pachydermoperiostosis
POEMS syndrome
Polycythemia
Primary hypertrophic osteoarthropathy[62]
Rendu-Osler-Weber syndrome
Seckel syndrome
Sprue

Cone-shaped epiphysis
Achondrophasia
Acrocephalosyndactyly, Apert type
Acrodysostosis
Acrodysplasia with retinitis pigmentosa and nephropathy (Saldino-Mainzer)
Acromesomelic dysplasia
Anorchia and cone-shaped epiphyses[210]
Asphyxiating thoracic dysplasia
Beckwith-Wiedemann syndrome
Bilginturan syndrome[22]
Brachydactyly syndrome, type E
Chondrodysplasia punctata
Chondroectodermal dysplasia
Christian syndrome[44]
Cleidocranial dysplasia
Cockayne syndrome
DOOR syndrome
Dyggve-Melchior-Clausen syndrome
Hyperthyroidism
Hypochondroplasia
Kashin-Beck disease[172]
Metaphyseal chondrodysplasia (McKusick)
Metaphyseal chondrodysplasia, type Jansen
Multiple epiphyseal dysplasia
Oro-facio-digital syndrome I
Osteoglophonic dysplasia
Osteopetrosis
Oto-palato-digital syndrome, type I
Peripheral dysostosis
Pseudoachondroplasia
Pseudohypoparathyroidism
Rualcaba syndrome
Seckel syndrome
Spondyloepiphyseal dysplasia
Tricho-rhino-phalangeal syndrome types 1 and 2

Vitamin A intoxication, chronic
Wedge-shaped epiphyses of the knees[16]
Weill-Marchesani syndrome

Contracture or joint stiffness
Aarskog syndrome
Aase-Smith syndrome
Acrocephalosyndactyly, Apert type
Acrocephalosyndactyly, Waardenburg type
Addison disease
Adducted thumb syndrome
Amyloidosis
Aplasia cutis congenita
Arthrogryposis—advanced skeletal maturation—unusual facies
Camptodactyly-ichthyosis syndrome
Cerebro-oculo-facio-skeletal syndrome
Chondroplasia ounctata
Chromosomal abnormalities (13, 18, XXXXY, etc.)
Chromosome 8 trisomy syndrome
Contractural arachnodactyly
Cockayne syndrome
de Lange syndrome
Dyschondrosteosis
Dysplasia epiphysealis hemimelica
Dyssegmented dysplasia
Dermo-chondro-corneal dystrophy of François
Diabetes mellitus
Diastrophic dysplasia
Digitotalar dysmorphism
Duchenne muscular dystrophy
Dyggve-Melchior-Clausen syndrome
Exostoses
Epidermolysis bullosa dystrophica
Fabry disease
Farber syndrome
Femoral-facial syndrome
Fetal alcohol syndrome
Fibrodysplasia ossificans progressiva
Fluorosis
Flynn-Aird syndrome
Freeman-Sheldon syndrome
Frontometaphyseal dysplasia
GM_1 gangliosidosis
German syndrome
Golden-Lakim syndrome
Goodman captodactyly syndrome B
Gordon syndrome
Hemophilia
Infantile multisystem inflammatory disease
Klein-Waardenburg syndrome
Kniest dysplasia
Kuskokwim syndrome
Kyphomelic dysplasia
Macrodystrophia lipomatosa
Mandibuloacral dysplasia
Marden-Walker syndrome
Melorheostosis
Metatropic dysplasia
Mietens-Weber syndrome
Moore-Federman syndrome
Mucolipidoses, mucopolysaccharidoses
Multiple epiphyseal dysplasia
Multiple synostosis syndrome
Myhre syndrome[224]
Nail-patella syndrome
Pachydermoperiostosis
Parastremmatic drawfism
Pelvic dysplasia—arthrogrypotic lower limbs
Pleonsoteosis (Léri)
Progeria
Progressive pseudorheumatoid chondroplasia

Psuedoachondroplasia
Pseudodiastrophic dysplasia
Pterygium syndromes
Rigid spine syndrome
Rutledge lethal congenital anomaly syndrome
Scleroderma
Schwartz-Jampel syndrome
Seckel syndrome
Shpritzen-Goldberg-syndrome
Sjögren-Larsson syndrome
Spondyloepiphyseal dysplasia
Spondylometaphyseal dysplasia
Stewart-Bergstrom syndrome
Stickler syndrome
Symphalangism surdity syndrome
Trismus pseudocamptodactyly syndrome (Hecht)
Tumoral calcinosis
Weill-Marchesani syndrome
Winchester syndrome
Zellweger syndrome

Cortical hyperostosis, thickening
Acromegaly
Anderson syndrome
Battered child syndrome
Bowed tubular bones
Caffey disease
Craniodiaphyseal dysplasia
Dentino-osseous dysplasia
Desmoid syndrome
Diaphyseal dysplasia (Engelmann)
Diaphyseal dysplasia—proximal myopathy[36]
Diaphyseal medullary stenosis—bone malignancy—Hardcastle
Distal osteosclerosis
Dubowitz syndrome
Endosteal hyperostosis (van Buchem)
Endosteal hyperostosis (Worth)
Erdheim-Chester disease
Fibrous dysplasia
Frontometaphyseal dysplasia
Gaucher disease
Gigantism
Histiocytosis
Hyperostosis generalisata with striation of the bones
Hyperostosis and hyperphosphatemia
Hyperparathyroidism
Hyperphosphatasia
Hypertrophic osteoarthropathy
Hypothyroidism
Koller syndrome
Klippel-Trenaunay-Weber syndrome
Lenz-Majewski hyperostotic dwarfism
Mannosidosis
McCune-Albright syndrome
Melorheostosis
Neurofibromatosis (hemorrhage)
Normal (neonatal)
Osteoarthropathy, familial idiopathic (Currarino)
Osteosclerosis, dominant-type, Stanescu
Pachydermoperiostosis
Pancreatitis
Prostaglandin-induced periostitis
Pycnodysostosis
Rickets
Scurvy
Sickle cell anemia
Thickened cortical bone and congenital neutropenia
Tricho-dento-osseous syndrome
Tuberous sclerosis
Tubular stenosis syndrome (Kenny-Caffey)
Tumoral calcinosis

Vitamin A intoxication
Vitamin D intoxication
Weismann-Netter syndrome

Cortical thinning
Anemias
Craniodiaphyseal dysplasia
Fibrogenesis imperfecta ossium
Fibrous dysplasia
GM_1 gangliosidosis
Hyperphosphatasemia
Membranous lipodystrophy
Niemann-Pick disease
Osteogenesis imperfecta, all types
Osteoporosis, various types and etiologies
Singleton-Merten syndrome
Stickler syndrome
Winchester syndrome

Coxa valga
Acrocephalopolysyndactyly, Carpenter syndrome
Archard syndrome
Arthrogryposis
Bencze syndrome
Caudal regression syndrome
Chromosome XO syndrome
Chromosome XXXXY syndrome
Cleidocranial dysplasia
Coffin-Lowry syndrome
Dyschondrosteosis
Dysplasia epiphysealis hemimelica
Frontometaphyseal dysplasia
Fucosidosis
Hypertrichosis-osteochondrodysplasia
Mannosidosis
Metaphyseal—sella turcica dysplasia—Rosenberg
Mucopolysaccharidoses
Muscular dystrophies
Myositis ossificans progressiva
Occipital horn syndrome
Ophthalmo-mandibulo-melic dysplasia
Osteodysplasty, Melnick-Needles
Osteopetrosis
Oto-palato-digital syndrome, type I
Prader-Willi syndrome
Progeria
Pseudohypoparathyroidism
Pycnodysostosis
Pyle disease
Schwartz-Jampel syndrome
Spondyloepiphyseal dysplasia-joint laxity
Stickler syndrome

Coxa vara
Achondroplasia
Arthrogryposis
Cleidocranial dysostosis
Diastrophic dysplasia
Dyggve-Melchior-Clausen syndrome
Enchondromatosis (Ollier)
Femoral-facial syndrome
Fibrous dysplasia
Frontometaphyseal dysplasia
Hyperparathyroidism
Hyperphosphatasemia
Hypophosphatasia
Hypothyroidism
Idiopathic
Kniest dysplasia
Legg-Calvé-Perthes disease
Metaphyseal chondrodysplasias
Metatropic dysplasia

Meyer dysplasia of femoral head
Multiple epiphyseal dysplasia
Osteogenesis imperfecta
Osteomalacia
Osteopetrosis
Patella aplasia—coxa vara-tassal synostosis
Pseudoachondroplastic dysplasia
Pseudohypoparathyroidism
Rickets
Schwartz-Jampel syndrome
Shwachman syndrome
Spondyloepimetaphyseal dysplasia—Irapa
Spondyloepimetaphyseal dysplasia—Strudwick
Spondyloepiphyseal dysplasia congenita
Spondyloepiphyseal dysplasia tarda
Spondylometaphyseal dysplasia—Kozlowski

Cubitus valgus
Chromosome 22 trisomy syndrome
Chromosome XO syndrome
Dyschondrosteosis
Pleoneostosis
Zellweger syndrome

Dactylitis
Chronic granulomatous disease of childhood
Phalangeal microgeodic syndrome
Sarcoidosis
Sickle cell disease

Dislocation, subluxation
Aminopterin fetopathy
Amyoplasia congenita
Arthrogryposis
Auriculo-osteodysplasia syndrome (Beals)
Campomelic dysplasia
Cat-eye syndrome
Chondrodysplasia punctata
Chromosomal abnormalities (21, XO, etc.)
Coffin-Siris syndrome
Cutis laxa
Dermo-chondro-corneal dystrophy of François
Diastrophic dysplasia
Dyschondrosteosis
Ehlers-Danlos syndrome
Fetal hydantoin syndrome
Fetal trimethadione syndrome
Fanconi anemia
Freeman-Sheldon syndrome
Frontometaphyseal dysplasia
Hajdu-Cheney syndrome
Humerospinal dysostosis
Keratoderma palmaris et plantaris familiaris (tylosis)
Larsen syndrome
Lenz-Majewski hyperostosis syndrome
Marfan syndrome
Mesomelic dysplasia (Werner)
Mucopolysaccharidoses
Nager syndrome
Nail-patella syndrome
Neurofibromatosis
Oculo-dento-osseous syndrome
Osteodysplasty, Melnick-Needles
Osteogenesis imperfecta, type I
Oto-palato-digital syndrome, type I
Oto-palato-digital syndrome, type II
Pallister-Hall syndrome
Pallister-Killian syndrome
Potter syndrome
Pterygium syndromes
Riley-Day syndrome
Robinow syndrome
Schwartz-Jampel syndrome

Seckel syndrome
Smith-Lemli-Opitz syndrome
Spondyloepimetaphyseal dysplasia
Spondyloepiphyseal dysplasia congenita
Stickler syndrome
TAR syndrome
Thevenard syndrome
Tricho-rhino-phalangeal dysplasia, type 2

Dumbbell-shaped tubular bones
Diastrophic dysplasia
Dissegmental dysplasia
Fibrochondrogenesis
Kniest dysplasia
Metatropic dysplasia
Oto-spondylo-megaepiphyseal dysplasia
Pseudoachondroplasia, severe form
Weissenbacher-Zweymüller syndrome

Dysostosis multiplex
Fucosidosis
Galactosialidosis
Mannosidosis
Mucolipidosis II
Mucolipidosis III
Mucopolysaccharidosis I-H
Mucopolysaccharidosis I-H/S
Mucopolysaccharidosis II
Mucopolysaccharidosis VII
Sialidosis

Elbow, dislocation
Aase-Smith syndrome
Acro-osteolysis, familial idiopathic
Acromesomelic dysplasia
Aminopterin fetopathy
Auriculo-osteodysplasia
C syndrome
Campomelic dysplasia
Cerebro-costo-mandibular syndrome
Chromosome 49 XXXXX syndrome
Chromosome XXXXY syndrome
Cloverleaf skull
Coffin-Siris syndrome
Congenital, isolated anomaly
Crouzon syndrome
Cutis laxa
de Lange syndrome
Dyschondrosteosis
Exostosis (multiple cartilaginous)
Familial dislocation of radial head[45]
Fanconi anemia
Frontometaphyseal dysplasia
Humerospinal dysostosis
Larsen syndrome
Mietens-Weber syndrome
Multiple epiphyseal dysplasia
Multiple synostosis syndrome
Nail-patella syndrome
Neurofibromatosis
Nievergelt syndrome
Noonan syndrome
Occipital horn syndrome
Ophthalmomandibulomelic dysplasia
Oto-palato-digital syndrome, type I
Oto-palato-digital syndrome, type II
Seckel syndrome
Spondyloepimetaphyseal dysplasia with joint laxity
W syndrome

Epiphysis, aseptic necrosis
Battered child syndrome
Cushing syndrome

Diabetes mellitus
Fabry disease
Gaucher syndrome
Gout
Hemophilia
Histiocytosis X
Hyperlipoproteinemia
Hypothyroidism
Meyer dysplasia of femoral head
Osteochondroses
Polycythemia vera
Sickle cell anemia
Steroid therapy
Tricho-rhino-phalangeal dysplasia, type 1
Winchester syndrome

Epiphysis, dense, sclerotic, ivory
Chromosome 21 trisomy syndrome
Cockayne syndrome
Coffin-Lowry syndrome
Coffin-Siris syndrome
Deprivation dwarfism
Dyggve-Melchior-Clausen syndrome
Homocystinuria
Hypercalcemia, idiopathic
Hypopituitarism
Hypothyroidism
Isolated phalangeal ivory epiphysis
Mucopolysaccharidosis IV A (Morquio)
Multiple epiphyseal dysplasia (Fairbank)
Renal osteodystrophy
Robinow syndrome
Seckel syndrome
Silver-Russell syndrome
Spondyloepiphyseal dysplasia
Stickler syndrome
Thiemann disease
Tricho-rhino-phalangeal syndrome, type 1

Epiphysis, large (megaepiphysis)
Hemophilia
Infantile multisystem inflammatory disease
Megepiphyseal dwarfism[89]
Osteoporosis-macroepiphyseal dysplasia[162]
Oto-spondylo-megaepiphyseal dysplasia
Spondyloepiphyseal dysplasia with macroepiphyses[126]
Spondylomegaepiphyseal-metaphyseal dysplasia (Silverman-Riley)

Epiphysis, premature fusion
Chromosome XO syndrome
Clinodactyly
Hyperthyroidism
Madelung deformity
Precocious puberty
Pseudohypoparathyroidism
Thalassemia
Tricho-rhino-phalangeal syndrome, type 1

Epiphysis, stippled or fragmented (children)
Deaf mutism−goiter−euthyroidism syndrome
DeBarsy syndrome (Cutis laxa−corneal clouding−mental retardation)
Dysplasia epiphysealis hemimelica
Homocystinuria
Hypopituitarism
Hypothyroidism
Kniest dysplasia
Meyer dysplasia of femoral head[246]
Mucolipidoses
Mucopolysaccharidoses
Multiple epiphyseal dysplasia
Osteochondroses

Osteopathia striata
Osteopetrosis
Osteopoikilosis
Smith-Lemli-Opitz syndrome
Spondyloepiphyseal dysplasia
Winchester syndrome
Wolcott-Rallison syndrome

Erlenmeyer flask deformity of metaphysis
Craniometaphyseal dysplasia
Dysosteosclerosis
Frontometaphyseal dysplasia
Gaucher disease
Hypertrichosis-osteochondrodysplasia
Lead poisoning, sequela
Membranous lipodystrophy
Niemann-Pick disease
Osteodysplasty, Melnick-Needles
Osteopetrosis
Oto-palato-digital syndrome, type I
Pyle disease
Schwarz-Lélek syndrome
Thalassemia

Femoral head, early ossification
Asphyxiating thoracic dysplasia
Chondroectodermal dysplasia
Short rib-polydactyly syndrome, type I (Saldino-Noonan)

Femoral head, flat and/or fragmented
Achondroplasia
Aseptic necrosis
Behçet syndrome
Chondrodysplasia punctata
Cushing disease
Diabetes mellitus
Diastrophic dysplasia
Enchondromatosis (Ollier)
Gaucher disease
Hemophilia
Histiocytosis X
Hypothyroidism
Legg-Calvé-Perthes disease
Meyer dysplasia of femoral head[246]
Mucopolysaccharidoses
Multipel endocrine neoplasia syndrome 2b
Renal osteodystrophy
Rickets
Sickle cell disease
Stickler syndrome
Thalassemia
Tricho-rhino-phalangeal syndrome, types 1 and 2
Winchester syndrome

Femoral head, slipped[161]
Acromegaly
Adiposogenital syndrome
Chemotherapeutic agents
Chorionic gonadotropin therapy
Chromosome 21 trisomy syndrome
Chromosome XXY syndrome (Klinefelter)
Coxa vara
Cushing syndrome (steroid therapy)
Gaucher disease
Gigantism
Growth hormone deficiency[198]
Growth hormone therapy
Hemosiderosis-panhypopituitarism
Hemophilia
Hyperparathyroidism
Hypoesterogenic states
Hypothyroidism

Idiopathic
Metaphyseal chondrodysplasia
Obesity
Pituitary tumors
Pseudohypoparathyroidism
Radiation therapy
Renal osteodystrophy
Rickets
Scurvy
Zellweger syndrome

Fibular defect (aplasia, hypoplasia, short)
Absent fibula-craniosynostosis[151]
Acrofrontofacionasal dysostosis syndrome
Campomelic dysplasia
Chondroectodermal dysplasia
Chromosomal abnormalities
de la Chapelle syndrome
Du Pan syndrome
Facio-auriculo-radial dysplasia
Femur-fibula-ulna syndrome
Limb deficiency—heart malformation syndrome[103]
Mietens-Weber syndrome
Ophthalmomandibulomelic dysplasia
Oto-onycho-peroneal syndrome
Polydactyly, syndactyly, and oligodactyly, aplasia or hypoplasia of fibula, hypoplasia of pelvis and bowing of femora
Seckel syndrome
Weyers syndrome (deficiency of ulnar and fibular rays)

Genu valgum
Achondroplasia
Acrocephalopolysyndactyly, Carpenter type
Bardet-Biedl syndrome
Chondrodysplasia punctata
Chondroectodermal dysplasia
Cohen syndrome
Diaphyseal dysplasia (Englemann)
Dyschondrosteosis
Hajdu-Cheney syndrome
Hypophosphatasia
Metaphyseal chondrodysplasias
Mucopolysaccharidoses
Multiple epiphyseal dysplasia
Nail-patella syndrome
Parastremmatic dwarfism
Physiologic
Pyle disease
Rickets
Spondyloepimetaphyseal dysplasia, Strudwick
Spondyloepiphyseal dysplasia

Genu varum
Blount disease
Campomelic dysplasia
Chromosome XO syndrome
Osteogenesis imperfecta
Rickets
Physiologic

Hand and foot, short/stubby
Aarskog syndrome
Achondrogenesis
Achondroplasia
Acrodysostosis
Acromesomelic dysplasia
Acro-osteolysis
Asphyxiating thoracic dysplasia
Börjeson-Forssman-Lehmann syndrome
Cephaloskeletal dysplasia (Taybi-Linder)
Chondroectodermal dysplasia
Chromosomal abnormalities (21, fragile X, etc.)

Cockayne syndrome
Diastrophic dysplasia
Enchondromatosis (Ollier)
Exostoses
Fountain syndrome
Hypochondroplasia
Hypopituitarism
Kabuki make-up syndrome
Metaphyseal chondrodysplasias
Metatropic dysplasia
Mucolipidoses
Mucopolysaccharidoses
Multiple epiphyseal dysplasia
Noonan syndrome
Oro-facio-digital syndrome I, II
Peripheral dysostosis
Pleonostosis (Léri)
Prader-Willi syndrome
Progeria
Pseudoachondroplasia
Pseudohypoparathyroidism
Ruvalcaba syndrome
Smith-Lemli-Opitz syndrome
Spondyloepimetaphyseal dysplasia
Spondylometaphyseal dysplasia
Tricho-rhino-phalangeal syndrome, types 1 and 2
Weill-Marchesani syndrome

Hand, large
Acromegaly
Beckwith-Wiedemann syndrome
Coffin-Lowry syndrome
Frontometaphyseal dysplasia
Gigantism
Hyperthyroidism
Kirghizian dermato-osteolysis
Lipodystrophy (lipoatrophic diabetes)
Marfan syndrome
Pachydermoperiostosis
Patterson syndrome
Precocious puberty
Sotos syndrome
Stickler syndrome
Wiedemann-Rautenstrauch syndrome

Hand, ulnar deviation
Digitotalar dysmorphism (ulnar drift)
Distal arthrogryposis[97]
Freeman-Sheldon syndrome
Metacarpotalar syndrome[7]

Hip, dislocation or subluxation
Aminopterin fetopathy
Auriculo-osteodysplasia syndrome
C syndrome
Campomelic dysplasia
Caudal dysplasia sequence
Cerebro-oculo-facio-skeletal syndrome
Cerebro-costo-mandibular syndrome
Chondrodysplasia punctata
Cloverleaf skull
Cutis laxa
Cutis laxa—growth deficiency syndrome
Ehlers-Danlos syndrome
Fanconi anemia
Farber syndrome
Fibrodysplasia ossificans progressiva
Gerodermia osteodysplastica hereditaria
Hallermann-Strieff syndrome
Indifference to pain (congenital)
Kniest dysplasia
Larsen syndrome

Limb/pelvis—hypoplasia/apalasia syndrome[196]
Marfan syndrome
Metacarpotalar syndrome[7]
Möbius syndrome
Mucolipidosis II
Mucopolysaccharidosis I-H
Nager syndrome
Oto-palato-digital syndrome, type I
Poland syndrome
Prader-Willi syndrome
Prune-belly syndrome
Rieger syndrome
Riley-Day syndrome
Silver-Russell syndrome
Spondyloepimetaphyseal dysplasia—joint laxity
Thalidomide embryopathy

Joint, ankylosis
Acrocephalosyndactyly, Apert type
Fibrodysplasia ossificans progressiva
Hemophilia
Mixed connective tissue disease
Osteogenesis imperfecta
Pena-Shokeir syndrome
Slceroderma
Winchester syndrome

Joints, degenerative changes
Acromegaly
Diabetes mellitus
Dyschondrosteosis
Fibrogenesis imperfecta ossium
Gaucher disease
Indifference to pain (congenital)
Lipoid dermatoarthritis
Macrodystrophia lipomatosa
Mediterranean fever
Metaphyseal chondrodysplasia (Schmid)
Multiple epiphyseal dysplasia
Osteogenesis imperfecta
Relapsing polychondritis
Riley-Day syndrome
Scleroderma
Thevenard syndrome

Joint laxity, hypermobility
Aarskog syndrome
Achard syndrome
Bannayan syndrome
Börjeson-Forssman-Lehmann syndrome
Chromosome 21 trisomy syndrome
Chromosome XXXXY syndrome
Coffin-Lowry syndrome
Coffin-Siris syndrome
Cohen syndrome
Cutis laxa
Cutis laxa—growth deficiency syndrome
Deafness and metaphyseal dysostosis
Ehlers-Danlos syndrome
FG syndrome
Gerodermia osteodysplastica hereditaria
Goltz syndrome
Hajdu-Cheney syndrome
Hallermann-Streiff syndrome
Hypermobility syndrome
Hypochondroplasia
Johanson-Blizzard syndrome
Joint laxity-idiopathic scoliosis[23]
Larsen syndrome
Lenz-Majewski hyperostatic dwarfism
LEOPARD syndrome
Lowe syndrome

Marfan syndrome
Marfanoid hypermobility syndrome
Megaepiphyseal dysplasia—wrinkled skin—aged appearance[162]
Metaphyseal chondrodysplasia, McKusick
Metatropic dysplasia
Mitral valve prolapse
Mucopolysaccharidosis IV A (Morquio)
Multiple endocrine neoplasia, type 2b
Nail-patella syndrome
Osteogenesis imperfecta
Osteoporosis-pseudoglioma syndrome
Pallister-Killian syndrome
Pseudoachondroplasia
Robinow syndrome
Rubinstein-Taybi syndrome
Seckel syndrome
Spondyloepimetaphyseal dysplasia—joint laxity
Spondyloepiphyseal dysplasia
Stickler syndrome
The 3-M syndrome
Tricho-rhino-phalangeal dysplasia, type 2
Velo-cardio-facial syndrome
Wrinkly skin syndrome
Zimmermann-Leband syndrome

Limb overgrowth
Hemangiomas
Hemihypertrophy
Klippel-Trenaunay syndrome
Lymphangioma
Macrodystrophia lipomatosa
Maffucci syndrome
Neurofibromatosis
Proteus syndrome
Sturge-Weber syndrome
Tuberous sclerosis
von Hippel-Lindau syndrome

Limb reduction
Acheiropody (Brazil type)
Aminopterin embryopathy
Amniotic band syndrome
Atelosteogenesis
CHILD syndrome
de Lange syndrome
EEC syndrome
Fetal varicella syndrome
Goltz syndrome
Grebe chondrodysplasia
Limb/pelvis—hypoplasia/aplasia syndrome[196]
Mermaid syndrome
Oromandibular-limb hypogenesis
Poland syndrome
Postaxial acrofacial dysostosis syndrome (Miller)
Prune-belly syndrome
Pterygium syndrome (popliteal)
Roberts syndrome
TAR syndrome
Tetra-amelia-multiple malformations[259]

Macrodactyly
Enchondromatosis (Ollier)
Fibrous dysplasia
Hemangioma
Klippel-Trenaunay-Weber syndrome
Lymphangioma
Macrodystrophia lipomatosa
Maffucci syndrome
Melorrheostosis
Neurofibromatosis
Plexiform neuroma
Proteus syndrome

Madelung deformity
Chromosome XO syndrome
Dyschondrosteosis (Leri-Weill)
Enchondromatosis (Ollier)
Exostosis (multiple cartilaginous)
LEOPARD syndrome
Maffucci syndrome

Medullary space stenosis
Aminopterin fetopathy
Endosteal hyperostosis (van Buchem)
Endosteal hyperostosis (Worth)
Diaphyseal medullary stenosis with bone malignancy—Hardcastle
Tubular stenosis (Kenny-Caffey)

Mesomelic limb shortness
Acromesomelic dysplasias[31]
Mesomelic dysplasias
Schinzel-Giedion syndrome

Metacarpal (first), short
Adducted thumb syndrome
de Lange syndrome
Diastrophic dysplasia
Dyggve-Melchior-Clausen syndrome
Triploidy syndrome

Metacarpal, long
Contractural arachnodactyly
Frontometaphyseal dysplasia
Homocystinuria
Marfan syndrome
Sotos syndrome

Metacarpal, short
Acrocephalosyndactyly, Saethre-Chotzen type
Brachydactyly (type E)
CHILD syndrome
Chondrodysplasia punctata (Conradi-Hünermann)
Chromosome XO syndrome
Coffin-Siris syndrome
Cohen syndrome
Dyschondrosteosis
Exostoses
Fetal alcohol syndrome
Grebe chondrodysplasia
Larsen syndrome
Nevoid basal cell carcinoma syndrome (Gorlin)
Oto-palato-digital syndrome, type I
Oto-palato-digital syndrome, type II
Pallister-Hall syndrome
Poland syndrome
Pseudohypoparathyroidism
Robinow syndrome
Ruvalcaba syndrome
Short rib-polydactyly syndromes
Tricho-rhino-phalangeal syndrome

Metaphyseal cupping
Achondrogenesis, type II
Achondroplasia
Cephaloskeletal dysplasia (Taybi-Linder)
Chondroectodermal dysplasia
Cone-shaped epiphyses
Copper deficiency
Dyssegmental dysplasia
Hypochondroplasia
Hypophosphatasia
Indifference to pain (congenital)
Menkes syndrome
Metaphyseal dysplasias
Mucolipidoses
Peripheral dysostosis

Phenylketonuria
Pseudoachondroplasia
Rickets
Scurvy (postfracture)
Thanatophoric dysplasia
Tricho-rhino-phalangeal syndromes
Vitamin A intoxication

Metaphyseal spur*
Copper deficiency
Hyperparathyroidism
Immune deficiency (severe combined) and adenosine deaminase deficiency
Menkes syndrome
Short rib-polydactyly syndrome, type 2
Short rib-polydactyly syndrome, type 3
Scurvy

Metatarsal, short
Achondrogenesis
Acromesomelic dysplasia
Acromicric dysplasia
Atelosteogenesis
Biemond syndrome I
Brachydactyly, type E
Chromosome 9 mosaic trisomy syndrome
Chromosome 9p syndrome
Chromosome XO syndrome
Cockayne syndrome
Cohen syndrome
Diastrophic dysplasia
Dyggve-Melchior-Clausen syndrome
Dyschondrosteosis
Dyssegmental dysplasia
Femoral-facial syndrome
Fetal alcohol syndrome
Grebe chondrodystrophy
Hand-foot-genital syndrome
Larsen syndrome
Multiple epiphyseal dysplasia
Nager syndrome
Opsismodysplasia
Oto-palato-digital syndrome, type 2
Pallister-Hall syndrome
Pseudohypoparathyroidism
Rothmund-Thomson syndrome
Ruvalcaba syndrome
Sjögren-Larsson syndrome
Spondyloepiphyseal dysplasia
Thanatophoric dwarfism
Tricho-rhino-phalangeal syndromes
Weaver syndrome
Weill-Marchesani syndrome

Oligodactyly
Acrorenal syndrome
Anonychia-ectrodactyly syndrome
Baller-Gerold syndrome
Charlie M syndrome
EEC syndrome
Glossopalatine ankylosis syndrome
Hanhart syndrome
Mesomelic dysplasia, type Werner
Polydactyly, syndactyly, and oligodactyly, aplasia or hypoplasia of fibula, hypoplasia of pelvis and bowing of femora
Postaxial Acrofacial Dysostosis (Miller)

Patella, aplasia, dysplasia, hypoplasia, dislocation
Arthrogryposis
Chromosome 8 trisomy

*Please also see "Exostosis, spur, horn" pp. 885, 895.

Coxo-podo-patellar syndrome[167]
Diastrophic dysplasia
Familial aplasia/hypoplasia[18, 32]
Familial dislocation[163]
Hypoplasia–dislocation of patella[212]
Kuskokwim syndrome
Mesomelic dysplasia, Werner type
Nail-patella syndrome
Neurofibromatosis
Patella aplasia–coxa vara–tarsal synostosis
Patella hypoplasia[32]
Pterygium syndrome (popliteal)
Seckel syndrome
Spondyloepimetaphyseal dysplasia
Spondyloepiphyseal dysplasia

Patella, double-layered or bipartite
Duplication in the coronal plane[80]
Multiple epiphyseal dysplasia
Ptergium syndrome

Phalanges, absent
Acheiropodia
Anonychia-ectrodactyly syndrome
Aplasia cutis congenita
Atelosteogenesis
Brachymesophalangy-nail dysplasia
Coffin-Siris syndrome
Goltz syndrome
Hand-foot-genital syndrome
Holt-Oram syndrome
Hypoglossia-hypodactylia syndrome
Poland syndrome
Pycnodysostosis

Polydactyly, postaxial
Acro-fronto-facio-nasal dysostosis syndrome
Acrorenal association
Acrocallosal syndrome
Acrocephalopolysyndactyly, Carpenter type
Asphyxiating thoracic dysplasia
Bardet-Biedl syndrome
Biemond II syndrome
C syndrome
Chromosome 13 trisomy syndrome
Goltz syndrome
Greig cephalopolysyndactyly syndrome
Hydrolethalus syndrome
Kaufman-McKusick syndrome
Meckel syndrome
Myopia-polydactyly[55]
Oro-facio-digital syndrome II
Pallister-Hall syndrome
Polydactyly, syndactyly, and oligodactyly, aplasia or hypoplasia of fibula, hypoplasia of pelvis and bowing femora
Rubinstein-Taybi syndrome
Short rib-polydactyly syndromes
Smith-Lemli-Opitz syndrome
Weyers acrodental dysostosis

Polydactyly, preaxial
Absent tibia–triphalangeal thumbs–polydactyly[135]
Acro-renal-ocular syndrome[94]
Bloom syndrome
Chromosome 21 trisomy syndrome
Cranio-fronto-nasal dysplasia
Diamond-Blackfan syndrome
Dubowitz syndrome
Fanconi anemia
Holt-Oram syndrome
Levy-Hollister syndrome
Nager syndrome

Poland syndrome
Short rib-polysyndactyly, type 2 (Majewski)
Townes-Brocks syndrome
VATER association

Pseudoarthritis
Amniotic band syndrome
Cleidocranial dysplasia
Congenital, isolated anomaly
Fibrous dysplasia
Kuskokwim syndrome
Neurofibromatosis
Osteogenesis imperfecta
Osteopetrosis

Radius/radial ray deficiency[85]
Aase syndrome
Aminopterin embryopathy
Baller-Gerold syndrome
Cat-eye syndrome
Chromosomal abnormalities (13, 18, etc.)
Craniosynostosis–radial defects
de la Chappele syndrome
de Lange syndrome
DR syndrome[154]
Dyschondrosteosis
Facio-auriculo-radial dysplasia
Fanconi anemia
Fetal varicella syndrome
Goldenhar syndrome
Hemifacial microsomia–Goldenhar radial defect syndrome
Holt-Oram syndrome
Ives-Houston syndrome[115]
IVIC syndrome
Juberg-Hayward syndrome
Klippel-Feil syndrome
Levy-Hollister syndrome
Mesomelic dysplasias
Mietens-Weber syndrome
Nager syndrome
Ophthalmo-mandibulo-melic dysplasia
Phocomelia
Radial hypoplasia–triphalangeal thumb–hypospadias–maxillary diastema
Radial ray aplasia–renal anomalies
Radial ray hypoplasia syndrome
Radio-digito-facial dysplasia
Roberts syndrome
Rothmund-Thomson syndrome
Seckel syndrome
TAR syndrome
Thalidomide embryopathy
Treacher Collins syndrome
Ulna-fibula duplication–absent radius-tibia
Upper limb-cardiovascular syndrome[147]
VATER association
WT syndrome[87]

Rhizomelic limb shortness
Achondroplasia
Chondrodysplasia punctata
Femoral dysplasia
Femoral-facial syndrome
Pseudoachondroplasia

Slender tubular bones
Arthrogryposis
Caudal dysplasia sequence
Cockayne syndrome
Contractural arachnodactyly
Fetal hypokinesia[93, 225]
Hallermann-Streiff syndrome

Hypopituitarism
Intrauterine dwarfism, peculiar facies, and thin bones with multiple fractures[128]
Lethal syndrome with thin bones[158]
Marshall-Smith syndrome
Muscular dystrophies
Neurofibromatosis
Neuromuscular disorders
Osteogenesis imperfecta, type I, II C, III, IV
Pena-Shokeir syndrome
Progeria
Pterygium syndrome (lethal multiple pterygium)
The 3-M syndrome
Winchester syndrome

Split hand, monodactyly, lobster claw hand

Absent ulna—split hand and foot deformity[13]
Acrorenal syndrome
Ankyloglossia superior
Autosomal dominant split hand—split foot malformation[226]
Ectrodactyly—absence of long bones[110]
Ectromelia-ichthyosis
EEC syndrome
EEC syndrome—growth hormone deficiency—absent septum pellucidum[124]
EEM syndrome (ectodermal dysplasia—ectrodactyly—muscular dystrophy)[178]
Familial split hand—split foot anomaly[247]
Hypoglossia-hypodactylia syndrome
Ives-Houston syndrome[115]
Karsch-Neugebauer syndrome
Möbius syndrome
Roberts syndrome
Scalp defects—ectrodactyly[27]
Treacher Collins syndrome
Ulnar aplasia—lobster claw deformity[13, 244]

Symphalangism

Brachydactyly B[15]
Brachydactyly C[15]
Diastrophic dysplasia
Facio-audio-symphalangism syndrome (WL)
Familial distal symphalangism[160]
Multiple synostosis syndrome
Pterygium syndrome
Short rib-polydactyly syndrome, type 1
Symphalangism with metacarpophalangeal fusion and elbow abnormalities

Syndactyly

Aarskog syndrome
Acrocephalopolysyndactyly, Carpenter type
Acrocephalopolysyndactyly, Goodman type
Acrocephalopolysyndactyly, Sakati type
Acrocephalosyndactyly, Apert type
Acrocephalosyndactyly, Hermann-Opitz type
Acrocephalosyndactyly, Pfeiffer type
Acrocephalosyndactyly, Saethre-Chotzen type
Acrocephalosyndactyly, Summit type
Acrocephalosyndactyly, Waardenburg type
Acrorenal syndrome
Aminopterin fetopathy
Amniotic band syndrome
Anonychia-ectrodactyly syndrome
Aplasia cutis congenita
Arthrogryposis
Bardet-Biedl syndrome
Bloom syndrome
Brachydactyly A-2
Brachydactyly B
C syndrome
Camptobrachydactyly[68]

Chondrodysplasia punctata
Chromosomal abnormalities (13, 18, 21, etc.)
Cloverleaf skull
Cohen syndrome
Cranio-fronto-nasal dysplasia
Cryptophthalmia syndrome
de Lange syndrome
DOOR syndrome
Dubowitz syndrome (toes)
EEC syndrome
Ehlers-Danlos syndrome
Epidermolysis bullosa dystrophica
F syndrome
Familial syndactyly with metacarpal and metatarsal fusion[204]
Fanconi anemia
Fetal hydantoin syndrome
FG syndrome
Fibrodysplasia ossificans progressiva
Filippi syndrome
Frontodigital syndrome
Goltz syndrome
Goodman camptodactyly syndrome A
Greig cephalopolysyndactyly syndrome
Hallermann-Streiff syndrome
Holt-Oram syndrome
Hypoglossia-hypodactylia syndrome
Hypomelanosis of Ito
Incontinentia pigmenti
Jarcho-Levin syndrome
Kaufman-McKusick syndrome
KBG syndrome
Lenz microphthalmia syndrome
Levy-Hollister syndrome
Meckel syndrome
Mesomelic dysplasia, Werner type
Möbius syndrome
Multiple synostosis syndrome
Nager syndrome
Neu-Laxova syndrome
Nevoid basal cell carcinoma syndrome (Gorlin)
Oculo-dento-osseous dysplasia
Oro-facio-digital syndrome I
Oromandibular-limb hypogenesis syndrome
Oto-palato-digital syndrome, type 1
Oto-palato-digital syndrome, type 2
Pallister-Hall syndrome
Poland syndrome
Polydactyly, syndactyly, and oligodactyly, aplasia or hypoplasia of fibula, hypoplasia of pelvis and bowing of femora
Postaxial acrofacial dysostosis syndrome (Miller)
Prader-Willi syndrome
Pterygium syndrome
Roberts syndrome
Robin syndrome
Rothmund-Thomson syndrome
Rubinstein-Taybi syndrome
Sclerosteosis
Short rib-polydactyly syndromes
Silver-Russell syndrome
Smith-Lemli-Opitz syndrome
Sorsby syndrome
TAR syndrome
Tricho-rhino-phalangeal dysplasia, types 1 and 2
Triploidy
Waardenburg anophthalmia syndrome
WT syndrome[87]

Synostosis, humeroradial/humeroulnar

Acrocephalosyndactyly, Pfeiffer type
Cloverleaf skull

Facio-audio-symphalangism syndrome
Familial humeroradial synostosis[119]
Femoral-facial syndrome
Holt-Oram syndrome
Humeroradial—multiple synostosis syndrome[202]

Synostosis, radioulnar[100]
Acrocephalosyndactyly, Pfeiffer type
Caffey disease
Chromosome 18 trisomy syndrome
Chromosome 49 XXXXX syndrome
Chromosome XXXXY syndrome
Chromosome XXXY syndrome
Chromosome XXY syndrome
Cloverleaf skull
Ehlers-Danlos syndrome
Exostosis, distal forearm
Facio-auriculo-radial dysplasia
Femoral-facial syndrome
Fetal alcohol syndrome
Holt-Oram syndrome
IVIC syndrome
Lacrimo-auriculo-dento-digital syndrome
Levy-Hollister syndrome
Multiple synostosis syndrome
Nager syndrome
Oculo-palato-skeletal syndrome
Thalidomide embryopathy
Thanatophoric dysplasia

Synostosis, tubular bones
Caffey disease
Cloverleaf skull
Exostosis (multiple cartilaginous)
Fetal alcohol syndrome
Holt-Oram syndrome
Humeroradial-humeroulnar synostosis (see this title)
Multiple synostosis syndrome
Radioulnar synosis (see this title)
Sensorineural deafness—hypospadias—synostosis of metacarpals[190]

Tarsal fusion
Arthrogryposis
Chromosome XO syndrome
Crouzon syndrome
F syndrome
Hand-foot-genital syndrome
Multiple synostosis syndrome
Patella aplasia—coxa vara—tarsal synostosis

Thumb, broad
Acrocephalopolysyndactyly, Carpenter type
Acrocephalosyndactyly, Apert type
Acrocephalosyndactyly, Pfeiffer type
Acromesomelic dysplasia
Chromosome 13 trisomy syndrome
Diastrophic dysplasia
FG syndrome
Fibrodysplasia ossificans progressiva
Frontodigital syndrome
Greig cephalopolysyndactyly syndrome
Hand-foot-genital syndrome
Larsen syndrome
Meckel syndrome
Oto-palato-digital syndrome, type 1
Oto-palato-digital syndrome, type 2
Pleonosteosis (Léri)
Robinow syndrome
Rubinstein-Taybi syndrome[174]
Sorsby syndrome
Weaver-Smith syndrome

Thumb, large
Klippel-Trenaunay-Weber syndrome
Macrodystrophia lipomatosa
Maffucci syndrome
Neurofibromatosis

Thumb, short, hypoplastic, or absent[255]
Acrocephalopolysyndactylies
Acrocephalosyndactylies
Acro-renal-ocular syndrome[94]
Aminopterin fetopathy
Baller-Gerold syndrome
Brachydactyly C
Brachydactyly, Christian
Brachydactyly D
Cephaloskeletal dysplasia (Taybi-Linder)
Chromosomal abnormalities (9, 18, etc.)
de Lange syndrome
Diastrophic dysplasia
Dyggve-Melchior-Clausen syndrome
Dyssegmental dysplasia
Ectodermal dysplasia
Facioaudiosymphalangism syndrome
Fanconi anemia
Fibrodysplasia ossificans progressiva
Hand-foot-genital syndrome
Holt-Oram syndrome
IVIC syndrome
Juberg-Hayward syndrome
Oto-palato-digital syndrome, type 1
Oto-palato-digital syndrome, type 2
Pterygium syndrome, popliteal
Radial hypoplasia syndromes
Rubinstein-Taybi syndrome
TAR syndrome
Thalidomide embryopathy
VATER association
Werner syndrome

Thumb, short proximal phalanx
Acrocephalopolysyndactyly, Carpenter type
Acrocephalosyndactyly, Apert type
Acrocephalosyndactyly, Pfeiffer type
Chromosome 18 trisomy syndrome
Diastrophic dysplasia
DOOR syndrome
Fibrodysplasia ossificans progressiva
Nevoid basal cell carcinoma syndrome (Gorlin)
Rubinstein-Taybi syndrome

Thumb, triphalangeal (TPT)[195, 255]
Aase syndrome
Absent tibias—triphalangeal thumb—polydactyly
Acrofacial dysostosis, cleft lip-palate—TPT
Agenesis of lung—congenital heart disease—TPT
Chromosome 13 trisomy syndrome
Chromosome 22 trisomy syndrome
Diamond-Blackfan syndrome
DOOR syndrome
Duane syndrome
Fanconi anemia
Fetal hydantoin syndrome
Goodman syndrome
Holt-Oram syndrome
Hypomelanosis of Ito
Isolated TPT
IVIC syndrome
Juberg-Hayward syndrome
Levy-Hollister syndrome
Poland syndrome
Radial hypoplasia—hypospadias—maxillary diastema

Radial   hypoplasia—thrombocytopathy—sensorineural   hearing
  impairment—TPT
Thalidomide embryopathy
Townes-Brocks syndrome
TPT—brachydactyly—ectrodactyly[223]
TPT—cleft palate—abnormal sternum
TPT—onychodystrophy—deafness
TPT—polydactyly
TPT—polydactyly—syndactyly
Tricho-rhino-phalangeal dysplasia, type 2
VATER association

Tibia, hemimelia[38, 135]
Carroro syndrome
Familial isolated tibial hemimelia[164]
Tibial hemimelia dipolodia syndrome
Tibial hemimelia—foot polydactyly—triphalangeal thumb (Werner
  syndrome)
Tibial hemimelia—micromelia—trigobrachycephaly syndrome
Tibial hemimelia—split hand-foot syndrome
Ulna and fibula duplication

Toe, broad
Acrocephalosyndactyly, Pfeiffer type
Chromosome XXXXY syndrome
Greig cephalopolydactyly syndrome
Oto-palato-digital syndrome, type 1
Oto-palato-digital syndrome, type 2
Rubinstein-Taybi syndrome

Toe, triphalangeal great toe (TGT)
Fetal hydantoin syndrome
Isolated anomaly
TGT—polydactyly
TGT—polydactyly—triphalangeal thumb—patella dislocation—short
  stature
TGT—triphalangeal thumb—onychodystrophy—deafness

Ulna/ulnar ray deficiency
Cardiomelic syndrome with ulnar agenesis[230]
Craniosynostosis-ulnar aplasia[37]
de la Chapelle syndrome
de Lange syndrome
Familial ulnar aplasia and lobster claw syndrome[13, 244]
Femur-fibula-ulna syndrome
Ive-Houston syndrome[115]
Klippel-Feil syndrome—absent ulna[43]
Mesomelic dysplasia, Nievergelt
Pallister syndrome[183]
Postaxial acrofacial dysostosis syndrome (Miller)
Roberts syndrome
Schinzel syndrome[104]
Symphalangism
Ulnar-mammary syndrome
Weyers syndrome of deficiency of ulnar and fibular rays

Vertical talus, congenital[99]
Caudal regression syndrome
Chromosomal abnormalities
Digitotalar dysmorphism
Idiopathic
Metacarpotalar syndrome[7]
neural tube defects
Neuromuscular disorders

PELVIS

Acteabular angle, small
Achondrogenesis, type I
Achondrogenesis, type II
Achondroplasia
Acrocephalopolysyndactyly, Carpenter type
Acrocephalosyndactyly, Waardenburg type

Aminopterin fetopathy
Arthrogryposis
Asphyxiating thoracic dysplasia
Caudal dysplasia
Cephaloskeletal dysplasia (Taybi-Linder)
Chondrodysplasia punctata
Chondroectodermal dysplasia
Chromosome 13 trisomy syndrome
Chromosome 21 trisomy syndrome
de Lange syndrome
Dyggve-Melchior-Clausen syndrome
Dyssegmental dysplasia
Hypothyroidism (cretinism)
Hypochondroplasia
Hypophosphatasia
Kniest dysplasia
Metaphyseal chondrodysplasia
Metatropic dysplasia
Mucopolysaccharidosis IVA (Morquio)
Nail-patella syndrome
Opsismodysplasia
Osteodysplasty, Melnick-Needles
Prune-belly syndrome
Pterygium syndrome
Rubinstein-Taybi syndrome
Schneckenbecken dysplasia
Spondyloepiphyseal dysplasia congenita
Thanatophoric dysplasia
Thoraco-laryngo-pelvic dysplasia

Iliac crest serration
Dyggve-Melchior-Clausen syndrome
Fluorosis
Parastremmatic dysplasia
Smith-McCort syndrome

Iliac wing, flared
Achondroplasia
Acro-cranio-facial dysostosis
Arthrogryposis multiplex congenita
Asphyxiating thoracic dysplasia
Caudal dysplasia sequence
Chondroectodermal dysplasia
Chromosome 21 trisomy syndrome
de Lange syndrome
Dyssegmental dysplasia
Frontometaphyseal dysplasia
Metatropic dysplasia
Mucolipidosis II
Mucolipidosis III
Mucopolysaccharidosis I-H
Mucopolysaccharidosis III
Mucopolysaccharidosis IV
Nail-patella syndrome
Osteodysplasty, Melnick-Needles
Prune-belly syndrome
Rubinstein-Taybi syndrome
Schneckenbecken dysplasia
Shwachman syndrome
Spondyloepiphyseal dysplasia congenita
Spondylometaphyseal dysplasia (Kozlowski)

Iliac wing, small
Barnes syndrome
Scapuloiliac dysostosis

Pelvis, small, hypoplasia
Achondrogenesis, type I
Achondrogenesis, type II
Asphyxiating thoracic dysplasia
Campomelic dysplasia
Chromosome 13 trisomy syndrome

Chromosome 18 trisomy syndrome
Chromosome 4p− syndrome
Coxo-podo-patellar syndrome[167]
Dyggve-Melchior-Clausen syndrome
Dyssegmental dwarfism
Fibrochondrogenesis
Goltz syndrome
Hypochondroplasia
Limb/pelvis−hypoplasia/aplasia syndrome[196]
Metaphyseal chondrodysplasia (McKusick)
Metatropic dysplasia
Molded baby syndrome
Osteodysplasty, Melnick-Needles
Pelvic dysplasia−arthrogrypotic lower limbs
Scapuloiliac dysostosis
Spondyloepimetaphyseal dysplasia−Irapa
Spondyloepiphyseal dysplasia
Stickler syndrome
Thanatophoric dysplasia
Thoracic-pelvic dysostosis
Thoraco-laryngo-pelvic dysplasia
Weaver syndrome

Protrusio acetabuli

Acrodysostosis and protrusio acetabuli[155]
Alkaptonuria
Chromosome XO syndrome
Familial protrusio acteabuli[245]
Hyperparathyroidism
Hyperphosphatasemia
Marfan syndrome
Mseleni joint disease[73]
Mucopolysaccharidoses
Osteogenesis imperfecta
Osteomalacia
Osteoporosis
Renal osteodystrophy
Rheumatoid arthritis
Rickets
Stickler syndrome

Pubis, wide "interpubic" distance or delayed ossification

Achondrogenesis
Boomerang dysplasia
Campomelic dysplasia
Caudal dysplasia sequence
Cephaloskeletal dysplasia (Taybi-Linder)
Chondrodysplasia punctata (Conradi-Hünermann)
Chondroectodermal dysplasia
Chromosome 4p− syndrome
Chromosome 9 (p+) trisomy syndrome
Cleidocranial dysplasia
Dyggve-Melchior-Clausen syndrome
Ehlers-Danlos syndrome
Familial pubic bone maldevelopment[222]
Fraser syndrome
Goltz syndrome
Hyperparathyroidism
Hypochondrogenesis
Hypophosphatasia
Hypothyroidism
Isolated symphyseal diastasis[228]
Larsen syndrome
Opsismodysplasia
Prune-belly syndrome
Pycnodysostosis
Renal, genital, and ear anomlies
Schinzel-Giedion syndrome
Sjögren-Larsson syndrome
Spondyloepimetaphyseal dysplasia, Strudwick
Spondylomegaepiphyseal-metaphyseal dysplasia

Spondyloepiphyseal dysplasia congenita
Symphyseal diastasis−genital anomaly[228]

Sciatic notch, small

Achondroplasia
Cephaloskeletal dysplasia (Taybi-Linder)
Dyggve-Melchior-Clausen syndrome
Dyssegmental dwarfism
Metatropic dysplasia
Parastremmatic dysplasia
Schneckenbecken dysplasia
Short rib-polydactyly syndrome, type I (Saldino-Noonan)
Smith-McCort dysplasia
Thanatophoric dysplasia
Thoracic-pelvic dysostosis
Thoraco-laryngo-pelvic dysplasia

SPINE

Absent or minimal ossification

Achondrogenesis, type I
Achondrogenesis, type II
Atelosteogenesis
Boomerang dysplasia
Dyssegmental dysplasia
Hypochondrogenesis
Opsismohysplasia
Spondylomegaepiphyseal−metaphyseal dysplasia

Atlantoaxial instability

Aarskog syndrome
Ankylosing spondylitis
Behçet syndrome
Calcium pyrophosphate dihydrate deposition disease (pseudogout)
Chondrodysplasia punctata
Chromosome 21 trisomy syndrome
Chromosome XO syndrome
CREST syndrome
Diastrophic dysplasia
Dyggve-Melchior-Clausen syndrome
Grisel syndrome
Hemophilia
Hypochondrogenesis
Klippel-Feil syndrome
Marfan syndrome
Metaphyseal chondrodysplasia (McKusick)
Metatropic dysplasia
Mucolipidosis III
Mucopolysaccharidoses
Neurofibromatosis
Opsismodysplasia
Patterson syndrome
Pseudoachondroplasia
Reiter syndrome
Spondylo-epi-metaphyseal dysplasia−Strudwick
Spondylo-epiphyseal dysplasia
Spondylometaphyseal dysplasia
Winchester syndrome

Beaked vertebral body

Achondroplasia
Aspartylglucosaminuria
Child abuse syndrome
Chromosome 21 trisomy
Diastrophic dysplasia
Dyggve-Melchior-Clausen syndrome
Fucosidosis
Hypothyroidism
Mannosidosis
Marshall syndrome
Mucolipidoses
Mucopolysaccharidoses
Niemann-Pick disease

Phenylketonuria
Pseudoachondroplasia
Spondyloepiphyseal dysplasia

Coronal cleft vertebrae
Atelosteogenesis
Chondrodysplasia punctata
Chromosome 13 trisomy syndrome
Dyssegmental dysplasia
Fibrochondrogenesis
Humerospinal dysostosis
Kniest dysplasia
Metatropic dysplasia
Oto-spondylo-megaepiphyseal dysplasia
Weissenbacher-Zweymüller syndrome

Disk calcification
Aarskog syndrome
Alkaptonuria
Ankylosing spondylitis
Calcium pyrophosphate dihydrate deposition disease
Cockayne syndrome
Gout
Hemochromatosis
Homocystinuria
Hypercalcemia
Hyperparathyroidism
Hypophosphatasia
Idiopathic
Klippel-Feil syndrome
Mucolipidosis II
Rheumatoid arthritis
Sickle cell disease
Spondyloepiphyseal dysplasia tarda
Vitamin D intoxication

Odontoid, aplasia or hypoplasia
Achondroplasia
Chromosome 21 trisomy
Diastrophic dysplasia
Dyggve-Melchior-Clausen syndrome
Fucosidosis
Klippel-Feil syndrome
Kniest dysplasia
Metaphyseal dysplasia, McKusick type
Metatropic dysplasia
Mucopolysaccharidoses
Multiple epiphyseal dysplasia
Smith-McCort syndrome
Spondylo-epi-metaphyseal dysplasia
Spondyloepiphyseal dysplasia congenita

Platyspondyly
Achondrogenesis
Achondroplasia, homozygous
Aspartylglucosaminuria
Atelosteogenesis
Brachyolmia
Cephaloskeletal dysplasia (Taybi-Linder)
Cushing syndrome
de la Chapelle syndrome
Diastrophic dysplasia
Dyggve-Melchior-Clausen syndrome
Dyschondrosclerosis
Ehlers-Danlos syndrome
Fibrochondrogenesis
Freeman-Sheldon syndrome
Fucosidosis
Gaucher disease
Gerodermia osteodysplastica hereditaria
GM$_1$ gangliosidosis
Hallermann-Streiff syndrome

Histiocytosis X
Homocystinuria
Hydrops—ectopic calcification—moth-eaten skeletal dysplasia
Hyperphosphatasemia
Hypertrichosis-osteochondrodysplasia
Hypochondroplasia
Hypophosphatasia
Hypopituitarism (anterior lobe)
Hypothyroidism
Immune deficiency (severe combined)
Kniest syndrome
Larsen syndrome
Marshall syndrome
Metaphyseal—sella turcica dysplasia—Rosenberg
Metatropic dysplasia
Mucopolysaccharidosis IV-A
Opsismodysplasia
Osteogenesis imperfecta
Osteoglophonic dwarfism
Osteoporosis (idiopathic juvenile)
Osteoporosis-pseudoglioma syndrome
Oto-spondylo-megaepiphyseal dysplasia
Parastremmatic dwarfism
Patterson syndrome
Progressive pseudorheumatoid chondrodysplasia
Pseudoachondroplasia
Pseudodiastrophic dysplasia
Rothmund-Thomson syndrome
Schwartz-Jampel syndrome
Short rib-polydactyly syndrome, type I (Saldino-Noonan)
Smith-McCort syndrome
Sotos syndrome
Spondylo-epi-metaphyseal dysplasias
Spondyloepiphyseal dysplasia congenita
Spondyloepiphyseal dysplasia tarda
Spondylometaphyseal dysplasia (Kozlowski)
Spondyloperipheral dysplasia
Thanatophoric dysplasia
Thanatophoric variant
Wolcott-Rallison syndrome

Spinal canal, narrow
Achondroplasia
Acrodysostosis
Acromegaly
Acromesomelic dysplasia
Alagille syndrome
Brachyolmia
Calcium phosphate dihydrate deposition disease (pseudogout)
Cauda equina syndrome
Cheirolumbar dysplasia[98, 248]
Chromosome XO syndrome
Congenital lumbar canal stenosis
Diastrophic dysplasia
Dyggve-Melchior-Clausen syndrome
Dyschondrosteosis
Gordon syndrome
Hypochondroplasia
Klippel-Feil syndrome
Kniest dysplasia
Osteoglophonic dwarfism
Pseudohypoparathyroidism
Rickets (hypophosphatemic)
Smith-McCort syndrome
Weill-Marchesani syndrome

Spinal canal, wide
Diastematomyelia
Distichiasis-lymphedema syndrome
Marfan syndrome
Meningomyelocele
Neurofibromatosis

Oto-palato-digital syndrome, type I
Tethered cord syndrome

Tail (caudal appendage)
Goltz syndrome
Metatropic dysplasia

Vertebrae, tall
Acrocraniofacial dysostosis
Chromosomal abnormalities
Freeman-Sheldon syndrome
Fuhrmann dysplasia[77, 205]
Infantile multisystem inflammatory disease
Osteodysplasty, Melnick-Needles
Proteus syndrome

Vertebrae, malsegmentation
Aicardi syndrome
Alagille syndrome
Binder syndrome
Caudal dysplasia sequence
CHILD syndrome
Chondrodysplasia punctata
Chromosomal abnormalities
de la Chapelle syndrome
Dyssegmental dysplasia
Femoral-facial syndrome
Fetal alcohol syndrome
Goldenhar syndrome
Goltz syndrome
Holt-Oram syndrome
Incontinentia pigmenti
Jarcho-Levin syndrome
Klippel-Feil syndrome[43]
Larsen syndrome
LEOPARD syndrome
MURCS association[67]
Nevoid basal cell carcinoma syndrome (Gorlin)
Noonan syndrome
Poland syndrome
Pterygium syndrome (multiple)
Robin sequence
Robinow syndrome
Split notocord syndrome
Spondylocostal dysostosis
Tethered conus syndrome
VATER association
Wildervanck syndrome

THORAX
Clavicle, aplasia or hypoplasia
CHILD syndrome
Cleidocranial dysplasia
Fucosidosis
Goltz syndrome
Holt-Oram syndrome
Mandibuloacral dysplasia
Osteodysplasty (Melnick-Needles)
Parietal "foramina"-clavicular hypoplasia
Progeria
Pycnodysostosis
Scapuloilac dysostosis
Yunis-Varón syndrome

Clavicle, broad or thickened
Distal osteosclerosis
Endosteal hyperostosis (van Buchem)
Endosteal hyperostosis (Worth)
Fucosidosis
Holt-Oram syndrome
Menkes syndrome
Mucolipidoses

Mucopolysaccharidoses
Oculo-dento-osseous dysplasia
Osteodysplasty (Melnick-Needles)
Pyle disease
Winchester syndrome

Clavicle, lateral hook
Camptomelic dysplasia
Chromosome 8 trisomy syndrome
de Lange syndrome
Diastrophic dysplasia
Facio-auriculo-radial dysplasia
Holt-Oram syndrome
Meckel syndrome
Osteogenesis imperfecta
Robin syndrome
Scapuloiliac dyssostosis
TAR syndrome

Clavicle, slender
Chromosome 18 trisomy syndrome
Chromosome XO syndrome
Cockayne syndrome
Fibrochondrogenesis
Larsen syndrome
Progeria

Glenoid fossa, shallow
Fucosidosis
Glenoid hypoplasia
Grant syndrome
Mucopolysaccharidoses
Ophthalmo-mandibulo-melic dysplasia
TAR syndrome

Pectus carinatum
Asphyxiating thoracic dysplasia
Coffin-Lowry syndrome
Dyggve-Melchior-Clausen syndrome
Ehlers-Danlos syndrome
Fetal alcohol syndrome
Homocystinuria
Hyperphosphatasemia
LEOPARD syndrome
Marfan syndrome
Mucopolysaccharidosis IV
Noonan syndrome
Osteogenesis imperfecta
Prune-belly syndrome
Schwartz-Jampel syndrome
Spondylo-epi-metaphyseal dysplasia, Strudwick type
Spondyloepiphyseal dysplasia congenita
The 3-M syndrome

Pectus excavatum
Aarskog syndrome
Coffin-Lowry syndrome
Cowden syndrome
Cutis laxa
Ehlers-Danlos syndrome
F syndrome
Fetal alcohol syndrome
Freeman-Sheldon syndrome
German syndrome
Golden-Lakim syndrome
Homocystinuria
LEOPARD syndrome
Marfan syndrome
Myotonic dystrophy
Noonan syndrome
Osteodysplasty (Melnick-Needles)
Osteogenesis
The 3-M syndrome

Rib anomalies

Baller-Gerold syndrome
C syndrome
Campomelic dysplasia
Cerebro-costo-mandibular syndrome
Chromosome 21 trisomy syndrome
Chromosome XXY syndrome
Costoiliac impingement syndrome
Femoral-facial syndrome
Fetal cytomegalovirus infection
Fetal hydantoin syndrome
Fetal varicella syndrome
Frontometaphyseal dysplasia
Goldenhar syndrome
Goltz syndrome
Holt-Oram syndrome
Incontinentia pigmenti
Jarcho-Levin syndrome
Klippel-Feil syndrome
Nager syndrome
Nevoid basal cell carcinoma syndrome
Noonan syndrome
Osteodysplasty (Melnick-Needles)
Poland syndrome
Pterygium syndromes
Scapuloiliac dysostosis
Spondylocostal dysostosis
TAR syndrome
Thoracic outlet syndrome
VATER association

Ribs, eleven pairs

Asphyxiating thoracic dysplasia
Atelosteogenesis
Campomelic dysplasia
Chromosome 1, partial deletion syndrome
Chromosome 18 trisomy syndrome
Chromosome 21 trisomy syndrome
Cleidocranial dysplasia
Femoral-facial syndrome
Short rib-polydactyly syndromes[137]

Ribs, flaring, cupping

Achondroplasia
Asphyxiating thoracic dysplasia
Copper deficiency
Farber syndrome
Fibrochondrogenesis
GM$_1$ gangliosidosis
Hypophosphatasia
Immune deficiency
Menkes syndrome
Metaphyseal chondrodysplasia (Jansen)
Metaphyseal chondrodysplasia (McKusick)
Metaphyseal chondrodysplasia (Schmid)
Metatropic dysplasia
Rickets
Scurvy
Short rib-polydactyly syndromes
Shwachman syndrome
Spondylometaphyseal dysplasia
Thalassemia
Thanatophoric dysplasia

Ribs, gap

Cerebro-costo-mandibular syndrome
Chromosome 8 trisomy (first rib)[127]

Ribs, notching or erosion

Hyperparathyroidism
Marfan syndrome
Neurofibromatosis

Osteodysplasty (Melnick-Needles)
Scleroderma
Superior vena cava syndrome
Takayasu arteritis
Thalassemia

Ribs, short

Achondrogenesis, type I
Achondrogenesis, type II
Achondroplasia
Asphyxiating thoracic dysplasia
Atelosteogenesis
Camptomelic dysplasia
Cerebro-costo-mandibular syndrome
Chondroectodermal dysplasia
Cleidocranial dysplasia
Dyssegmental dysplasia
Enchondromatosis (Ollier)
Fibrochondrogenesis
Hypochondrogenesis
Hypophosphatasia
Immune deficiency (severe combined) and adenosine deaminase
 deficiency
Jarcho-Levin syndrome
Mandibuloacral dysplasia
Metatropic dysplasia
Mucopolysaccharidoses
Osteodysplasty (Melnick-Needles)
Osteogenesis imperfecta, type 2
Pseudoachondroplasia
Rickets
Short rib-polydactyly syndromes
Spondylocostal dysplasia
Spondyloepiphyseal dysplasia congenita
Thanatophoric dysplasia
Thantophoric variants
Thoracic-pelvic dysostosis
Thoracolaryngopelvic dysplasia

Ribs, slender, thin or twisted

Achondrogenesis, type I
Achondrogenesis, type II
Aminopterin fetopathy
Anderson syndrome
Antley-Bixler syndrome
Campomelic dysplasia
Chondrodysplasia punctata
Chromosome 13 trisomy syndrome
Chromosome 18 trisomy syndrome
Chromosome 21 trisomy syndrome
Chromosome 8 trisomy syndrome
Chromosome XO syndrome
Cockayne syndrome
Contractural arachnodactyly
Floppy infant
Hallermann-Streiff syndrome
Hyperparathyroidism
Larsen syndrome
Lethal syndromes with thin bones[128, 158]
Metaphyseal chondrodysplasia (Jansen)
Myotonic dystrophy
Myotubular myopathy
Neurofibromatosis
Nevoid basal cell carcinoma syndrome (Gorlin)
Osteodysplasty (Melnick-Needles)
Osteogenesis imperfecta, types 1, 3, and 4
Osteoporosis
Progeria
Scleroderma
The 3-M syndrome
Werdnig-Hoffmann disease

Ribs, supernumerary
Chromosome 8 trisomy syndrome
Chromosome XO syndrome
Incontinentia pigmenti

Ribs, wide or thickened
Achondroplasia
Acromegaly
Caffey disease
Chromosome 8 trisomy syndrome
Craniodiaphyseal dysplasia
Dysosteosclerosis
Endosteal hyperostosis (van Buchem)
Endosteal hyperostosis (Worth)
Erdheim-Chester disease
Fibrous dysplasia
Fluorosis
Fucosidosis
Gaucher disease
Geleophysic dysplasia
Hyperphosphatasia
Hypochondroplasia
Mannosidosis
Mucolipidosis II
Mucolipidosis III
Mucopolysaccharidoses
Myhre syndrome
Nevoid basal cell carcinoma syndrome (Gorlin)
Niemann-Pick disease
Oculo-dento-osseous dysplasia
Osteogenesis imperfecta, type II
Osteopetrosis
Pachydermoperiostosis
Proteus syndrome
Pseudoachondroplastic dysplasia
Pyle disease
Sickle cell disease
Thalassemia
Tuberous sclerosis
Weill-Marchesani syndrome

Scapula, abnormal
Achondrogenesis
Auriculo-osteodysplasia
Campomelic dysplasia
Cleidocranial dysplasia
Cloverleaf skull deformity
de la Chapelle dysplasia
Dyggve-Melchior-Clausen syndrome
Dyssegmental dysplasia
Fetal varicella syndrome
Fucosidosis
Geoderma osteodysplastica hereditaria
Glenoid hypoplasia
Hallermann-Streiff syndrome
Holt-Oram syndrome
Hypophosphatasia
Klippel-Feil syndrome
LEOPARD syndrome
Menkes syndrome
Mucopolysaccharidoses
Mucolipidosis II
Nail-patella syndrome
Nevoid basal cell carcinoma syndrome (Gorlin)
Poland syndrome
Proteus syndrome
Robin sequence[21]
Scapuloiliac dysostosis
Short rib-polydactyly syndromes
Sprengel shoulder deformity[108]
TAR syndrome
Wrinkly skin syndrome

Shield-like thorax
Chromosome 18 trisomy syndrome
Chromosome XO syndrome
Noonan syndrome

Sternal anomaly
Achondrogenesis, type I
Achondrogenesis, type II
C syndrome
Cantrell syndrome
Chromosome 18 trisomy syndrome
Chromosome 21 trisomy syndrome
Chromosome XO syndrome
Chromosome XXXXY syndrome
Cleidocranial dysplasia
de Lange syndrome
Dysosteosclerosis
Hypothyroidism
Metaphyseal chondrodysplasia (McKusick)
Metatropic dysplasia
Noonan syndrome
Poland syndrome
Rubinstein-Taybi syndrome
Seckel syndrome
Sternal malformation–vascular dysplasia association
Sternal-cardiac malformation association

Thoracic dysplasia, small thorax
Achondrogenesis, type I
Achondrogenesis, type II
Achonroplasia (severe form)
Antley-Bixler syndrome
Asphyxiating thoracic dysplasia
Atelosteogenesis
Barnes syndrome
Campomelic dysplasia
Cerebro-costo-mandibular syndrome
Chondrodysplasia punctata
Chondroectodermal dysplasia
Cleidocranial dysplasia
de la Chapelle syndrome
Diastrophic dysplasia
Dyssegmental dysplasia
Fibrochondrogenesis
Hypochondrogenesis
Hypophosphatasia
Jarcho-Levin syndrome
Metatropic dysplasia
Metaphyseal chondrodysplasia (Jansen)
Noonan syndrome
Osteodysplasty (Melnick-Needles)
Osteodysplasty, precocious
Osteogenesis imperfecta, type 2
Progeria
Pseudoachondroplasia
Pterygium syndrome (lethal form)
Short rib-polydactyly syndromes
Shwachman syndrome
Spondylo-epi-metaphyseal dysplasia with joint laxity
Spondyloepiphyseal dysplasia congenita
Thanatophoric dysplasia
Thantaophoric variants
Thoracic-pelvic dysostosis

MISCELLANEOUS (SKELETAL SYSTEM)
Arthropathy, arthritis[41, 187]
Acromegaly
Agammaglobulinemia
Alkaptonuria
Amyloidosis
Behçet syndrome

Calcium pyrophosphate dihydrate deposition disease (pseudogout)
Caplan syndrome
Cystic fibrosis
Diabetes mellitus
Fabry disease
Familial hypertrophic synovitis[41]
Fetal alcohol syndrome
Fetal rubella syndrome
Fluorosis
Glycogenesis, type I
Gout
Hemochromatosis
Hydroxyaptite deposition disease
Hyperlipoproteinemia
Hyperparathyroidism (secondary)
Hypertrophic osteoarthropathy
Hypothyroidism
Infantile multisystem inflammatory disease
Inflammatory bowel disease
Intestinal bypass syndrome
Irritable hip syndrome
Jadhassohn-Lewandowksy syndrome
Juvenile ankylosing spondylitis
Kashin-Beck disease[172]
Lipoid dermatoarthritis
Macrodystrophia lipomatosa
Mediterranean fever
Mixed connective tissue disease
Osteoarthropathy, familial idiopathic (Curranino)
Osteolysis without nephropathy
Pancreatic disease, subcutaneous fat necrosis, and polyserositis
Pancreatitis with arthritis[41]
Progressive pseudorheumatoid chondrodysplasia
Psoriatic arthritis
Reiter syndrome
Relapsing polychondritis
Rheumatoid arthritis
Sarcoidosis
Sickle cell disease
Sjögren syndrome
Stagnant small bowel syndrome
Weber-Christian syndrome
Wilson syndrome
Winchester syndrome
Wissler syndrome

Bone age, advanced
Acrodysostosis
Adrenal hyperplasia, congenital
Adrenocortical tumor
Aldosteronism, primary
Arthrogryposis—advanced skeletal maturation—unusual facies
Beckwith-Wiedemann syndrome
Cerebral tumor
Chromosome 8 trisomy syndrome
Cockayne syndrome
Contractural arachnodactyly
Cushing syndrome
Diastrophic dysplasia (hands)
Ectopic gonadotropin production
Gigantism
Homocystinuria
Hyperthyroidism
Idiopathic familial advanced bone age
Idiopathic isosexual precocious puberty
Lipodystrophy
Marshall-Smith syndrome
McCune-Albrigt syndrome
Neurofibromatosis
Obesity
Peripheral dysostosis (Brailsford)

Pseudohypoparathyroidism
Sexual precocity (various etiologies)
Sotos syndrome
Tuberous sclerosis
Weaver syndrome

Bone age, advanced, newborn
Asphyxiating thoracic dysplasia (hips)
Beckwith-Wiedemann syndrome
Chondroectodermal dysplasia (hips)
Greig cephalopolysyndactyly syndrome
Hyperthyroidism (maternal)
Larsen syndrome
Lethal congenital dwarfism—accelerated skeletal maturation[26]
Marshall-Smith syndrome
Spondylometaphyseal abnormalities, advanced bone age[14]
Weaver syndrome

Bone age, retarded
Addison disease
Aminopterin fetopathy
Anemias
Aspartylglucosaminuria
C syndrome
Celiac disease
Chromosomal abnormalities (XO, 21, etc.)
Cleidocranial dysplasia
Coffin-Lowry syndrome
Coffin-Siris syndrome
Copper deficiency
Cushing syndrome
Cystic fibrosis
Cystinosis
de Lange syndrome
de Morsier syndrome
De Sanctis-Cacchione syndrome
Deaf mutism—goiter—euthyroidism syndrome
Deprivation dwarfism
Diabetes mellitus
Dubowitz syndrome
Fanconi anemia
Fetal rubella syndrome
Freeman-Sheldon syndrome
Fucosidosis
GAPO syndrome
Geophagia-dwarfism hypogonadism syndrome
Gigantism
Glycogenosis, type I
Histiocytosis X
Hypoadrenalism
Hypogonadism
Hypoparathyroidism
Hypopituitarism (anterior lobe)
Hypothyroidism
Incontinentia pigmenti
Intrauterine growth retardation
Johanson-Blizzard syndrome
KBG syndrome
Kocher-Debré-Sémélaigne syndrome
Laron dwarfism
Larsen syndrome
Legg-Calvé-Perthes disease
lenz-Majewski hyperostotic dwarfism
Lesch-Nyhan syndrome
Malnutrition
Marinesco-Sjögren syndrome
Mauriac syndrome
Metatropic dysplasia
Meyer dysplasia of femoral head
Mucolipidosis III
Mucopolysaccharidoses

Nephrotic syndrome
Noonan syndrome
Osteodysplasty, Melnick-Needles
Osteoporosis (idiopathic juvenile)
Papillon-Lefèvre syndrome
Patterson syndrome
Phenylketonuria
Pleonosteosis
Prader-Willi syndrome
Renal failure
Renal tubular acidosis
Rickets
Riley-Day syndrome
Rubinstein-Taybi syndrome
Silver-Russell syndrome
Skeletal dysplasias (majority)
Thalassemia
The 3-M syndrome
Trichorhexis nodosa syndrome
Weill-Marchesani syndrome
Wilson disease
Zellweger syndrome

Calcification, chondral and/or periarticular

Acromegaly
Alkaptonuria
Arterial calcification of infancy
Calcinosis interstitialis universalis
Calcium pyrophosphate dihydrate deposition disease
Chondrodysplasia punctata
CREST syndrome
Dermatomyositis
Diabetes mellitus
Dysplasia epiphysealis hemimelica
Fluorosis
GM$_1$ gangliosidos
Gout
Hemochromatosis
Hydroxyaptite deposition disease
Hyperparathyroidism
Hypoparathyroidism
Hypophosphatasia
Hypothyroidism
Idiopathic hip calcification in infants and children[214]
Metastatic calcification
Milk-alkali syndrome
Mixed connective tissue disease
Multiple endocrine neoplasia, type 2a
Niemann-Pick disease
Oxalosis
Progressive pseudorheumatoid chondrodysplasia
Renal osteodystrophy
Sarcoidosis
Scleroderma
Tumoral calcinosis
Vitamin D intoxication
Warfarin embryopathy
Werner syndrome
Wilson disease
Zellweger syndrome

Dwarfism with neonatal death

Achondrogenesis, type I
Achondrogenesis, type II
Achondroplasia (homozygous)
Asphyxiating thoracic dysplasia
Atelosteogenesis
Boomerang dysplasia
Campomelic dysplasia
Cephaloskeletal dysplasia (Taybi-Linder)
Chondrodysplasia punctata

Dappled diaphyseal dysplasia[40]
de la Chapelle dysplasia
Diastrophic dysplasia (rarely lethal)
Dyssegmental dwarfism
Fetal cytomegalovirus infection
Fetal herpes simplex infection
Fetal rubella syndrome
Fibrochondrogenesis
Hydrops—ectopic calcification—moth-eaten skeletal dysplasia
Hypochondrogenesis
Hypophosphatasia
Intrauterine dwarfism, peculiar facies, and thin bones with multiple fractures[128]
Jarcho-Levin syndrome
Lethal congenital dwarfism with accelerated skeletal maturation[26]
Metatropic dysplasia
Neu-Laxova syndrome
Osteodysplasty, Melnick-Needles (lethal male)
Osteogenesis imperfecta, type II
Osteopetrosis
Potter syndrome
Round femoral distal epiphyseal micromelic dysplasia—Maroteaux
Schneckenbecken dysplasia
Sedaghatian congenital lethal metaphyseal chondrodysplasia[181]
Short rib syndrome, type Beemer
Short rib-polydactyly, type 1
Short rib-polydactyly, type 2
Short rib-polydactyly, type 3
Spondyloepiphyseal dysplasia congenita
Spondylometaphyseal abnormalities—advanced bone age[14]
Thanatophoric dysplasia
Thanatophoric variants
Warfarin embryopathy

Exostosis, spur, horn*

Acrodysostosis (proximal tibia)
Alagille syndrome
Chondroectodermal dysplasia
Chromosome XO syndrome
Dentino-osseous dysplasia
Dysplasia epiphysealis hemimelia
Exostosis (multiple cartilaginous)
Fibrodysplasia ossificans progressiva
Frontometaphyseal dysplasia
Iso-Kikuchi syndrome
Median cervical webbing/cleft—micrognathia—symphyseal spur
Metachondromatosis
Nail-patella syndrome (iliac horn)
Occipital horn syndrome
Spondylo-epi-metaphyseal dysplasia with joint laxity
Suprachondylar humeral process
Tricho-rhino-phalangeal dysplasia, type 2
Tuberous sclerosis
Unusual facies—arthrogryposis—advanced skeletal maturation syndrome[116]

Fragile Bones, Pathologic Fracture

Achondrogenesis
Aluminum intoxication
Amyoplasia
Anderson syndrome
Arthrogryposis
Aspartylglucosaminuria
Cleidocranial dysplasia
Copper deficiency
Cushing syndrome
Cutis laxa
Cystinosis
Dysosteosclerosis

*Please see **metaphyseal spur,** p. 874.

Enchondromatosis (Ollier)
Fibrous dysplasia
Gaucher disease
Gerodermia osteodysplastica hereditaria
Glycogenosis, type I
GM₁ gangliosidosis I
Homocystinuria
Hyperparathyroidism
Hyperphosphatasemia
Hyperthyroidism
Hypophosphatasia
Koller syndrome
Lethal syndromes with thin bones[128, 158]
Lichtenstein syndrome
Lowe syndrome
McCune-Albright syndrome
Membranous lipodystrophy
Menkes syndrome
Metaphyseal chondrodysplasia, type Jansen
Milkman syndrome
Mucolipidosis II
Niemann-Pick disease
Osteogenesis imperfecta, all types
Osteopetrosis
Osteoporosis (refer to the list)
Osteoporosis (idiopathic juvenile)
Osteoporosis-megaepiphyseal dysplasia[162]
Osteoporosis-pseudoglioma syndrome
Oxalosis
Pena-Shokeir syndrome
Progeria
Pycnodysostosis
Pyle disease
Renal tubular acidosis
Rickets
Riley-Day syndrome
Scurvy
Stiff-man syndrome
Thalassemia
Thevenard syndrome
Tricho-rhino-phalangeal dysplasia, type 2
Werdnig-Hoffmann syndrome
Wilson disease

Gout
Hyperlipoproteinemia
Glycogenesis, type I
Lesch-Nyhan syndrome
Thalassemia
Vaquez-Osler syndrome

Hemihypertrophy (localized or generalized)
Beckwith-Wiedemann syndrome
Hemihypertrophy
Klippel-Trenaunay syndrome
Macrodystrophia lipomatosa
Proteus syndrome

Lytic lesions, radioluent defects
Amyloidosis
Calcium hydroxyapatite crystal deposition disease
Enchondromatosis
Farber syndrome
Fibromatosis
Fibrous dysplasia
Gaucher disease
Gout
Hemochromatosis
Hemophilia
Histiocytosis X
Hyperlipoproteinemia

Hyperparathyroidism (brown tumor)
Kasabach-Merritt syndrome
Kirghizian dermato-osteolysis
Lipoid dermatoarthritis
Lymphangiomatosis
Macrodystrophia lipomatosa
Maffucci syndrome
Membranous lipodystrophy
Mixed connective tissue disease
Mucolipidoses
Neurofibromatosis
Oro-facio-digital syndrome I
Osteogenesis imperfecta
Osteoglophonic dwarfism
Osteolyses
Osteolysis, familial expansile
Pancreatitis
Phalangeal microgeodic syndrome of infancy
POEMS syndrome
Pseudohypoparathyroidism
Reflex sympathetic dystrophy syndrome
Relapsing polychondritis
Rothmund-Thomson syndrome
Sarcoidosis
Scleroderma
Sickle cell anemia
Sjögren syndrome
Tuberous sclerosis
Winchester syndrome
Xanthomatosis

Osteolysis
Acro-osteolysis (refer to the list)
Ehlers-Danlos syndrome
Hajdu-Cheney syndrome
Hyperparathyroidism
Keratoderma palmaris et plantaris familiaris
Kirghizian dermato-osteolysis
Kuskokwim syndrome
Mixed connective tissue disease
Osteolysis (Gorham disease)
Osteolysis, familial expansile
Osteolysis with nephropathy
Osteolysis without nephropathy
Pachydermoperiostosis
Paget disease[166]
Progeria
Pseudoxanthoma elasticum
Rothmund-Thomson syndrome
Sarcoidosis
Scleroderma
Singleton-Merten syndrome
Thevenard syndrome
Wegener granulomatosis
Winchester syndrome

Osteoporosis
Acromegaly
Addison, disease
Alkaptonuria
Aluminum intoxication
Anemias
Arthrogryposis
Aspartylglucosaminuria
Asphyxiating thoracic dysplasia
Calcium hydroxyapatite crystal deposition disease
Calvarial doughnut lesions–osteoporosis–dentinogenesis imperfecta
Celiac disease
Cerebro-oculo-facio-skeletal syndrome
Chromosomal abnormalities (13, 18, 21, XO, etc.)

Cockayne syndrome
Contractural arachnodactyly
Copper deficiency
Cranioectodermal dysplasia
CREST syndrome
Cushing syndrome
Cystic fibrosis
Deprivation dwarfism
Diabetes mellitus
Duchenne muscular dystrophy
Ehlers-Danlos syndrome
Epidermolysis bullosa dystrophica
Estrogen deficiency (postmenopausal)
Fanconi syndrome
Farber disease
Fibrodysplasia ossificans progressive
Fibrogenesis imperfecta ossium
Flynn-Aird syndrome
Focal scleroderma
Gaucher disease
Gerodermia osteodysplastica hereditaria
Glycogenosis, type I
GM$_1$ gangliosidosis
Goltz syndrome
Gout
Grant syndrome
Hajdu-Cheney syndrome
Hallermann-Streiff syndrome
Hemochromatosis
Hemophilia
Homocystinuria
Hypercalcemia, idiopathic
Hyperparathyroidism
Hyperphosphatasemia
Hyperthyroidism
Hypogonadism
Hypoparathyroidism
Hypophosphatasia
Hypopituitarism
Hypothyroidism
Infantile multisystem inflammatory disease
Kawasaki syndrome
Keratosis palmaris et plantaris familiaris
Laron syndrome
Liver disease
Lowe syndrome
Malabsorption syndrome
Mannosidosis
Mauriac syndrome
Mediterranean fever
Membranous lipodystrophy
Menkes syndrome
Metachromatic leukodystrophies
Metaphyseal chondrodysplasia, Jansen type
Mixed connective tissue disease
Mucolipidosis
Mucopolysaccharidoses
Muscular dystrophies
Myotonia congenita
Niemann-Pick disease
Osteogenesis imperfecta, all types
Osteolysis (Gorham)
Osteolysis with nephropathy
Osteoporosis (idiopathic juvenile)
Osteoporosis of the hip (transient)
Osteoporosis-megaepiphyseal dysplasia[162]
Osteoporosis-pseudoglioma syndrome
Pancreatitis
Papillon-Lefèvre syndrome
Parastremmatic dwarfism
Phenylketonuria

Prader-Willi syndrome
Progeria
Pseudohypoparathyroidism
Pyruvate kinase deficiency
Reflex sympathetic dystrophy syndrome
Refsum disease
Regional migratory osteoporosis[121]
Renal tubular acidosis
Rickets
Rothmund-Thomson syndrome
Scleroderma
Scurvy
Sickle cell anemia
Singleton-Merten syndrome
Spherocytosis
Thalassemia
Thevenard syndrome
Thoracic outlet syndrome
Trichorrhexis nodosa syndrome (peripheral osteopenia)
Vitamin D intoxication
Waldenström syndrome
Wegener granulomatosis
Werner syndrome
Wilson syndrome
Winchester syndrome
Wolman disease

Osteosclerosis

Anderson syndrome
Caffey disease
Calcium hydroxyapatitie crystal deposition disease
Central osteosclerosis–bamboo-hair
Côté-Katasantoni syndrome
Craniodisphyseal dysplasia
Craniometaphyseal dysplasia
Dentino-osseous dysplasia
Diaphyseal dysplasia (Engelmann)
Diaphyseal dysplasia–anemia[83]
Diaphyseal dysplasia–proximal myopathy[36]
Distal osteosclerosis
Dysosteosclerosis
Endosteal hyperostosis (van Buchem)
Endosteal hyperostosis (Worth)
Epidermal nevus syndrome
Erdheim-Chester disease
Fibrogenesis imperfecta ossium
Fibrous dysplasia
Fluorosis
Frontometaphyseal dysplasia
Fucosidosis
Gardner syndrome
Gaucher disease
Hyperostosis-hyperphosphatemia syndrome
Hyperparathyroidism (treated)
Hyperthyroidism (thyroid acropathy)
Hypertrophic osteoarthropathy, idiopathic
Hypoparathyroidism
Hypoparathyroidism-skeletal hyperostosis[136]
Hypothyroidism (infants, juvenile)
Lead intoxication
Lenz-Majewski hyperostotic dwarfism
Lipodystrophy (lipoatrophic diabetes)
Mixed sclerosing bone dystrophy with angiodysplasia
Mixed sclerosing bone dystrophies
Neurofibromatosis
Oculo-dento-osseous dysplasia
Osteoarthropathy, familial idiopathic (Currarino)
Osteomalacia, healing
Osteomesopyknosis
Osteopathia striata
Osteopetrosis

Osteopoikilosis
Osteosclerosis, dominant-type Stanescu
Oxalosis
Pachydermoperiostosis
Patterson syndrome
Peripheral osteosclerosis
Physiologic, newborns
POEMS syndrome
Prostaglandin-induced periostitis
Pseudohypoparathyroidism
Pycnodysostosis
Pyle disease (infants)
Renal osteodystrophy
Robinow syndrome
Rothmund-Thomson syndrome
Schwarz-Lélek syndrome
Sclerosteosis
Sickle cell anemia
Sterno-costo-clavicular hyperostosis
Thickened cortical bone and congenital neutropenia
Tricho-dento-osseous syndrome
Trichorrhexis nodosa syndrome (axial osteosclerosis)
Tuberous sclerosis

Tubular stenosis (Kenny-Caffey) dysplasia
Vitamin A intoxication
Vitamin D intoxication
Weismann-Netter syndrome
Williams syndrome

Rickets
Bartter syndrome
Cystinosis
Epidermoid nevus syndrome
Fanconi syndrome
Fibrous dysplasia
Lowe syndrome
McCune-Albright syndrome
Melorheostosis[141]
Neurofibromatosis
Osteopetrosis
Paraneoplastic syndromes
Renal tubular acidosis
Sjögren syndrome
Tyrosinemia
Wilson syndrome

SKIN, HAIR, AND NAILS

Adipose tissue absence
Diencephalic syndrome
Lipodystrophy

Alopecia, sparse hair
Acrocephalopolysyndactyly, Sakati type
Acrodermatitis enteropathica
CHILD syndrome
Chondrodysplasia punctata
Chondroectodermal dysplasia
Chromosome 18p− syndrome
Chromosome 21 trisomy syndrome
Clouston syndrome
Cockayne syndrome
Cronkhite-Canada syndrome
Dubowitz syndrome
Dyskeratosis congenita
Ectodermal dysplasia (hypohidrotic)
Encephalo-cranio-cutaneous lipomatosis
Endocrine-moniliasis syndrome
Epidermal nevus syndrome
Flynn-Aird syndrome
GAPO syndrome
Goltz syndrome
Hallermann-Streiff syndrome
Hay-Wells syndrome[102]
Homocystinuria
Hypomelanosis of Ito
Hypoparathyroidism
Hypopituitarism (anterior lobe)
Incontinentia pigmenti
Keratoderma hereditaria mutilans
Laron dwarfism
Mandibuloacral dysplasia
Marinesco-Sjögren syndrome
Menkes syndrome
Metaphyseal chondrodysplasia (McKusick)
Myotonic dystrophy
Neu-Laxova syndrome
Oculo-dento-osseous syndrome
Odonto-tricho-melic hypohidrotic dysplasia
Oro-facio-digital syndrome I
Pallister-Killian syndrome

Polyglandular autoimmune disease
Progeria
Pterygium syndrome
Rosselli-Gulienetti syndrome
Rothmund-Thomson syndrome
Seckel syndrome
Senter syndrome[220]
Tricho-odonto-onychial dysplasia
Tricho-rhino-phalangeal dysplasia, types 1 and 2
Werner syndrome
Yunis-Varón syndrome

Aplasia or hypoplasia of skin
Aplasia cutis congenita
Chromosome 4p− syndrome
Chromosome 13 trisomy syndrome
Oculo-cerebro-cutaneous syndrome

Café au lait spots
Ataxia-telangiectasia
Bloom syndrome
Dubowitz syndrome
Gastrocutaneous syndrome
Hemihypertrophy
Jaffe-Campanacci syndrome
McCune-Albright syndrome
Multiple endocrine neoplasia, type 3
Neurofibromatosis
Ring chromosome 11[72]
Silver-Russell syndrome
Tuberous sclerosis

Cutis gyrata
Cutis verticis gyrata
Pachydermoperiostosis

Cutis laxa
C syndrome
Chromosome XO syndrome
Cutis laxa
Cutis laxa/Ehlers-Danlos syndrome[242]
Diastrophic dysplasia
Ehlers-Danlos syndrome
Gerodermia osteodysplastica hereditaria

Marfanoid hypermobility syndrome
Occipital horn syndrome
Osteogenesis imperfecta
Patterson syndrome
Potter syndrome
Weaver syndrome

Dimple, skin
Amyoplasia congenita disruptive sequence
Campomelic dysplasia
Caudal dysplasia sequence
Chromosome 18q− syndrome
Chromosome 9p trisomy syndrome
Distal arthrogryposis[97]
Freeman-Sheldon syndrome
Hypophosphatasia
Kyphomelic dysplasia
Mesomelic dysplasia (Nievergelt)
Pena-Skokeir syndrome
Smith-Lemli-Opitz syndrome
Zellweger syndrome

Ectodermal dysplasia
Chondroectodermal dysplasia
Clouston syndrome
Côté-Katasantoni syndrome
Ectodermal dysplasia (hypohidrotic)
EEC syndrome
EEM syndrome (ectodermal dysplasia, ectrodactyly, macular dystrophy)[178]
Hay-Wells syndrome[102]
Marshall syndrome
Rosselli-Gulienetti syndrome

Eczema, eczematoid lesion
Acrodermatitis enteropathica
Ataxia-telangiectasia
Chromosome 18q− syndrome
Chronic granulomatous disease of childhood
Dubowitz syndrome
Ectodermal dysplasia, hypohidrotic
Hyperimmune E syndrome
Hypoparathyroidism
Incontinentia pigmenti
Osteoarthropathy, familial idiopathic (Currarino)
Phenylketonuria
Shwachman syndrome
Wiskott-Aldrich syndrome

Hair abnormality, miscellaneous
Aminopterin fetopathy
Chromosome 21 trisomy syndrome
Cutis verticis gyrata
Hemihypertrophy
Hypothyroidism
Menkes syndrome
Mucopolysaccharidosis I-H
Noonan syndrome
Occipital horn syndrome
Odonto-tricho-melic hypohidrotic dysplasia
Romberg syndrome
Rubinstein-Taybi syndrome
Treacher Collins syndrome
Tricho-dento-osseous syndrome
Trichorrhexis nodosa syndrome
Yunis-Varón syndrome

Hair, color abnormalities
Cystinosis
Klein-Waardenburg syndrome
Kwashiorkor
Metaphyseal chondrodysplasia (McKusick)

Smith-Lemli-Opitz syndrome
Waardenburg syndrome
Werner syndrome

Hairline, low
Chromosome 4p trisomy syndrome
Chromosome XO syndrome
de Lange syndrome
Fetal hydantoin syndrome
Fraser syndrome
Goldenhar syndrome
Klippel-Feil syndrome
Noonan syndrome

Hirsutism
Adrenal hyperplasia
Bardt-Biedl syndrome
Bloom syndrome
Cerebro-oculo-facio-skeletal syndrome
Chromosome 18 trisomy syndrome
Chromosome XO syndrome
Coffin-Siris syndrome
de Lange syndrome
Mucopolysaccharidoses
Endocrinopathies in female (androgenic-mediated, drug-induced)[203]
Epidermal nevus syndrome
Fetal alcohol syndrome
Fetal hydantoin syndrome
Frontometaphyseal dysplasia
Hajdu-Cheney syndrome
Hemihypertrophy
Hypertrichosis-osteochondrodysplasia
Leprechaunism syndrome
Lipodystrophy (lipoatrophic diabetes)
Marshall-Smith syndrome
Morgagni-Stewart-Morel syndrome
Mucopolysaccharidoses
Patterson syndrome
POEMS syndrome
Polycystic ovary syndrome (Stein-Leventhal)
Rubinstein-Taybi syndrome
Schinzel-Giedion syndrome
Thevenard syndrome
Unusual facies−arthrogryposis−advanced skeletal maturation[116]
Winchester syndrome
Zimmerman-Laband syndrome

Hyperhidrosis
Böök syndrome
Chédiak-Higashi syndrome
Dyskeratosis congenita
Jadassohn-Lewandowsky syndrome
Keratosis palmaris et plantaris familiaris
Osteoarthropathy, familial idiopthic (Currarino)
Pachydermoperiostosis
POEMS syndrome
Reflex sympathetic dystrophy syndrome
Shapiro syndrome
Silver-Russell syndrome
TAR Syndrome

Hypohidrosis/anhidrosis
Cokayne syndrome
Ectodermal dysplasia (hypohidrotic)
Hay-Wells syndrome
Menkes syndrome
Rapp-Hodgkin ectodermal dysplasia
Rosselli-Gulienetti syndrome
Shy-Drager syndrome
Sjögren-Larsson syndrome

Icthyosis, ichthyosiform lesion, thick skin

Bloom syndrome
Camptodactyly-ichthyosis syndrome
CHILD syndrome
Chondrodysplasia punctata
Clouston syndrome
Epidermal nevus syndrome
Geleophysic dysplasia
Hypomelanosis of Ito
Jadasshon-Lewandowsky syndrome
Keratoderma hereditaria mutilans
Koller syndrome
Menkes syndrome
Metachromatic leukodystrophies
Mucolipidosis II
Mucopolysaccharidosis I-H/S
Neu-Laxova syndrome
Pachydermoperiostosis
Refsum syndrome
Senter syndrome[220]
Sjögren-Larsson syndrome
Trichorrhexis nodosa syndrome
Werner syndrome

Keratosis

Darier disease
Dyskeratosis congenita
Jadassohn-Lewandowsky syndrome
Keratoderma hereditaria mutilans
Keratosis palmaris et plantaris familiaris (tylosis)
Mal de Meleda
Papillon-Lefèvre syndrome
Proteus syndrome

Nail aplasia, hypoplasia, deformity

Acro-fronto-facio-nasal dysostosis syndrome
Acrodysostosis
Acromesomelic dysplasia
Amniotic band syndrome (Adams-Oliver)
Anonychia-ectrodactyly of foot[182]
Anonychia-ectrodactyly syndrome
Antley-Bixler syndrome
Aplasia cutis congenita
Asphyxiating thoracic dysplasia
Brachydactyly−ectrodactyly−onychodystrophy and anonychia[130]
Brachymesophalangy-nail dysplasia
CHILD syndrome
Chondroectodermal dysplasia
Chromosomal abnormalities (4, 8, 9, 13, 18, XO, etc.)
Clouston syndrome
Coffin-Siris syndrome
Cronkhite-Canada syndrome
DOOR syndrome
Dyskeratosis congenita
Ectodermal dysplasia, hereditary
EEC syndrome
Epidermolysis bullosa dystrophica
Familial acrogeria (Grottron)
Fetal alcohol syndrome
Fetal hydantoin syndrome
Fetal primidone syndrome
Fetal valproate syndrome
Fibrochondrogenesis
Fryns syndrome
Goltz syndrome
Hajdu-Cheney syndrome
Hallermann-Streiff syndrome
Hypothyroidism (infants)
Incontinentia pigmenti
Iso-Kukuchi syndrome
Isolated anonychia, familial

Jadassohn-Lewandowsky syndrome
Kirghizian dermato-osteolysis
Larsen syndrome
LEOPARD syndrome
Mandibuloacral dysplasia
Metaphyseal chondrodysplasia (McKusick)
Multiple synostosis syndrome
Nail-patella syndrome
Onychonychia and absence or hypoplasia of distal phalanges
Oto-onycho-peroneal syndrome
Oto-palato-digital syndrome, type 1
Pallister-Hall syndrome
Progeria
Pterygium syndrome
Pycnodysostosis
Rapp-Hodgkin ectodermal dysplasia syndrome
Roberts syndrome
Robinow syndrome
Rosselli-Gulienetti syndrome
Rothmund-Thomson syndrome
Rubinstein-Taybi syndrome
Schinzel-Giedion syndrome
Sclerosteosis
Short rib-polydactyly syndrome, type 1
Sorsby syndrome
Sotos syndrome
Tricho-dento-osseous syndrome
Tricho-odonto-onychial dysplasia
Tricho-rhino-phalangeal dysplasia, types 1 and 2
Trichorrhexis nodosa syndrome
Triphalangeal thumb−onychodystrophy−deafness
Warfarin embryopathy
Weaver syndrome
Williams syndrome
Yellow nail syndrome
Zimmerman-Laband syndrome

Nail discoloraton[12]

Bacterial and fungal infections
Dermatoses
Malnutrition
Nevi
POEMS syndrome
Shell nail syndrome (bronchiectasis)
Trichorhinophalangeal syndrome
Wilson disease
Yellow nail syndrome

Onycholysis[12]

Congenital, isolated abnormality
Dermatoses
Drug-induced
Hyperthyroidism
Incontinentia pigmenti
Iron deficiency anemia
Onychodystrophy
Onychomycosis
Pellagra
Porphyria
Stevens-Johnson syndrome
Yellow nail syndrome

Pigmentary abnormalities of skin

Acrodysostosis
Acrodysplasia with retinitis pigmentosa and nephropathy (Saldino-Mainzer)
Acrogeria
Addison disease
Alkaptonuria
Ataxia-telangiectasia
Bloom syndrome
Chédiak-Higashi syndrome

Chondrodysplasia punctata
Chromosome XO syndrome
Clouston syndrome
Copper deficiency
Cronkhite-Canada syndrome
DeSanctis-Cacchione syndrome
Dyskeratosis congenita
Ectodermal dysplasia (hypohidrotic)
EEC syndrome
Epidermal nevus syndrome
Fanconi anemia
Farber syndrome
Gastrocutaneous syndrome
Gaucher disease
Goltz syndrome
Hay-Wells syndrome[102]
Hemihypertrophy
Hemochromatosis
Homocystinuria (malar flush)
Hyperphosphatasemia
Hypomelanosis of Ito
Incontinentia pigmenti
Klein-Waardenburg syndrome
Klippel-Trenaunay-Weber syndrome
Kuskokwim syndrome
LAMB syndrome
LEOPARD syndrome
Lipodystrophy
Maffucci syndrome
McCune-Albright syndrome
Melorheostosis
Myxoma—spotty pigmentation—endocrine overactivity
Neurocutaneous melanosis sequence
Neurofibromatosis
Nevoid basal cell carcinoma syndrome (Gorlin)
Noonan syndrome
Patterson syndrome
Peutz-Jeghers syndrome
Piebaldism-Waardenburg syndrome[118]
POEMS syndrome
Polyglandular autoimmune disease
Prader-Willi syndrome
Progeria
Proteus syndrome
Reflex sympathetic dystrophy syndrome
Romberg syndrome
Rothmund-Thomson syndrome
Ruvalcaba-Myhre-Smith syndrome
Senter syndrome[220]
Silver-Russell syndrome
Tricho-rhino-phalangeal dysplasia, type 2
Tuberous sclerosis
Tuomaala syndrome
Vitamin A intoxication
Waardenburg syndrome
Weber-Christian syndrome
Wilson disease
Winchester syndrome

Skin atrophy
Acrocephalopolysyndactyly, Sakati type
Acrogeria
Ataxia-telangiectasia
Flynn-Aird syndrome
Hallermann-Streiff syndrome
Incontinentia pigmenti
Mandibuloacral dysplasia
Progeria
Rothmund-Thomson syndrome
Scleroderma
Weber-Christian syndrome

Skin eruption, erythema, rash
De Sanctis-Cacchione syndrome
Degos syndrome
Dermatomyositis
Dermo-chondro-corneal dystrophy of François
Dubowitz syndrome
Epidermal nevus syndrome
Epidermolysis bullosa dystrophica
Fabry syndrome
Farber syndrome
Fetal cytomegalovirus infection
Fetal herpes simplex infection
Glucogonoma syndrome
Hemolytic uremic syndrome
Henoch-Schönlein syndrome
Histiocytosis X
Homocystinuria
Horner syndrome
Hyperlipoproteinemia
Infantile multisystem inflammatory disease
Juvenile xanthogranuloma
Kawasaki syndrome
LEOPARD syndrome
Lipoid dermatoarthritis
Macrodystrophia lipomatosa
Mediterranean fever
Mixed connective tissue disease
Oro-facio-digital syndrome
Osteoarthropathy, familial idiopathic (Currarino)
Phenylketonuria
Pseudoxanthoma elasticum
Reiter syndrome
Relapsing polychondritis[29]
Rothmund-Thomson syndrome
Sea-blue histiocyte syndrome
Sézary syndrome
Stevens-Johnson syndrome
Sweet syndrome
Toxic shock syndrome
Vitamin A intoxication
Wegener granulomatosis
Wiskott-Aldrich syndrome
Wissler syndrome

Skin lesions in metabolic disorders[140]
Alkaptonuria
Arginosuccinic aciduria
Biotin deficiency
Homocystinuria
Phenylketonuria
Tyrosinemia II (Richner-Hanhart syndrome)

Telangiectasia
Ataxia-telangiectasia
Bloom syndrome
Carcinoid syndrome
Chromosome XO syndrome
CREST syndrome
Dyskeratosis congenita
Fetal alcohol syndrome
Fetal hydantoin syndrome
Hemihypertrophy
Klippel-Trenaunay syndrome
Rendu-Osler-Weber syndrome
Rothmund-Thomson syndrome
Wegener granulomatosis

Tumor, cutaneous
Cowden syndrome
Epidermal nevus syndrome
Gardner syndrome

Gastrocutaneous syndrome
LAMB syndrome
Myxoma—spotty pigmentation—endocrine overactivity
Nevoid basal cell carcinoma syndrome (Gorlin)
Osteoma cutis, familial
Osteopoikilosis

Wrinkled skin
Acrogeria
Cutis verticis gyrata (scalp)
Megaepiphyseal dysplasia—wrinkled skin and aging[162]
"Michelin tire baby" syndrome (skin folds)[131]
Wrinkly skin syndrome

TUMORS

Cancer, propensity to develop
Alagille syndrome[65]
Aniridia
Ataxia-telangiectasis
Bannayan syndrome
Beckwith-Wiedemann syndrome
Behçet syndrome
Bloom syndrome
Blue rubber bleb nevus syndrome
Carney syndrome
Celiac disease
Chédiak-Higashi syndrome
Chromosomal abnormalities (21, XXY, etc.)
Cowden syndrome
Cronkhite-Canada syndrome
De Sanctis-Cacchione syndrome
Diamond-Blackfan syndrome
Diaphyseal medullary stenosis with bone malignancy—Hardcastle
Drash syndrome
Dubowitz syndrome
Dyskeratosis congenita
Enchondromatosis (Ollier)
Epidermal nevus syndrome
Epidermolysis bullosa
Exostosis
Familial atypical multiple mole-melanoma syndrome (FAMMM)[152]
Fanconi anemia
Fetal alcohol syndrome
Fetal hydantoin syndrome
Fibrous dysplasia
Gardner syndrome
Glycogenosis, type I
Goldenhar syndrome
Hemihypertrophy
Hemochromatosis
Hepatic fibrosis—renal cystic disease
Incontinentia pigmenti
Li-Fraumeni cancer family syndrome[153, 184]
Lymphoproliferative syndrome
Lynch syndrome I
Lynch syndrome II
Maffucci syndrome
McCune-Albright syndrome
Multiple endocrine, type 1
Multiple endocrine, type 2a
Multiple endocrine, type 2b
Myxoma—spotty pigmentation—endocrine overactivity
N syndrome
Neurocutaneous melanosis sequence
Neurofibromatosis
*OSLAM syndrome[168]
Osteopoikilosis
Paraneoplastic syndromes
Perlman syndrome[171]
Persistent Müllerian duct syndrome

Peutz-Jegher syndrome
Rothmund-Thomson syndrome
Shwachman syndrome
Sjögren syndrome
Sotos syndrome
Stewart-Treves syndrome
Sweet syndrome
Thymic tumor syndromes
Torre syndrome[91]
Trousseau syndrome
Tuberous sclerosis
Turcot syndrome
Tyrosinemia, type I
von Hippel-Lindau syndrome
WDHA syndrome
Werner syndrome
†Weinberg-Zumwalt syndrome[251]
Wilms tumor—multiple lung hamartomas[149]
Wiskott-Aldrich syndrome
Xeroderma pigmentosa syndrome
Yellow nail syndrome
Zollinger-Ellison syndrome

Hamartomatous lesions
Cystic hamartoma of lung and kidney
Epidermal nevus syndrome
LEOPARD syndrome
Multiple endocrine neoplasia syndrome, type 2b
Neurofibromatosis
Nevoid basal cell carcinoma syndrome (Gorlin)
Oculo-cerebro-cutaneous syndrome
Perlman syndrome[171]
Peutz-Jeghers syndrome
Proteus syndrome
Sturge-Weber syndrome
Tuberous sclerosis
von Hippel-Lindau syndrome
Wilms tumor-multiple lung hamartomas[149]

Hemangioma, vascular stain
Aplasia cutis congenita
Baller-Gerold syndrome
Bannayan syndrome
Beckwith-Wiedemann syndrome
Blue rubber bleb nevus syndrome
Chromosome 13 trisomy syndrome
Cobb syndrome (cutaneo-meningio-spinal angiomatosis)[70]
Diastrophic dysplasia
Familial nevus flammeus
Fetal alcohol syndrome
Hemangiomatous branchial clefts, lip pseudoclefts, unusual facies[96]
Hemihypertrophy
Kasabach-Merritt syndrome
Klippel-Trenaunay-Weber syndrome
Maffucci syndrome
Mucolipidosis II
Opitz syndrome
Osteolysis (Gorham)
Pallister-Hall syndrome
Proteus syndrome

---

*Osteosarcoma, limb anomalies, and erythroid macrocytosis with megaloblastic marrow
†Nephromegaly and multiple pulmonary cysts

Pseudoxanthoma elasticum
Pterygium syndrome
Rendu-Osler-Weber syndrome
Riley-Smith syndrome
Roberts syndrome
Robinow syndrome
Rubinstein-Taybi syndrome
Sacral hemangiomas and multiple congenital anomalies[70]
Schinzel-Giedion syndrome
Sternal malformation–vascular dysplasia syndrome[106]
Sturge-Weber syndrome
Vascular syndromes

von Hippel-Lindau syndrome
Xeroderma pigmentosa syndrome

Wilms tumor, association with
Aniridia-Wilms tumor association
Beckwith-Wiedemann syndrome
Drash syndrome
Hemihypertrophy
Horseshoe kidney malformation
Perlman syndrome[171]
Wilms tumor–multiple lung hamartomas[149]

MISCELLANEOUS

Adipose tissue, absent or deficient
Chondrodysplasia punctata, dominant type
Cockayne syndrome
Diencephalic syndrome
Fetal alcohol syndrome
Leprechaunism syndrome
Lipodystrophy (lipoatrophic diabetes)[241]
Progeria
Rothmund-Thomson syndrome
Werner syndrome
Wiedemann-Rautenstrauch syndrome

Asymmetry
Acrocephalosyndactyly, Saethre-Chotzen type (face)
Angiodysplasias
Bannayan syndrome
Beckwith-Wiedemann syndrome
Cerebral palsy
CHILD syndrome
Chondrodysplasia punctata
Chromosomal abnormalities
Coffin-Lowry syndrome
Enchondromatosis (Ollier)
Exostosis (multiple cartilaginous)
Fibrous dysplasia
Goldenhar syndrome (face)
Goltz syndrome
Hemiatrophy
Hemihypertrophy
Hemophilia (sequela to bleeding)
HHHH syndrome
Hypomelanosis of Ito
Incontinentia pigmenti
Klippel-Feil syndrome (face)
Klippel-Trenaunay syndrome
Lipomatosis
Lymphatic abnormalities
Macrodystrophia lipomatosa
Maffucci syndrome
Marfan syndrome (asymmetric form)
McCune-Albright syndrome
Melorheostosis
MURCS association (face)[67]
Neurofibromatosis
Noonan syndrome (head)
Opitz syndrome (head)
Oromandibular-limb hypogenesis (face)
Poland syndrome
Prader-Willi syndrome
Proteus syndrome
Romberg syndrome
Scurvy (sequela)
Seckel syndrome
Silver-Russell syndrome

Sturge-Weber syndrome
Tuberous sclerosis

Breast abnormalities
Cowden syndrome
Neurofibromatosis
Polycystic ovary syndrome (Stein-Leventhal)

Calcification, fingertip
Calcinosis circumscripta universalis
CREST
Dermatomyositis
Epidermolysis bullosa
Mixed connective tissue disease
Raynaud disease
Rothmund-Thomson syndrome
Scleroderma

Calcification, soft tissue[235]
Alkaptonuria
Anterior tibial compartment syndrome
Calcinosis universalis
Calcium pyrophosphate dihydrate deposition disease
Chondrodysplasia punctata
Compartmental syndrome
Copper deficiency
CREST syndrome
Dermatomyositis
Ehlers-Danlos syndrome
Epidermal nevus syndrome
Epidermolysis bullosa
Fat necrosis
Fibrodysplasia ossificans progressive
Fibrogenesis imperfecta ossium
Fluorosis
Focal scleroderma
Gout
Granulomatous disease of childhood
Homocystinuria (vascular calcification)
Hydrops–ectopic calcification–moth-eaten skeletal dysplasia
Hypercalcemia (idiopathic, etc.)
Hyperlipoproteinemia
Hyperparathyroidism
Hypoparathyroidism[136]
Hypophosphatasia
Klippel-Trenaunay-Weber syndrome
Lupus erythematosus
Madelung disease
Maffucci syndrome
Mandibuloacral dysplasia
Melorheostosis
Milk-alkali syndrome
Mixed connective tissue disease
Multiple endocrine neoplasia, type 2a
Myositis ossificans

Nevoid basal cell carcinoma syndrome (Gorlin)
Niemann-Pick disease
Osteodysplasty, Melnick-Needles
Osteoma cutis, familial
Oxalosis
Pachydermoperiostosis
Porphyria
Progeria (vascular calcification)
Pseudohypoparathyroidism
Pseudoxanthoma elasticum
Renal osteodystrophy
Rothmund-Thomson syndrome
Scleroderma
Singleton-Merten syndrome
Takayasu arteritis (vascular calcification)
Tietze syndrome
Tumoral calcinosis
Vitamin A intoxication (ligament calcification)
Vitamin D intoxication
Weber-Christian syndrome
Werner syndrome
Williams syndrome
Wilson disease
Xanthomas

Calcification, stippled (infants)
Acheiria
CHILD syndrome
Chondrodysplasia punctata
Chromosome 18 trisomy syndrome
Chromosome 21 trisomy syndrome
Chromosome X; Y translocation[2]
Cutis laxa
Fetal alcohol syndrome
GM_1 gangliosidosis
Hypopituitarism (anterior lobe)
Hypothyroidism
Infantile multisystem inflammatory disease
Keutel syndrome
Listeria monocytogenesis infection
Metachromatic leukodystrophy
Mucolipidosis II
Smith-Lemli-Opitz syndrome
Warfarin embryopathy
Zellweger syndrome

Chromosomal abnormality
Aniridia-Wilms tumor association
Aplasia cutis congenita
Ataxia-telangiectasia
Barter syndrome
Bloom syndrome
Campomelic dysplasia
Cat-eye syndrome
Caudal dysplasia syndrome
Chondrodysplasia punctata[2]
Cloverleaf skull-limb anomalies
de Lange syndrome
DiGeorge syndrome
Diamond-Blackfan syndrome
Fanconi anemia
Fetal rubella syndrome
Gardner-Silengo-Wachtel syndrome
Goldenhar syndrome
Greig cephalopolysyndactyly syndrome
Holoprosencephaly
Hypereosinophilic syndrome (idiopathic)
Hyperthyroidism
Hypomelanosis of Ito
Hypoparathyroidism
Hypothyroidism (infant)

Incontinentia pigmenti
Mayer-Rokitansky-Küster syndrome
Multiple endocrine neoplasia syndrome, type 1
Multiple endocrine neoplasia syndrome, type 2a
Osteogenesis imperfecta[123]
Pachydermoperiostosis
Pallister-Killian syndrome
Pendred syndrome
Potter syndrome
Prader-Willi syndrome
Pterygium syndrome
Retinoblastoma, chromosome 13q−
Rieger syndrome
Roberts syndrome
Robin sequence
Shwachman syndrome[74]
Silver-Russell syndrome
Smith-Lemli-Opitz syndrome
Treacher Collins syndrome
Werner syndrome
Zellweger syndrome

Edema
Boomerang dysplasia
Budd-Chiari syndrome
Chromosome XO syndrome
Copper deficiency
Cronkhite-Canada syndrome
Cutis laxa
Cyclical edema syndrome
Distichiasis-lymphedema syndrome
G syndrome
Henoch-Schönlein syndrome
Hydrops−ectopic calcification−moth-eaten skeletal dysplasia
Hyperthyroidism
Johanson-Blizzard syndrome
Kwashiorkor
Ménétrier disease
Nephrotic syndrome
Neu-Laxova syndrome
POEMS syndrome
Schneckenbecken dysplasia
TAR syndrome
Wilson disease

Gigantism, early macrosomia
Acromegaly
Adrenal hyperplasia, congenital
Beckwith-Wiedemann syndrome
Chromosome XXY syndrome (Kleinfelter)
Homocystinuria
Hyperpituitarism (gigantism)
Hypertrichosis-osteochondrodysplasia
Lipodystrophy (lipoatrophic diabetes)
Marshall-Smith syndrome
McCune-Albright syndrome
Neurofibromatosis
Pallister-Killian syndrome
Perlman syndrome
Ruvalcaba-Myhre-Smith syndrome
Sclerosteosis
Simpson-Golabi-Behmel syndrome
Sotos syndrome
Tuberous sclerosis
Weaver syndrome

Gynecomastia
Chromosome XXY syndrome
Cowden syndrome
Hyperthyroidism
Hypothyroidism (juvenile)

McCune-Albright syndrome
Nevoid basal cell carcinoma syndrome (Gorlin)
Paraneoplastic syndromes
POEMS syndrome
Reifenstein syndrome

"Horn" (exostosis)

Calvarial hyperostosis, familial
Nail-patella syndrome
Occipital horn syndrome
Proteus syndrome

"Hurler-like" features

Fucosidosis
GM[1] gangliosidosis
Mucolipidoses
Mucopolysaccharidosis I-H/S
Mucopolysaccharidosis II

Hydrops fetalis (nonimmune)[107]

Abdominal
Achondrogenesis
Achondroplasia
Anemias
Cardiovascular diseases
Central nervous system anomalies
Chondrodysplasia punctata (Conradi-Hünermann)
Chorioangioma
Chromosome 13 trisomy syndrome
Diabetes mellitus
Diaphragmatic hernia
Fetal infections (TORCH)
Hydrolethalus syndrome
Hydronephrosis
Hydrops—ectopic calcification—moth-eaten skeletal dysplasia
Idiopathic
Intestinal obstruction
Lung-mediastinal masses obstructing venous return
Meconium peritonitis
Mucopolysaccharidosis VII
Myotonic dystrophy
Noonan syndrome
Osteogenesis imperfecta, type II
Posterior urethral valve
Pterygium syndrome (lethal, multiple)
Short rib-polydactyly syndromes
Soft tissue tumors
Thanatophoric dysplasia
Toxemia (mother)
Tuberous sclerosis
Twin-to-twin transfusion syndrome

Jaundice

Alagille syndrome
Alpha[1]-antitrypsin deficiency
Bile plug syndrome
Budd-Chiari syndrome
Dubin-Johnson syndrome
Fetal herpes simplex infection
Galactosemia
Gilbert syndrome
Hypopituitarism (anterior lobe)
Hypothyroidism
Kawasaki syndrome
Mirizzi syndrome
Osteopetrosis
Paroxysmal nocturnal hemoglobulinuria
Pyruvate kinase deficiency
Renal-hepatic-pancreatic dysplasia
Rotor syndrome
Sickle cell anemia
Spherocytosis

Thalassemia
Tyrosinemia, type 1
Wilson disease

Lipomatosis

Encephalo-cranio-cutaneous lipomatosis
Macrodystrophia lipomatosa
Madelung syndrome
Opitz syndrome
Proteus syndrome

Marfanoid features

Frontometaphyseal dysplasia
Homocystinuria
Marfanoid habitus—X-linked mental retardation[75]
Marfanoid hypermobility syndrome
Marfanoid phenotype-congenital contracture[232]
Marfanoid syndrome with craniosynostosis[78]
Multiple endocrine neoplasia, type 1
Multiple endocrine neoplasia, type 2b
Nevoid basal cell carcinoma syndrome (Gorlin)

Neurocutaneous syndromes[92]

Ataxia-telangiectasia[92]
Encephalo-cranio-cutaneous lipomatosis
Hypomelanosis of Ito
Incontinentia pigmenti[92]
Neurocutaneous angiomatosis, hereditary[113]
Neurocutaneous melanosis (Rokitansky-van Bogaert syndrome)[112]
Neurofibromatosis
Oculocerebral angiomatosis (Brégeat syndrome)
Sjögren-Larsson syndrome
Sturge-Weber syndrome
Systemic angiomatosis (Ullmann syndrome)
Tuberous sclerosis
von Hippel-Lindau syndrome

Nipple anomalies

Aplasia cutis congenita (Adams-Oliver syndrome)
Cerebro-oculo-facio-skeletal syndrome
Chromosomal abnormalities (others)
Cryptophthalmia syndrome
de Lange syndrome
Ectodermal dysplasia (hypohidrotic)
EEC syndrome
Familial supernumerary nipples[145]
Fetal hydantoin syndrome
Fraser syndrome
Hay-Wells syndrome[102]
Johanson-Blizzard syndrome
Leprechaunism
Mucolipidosis II
Noonan syndrome
Poland syndrome
Postaxial acrofacial dysostosis syndrome (Miller)
Progeria
Pterygium syndrome (Escobar)
Ruvalcaba-Myhre-Smith syndrome
Schinzel-Giedion syndrome
Smith-Lemli-Opitz syndrome
Supernumerary nipple and urinary system anomalies (possible association)
Tricho-rhino-phalangeal dysplasia, type 2
Ulnar-mammary syndrome
Weaver syndrome

Obesity

Acrocephalopolysyndactyly, Carpenter type
Bardet-Biedl syndrome
Biemond syndrome II
Börjeson-Forssman-Lehmann syndrome
Chromosomal abnormalities (4, 21, XO, XXY, XXXXY)

Cohen syndrome
Cushing syndrome
Gonadal dysfunction—obesity[42]
Grebe chondrodysplasia
Morgagni-Stewart-Morel syndrome
Pallister-Killian syndrome
Pickwickian syndrome
Polycystic ovarian syndrome (Stein-Leventhal syndrome)
Prader-Willi syndrome
Pseudohypoparathyroidism
Sleep apnea syndrome
Ulnar-mammary syndrome

Ossification, soft tissue
Ehlers-Danlos syndrome
Fibrochondrogenesis
Fibrodysplasia ossificans progressiva
Melorheostosis
Osteoma cutis, familial
Pachydermoperiostosis
Pseudohypoparathyroidism

Peroxisomal disorders[169, 253]
Acatalasemia
Adrenoleukodystrophy, neonatal
Chondrodysplasia punctata, rhizomelic type
Hyperoxaluria type I
Hyperpipecolic acidemia
"Pseudo-Zellweger syndrome" (3-oxoacyl-coenzyme A thiolase deficiency
Refsum disease, infantile
Zellweger syndrome

Premature aging/progeroid appearance
Acrogeria[59]
Chromosome 21 trisomy syndrome
Cockayne syndrome
Congenital dyskeratosis (X-linked)
Cutis laxa
Flynn-Aird syndrome
Gerodermia osteodysplastica hereditaria
Hallermann-Streiff syndrome

Lipodystrophy (Berardinelli-Seip syndrome)
Megaepiphyseal dysplasia—wrinkled skin and aged appearance[162]
Progeria
Rothmund-Thomson syndrome
Werner syndrome
Wiedemann-Rautenstrauch syndrome

Pterygium
Acrocephalosyndactyly, Hermann-Opitz type
Chromosome XO syndrome
Klippel-Feil syndrome
Mental retardation with pterygia, shortness, and distinct facial features[218]
Nail-patella syndrome
Noonan syndrome
Pterygium syndromes

Voice abnormality
Cardiovocal syndrome
Chromosome 5p− syndrome (cri due chat)
Cutis laxa
de Lange syndrome
Farber syndrome
G syndrome
Geleophysic dysplasia
Hajdu-Cheney syndrome
Hypopituitarism
Hypothyroidism
Jadassohn-Lewandowsky syndrome
Lipoid proteinosis
Lowe syndrome
Moore-Federman syndrome
Mucopolysaccharidosis I-H
Pelizaeus-Merzbacher syndrome
Progeria
Relapsing polychondritis
Rüdiger syndrome
Sarcoidosis
Schwartz-Jampel syndrome
Smith-Lemli-Opitz syndrome
Weaver syndrome
Werner syndrome

REFERENCES

1. Acquafredda A et al: Rudimentary testes syndrome revisited. *Pediatrics* 1987; 80:209.
2. Agematsu K et al: Chondrodysplasia punctata with X;Y translocation. *Hum Genet* 80:105, 1988.
3. Andermann F et al: Familial agenesis of the corpus callosum with anterior horn cell disease: A syndrome of mental retardation, areflexia, and paraparesis. *Trans Am Neurol Assoc* 1972; 97:242.
4. Anuras S et al: Recurrent or chronic intestinal pseudo-obstruction. *Clin Gastroenterol* 1981; 10:177.
5. Araki Y et al: Congenital hemicerebral arterial ectasia complicating unilateral megalencephaly. *Br J Radiol* 1987; 60:395.
6. Arnold R et al: The psychological characteristics of infantile hypercalcemia: A preliminary investigation. *Dev Med Child Neurol* 1985; 27:49.
7. Ashley RK et al: Congenital metacarpotalar syndrome. *Ann Acad Med Singapore* 1981; 10:434.
8. Avasthey P et al: Primary pulmonary hypertension, cerebrovascular malformation and lymphedema feet in a family. *Br Heart J* 1968; 30:769.
9. Baraitser M: A new camptodactyly syndrome. *J Clin Genet* 1982; 19:40.
10. Barakat AY et al: Urogenital abnormalities in genetic disease. *J Urol* 1986; 136:778.
11. Barkovich AJ et al: Absence of the septum pellucidim: A useful sign in the diagnosis of congenital brain malformations. *AJNR* 1988; 9:107.
12. Barth JH et al: Diseases of the nails in children. *Pediatr Dermatol* 1987; 4:275.
13. Beck RB et al: Bilateral absence of the ulna in twins as a manifestation of the split hand-split foot deformity. *Am J Perinatol* 1989; 6:1.
14. Beemer FA et al: A new syndrome of dwarfism, neonatal death, narrow chest, spondylometaphyseal abnormalities, and advanced bone age. *Am J Med Genet* 1985; 20:555.
15. Bell J: On brachydactyly and symphalangism, in Penrose LS (ed): *Treasury of Human Inheritance*, vol 5, part 1. Cambridge, England, University Press, 1951, pp 1–31.
16. Bellini F et al: Wedge-shaped epiphyses of the knees in two siblings: A new recessive rare dysplasia? *Helv Paediatr Acta* 1984; 39:365.
17. Bennett CP et al: Exclusion of calcitonin as a candidate gene for the basic defect in a family with autoso-

mal dominant supravalvular aortic stenosis. *J Med Genet* 1988; 25:311.

18. Berhang Am et al: Familial absence of the patella. *J Bone Joint Surg [Am]* 1973; 55A:1088.

19. Berkenstadt M et al: Partial duplication of the eyebrows with other congenital malformations: A new syndrome. *Clin Genet* 1988; 33:207.

20. Bertino RE et al: Prenatal diagnosis of agenesis of the corpus callosum. *J Ultrasound Med* 1988; 7:251.

21. Bezirdjian DR et al: Sickle-shaped scapulae in a patient with Pierre Robin syndrome. *Br J Radiol* 1989; 62:171.

22. Bilginturan N et al: Hereditary brachydactyly associated with hypertension. *J Med Genet* 1973; 10:253.

23. Binns M: Joint laxity in idiopathic adolescent scoliosis. *J Bone Joint Surg [Br]* 1988; 70-B:420.

24. Bird AR, et al: Type IV congenital dyserythropoietic anemia with an unusual response to splenectomy. *Am J Pediatr Hematol Oncol* 1985; 7:199.

25. Bisset GS III et al: MR imaging of coronary artery aneurysms in a child with Kawasaki disease. *AJR* 1989; 152:805.

26. Blomstrand S et al: A case of lethal congenital dwarfism with accelerated skeletal maturation. *Pediatr Radiol* 1985; 15:141.

27. Bonafede RP et al: Autosomal dominant inheritance of scalp defects with ectrodactyly. *Am J Med Genet* 1979; 3:35.

28. Boocock GR et al: Anorectal malformation: Familial aspects and associated anomalies. *Arch Dis Child* 1987; 62:576.

29. Booth A et al: The radiological manifestations of relapsing polychondritis. *Clin Radiol* 1989; 40:147.

30. Bourgeois MJ et al: Micropenis and congenital adrenal hypoplasia. *Am J Perinatol* 1989; 6:69.

31. Brahimi L et al: Acromesomelic dysplasia: A new type. Report of two siblings. *Pediatr. Radiol* 1988; 18:67.

32. Braun H-St: Familial aplasia or hypoplasia of the patella. *Clin Genet* 1978; 13:350.

33. Brenbridge AN et al: Pathologic significance of nephromegaly in pediatric disease. *Am J Dis Child* 1987; 141:652.

34. Bronspriegel N et al: Aplasia cutis congenita and intestinal lymphangiectasia. An unusual association. *Am J Dis Child* 1985; 139:509.

35. Burton BK et al: A new skeletal dysplasia: Clinical, radiologic, and pathologic findings. *J Pediatr* 1986; 109:642.

36. Bye AME et al: Progressive diaphyseal dysplasia and a low muscle carnitine. *Pediatr Radiol* 1988; 18:340.

37. Calabro A et al: Craniosynostosis and unilateral ulnar aplasia. *Am J Med Genet* 1985; 20:203.

38. Cantu J-M et al: Lethal faciocardiomelic dysplasia: A new autosomal recessive disorder. *Birth Defects* 1975; 11(5):91.

39. Carter CO et al: A family study of craniosynostosis, with probable recognition of a distinct syndrome. *J Med Genet* 1982; 19:280.

40. Carty H et al: Dappled diaphyseal dysplasias. *Frotschr Röntgenstr* 1989; 150:228.

41. Cassidy JT: Miscellaneous conditions associated with arthritis in children. *Pediatr Clin N Am* 1986; 33:1033.

42. Castro-Magana M: Hypogonadism and obesity. *Pediatr Ann* 1984; 13:491.

43. Chemke J et al: Absent ulna in the Klippel-Feil syndrome: An unusual associated malformation. *Clin Genet* 1980; 17:167.

44. Christian JC et al: Dominant preaxial brachydactyly with hallux varus and thumb abduction. *Am J Hum Genet* 1972; 24:694.

45. Cockshott WP et al: Familial congenital posterior dislocation of both radial heads. *J Bone Joint Surg [Br]* 1958; 40B:483.

46. Cohen MM Jr. in Emery AEH, Rimoin DL (eds): *Principles and Practice of Medical Genetics*. New York, Churchill Livingston, Inc, 1983, pp 591–592.

47. Cohen MM Jr in Emery AEH, Rimoin DL (eds): *Principles and Practices of Medical Genetics*. New York, Churchill Livingstone, 1983, pp 580–589.

48. Cooper LF et al: Aural atresia associated with multiple congenital anomalies and mental retardation: A new syndrome. *J Pediatr* 1987; 110:747.

49. Cornel G et al: Familial coarctation of the aortic arch with bilateral ptosis: A new syndrome? *J Pediatr Surg* 1987; 22:724.

50. Couch RM et al: Autosomal dominant form of adolescent multinodular goiter. *Am J Hum Genet* 1986; 39:811.

51. Cowchock FS et al: Brief clinical report; Not all cystic hygromas occur in the Ulrich-Turner syndrome. *Am J Med Genet* 1982; 12:327.

52. Cremin B et al: Wormian bones in osteogenesis imperfecta and other disorders. *Skeletal Radiol* 1982; 8:35.

53. Currarino G et al: Severe craniofacial sclerosis and multiple anomalies in a boy and his mother. *Pediatr Radiol* 1986; 16:441.

54. Czeizel A et al: A family study of congenital diaphragmatic defects. *Am J Med Genet* 1985; 21:105.

55. Czeizel A et al: A postaxial polydactyly and progressive myopia syndrome of autosomal dominant origin. *Clin Genet* 1986; 30:406.

56. Daneman D et al: Association of multinodular goiter, cystic renal disease and digital anomalies. *J Pediatr* 1985; 107:270.

57. Danon YL et al: Cholelithiasis in children with immunoglobulin A deficiency: A new gastroenterologic syndrome. *J Pediatr Gastroenterol Nutr* 1983; 2:663.

58. Day RE et al: Normal children with large heads: Benign familial megalencephaly. *Arch Dis Child* 1979; 54:512.

59. De Groot WP et al: Familial acrogeria (Gottron). *Br J Dermatol* 1980; 103:213.

60. De Myer W: Megalencephaly in children: Clinical syndromes, genetic patterns and differential diagnosis from other causes of megalocephaly. *Neurology* 1972; 22:634.

61. Dionisi Vici C et al: Agenesis of the corpus callosum, combined immunodeficiency, bilateral cataract, and hypopigmentation in two brothers. *Am J Med Genet* 1988; 29:1.

62. Diren HB et al: Primary hypertrophic osteoarthropathy. *Pediatr Radiol* 1986; 16:231.

63. Doyle AJ: Demonstration on computed tomography of tracheomalacia in tracheobronchomegaly (Mounier-Kuhn syndrome). *Br J Radiol* 1989; 62:176.

64. Draper MW et al: Distinct form of osteosclerosis in identical twins with mental retardation. *AJR* 1982; 139:1205.

65. du Cret RP et al: Hepatocarcinoma in association with Alagille syndrome. *Clin Nucl Med* 1988; 13:920.

66. Duke RA et al: Acro-osteolysis secondary to pityriasis rubra pilaris. *AJR* 1987; 149:1082.

67. Duncan PA et al: The MURCS association: Muellerian duct aplasia, renal aplasia, and cervicothoracic somite dysplasia. *J Pediatr* 1979; 95:399.

68. Edwards JA et al: Camptobrachydactyly: A new autosomal dominant trait with two probable homozygotes. *Am J Hum Genet* 1972; 24:464.

69. Elejalde BR et al: Nuchal cysts syndromes: Etiology, pathogenesis, and prenatal diagnosis. *Am J Med Genet* 1985; 21:417.

70. Esterly NB: Cutaneous hemangiomas, vascular stains, and associated syndromes. *Curr Probl. Pediatr.* 1987; 17:1.

71. Exner GU: Serpentine fibula-polycystic kidney syndrome: A variant of the Melnick-Needles syndrome or a distinct entity? *Eur J Pediatr* 1988; 147:544.

72. Fagan K et al: Ring chromosome 11 and café-au-lait spots. *Am J Med Genet* 1988; 30:911.

73. Fincham JE et al: Mseleni joint disease: A manganese deficiency? *South Afr Med J* 1981; 60:445.

74. Fraccaro M et al: Shwachman syndrome and chromosome breakage. *Hum Genet* 1988; 79:194.

75. Fryns JP et al: X-linked mental retardation with marfanoid habitus. *Am J Med Genet* 1987; 28:267.

76. Fryns JP et al: Oculocerebral syndrome with hypopigmentation (Cross syndrome). *Clin Genet* 1988; 34:81.

77. Fuhrman W et al: Dwarfism with disproportionately high vertebral bodies. *Humangenetik* 1972; 16:271.

78. Furlong J et al: New marfanoid syndrome with craniosynostosis. *Am J Med Genet* 1987; 26:599.

79. Gardner RJM et al: A syndrome of congenital thrombocytopenia with multiple malformations and neurologic dysfunction. *J Pediatr* 1983; 102:600.

80. Gasco J et al: Double patella: A case of duplication in the coronal plane. *J Bone Joint Surg [Br]* 1987; 69B:602.

81. Ge K et al: Keshan disease: An endemic cardiomyopathy in China. *Virchows Arch Pathol Anat* 1983; 401:1.

82. GENčik A et al: Familial occurrence of congenital diaphragmatic defect in three families. *Helv Paediatr Acta* 1982; 37:289.

83. Ghosal SP et al: Diaphysial dysplasia associated with anemia. *J Pediatr* 1988; 113:49.

84. Gilgenkrantz S et al: Association of del (11) (p 15.1 p 12), aniridia, catalase deficiency, and cardiomyopathy. *Am J Med Genet* 1982; 13:39.

85. Goldberg MG et al: Congenital hand anomaly, etiology and associated malformations. *Hand Clin* 1985; 1:405.

86. Gollop TR et al: Frontofacionasal dysplasia: Evidence for autosomal recessive inheritance. *Am J Med Genet* 1984; 19:301.

87. Gonzalez CH et al: The WT syndrome: A "new" autosomal dominant pleiotropic trait of radial/ulnar hypoplasia with high risk of bone marrow failure and/or leukemia. *Birth Defects* 1977; 13(3B):31.

88. Gorlin RJ et al: Cryptodontic brachymetacarpalia. *Birth Defects* 1971; 7:200.

89. Gorlin RJ et al: Megaepiphyseal dwarfism. *J Pediatr* 1973; 83:633.

90. Gorman CA et al: Significance of some skeletal singularities: Preliminary observations. *Mayo Clin Proc* 1962; 37:530.

91. Graham R et al: Torre-Muir syndrome: An association with isolated sebaceous carcinoma. *Cancer* 1985; 55:2868.

92. Greenwald MJ et al: Ocular manifestations of the neurocutaneous syndromes. *Pediatr Dermatol* 1984; 2:98.

93. Hageman G et al: The pathogenesis of fetal hypokinesia: A neurological study of 75 cases of congenital contractures with emphasis on cerebral lesions. *Neuropediatrics* 1987; 18:22.

94. Halal F et al: Acro-renal-ocular syndrome. Autosomal dominant thumb hypoplasia, renal ectopia, and eye defect. *Am J Med Genet* 1984; 17:753.

95. Hall BD et al: Familial congenital bowing with short bones. *Radiology* 1979; 132:611.

96. Hall BD et al: Brief clinical report: A new syndrome of hemangiomatous branchial clefts, lip pseudoclefts, and unusual facial appearance. *Am J Med Genet* 1983; 14:135.

97. Hall JG et al: The distal arthrogryposis: Delineation of new entities. Review and nosologic discussion. *Am J Med Genet* 1982; 11:185.

98. Halloran SI et al: Cheirolumbar dysostosis: A phenotype of pseudohypoparathyroidism. *Skeletal Radiol* 1983; 10:61.

99. Hamanishi C: Congenital vertical talus: Classification with 69 cases and new measurement systems. *J Pediatr Orthop* 1984; 4:318.

100. Hansen OH et al: Congenital radio-ulnar sysnostosis. *Acta Orthop Scand* 1970; 41:225.

101. Hartley JW et al: Diagnosis and treatment of the inferior vena cava syndrome in advanced malignant disease. *Am J Surg* 1986; 152:70.

102. Hay RJ, Wells RS: The syndrome of ankyloblepharon, ectodermal defects, and cleft lip and palate: An autosomal dominant condition. *Br J Dermatol* 1976; 94:277.

103. Hecht JT et al: Limb deficiency syndrome in half-sibs. *Clin Genet* 1981; 20:432.

104. Hecht JT et al: The Schinzel syndrome in a mother and daughter. *Clin Genet* 1984; 25:63.

105. Hendrix GH: Familial pulmonary hypertension. *South Med J* 1974; 67:981.

106. Hersch JH et al: Sternal malformation/vascular dysplasia association. *Am J Hum Genet* 1985; 21:177.

107. Hill MC et al: Prenatal diagnosis of fetal anomalies using ultrasound and MRI. *Radiol Clin N Am* 1988; 26:287.

108. Hodgson SV et al: Dominant transmission of Springel's shoulder and cleft palate. *J Med Genet* 1981; 18:263.

109. Hollister DW, Hollister WG: The "long-thumb" brachydactyly syndrome. *Am J Med Genet* 1981; 8:5.

110. Hoyme HE et al: Autosomal dominant ectrodactyly and absence of long bones of upper or lower limbs: Further clinical delineation. *J Pediatr* 1987; 111:538.

111. Hudson CD et al: Autosomal dominant hypodontia with nail dysgenesis: Report of twenty-nine cases in six families. *Oral Surg* 1975; 39:409.

112. Humes RA et al: Melanosis and hydrocephalus. *J Neurosurg* 1984; 61:365.

113. Hurst J et al: Hereditary neurocutaneous angiomatous malformations: Autosomal dominant inheritance in two families. *Clin Genet* 1988; 33:44.

114. Ionasescu V et al: Late onset oculogastrointestinal muscular dystrophy (letter). *Am J Med Genet* 1984; 18:781.

115. Ives EJ, Houston CS: Autosomal recessive microcephaly and micromelia in Cree Indians. *Am J Med Genet* 1980; 7:351.

116. Jequier S et al: Unusual facies, arthorgryposis, advanced skeletal maturation and unique bone changes. A new congenital malformation syndrome. *Pediatr Radiol* 1987; 17:405.

117. Jones SN et al: Radiology at your fingertips: Lesions of the terminal phalanx. *Clin Radiol* 1988; 39:478.

118. Kaplan P et al: Piebaldism-Waardenburg syndrome: Histologic evidence of a neural crest syndrome. *Am J Med Genet* 1988; 31:679.

119. Keutel J et al: Eine wahrscheinlich autosomal recessive vererbte Skeletmissbildung mit Humeroradialsynostose. *Humangenetik* 1970; 9:43.

120. Khoo-Boo-Chai: The bifid nose, with report of 3 cases in siblings. *Plast Reconstr Surg* 1965; 36:626.

121. Kim SM et al: Scintigraphic evaluation of regional migratory osteoporosis. *Clin Nucl Med* 1989; 14:36.

122. Klene C et al: Sclérodermie "en coup de sabre" et hemi-atrophie faciale de Parry-Romberg. Problème nosologique. Complication neurologique. *Ann Pediatr* 1989; 36:123.

123. Knisely AS et al: Lethal osteogenesis imperfecta associated with 46, XY, inv (7) (p13q22) karyotype. *J Med Genet* 1988; 25:352.

124. Knudtzon J et al: Growth hormone deficiency associated wtih the ectrodactyly—ectodermal dysplasia—clefting syndrome and isolated absent septum pellucidum. *Pediatrics* 1987; 79:410.

125. Koletzko B et al: Congenital anomalies in patients with choanal atresia: CHARGE association. *Eur J Pediatr* 1984; 142:271.

126. Kozlowski K: Unclassified type of spondyloepiphyseal dysplasia with macroepiphyses. *Australas Radiol* 1972; 16:73.

127. Kozlowski K et al: The rib gap anomaly in partial or mosaic trisomy 8. *Skeletal Radiol* 1988; 17:251.

128. Kozlowski K et al: Intrauterine dwarfism, peculiar facies, and thin bones with multiple fractures: A new syndrome. *Pediatr Radiol* 1988; 18:394.

129. Kufs WM et al: Familial thyrotoxic periodic paralysis. *West J Med* 1989; 150:461.

130. Kumar D et al: Autosomal dominant onychodystrophy and anonychia with type B brachydactyly and ectrodactyly. *Clin Genet* 1986; 30:219.

131. Kunze J: The "Michelin tire baby syndrome": An autosomal dominant trait (letter). *Am J Med Genet* 1986; 25:169.

132. Kurczynski TW et al: Auralcephalosyndactyly: A new hereditary craniosynostosis syndrome. *J Med Genet* 1988; 25:491.

133. Küster W et al: Cleft lip and palate, lower lip pits, and limb deficiency defects. *J Med Genet* 1988; 25:565.

134. Lachiewicz AM et al: Hereditary renal disease and preauricular pits: Report of a kindred. *J Pediatr* 1985; 106:948.

135. Lamb DW et al: Five-fingered hand associated with partial or complete tibial absence and pre-axial polydactyly. A kindred of 15 affected individuals in five generations. *J Bone Joint Surg [Br]* 1983; 65-B:60.

136. Lambert RGW et al: Diffuse skeletal hyperostosis in idiopathic hypoparathyroidism. *Clin Radiol* 1989; 40:212.

137. Landing BH: Personal communication, 1989.

138. Larned DC et al: The association of congenital ptosis and congenital heart disease. *Ophthalmol* 1986; 93:492.

139. Law WM et al: High resolution parathyroid ultrasonography in familial benign hypercalcemia (familial hypercalciuric hypercalcemia). *Mayo Clin Proc* 1984; 59:153.

140. Lee EB: Metabolic diseases and the skin. *Pediatr Clin N Am* 1983;30:597.

141. Lee SH et al: Hypophosphatemic rickets and melorheostosis. *Clin Radiol* 1989; 40:209.

142. Leenders KL et al: Steele-Richardson-Olszewski syndrome. *Brain* 1988; 111:615.

143. Lehrer HZ et al: A concordant craniofacial dysostosis with enlarged parietal foramina in twins. *Radiology* 1969; 92:127.

144. Leung AKC: Natal teeth. *Am J Dis Child* 1986; 140:249.

145. Leung AKC: Familial supernumerary nipples. *Am J Med Genet* 1988; 31:631.

146. Leupold D et al: 3-Hydroxy-3 methyglutaryl-CoA Lyase deficiency in an infant with macrocephaly and mild metabolic acidosis. *Eur J Pediatr* 1982; 138:73.

147. Lewis KB: The upper limb cardiovascular syndrome. *JAMA* 1965; 193:1080.

148. Liebenberg F: A pedigree with unusual anomalies of the elbows, wrists, and hands in five generations. *S Afr Med J* 1973; 47:745.

149. Linder H et al: Simultaneous occurrence of Wilms' tumours and multiple hamartomas of the lung in a 15 year old girl. *Z Kinderchir* 1987; 42:123.

150. Linterman JP: Echocardiography in neurological disorders. *Eur J Pediatr* 1987; 146:15.

151. Lowry RB: Congenital absence of the fibula and craniosynostosis in sibs. *J Med Genet* 1972; 9:227.

152. Lynch HT et al: Phenotypic variation in the familial atypical multiple mole-melanoma syndrome (FAMMM). *J Med Genet* 1983; 20:25.

153. Lynch HT et al: The sarcoma, breast cancer, lung cancer, and adrenocortical carcinoma syndrome revisited. Childhood Cancer *Am J Dis Child* 1985; 139:134.

154. MacDermot KD et al: Radial ray defect and Duane anomaly: Report of a family with autosomal dominant transmission. *Am J Med Genet* 1987; 27:313.

155. Macnicol MF et al: Acrodysostosis and protrusio acetabuli: An association. *J Bone Joint Surg* 1988; 70-B:38.

156. Mafee MF et al: Congenital sensorineural hearing loss. *Radiology* 1984; 150:427.

157. Marchal JL et al: Néphronophtise, dégénérescence tapeto-retinienne, encéphalopathie et agénésie vermienne: Une nouvelle association. A propos de trois cas familiaux. *Ann Pediatr* 1989; 36:126.

158. Maroteaux P et al: Syndromes létaux avec gracilité du squelette. *Arch Fr Pediatr* 1988; 45:477.

159. Martin NDT et al: Idiopathic infantile hypercalcemia: A continuing enigma. *Arch Dis Child* 1984; 59:605.

160. Matthews S et al: Distal symphalangism with involvement of the thumbs and great toes. *Clin Genet* 1987; 32:375.

161. McAfee PC et al: Endocrinologic and metabolic factors in atypical presentations of slipped capital femoral epiphysis. Report of four cases and review of the literature. *Clin Orthop* 1983; 180:188.

162. McAlister WH et al: Macroepiphyseal dysplasia with symptomatic osteoporosis, wrinkled skin, and aged appearance: A presumed autosomal recessive condition. *Skeletal Radiol* 1986; 15:47.

163. McCall RE et al: Bilateral congenital dislocation of the patella. *J Pediatr Orthop* 1987; 7:100.

164. McKay M et al: Isolated tibial hemimelia in sibs: An autosomal-recessive disorder? *Am J Med Genet* 1984; 17:603.

165. Memberg A et al: Three different manifestations of congenital muscular aplasia in a family. *Acta Paediatr Scand* 1987; 76:375.

166. Mitchell ML et al: Case report 438. *Skeletal Radiol* 1987; 16:498.

167. Morin P et al: Le syndrome coxo-podo-patellaire. *J Radiol* 1985; 66:441.

168. Mulvihill JJ et al: Multiple childhood osteosarcomas in an American Indian family with erythroid macrocytosis and skeletal anomalies. *Cancer* 1977; 40:3115.

169. Naïdu S et al: Phenotypic and genotypic variability of generalized peroxisomal disorders. *Pediatr Neurol* 1988; 4:5.

170. Natowicz M et al: Mendelian etiologies of stroke. *Ann Neurol* 1987; 22:175.

171. Neri G et al: The Perlman syndrome: Familial renal dysplasia with Wilms tumor, fetal giantism, and multiple congenital anomalies. *Am J Med Genet* 1984; 19:195.

172. Nesterov AI: The clinical course of Kashin-Beck disease. *Arthritis Rheum* 1964; 7:29.

173. Neufeld M et al: Two types of autoimmune Addison's disease associated with different polyglandular autoimmune (PGA) syndromes. *Medicine* 1981; 60:355.

174. Neuhold VA et al: Taybi-Rubinstein syndrom: Der Stellenwert des Röntgenbildes. *Fortschr Rontgenstr* 1989; 150:49.

175. Nishi Y et al: The Perrault syndrome: Clinical report and review. *Am J Med Genet* 1988; 31:623.

176. Oates E: Spectrum of appearance of hyperostosis frontalis interna on In 111 leukocyte scans. *Clin Nucl Med* 1988; 13:922.

177. Oggero R et al: Transient hyperphosphatemia of infancy: Fifteen new cases. *Acta Paediatr Scand* 1988; 77:257.

178. Ohdo S et al: Association of ectodermal dysplasia, ectrodactyly, and macular dystrophy: The EEM syndrome. *J Med Genet* 1983; 20:52.

179. Okihiro MM et al: Duane syndrome and congenital upper limb anomalies. A familial occurrence. *Arch Neurol* 1977; 34:174.

180. Oley C et al: Blepharophimosis, ptosis, epicanthus inversus syndrome (BPES syndrome). *J Med Genet* 1988; 25:47.

181. Opitz JM et al: Sedaghatian conenital lethal metaphyseal chondrodysplasia: Observations in a second Iranian family and histopathological studies. *Am J Med Genet* 1987; 26:583.

182. Ortonne J-P et al: Anonychia with ectrodactyly of one foot. *Int J Dermatol* 1986; 25:188.

183. Pallister PD et al: Studies of malformation syndromes in man XXXXII: a pleiotropic dominant mutation affecting skeletal, sexual, and apocrine-mammary development. *Birth Defects* 1976; 12(5):247.

184. Pearrson ADJ et al: Two families with the Li-Fraumeni cancer family syndrome. *J Med Genet* 1982; 19:362.

185. Perri G: The radiological features of a new bone dysplasia. *Pediatr Radiol* 1981; 11:109.

186. Pettit RE et al: Macrocephaly with head growth parallel to normal growth pattern. *Arch Neurol* 1980; 37:518.

187. Petty RE et al: Spondyloarthropathies of childhood. *Pediatr Clin N Am* 1986; 33:1079.

188. Pfeiffer RA, Weber U: Kongenitales Glaukom, Brachymetapodie, Minderwuchs, Debilität, und Aortenstenose bei 2 nicht verwandten Kindern. Ein neues syndrom? *Klin Paediatr* 1974; 186:148.

189. Pfeiffer RA et al: Sagittal craniosynostosis, congenital heart disease, mental deficiency, and various dysmorphies in two sibs: A "new" syndrome? *Eur J Pediatr* 1987; 146:75.

190. Pfeiffer RA et al: Sensorineural deafness, hypospadias, and synostosis of metacarpals and metatarsals 4 and 5: A previously apparently undescribed MCA/MR syndrome. *Am J Med Genet* 1988; 31:5.

191. Polinky MS et al: Urolthiasis in childhood. *Pediatr Clin N Am* 1987; 34:683.

192. Pressly TA et al: Ocular complications of Tangier disease. *Am J Med* 1987; 83:991.

193. Protonotarios N et al: Cardiac abnormalities in familial palmoplantar keratosis. *Br Heart J* 1986; 56:321.

194. Qazi QH et al: Inheritance of posterior choanal atresia. *Am J Med Genet* 1982; 13:413.

195. Qasi Q et al: Triphalangeal thumb. *J Med Genet* 1988; 25:505.

196. Raas-Rothschild A et al: Pathological features and prenatal diagnosis in the newly recognized limb/pelvis-hypoplasia/aplasia syndrome. *J Med Genet* 1988; 25:687.

197. Raghavan N et al: MR imaging in the tethered spinal cord syndrome. *AJR* 1989; 152:843.

198. Rappaport EB et al: Slipped capital femoral epiphysis in growth hormone-deficient patients. *Am J Dis Child* 1985; 139:396.

199. Razavi-Encha F et al: Infantile familial encephalopathy with cerebral calcification and leukodystrophy. *Neuropediatr* 1988; 19:72.

200. Reynolds JF et al: Familial Hirschsprung's disease and type D brachydactyly: A report of four affected males in two generations. *Pediatrics* 1983; 71:246.

201. Reynoso M et al: Autosomal dominant macroglossia in two unrelated families. *Hum Genet* 1986; 74:200.

202. Richieri-Costa A et al: Humeroradial multiple synostosis syndrome in a Brazilian child with consanguineous parents: A new multiple synostosis syndrome? *Rev Brasil Genet* 1986; 9:115.

203. Rittmaster RS et al: Hirsutism. *Ann Intern Med* 1987; 106:95.

204. Robinow M et al: Syndactyly type V. *Am J Med Genet* 1982; 11:475.

205. Rochiccioli P et al: Nanisme avec vertèbres hautes et étroites. Deux nouvelles observations. *Ann Pediatr* 1983; 30:709.

206. Rossi LN et al: Autosomal dominant microcephaly without mental retardation. *Am J Dis Child* 1987; 141:655.

207. Rozin MM et al: A new syndrome with camptodactyly, joint contractures, facial anomalies, and skeletal defects: A case report and review of syndromes with camptodactyly. *Clin Genet* 1984; 26:342.

208. Rozycki DL et al: Autosomal recessive deafness associated with short stature, vitiligo, muscle wasting and achalasia. *Arch Otolaryngol* 1971; 93:194.

209. Sackey K et al: Multiple dysmorphic features and pancytopenia: A new syndrome? *Clin Genet* 1985; 27:606.

210. Saldino RM et al: Cone-shaped epiphyses in the distal phalanges. Case report of a child with anorchia. *Radiol Clin Biol* 1972; 41:449.

211. Sanchis A et al: Duplication of hands and feet, multiple joint dislocation, absence of corpus callosum and hypsarrhythmia: Acrocallosal syndrome? *Am J Med Genet* 1985; 20:123.

212. Sandhaus YS et al: A new patella syndrome. *Clin Genet* 1987; 31:143.

213. Sartoris DJ et al: The horn: A pathognomonic feature of paediatric bone dysplasias. *Aust Paediatr J* 1987; 23:347.

214. Sauvegrain J et al: Calcification of the hip in infants and children. New cases and long-term follow-up. *Pediatr Radiol* 1981; 11:29.

215. Say B, Meyer J: Familial trigonocephaly associated with short stature and developmental delay. *Am J Dis Child* 1981; 135:711.

216. Schanker HMJ et al: Recurrent respiratory disease, azoospermia, and nasal polyposis. A syndrome that mimics cystic fibrosis and immotile cilia syndrome. *Arch Intern Med* 1985; 145:2201.

217. Schinzel A et al: The Van der Woude syndrome (dominantly inherited lip pits and clefts). *J Med Genet* 1986; 23:291.

218. Schrander-Stumpel C et al: Mental retardation with pterygia, shortness, and distinct facial appearance: Confirmation of a new MCA/MR syndrome. *Clin Genet* 1988; 34:279.

219. Schuman JS et al: Senior-Loken syndrome (familial renal-retinal dystrophy) and Coats disease. *Am J Ophthalmol* 1985; 100:822.

220. Senter TP et al: Atypical ichtyosiform erythroderma and congenital sensorineural deafness: A distinct syndrome. *J Pediatr* 1978; 92:68.

221. Serur D: Agenesis of the corpus callosum: Clinical, neuroradiological, and cytogenetic studies. *Neuropediatr* 1988; 19:87.

222. Shey WL et al: Familial pubic bone maldevelopment. *Radiology* 1971; 101:174.

223. Silengo MC et al: Triphalangeal thumb and brachyectrodactyly syndrome. *Clin Genet* 1987; 31:13.

224. Soljak MA et al: A new syndrome of short stature, joint limitation, and muscle hypertrophy. *Clin Genet* 1983; 23:441.

225. Spranger JW et al: Cerebroarthrodigital syndrome. *Am J Med Genet* 1980; 5:13.

226. Spranger M et al: Anomalous inheritance in a kindred with split hand, split foot malformation. *Eur J Pediatr* 1988; 147:202.

227. Sreeram N et al: Cardiac abnormalities in the fragile X syndrome. *Br Heart J* 1989; 61:289.

228. Steidle CP et al: Symphyseal diastasis in the absence of the exstrophy-epispadias complex. *J Urol* 1988; 140:349.

229. Stoll C et al: Hypoplasie cerébélleuse congénitale avec lésions osseuses. *Ann Pediatr* 1986; 33:417.

230. Stratton RF et al: An unusual cardiomelic syndrome. *Am J Med Genet* 1988; 29:333.

231. Sybert VP et al: Variable expression in a dominantly inherited skeletal dysplasia with similarities to brachydactyly E and spondyloepiphyseal-spondyloperipheral dysplasia. *Clin Genet* 1979; 15:160.

232. Tamminga P et al: An infant with marfanoid phenotype and congenital contractures associated with ocular and cardiovascular anomalies, cerebral white matter hypoplasia, and spinal axonopathy. *Eur J Pediatr* 1985; 143:228.

233. Tanner MS et al: Functional intestinal obstruction due to deficiency of argyrophil neurones in the myenteric plexus: Familial syndrome presenting with short small bowel malrotation and pyloric hypertrophy. *Arch Dis Child* 1976; 51:837.

234. Taheri SA et al: Iliocaval compression syndrome. *Am J Surg* 1987; 154:169.

235. Taybi H: Thoracic and abdominal calcification in children: A review. *Perspectives in Radiology* (in press).

236. Taybi H: Ocular calcification and retrolental fibrodysplasia. *Am J Roentgenol* 1956; 76:583.

237. Teodori JB et al: Basilar impression in children. *Pediatrics* 1984; 74:1097.

238. Terrafranca RJ et al: Congenital hereditary cranium bifidum occultum frontalis. *Radiology* 1953; 61:60.

239. Tolmie JL et al: Congenital anal anomalies in two families with Opitz G syndrome. *J Med Genet* 1987; 24:688.

240. Toriello HV et al: Corpus callosum agenesis, facial anomalies, Robin sequence, and other anomalies: A new autosomal recessive syndrome? *Am J Med Genet* 1988; 31:17.

241. Tsui-Chun K et al: Scintographic findings in congenital lipodystrophy. *Clin Nucl Med* 1989; 14:30.

242. Tsukahara M et al: A disease with features of cutis laxa and Ehlers-Danlos syndrome: Report of a mother and daughter. *Hum Genet* 1988; 78:9.

243. Turner G: A second family with renal, vaginal, and middle ear anomalies. *J Pediatr* 1970; 76:641.

244. Van den Berghe H: Familial ulnar aplasia and lobster claw deformity. *Clin Genet* 1978; 13:106.

245. Ventruto V et al: Primary protrusio acetabuli in four generations of an Italian family. *J Med Genet* 1980; 17:404.

246. Vila JHG et al: La dysplasia de Meyer. *Radiologia* 1984; 26:113.

247. Viljoen DL et al: The split-hand and split-foot anomaly in a central African negro population. *Am J Med Genet* 1984; 19:545.

248. Wackenheim A et al: Cheirolumbar dysostosis: A mono-osseous form (monovertebral and monophalangeal). *Neuroradiol* 1987; 29:589.

249. Wade JL et al: Neurocrest and colonic tumors: New clinical syndrome. Report of three cases. *Am J Med* 1984; 77:725.

250. Weaver RG et al: Optic nerve coloboma associated with renal disease. *Am J Med Genet* 1988; 29:597.
251. Weinberg AF, Zumwalt RE: Bilateral nephromegaly and multiple pulmonary cysts. *Am J Clin Pathol* 1977; 67:284.
252. Weisberg LA et al: Computed tomographic findings and differential diagnostic considerations in subcortical arteriosclerotic encephalopathy (Binswanger's disease). *Comput Med Imag Graph* 1988; 12:249.
253. Wilson GN et al: Peroxisomal disorders: Clinical commentary and future prospects. *Am J Med Genet* 1988; 30:771.
254. Wise JE et al: Phenotypic features of patients with congenital adrenal hypoplasia and glycerol kinase deficiency. *Am J Dis Child* 1987; 141:744.
255. Wood VE: Congenital thumb deformities. *Clin Orthop* 1985; 195:7.
256. Woodring JH et al: Acquired tracheomegaly in adults as a complication of diffuse pulmonary fibrosis. *AJR* 1989; 152:743.
257. Young ID et al: Agenesis of the corpus callosum and macrocephaly in siblings: *Clin Genet* 1985; 28:225.
258. Zerres K et al: Cystic kidneys. *Hum Genet* 1984; 68:104.
259. Zimmer EZ et al: Tetra-amelia with multiple malformations in six male fetuses of one kindred. *Eur J Pediatr* 1985; 144:412.

Appendix B

International Nomenclature of Constitutional Diseases of Bone*

I. **Skeletal dysplasias (osteochondrodysplasias): abnormalities of cartilage and/or bone growth and development.**
  A. **Defects of growth of tubular bones and/or spine**
    Identifiable at birth
    Usually lethal before or shortly after birth
    1. Achondrogenesis type I (Parenti-Fraccaro)
    2. Achondrogenesis type II (Langer-Saldino)
    3. Hypochondrogenesis
    4. Fibrochondrogenesis
    5. Thanatophoric dysplasia
    6. Thanatophoric dysplasia with clover-leaf skull
    7. Atelosteogenesis
    8. Short rib syndrome (with or without polydactyly)
      a. type I (Saldino-Noonan)
      b. type II (Majewski)
      c. type III (Verma-Naumoff)
      d. type Beemer
    9. Schneckenbecken dysplasia
    10. Hydrops—ectopic Calcification—moth-eaten skeletal dysplasia
    11. de la Chapelle dysplasia
    12. Boomerang dysplasia
    13. Opsismo dysplasia
    14. Thanatophoric varients
    15. Antley Bixler
    16. Lethal skeletal dysplasia—round inferior femoral epiphyseal type—Maroteaux
    Usually nonlethal dysplasia
    17. Chondrodysplasia punctata
      a. rhizomelic form autosomal recessive
      b. dominant X-linked form
      c. Conradi Hunermann
      d. X-linked recessive
      e. common mild form (Sheffield)
    18. Campomelic dysplasia
    19. Kyphomelic dysplasia
    20. Achondroplasia
    21. Diastrophic dysplasia
    22. Metatropic dysplasia (several forms)
    23. Chondro-ecto-dermal dysplasia (Ellis-Van Creveld)
    24. Asphyxiating thoracic dysplasia (Jeune)
    25. Spondyloepiphyseal dysplasia congenita
      a. autosomal dominant form
      b. autosomal recessive form
    26. Kniest dysplasia
    27. Dyssegmental dysplasia
      a. type Rolland-Desbuquois
      b. type Silverman-Handmaker
    28. Mesomelic dysplasia
      a. type Nievergelt
      b. type Langer (probable homozygous dyschondrosteosis)
      c. type Robinow
      d. type Rheinardt
      e. type Werner
      f. Osebold-Remondini dysplasia
    29. Acromesomelic dysplasia
    30. Cleidocranial dysplasia
    31. Oto-palato-digital syndrome
      a. type II (Andrè)
    32. Pseudodiastrophic dysplasia
    33. Spondylomegaepiphyseal-metaphyseal dysplasia (SMMD)
    34. Geleophysic dysplasia
    35. Yunis-Varón
    36. Grebe dysplasia
    37. Thoraco-laryngo-pelvic dysplasia
    Identifiable in later life
    38. Hypochondroplasia
    39. Dyschondrosteosis
    40. Metaphyseal chondrodysplasia type Jansen
    41. Metaphyseal chondrodysplasia type Schmid
    42. Metaphyseal chondrodysplasia type McKusick
    43. Metaphyseal chondrodysplasia with exocrine pancreatic insufficiency and cyclic neutropenia (Shwachman)
    44. Spondylo-metaphyseal dysplasia
      a. type Kozlowski
      b. other forms
    45. Multiple epiphyseal dysplasia
      a. type Fairbank
      b. type Ribbing
    46. Multiple epiphyseal dysplasia with early diabetes (Wolcott-Rallisson)

*Modified from International Nomenclature of Constitutional Diseases of Bone, revision May 1983. *Ann Radiol* 1983; 26:457.

903

47. Pseudo-achodoplasia
    a. dominant
    b. recessive
48. Spondylo-epiphyseal dysplasia tarda
49. Progressive pseudo-rheumatoid chondrodysplasia
50. Brachyolmia
    a. autosomal recessive
    b. autosomal dominant
51. Dyggve-Melchior-Clausen dysplasia
52. Spondylo-epi-metaphyseal dysplasia
    a. type Irapa
    b. type Strudwick
53. Spondylo-epi-metaphyseal dysplasia with joint laxity
54. Oto-spondylo-megaepiphyseal dysplasia (OSMED)
55. Parastremmatic dysplasia
56. Tricho-rhino-phalangeal dysplasia, type 1
57. Acrodysplasia with retinitis pigmentosa and nephropathy (Saldino-Mainzer)
58. Spondyloperipheral dysplasia
59. Acromicric dysplasia
60. Metaphyseal—Sella turcica dysplasia—Rosenberg
61. Dolichospondylic dysplasia
62. ADA deficiency (with metaphyseal dysplasia)
63. Weissenbacher—Zweymuller
64. Acrodysostosis

B. **Disorganized development of cartilage and fibrous components of skeleton**
   1. Dysplasia epiphysealis hemimelica
   2. Multiple cartilaginous exostoses
   3. Acrodysplasia with exostoses (Giedion-Langer)
   4. Enchondromatosis (Ollier)
   5. Enchondromatosis with hemangioma (Maffucci)
   6. Metachondromatosis
   7. Spondyloenchondroplasia
   8. Osteoglophonic dysplasia
   9. Fibrous dysplasia (many types)
   10. Cherubism (familial fibrous dysplasia of the jaws)

C. **Abnormalities of density of cortical diaphyseal structure and/or metaphyseal modeling**
   1. Osteogenesis imperfecta (several forms)
   2. Osteoporosis with pseudo-glioma
   3. Osteopetrosis
      a. autosomal recessive lethal
      b. intermediate recessive
      c. autosomal dominant
      d. recessive with tubular acidosis
   4. Pycnodysostosis
   5. Dominant osteoclerosis type Stanescu
   6. Osteomesopycnosis
   7. Osteopoikilosis
   8. Osteopathia striata
   9. Osteopathia striata with cranial sclerosis
   10. Melorheostosis
   11. Diaphyseal dysplasia (Camurati-Engelmann)
   12. Craniodiaphyseal dysplasia

13. Endosteal hyperostosis
    a. autosomal dominant (Worth)
    b. autosomal recessive (Van Burchem)
    c. autosomal recessive (sclerosteosis)
14. Tubular stenosis (Kenny-Caffey)
15. Osteodysplasty (Melnick-Needles)
16. Frontometaphyseal dysplasia
17. Craniometaphyseal dysplasia (several forms)
18. Metaphyseal dysplasia (Pyle)
19. Dysosteosclerosis
20. Diaphyseal medullary stenosis with bone malignancy—Hardcastle
21. Osteoplasty, precocious
22. Sponastrime dysplasia
23. Lenz-Majewski dysplasia
24. Mixed sclerosing bone dysplasia
25. Hyperostosis generalisata with striations
26. Distal osteosclerosis

II. **Dysostoses: Malformation of individual bones, singly or in combination.**
   A. **Dysostoses with cranial and facial involvement**
      1. Craniosynostosis (several forms)
      2. Craniofacial dysostosis (Crouzon)
      3. Acrocephalosyndactyly
         a. type Apert
         b. type Chotzen
         c. type Pfeiffer
         d. other types
      4. Acrocephalopolysyndactyly (Carpenter and others)
      5. Cephalopolysyndactyly (Greig)
      6. First and second branchial arch syndromes
         a. mandibulofacial dysostosis (Treacher Collins, Franceschetti)
         b. acro-facial dysostosis (Nager)
         c. oculo-auriculo-vertebral dysostosis (Goldenhar)
         d. hemifacial microsomia
         e. others
            (probably parts of a large spectrum)
      7. Oculo-mandibulo-facial syndrome (Hallermann-Streiff-Francois)
   B. **Dysostoses with predominant axial involvement**
      1. Vertebral segmentation defects (including Klippel-Feil)
      2. Cervico-oculo-acoustic syndrome (Wildervanck)
      3. Sprengel anomaly
      4. Spondylocostal dysostosis
         a. dominant form
         b. recessive forms
      5. Oculovertebral syndrome (Weyers)
      6. Osteo-onychodysostosis
      7. Cerebro-costo-mandibular syndrome
   C. **Dysostoses with predominant involvement of extremities**
      1. Acheiria
      2. Apodia

3. Tetraphocomelia syndrome (Roberts) (SC pseudo thalidomide syndrome)
4. Ectrodactyly
   a. isolated
   b. ectrodactyly-ectodermal dysplasia cleft-palate syndrome
   c. ectrodactyly with scalp defects
5. Oro-acral syndrome (aglossia syndrome, Hanhart syndrome)
6. Familial radioulnar synostosis
7. Brachydactyly, types A, B, C, D, E (Bell's classification)
8. Symphalangism
9. Polydactyly (several forms)
10. Syndactyly (several forms)
11. Poly-syndactyly (several forms)
12. Camptodactyly
13. Manzke syndrome
14. Poland syndrome
15. Rubinstein-Taybi syndrome
16. Coffin-Siris syndrome
17. Pancytopenia-dysmelia syndrome (Fanconi)
18. Blackfan-Diamond anemia with thumb anomalies (Aase syndrome)
19. Thrombocytopenia-radial aplasia syndrome
20. Oro-digito-facial syndrome
    a. type Papillon-Leage
    b. type Mohr
21. Cardiomelic syndromes (Holt-Oram and others)
22. Femoral focal deficiency (with or without facial anomalies)
23. Multiple synostoses (includes some forms of symphalangism)
24. Scapuloiliac dysostosis (Kosenow-Sinios)
25. Hand-foot-genital syndrome
26. Focal dermal hypoplasia (Goltz)

III. **Idiopathic osteolyses**
1. Phalangeal (several forms)
2. Tarsocarpal
   a. including Francois form and others
   b. with nephropathy
3. Multicentric
   a. Hajdu-Cheney form
   b. Winchester form
   c. Torg form
   d. other forms

IV. *Miscellaneous disorders* **with osseous involvement**
1. Early acceleration of skeletal maturation
   a. Marshall-Smith syndrome
   b. Weaver syndrome
   c. other types
2. Marfan syndrome
3. Congenital contractural arachnodactyly
4. Cerebro-hepato-renal syndrome (Zellweger)
5. Coffin-Lowry syndrome
6. Cockayne syndrome
7. Fibrodysplasia ossificans congenita
8. Epidermal nevus syndrome (Solomon)

9. Nevoid basal cell carcinoma syndrome
10. Multiple congenital fibromatosis
11. Neurofibromatosis

V. **Chromosomal aberrations**
VI. **Primary metabolic abnormalities**
A. Calcium and/or phosphorus
1. Hypophosphatemic rickets
2. Vitamin D dependency or pseudodeficiency rickets
   a. type I with probable deficiency in 25 hydroxy vitamin D-1-alpha-hydroxylase
   b. type II with target-organ resistance
3. Late rickets (McCance)
4. Idiopathic hypercalciuria
5. Hypophosphatasia (several forms)
6. Pseudo-hypoparathyroidism (normocalcemic and hypocalcemic forms)

B. Complex carbohydrates
1. Mucopolysaccharidosis type I (alpha-L-iduronidase deficiency)
   a. Hurler form
   b. Scheie form
   c. other forms
2. Mucopolysaccharidosis type II—Hunter (sulfoiduronate sulfatase deficiency)
3. Mucopolysaccharidosis type III—Sanfilippo
   a. type III A (heparin sulfamidase deficiency)
   b. type III B (N-acetyl-alpha-glucosaminidase deficiency)
   c. type III C (alpha-glucosaminide-N-acetyl transferase deficiency)
   d. type III D (N-acetyl-glucosamine-6 sulfate sulfatase deficiency)
4. Mucopolysaccharidosis type IV
   a. type IV A—Morquio (N-acetyl-galactosamine-6 sulfate-sulfatase deficiency)
   b. type IV B (beta-galactosidase deficiency)
5. Mucopolysaccharidosis type VI—Maroteaux-Lamy (aryl-sulfatase B deficiency)
6. Mucopolysaccharidosis type VII (beta-glucuronidase deficiency)
7. Aspartylglucosaminuria (Aspartyl-glucosaminidase deficiency)
8. Mannosidosis (alpha-mannosidase deficiency)
9. Fucosidosis (alpha-fucosidase deficiency)
10. GM1-Gangliosidosis (beta-galactosidase deficiency) (several forms)
11. Multiple sulfatases deficiency (Austin-Thieffry)
12. Isolated neuraminidase deficiency, several forms. Includes:
    a. mucolipidosis I
    b. nephrosialidosis
    c. cherry red spot myoclonia syndrome
13. Phosphotransferase deficiency, several forms. Includes:
    a. mucolipidosis II (I cell disease)
    b. mucolipidosis III (pseudo-polydystrophy)

14. Combined neuraminidase beta-galactosidase deficiency
15. Salla disease
C. Lipids
   1. Niemann-Pick disease (sphingomyelinase deficiency) (several forms)
   2. Gaucher disease (beta-glucosidase deficiency) (several types)

   3. Farber disease—lipogranulomatosis (ceraminidase deficiency)
D. Amino acids
   1. Homocystinuria and others
E. Metals
   1. Menkes syndrome (Kinky hair syndrome and others)

Appendix C*

Requiem for the Eponym

(Eponymomania)
(For the International Skeletal Society)

The names of good doctors are commonly shown,
Describing disorders marked down as their own.
Afflictions of others they blatantly named,
Though personal suffering never was claimed.
James Paget was healthy as far as is known,
And never complained of his nipple or bone,
But lending his name as a possessive noun,
Instead of an adjective, he gained renown.

Both *Colles* and *Bennett* wrist fractures begot,
But ankles were cornered by *Percival Pott*.
Already he'd claimed the tuberculous spine,
The time *Perthes* pulled *Calve's Legg* into line,
And earlier *Ollier* earned some respect
Concerning a cartilage bony defect.
No mention of malaise maligned *Morquio*
And *Hurler* was happily having a throw.

Was *Klippel* stiff necked, did he ponder a while
On how he would fare in the absence of *Feil?*
Was *Brodie* obsessed, who inflammed poor *Garré,*
Did *von Recklinghausen* drink *Caffey* au lait?
The horns of dilemma we credit to *Fong,*
And *Sudeck's* ghost *Reiter* said *Ewing* was wrong.
To *Needle* poor *Melnick* in *Burkitt's* bush shack,
And *Scheuermann Still* had a pain in the back.

Soon osteochondritis won lasting acclaim,
Because of those chaps with a Teutonic name,
But *Engelmann's* bones were sclerotic and thick,
And *Gaucher's* expanded, upstaged *Niemann-Pick,*
Fanconi and *Hodgkin* were hard to resist,
With *Kienböck* and *Madelung* grabbing a wrist,
While *Letterer-Siwe* led *Wilson* a dance,
Both *Lobstein* and *Larsen* were *Pyled* up by *Chance.*

San Filipo offered to *Hunter* a loan,
And *Keith* quite aclastic was short of a bone.
The *Milkman,* malacic found cracks in his *Van,*
Just borrowed from *Buchem* a friend of *Marfan.*
A picnic was painted by *Toulouse-Lautrec,*

And *Chester* called *Erdheim* a pain in the neck.
Maffuci and *Crouzon* were feeling the strain,
And *Taybi* was asked to come up and explain.

McKusick and *Jansen* and *Schmid,* it is said,
Preceded *Kozlowski,* now shooting ahead.
Was *Schlatter-Osgood* as his word on his knees?
Did *Harris* displace *Salter's* epiphyses?
Should *Fairbank* tell *Brailsford* he'd not give a hang
What happened to *Trevor, Cornelia de Lange*
Since early pathologists were not *Albright*
Till *Jaffe* arrived to start shedding some light.
Would *Schüller* and *Christian* please lend us a *Hand,*
To render assistance to *Grave's* thyroid gland?
With *Albers-Schönberg* on his marble commode,
While *Schmorl* was excitedly picking his node,
It seemed that men's names were of no more account,
Like *Koehler* and *Cushing* and *Cooley* and *Blount.*
So *Murray* and *Jacobson* aren't nominees
And not even *Resnick* has claimed a disease.

Well now I shall offer the lot some redress,
By simply removing apostrophe-"S",
Enabling colleagues to take up the cure,
And cast aside ailments they cannot endure.
Now learned researchers are happy to speak
Of troubles derived from the Latin or Greek.
Or else from vernacular, titles they cull,
Though generic names may be mundane and dull.

I'm bound to confess to a pedantic streak,
Affording our jargon this semantic tweak,
But sooner or later these facts you should face,
To strike from the journals the genitive case,
Permitting eponymous ailments hallowed,
To enter the books in anonymous mode.
Then medical parlance will show due restraint
When doctors no longer will own their complaint.

Len Green†
Sydney
September 1988

*From Green L: Requiem for the eponym. *Skeletal Radiol* 1989; 17:589. Used with permission.

†Dr Green is Visiting Radiologist to Prince Henry, Prince of Wales and Royal South Sydney Hospitals (Sydney), and Lecturer in Bone Diseases for the Royal Australasian College of Radiologists.

INDEX